PRINCIPLES OF
ORAL AND MAXILLOFACIAL SURGERY

EDITOR

Larry J. Peterson, D.D.S.

EDITORIAL BOARD

A. Thomas Indresano, D.M.D.
Robert D. Marciani, D.M.D.
Steven M. Roser, D.M.D., M.D.

SECTION EDITORS

O. Ross Beirne, D.D.S.
Arthur A. Gonty, D.D.S.
John F. Helfrick, D.D.S.
James R. Hupp, D.M.D., M.D.
Michael C. Kinnebrew, D.D.S., M.D.
Daniel Lew, D.D.S.
Joseph E. Van Sickels, D.D.S.
Thomas P. Williams, D.D.S.

Illustrated by William M. Winn

PRINCIPLES OF

ORAL AND MAXILLOFACIAL SURGERY

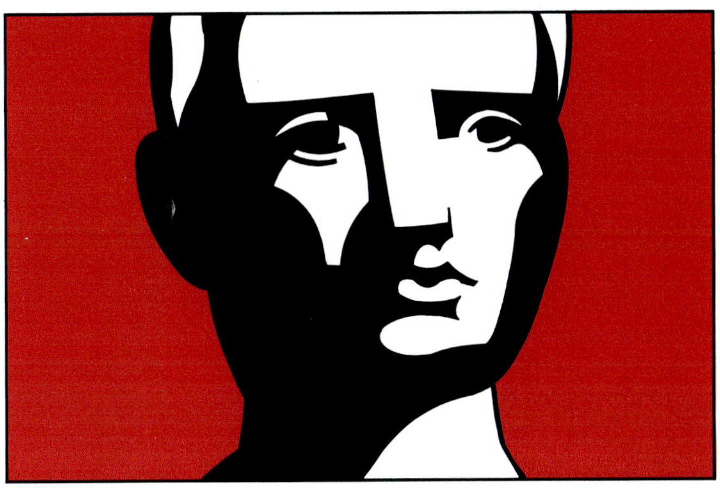

VOLUME ONE

J. B. LIPPINCOTT COMPANY
Philadelphia

Acquisitions Editor: Darlene Barela Cooke
Developmental Editor: Delois Patterson
Project Editor: Dina K. Rubin
Indexer: Victoria Boyle
Designer: Doug Smock
Production Manager: Caren Erlichman
Production Coordinator: Sharon McCarthy
Compositor: G&S Typesetters, Inc.
Printer/Binder: Halliday Lithograph

Library of Congress Cataloging-in-Publication Data

Principles of oral and maxillofacial surgery / editor, Larry J. Peterson ; editorial board, A. Thomas Indresano . . . [et al.] ; illustrated by William M. Winn.
p. cm.
Includes bibliographical references and index.
ISBN 0-397-51011-X (set: v. 1, 2, and 3)
ISBN 0-397-51232-5 (v. 1)
ISBN 0-397-51233-3 (v. 2)
ISBN 0-397-51234-1 (v. 3)
1. Mouth—Surgery. 2. Maxilla—Surgery. 3. Face—Surgery.
I. Peterson, Larry J., 1942–
[DNLM: 1. Face—surgery. 2. Maxilla—surgery. 3. Surgery, Oral.
WU 600 P957]
RK529.P75 1992
617.5′2059—dc20
DNLM/DLC
for Library of Congress 91-25360
CIP

6 5 4 3 2

The authors and publisher have exerted every effort to ensure that drug selection and dosage set forth in this text are in accord with current recommendations and practice at the time of publication. However, in view of ongoing research, changes in government regulations, and the constant flow of information relating to drug therapy and drug reactions, the reader is urged to check the package insert for each drug for any change in indications and dosage and for added warnings and precautions. This is particularly important when the recommended agent is a new or infrequently employed drug.

To Sue, Brie, and Tucker, who endured my absence and bad humor; and to my teachers and residents (who were, and continue to be, my real teachers) who have given me the opportunity to learn about and fall in love with this, the greatest of all specialties.

LJP

To my wife, Rita, and my children Kim, Scott, Jeff, Andy, and Joey, who tolerate my behavior and love me in spite of it. To Nita Bonnell and Mary Remner who worked tirelessly to make the deadlines. To my residents and faculty for letting me take the time away from them to work on this project.

ATI

To the most important person in my life, my wife, Hendra, and my daughters, Marisa, Kara, and Cristina for their tolerance and patience. My contributions to this text would not have been possible without the continuous support of my loyal friend, Elizabeth Readnower and the persistent efforts of Tina Mattox for wordprocessing my chapters.

RDM

To my wife Susan and my children Meredith, Craig, and Melissa. To Ms. Vicky Leung for her tireless assistance and my colleagues for their excellent manuscripts; and to Dr. Walter Guralnick who has continued to inspire me in every phase of my professional life.

SMR

CONTRIBUTORS

Robert W. Alexander, M.D., D.M.D.
Stevens Memorial Hospital
Department of Surgery
Division of Maxillofacial/Plastic Surgery
Edmonds, Washington

Leon A. Assael, D.M.D.
Associate Professor and Residency Program Director
Oral and Maxillofacial Surgery
The University of Connecticut Health Center
School of Dental Medicine
Farmington, Connecticut

Robert A. Bays, D.D.S.
Chairman
Division of Oral and Maxillofacial Surgery
Department of Surgery
Emory University School of Medicine and Affiliated Hospitals
Atlanta, Georgia

O. Ross Beirne, D.D.S.
Associate Professor and Director of Residency Training
University of Washington
School of Dentistry
Department of Oral and Maxillofacial Surgery
Seattle, Washington
Associate Adjunct Professor
University of California, San Francisco
Department of Oral and Maxillofacial Surgery
School of Dentistry
San Francisco, California

Stanley A. Berman, D.D.S.
Clinical Instructor
Metrohealth Medical Center
and The Case Western Reserve University
Cleveland, Ohio

Charles N. Bertolami, D.D.S., D.Med.Sc.
Professor and Chairman
Section of Oral and Maxillofacial Surgery
University of California—Los Angeles
School of Dentistry
Chief, Dental Service
University of California—Los Angeles
Medical Center
Los Angeles, California

Michael S. Block, D.M.D.
Associate Professor
Department of Oral and Maxillofacial Surgery
LSU School of Dentistry
New Orleans, Louisiana

Dale S. Bloomquist, D.D.S.
Associate Professor
Department of Oral and Maxillofacial Surgery
School of Dentistry
University of Washington
Seattle, Washington

Jon P. Bradrick, D.D.S.
Assistant Professor of Surgery
Division of Oral and Maxillofacial Surgery
Case Western Reserve University College of Medicine
Cleveland Metropolitan General Hospital
Cleveland, Ohio

Ralph D. Buoncristiani, D.D.S.
Lecturer, Section of Oral and Maxillofacial Surgery;
Clinical Instructor
Continuing Education in Dentistry
UCLA School of Dentistry;
Staff Surgeon, UCLA Medical Center
Los Angeles, California;
Staff Surgeon, St. John's Hospital and Health Center
Santa Monica, California

Robert L. Campbell, D.D.S.
Professor of Oral and Maxillofacial Surgery and Anesthesiology
Medical College of Virginia
Richmond, Virginia

Joseph Canzona, D.D.S., M.D.
Clinical Assistant Professor
Division of Oral and Maxillofacial Surgery
Northwestern University Dental School
Chicago, Illinois

Robert Chuong, M.D., D.M.D.
Assistant Clinical Professor in Plastic and Maxillofacial Surgery
University of South Florida
Tampa, Florida

Arthur W. Curley, J.D.
Associate Professor, Dental Jurisprudence
University of the Pacific School of Dentistry
San Francisco, California

John A. Dean, M.D.
Chief Resident, Department of Plastic Surgery
Eastern Virginia Medical School
Norfolk, Virginia

Bruce N. Epker, D.D.S., Ph.D.
Director, Oral and Maxillofacial Surgery
Director, Center for Correction of Dentofacial Deformities
Director, Fort Worth Cleft Palate Program
John Peter Smith Hospital
Fort Worth, Texas

Mark F. Erickson, D.D.S.
Clinical Instructor
Division of Oral and Maxillofacial Surgery
Northwestern University Dental School
Chicago, Illinois

Stephen E. Feinberg, D.D.S., Ph.D.
Associate Professor and Chairman
Department of Oral Medicine, Pathology, and Maxillofacial Surgery
University of Michigan
School of Dentistry
Ann Arbor, Michigan

Michael W. Finkelstein, D.D.S.
Department of Oral Pathology & Diagnosis
College of Dentistry
University of Iowa
Iowa City, Iowa

David E. Frost, D.D.S.
Clinical Associate Professor for Research
University of North Carolina at Chapel Hill
Attending Staff
Durham County General Hospital
Chapel Hill, North Carolina

Thomas S. Golec, D.D.S., FACD
Private Practice
Escondido, California

Arthur A. Gonty, D.D.S.
Associate Professor
Section of Oral and Maxillofacial Surgery
Department of Oral Health Practice
University of Kentucky
College of Dentistry
Lexington, KY

Brian K. Hall, Ph.D.
Professor of Biology
Dalhousie University
Halifax, Nova Scotia, Canada

Richard E. Hall, D.D.S., Ph.D.
Associate Professor
Department of Oral and Maxillofacial Surgery and Oral Biology
School of Dental Medicine and Biomedical Sciences
State University of New York at Buffalo
Attending Oral Surgeon—Buffalo General Hospital and Erie County Medical Center
Buffalo, New York

Richard H. Haug, D.D.S.
Attending Surgeon, Department of Surgery
Division of Oral and Maxillofacial Surgery
Cleveland Metropolitan General Hospital
Assistant Professor of Surgery
Cleveland Metropolitan General Hospital and the Case Western Reserve University
Cleveland, Ohio

Michael S. Hauser, D.M.D., M.D.
Chief, Division of Dentistry and Oral and Maxillofacial Surgery
Mt. Sinai Medical Center
Cleveland, Ohio

Leslie B. Heffez, D.M.D, FRCD
University of Illinois
TMJ & Facial Pain Clinic
Department of Oral and Maxillofacial Surgery
Associate Professor & Associate Head
Attending, Humana Hospital—Michael Reese
Cook County Hospital
West Side Veteran's Administration
Highland Park, Illinois

Arden K. Hegtvedt, D.D.S.
Assistant Professor
Oral and Maxillofacial Surgery
College of Dentistry
The Ohio State University
Columbus, Ohio

John F. Helfrick, D.D.S.
Professor and Chairman
Department of Oral and Maxillofacial Surgery
University of Texas Health Science Center at Houston
Dental Branch
Houston, Texas

Robert M. Hinkle, D.D.S.
Private Practice in Oral and Maxillofacial Surgery
Columbus, Ohio

P. Craig Hobar, M.D.
Assistant Professor of Plastic Surgery
University of Texas Southwestern Medical Center
Dallas, Texas

James R. Hupp, D.M.D., M.D.
Associate Professor and Chairperson
Department of Oral/Maxillofacial Surgery
University of Medicine and Dentistry of New Jersey
Newark, New Jersey

A. Thomas Indresano, D.M.D.
Director, Division of Oral and Maxillofacial Surgery
MetroHealth Medical Center
Associate Professor
Case Western Reserve University
Cleveland, Ohio

Howard A. Israel, D.D.S.
Associate Professor
Division of Oral and Maxillofacial Surgery
Columbia University
School of Dental and Oral Surgery
New York, New York

Jonathan S. Jacobs, D.M.D., M.D., FACS
Associate Professor, Department of Plastic Surgery
Eastern Virginia Medical School
Norfolk, Virginia

Jerry L. Jones, D.D.S., M.D.
Clinical Associate Professor
Department of Surgery
University of New Mexico Medical School
Albuquerque, New Mexico

Leonard B. Kaban, D.M.D., M.D.
Professor and Chairman
University of California, San Francisco
Department of Oral and Maxillofacial Surgery
San Francisco, California

David A. Keith, D.M.D.
Associate Professor of Oral and Maxillofacial Surgery
Harvard School of Dental Medicine
Chief of Oral Surgery
Harvard Community Health Plan
Boston, Massachusetts

Brent D. Kennedy, D.D.S., M.D.
Associate Clinical Professor
Division of Oral and Maxillofacial Surgery
University of Texas Southwestern Medical School
Dallas, Texas
Director, Facial Surgical Institute
Salt Lake City, Utah

John N. Kent, D.D.S.
Boyd Professor and Head
Department of Oral and Maxillofacial Surgery
Louisiana State University Medical Center
New Orleans, Louisiana

Michael C. Kinnebrew, D.D.S., M.D.
Clinical Associate Professor
Department of Oral and Maxillofacial Surgery
Louisiana State University Medical Center
New Orleans, Louisiana

John P. LaBanc, D.D.S.
Associate Professor
Oral and Maxillofacial Surgery
University of Florida
Gainesville, Florida

Peter E. Larsen, D.D.S.
Assistant Professor
Department of Oral and Maxillofacial Surgery
The Ohio State University
College of Dentistry
Columbus, Ohio

Harry L. Legan, D.D.S.
Professor and Chairman
Department of Orthodontics
West Virginia University
School of Dentistry
Morgantown, West Virginia

Daniel Lew, D.D.S.
Professor of Surgery and Chief
Section of Oral and Maxillofacial Surgery
Louisiana State University Medical Center
Shreveport, Louisiana

Stuart E. Lieblich, D.M.D.
Attending Staff
Hartford Hospital
Hartford, Connecticut
Attending Staff
Newington Children's Hospital
Newington, Connecticut

Gilbert E. Lilly, D.D.S.
Professor and Head, Department of Oral Pathology and Diagnosis
College of Dentistry, The University of Iowa
Director, Diagnosis and Oral Pathology
University of Iowa Hospitals and Clinics
Iowa City, Iowa

Neil H. Luyk, B.D.S., M.S., FRACDS, FDSRCS, FRACDS(OMS)
Senior Lecturer in Oral and Maxillofacial Surgery
University of Otago, Consultant Oral & Maxillofacial Surgeon
Otago Area Health Board
Dunedin, New Zealand

Robert Bruce MacIntosh, D.D.S.
Clinical Professor, Director of Graduate Education
University of Detroit
Detroit, Michigan

Robert D. Marciani, D.M.D.
Professor, Oral and Maxillofacial Surgery
University of Kentucky
College of Dentistry
Lexington, Kentucky

Joseph E. Margarone, D.D.S.
Associate Professor and Chairman
Department of Oral and Maxillofacial Surgery
State University of New York at Buffalo School of Dental Medicine
Chief, Division of Oral and Maxillofacial Surgery
Buffalo General Hospital
Buffalo, New York

Ronald B. Marks, D.D.S.
Clinical Associate Professor of Oral and Maxillofacial Surgery
Louisiana State University Medical Center
Shreveport and New Orleans, Louisiana
Clinical Assistant Professor OMS
Tulane Medical School
New Orleans, Louisiana

Louis G. Mercuri, D.D.S., M.S.
Head, Department of Oral and Maxillofacial Surgery
University of Illinois
College of Dentistry
Chief of Service
Department of Dentistry
Humana Hospital—Michael Reese
Chicago, Illinois

Ralph G. Merrill, D.D.S.
Professor and Chairman
Oral and Maxillofacial Surgery
Oregon Health Sciences University
Portland, Oregon

Dale J. Misiek, D.M.D.
Associate Professor
Department of Oral and Maxillofacial Surgery
Louisiana State University Medical Center
New Orleans, Louisiana

Don M. Morris, M.D.
Professor of Surgery
University of New Mexico
Director of Surgical Oncology
UNM Cancer Center
Chief, Surgical Service
VAMC
Albuquerque, New Mexico

Bernard C. Pecaro, D.D.S., M.D.
Professor and Director
Division of Oral and Maxillofacial Surgery
Northwestern University Dental School
Chicago, Illinois

David H. Perrott, D.D.S., M.D.
Assistant Professor
University of California, San Francisco
Department of Oral and Maxillofacial Surgery
San Francisco, California

Larry J. Peterson, D.D.S.
Professor and Chairman
Oral and Maxillofacial Surgery
College of Dentistry
The Ohio State University
Columbus, Ohio

Joseph F. Piecuch, D.M.D., M.D.
Attending Staff
Hartford Hospital
Hartford, Connecticut
Attending Staff
Newington Children's Hospital
Newington, Connecticut

J.C. Posnick, D.M.D., M.D., FRCS(C)
Medical Director
Craniofacial Program and Consultant
Plastic Surgery Division
Department of Surgery
The Hospital for Sick Children
Assistant Professor
Department of Surgery
University of Toronto
Toronto, Canada

Michael Powers, D.D.S.
Assistant Professor
Department of Oral and Maxillofacial Surgery
Case Western Reserve University
School of Dentistry
Cleveland, Ohio

David S. Precious, D.D.S., FRCD(C)
Professor and Head
Oral and Maxillofacial Surgery
Dalhousie University
Halifax, Nova Scotia, Canada

Peter D. Quinn, D.M.D., M.D.
Chairman, Oral and Maxillofacial Surgery
University of Pennsylvania
School of Dental Medicine
Chief, Oral and Maxillofacial Surgery Service
Hospital of the University of Pennsylvania
Philadelphia, Pennsylvania

Rod J. Rohrich, M.D.
Chief of Plastic Surgery
Parkland Memorial Hospital
Associate Professor
University of Texas Southwestern Medical Center
Dallas, Texas

Steven M. Roser, D.M.D., M.D.
Associate Professor and Director
Oral and Maxillofacial Surgery
School of Dental and Oral Surgery
Columbia University
Acting Director
Dental Service
Presbyterian Hospital
New York, New York

Kenneth S. Rotskoff, D.D.S., M.D.
Assistant Professor
Oral and Maxillofacial Surgery
St. Louis University School of Orthodontics
Director of Oral and Maxillofacial Surgery Fellowship
Missouri Baptist Hospital
St. Louis, Missouri

Bruce Sanders, D.D.S.
Adjunct Professor
Section of Oral and Maxillofacial Surgery
University of California School of Dentistry
Senior Staff
Saint John's Hospital and Health Center
Santa Monica, California

David W. Shelton, D.M.D., FICD
Professor, Department of Oral and Maxillofacial Surgery
School of Dentistry
Professor, Department of Surgery
School of Medicine
Medical College of Georgia
Augusta, Georgia

Vivek Shetty, D.M.D.
Adjunct Assistant Professor
Section of Oral & Maxillofacial Surgery
University of California Los Angeles
School of Dentistry
Los Angeles, California

Samuel Stal, M.D.
Associate Professor of Plastic Surgery
Baylor College of Medicine
Houston, Texas

Mark J. Steinberg, D.D.S., M.D.
Director, Division of Oral and Maxillofacial Surgery
Humana Hospital—Michael Reese
Clinical Assistant Professor, Department of Oral and Maxillofacial Surgery
Northwestern University
School of Dentistry
Chicago, Illinois

Paul J.W. Stoelinga, M.D., D.D.S., Ph.D.
Affiliate Professor, Department of Oral and Maxillofacial Surgery
University of Washington
Seattle, Washington

Steven B. Syrop, D.D.S.
Assistant Clinical Professor
Director, TMJ Facial Pain Clinic
Columbia Presbyterian Medical Center
Columbia University School of Dental and Oral Surgery
New York, New York

David P. Timmis, D.D.S.
Assistant Professor
Division of Oral and Maxillofacial Surgery
Department of Surgery
Emory University School of Medicine
Oral and Maxillofacial Surgeon
Emory Clinic
Robert Woodruff Health Science Center
Augusta, Georgia

B.D. Tiner, D.D.S., M.D.
Assistant Professor
Department of Oral and Maxillofacial Surgery
University of Texas Health Science Center
San Antonio, Texas

Myron R. Tucker, D.D.S.
Associate Director and Director of Graduate Training
Department of Oral and Maxillofacial Surgery
School of Dentistry and University of North Carolina Hospitals
Chapel Hill, North Carolina

Timothy A. Turvey, D.D.S.
Professor
Department of Oral and Maxillofacial Surgery
University of North Carolina
Chapel Hill, North Carolina

Gerald P. Unhold, D.M.D., M.D.
General Surgery Resident
University of Illinois
Peoria, Illinois

Joseph E. Van Sickels, D.D.S.
Professor and Director
Dentofacial Deformity Clinic
The University of Texas Health Science Center at San Antonio
San Antonio, Texas

Steven D. Vincent, D.D.S.
Associate Professor
Oral Pathology and Diagnosis
University of Iowa
Iowa City, Iowa

Stepen A. Wagner, D.D.S.
Adjunct Assistant Professor
University of New Mexico Medical School
Albuquerque, New Mexico

Peter D. Waite, M.P.H., D.D.S., M.D.
Associate Professor
Vice Chairman, Program Director
Department of Oral and Maxillofacial Surgery
School of Dentistry
University of Alabama
Birmingham, Alabama

R. P. Ward-Booth, MBChB, FDS, RCS, FRCS(Ed)
Consultant Oral & Maxillofacial Surgeon
Sunderland District General Hospital
Sunderland, England

Joel M. Weaver, D.D.S., Ph.D.
Associate Professor and Director
Dental Anesthesiology Residency Program
Section of Oral and Maxillofacial Surgery
College of Dentistry
Associate Professor
Department of Anesthesiology
College of Medicine and University Hospitals
The Ohio State University
Columbus, Ohio

Roger A. West, D.M.D.
Private Practice
Northwest Center for Corrective Jaw Surgery
Seattle, Washington

Thomas P. Williams, D.D.S.
Adjunct Associate Professor of Oral Pathology and Oral and Maxillofacial Surgery
University of Iowa
Dubuque, Iowa

George A. Zarb, D.D.S., FRCD(C), Dr. Odont. (H.C.)
Professor and Chairman, Department of Prosthodontics
Faculty of Dentistry
University of Toronto
Toronto, Ontario, Canada

Deborah L. Zeitler, D.D.S.
Associate Professor
Director of Graduate Education
Oral and Maxillofacial Surgery
University of Iowa Hospitals and Clinics
College of Dentistry
Iowa City, Iowa

Michael F. Zide, D.D.S.
Associate Director
Oral and Maxillofacial Surgery
John Peter Smith Hospital
Fort Worth, Texas

PREFACE

The specialty of Oral and Maxillofacial Surgery has advanced dramatically over the last 15 years. Significant innovations in a number of areas have broadened the scope of practice for the oral and maxillofacial surgeon into surgical arenas unknown and unexplored only a short time ago. Many factors have contributed to this dynamic change, but the fact remains that much of the surgery that the individual practitioner is called on to do today was learned after formal residency training. Thus, it has become increasingly necessary for the oral and maxillofacial surgeon to have a reference that can be consulted to obtain an organized, systematic discussion of a specific problem and potential surgical solutions.

Such a reference must be complete and comprehensive, but also practical and readable. *Principles of Oral and Maxillofacial Surgery* fills this need. The primary purpose of this work is to present treatment modalities and surgical techniques of all of the broad range of patient-related problems with which the contemporary oral and maxillofacial surgeon is faced. This book discusses traditional management, but also emphasizes new and innovative methods and techniques. This reference is designed principally for use by the oral and maxillofacial surgeon with basic skills and knowledge who is looking for "state-of-the-art" information.

Some of the material discussed may be beyond the scope of individual oral and maxillofacial surgeons, but clearly is included within the scope of the specialty. The authors are primarily oral and maxillofacial surgeons who have broad experience and who have been especially innovative in the expansion of the specialty of oral and maxillofacial surgery. Each chapter emphasizes the underlying principles on which diagnosis, treatment planning, and surgery are based.

Principles of Oral and Maxillofacial Surgery is divided into 12 sections, each of which discusses a general topic. Each section is further divided into chapters that present detailed information in specific topic areas.

This reference is the first of its kind in the specialty of oral and maxillofacial surgery. Certainly there have been other books written that have discussed many of the same topics presented in this work. However, no previous or contemporary book discusses the topics that are relatively recent additions to the specialty. Therefore, this work meets a very specific need of the specialty and of its individual members.

CONTENTS

VOLUME ONE

VOLUME TWO

Part VII
RECONSTRUCTION OF THE SOFT AND HARD TISSUE OF THE MAXILLOFACIAL REGION 917

A. Thomas Indresano, Editorial Board
Daniel Lew, Section Editor

Part VIII
IMPLANTS AND PREPROSTHETIC RECONSTRUCTION SURGERY 1089

Steven M. Roser, Editorial Board
O. Ross Beirne, Section Editor

VOLUME THREE

Part IX
PRINCIPLES OF ORTHOGNATHIC SURGERY 1209

Robert D. Marciani, Editorial Board
Joseph Van Sickels, Section Editor

PRINCIPLES OF
ORAL AND MAXILLOFACIAL SURGERY

VOLUME ONE

I

PRINCIPLES OF SURGERY

1

The Physiology of Wound Healing

Vivek Shetty
Charles Bertolami

Surgery is based on the presumption of efficient wound healing. Accordingly, surgeons require a sound understanding of the mechanisms that influence healing if they are to tackle the problems of infection and incomplete or excessive repair. Confronted by the explosion of new information as advances in the biologic sciences unravel the complexities of wound healing, surgeons need to focus on the practical implications for wound care as a basis for building a clinical approach that will promote optimal tissue repair.

HEALING TERMINOLOGY

A *wound* represents an anatomic or functional interruption in the continuity of a tissue that is accompanied by cellular damage and death. It may be inflicted by physical, chemical, or biologic injury. Every injury initiates a series of coordinated processes directed toward restoring the injured tissues of the body to as near normal as possible. This process of restitution represents healing. Replacement of lost tissue can be accomplished by two distinct processes: regeneration and repair.

As an initial approximation, healing can be characterized according to a tissue's capacity either to regenerate or to repair. When the end product of the healing process is a tissue which is structurally and functionally indistinguishable from its preinjury state, regeneration has taken place. In contrast, when tissue integrity is reestablished through the formation of a fibrous, connective-tissue scar, healing has occurred through repair. Dead or missing tissue cells are replaced by tissues that resemble the original but are nonetheless readily distinguishable, possessing a markedly distorted architecture. Unlike regeneration, the tissues in repair are functionally inferior to normal, uninjured tissue.

The features that determine the regenerative potential of a tissue are defined at the cellular level. The nature of clinical healing evident to the practitioner simply reflects the capacity of the tissue's constituent cells to actualize this potential. Based on their ability to regenerate, cells are classified as labile, stable, or permanent. *Labile cells,* such as keratinocytes of the epidermis and epithelial cells of the oral mucosa, divide throughout their life span. *Stable cells* such as fibroblasts exhibit a low rate of duplication, but can undergo rapid proliferation in response to injury. For example, bone injury causes pluripotential mesenchymal cells to differentiate into osteoblasts and osteocytes. *Permanent cells* do not divide in postnatal life and include specialized nerve and cardiac muscle cells. This differing ability to regenerate accounts for variability in the extent of regeneration, depending on the area of the body injured. As the end product of the healing process is contingent on the types of cells involved, the surgeon's expectations of "normal" healing must be realistic. In ordinary circumstances, healing of bone (regeneration) differs from that of dermis (repair). Consequently, a fibrous scar should be perceived as normal healing for certain tissues; whereas, in those tissues capable of regeneration, fibrosis must be viewed as suboptimal.

From a clinical standpoint wound healing can be categorized as first, second, and third intention. Healing by *first intention*, or primary healing, occurs when a sharply made wound is accurately reapproximated within hours of the incision and heals with minimum space between its edges. Surgical incisions closed by suturing and fractures accurately reduced with compression bone plates are examples of primary healing. Healing by *secondary intention* (secondary healing) involves filling a tissue defect through formation of new connective tissue. This type of healing is seen after excisional and avulsive injury, which leaves a residual defect, and in the spontaneous healing of compound fractures. Healing by *third intention* occurs when a wound is surgically closed after secondary intention healing has begun or when tissue grafts are used to assist in the healing of a wound. This type of closure is also known as delayed primary closure.

COMPONENTS OF CUTANEOUS HEALING

Like wound healing in general, cutaneous repair comprises a complex constellation of overlapping phases. A paradigm of the healing process, the healing cutaneous wound offers an opportunity to study the many distinct biologic phenomena that constitute healing. Moreover, virtually every tissue heals by the same process that occurs in skin, with minor variations.

Inflammatory Phase

Inflammation is the initial response to injury. The inflammatory response impels the healing process and provides the milieu for the restoration of structural integrity. Tissue trauma and local bleeding result in activation of the Hageman factor (XII), which in turn initiates various biochemical systems such as the clotting, complement, and kinin cascades, releasing mitogens and chemoattractants. Platelets (thrombocytes) aggregate and adhere to the damaged surfaces. Degranulation of these platelets releases serotonin (5-hydroxytryptamine), catecholamines, and histamines, which further amplify the clotting mechanism and ensure complete activation of the complement-kinin cascades. Initial vasoconstriction is caused in part by arachidonic acid metabolites and serves to minimize the blood loss by effecting hemostasis. Subsequent vasodilation is pronounced, especially of the venules. These vascular changes are partly due to prostaglandins and histamine, which are synthesized and released by damaged tissue. Platelets and erythrocytes begin to adhere to the endothelial lining of the capillaries, and the blood clot that forms serves as a matrix for the influx of inflammatory cells. Agents such as bradykinin and histamine cause a reversible separation of the vascular endothelial cells. Increased margination is closely followed by migration of leukocytes between endothelial cells by diapedesis. The leukocytes are drawn to the site of injury by chemotactic stimuli, accompanied by the egress of plasma proteins and erythrocytes into the interstitial space.

Neutrophils are the first cells to populate the wound site and serve to control infection by phagocytizing and killing bacteria and lysing devitalized tissue. Neutrophilic activity is accentuated by opsonic antibodies leaking into the wound from altered vasculature. Predominant in the wound during the first 2 to 3 days postinjury, neutrophils gradually decrease in number and are replaced by other inflammatory cell types.

Complement chemotactic factors also mobilize a large number of lymphocytes, leading to a dense infiltration of the wound area by these cells. Thymus (T) and bursa (B) lymphocytes attracted to the site of injury secrete lymphokines that contribute to wound antibacterial defenses. By day 5 or 6 macrophages become the predominant phagocytic cells in the inflammatory tissue. They come from macrophages resident in the tissue at the site of injury or from circulating blood monocytes that reach the site of injury. Attracted to the wound by chemoattractants like fibrin degradation products, the actively phagocytic macrophages continue the process of wound microdebridement initiated by the neutrophils.

In addition to killing bacteria and producing vasoactive mediators, macrophages also release a series of monokines like fibroblast chemotactic and fibroblast stimulation factors that are believed to direct subsequent healing activity. Concomitant activation of platelets by thrombin results in the release of growth factors, including the platelet-derived growth factor (PDGF) and basic fibroblast growth factor (bFGF).

These growth factors serve as mitogens and stimulants for subsequent fibroplasia and neovascularization. Acting in concert with other chemoattractants present in the injured area, growth factors modulate wound healing by ensuring that adequate numbers of wound healing cells are attracted to the site of injury. The presence of a chemoattractant-specific receptor mechanism is strongly insinuated by the specificity of cell types at the different stages of healing.

Although the inflammatory response mainly serves to debride the site of injury and prepare it for repair, it also has the potential for destroying more than is necessary if not regulated. In the case of normal repair, the inflammatory component automatically regresses and eventually ceases as its stimuli fade. Factors that provoke persistent inflammation tend to interfere with the subsequent phases of wound healing by exaggerating the destructive component of the healing response beyond the capacity of the injured tissue for repair. Hence, the degree and duration of the inflammatory response is often a predictor of the extent of morbidity and incidence of failure to heal.

Neovascularization

Wound neovascularization, or angiogenesis, begins within the first few days after injury. Being metabolically active, inflammatory cells and fibroblasts are dependent on adequate perfusion and oxygen supply. During phagocytosis, some of the oxygen consumed by the granulocytes and macrophages is reduced by specific enzymes to bactericidal free radicals and other reactive oxygen species capable of killing phagocytosed organisms. Hypoxia depletes these enzymes through substrate deprivation and causes granulocytes to lose up to half of their antimicrobial activity. Impaired circulation of the injured tissue, along with the increased metabolic demands of the actively metabolizing leukocytes, creates a local "energy crisis." An oxygen gradient is established with the lowest tensions at the wound margins. This hypoxic state along with factors released from injured cells are responsible for stimulating angiogenesis. By restoring blood flow to the relatively ischemic wound site, revascularization supplies nutrition necessary for tissue healing.

In addition to initiating angiogenesis, local acidosis and lactate accumulation also determine fibroplasia and collagen synthesis by regulating the wound microenvironment. Activated macrophages react to the "energy crisis" present in the wound area by secreting angiogenic factors like bFGF which, along with PDGF, serve as a chemoattractant for the vascular endothelial cells. The bFGF activates hydrolytic enzymes like stromelysin, collagenase, and plasminogen, which help dissolve the basement membranes surrounding the existing blood vessels. Thus, a stage is set for endothelial budding and formation of new vessels and ingrowth of surrounding poorly vascularized tissue by migrating capillary buds. Endothelial buds, migrating along the chemotactic gradient established in the wound, fuse with adjoining buds to form new capillary loops. Once new vascular anastomoses are established, rising oxygen tensions depress further release of these angiogenic factors.

Provided wound edges are well approximated, capillaries can readily bridge the wound to unite with a vessel from the other side. However, large tissue defects, as in avulsive injuries, necessitate the development of an entirely new vascular network. Newly formed capillaries are fragile and will tear if mechanically disturbed. Eventually, these new vessels find external support in the collagen layer secreted by perivascular cells. Once the capillary network connects with existing vessels in the tissues subjacent to the wound site, the flow of erythrocytes and plasma can begin through the new microvessels. This dense layer of new vessels in combination with accompanying fibroplasia is referred to as *granulation tissue*, the provisional tissue of repair. Granulation tissue is an expression of the increased metabolic demands of the healing wound and is very sensitive to changes in wound perfusion. As wound healing progresses, its metabolic demands alter correspondingly, resulting in an extensive remodeling of this capillary network.

Fibroblastic Proliferation

Fibroblasts begin to proliferate in the wound area around the second day after injury. They appear to originate primarily from perivascular connective tissue. Mesenchymal cells, stimulated by local tissue hypoxia and macrophage and platelet growth factors, are believed to be the precursors for wound fibroblasts. An interdependency of fibroplasia and angiogenesis is established early in the healing process and is choreographed by the physicochemical environment within the wound. The role of the metabolic gradients in the wound and their role in stimulating fibroblastic activity has been elucidated by Hunt (1976) in his description of tissue repair as a "healing module." Actively dividing fibroblasts followed by mature fibroblasts appear after the macrophages that form the vanguard of the advancing wound front. Because they are metabolically active, the maturing fibroblasts require fresh nutrients, which are provided by the new vasculature. By producing the primary extracellular components of the connective tissue matrix, namely collagen and proteoglycans, fibroblasts facilitate the angiogenic process by providing support to developing vessels. Cellular ingrowth is also aided by fibrin strands of the blood clot, which serve as substrate and attachment for invading fibroblasts and neovasculature. The end result of fibroblastic invasion is the bridging of the wound edges by collagen strands.

Connective Tissue Restitution

Restoration of connective tissue is first evidenced by the appearance of invading fibroblasts and developing blood vessels. Synthetic activity of these fibroblasts includes glycosaminoglycans (GAGs): large, linear, polyanionic polysaccharides that are covalently linked to a core protein to form large sugar-protein complexes termed proteoglycans. These GAGs are hydrated to an amorphous gel as they are secreted and influence the subsequent aggregation of collagen fibers. Production of collagen by the fibroblasts is stimulated by the growth factors and the high tissue lactate levels produced by the inflammatory cells. Building blocks, including proline, glycine, and hydroxyproline, are absorbed by fibroblasts by micropinocytosis and synthesized into polypeptide chains. Three of these polypeptide chains unite to form a molecule of collagen precursor tropocollagen, which is subsequently extruded into the extracellular matrix. Once in the extracellular compartment, tropocollagen molecules align themselves to form collagen fibers, and the final structure is stabilized by both inter- and intramolecular cross-linking.

Cross-linking, which gives the collagen polymer rigidity, is usually mediated through reactive aldehyde groups associated with the amino acids lysine and hydroxylysine. Abnormal deposition of collagen fibers has been attributed to alterations in cross-linking and maturation of the collagen molecule, or to the effect of cross-link inhibitors such as β-aminopropionitrile and penicillamine. Newly formed collagen is able to interact with other interstitial matrix components such as the proteoglycans to form an extracellular matrix that contributes significantly to the functional and structural integrity of the wound. In the initial stages of repair, collagen synthesis and collagenolysis are simultaneous, and the healing of the wound can be thought of as a regulated disequilibrium between synthesis and lysis. Modulating factors like vitamin C and zinc can cause either an increase in the lytic activity or decrease in collagen formation leading to wound dehiscence. However, once collagen is stabilized, it becomes more resistant to degradation by tissue collagenases. The increasing strength of the wound over time is a manifestation of continued cross-linking and remodeling of the newly formed collagen.

Epithelialization

Satisfactory cutaneous healing requires that newly synthesized connective tissue components be resurfaced with epithelium. Epithelialization seals off the wounded area, permitting fibrous protein and ground substance synthesis to bridge the tissue defect and provide structural integrity. Failure to reepithelialize may also render the wound susceptible to continued contamination. Loss of the squamous epithelium following avulsive or excisional injury leads to a response of the marginal basal epithelial cells within 24 to 48 hours. Mitosis of the basal cells is remarkably increased; they enlarge, flatten, and migrate across the wound while remaining in contact with mesenchymal tissue. Their responses are apparently initiated by epidermal growth factors released by macrophages and platelets. However, the presumptive keratinocytes will only migrate over viable tissues. Collagenase released by the migrating layer of epithelial cells allows them to advance deep to dead or damaged dermis (eschar) by cleaving the collagen connecting viable and nonviable tissue.

Resurfacing by proliferating epithelial cells continues until apposition between epithelial sheets occurs. Once a single layer develops, more layers are formed by mitotic division of the epidermal cells. The thin epidermis formed initially is vulnerable to avulsion and slough because of the absence of rete pegs anchoring the epidermis to the wound surface. Once confluent, the cells begin to mature and keratinize but may never attain the characteristics of normal epithelium. This is especially true for a full-thickness loss of the epidermis in which healing proceeds from the margins. In the case of partial loss of epidermis, reepithelialization may proceed from epithelial cells of dermal appendages.

Wound Contraction

Contraction is a complex process that produces a dramatic spatial decrease of the wound area and, together with reepithelialization, accounts for a significant proportion of wound closure. Clinically, an active centripetal movement of the wound margins is observed during the first 5 to 10 days after injury. Contractile elements resident within the wound granulation tissue are believed to be responsible for contraction. Ironically, the benefits of rapid wound closure can be mitigated by the generation of powerful tensile forces attendant to the contractile process. Wound contractile forces on the order of 3.2×10^4 dynes/cm^2 have been measured.

The exact cause of contraction remains unknown and the motive forces for the process are the subject of some controversy. A popular but as yet unsubstantiated theory for skin contraction envisages the existence of specialized fibroblasts known as "myofibroblasts." The identifying features of myofibroblasts include the presence of microfibrillar arrangements of the contractile proteins actin and myosin, highly indented nuclei (reminiscent of smooth muscle cells), and desmosomes and hemidesmosomes between cells providing for a syncytial arrangement of contractile cells throughout the wound sites. Like smooth muscle cells, myofibroblasts are thought to be capable of contraction, and their extracellular extensions allow transmission of contractile forces between cells. Central contraction of open wound margins has been attributed to these myofibroblasts within the collagen matrix. Unfortunately, not all of the work leading to the development of a theory of myofibroblastic contraction has been substantiated by independent investigators. Hence, the fundamental causes of the contractile phenomena must still be viewed as uncertain. Certainly, many other, equally plausible hypotheses exist.

From a clinical perspective, at least two factors seem to be important for wound contraction: the formation of a significant quantity of granulation tissue and the presence of movable wound edges. Any process that inhibits granulation tissue formation reduces contraction, as exemplified by open wounds that have received a skin graft. Wounds made entirely in soft tissue generally have highly mobile edges and characteristically experience rapid and extensive contraction; those with a periosteal base have less movable edges and correspondingly exhibit less contraction. Because rapidly contracting mucosal wounds require minimal reepithelialization and characteristically form small scars, intraoral healing has sometimes been attributed erroneously to true regeneration rather than to true repair.

Although contraction occurs following tissue injury in all parts of the body, it generates adverse effects only in certain clinical situations. Depending on the site and extent of injury, contraction can limit motion, cause unsightly contractures, or even inhibit the growth of skeletal structures. Desirable in some sites, contraction can be devastating in others. The rapid rate of buccal wound closure and the rapid restoration of mucosal integrity make the buccal mucosa a highly suitable donor site for mucosal grafts. On the other hand, contraction-induced tissue distortion may produce strictures of the salivary gland ducts or may hinder tissue mobility at the base of the tongue. The magnitude of tensile forces generated by progressive wound contraction, as in burns of the anterior neck, may be sufficient to severely deform osseous structures. These contractile forces have also been implicated in the relapse of corrective surgical procedures including diminution in maxillary growth after cleft palate surgery. Hence, wound contraction should be viewed as an undesirable process that has the potential to deleteriously affect healing by rendering otherwise normal uninjured structure less functional or dysmorphic.

Scar Remodeling

Increased collagenase activity at the site of injury observed within the first week postinjury marks the initiation of wound remodeling. The process of scar remodeling persists for a prolonged period and results in reduction of scar size and reorganization of collagen fibers. When first extruded from the fibroblasts, the collagen fibers are deposited in a haphazard fashion. A gradual orientation of the fibers occurs over time, with reorganization resulting in closely aligned collagen fibers that allow for increased intermolecular bonding and concomitant increase in tensile strength. Collagen homeostasis in the scar is regulated to a large extent by tissue collagenases, which carry out collagenolysis and prevent excessive buildup of collagen. Increased tissue collagenase at the site of injury can be measured for as long as 20 years in human scar tissue. As wound healing progresses, there is a gradual transition from increased collagen synthesis and limited lysis to increased collagenolysis and decreased synthesis. Hence, at any given time, the healing wound can be considered to exist as a regulated disequilibrium between synthesis and lysis.

Changes in the kinetics of collagen synthesis or breakdown are responsible for a whole spectrum of healing aberrations ranging from wound dehiscence to hypertrophic scar and keloid formation. For example, excessive collagenolysis decreases scar strength so that it is unable to withstand even ordinary tissue tensile forces. As the metabolic demands of the healing wound decrease, the rich network of capillaries begins to regress. An equilibrium between collagenolysis and continuing collagen deposition is ultimately achieved. Despite the protracted remodeling phase, scar tissue is never as elastic as normal tissue.

HEALING OF SPECIALIZED TISSUES

Nerves

Peripheral nerve injury encountered in surgical practice often results from trauma, either accidental or iatrogenic. Injury may range from simple compression to transection of the nerve; the conduction of impulses to and from the central nervous system may be disrupted. Most nerve injuries resolve spontaneously. However, from a therapeutic viewpoint the clinician should understand the types of nerve injury, whether neurapraxia, axonotmesis, or neurotmesis, and their prognoses.

Neuropraxia denotes a simple contusion of the nerve and is the mildest form of peripheral nerve damage. The continuity of both the epineural sheath and the axons is maintained. Blunt trauma, traction, or even inflammation causes a disintegration and resorption of a segment of the myelin sheath investing the axon. However, the portion of nerve proximal to the site of injury retains its capacity to respond to stimulation. Loss in continuity results in a transient block in impulse conduction. In cases of neuropraxia, function usually returns spontaneously within a few days or weeks. *Axonotmesis* is characterized by destruction of both axon and myelin sheath while the endoneurium remains intact. Such lesions are commonly produced by crushing or compression injuries or even extreme traction exerted on the nerve. As nerve continuity is maintained by the intact endoneurium, axonal regeneration may occur with a return of function. Regeneration is incumbent on a number of factors such as age, proximity to cell body, and fiber caliber, and may take from 2 to 6 months. Complete transaction of the nerve trunk is known as *neurotmesis*, for which there is little hope for repair without microsurgery.

Following transection or even crush injury, the myelin sheath of the nerve segment distal to the site of injury starts breaking down. At the same time, the severed axonal segment undergoes wallerian degeneration, which extends as far as the peripheral nerve endings. Similar degeneration is also seen in the proximal nerve segment up to the first node of Ranvier. Breakdown products of myelin sheath degeneration are removed by macrophages and Schwann cells. At a central level, axonal injury manifests as a swelling of the nerve cell body. Chromatolysis, or disappearance of the Nissl granules, and displacement of the nucleus to the periphery is observed. Unlike myelin sheath and axon, the investing Schwann cells do not degenerate. Schwann cells close to the injury site begin to proliferate within the first week postinjury and grow toward one another. The result is the formation of tubular glial bands known as Hanke-Bünger bands, which bridge the gap formerly occupied by the transected axon. Axonal sprouts arising from the severed end of the proximal axon use these Hanke-Bünger bands as a bridge to locate the end-organ. While numerous axonal sprouts enter the distal segment, only some make contact with an end-organ and form a new axon, whereon the other sprouts degenerate. As the axon bud advances at the rate of 1 mm to 3 mm a day, the investing Schwann cells cause a new myelin sheath to form around it. The regeneration phase lasts up to 3 months and ends on contact with the end-organ by a thin, myelinated axon. In the concluding maturation phase, both the diameter and performance of the regenerating nerve fiber increases.

In contrast to axonotmesis, in which the undamaged endoneural tube confines and guides the regenerating axonal sprout, neurotmesis provides an unfavorable environment for axonal regeneration. Lack of endoneurial tube continuity hinders the entry of axonal sprouts into their original or related tubules. The presence of a large gap between the cut nerve ends causes the proliferating Schwann cells and outgrowing axonal sprouts of a sensory nerve to get lost in scar tissue growing in between the stumps. The corollary is often an amputation neuroma that is very sensitive to mechanical stimulation.

Superior functional results of neural regeneration are facilitated by microscopic repair of transected nerves. Microsurgical repair is carried out by direct reanastomosis of the severed ends or by interposition of a sural or greater auricular nerve graft. Many of the Schwann cells in the interpositional autologous nerve graft may survive and proliferate. Provided surgical repair is carried out early and under favorable conditions, a regenerating axon may cross the suture line and enter the distal stump within 3 to 20 days after repair.

While nerve fibers are regenerating, muscle fibers and other effectors supplied by them can atrophy due to inactivity. Although denervation changes are reversible following successful nerve regeneration, failure of axons to regenerate makes these changes permanent. Hemifacial atrophy subsequent to permanent facial nerve damage is a clinical manifestation of this phenomenon.

Bone

Bone is a specialized connective tissue that heals in a manner analogous to soft tissue, except that it also involves calcification of the connective tissue matrix. Osseous healing can be considered regeneration rather than repair because the characteristic structure of bone is restored. The initial biologic response to a disruption in the continuity of bone is bleeding from ruptured vessels in the haversian canals, marrow, and periosteum. As in soft tissue, the interrupted vessels are sealed off by thrombus formation. A hematoma forms between the fragments and is accompanied by a typical inflammatory response. Border zones at the fragment ends are left without blood supply, which sets up an oxygen gradient. The pattern of healing thereafter is determined to a large extent by the degree of anatomic repositioning of the fragments and by the amount of movement across the fracture line. As fractured bone has a strong tendency to unite, bony union usually occurs after realignment and fixation, provided there are no complicating factors like infection or repeated trauma. Given the regenerative potential of bone, it is inapt to consider osseous healing in terms of primary or secondary, because secondary healing bears a negative connotation. Current practice is to describe osseous healing as either "direct" or "indirect," based on the morphologic aspects. Bone healing by callus and cartilage formation is considered indirect; direct healing takes place by intracortical remodeling.

Spontaneous *indirect healing* of bone follows a routine histologic cascade involving the sequential formation of granulation tissue, fibrous tissue, fibrocartilage, and bone. The initial hematoma is replaced by granulation tissue stimulated by the hypoxic tissue environment around the fractured zone. Endosteal cells of viable marrow and haversian nutrient canals contribute to synthesis of the granulation tissue. Present in the granulation tissue are capillary sprouts, mononuclear cells, fibroblasts, and fibrocytes. Capillaries grow into the wound site from blood vessels of the periosteum, endosteum, and bone marrow. The increase in blood supply causes a corresponding reduction in tissue hypoxia. The mobilization of minerals and active metabolites to the fracture site enables mineralization to proceed. Hence, the granulation tissue formed initially acts as a skeletal blastema, which increases in stiffness as it matures.

Increases in alkaline phosphatase, inorganic pyrophosphatase, and glycosaminoglycans at the fracture site are consistent with increased bone turnover. In areas of hydrostatic pressure, chondroblasts differentiate within the granulation tissue to form a fibrocartilaginous callus that bridges the fracture gap. This callus acts as a biologic splint, decreasing the mobility of the fragments by damping interfragmentary motion. Reduced mobility, in turn, facilitates initial mineralization of the callus, with the mineralization front progressing through the fibrocartilage from the fragment ends to the center. By the third week woven bone starts forming by endochondral ossification within the callus and by subperiosteal deposition at its periphery. Early immature bone consists of coarse, irregularly arranged collagen fibers. Through continuous remodeling, mature lamellar bone forms, consisting of regularly arranged collagen fibers. The remodeling process ensures that the new bone tissue is arranged in the most efficient way to resist functional stresses.

The histologic cascade observed in fracture healing reflects the unique capacity of the forming osseous tissue to adapt to constantly changing interfragmentary strains. The granulation tissue that forms initially has minimal strength but can tolerate the highly deforming forces found in the interfragmentary zone in the early stages of fracture healing. Granulation tissue helps splint the bone segments and dampens interfragmentary movement. Decreased interfragmentary movement, in turn, permits the subsequent replacement of the granulation tissue by fibrous tissue. By enhancing stabilization of the bone segments, fibrous tissue facilitates successive formation of fibrocartilage. Once the strain levels are within viable tissue limits, the fibrocartilage mineralizes and bone forms. The complex interplay of mechanical and biologic processes at the fracture site results in a gradual transition from an elastic tissue of high energy-absorbing capacity (granulation tissue) to stiff tissue (bone). Each succeeding tissue type gently and progressively limits interfragmentary motion, thus permitting replacement by tissue with decreasing tolerance to deformation and increasing strength.

In contrast to indirect healing, which occurs by callus and cartilage formation, *direct healing* takes place through intracortical remodeling. Under absolute stability the healing process is abbreviated as the interfragmentary strains are reduced to an extremely low level. Intermediate connective tissue, callus, and cartilage stages are thus absent, with lamellar bone being laid down right from the beginning. Direct bone healing follows excellent anatomic apposition and rigid maintenance of the fragments in this position until the fracture has consolidated. The absolute stability afforded by compression bone plates precludes even microscopic movements in the fracture zone, and there is no room for a hematoma due to the accurate coaptation of the fragments. Local destruction of the osteons close to the fracture site stimulates an intensive regeneration of new haversian systems in that area. Osteoclasts form "cutting cones" at the ends of haversian canals close to the fracture site. These spearheads tunnel across the fracture line to form enlarged haversian canals. Each osteoclast spearhead is followed immediately by vessels and a front of osteoblasts, forming a new osteon which traverses the fracture line replacing the old osteon. New osteoid is deposited in the canals, which eventually matures into lamellar bone. This form of direct healing is known as *contact healing*.

This repair sequence cannot always be assured, even after clinically optimal anatomic reduction, inasmuch as there may not be an ideal meshing of the fractured ends. Interfragmentary compression is not always homogeneously distributed, with minute gaps remaining between the fracture ends. Fibrous bone may fill the gaps and is eventually replaced by lamellar bone under stable conditions. The repair tissue is gradually restructured by haversian remodeling, resulting in longitudinally arranged osteons. This form of direct healing is known as *gap healing*. In both contact and gap healing, rigid internal fixation helps keep interfragmentary stresses below critical limits.

Complications of Fracture Healing

Despite the excellent ability of bone to heal, complications do develop. These complications range from malunion caused by poorly aligned bone ends to nonunion and osteomyelitis. Although malunion does not reflect an aberrant healing process, it can be devastating in the dentulous patient. Disturbed occlusion necessitates extensive occlusal rehabilitation postoperatively. Mismatch between structure and function caused by occlusal discrepancies has deleterious effects on facial skeletal structure.

NONUNION. Nonunion is failure of the fracture to heal. As alluded to earlier, mineralization of the fibrocartilage can proceed only when there is relative stability across the fracture line. Excessive interfragmentary motion results in a nonunion with the fibrocartilage persisting. A well vascularized nonunion is essentially callus tissue, and stabilizing it with a bone plate often may suffice to enable the ossification process to progress to completion. On the other hand, poorly vascularized atrophic nonunion may prove difficult to treat, especially if infected. Soft tissue, such as muscle and fascia, interpositioned between the fractured ends is another possible cause of nonunion.

Osteomyelitis. The infectious process of osteomyelitis usually begins in the marrow spaces and spreads to the cortical bone. Medullary spaces are filled with inflammatory exudate, which may progress to the formation of pus. Osteoblasts bordering the trabeculae are generally destroyed and adjoining trabeculae become nonviable and begin to undergo slow resorption. Fragment ends separate and remain as sequestra in the site of infection. Factors such as poor host resistance, impaired vascularity of bone, and poor immobilization of the fracture are all conducive to the establishment of osteomyelitis.

Extraction Wounds

Healing of an extraction wound is a specialized example of healing by secondary intention. Following extraction, there is bleeding from exposed periodontal ligament vessels which causes the socket to fill with blood. The unsupported gingiva collapses into the opening of the extraction wound, helping maintain the clot in its position and reducing the size of the mucosal wound.

Organization of the clot begins within the first 24 hours with leukocytic migration, capillary budding, and fibroblastic proliferation. The clot acts as a scaffold on which cells associated with the healing process may migrate. It is gradually replaced by granulation tissue. At the same time epithelium grows from the mucosal edges over the surface of the organizing clot. Osteoclasts accumulate along the crestal bone to set the stage for active crestal resorption. By the second week the clot is highly organized with new capillaries extending to the center of the clot. Epithelial proliferation over the surface of the wound may be complete around this time in the case of small sockets. Trabeculae of osteoid slowly start growing into the clot from the walls of the alveolus accompanied by concomitant remodeling of the cortical bone of the alveolar socket. This is evidenced on radiographs as a diminishing radio-opacity of the lamina dura. The socket is completely epithelialized and filled with osteoid tissue by the fourth week. However, osteoid tissue being poorly calcified is not visible on the radiographs at this time. Maturative remodeling of bone is accompanied by crestal resorption of the alveolar bone causing it to lie below that of the adjacent teeth. Due to active remodeling, the extraction site may not be discernible on radiographs after 4 to 6 months.

Occasionally the blood clot fails to form or may disintegrate, which causes a localized alveolar osteitis. In such instances, healing proceeds slowly and the socket eventually fills with granulation tissue from the alveolar wall.

Root Fractures

If the fractured root of a tooth is reduced and splinted well and providing the pulp recovers from the trauma, the fracture crevice will fill with granulation tissue from the periodontium. Mineralization of this granulation tissue leads to the formation of osteocementum, which cements the root fragments to each other. A layer of secondary dentin is also deposited on the pulpal side of the fracture. If splinting is not carried out the gap may remain filled only with connective tissue. Occasionally, a resorptive process begins at the fracture gap and the dentin and cementum are replaced by bone. Usually, trauma sufficient to fracture a root also causes the tooth to be devitalized, which impedes healing of the fracture gap.

Free Skin Grafts

Skin grafts may be either full thickness or split thickness. A *full-thickness graft* is composed of epidermis and the entire dermis; a *split-thickness graft* is composed of the epidermis and varying amounts of dermis. Depending on the amount of underlying dermis included, split-thickness grafts are described as thin, intermediate, or thick. Following grafting, nutritional support for a free skin graft is initially provided by plasma that exudes from the dilated capillaries of the host bed. A fibrin clot forms at the graft-host interface, fixing the graft to the host bed. There is accompanying infiltration of host leukocytes into the graft, with the leukocytes invading the lower layers of the graft initially. Graft survival depends on the ingrowth of blood vessels from the host into the graft (neovascularization) and direct anastomoses between the graft and the host vasculature (inosculation). The endothelial capillary buds from the host invade the graft, reaching the dermoepidermal junction by 48 hours. Concomitantly, vascular connections are established between host and graft vessels. However, only a few of the ingrowing capillaries succeed in developing a functional anastomosis. Formation of vascular connections between recipient bed and transplant is signaled by the pink appearance of the graft, which appears between days 3 and 5 after transfer. Fibroblasts from the recipient bed begin to invade the layer of fibrin and leukocytes by the fourth day after transplantation. The fibrin clot is slowly resorbed and organized as the fibroblastic infiltration continues. By the ninth day the new blood vessels and fibroblasts have achieved a firm union, anchoring the deep layers of the graft to the host bed.

Reinnervation of the skin graft occurs by nerve fibers entering the graft through its base and sides, and following the vacated neurilemmal cell sheaths to reconstruct the innervation pattern of the donor skin. Recovery of sensation usually begins within 2 months after transplantation. Grafts rarely attain the sensory qualities of normal skin, because the extent of reinnervation depends on how accessible the neurilemmal sheaths are to the entering nerve fibers. Because split-thickness grafts are thinner than full-thickness grafts, they are susceptible to trauma and undergo considerable contraction, but clinically they exhibit increased survival rates. In contrast, the "take" of full-thickness grafts is not as good and they are more slowly revascularized. However, full-thickness grafts are less susceptible to trauma and undergo minimal shrinkage.

NEUROENDOCRINE RESPONSE TO INJURY

Any form of injury evokes an immediate neuroendocrine response, which represents a coordinated defensive reaction by the central nervous system to a variety of signals elicited by tissue damage and its consequences. Neural input arising from damaged tissues and from receptors detecting fluid loss stimulates various hypothalamic nuclei, which in turn alters pituitary hormone secretion and activation of the sympathoadrenal system. Corresponding changes in the secretion of adrenal, pancreatic, and thyroid hormones occurs. Alteration in hormone concentrations induced by injury are regarded to occur in phases: an early postinjury phase that may last up to 24 to 72 hours and a late phase that may be complete by 2 weeks (brief) or last up to 8 weeks or longer (protracted). Although the precise effects of injury on the hypothalamopituitary axis are not yet ascertained, the flux in the hormonal levels attendant to injury is believed to induce metabolic alterations with important nutritional and therapeutic implications.

Increased secretion of hormones like adrenocorticotropic hormone (ACTH), growth hormone, prolactin, and vasopressin is a direct result of trauma. Adrenaline and nonadrenaline concentrations exhibit corresponding increases and their levels rise exponentially with the severity of injury. Secondary changes include stimulation of cortisol and aldosterone and an inhibition of insulin and somatomedin secretion. Rapid increases in plasma cortisol following trauma have been attributed to the increased concentrations of ACTH that accompany injury. Although the exact role of ACTH in the maintenance of cortisol levels is not definitive, the duration of cortisol response seems to increase fairly consistently with the severity of injury. Analogous changes in the plasma growth hormone concentration are also observed, although the elevated levels are generally confined to the initial postinjury phase. Conversely, plasma somatomedin activity tends to fall within hours of injury, only to rise again over the next few days. Elevated prolactin levels, albeit transient, also reflect a neuroendocrine response to injury. Basal thyrotropic-stimulating hormone (TSH) concentration is consistent throughout the postinjury intervals. In contrast, plasma triiodothyronine (T_3) levels tend to fall and can remain depressed for a few days to even weeks after major injury. The kinetics of these hormone level changes is unclear at the present time. Vasopressin demonstrates a neuroendocrine response to injury that is similar to ACTH in that its levels rise rapidly in the early postinjury phase and gradually return to normal. Postinjury elevations in plasma glucagon concentration also occur, either immediately or after a delay, and begin to fall after about 3 days. However, elevated glucagon levels may still be detected 10 days after injury.

As a rule, the duration of the neuroendocrine responses generally depends on the severity of the injury. Nevertheless, there is considerable variability among hormones, for reasons that are not yet elucidated. The only endocrine changes consistently seen at later times after trauma are an increase in insulin secretion, which supersedes the initial suppression, and decreases in the concentrations of T_3 and gonadal steroids. The complex constellation of overlapping effects of the various hormones makes it difficult to attribute roles to specific hormones. As a simplifying assumption, the initial neuroendocrine response to injury can be construed as playing a defensive role. It helps the body withstand the effects of injury through a complex regulatory mechanism that influences inflammatory and immunologic processes, carbohydrate mechanism, shock, and water balance. Initial vasoconstriction caused by sympathetic activity and also increased levels of adrenaline and vasopressin helps compensatory fluid movement into circulation and limits blood loss from the wound.

Neuroendocrine stimulus is also responsible for the mobilization of body fuels for coping with the injury. Postinjury hyperglycemia caused by a combination of glycogen breakdown and impairment of insulin secretion is believed to contribute to the body's defenses, although the evidence is still conjectural at present. Peripheral insulin resistance, which is another early metabolic effect of injury, inhibits the use of glucose. By preventing mobilized glycogen from being squandered, insulin resistance helps the body to withstand a period of forced starvation. Neuroendocrine responses that occur in the late phase are believed to have a more adaptive function. Due to the putative understanding of the function of the neuroendocrine response, the scope for therapeutic intervention remains unclear at the present time.

FACTORS AFFECTING HEALING

Wound Infection

Gross bacterial contamination is a major cause of impaired wound healing. All wounds have some degree of bacterial contamination; however, this must be distinguished from true infection. The approximate number of organisms required to classify a wound as infected ranges from 10^5 to 10^6 organisms per gram of tissue. Bacteria provoke varying degrees of inflammation in the wounded tissue by releasing neutrophil proteases and endotoxins as they are destroyed by host defense mechanisms. Newly formed cells, and their collagen matrix, are susceptible to these breakdown products of wound infection, and the attendant cell and collagen lysis contribute to impaired healing. Resistance of the wound to infection depends on a number of factors including perfusion of the healing wound and the magnitude and nature of contamination. Inadequate tissue perfusion and oxygenation of the wound during the postoperative period will allow infection to be established. Transformation of contaminated wounds into infected wounds is also facilitated by necrotic tissue, foreign bodies, or compromised host defenses. The most important factor in minimizing the risk of infection is meticulous surgical technique, including thorough debridement, adequate hemostasis, and elimination of dead space. Careful technique must be augmented by proper postoperative care, which includes keeping the wound site clean and protecting it from trauma.

Tissue Perfusion

Oxygen is fundamental for normal cell function and proliferation. Relative hypoxia in a region of injury stimulates a fibroblastic response and helps to mobilize other cellular elements of repair. However, very low oxygen levels acting together with lactic acid production by bacteria lower tissue pH and contribute to tissue breakdown. Cell lysis follows, with releases of proteases and glycosidases and with subsequent digestion of extracellular matrix. Impaired local circulation also hinders delivery of nutrients and oxygen to the wound. Delayed movement of neutrophils, opsonins, and the other mediators of inflammation to the wound site diminishes the effectiveness of the phagocytic defense system and allows the bacteria to proliferate. Wounds in hypoxic tissue are more easily infected and heal poorly because both leukocytes and fibroblastic proliferation are depressed by hypoxia. Poor oxygenation also interferes with collagen synthesis because it requires high levels of molecular oxygen. Most healing problems associated with diabetes mellitus, irradiation, small vessel atherosclerosis, and chronic infection can be largely ascribed to a faulty oxygen delivery system.

The state of the microcirculation in the wound after surgery is an indicator of the wound's ability to resist the inevitable bacterial contamination. Tissue rendered ischemic by improper scalpel use, or desiccated by cautery or prolonged air drying, tends to be poorly perfused and susceptible to infection. Similarly, strangulation of tissue by use of too many or constricting sutures, tissue edema, remaining dead tissue or a systemic perfusion defect like hypovolemia, all adversely affect wound healing. Although careful surgical technique is imperative for ensuring adequate wound perfusion, the natural resistance of the wound can also be enhanced by maintaining good body fluid volume and adequate arterial oxygen tension. The use of hyperbaric oxygen to maintain the wound in a state of hyperoxia is based on this rationale.

Hematomas and Foreign Bodies

Poor hemostasis at the time of surgery is a common cause of hematomas. Every hematoma has potential for becoming infected or fibrotic as healing progresses, which can impede the healing process. Hematomas can cause necrosis of an overlying flap, as sometimes seen in ablative head and neck surgery. Careful hemostasis accompanied by adequate surgical drainage helps to alleviate this problem. Foreign bodies including sutures can potentiate infection and that is why sutures should be used sparingly and far enough apart to achieve a satisfactory sealed wound. Prosthetic grafts including implants used for aesthetic augmentation incite varying degrees of foreign body reaction and adversely impact the healing process. Dirt and tar located in dermal wounds not only jeopardize healing but may result in a "tattoo" deformity. Hence, traumatic soft tissue wounds, especially abraded ones, should be cleaned thoroughly after adequate anesthesia.

Radiation Injury

Therapeutic radiation produces structural damage in undiseased tissue adjacent to the targeted tissue, reducing its capacity for regeneration and repair. The intensity of the effect of radiation on tissue is dose dependent and these effects may be acute or chronic. Acute changes primarily affect the cells with a high turnover rate and manifest clinically as mucositis, desquamation, erythema, and depression of the bone marrow. Fibroblastic and endothelial cell proliferation are also depressed. Hence, surgeons operating in an irradiated area should allow the acute effects to subside before proceeding (3–4 weeks). With small to moderate doses of radiation, the acute reactions will begin to subside and the wound becomes morphologically normal. Late effects of radiation are permanent, directly related to total dose, and are typically manifested in connective tissues of skin as well as the walls of the blood vessels. Collagen hyalinizes and tissues become fibrotic and hypoxic due to obliterative vasculitis, and tissue susceptibility to infection increases dramatically. Once these changes occur they are irreversible and do not change with time.

Due to the propensity of obliterative vasculitis to seriously impair capacity for repair, the surgeon must always anticipate the possibility of a complicated healing following surgery or traumatic injury in an irradiated area. Wound dehiscences are common and supervening open wounds heal slowly or incompletely. Even minor trauma may result in ulceration and colonization by opportunistic bacteria. If the patient cannot mount an effective inflammatory response, progressive necrosis of the tissues may follow. Such complications may occur as early as a few months to even years after irradiation. Healing can often be achieved only by excising all nonvital tissue and covering the bed with a well vascularized skin or myocutaneous flap. For purposes of repair, tissue with intact normal blood supply is brought in to provide both oxygen and the cells necessary for inflammation and healing. Just as in other tissues, irradiation renders bone relatively avascular. Following trauma or disintegration of the soft tissue cover due to inflammatory reaction (e.g., periodontal disease in an irradiated jaw) healing does not occur because irradiated marrow cannot form granulation tissue. In such instances, the nonreactive bone substance must be removed down to the healthy portion and the osseous defect reconstructed with a vascularized osteomyocutaneous flap.

Age

Healing is generally faster in young persons but may be protracted in elderly persons. Impaired healing in the elderly probably results from the general reduction in the rate of tissue metabolism as the person ages, which itself may be a manifestation of decreased circulatory efficiency. In the absence of compromising systemic conditions, differences in healing as a function of age seem to be small.

Nutritional Factors

Adequate nutrition is important for normal repair. Malnourishment adversely alters the body's metabolism, hindering the normal wound healing process. This is particularly true for patients with chronic illnesses. Dietary protein and vitamin C have received special emphasis with respect to healing. When the serum protein concentration is below 2 g/dL, significant impairment occurs in the rate at which wound tensile strength is gained. The cause of this effect is not clear, but hypoproteinemia apparently impairs fibroplasia. An absence of essential building blocks obviously thwarts normal repair, but the reverse is not necessarily true. The availability of methionine and the subsequent conversion of methionine to cystine seem to be important for healing and necessitate a minimum protein intake. However, a high protein diet does not shorten the time required for healing.

Several vitamins play an important role in wound healing. Vitamin A stimulates fibroplasia, collagen cross-linking, and epithelialization, and it will restimulate these processes in the steroid-retarded wound. Vitamin C deficiency impairs collagen synthesis by fibroblasts, because it is an important cofactor, along with alpha-ketoglutarate and ferrous iron, in the hydroxylation process of proline and lysine. Healing wounds appear to be more sensitive to absorbate deficiency than uninjured tissue. Increased rates of collagen turnover persist for a long time, and healed wounds may rupture when the individual becomes scorbutic. Local antibacterial defenses are also impaired because ascorbic acid is also necessary for neutrophil superoxide production. Vitamin D, thiamine, and riboflavin deficiencies also result in poor repair.

Depleted serum levels of metals such as zinc result in impaired epithelial and fibroblastic proliferation; cells migrate normally but do not undergo mitosis. Numerous enzymes are zinc-dependent, particularly DNA-polymerase and reverse-transcriptase. On the other hand, exceeding the zinc levels can exert a distinctly detrimental effect on healing by inhibiting macrophage migration and interfering with collagen cross-linking. Copper is also essential for covalent cross-linking of collagen.

Diabetes

Patients with severe diabetes heal poorly; however, the precise effects of insulin deficiency and hyperglycemia are not yet understood. Small vessel occlusive disease leading to impaired circulation and wound ischemia is a major contributing factor. Poor healing has also been related to the metabolic problems related to hyperglycemia, insulin deficiency, and insulin resistance. Insulin deficiency is believed to contribute to the defective leukocyte function in diabetes, and this may manifest clinically as an increased incidence of infection. Control of blood sugar is essential in the diabetic patient undergoing surgery.

Drug Therapy

Therapeutic drugs have the potential for altering both inflammatory reactions and cell metabolism and, as such, can alter the healing process both in rate and quality. Nonsteroidal antiinflammatory drugs such as indomethacin decrease collagen synthesis to some extent. Exogenous corticosteroids diminish propylhydroxylase and lysyl oxidase activity, depressing both fibroplasia and neovascularity. They reduce the tensile strength of closed wounds, especially if given within the first 3 days after injury. Besides a reduction in the inflammatory reaction and collagen synthesis, epithelialization and contraction are also impaired. The inhibitory effects of glucocorticosteriods are attenuated to some extent by vitamin A given concurrently. Most of the antineoplastic agents exert their cytotoxic effect by interfering with DNA or RNA production. Reduction in protein synthesis or cell division manifests as impaired proliferation of fibroblasts and collagen formation. Neutropenia attendant to chemotherapy predisposes to wound infection and prolongs the inflammatory phase of wound healing. Because of their deleterious effect on wound healing when given in the perioperative stage, it would seem reasonable to withhold administration of antineoplastic drugs until the time for potential postoperative complications has passed.

ABERRANT HEALING

Aberrant healing results from an abnormal mechanism that leads to the formation of excess scar tissue, contractures, constrictions, or adhesions. An imbalance between collagen deposition and degradation may manifest an excessive scarring in the form of a hypertropic scar or keloid. These lesions are characterized by overabundant collagen deposition. Although the exact pathogenesis of hypertrophic scars and keloids is not known, they probably result from an inadequate lysis of collagen by collagenase or are due to elevated levels of propylhydroxylase, which contributes to collagen formation. Although healing appears to be proceeding normally initially, the control mechanisms of normal repair are deficient and connective tissue synthesis and accumulation continues well beyond the bounds of the original injury. The biologic and clinical differences between hypertrophic scars and keloids are still not clearly established. Hypertrophic scars generally remain within the boundaries of the wound, arise soon after the injury, and eventually subside. In contrast, keloids outgrow their boundaries, appear months after injury, and rarely subside. They mostly appear on the face, ear lobes, and anterior chest. There is a clear familial and racial predilection for keloid formation, and dark-skinned individuals and those younger than age 30 have a propensity to develop these abnormalities. Numerous methods for preventing or treating these lesions have been attempted but no effective therapy has emerged.

At a clinical level, a side effect of the anticonvulsant drug phenytoin (Dilantin) is the production of a form of gingival hyperplasia that may resemble hypertrophic repair. Increases occur in collagen content, glycosaminoglycan synthesis, and the number of fibroblasts present. The mechanism of phenytoin action is not known, but it has been described to increase the growth rate of human gingival fibroblasts, to suppress collagen hydroxylation, and to enhance protein synthesis. Whatever the mode of action, phenytoin seems to exert effects on connective tissue elements that are modulated by trauma and inflammation.

RECENT ADVANCES

An enhanced understanding of wound healing pathophysiology, coupled with attempts to favorably influence the healing process, has impelled the search for substances to promote healing. Recently, certain polypeptide molecules were discovered within the healing wound. These peptides, called *growth factors*, exhibit special properties important to the process of repair. Although anachronistically named after the biologic activity that led to their discovery, the ubiquitous growth factors demonstrate a whole spectrum of effects ranging from promotion of cell proliferation and differentiation to immunomodulation. An intrinsic part of the repair mechanism, these endogenous polypeptides are believed to exert their specific effects through a receptor mechanism present on the surfaces of the target cells.

Platelet-derived growth factor (PDGF) was so termed because it was first detected in the alpha granules of circulating platelets. It has been discovered subsequently that PDGF is also elaborated by fibroblasts, macrophages, smooth muscle cells, and vascular endothelial cells. PDGF stimulates mitogenesis and protein synthesis in cells of mesenchymal origin, such as fibroblasts and smooth muscle cells. Endothelial or epithelial cells that lack specific PDGF receptors are not affected by it. Another polypeptide found to be mitogenic for a number of cell types, including epithelial, fibroblastic, and endothelial cells, is the epidermal growth factor (EGF). Accelerated epidermal regeneration and stimulation of collagen and glycosaminoglycan deposition occurs when EGF is applied to dermal wounds. Similar biologic activity is demonstrated by transforming growth factor-α (TGF-α), which shares the same receptor as EGF.

Other wound healing factors that have been isolated include an aggregation of growth factors termed transforming growth factor-β (TGF-β). This group encompasses a number of homodimeric forms which share several biologic features while differing in biologic activity. The TGF-β can stimulate or retard the growth of many cell types and act synergistically with EGF or PDGF. Addition of TGF-β has been demonstrated to increase granulation tissue formation and the tensile strength of healing dermal wounds. Also belonging to the TGF-β family are the bone morphogenetic proteins (BMP), a group of polypeptides involved in the induction of cartilage and bone formation. The target cells for BMP activity are the undifferentiated, perivascular mesenchymal type cells. Although the nature of the BMP receptor mechanism is unknown, it is believed that once the BMP is bound to the mesenchymal cells, the genome of the cells is reprogrammed in favor of chondroosteogenetic DNA sequences.

Currently there is sufficient evidence that growth factors are cardinal to the initial events following injury and throughout the later stages of wound repair including wound remodeling. The efficacy of wound healing factors in reversing defective wound repair induced by chemotherapy and steroids has been demonstrated in animal models. Preliminary human clinical data show that growth factors acting alone or synergistically can restore healing in patients with chronic, nonhealing ulcers due to diabetes, chronic venous stasis, or rheumatoid arthritis. This connotes exciting therapeutic potential for these modulators of the healing process. Due to their ability to enhance the repair mechanism, exogenously added growth factors help the tissues of nonhealing wounds to regain their reparative potential. It is feasible that surgeons eventually may be able to influence the healing process by adding exogenous growth factors, although a controlled release of growth factors into the injury site will probably be necessary to prevent overstimulation and excessive scarring. Continued isolation of more growth factors and definition of their properties, coupled with the ability to produce them with the help of recombinant DNA methods, portends exciting possibilities in the field of wound healing research.

BIBLIOGRAPHY

Book Chapters

Barratt GE, Koopmann CF Jr. Skin grafts: Physiology and clinical considerations. In: Symposium on Wound Healing. Otolaryngol Clin North Am 1984: 17; 335.

Bertolami C. Oral wound repair. In: Clark JW, ed. Clinical Dentistry, vol. 3 New York: Harper & Row, 1982: 1.

Cuthbertson DP. Surgical metabolism: Historical and evolutionary aspects. In: Wilkinson AW, Cuthbertson D, eds. Metabolism and the Response to Injury. London: Pitman Medical, 1976: 1.

Hunt TK, ed. Wound Healing and Wound Infections: Theory and Surgical Practice. New York: Appleton-Century-Crofts, 1980.

Hunt TK. Wound healings: Disorders of repair. In: Fundamentals of Wound Management in Surgery. South Plainfield: Chirurgecom, 1976.

Hunt TK, Knighton DR, Goodson WH. Wound healing. In: Way LW, ed. Current Surgical Diagnosis and Treatment, ed 7. Los Altos, CA: Lange Medical Publications, 1988: 86.

Krstic RV. General Histology of the Mammal. New York: Springer-Verlag, 1985.

Müller ME, Allgöwer M, Schneider R, Willenegger H. Manual of Internal Fixation, ed 2. New York: Springer-Verlag, 1979.

Peacock EE. Wound healing and care. In: Schwartz SI, et al, eds. Principles of Surgery, ed 4. New York: McGraw-Hill, 1984: 289.

Peacock EE: Wound Repair, ed 3. Philadelphia: WB Saunders, 1984.

Rahn BA. Bone healing: Histologic and physiologic concepts. In: Sumner-Smith G, ed. Bone in Clinical Orthopaedics—A Study in Comparative Osteology. Philadelphia: WB Saunders, 1982: 335.

Stoner HB. An integrated neuro-endocrine response to injury. In: Wilkinson AW, Cuthbertson D, eds. Metabolism and the Response to Injury. London: Pitman Medical, 1976: 194.

Stoner HB. Causitive factors and afferent stimuli involved in the metabolic response to injury. In: Wilkinson AW, Cuthbertson D, eds. Metabolism and the Response to Injury. London: Pitman Medical, 1976: 202.

Journal Articles

Barton RN. Neuroendocrine mobilization of body fuels after injury. Brit Med Bull 1985; 41: 218.

Barton RN. The neuroendocrinology of physical injury. Baliere's Clin Endocrinol Metab 1987; 1: 355.

Carter DM, Balin AK., Gottlieb AB, Eisinger M, Lin A, Pratt L, Sherbany A, Caldwell D. Clinical experience with crude preparation of growth factors in healing of chronic wounds in human subjects. Prog Clin Res 1988; 266: 303.

Clark RAF. Cutaneous tissue repair: Basic biologic considerations—I. Dermatol 1985; 13: 701.

Clark RAF. Cutaneous tissue repair: Practical implications of current knowledge—II. J Am Acad Dermatol 1985; 13: 919.

Dayer JM, Breard J, Chess L, Krane SM. Participation of monocyte-macrophages and lymphocytes in the production of a factor that stimulates collagenase and prostaglandin release by rheumatoid synovial cells. J Clin Invest 1979; 64: 1380.

Diegelmann RF, Cohen IK, Kaplan AM. The roles of macrophages in wound repair: A review. Plast Reconstr Surg 1981; 68: 107.

Gabbiani G, Hirschel BJ, Ryan GB, Statkov PR, Majno G. Granulation tissue as a contractile organ: A study of structure and function. J Exper Med 1972; 135: 719.

Gann DS, Lilly MP. The endocrine response to injury. Prog Crit Care Med 1984; 1: 15.

Jensen JA, Hunt TK, Scheuenstuhl H, Banda M. Effect of lactate, pyruvate and pH on secretion of angiogenesis and mitogenesis factors by macrophages. Lab Inv 1986; 54(5): 574.

Knighton DR, Fiegel VD, Austin LL, Ciresi KF, Butler EL. Classification and treatment of chronic non-healing wounds. Ann Surg 1986; 204: 322.

Kostyo JL. CNS peptides that regulate pituitary function. Ann Rev Phys 1986; 48: 473.

Kremenak CR, Pratt S, Koopmann C, Morris J, Murray R. Reduction of wound contraction after palatal surgery in weaning beagles. J Dent Res 1974; 53 (Special Issue): 149.

Laato M. The effect of epidermal growth factor or granulation tissue formation in the rat. Acta Chir Scand Suppl 1988; 546: 1.

Lawrence WT, Sport MB, Groschboth C, Norton JA, Grotendorst GR. The reversal of an adriamicin induced healing impairment with chemoattractants and growth factors. Ann Surg 1986; 203: 142.

Lunch SE, Colvin RB, Antoniades HN. Growth factors in

wound healing. Single and synergistic effects on partial thickness porcine skin wounds. J Clin Invest 1989; 84:640.

Mustoe TA, Pierce GF, Thomason A, Gramates P, Sporn MB, Deuel TF. Accelerate healing of incisional wounds in rats induced by transforming growth factor beta. Science 1987; 237:1333.

Nakagawa S, Yoshida S, Hirao Y, Kasuga S, Fuwa T. Biological effects of biosynthetic human EGF on the growth of mammalian cells in vitro. Differentiation 1985; 29:284.

Orgill D, Demling RH. Current concepts and approaches to wound healing. Crit Care Med 1988; 16(9):899.

Ross R, Raines EW, Bowen-Oope DF. The biology of platelet-derived growth factor. Cell 1986; 45:155.

Rudolph R. Contraction and the control of contraction. World J Surg 1980; 4:279.

Rudolph R, Guber S, Suzuka M, et al. The life cycle of the myofibroblast. Surg Gynecol Obstet 1977; 145:389.

Sato K, Urist MR. Bone morphogenetic protein-induced cartilage development in tissue culture. Clin Orthop 1978; 134:342.

Todaro GJ, Fryling C, Delarco JE. Transforming growth factors produced by certain human tumor cells: Polypeptides that interact with epidermal growth factor receptors. Proc Natl Acad Sci USA 1980; 77:5258.

Urist MR, DeLange RJ, Finerman GAM. Bone cell differentiation and growth factors. Science 1983; 22:680.

Wozney JM, Rosen V, Celeste AJ, Mitsock LM, Whitters MJ, Kriz RW, Hewick RM, Wang EA. Novel regulations of bone formation: Molecular clones and activities. Science 1988; 242:1528.

2

Medical Management of the Surgical Patient

James R. Hupp

Oral and maxillofacial surgery frequently causes temporary but significant alteration of the anatomy and physiology of the upper aerodigestive tract but has little direct impact on vital organ systems. Therefore, the surgery itself is safe to perform even on relatively unhealthy individuals. However, the physiologic stresses produced by surgery and the general anesthetic techniques necessary for these procedures can lead to serious morbidity and mortality. This is especially true in patients with various organs on the brink of decompensation due to disease.

This chapter presents the common medical situations with potential to compromise the successful outcome of oral or maxillofacial surgery. Emphasis is given to the means of detecting health problems preoperatively and of preparing patients with various medical disorders so that complications in the perioperative period are avoided. The liberal use of medical consultations is highly recommended for all situations in which the surgeon has concerns for the medical well-being of a surgical patient.

SURGERY IN THE PATIENT WITH CARDIAC DISEASE

Preservation of cardiac health is an essential element of any perioperative protocol. The proper match of oxygen supply to oxygen use in myocardial tissue is the key to maintaining proper contractility and electrical activity. In the patient with a healthy heart and lungs, the myocardium is protected in the perioperative period by avoiding hypovolemia, ensuring adequate oxygen-carrying capacity of the blood, keeping serum electrolytes within physiologic limits, and supplying the lungs with adequate oxygen. Cardiac output also depends on properly functioning valves. Finally, the load against which the ventricles must work must stay within reasonable limits to preserve myocardial function.

Several cardiac conditions can exist preoperatively which have the potential to compromise the heart's ability to maintain adequate blood pressure intra- or postoperatively. These conditions include coronary artery disease, valvular disease, various processes predisposing the heart to congestive failure, and abnormalities of electrical impulse generation or conduction. In the discussion of these four conditions that follows, emphasis is on the means of assessing the degree of cardiac compromise and reserve, of improving the situation preoperatively, and of managing the condition perioperatively.

Coronary Artery Disease

The two principal processes that cause an insufficient blood supply to the myocardium are coronary artery obstruction and spasm. Myocardial ischemia will occur when the supply of oxygen is inadequate to meet the demand for oxygen. Myocardial oxygen need is increased when the heart has increased rate or mass, has decreased contractility, or is forced to work against an increased afterload which increases end-diastolic wall tension. In these situations symptoms of ischemia will occur if oxygen supply to the myocardium cannot be increased because the coronary arteries are critically narrowed by fixed atheromatous lesions or spasm; clinically this is manifested by exercise-induced angina pectoris. The myocardial oxygen supply also can be acutely decreased by a long-ago described, but only recently understood, process in which thrombosis of a coronary artery occurs at the site of an atheromatous plaque that has ulcerated or been torn. Because this circumstance is not related to myocardial work, it can occur at any time. The development of an acute myocardial infarct while a patient is at rest is a clinical example of such an event. Spasm of coronary arteries is a less well understood phenomena but is commonly visualized during coronary angiography. Spasms can occur in the absence of significant atheromatous lesions, producing Prinzmetal's (variant) angina, which can occur at rest.

Myocardial ischemia produces decreased myocardial contractility rapidly leading to systemic hypotension and pulmonary vascular congestion. Patients may complain of a squeezing, choking, or tight feeling in the substernal region radiating to the throat, jaws, shoulders, or arms. The patient may also experience dyspnea, diaphoresis, and nausea. Anginal symptoms will regress soon after the provoking activity ceases or after transoral mucosal nitroglycerin is administered. Infarction symptoms will persist despite nitroglycerin use or rest.

There are no standard physical signs of coronary artery insufficiency so preoperative screening relies on historic information and electrocardiography. Symptoms of compromised coronary arteries should be sought preoperatively in all adult males and menopausal and postmenopausal females. A heightened index of suspicion should be used with patients with known risk factors including obesity, tobacco smoking, diabetes, hyperlipidemia, age over 70, hypertension, and family history of coronary disease. Specific questioning about problems occurring during physical activity or postprandially should be included.[1]

Electrocardiograms (ECG) should be done within a month of a planned elective general anesthetic and surgery in all males age 35 and older, females age 45 and older, and all other patients with a history suggestive of cardiac disease.[2] Although it is unlikely to see resting ECG changes suggestive of acute ischemia, old silent infarcts (representing 20% to 60% of all infarctions) or conduction blocks due to coronary disease may be detected.[3] It should be noted that 30% of patients with a history of MI have a normal resting ECG.[4] ECG after controlled treadmill exercise is a more sensitive means of detecting ischemic tendencies as evidenced by ST depression or T-wave inversion. Patients with a past history of cardiac disease should have preoperative posteroanterior and lateral chest radiographs to detect early signs of congestive heart failure. Finally, coronary angiography can be performed to identify areas of narrowing, which predispose the patient to perioperative myocardial ischemia.

All patients with a documented history of angina may have an increased risk of perioperative infarction. The risk varies with the severity of the coronary disease and the degree of physiologic stress in the perioperative period. Angina that is worsening with respect to frequency, duration, response to medication, or ease of production is, by definition, unstable angina. Surgery in such a situation should only proceed if needed emergently. Patients with stable but poorly controlled angina need medical intervention to improve their cardiac status before any elective surgery. This intervention may include the administration of long-acting vasodilators or sympathetic nervous system or calcium channel antagonists. Angiographic results may indicate that preoperative transluminal coronary angioplasty (TCA) or coronary artery bypass grafting (CABG) should predate elective surgery. Surgery can follow successful TCA within weeks, whereas 6 months should elapse between elective surgery and prior CABG.[5,6]

Patients with a known history of myocardial infarction should be carefully questioned concerning the presence of any symptoms of poor cardiac output and dysrhythmias. The amount and location of myocardial scar tissue following a healed infarction will dictate the degree of myocardial dysfunction. Elective surgery should be delayed 6 months until the risk of perioperative infarction drops to its lowest point, about 5%. In comparison, the risk of reinfarction is 15% in those operated on less than 6 months after an infarction and 0.13% in patients without a history of infarction.

Patients with stable, well controlled angina or who

have delayed surgery 6 months since an uncomplicated myocardial infarction can usually undergo elective maxillofacial procedures safely if agreement is obtained from the physician managing their cardiac problem and if intraoperative hyper- or hypotension is avoided. Although some studies indicate the risk of infarction increases with the duration of surgery, this has only been well documented in the case of major thoracic or upper abdominal procedures. Modern day general anesthesia may actually be protective of the myocardium, because supraphysiologic levels of oxygen are administered and cardiac work is minimized through maintenance of muscle relaxation, sympathetic nervous system antagonism, blood pressure control, and prompt dysrhythmia recognition and management. To assist with these goals, consideration should be given to radial artery cannulation for blood gas and pH measurement and precise blood pressure monitoring.[2,7]

Patients on nitrate vasodilators can be switched to intravenous nitroglycerin for surgery.[8] Patients on preoperative sympathetic or calcium channel antagonists should have them continued in the perioperative period. Some clinicians advocate digitalizing patients with coronary artery disease (CAD) perioperatively. If this is done, serum digoxin and potassium levels should be carefully monitored. Digoxin levels should be kept on the low side of the therapeutic range, because digoxin toxicity may be difficult to detect in the early postoperative period. For patients on low-dose aspirin, the physician managing their cardiac problems should be consulted before stopping the aspirin perioperatively.

The presence of signs of chronic congestive failure following a myocardial infarction increases operative risk, as is discussed later in this chapter.

Patients with CAD have their greatest risk of cardiac problems in the early postoperative period. The cardiorespiratory system is no longer controlled by general anesthesia, and the normal stresses which occur in the early recovery period exist. There is usually a need for increased cardiac output, which the diseased heart may not be able to provide or tolerate, and ischemia can result. Therefore, these patients need frequent cardiopulmonary physical examinations and close monitoring of vital signs, urine output, jugular venous pressure, electrolytes, and, if indicated, digoxin levels postoperatively for up to 3 days. An immediate postoperative ECG should be obtained in patients with a history of CAD, particularly if they show any of the following:

Unexplained hypotensive episode
Signs of heart failure
Dysrhythmias
Angina
Unexplained syncope

In the absence of ECG changes clinicians should also consider obtaining serial cardiac enzymes and possibly a radionuclide scan.

Care in the postoperative period should be taken to maintain normal intravascular volume, avoid hyper- or hypotension, keep serum electrolytes in their physiologically normal ranges, manage patient anxiety and pain, give supplemental oxygen when needed, and resume preoperative cardiac medications. Signs of infections or pulmonary problems should be pursued aggressively.

Valvular Heart Disease

Most patients with valvular heart disease who have few symptoms or limitations of activity can safely undergo most elective maxillofacial surgery. Diseased cardiac valves pose two general risks: precipitation of cardiac failure and susceptibility to infective endocarditis. The likelihood of causing failure or worsening preexisting cardiac failure is dependent on the location and severity of valve pathology. Prophylactic antibiotics should be used for all patients with a cardiac valve abnormality who undergo maxillofacial procedures in which bleeding occurs[9] (Table 2–1).

Mitral Stenosis

Mitral stenosis is almost always a sequela of childhood rheumatic heart disease, although a definite history can be obtained in only half of such cases. The rheumatic disease process causes valve fibrosis, fusion, and calcification. These changes limit valve motion, thus restricting the flow of blood into the left ventricle. The latency period is usually 15 to 20 years. Once valve obstruction occurs the patient will begin to suffer gradually worsening exertional dyspnea and fatigue due to pulmonary vascular congestion and progressive right heart failure. Left arterial enlargement may lead to the appearance of arterial fibrillation (AF)

Table 2–1. *Recommended Standard Antibiotic Prophylactic Regimen for Dental, Oral, or Upper Respiratory Tract Procedures in Patients at Normal Risk**

Patient Type	Drug	Dosage
PATIENTS NOT ALLERGIC TO PENICILLINS		
	Amoxicillin	3 g PO 1 h before procedure, then 1.5 g 6 h later
PATIENTS ALLERGIC TO PENICILLINS		
	Erythromycin	Either 800 mg erythromycin ethylsuccinate or 1 g erythromycin stearate PO 2 h before procedure, then half the dose 6 h later
	Clindamycin	300 mg PO 1 h before procedure, then 150 mg 6 h later
PATIENTS UNABLE TO TAKE PO MEDICATIONS, NOT ALLERGIC TO PENICILLINS		
	Ampicillin	2 g IM or IV 30 min before procedure, then either 1 g IM or IV or 1.5 g PO, 6 h later
PATIENTS UNABLE TO TAKE PO MEDICATIONS, ALLERGIC TO PENICILLINS		
	Clindamycin	300 mg IV 30 min before procedure, then 150 mg PO or IV 6 h later
PATIENTS AT ESPECIALLY HIGH RISK,† NOT ALLERGIC TO PENICILLINS		
	Ampicillin/gentamicin	2 g IM or IV ampicillin plus 1.5 mg/kg IM or IV gentamicin 30 min before procedure, then either repeat same regimen 8 h later, or give 1.5 g PO amoxicillin 6 h later
PATIENTS AT ESPECIALLY HIGH RISK,† ALLERGIC TO PENICILLINS		
	Vancomycin	1 g IV over 1 h, starting 1 h before procedure with no repeat dose

* *Patients with prosthetic heart valves (either bioprosthetic or homografts), most congenital heart malformations, rheumatic and other acquired valvular dysfunctions, hypertrophic myopathies, and mitral valve prolapse with vulvular regurgitation*

† *Patients with history of previous endocarditis, surgically created systemic-pulmonary shunts or conduits, or patients with prosthetic heart valves for which some practitioners prefer to use a parenteral regimen*

with possible atrial thrombus formation and systemic arterial embolization.[10]

Examination of the patient with clinically significant mitral stenosis may reveal an early diastolic opening snap followed by a low-pitched murmur and a loud first heart sound. Patients in AF will characteristically have an irregularly irregular pulse. A chest radiograph will reveal an enlarged left atrium, pulmonary vascular enlargement, and, in more severe cases, right ventricular hypertrophy. An ECG may reveal AF, left atrial enlargement, or right ventricular hypertrophy. An echocardiogram is usually the definitive test used to detect and characterize mitral stenosis.

Patients with severe mitral stenosis who require elective surgery may need preoperative mitral valve commissurotomy or valve replacement. AF may be managed by preoperative digitalization or β-sympathetic blockade; pulmonary congestion is treated with diuretic therapy. Patients with a known or suspected atrial thrombus are usually on chronic anticoagulant therapy, which may need temporary alteration. Surgeons should note the compromised cardiac output of patients with mitral stenosis.

Acute pulmonary edema is not uncommon following noncardiac surgery on patients with significant mitral stenosis, particularly if excess fluid replacement was given. An additional problem these patients can have is diminished pulmonary compliance that may require that they remain on mechanical ventilation longer than is usually necessary postoperatively.

Mitral Regurgitation

Mitral regurgitation or insufficiency is most commonly the result of rheumatic heart disease or chronic CAD. The incompetent valve forces left ventricular enlargement as the heart works to maintain cardiac output. Symptoms of congestive failure appear as regurgitation worsens and the enlarging heart moves to the decompensation side of the Starling curve.

Physical examination of the patient with significant mitral regurgitation will reveal an apical point of maximal impact (PMI) displaced inferolaterally, an apical high-pitched holosystolic murmur, and a third heart sound (gallup rhythm). Left ventricular hypertrophy and AF may appear on ECG. Echocardiography will help define the extent of valve disease and, with a measurement of end-systolic left ventricular dimension, prognosis can be determined (a dimension of more than 55 mm would indicate left ventricular dysfunction). Doppler studies or cardiac angiography can be used to determine the severity of dysfunction.

Patients with failure secondary to initial regurgitation are medically managed with sodium restriction, digoxin, diuretics, and preload and afterload reducing vasodilators. Eventually surgical valve repair or replacement may be necessary.

There is little increased risk during maxillofacial surgery for patients with well controlled mitral regurgitation. The surgeon and anesthesiologist must guard against the pulmonary edema for which these patients are prone. Monitoring of pulmonary capillary wedge pressure will help guide therapy.

Mitral Valve Prolapse

Mitral valve prolapse is a common form of mitral regurgitation, most frequently seen in young women, in which one or both of the mitral valve leaflets prolapse into the left atrium during systole, allowing varying degrees of regurgitation to occur. It is characterized by a midsystolic click followed by a late systolic murmur. Symptoms include palpitations and chronic fatigue; echocardiography is diagnostic. Mitral valve prolapse is usually treated symptomatically, using β-sympathetic antagonists to control palpitations.[12]

As with other causes of mitral regurgitation, with medical management there is little increased risk for anesthesia and surgery. Patients should have ECG monitoring to detect intraoperative dysrhythmias, and those with a murmur should be given antibiotics to prevent infective endocarditis.

Aortic Regurgitation

Aortic regurgitation or insufficiency occurs when the aortic valve becomes partially incompetent, which results in a backflow of aortic blood into the left ventricle during diastole. This causes left ventricular volume overload resulting in hypertrophy and increased wall thickness, all of which increase myocardial oxygen requirements.

Patients with clinically significant aortic regurgitation will report unusual awareness of their heart beat, prominent neck pulsations, and symptoms of pulmonary congestion at rest that resolve during exercise. Examination reveals a widened pulse pressure, a bisferious (bifid) carotid pulse, an inferolaterally displaced and prolonged apical PMI, and diastolic decrescendo murmur at the base. In severe cases, there may be a third heart sound and apical low-pitched diastolic (Austin-Flint) murmur.

The ECG will reveal left ventricular hypertrophy, and a chest film will show left ventricular and aortic root enlargement. Echocardiography with or without Doppler is used to diagnose and characterize aortic regurgitation.

Patients who show signs of failure will be medically managed with drugs similar to those used in any form of congestive heart failure. Eventually aortic valve replacement may be necessary. Typically bradycardia or vasodilation cannot be tolerated, thus measures to prevent these changes should be used. The ECG lead V_5 should be monitored perioperatively for signs of subendocardial ischemia. Pulmonary artery catheterization is useful in the perioperative period for measuring left-sided pressure and cardiac output. Afterload reduction may be helpful in patients with normal left ventricular function by reducing the regurgitant fraction, increasing stroke volume, and decreasing left ventricular end-diastolic volume and pressure. Care must be taken when using afterload reducers to not allow aortic diastolic pressure to drop so low as to compromise coronary perfusion.[13]

Aortic Stenosis

Aortic stenosis can involve the valve itself or be supra- or infravalvular. Valve stenosis is most often due to either a congenitally bicuspid valve (which occurs in about 2% of the population) or an aging-related degeneration of a normal trileaflet valve. In either situation valve fibrosis and calcification occur and cause varying degrees of left ventricular outflow obstruction.

Symptoms classically include exertional angina or syncope and dyspnea. However, many patients can be asymptomatic until surgical stress unmasks problems. Physical examination of the patient with significant aortic stenosis will typically reveal a weak pulse, narrow pulse pressure, and a nondisplaced but accentuated and prolonged PMI. A diamond-shaped systolic murmur is heard at the base while a fourth heart sound is heard at the apex. Patients typically have little pulmonary hypertension so that many of the classic noncardiac symptoms and signs of heart failure are not present. But because the left ventricle depends on the end-diastolic boost from the left atrium, the development of AF can be catastrophic and should be suspected in a patient with aortic stenosis who suddenly deteriorates.

The ECG shows left ventricular hypertrophy; the chest radiograph reveals left ventricular and ascending aortic enlargement and calcification. Echocardiography can be used to define the valvular pathology, and cardiac angiography is used to determine the pressure gradient across the valve and to check the status of the coronary arteries. Severely stenotic valves may require surgical replacement.[11]

Patients with mild to moderate dysfunction requiring maxillofacial surgery typically require little alteration in surgical or anesthetic management. The aortic valve opening must be narrowed to 75% of its normal size before obstructive signs occur. If aortic and mitral stenosis coexists, the problems due to mitral stenosis will predominate. Perioperative risks in patients with isolated aortic stenosis are highest if the history includes exertional dizziness, syncope, or angina and the presence of CAD.[11]

The preservation of sinus rhythm is important in these patients. Tachydysrhythmias are to be avoided. Digitalization in the perioperative period should be strongly considered, along with normalization of serum potassium; and ECG monitoring is essential. Supraventricular tachycardias should be treated immediately with direct current cardioversion. Sinus tachycardia may require administration of a β-sympathetic antagonist. Bradycardia is also harmful, and rates below 45 should be increased with atropine. Anesthetics which cause myocardial depression should be used cautiously, if at all. The ECG lead V_5 should be monitored for signs of ischemia; if detected, coronary obstruction must be differentiated from insufficient coronary filling pressure due to aortic stenosis. Nitroglycerin will help the former condition whereas it can actually worsen the latter.

Prosthetic Heart Valves

Patients with prosthetic heart valves represent a special situation in which properly functioning valves have essentially normal cardiac function but may have new problems directly related to the artificial valve itself. These patients are susceptible to staphylococcal endocarditis, red cell destruction by the valve, prosthetic valve obstruction by thrombosis or pannus formation, and paravalvular regurgitation. Serum bilirubin, lactate dehydrogenase, and reticulocytes should be measured to detect occult hemolysis. These patients are all on chronic anticoagulant therapy, which needs perioperative management. Patients with prosthetic valves should be given antibiotics to prevent infective endocarditis.

Congestive Heart Failure

The normal myocardium responds to increased physiologic demands by increasing the frequency of contractions and by dilating, which, through the Starling mechanism, increases contractility (the end-diastolic wall tension). Heart failure occurs when the heart's compensatory mechanisms fail to handle the hemodynamic load, causing blood to back up into the pulmonary vasculature, right heart, and major venous beds such as the portal system.

Failure can be produced in two basic ways. First, the heart can be overwhelmed by excessive loads, such as elevated preload (venous return) produced, for example, by hypervolemia, or increased afterload (resistance to ejection) produced, for example, by elevated total peripheral resistance or aortic stenosis. Second, the heart's ability to compensate for increased demands can be compromised, such as by myocardial infarction or cardiomyopathy.

Long-term management requires that both excessive preload and afterload be modulated. Preload is lessened by limiting intravascular volume through the use of dietary sodium restriction and diuretics and by venodilation with drugs such as nitrates. Afterload is reduced through the administration of vasodilators. Cardiac contractility is augmented by digoxin. Finally, physiologic demands on the heart are controlled by advising the patient to get adequate rest and avoid strenuous exercise.

A failing heart produces many signs and symptoms that vary according to the severity of the decompensation. Dilation of the heart as it tries to compensate can be detected on a posteroanterior chest radiograph. The chest film will also show increased pulmonary vascular markings, which occur as pressure forces fluid into interstitial spaces and alveoli, producing pulmonary edema. The signs of rales and decreased breath sounds in dependent portions of the lungs, and symptoms such as dyspnea at rest or on exertion, paroxysmal nocturnal dyspnea, and orthopnea commonly occur. Failure of the heart to propel blood out of the systemic venous system can produce increased interstitial fluid in the lower legs which is revealed as pitting edema, increased central venous pressure giving jugular venous distention, and portal hypertension causing hepatomegaly.

When surgery is contemplated for a patient with a history of congestive heart failure steps should be taken to optimize the patient's physical status preoperatively. The patient should be questioned about the amount of exertion necessary to produce dyspnea and about how many pillows are necessary while sleeping to prevent orthopnea in order to quantitate the severity of the cardiac disability. Nocturnal cough and restlessness and easy fatigability can be early symptoms of problems. Signs of congestive failure include jugular venous distention, presence of a third heart sound (gallup rhythm), pulsus alternans, basilar rales, and pitting edema. A chest radiograph and ECG should be used to measure heart size, to visualize the lung fields, and to help detect AF. If poorly compensated failure is detected the risk of postoperative pulmonary edema is raised by 25%.[14]

Patients prone to failure can be improved by increased attention to sodium and water restriction and to compliance with taking medications such as diuretics, digoxin, and preload and afterload reducers. Potassium levels should be normalized. Mild preoperative hypokalemia can be managed by oral replacement therapy or intravenous administration at a rate of up to 10 mEq/h in concentrations up to 30 mEq/L. Patients taking digoxin should have serum levels measured. Signs and symptoms of digoxin toxicity such as nausea, diarrhea, anorexia, and dysrhythmias should prompt postponement of surgery until levels are normalized. Consideration should be given to placement of a central venous line for monitoring perioperative central venous pressure or for placing a Swan-Ganz catheter. An indwelling arterial line can also be useful for monitoring mean arterial pressure and for obtaining samples for blood gas analysis. After intubation the patient's lung compliance should be monitored closely, because decreasing compliance is an early sign of pulmonary edema. Minidose heparin and elastic stockings can be used postoperatively to decrease the likelihood of deep vein thrombosis and pulmonary embolization. Passive leg exercises and early ambulation postoperatively also help prevent these problems. An early postoperative chest radiograph can reveal early signs of pulmonary edema, as does an elevation of pulmonary capillary wedge pressures. During recovery the patient's physical activity and emotional stress should be kept low to reduce unnecessary demands on the heart.

Cardiac Dysrhythmias

Patients with diagnosed or occult cardiac rhythm disturbances present a management challenge to the surgeon and anesthesiologist in the perioperative period. Dysrhythmias can compromise cardiac output leading to myocardial ischemia, cerebral ischemia, congestive failure, or shock. In addition, dysrhythmias can predispose towards the formation of intracardiac thrombi and subsequent systemic embolization.[15]

Patients with significant dysrhythmias may or may not have symptoms. The tendency of dysrhythmias to compromise cardiac function frequently depends on overall cardiac health. For example, an otherwise healthy individual can easily tolerate heart rates at the extremes of the range of 40 to 180, whereas a diseased heart would be less tolerant.

Anesthesia and surgery are capable of unmasking a tendency toward dysrhythmias through vagal stimulation, stress-related release of catecholamines, drug-induced histamine release, dysrhythmogenic drugs such as inhalational anesthetics, and by hypoxia due to inadequate ventilation. Statistically, perioperative dysrhythmias are most common in patients with preexisting dysrhythmias or heart disease, particularly during intubation, or who are on digoxin medication or undergo surgery and anesthesia for longer than 3 hours. In addition, surgery near the carotid sinus can cause atrioventricular conduction disturbances due to the stimulation of intercostal nerves.[16]

The presence of significant cardiac dysrhythmias can often be detected based on symptoms reported during a medical history, such as intermittent palpitations, unexplained syncopal episodes, and transient ischemic attacks. Determination of pulse rate and rhythm should be obtained during the physical examination. An ECG should be obtained in all patients with either suspected or diagnosed dysrhythmias.

Sinus Tachycardia

The most common dysrhythmia is sinus tachycardia with a heart rate of 100 to 180. An elevated rate compromises cardiac output by lessening diastolic filling time and increasing myocardial oxygen consumption. Sinus tachycardia can have many etiologies including fever, hypovolemia, anemia, hypoxia, drug use, and hyperthyroidism. Therapy is directed at the underlying cause.[17]

Paroxysmal Atrial Tachycardia

Paroxysmal atrial tachycardia (PAT) is a frequent dysrhythmia that can indicate poor cardiac health and commonly heralds the development of atrial fibrillation. The atrial rate in PAT is usually 140 to 240 with a variable ventricular response rate. PAT can be due to digoxin toxicity or myocardial ischemia.

Although PAT can be well tolerated, attempts should be made preoperatively to control it. Drugs such as digoxin, β-sympathetic antagonists or calcium channel antagonists can be used. Direct-current cardioversion can be tried as well. Symptomatic PAT, if not controllable by medical management, may be treated by a cardiac pacemaker.[18]

Atrial Flutter

Atrial flutter (rate 250 to 300) commonly appears with a 2:1 block producing a ventricular rate of 125 to 150. Patients in atrial flutter who undergo surgery have a 50% mortality rate. It is therefore incumbent on the surgeon to correct the dysrhythmia preoperatively with direct current, low-energy (25 to 50 watt-seconds) cardioversion.

Atrial Fibrillation

Atrial fibrillation (AF) is the second most common cardiac dysrhythmia. It is usually asymptomatic but characteristically produces an irregularly irregular pulse rhythm and a fibrillation pattern on ECG. The atrial rate is greater than 350, whereas the ventricular rate varies from 140 to 180. Etiologies include any cause of left atrial hypertrophy, thyrotoxicosis, CAD, and excessive use of caffeine, cocaine, ethanol, or nicotine even in healthy hearts.[19]

The physiologic compromise produced by AF depends on the ventricular response, myocardial health, and duration of the dysrhythmia. A rapid ventricular response increases perioperative mortality about 15%. Congestive heart failure or myocardial ischemia can appear abruptly in susceptible patients going into AF. Long-standing AF can allow the formation of an atrial thrombus and subsequent thromboembolic complications.

Preoperative management of patients with a history of AF should include consideration of digitalization, which by itself may convert AF to a normal sinus rhythm. Intravenous verapamil can also be used but is less successful in converting AF. Both digoxin and calcium channel antagonists decrease dromotropy, thus helping to slow the ventricular response rate to more physiologic levels. Care should be taken to not allow the ventricular rate to fall below 70. Acute onset of AF is most effectively managed with direct current cardioversion starting at about 200 watt-seconds. Patients with chronic AF should be on anticoagulants, which must be adjusted perioperatively.

Premature Ventricular Contractions

Premature ventricular contractions (PVCs) can be due to many causes including fever, hypoxia, drugs including digoxin, aminophylline, and inhalational anesthetics, pulmonary artery catheters, electrolyte disturbances, and myocardial ischemia, or they may be idiopathic. An occasional asymptomatic PVC seen in an otherwise healthy individual requires no therapy, but other configurations of PVCs should cause concern, particularly in the perioperative period. These include those occurring more than six times per minute, those occurring on or close to the peak of the T wave (R-on-T phenomenon), those with varying QRS forms, and those occurring in pairs or triplets. PVCs in these patterns are commonly associated with severe underlying heart disease.

The discovery of significant PVC activity on a preoperative ECG warrants a complete cardiac evaluation and identified causes of PVCs should be corrected preoperatively. When a cause for PVCs cannot be discovered and surgery must proceed, lidocaine or procainamide can be used to suppress ectopic activity.

Ventricular Tachycardia

The appearance of three or more PVCs in a row is defined as *ventricular tachycardia*. It has a variety of etiologies including hypoxia, acidosis, myocardial ischemia, digoxin toxicity, hyper- or hypokalemia, and hypercalcemia. Prompt therapy consists of intravenous lidocaine or low-energy, direct current cardioversion.[16, 20]

Heart Blocks

Atrioventricular blocks take several forms. A PR interval greater than 20 ms constitutes first-degree AV block and is of little significance perioperatively in the absence of other cardiac abnormalities. In second-degree block some atrial impulses are not conducted into the ventricles. The Mobitz I (Wenckebach) second-degree block has a PR interval that progressively lengthens until a nonconducted P wave occurs and the cycle begins again. Mobitz I rhythms are usually due to digoxin excess, myocardial ischemia, or degeneration of cardiac conduction tissue. Treatment with atropine is necessary only for excessively slow ventricular rates. Mobitz II second-degree block has a constant PR interval but frequent P waves without a ventricular response. This is a worrisome dysrhythmia and perioperative ventricular pacing should be considered.[21, 22]

Third-degree atrioventricular block implies a complete block of atrial impulses into the ventricle. The ventricles therefore beat at their low intrinsic rate of about 45. Therapy usually requires the use of a pacemaker.

Bundle-branch blocks present no direct contraindication to anesthesia and surgery but usually signal some underlying cardiac disease. Pacing for bundle-branch blocks is necessary only if symptomatic bradycardia or complete heart block occurs.

Patients who have permanent cardiac pacemakers pose little increased risk during surgery over and above the underlying cardiac problem. If electrocautery is necessary special care should be taken to ensure that it is properly grounded. A magnet to convert a demand pacemaker to the fixed rate mode should be available in the operating suite.[19]

SURGERY IN THE PATIENT WITH RESPIRATORY PROBLEMS

General Assessment of Airways and Lungs

Maxillofacial surgery itself has little effect on pulmonary function compared with general thoracic or abdominal surgery, except when tissue is being transferred from the thorax to the maxillofacial region. However, maxillofacial surgery does commonly involve prolonged general anesthesia and may cause compromised upper airways. Therefore, it is important to discover and treat airway and lung abnormalities preoperatively or, when not possible, to make necessary compensations in surgical and anesthetic plans.

The medical history should ascertain the following about the status of the ventilatory system: The presence of symptoms such as wheezing, productive cough, and low exercise tolerance; the use of pulmonary medications; cigarette smoking; prior thoracic surgery or trauma; and previously diagnosed pulmonary diseases including asthma, pneumonia, chronic obstructive pulmonary disease (COPD), or tuberculosis. Points of the physical examination of significance to the assessment of the respiratory system include a careful inspection of the nasal airways, auscultation of lung fields for abnormal sounds, inspection of mucosa and nail beds for signs of cyanosis or clubbing, and measurement of the respiratory rate.[29–31]

A plain chest radiograph is useful for detecting diffuse or localized parenchymal disease, pulmonary edema, hyperinflation, and consolidations such as pneumonia or neoplasms. But the yield from routine preoperative chest radiographs is low in patients without a history or examination suggestive of pulmonary disease.

Some pulmonary function testing can be performed at bedside, such as the breath-holding test. The breath-holding test involves having a patient make a maximum inspiration and then hold the breath for as long as possible. Inability to hold it for at least 15 seconds is indicative of significant pulmonary problems. Spirometry is another bedside test for assessing pulmonary function. Surgeons should request formal pulmonary function testing (PFT) for all patients in whom lung disease is suspected. PFTs help gauge respiratory reserve and measure their response to measures taken to improve lung function.[32–34]

Measurement of arterial blood gases (ABGs) is frequently a part of pulmonary function testing. ABG determination serves both as a baseline for intra- and postoperative measurements and helps assess the status of pulmonary gas exchange. A low PaO_2 can be due to hypoventilation, diffusion impairment, shunting, or a ventilation-perfusion inequality; the last being the most common cause. An elevated $PaCO_2$ is a sign of hypoventilation either due to an inadequate respiratory rate or depth or to a ventilation-perfusion inequality. Intraoperative capnography and intra- and postoperative oximetry have reduced the need for frequent ABG sampling. Oximetry is also beneficial during the first few hours after maxillofacial surgery when respiratory insufficiency is most likely to occur.[31, 35]

Asthma

The patient with a recent history of problematic asthma is at significant risk when having general anesthesia and surgery. The bronchospasm that characterizes asthma can develop precipitously and compromise ventilation, even with positive pressure, and may be difficult to reverse in time to prevent complications. As with most conditions of this nature, recognition and prevention are the best management strategies.

Asthma is divided into intrinsic and extrinsic forms based on which factors trigger the bronchospasm. The factors causing *extrinsic asthma* stimulate the production of IgE antibody and include environmental pollutants, pollens, drugs, foods, insects, and animals. This type of asthma usually has its onset early in life, symptoms tend to occur seasonally, serum IgE levels are elevated, and the process tends to disappear in later life. *Intrinsic asthma* is characterized by the absence of specific external triggers of bronchoconstriction, the onset tends to be later in life, IgE levels are normal, and the disease process tends to be persistent and progressive. Factors such as emotional stress, infections, exercise, and surgery can trigger intrinsic asthma. Because of its resistance to preventive measures, intrinsic asthma has a much greater propensity for causing perioperative problems as compared to the extrinsic form.[30]

The airway narrowing in asthma is due to smooth muscle contraction, edema in airway walls, or mucus plugging of airways. Whereas bronchospasm is rapidly reversible with muscle relaxants, edema and plugging are not. Clinicians can test the degree of hyperresponsiveness by using inhaled methacholine to stimulate bronchospasm, then measuring the forced expiratory volume in one second (FEV_1). The concentration of methacholine that produces a 20% decrease in FEV_1 is called the *provocative concentration 20%* (PC20). A PC20 less than 2 mg/mL is diagnostic of asthma; between 2 and 8 mg/mL is suggestive of the disease; and values over 16 mg/mL effectively rule out asthma in a patient.[36]

The likelihood of an asthmatic episode occurring during surgery can be judged by a few pieces of historic information. The frequency, severity, duration, and response to therapy of recent asthma attacks will help gauge how well an individual's asthma is controlled and therefore the safety of proceeding with surgical plans. In addition, the patient should be queried concerning the occurrence of nocturnal symptoms and which external agents seem to trigger episodes. The patient should be asked in particular about any problems with wheezing when any nonsteroidal anti-inflammatory drugs are used, because many asthmatics are sensitive to these drugs.

Patients with asthma being prepared for anesthesia and surgery should have their disease maximally controlled pharmacologically and should avoid triggering agents and circumstances. The patient should be free of infection and kept away from known environmental irritants. Anxiety reduction techniques are useful as well. During the physical examination the presence of wheezing should be sought. A chest radiograph can be used to detect hyperinflation or atelectasis. Formal PFTs may be useful, particularly when a response to bronchodilators is measured. The serum IgE level can be measured if indicated by clinical circumstances.[37]

Many asthmatics use various medications to prevent their asthmatic episodes. β-2 sympathetic antagonists have become a cornerstone of pharmacologic management of asthma. Although available to be given systemically, topical use of β-2 antagonists by aerosolization from metered dose inhalers avoids the side effects of systemic administration.[38]

Up to recent times methylxanthines were the mainstay of asthma treatment but the side effects of these drugs, as well as the appearance of β-2 antagonists, has prompted many clinicians to revise their thinking about methylxanthines. Some clinicians now reserve their use for more refractory asthmatics. Patients on methylxanthines, such as theophylline, who are going to surgery should have the drug's serum level checked to ensure that it is within the therapeutic range of 10 to 20 mg/mL. But even levels between 15 and 20 mg/mL can cause side effects such as nausea, tremors, and palpitations. In addition, the patient will be predisposed to the development of seizures or serious dysrhythmias.

Corticosteroids are generally reserved for use in asthma only when acute episodes occur or the patient is not adequately controlled by other drugs. Prolonged corticosteroid use carries its own risks as is discussed later in this chapter. The surgeon should confer with the physician managing a patient's asthma to ensure that the patient has recently been evaluated and that the steroid regimen provides the least amount of drug that is still effective. If possible, the patient may benefit from a switch to topical corticosteroid use through metered-dose inhalers, which may help minimize systemic effects.

Several drugs that help protect against asthmatic episodes are under development. In the United States, cromolyn sodium is the only agent in wide use. This drug stabilizes mast cells and prevents degranulation. The drug is most effective in children with asthma but is also useful in adults. It must be used prior to a challenge by a triggering agent in order to be effective and has been given in the past in the form of a dry powder placed in a spinhaler that facilitates inhalation of the drug. Newly available metered-dose inhalers and nebulizer solutions make dosing easier for patients.[38]

Intra- and postoperatively, asthmatic patients should be monitored for the appearance of increased airway resistance, wheezing, pulsus paradoxus, tachycardia, fever, hyoxemia, hypercapnea, and acidosis. Atelectasis is common in asthmatics, and they have an increased risk of bacterial pneumonia, which is why thorough pulmonary examinations must be given at frequent intervals during recovery.

Chronic Obstructive Pulmonary Disease

Chronic obstructive pulmonary disease (*COPD*) is an all-encompassing nonspecific term used to describe pulmonary problems that involve varying degrees of obstructive airway disease versus changes in interstitial tissues restricting proper inflation and diffusion of gases at the air–blood interface. *Chronic obstructive bronchitis* is used to designate patients with chronic cough, excessive pulmonary secretions, and obstructed airways not responsive to bronchodilators; *asthmatic bronchitis* patients have the same problems but have significant reversibility of their airway disease with bronchodilators. Clinicians use *emphysema* to describe patients with varying severity of dyspnea on exertion and who show irreversible airway changes with hyperinflation of the lungs and impaired diffusion across the pulmonary membranes. Because most patients have components of all three of these disease categories simultaneously, the term COPD is believed by clinicians to be most descriptive.[39]

Surgery and anesthesia for patients with significant COPD usually incurs few intraoperative risks due to the lung disease itself. However, the likelihood of postoperative pulmonary complications is high in COPD patients. Therefore, proper preoperative identification and preparation are important.[40]

COPD produces a chronic productive cough, dyspnea on exertion, wheezing, and susceptibility to lung infections. The history usually reveals a long history of cigarette smoking or exposure to environmental or occupational pollutants.

Examination of patients with COPD typically reveals signs of hyperinflation including an increased anteroposterior dimension of the chest, depression of the hemidiaphragms, and hyperresonance to percussion. Airway obstruction is signaled by wheezing. In milder forms of COPD wheezing may only be detectable during forced expiration, but more severe cases have more prominent wheezing audible earlier in the expiratory phase of breathing.[39]

Chest radiographs reveal hyperlucency due to overinflation and depressed diaphragms and increased anteroposterior diameter in lateral views. PFTs help demonstrate obstructive changes by an FEV_1 of less than 80% of the vital capacity. The maximum mid-expiratory flow rate is also decreased in COPD and is less sensitive to changes in patient cooperation compared with FEV_1. Repetition of these tests after use of bronchodilators helps determine the reversibility of the lung pathology. A good estimate of FEV_1 can be made at bedside by asking the patient to take a deep breath and blow it out as completely and fast as possible. Continued audible air flow for longer than 6 seconds reveals significant airway obstruction. An expiratory time of 10 to 12 seconds corresponds with an FEV_1 of 1.5 L; 12 to 16 seconds roughly translates to an FEV_1 of 1 L. Restrictive components of COPD cause reduced volumes on pulmonary function testing. Diffusion tests (carbon monoxide uptake) help further define the lung pathology.[41, 42]

Measurement of arterial blood gases in COPD show varying amounts of carbon dioxide retention, hypoxia, and respiratory acidosis with metabolic compensation.

Preparing COPD patients for surgery usually involves reversing pathology able to be altered medically. Theophylline is standard treatment for chronic bronchospasm. β-2 agonists such as metaproterenol or albuterol also stimulate bronchodilation and can be used before and during anesthesia. Many patients with severe COPD need corticosteroids administered. Production of mucopurulent sputum may indicate the need for preoperative antibiotics to help improve COPD symptoms. Ampicillin, trimethoprim/sulfa combinations, tetracyclines, or erythromycin are used most commonly and are given in 7- to 10-day courses. Elderly patients with COPD frequently improve when given inhaled anticholinergic agents, such as ipratropium bromide, which reverse the parasympathetically mediated elevation of bronchomotor tone. Patients with a $Pa O_2$ of consistently less than 60 mm Hg improve when supplemental oxygen is administered in quantities sufficient to keep the $Pa O_2$ between 60 to 65 mm Hg. Attempts to raise arterial oxygen above this level are hazardous because patients with chronic hypercapnea come to depend on their hypoxemia to provide their respiratory drive.[31,42,43]

Cigarette smoking is the most common cause of COPD and further exacerbates symptoms if continued after lung pathology occurs. Reversible problems that smoking causes include the release of nicotine, production of carbon monoxide, mucus hypersecretion, impaired ciliary function, and impaired local lung immunity. Preoperative cessation of smoking for 24 hours allows a significant decline in plasma carboxyhemoglobin and nicotine levels, but the rate of pulmonary complications due to smoking takes weeks to fall after smoking is stopped. In the case of coronary artery bypass grafting, the percentage of postoperative pulmonary complications in former smokers does not begin to approach the rate seen in nonsmokers until after at least 8 weeks of abstinence from smoking.[39]

Other preoperative measures that can prevent postoperative problems in patients with COPD include good nutrition and correction by hypokalemia to improve respiratory muscle strength and familiarization of the patient with incentive spirometry. Preoperative pulmonary therapy techniques such as positive pressure breathing treatments and percussion with postural drainage have not been shown to reduce postoperative problems.

There are several anesthetic considerations for patients with COPD. Volatile anesthetics provide bronchodilatory effects and thus are useful. Nitrous oxide, on the other hand, may cause problems due to its accumulation in bullae potentiating rupture and production of pneumothorax. The respiratory depressive effects of narcotics makes their use in COPD patients hazardous, especially if it is likely that their effects will outlast the duration of needed anesthesia.

The techniques of controlled ventilation must be altered in patients with obstructive airway disease. Ventilatory rates need to be slow enough (typically 6 to 10/min) to allow sufficient exhalation time and to compensate for slower diffusion of gases across membranes. Care should be taken to avoid high pressures to lessen the potential of ruptured bullae. Generally COPD patients do best with large tidal volumes at slow rates and will not need positive end-expiratory pressure.[43]

SURGERY IN PATIENTS WITH RENAL AND URINARY TRACT DISEASE

The kidneys play several roles in helping maintain physiologic normalcy; they are therefore important for continuing or regaining homeostasis during and after surgery and anesthesia. The renal system is necessary to support the processes of fluid, electrolyte, and acid-base balance, drug metabolism and elimination, blood pressure control through the renin-angiotension system, red blood cell production through erythropoietin production, and vitamin D hydroxylation.

There are several diseases that can affect one or more of the kidneys' functions. However, for the maxillofacial surgeon a better gauge of the degree to which the patient's ability to tolerate anesthesia and surgery is compromised is the adequacy of renal function. The glomerular filtration rate (GFR), normally 100 to 125 mL/min per 1.73 m^2 of body surface area in an adult, is the single most useful measure of renal health. The GFR is measured clinically by determining the clearance of endogenous creatinine. The body's serum creatinine (SC) load is highly dependent on muscle mass, and the clearance of creatinine from the serum depends on the number of functioning glomeruli, a number which gradually decreases with age. Also, SC varies inversely with creatinine clearance (CCR). Thus, an estimation of the CCR in males involves obtaining the level of SC and then multiplying its reciprocal by factors which correct for muscle mass and age.[42]

$$\text{CCR} = \frac{(140 - \text{age in years})\,(\text{weight in kg})}{(\text{SC})\,(72\ \text{kg})}$$

For females, the above result is multiplied by 0.85.

Although much less accurate, measurement of SC (normal is less than 1.5 mg/dL) can be used to help gauge renal function. Although measurement of blood urea nitrogen (BUN) is used commonly to test renal health, it is a crude measure and may be misleading, especially in patients with poor nutrition or with hepatic disease.

Serum electrolyte abnormalities can signal significant renal disease. Poor renal function will often result in decreased secretion of potassium causing hyperkalemia or a concentrating defect leading to urinary sodium wasting and hydrogen ion retention with resultant hyperchloremic metabolic acidosis. Other indications of renal problems include proteinuria, pyuria, and hematuria, all detectable on routine urinalysis.

Chronic Renal Insufficiency

The risks of anesthesia and surgery in the patient with known renal insufficiency vary according to the severity of renal compromise. Patients with mild to moderately severe renal insufficiency (GFR of 25–50 mL/min) usually tolerate the perioperative period well if properly managed. When renal function is severely impaired (GFR of 10–25 mL/min) or frank failure is present (GFR $<$ 10 mL/min) complications of renal origin are much more likely. Patients with severe renal insufficiency have a 60% increase in perioperative morbidity and a 2% to 4% increased mortality compared to healthy patients.

One of the earliest manifestations of severe renal insufficiency is the accumulation of nitrogen metabolites and disturbances in fluid and electrolyte balance. Disordered handling of sodium and water by the kidneys frequently causes excessive fluid retention. Potassium balance can usually be maintained until the GFR falls below 10 mL/min when it will begin to accumulate. A high anion-gap metabolic acidosis occurs when the GFR falls below 25 mL/min, when compensatory hyperventilation may be triggered.[44]

Extrarenal problems are produced by renal insufficiency. Normochromic or normocytic anemia frequently occurs due to several factors, including decreased erythropoietin, decreased red cell survival time, and bone marrow depression. In addition, uremia also can cause decreased platelet aggregating ability and depressed platelet factor-3 release.[45]

Pericardial inflammation or effusion is commonly associated with chronic uremia or hemodialysis, as is myocardial dysfunction. End-stage renal disease is almost always complicated by systemic hypertension. Patients with renal insufficiency have impairment of their immune systems with heightened susceptibility to bacterial, viral, and fungal infections. The cause seems to be faulty neutrophil and lymphocyte production and function. Many of the other problems caused by renal dysfunction affect the gastrointestinal tract. Symptoms of nausea, vomiting, diarrhea, and anorexia frequently accompany uremia. Acute stomatitis and salivary adentitis can occur, as can pancreatitis. The stomach and intestine linings may undergo inflammatory changes. Although liver disease is often present in renal failure patients, this association is believed to be due to hemodialysis-associated hepatitis.

Preparation of patients with chronic renal insufficiency for anesthesia and surgery usually involves maximizing the patient's physiologic status using techniques or drugs to reverse the changes due to poor renal function. Baseline information should be obtained such as eliciting any symptoms of renal problems including water retention and leg edema, easy fatigability, lethargy, and anorexia. The results of laboratory testing will help confirm the presence and severity of renal compromise.[8]

Excessive water retention is most easily managed by fluid restriction, which usually helps improve the hypo-osmolar state and the sodium and hydrogen ion balance. Hyperkalemia before elective surgery can be managed with dietary potassium restriction and potassium wasting diuretics. More acute potassium control may necessitate the use of cation-exchange resins, strategies to drive potassium intracellularly, or dialysis. Hypertension and fluid retention may necessitate diuretic use preoperatively. In cases of renal failure, hemodialysis is recommended to reverse fluid, electrolyte, and acid-base problems, as well as extrarenal disorders such as uremic immunodepression. Dialysis should be performed no more than 24 hours preoperatively. The lower heparin requirements in newer dialysis techniques prevent many of the anticoagulation problems of the past. Preoperative chest radiographs and an ECG can be used to detect myocardial dysfunction or pericardial problems due to uremia or chronic fluid overload. Plans should include the use of prophylactic antibiotics even for minimally invasive procedures.[46, 47]

Intraoperative management of the patient with severe renal insufficiency should include careful cardiac monitoring for dysrhythmias and fluid overload. Intravenous fluids should be administered in quantities only sufficient to replace insensible fluid and blood losses, and be free of potassium. If a hemodialysis vascular access (shunt) is in place it should be protected from trauma. Hemostasis should be especially meticulous if the patient will be dialyzed immediately after surgery.[48]

After surgery steps should be taken to maintain proper fluid and electrolyte balance particularly until dialysis can be done. Most surgeons delay postoperative hemodialysis for at least 2 to 3 days to lessen the chance of wound bleeding during heparinization. However, patients with oral or nasal procedures commonly swallow a significant amount of blood, which increases the blood's nitrogen load and may prompt earlier dialysis than would otherwise be necessary. Extended nasogastric suctioning may help prevent blood swallowing when the likelihood of swallowing large amounts is high.

A significant problem the anesthesiologist and surgeon face when managing a patient with renal insufficiency is drug elimination and the toxic effects of some drugs on the kidney. Drugs commonly used during maxillofacial surgery that need to be avoided or used with care in the patient with renal compromise include cephalosporins, penicillin, and sulfa antibiotics, nonsteroidal antiinflammatory drugs, nondepolarizing muscle relaxants, and enflurane. Many references are available which list drugs and dosing modifications needed in renal failure patients.[49]

Hypertension

Essential hypertension is one of the most common disorders of adults, so it is not surprising that a large percentage of adult patients who require surgery have hypertension. With more people aware of the hazards of allowing hypertension to go untreated, most patients seeking the type of care offered by specialty surgeons have had their hypertensive status evaluated and a management regimen prescribed.

Two basic problems can arise in the hypertensive patient requiring anesthesia and surgery. The first is that untreated chronic hypertension can damage many organ systems particularly the heart, kidneys, and brain. The damaged organs may be less able to tolerate demands placed on them during the perioperative period. The second problem is that for many hypertensive patients the medications prescribed for controlling hypertension may dull some of the natural responses the body uses to counteract anesthetic and surgical challenges.

Statistically there is no increase in the incidence of adverse effects from untreated hypertension as long as the diastolic pressure is less than 110 mm Hg and no concurrent medical problems exist. When conferring with a patient the surgeon can usually gain an idea of the likelihood of hypertensive organ damage by attempting to learn of the patient's compliance with antihypertensive regimens. The patient's physician can often supply this information. Target organ damage can also be detected by various physical and laboratory examinations. Cardiac damage usually manifests initially with left ventricular hypertrophy (LVH). This causes a prolonged and displaced point of maximal impact of the heart apex on palpation. In addition, LVH shows on ECG, chest radiographs, and echocardiograms. With time, signs and symptoms of congestive heart failure arise predisposing the heart to dysrhythmias, ischemia, and the appearance of pulmonary edema.[23–25]

The renal damage caused by chronic high blood

pressure usually consists of nephrosclerosis. This may be detectable by routine urinalysis on which proteinuria, hematuria, or pyuria is seen. Renal damage may also cause serum creatinine levels to rise.

Cerebral damage due to hypertension usually manifests later in life with an increased incidence of stroke. In addition, the cerebral vascular system's ability to autoregulate is impaired so that a greater perfusion pressure must be maintained than would otherwise be necessary. Some clinicians also believe chronic hypertension promotes the progress of carotid atherosclerosis and therefore recommend that the surgeon ascultate for carotid bruits.[26]

Many of the vascular changes that occur because of chronic hypertension can easily be seen in the one site where the small vessels are visible, that is, the fundus of the eye. Hemorrhages and exudates seen on fundoscopic examination indicate similar changes in other vascular beds.

For the patient with poorly controlled hypertension (systolic pressure over 200mm Hg, diastolic pressure over 110mm Hg) the surgeon should defer elective surgery until better control is obtained and any end-organ damage is detected; appropriate compensations should be made in the treatment plan.

The patient whose hypertension is already controlled by antihypertensive regimens requires additional considerations. The potential for adverse drug interactions and alterations of normal cardiovascular protective reflexes caused by many hypertensive agents need to be evaluated.[27]

Characteristically the first type of drug used to control blood pressure are diuretics. These agents usually decrease intravascular volume and, in the case of non-potassium-sparing diuretics, can cause hypokalemia if inadequate potassium replacement occurs. Problems due to diuretic-induced hypovolemia can be reversed intraoperatively by volume expansion, which is usually necessary to support the blood pressure at acceptable levels intraoperatively. But intraoperative volume expansion in this situation predisposes the patient toward marked postoperative hypertension, which commonly requires quick attention in the postanesthetic care unit. Diuretic-induced hypokalemia can cause several problems perioperatively, including cardiac dysrhythmias (particularly in the presence of excessive digoxin), paralytic ileus, and accentuated action of nondepolarizing muscle relaxants.

Sympathetic β-antagonists are commonly the second-line drug used for control of hypertension. Newer cardioselective (they selectively antagonize β-1 receptors) blockers are replacing nonselective antagonists such as propranolol. Past recommendations to interrupt β-antagonist administration during the perioperative period have been replaced by regimens that continue them through this period. In fact, abrupt discontinuance of these drugs is associated with dysrhythmias, unstable angina, and myocardial infarction. The cardiodepressant effects of β-blockade must be borne in mind during general anesthesia to avoid episodes of inadequate cardiac output due to insufficient heart rate and contractility. Similar concerns are present with calcium channel antagonists which were commonly used as a third-line antihypertensive but recently have been promoted as first-line drugs. But again these agents do not need to be discontinued perioperatively.[24]

Other categories of antihypertensive agents include α-antagonists (prazosin, terazosin), direct vasodilators (hydralazine, minoxidil), and the angiotensin-converting enzyme inhibitors (captopril, enalapril). None of these drugs appears to increase the risk of perioperative complications and thus they do not need to be stopped preoperatively. Three drugs that do have an interesting effect on anesthesia are methyldopa, reserpine, and clonidine. These agents seem to lower the minimal alveolar concentration of halothane necessary to produce a given plane of general anesthesia. However, this effect does not warrant the cessation of their administration perioperatively.

Patients whose blood pressure is well controlled preoperatively usually exhibit large swings in their blood pressure during and after surgery. Hypotension usually responds to fluid administration. Hypertension usually can be tolerated if it does not reach severe levels. Excessive increases in blood pressure can be managed with short courses of additional antihypertensive medications until anesthetic drugs or surgery-related stresses have stopped, allowing patients to return to their preoperative status.[28]

SURGERY IN PATIENTS WITH ENDOCRINE DISORDERS

Diabetes Mellitus

The impact of diabetes mellitus on the anesthetic and surgical management of a patient is highly dependent on the type, severity, and degree of control of the diabetes. *Type I*, or *insulin dependent diabetes mellitus* (*IDDM*), is due to impaired production by or an insufficient mass of pancreatic islet β-cells. *Type II*, or *noninsulin dependent diabetes mellitus* (*NIDDM*), occurs due to altered number and affinity of peripheral insulin receptors. Total insulin production may also be depressed.

Three criteria are commonly used to diagnose diabetes:

Two fasting plasma glucose measurements of greater than 140 mg/dL, or
Two-hour plasma glucose measurement after 75 g of oral glucose of greater than 200 mg/dL, with one other value during glucose tolerance test exceeding 200 mg/dL, or
Presence of diabetic ketoacidosis

The usual daily production of insulin by a lean adult is 33 units; approximately 3 to 5 units are needed for each meal whereas the basal insulin requirement is about 1 U/h. The ketosis-prone diabetic produces less than 10% of the average daily insulin requirement, but the typical NIDDM patient produces an average of 15 U/24 h.[50]

Type I diabetes presents the more significant challenge to the well-being of a surgical patient. Patients are usually lean and have had this disease since their youth. Those with long-standing IDDM cannot go without their insulin for more than 48 hours without diabetic ketoacidosis (DKA) occurring. Hormones that increase during periods of physiologic stress, including cortisol, catecholamines, and glucagon, act to counter the effects of insulin, producing a stress-induced glucose intolerance, even in many healthy nondiabetic patients. This is why IDDM patients who depend on exogenous administration of their insulin commonly have increased insulin requirements from preoperative emotional stress, intraoperative anesthetic stress, and postoperative wound and emotional stress. Studies have shown that elevated blood glucose not only impairs wound healing but also can depress leukocyte and pancreatic β-cell function, which are reasons, in addition to prevention of DKA, for appropriate insulin supplementation during and after surgery.

IDDM patients, in contrast to those with NIDDM, have a high rate of systemic problems. Peripheral neuropathies are common, predisposing these individuals to chronic foot and leg lesions, which should be detected and noted preoperatively and prevented perioperatively. Long-standing diabetics are also at increased risk for coronary artery disease and may suffer silent (painless) ischemic episodes due to myocardial neuropathy. Insulin dependent diabetics, particularly those with poor control, handle infections poorly. Therefore, vigilance should be especially high for breaks in aseptic techniques and consideration be given to the use of prophylactic antibiotics. IDDM patients also have enhanced platelet stickiness which may promote unwanted clotting in surgical flaps. The formation of glycosated hemoglobin (A-1C) interferes with oxygen release into tissues.[51, 52]

Many regimens have been proposed to help diabetics maintain plasma glucose levels within acceptable ranges during the perioperative period. As during nonoperative periods of a diabetic person's life, insulin requirements vary according to the balance, or lack thereof, of glucose intake and use. Procedures that produce little physiologic or emotional stress and do not interfere significantly with appetite, ability to eat, or general patient activity need not change their usual insulin regimen. More involved procedures may be managed more safely by an insulin regimen that protects against hypoglycemia. This would involve decreasing the usual morning insulin by one-third to one-half to allow plasma glucose to rise during the surgery. This is a useful regimen for procedures lasting less than 1 hour done under local anesthesia.

If a patient is to have relatively short duration, ambulatory surgery and is required to consume nothing by mouth the morning of surgery, only half the usual morning dose of insulin should be given at the time when intravenous access is gained. Surgery should be early in the morning and intravenous glucose should be given intraoperatively. During surgery the clinician should watch for signs of hypoglycemia such as tachycardia and diaphoresis. The patient should then be encouraged to consume some calorie source by mouth within 3 hours after surgery is completed.

Patients requiring more major surgery and longer duration general anesthesia are usually best managed in a setting in which an anesthesiologist can monitor blood glucose levels in the operating room and administer insulin on an as-needed basis. The morning insulin should be withheld until intravenous glucose is available; then one half to three quarters of the usual dose can be administered and supplemented intraoperatively by the anesthesiologist.

When patients are unlikely to enterally receive their usual caloric supply postoperatively their insulin should be given based on periodic (every 6 h) plasma glucose sampling. Insulin doses should be gauged to keep the plasma glucose at 150 to 250 mg/dL until normal dietary habits and activity levels return. The patient's primary care physician can help guide dietary decisions.[53–55]

The NIDDM patients usually have fewer systemic abnormalities due to diabetes and are less likely to suffer perioperative complications. But when major surgery and general anesthesia are performed these patients usually become hyperglycemic. Not uncommonly, patients who are well managed on diet and oral hypoglycemics will need temporary insulin supplementation in the intra- and postoperative periods. As in IDDM patients, blood glucose should be kept at 150 to 250 mg/dL, with insulin supplementation based on periodic sampling.

Thyroid Disorders

The need for normal levels of thyroid hormones to maintain the function of many of the body's physiologic functions makes proper thyroid gland function important to the surgeon. The gland is composed of follicles, each of which is a lumen filled with thyroglobulin, which is produced by a single layer of epithelial cells lining the follicle. Thyroid hormones, thyroxine (T_4) and triiodothyronine (T_3), are produced and stored in the gland in a ratio of 10 to 15:1 (T_4:T_3) and are released on stimulation by thyroid-stimulating hormone, an anterior pituitary hormone. Between the follicles parafollicular cells exist which secrete calcitonin, whose function is to help lower serum calcium by blocking its release from bone.[56]

The majority of T_4 and T_3 released from the gland is bound to various carrier proteins. Most circulating T_3 is produced by conversion from T_4 in the liver and kidney. T_3 is much more potent than T_4 but only the unbound form of either hormone is active and, in the case of T_3, an inactive form called reverse T_3 (rT_3) can be formed. In normal states 35% of T_4 is converted to T_3, 40% to rT_3. But in times of physical illness or emotional stress, or if certain drugs (such as corticosteroids) are used, a higher percentage of T_4 conversion to rT_3 can occur.

The most common laboratory tests of thyroid function are measurements of total T_4 by radioimmunoassay (normal is 5–12 μg/dL) in which high values indicate hyperthyroidism and low values hypothyroidism, and T_3 resin uptake in which unoccupied thyroid hormone binding sites on thyroid-binding globulin are measured. High values of T_3 resin uptake are associated with hypothyroidism whereas low values are consistent with hyperthyroidism.[57]

Hyperthyroidism

Symptoms of hyperthyroidism include weight loss, palpitations, and restlessness. Exophthalmos occurs in more severe cases owing to increased amounts of retroorbital fat. Once diagnosed, therapy usually begins with antithyroid drugs such as propylthiouracil or methimazole. Beta adrenergic antagonists can be used to control symptoms until thyroid hormone levels decrease. Thyroid hormone secreting adenomas may require thyroid surgery to remove portions or all of the gland, with exogenous thyroid supplementation then necessary.[58]

Surgery in the face of hyperthyroidism carries high risks of cardiac dysrhythmias or failure and the potential for causing a thyroid crisis. Therefore, elective surgery should be deferred until thyroid hormone levels are properly managed. If emergency surgery is necessary on a patient with poorly controlled hyperthyroidism, β-sympathetic antagonists can be used to help control the effects of thyroid hormones on the heart while intravenous sodium iodide (1 g) can be administered to help block hormone release from the thyroid gland. The β-antagonist should be continued postoperatively until administered antithyroid drugs take effect. Palpation of the thyroid gland should be gentle in patients with known hyperthyroidism to avoid increasing hormone release, and infections should be aggressively managed because they, too, may precipitate a thyroid crisis.[59,60]

Hypothyroidism

The hypothyroid patient presents a lesser surgical and anesthetic risk when compared with the hyperthyroid patient. The insufficiency of thyroid hormones causes cardiac depression, respiratory depression with weakening of the muscles of respiration, hyponatremia, constipation, neurologic problems with memory loss and depression, and several other metabolic problems. Signs of hypothyroidism include weight gain, periorbital edema, bradycardia, slowed deep tendon reflexes, generalized muscle weakness, and hair loss.[58]

The potential surgical problems in a patient with untreated hypothyroidism include intra- or postoperative heart failure, hypotension, ileus, mental confusion, and delayed wound healing. Therefore, thyroid replacement therapy is advisable prior to elective surgery. In an emergency the surgeon must remain alert to potential problems due to the hypothyroidism and compensate for them if they occur.

Adrenal Gland Disorders

The adrenal gland, responsible for the production of a variety of hormones including cortisol, aldosterone, and androgens, plays a central role in regulating many metabolic processes. Usually it comes to the attention of surgeons because of abnormalities in cortisol production. The average daily secretion of cortisol in the adult is 15 to 17 mg (range 8 to 28 mg). Secretion follows a diurnal pattern, peaking at about 3 or 4 AM and falling to low levels at about 8 or 9 PM. Release of cortisol is regulated by corticotropin (ACTH) secreted by the pituitary, with ACTH release normally increased in time of physiologic stress. It is not unusual for plasma cortisol levels to remain elevated for 10 days after major surgery.

Excessive release of cortisol from the adrenal cortex (Cushing's disease) is rare. These patients show truncal obesity, hypertension, thin skin which heals poorly, and glucose intolerance. These problems can also be seen in patients on long-term therapeutic corticosteroids for problems such as inflammatory joint or bowel disease. Increased surgical risks faced by patients with hypercortisolism include delayed wound healing and a tendency for infections. Delay of elective surgery is warranted until excessive cortisol levels are under control. If surgery cannot wait, techniques designed to compensate for poor wound healing such as better vasularized flaps and the use of prophylactic antibiotics will be helpful.[61]

Adrenal insufficiency is more commonly seen due to exogenous therapeutic steroid administration than to primary adrenal glandular disease. Exogenous corticosteroids will inhibit ACTH release. If this inhibition continues for even as brief a period as 10 days, prolonged adrenal suppression can occur. Once adrenal suppression has occurred, a patient is at great risk for problems during major surgery due to their inability to mount a significant cortisol response to the stress. This may precipitate an adrenal crisis, signaled by the onset of lethargy, tachycardia, flank or abdominal pain, vomiting, fever, restlessness, delirium, hypotension, or coma. Because mineralocorticoid production is not controlled by ACTH, its levels remain normal.[59,62]

Prevention of problems remains the focus of management of patients prone to adrenal insufficiency. Any patient having received pharmacologic amounts of glucocorticoids for more than 10 days in the year preceding a major surgical procedure should be evaluated with a cortrosyn stimulation test or be given supplemental corticosteroids empirically perioperatively. In the cortrosyn stimulation test, a synthetic ACTH is administered to the patient. Plasma cortisol levels are measured before and afterward to check adrenal responsiveness. If a decision is made to give supplemental steroids, an equivalent to 100 mg of hydrocortisone sodium succinate can be given intravenously immediately before surgery and every 8 hours intraoperatively. The drug dosage should be tapered over the next 5 to 7 days. The anesthesiologist should closely monitor blood pressure intraoperatively and consider adrenal insufficiency as a likely cause of unexpected hypotension.[62,63]

SURGERY FOR THE PATIENT WITH HEPATOGASTROINTESTINAL DISORDERS

Liver Disease

Surgeons are well aware of the liver's vital roles in processing nutrients, synthesizing protein, and metabolizing drugs. Fortunately, the liver has a tremendous reserve capacity for maintaining function in the face of even severe hepatic pathology.

Protein synthesis is one of the principal liver activities. Of proteins produced, the ones of particular concern to surgeons and anesthesiologists are albumin and several of the clotting factors. Hepatic production of albumin is in the range of 10 to 15 g daily. Albumin helps maintain the oncotic force necessary to restrict excessive loss of intravascular fluid into the interstitium. Albumin also has a large number of reactive sites and can therefore reversibly bind to most drugs. If albumin production slows sufficiently that serum levels fall below 2.5 g/dL, the results are edema and ascites and an elevation in the free-to-bound ratio of administered drugs.

The vitamin K–dependent coagulation factors II, VII, IX, and X are made in the liver. A significant fall in their levels can be seen with either severe hepatocellular disease or with impaired vitamin K absorption due to biliary problems.

The liver is responsible for the proper function of several enzyme systems that help to limit drug actions. Plasma cholinesterase is produced by the liver; by breaking ester linkages it inactivates drugs such as succinylcholine and ester-type local anesthetics. The hepatic microsomal enzyme system converts lipid-soluble drugs into more water soluble ones that can be excreted by the kidney. Agents such as some benzodiazepines, lidocaine, meperidine, morphine, and alfentanil depend on this system for elimination.[64]

The most common insults to the liver that affect the performance of maxillofacial surgery are ethanol and infectious hepatitis. In the first case many liver functions can be compromised; whereas in the second case not only is proper liver function jeopardized but the surgeon must also help prevent the spread of the infection to others.

Other important consequences of liver disease include impaired glycogen storage and gluconeogenesis, hypersplenism, due to obstructed portal blood flow, causing thrombocytopenia, and poor handling of large gastrointestinal nitrogen loads such as swallowed blood, which alters the level of consciousness in patients with severe liver dysfunction.

Significant liver problems cause a large number of signs and symptoms so that detection is usually straightforward. Laboratory tests of liver function tend to be nonspecific indicators of tissue damage but are commonly used to evaluate patients with suspected liver disease. Serum aspartate aminotransferase (AST, SGOT) levels rise because of damage to either liver, heart, kidney, or skeletal muscles. Changes in serum alanine aminotransferase (ALT, SGPT) levels, on the other hand, are more specific for hepatocellular disease. Lactate dehydrogenase (LDH) is commonly measured but is another nonspecific indicator of tissue damage, although its isoenzyme-5 fraction is believed to be more specific for liver damage. Elevations in serum alkaline phosphatase indicate obstructed bile ducts. Measurement of serum albumin helps gauge the severity of liver disease, with levels of less than 2.5 g/dL being significant; however, malnutrition can also cause hypoalbuminemia. Severe liver disease is indicated by a prolonged prothrombin time (PT) and a decreased platelet count. Suspicion of an infectious cause of hepatic disease mandates the use of immunologic tests for signals of viral disease. Hepatitis A, typically due to fecal contamination of food and water, is evidenced by hepatitis A antibodies. Acute hepatitis B, transmitted parenterally or venereally, will stimulate production of surface and core antigen antibodies; the chronic form is revealed by the presence of only surface antigen antibodies. Non-A, non-B hepatitis, caused by several different viruses and usually transmitted by infected blood products, causes elevated ALT but no hepatitis A or B antibodies. Finally, hepatitis D (δ agent), seen most commonly in illicit drug users and multiply transfused patients, causes the appearnce of δ agent antibodies and, in its acute form, coexists with hepatitis B.[64]

Maxillofacial surgery in the patient with mild to moderate liver disease usually presents few problems because of hepatic reserve. Borderline severe cases require special perioperative attention to prevent complications or a deterioration of liver function. Liver function tests, especially serum ALT measurement, are useful. A PT and platelet count are necessary to detect a potential coagulopathy. Intravenous vitamin K (5–10 mg over 3–5 min) can be administered if a deficiency is suspected and will shorten an abnormal PT in 4 to 12 hours. Fresh frozen plasma can be used temporarily to make up for a vitamin K deficiency until the parenterally administered vitamin is effective. Many clinicians recommend administration of H_2 blockers to patients with liver disease requiring surgery to lessen the chances of gastrointestinal hemorrhage. Prolonged use of nasogastric tubes is avoided for the same reason, and also to avoid traumatizing esophageal varices.[65]

Because patients with severe liver disease have problems with improper gluconeogenesis, the surgeon should closely monitor serum glucose levels. Patients likely to handle nitrogen poorly, particularly those with a history of hepatic encephalopathy, should be placed on dietary protein restriction. If it is likely that blood will be swallowed the patient may need measures to reduce nitrogen absorption in the intestines, such as administration of nonabsorbable antibiotics or the use of a cathartic such as lactulose; consciousness should be closely monitored.

Drugs used for anesthesia and analagesia may need to be modified in the patient with hepatic disease. Drugs to avoid in patients with severe liver disease include all nonsteroidal antiinflammatory drugs, tetracyclines, pentazocine, and atenolol. Drugs for which dosages need to be reduced include diazepam, chlordiazepoxide, meperidine, morphine, propoxyphene, theophylline, lidocaine, verapamil, and most β-sympathetic antagonists. Most anesthetics are generally safe to use in patients with hepatic disease, although some feel halothane, fentanyl, and nitrous oxide should be avoided because of their potential for causing liver toxicity.

Peptic Ulcer Disease

Peptic ulcers and gastritis are two of the most common afflictions of adults, but they are usually easily controlled with H_2-receptor antagonists, which reduce acid secretion, or sucralfate which forms a protective coat over lesions protecting them from the effects of pepsin and acid. Although many patients still use antacids, side effects such as diarrhea (in magnesium-based antacids), constipation (in aluminum-based antacids), and sodium overload make them less desirable.

Signs of active gastrointestinal bleeding include unexplained anemia and guaiac-positive stools, but the process is usually diagnosed based on the presence of epigastric pain temporarily relieved by food or antacids. Endoscopy is used to confirm clinical suspicions.

Before maxillofacial surgery can be performed in patients with a history of gastritis or peptic ulcer disease or predisposed to these problems due to prolonged physiologic stress, the surgeon must ensure that the patient's gastrointestinal problem is being addressed properly. The clinician should verify that the patient is compliant with either their H_2-receptor antagonist regimen (cimetidine, 800 mg qdhs; ranitidine, 150 mg bid; or famotidine, 40 mg qdhs) or with sucralfate (1 g qid). When the patient is unable to take oral medication, cimetidine (300 mg q8h), ranitidine (50 mg q8h), or famotidine (20 mg q12h) can be given intravenously or intramuscularly.[66]

Patients with a predisposition to gastritis or peptic ulcer disease should not be given nonsteroidal antiinflammatory drugs (NSAIDs). The use of corticosteroids in these patients is controversial.[67,68] There is no strong scientific evidence that corticosteroids can cause peptic ulcers in most patients, but many clinicians avoid their use in these patients.

SURGERY IN PATIENTS WITH DISORDERS OF CONNECTIVE TISSUE AND JOINTS

Rheumatoid Arthritides

Rheumatoid arthritis (RA) is a chronic disease causing not only polyarthritis but also problems in serosal surfaces, blood vessels, muscle, skin, and bone marrow. Maxillofacial surgery in patients with RA requires careful evaluation to discover the extent of the patient's abnormalities and to attempt to have those problems under reasonable control. Classic signs and symptoms of RA include morning stiffness of involved joints, symmetric involvement of proximal hand joints, subcutaneous (rheumatoid) nodules over bony prominences or extensor surfaces, elevated serum rheumatoid factor, and marked bony erosions visible on radiographs.

Nonarticular problems seen with RA include pericarditis, pleuritis, pneumonitis, myopathies, vasculitides, bone marrow depression, and skin ulcers.

Patients with RA are usually given several medications to help control their disease. These include salicylates, corticosteroids, gold, penicillamine, antimalarials, azathioprine, methotrexate, and cyclophosphamide. The surgeon therefore must get an accurate list of the medications the patient receives and modify perioperative care appropriately.

The patient on NSAIDs should be on or given drugs to prevent GI side effects. The H_2-receptor antagonists antacids or sucralfate are adequate. The surgeon may also want to stop NSAIDs a week to 10 days before surgery to allow their antiplatelet aggregation effects to abate. If long-term discontinuance of NSAIDs is necessary, consideration may be given to substituting NSAIDs such as salicylate or choline salicylate during the perioperative period, since they cause fewer platelet effects. Patients temporarily unable to take NSAIDs after the immediate postoperative period can be administered rectal formulations of salicylate or indomethacin.

Corticosteroids are used in RA to control severe flares of joint disease, vasculitis, pleural or pericardial disease, or ocular involvement. In this case perioperative steroid supplementation will be necessary.

Cytotoxic agents and penicillamine show evidence of impairment of wound healing in animal models but clinically their effects seem to be minor.[69,70]

Patients with RA who require endotracheal intubation should be evaluated preoperatively for ability to extend at the neck, open their mandible, and move their cricoarytenoid joints. The surgeon needs to remain more vigilant than usual to prevent long periods of overextension or flexion of involved joints. Patients with Raynaud's phenomena need their fingers and toes kept warm intraoperatively. Patients with Sjögren's syndrome will require special care to prevent eye desiccation. The skin of RA patients is commonly thin and easily damaged, so additional padding of pressure points is indicated. Preoperative PT and PTT measurement will help detect circulating anticoagulants due to the RA. Early postoperative ambulation, heat treatments and, possibly, physical therapy of affected joints will help prevent prolonged stiffness.[71]

Systemic Lupus Erythmatosis

Systemic lupus erythmatosis (SLE) is a disorder of connective tissue that can produce dermatitis, arthritis, serositis, myositis, renal disease, neurologic problems, and hematologic dysfunction. Patients with SLE will be managed with many of the same medications that are used for RA including corticosteroids and cytotoxic agents.

In the case of SLE patients, surgeons must choose incision sites free of involved skin, keep extremities warm if Raynaud's phenomena is present, keep photosensitive patients from prolonged exposure to fluorescent lights, and give steroid supplementation perioperatively. SLE-induced renal damage frequently causes a nephrotic syndrome and altered drug elimination.[72]

Preoperative assessment of patients with SLE should include a complete blood count to check for anemia and for depressed leukocyte and platelet counts, a PT and PTT to check for circulating anticoagulants, and either a sedimentation rate or antinuclear antibody to check the activity of the SLE. Blood typing may be a problem due to multiple autoerythrocyte antibodies. A chest radiograph and ECG are indicated to look for evidence of pleural or pericardial disease.

The medications specific to SLE may cause a number of problems including a higher than normal incidence of ibuprofen allergy, frequent occurrence of rashes and fever when ampicillin is used, and the potential exacerbation of the SLE by sulfa-containing drugs.

SURGERY IN PATIENTS WITH NEUROLOGIC AND NEUROMUSCULAR DISORDERS

Seizure Disorders

Seizures are typically recurrent transient paroxysms of hyperactive brain function, which can appear as impaired consciousness, involuntary movement, autonomic disturbance, or psychic experiences. They can result from known causes such as fever, ethanol withdrawal, hypoglycemia, hypoxia, or brain damage or be idiopathic. Most investigators feel the fundamental site of pathology is in the cerebral cortex, which can be detected by electroencephalography (EEG).

The reconstructive maxillofacial surgeon is likely to encounter patients who suffer seizures secondary to head trauma. (Chronic recurrent seizures occur in 30% of patients with cerebral hematomas, 15% of those with depressed skull fractures, and 5% of patients hospitalized with closed head injuries.) Chronic post–head trauma seizures usually do not occur until 6 to 12 months from the time of injury.

Patients giving a past history of any form of seizure disorder (except perhaps febrile seizures in childhood) should be under the care of or evaluated by a neurologist before undergoing major elective surgery. Patients with well-documented seizures and under good control can safely have general anesthesia and surgery. Control is usually obtained by the use of antiseizure medications such as dilantin, phenobarbital, valproic acid, carbameazepine, ethosuximide, and clorazepate. Most of these drugs can cause sedation, which can be additive with anesthetic drugs. Side effects of carbamazepine and dilantin include nausea, dizziness, diplopia, and, rarely, bone marrow depression. Valproic acid can inhibit liver enzymes, potentially causing oversedation with barbiturates.

When evaluating a patient with a seizure disorder for surgery the clinician should learn of the frequency, type, duration, and sequellae of seizures to gauge the degree to which control of the seizures has been obtained. Serum drug levels of these agents can be obtained to help check compliance and to help predict the appearance of seizures, if subtherapeutic, or possible toxic reactions.

Cerebrovascular Disease

Patients with a history of cerebrovascular accidents (transient ischemic attacks [TIAs] or strokes) who require maxillofacial surgery need evaluation by their primary physician before surgery. In most cases little can be done preoperatively to diminish the risk of a stroke during surgery. A careful neurologic examination should be performed preoperatively to document residual damage and again postoperatively to detect evidence of intraoperative problems.

Two situations in which preoperative improvement may be possible are in the patient with either poorly controlled hypertension or severe carotid stenosis. Essential hypertension is a known risk factor for the development of a stroke; therefore, institution of successful antihypertensive therapy before elective surgery is recommended. The preoperative management of patients with carotid lesions is controversial. Part of the problem is that the finding of a carotid bruit by itself does not correlate with the degree or even presence of carotid stenosis. Thus, angiography is necessary if stenosis is suspected to document the severity of the process. The question of whether to perform a carotid endarterectomy before elective surgery continues to be debated, but one recommended guideline is that endarterectomy be performed only if a TIA occurs or if carotid artery occlusion is greater than 80%.[73,74]

Patients with a history of symptomatic cerebrovascular disease are often placed on inhibitors of platelet aggregation such as aspirin or dipyridamole. Most physicians will permit these drugs to be stopped at least 1 week preoperatively to prevent bleeding problems perioperatively.

Myositis

Polymyositis and dermatomyositis both involve weakening of the proximal musculature over several weeks or months. Dermatomyositis includes a rash that extends over the face, shoulders, and arms. These processes commonly occur in association with RA, SLE, and carcinomas of various organs. The diagnosis is based on the finding of elevated serum creatinine phosphokinase levels, abnormal electromyographic studies, and muscle biopsy.

Preoperative considerations for these patients include PFTs to detect problems due to weak muscles of respiration, ECG to detect cardiac conduction disturbances, and questioning of swallowing ability to detect weakness of pharyngeal or esophageal muscles. Patients with myositis are commonly on corticosteroid therapy, which will need supplementation during the operative period.

Myotonic Dystrophy

Myotonic dystrophy is an autosomal dominant process which usually has its onset about age 20 to 25. Affected patients are unable to relax affected muscles (myotonia). This disease can cause several problems of significance to surgeons, including frequent dysphagia, cardiac conduction disorders, pulmonary disease due to abnormal diaphragm activity, and gastrointestinal hypomobility. Prolonged apnea frequently occurs after anesthesia.

Perioperative care should include evaluation of pulmonary and cardiac health with PFTs and an ECG, and vigilance for intra- or postoperative pulmonary, cardiac, and gastrointestinal motility disorders.

Malignant Hyperthermia

Malignant hyperthermia is the leading cause of unexpected anesthetic death in North America. Three types of myopathy can instigate the disorder:

1. An autosomal dominant form occurring in normal-appearing patients (most frequent type)
2. A probably recessive form affecting young males with short stature, neck webbing, scapular winging, kyphoscoliosis, undescended testes, and subnormal intelligence
3. A form featuring central core myopathy with autosomal dominant inheritance characterized by congenital muscle weakness especially of the legs

In all types of malignant hyperthermia the pathophysiology involves an acute rise in calcium release and re-uptake by muscle sarcoplasmic reticulum.[75]

Typically it presents soon after induction of anesthesia with a rapid rise in body temperature and muscle rigidity. Difficulty in ventilating the patient or opening the mandible for intubation are common early manifestations. Other signs include diaphoresis, tachypnea, tachycardia, hyperkalemia, hypocalcemia, elevated temperature and carbon dioxide content of expired air, and cardiac dysrhythmias. Renal failure can occur due to rhabdomyolysis and myoglobinuria. Consumptive coagulopathy can also be triggered. Mortality in patients in which the disorder was not suspected before anesthesia ranges from 63% to 73%.[76]

A predisposition of malignant hyperthermia should be suspected in patients with the following characteristics:[77]

Unusual muscle hypertrophy
Ptosis, ophthalmoplegia, strabismus
Pectus deformities or kyphoscoliosis
Limb girdle weakness
Hip dislocation, dislocated patella, malaligned feet
Known central core myopathy
Young males with previously described appearance
Any history of myopathy of unknown etiology

Patients with a known or suspected tendency should be considered for local or regional anesthetic techniques. If general anesthesia is necessary, a technique that uses nitrous oxide, barbiturates, benzodiazepines, narcotics, or neuroleptic drugs is advisable. Nondepolarizing muscle relaxants should be used if necessary. Drugs such as succinylcholine, amide local anesthetics, ketamine, and volatile anesthetics should be avoided. Premedication with dantrolene (1 mg/kg) orally the day before surgery or as an intravenous bolus the day of surgery is appropriate when malignant hyperthermia is a high probability. In addition, a set protocol for its management, should it occur, must be in place before starting anesthesia for patients at risk for malignant hyperthermia.[78–80]

Myasthenia Gravis

Myasthenia gravis is a disorder of the muscle endplate in which insufficient acetylcholine acts postsynaptically to permit proper muscle function. These patients have fluctuating weakness, with weakness worsening during periods of constant muscle activity. Ocular and oropharyngeal muscles are involved in almost all cases. The diagnosis is confirmed by unequivocal improvement of muscle weakness in response to anticholinesterase administration (neostigmine, pyridostigmine, edrophonium). Peak incidence is ages 20 to 30 for females and ages 50 to 60 for males.

Perioperative considerations include the need to check for signs of pulmonary or cardiac problems. Signs of thyroid disorder (a frequent finding) should also be sought. Maintenance medications should be continued perioperatively, and steroids should be augmented if in use. Drugs that aggravate myasthenia gravis such as streptomycin, tetracyclines, beta-sympathetic antagonists, procainamide, and quinidine should also be avoided. Surgeons should note that myasthenia gravis patients who are not already taking corticosteroids may experience an exacerbation of their disease when steroids are first administered.

Spinal Cord Disorders

Paraplegia due to spinal cord damage can cause a number of problems of which the surgeon needs to be cognizant. Abnormal bladder emptying predisposes these patients to urinary tract infections and chronic pyelonephritis. Paraplegia affecting the diaphragm can lead to pneumonia, and inability to exercise the lower extremities and pelvic region sets up a situation in which thromboembolism to the lungs is common. Inability to move can also cause the development of decubitus ulcers. Renal and adrenal function are often impaired due to amyloidosis, and anemia of chronic disease is frequent in paraplegics.

Maxillofacial surgery for these individuals can be accomplished safely with good patient preparation.

Preoperative checks of pulmonary and renal function will reveal patients at high risk for perioperative complications. The sputum and urine should be checked for evidence of infection and blood count obtained to discover if anemia is present. Special care needs to be taken to properly position and pad vulnerable parts of the body during and after surgery. Minidose heparin will help prevent pulmonary embolism, as will keeping the legs elevated during surgery and providing proper physical therapy after surgery. Physical therapy is also necessary to the upper extremities to prevent contractures. Continuous urinary catheterization is needed during surgery, returning to the intermittent bladder catheterization regimen in place preoperatively as soon as possible after surgery.

SURGERY IN THE PATIENT WITH A PSYCHIATRIC DISORDER

Affective Disorders

Affective disorders such as depression are common problems in modern society. Patients with this disorder need special care during any surgical treatment.

Major depression is characterized by a depressed mood and an inability to enjoy life. Symptoms include sleep disturbance such as early morning wakening, appetite disturbance, fatigue, decreased libido, low self-esteem, and a feeling of hopelessness. Many patients are able to mask or deny their symptoms when under no undue stress, but facing a surgical procedure will usually uncover hidden symptoms of depression.

In addition to the emotional problems patients with depression incur in the perioperative period, problematic drug interactions can occur between anesthetic agents and many of the agents used to control depression. Tricyclic antidepressants are in common use. They carry unwanted anticholinergic and hypotensive side effects, which should be remembered when anesthesia is given. An additional problem with tricyclic antidepressants is their tendency to cause increased conduction delays in patients with preexisting heart blocks.

Monoamine oxidase inhibitors (MAOI) are also used to manage depressive symptoms. They also have anticholinergic and orthostatic hypotensive effects. Drugs with sympathomimetic action should be avoided in patients on MAOI.

Lithium carbonate is used for patients with bipolar (manic-depressive) disorders. It induces the characteristic ECG changes of inverted and flattened T waves. It can also produce sinus node dysfunction and ventricular irritability. Serum levels should be checked preoperatively in these patients.

Benzodiazepines used for depression pose little risk for safe anesthesia as long as the anesthesiologist is aware of their use. Abrupt discontinuation should be avoided to prevent the appearance of a withdrawal phenomena.

Psychotic Disorders

Psychotic disorders are characterized by delusions and hallucinations. Psychotic patients are usually easily recognized by the results of a comprehensive mental status examination. Antipsychotic drugs such as phenothiazines, thioxanthenes, butyrophenones, and indalones control many of the symptoms of psychosis and cause little increased risk of problems with anesthesia. They do have the tendency to cause sedation and extrapyramidal symptoms in many patients.

Surgery in psychotic patients carries no increased risk of complication as long as the disorder is well controlled.

Substance Abuse

Ethanolism

Patients who regularly consume large amounts of ethanol must be allowed to withdraw from the effects of ethanol before they undergo elective surgery and anesthesia. Failure to follow this strategy risks the appearance of minor alcohol withdrawal syndrome, with its compensatory neuronal excitability and catecholamine release, or the severe syndrome (*delirium tremens*) with hallucinosis, hyperpyrexia, hypertension, and life-threatening cardiac dysrhythmias and seizures.

Most of the anesthetic hazards in the sober ethanolic patient are due to ethanol-induced hepatic changes (see section on liver disorders). Chronic ethanol use increases anesthetic requirements for halothane and isoflurane. Clearance of benzodiazepines is also increased, so that larger doses may be necessary in ethanolic patients. Patients with ethanol-induced liver disease are prone to hypoglycemia and need frequent serum glucose determinations during and after surgery.[81]

Ethanolic patients may be treated with disulfiram to discourage ethanol intake. Anesthesia in patients taking disulfiram can be complicated by its tendency to produce sedation and hepatotoxicity. Disulfiram can also induce hypotension. Finally, alcohol-containing preparation solutions should be avoided in these patients.

Opioid Abusers

If surgery is urgently necessary in opioid-dependent patients it is usually prudent for the surgeon to avoid precipitating the withdrawal syndrome by substituting methadone (2.5 mg equals 10 mg of morphine) for the abused opioid. Usually 20 to 40 mg of methadone is needed daily, administered orally or intramuscularly in four to six divided doses. Clonidine has also been found useful for helping prevent symptoms of opioid withdrawal.

Hypotension is a common problem in opioid abusers during the perioperative period. They also are likely to have difficult veins in which to gain access, necessitating placement of central lines. Intravenous illicit drug abusers also have a high incidence of hepatitis B and human immunodeficiency virus positivity.

SURGERY IN SPECIAL PATIENT GROUPS

Obese Patients

Obesity is a common affliction in modern society due to a combination of poor dietary habits and general lack of physical activity. The excessive weight in an obese individual is due to an overabundance of adipose tissue. *Morbid obesity* is defined as when a patient is 100% over ideal body weight due to fat accumulation.

Obesity by itself does not increase surgical mortality until it becomes severe, but then the risk rises exponentially. The *ponderal index* has been used to quantitate the increased risk faced by obese individuals. The index is calculated by dividing an individual's height in inches by the cube root of their weight in pounds. A result greater than 12.5 correlates highly with a significantly heightened risk of complications in the perioperative period. The *Chase method* is another means of gauging risk in obese individuals in which surgical risk is determined by the ratio of weight versus height.[82]

Pulmonary problems are the most frequent complications in the perioperative period in obese patients. These include pulmonary embolism, bronchospasm, atelectasis, and pneumonia. Obesity creates a form of restrictive lung disease, especially when these patients are supine, due to the excessive weight on the thorax and abdomen that restricts full inspiration.[83,84]

Before elective surgery in obese patients a careful history and physical examination are necessary to determine how the obesity may affect anesthesia and to detect a concurrent disease. Specific questions about a history of daytime somnolence and snoring are needed to find if a patient's airway is easily compromised. Past history of lung disease, heart problems, thrombophlebitis, or pulmonary embolism should also be elicited. Obese patients should also be asked about any previous problems in the establishment of venous access. The usefulness of physical examination of the chest and abdomen is commonly limited in obese patients. Therefore, ancillary examination techniques such as PFTs, ECG, and plain chest radiography are usually warranted.

Because obese patients have heightened risks of pulmonary problems, those who smoke should be helped to quit, hopefully for as long as possible before surgery. A reasonable program of weight reduction should also be recommended. When planning surgery the possibility of regional anesthesia should be considered. Deep sedation should be avoided if the airway is likely to be difficult to maintain. If general anesthesia is selected as the method of pain and anxiety control the patient can be given preoperative instruction in incentive spirometry techniques. Prophylactic bronchodilators may be useful, especially if PFTs reveal improvement after their use. The increased risk of thrombophlebitis in these patients can be lessened by the use of a minidose heparin regimen. Finally, a lowered threshold is appropriate for placement of invasive monitors such as a central venous pressure line or a Swan-Ganz catheter.[85]

Obese patients are difficult anesthetic cases. They are typically more of a problem to mask ventilate during the induction of anesthesia. This should be anticipated by being ready to quickly intubate the patient if necessary. The excess weight usually decreases pulmonary compliance and the functional residual and vital capacities. It should be kept in mind that squeezing the bag connected to the endotracheal tube will not give an accurate feel of pulmonary compliance due to the weight of the chest wall. And the lowered lung capacities will cause an increased shunt fraction, which should be monitored by frequent measurements of arterial blood gases. Chest weight effects on the lungs can be lessened by elevating the upper body 15 to 20 degrees from horizontal.

The pharmacokinetics of drugs differ in obese versus lean individuals. The washout of fat-soluble anesthetic agents needs to begin earlier in the surgery to allow the patient to be awakened when desired. When calculating the dose of water-soluble drugs, the estimated lean body mass of the obese individual should be used.

Postoperative management of obese patients should include elevation of the head of the bed, early ambulation, incentive spirometry, minidose heparin, and frequent physical examination for signs of pulmonary problems or deep-vein thrombophlebitis.[86]

Geriatric Patients

Although many clinicians are concerned when treating elderly patients that there will be complications, studies substantiate the fact that most elective surgery is safe in healthy geriatric patients. However, geriatric patients with chronic diseases such as COPD, diabetes, and coronary artery disease are certainly susceptible to the same problems as younger individuals with these same processes. So when older patients have chronic diseases, preoperative preparation should include efforts to minimize the detrimental effects of the disease process on the patient's physiology.

Even though elderly patients can appear frail and sick, a large percentage are actually well. Conversely the appearance of health can be deceiving, because all older individuals experience various changes in physiologic function that can affect their response to the stress of an operation.

Statistically the most common complications that follow major surgery in the elderly are pulmonary embolism, myocardial infarction, pneumonia, and congestive heart failure. The surgeon should be especially vigilant for a past history or perioperative signs of these problems. Also, although geriatric patients usually are able to withstand the initial physiologic stresses of surgery, if a complication occurs they have less reserve to aid with recovery.

The heart undergoes age-related changes that decrease the maximal heart rate (220 minus the age in years). Cardiac output falls (about 1% each year after age 20) because of increased afterload and decreased elasticity of arteries secondary to atherosclerosis. This decreased elasticity also causes any small increase in blood volume to cause sharp increases in blood pressure. Total circulation time at age 20 is 48 seconds; this rises to 65 seconds at age 70. The cardiovascular system also loses much of its responsiveness to catecholamines with age, so that postural hypotension is common. Maximum coronary flow capacity in the elderly is about 65% of that in teenagers.[87–89]

Pulmonary function also falls as people get older. Loss of lung elasticity and increased stiffness of the chest wall predispose lungs to atelectasis and ventilation-perfusion imbalances, as does the increased residual volume in older lungs. Whereas the PaO_2 on room air at age 30 averages about 94 mm Hg, it normally falls to about 74 mm Hg above age 60. Vital capacity and expiratory flow rate begin to fall when individuals reach age 30. Muscle weakness prevents forceful coughing, and degeneration of bronchial epithelium leads to less efficient lung cleansing. All of these changes help to account for the relatively high incidence of pulmonary complications following surgery in older patients.[90]

Renal function decreases 20% to 30% between the ages of 30 and 80 because of natural loss of glomeruli and fibrosis of interstitial tissue. Creatinine clearance falls, but because lean body mass also decreases there is usually no change in measured serum creatinine. An approximation of expected age-related changes in renal function can be gained by the following equation:

$$\text{Creatinine clearance (mL/min)} = 135 - (0.84 \times \text{age})$$

This formula can be used to judge dosages of drugs depending on renal clearance. Geriatric patients also suffer a loss of renal concentrating and diluting ability as tubules become less responsive to antidiuretic hormone. For that reason they can easily have intravascular volume disturbances and electrolyte abnormalities. Thirst perception also becomes a problem and thirst cannot be relied on to help gauge fluid requirements in these patients. Prostatic hypertrophy occurs in 80% of men with age causing urinary problems that are commonly worsened by general anesthesia.[91]

The loss of muscle mass and plasma volume with age may affect drug actions and necessitate changes in drug doses. Older white females are also predisposed to loss of bone strength owing to osteoporosis; extra care should be taken when transporting these patients to and from the operating table. Thinning of skin in older patients also makes them more susceptible to pressure damage, heightening the need for proper intraoperative padding.

Geriatric patients tend to mount poor fever responses to pyrogens. Therefore, other signs of problems such as malaise or altered states of consciousness may need to be used to detect infections. The hearing and visual problems of older patients predispose them to states of confusion owing to sensory deprivation; providing appropriate sensory stimulation helps prevent this problem.

A decrease in gastrointestinal motility leads to frequent constipation, and aging often causes impaired glucose tolerance.

Evaluation of elderly patients before elective maxillofacial surgery should begin with a careful medical history. Old records and consultation with the patient's primary care provider are usually excellent sources of needed information. During the physical examination specific note should be made of the patient's state of hydration, signs of age-related problems such as carotid or aortic stenosis, and any pulmonary and mental status problems. An ECG and chest radiograph are useful for detecting occult problems and provide a baseline for later comparisons.

Intraoperatively the patient should be kept from excessive loss of heat and over- or underhydration. Postoperatively, the clinician should be alert to possible respiratory depression due to narcotics and signs of myocardial damage such as sudden dyspnea or worsening of congestive heart failure.

Drug modifications in the elderly include halving benzodiazepine dosages, recognizing the dysrhythmogenic potential of atropine, being aware that narcotics such as morphine and meperidine have prolonged duration of action, and that water-soluble drugs will have a heightened pharmacologic effect while lipid soluble drugs such as barbiturates will have a long α elimination time.[92, 93]

Pediatric Patients

The surgical challenges in pediatric patients are usually due to their small size. However, it is hazardous to consider children as just small adults when considering their anesthetic needs for surgery.[94, 95]

The physiology of pediatric patients is what makes them differ from adults in their response to drugs and anesthesia. Newborns and infants are obligate mouth breathers. Children have relatively small nasal airways, large tongues, small mandibles, short necks, and abundance of pharyngeal lymphoid tissue, all of which serve to create an airway that is easily compromised. Dead space in children is about 2 mL/kg, and tidal volume is about three times the dead space.

The heart of infants has a fixed stroke volume, so that cardiac output is entirely dependent on heart rate. Blood volume in relation to body weight is high in infants, but the ratio decreases with age. Fluid requirements of children vary with weight:

1–10 kg	100 mL/kg daily
10–20 kg	100∅ mL + 50 mL/kg over 10 kg daily
20 kg	1500 mL + 20 mL/kg over 20 kg daily

Normal urine output also varies:

Age 0–2 years	3 mL/kg/h
2–5 years	2 mL/kg/h
5 years to adult	1 mL/kg/h

Children have relatively large surface areas, which can quickly allow excessive heat loss if they are left uncovered in an operating room.

Dosing of drugs to children is usually best decided based on the manufacturer's recommendations.

Pregnant and Lactating Patients

Pregnancy and lactation are contraindications to elective maxillofacial surgery because of the negative effects on the mother and developing child of various drugs, irradiation from imaging studies, and psychologic stress associated with surgery.

If surgery cannot be deferred, the patient's obstetrician should be consulted for guidance with respect to safe drugs to use (Table 2–2). When feasible the surgery should be conducted under local anesthesia. Steps to minimize anxiety are also appropriate. During later stages of pregnancy patients cannot tolerate

Table 2–2. *Medications to Avoid During Pregnancy*

Aspirin and other nonsteroidal antiinflammatory agents
Carbamazepine
Chloral hydrate (if chronically used)
Chlordiazepoxide
Corticosteroids
Diazepam and other benzodiazepines
Diphenhydramine hydrochloride
Morphine
Nitrous oxide (if exposure greater than 9 h/week)
Pentazocine hydrochloride
Phenobarbital
Promethazine
Propoxyphene
Tetracyclines

Note: All medications should be used with care in pregnant patients. The involved obstetrician should be consulted if there is any question concerning the safety of a drug for a pregnant patient.

long procedures without being allowed to empty their bladder. In addition, pressure from the uterus compromises venous return to the heart by placing pressure on the vena cava when patients are in a supine position. Therefore, allowing patients to assume a more lateral position is necessary.

Lactating patients need to avoid the use of drugs capable of passing into breast milk and potentially harming the infant (Table 2–3).

Table 2–3. *Medications for Breast-feeding Mothers*

Safe	*Potentially Harmful*
Acetaminophen	Ampicillin
Antihistamines	Aspirin
Cephalexin	Barbiturates
Codeine	Chloral hydrate
Erythromycin	Corticosteroids
Fluoride	Diazepam
Lidocaine	Metronidazole
Meperidine	Penicillin
Oxacillin	Propoxyphene
Pentazocine	Tetracyclines

REFERENCES

1. Owslander JG. Drug prescribing for the elderly. West J Med 1981; 135:455.
2. Felner JM, Arensberg D. Perioperative management of the cardiac patient. In: Lubin MF, Walker HK, Smith RB, eds. Medical Management of the Surgical Patient, ed 2. Boston: Butterworths, 1988:91.
3. Miller R, Silvoy G, Lumb PD. Anesthesia, surgery and myocardial infarction: A review. Anesth Rev 1979; 6:14.
4. Mauney FM, Ebert PA, Salistan DC. Postoperative myocardial infarction. A study of predisposing factors, diagnosis and mortality in a high-risk group of surgical patients. Ann Surg 1970; 172:497.
5. Goldman L, Caldera DL, Southwick FS, et al. Multifactorial index of cardiac risk in noncardiac surgical procedures. N Engl J Med 1977; 297:845.
6. Hupp JR. Myocardial infarction: Current management strategies. J Oral Maxillofac Surg 1989; 47:1070.
7. Chariker FG, Mahaffey JE. Anesthesia for dentistry in children. In: Smith R, ed. Anesthesia for infants and children. St. Louis: CV Mosby, 1980.
8. Coriat P, Daloz M, Bousseau D, et al. Prevention of intraoperative myocardial ischemia during noncardiac surgery with intravenous nitroglycerin. Anesthesiology 1984; 61:193.
9. Shulman ST, Amren DP, Bisno AL. Prevention of bacterial endocarditis. Circulation 1984; 70:1123A.
10. Rackley CE, Edwards JE, Karp RB. Mitral valve disease. In: Hurst JW, ed. The Heart, ed 7. New York: McGraw-Hill, 1990:820.
11. Rahimtoola SH. Valvular heart disease. In: Kelley WN, ed. Textbook of Internal Medicine. Philadelphia: JB Lippincott, 1989:205.
12. Cheitlin MD, Byrd RC. Prolapsed mitral valve. Curr Probl Cardiol Dis 1984; 8:1.
13. Felner JM. Valvular heart disease. In: Lubin MF, Walker HK, Smith RB, eds. Medical Management of the Surgical Patient, ed 2. Boston: Butterworths, 1988:108.
14. Felner JM. Congestive heart failure. In: Lubin MF, Walker HK, Smith RB, eds. Medical Management of the Surgical Patient, ed 2. Boston: Butterworths, 1988:133.
15. McIntosh HD, Morris J Jr. The hemodynamic consequences of arrhythmias. Prog Cardiovasc Dis 1966; 8:330.
16. Zipes DP. Cardiac arrhythmias. In: Kelley WN, ed. Textbook of Internal Medicine. Philadelphia: JB Lippincott, 1989:176.
17. Kaufman L. Unforeseen complications encountered during dental anaesthesia. Proc Royal Soc Med 1966; 59:731.
18. Ditchey RV, Karliner JS. Safety of electrical cardioversion without digitalis toxicity. Ann Intern Med 1981; 95:676.
19. Felner JM. Arrhythmias and conduction disturbances.

In: Lubin MF, Walker HK, Smith RB, eds. Medical Management of the Surgical Patient, ed 2. Boston: Butterworths, 1988:125.
20. Lown B, Graboys TB. Management of patients with malignant ventricular dysrhythmias. Am J Cardiol 1977; 39:910.
21. Belocci F, Sontarelli P, Di Gennaro M, et al. The risk of cardiac complications in surgical patients with bifascicular block. Chest 1980; 77:343.
22. Pastore JO, Yurchak PM, Janis KM, et al. The risk of advanced heart block in surgical patients with right bundle branch block and left axis deviation. Circulation 1978; 57:677.
23. Edwards WJ. Preanesthetic management of the hypertensive patient. N Engl J Med 1979; 301:158.
24. Goldman L, Caldera DL. Risks of general anesthesia and elective operation in the hypertensive patient. Anesthesiology 1979; 50:285.
25. Hall WD. Preoperative hypertension. In: Lubin MF, Walker HK, Smith RB, eds. Medical Management of the Surgical Patient, ed 2. Boston: Butterworths, 1988:139.
26. Ropper AH, Wechsler LR, Wilson LS. Carotid bruit and the risk of stroke in elective surgery. N Engl J Med 1982; 307:1388.
27. Vertes V, Goldberg G. The preoperative patient with hypertension. Med Clin North Am 1979; 63:1299.
28. Martin DE, Kommerer WS. The hypertensive surgical patient. Surg Clin North Am 1983; 63:1017.
29. Hodgkin JD. Preoperative assessment of respiratory function. Respir Care 1984; 29:496.
30. Tisi GM. Preoperative identification and evaluation of the patient with lung disease. Med Clin North Am 1987; 71:399.
31. Wellman JJ, Smith BA. Preoperative respiratory evaluation. In: Lubin MF, Walker HK, Smith RB, eds. Medical Management of the Surgical Patient, ed 2. Boston: Butterworths, 1988:161.
32. Ford GT, Guenter CA. Toward prevention of postoperative pulmonary complications. Am Rev Respir Dis 1984; 130:4.
33. Gass GD, Olsen GN. Preoperative pulmonary function testing to predict postoperative morbidity and mortality. Chest 1986; 89:127.
34. Stein M, Cassara EL. Preoperative pulmonary evaluation and therapy for surgery patients. JAMA 1970; 211:787.
35. Saunders NA, Powles AC, Rebuck AJ. Ear oximetry: Accuracy and practicability in the assessment of arterial oxygenation. Am Rev Respir Dis 1976; 113:745.
36. Parc PD, Gonzalez Montoner JS. Asthma. In: Kelley WN, ed. Textbook of Internal Medicine. Philadelphia: JB Lippincott, 1989:1873.
37. McFadden ER Jr. Asthma. In: Wilson JD, Braunwald E, Isselbacher KJ, et al, eds. Harrison's Principles of Internal Medicine, ed 10. New York: McGraw-Hill, 1990.
38. Newhouse MT, Dolovich MF. Control of asthma by aerosols. N Engl J Med 1986; 315:870.
39. Petty TL. Chronic obstructive pulmonary disease. In: Kelley WN, ed. Textbook of Internal Medicine. Philadelphia: JB Lippincott, 1989:1884.
40. Tarhan S, Moffitt EA, Sessler AD, et al. Risk of anesthesia and surgery in patients with chronic bronchitis and chronic obstructive pulmonary disease. Surgery 1973; 74:720.
41. Bartlett RH. Pulmonary pathophysiology in surgical patients. Surg Clin North Am 1980; 60:1323.
42. Gracey DR, Divertie MB, Didier EP. Preoperative pulmonary preparation of patients with chronic obstructive pulmonary disease. Chest 1979; 76:123.
43. Rehder K, Sessler AD, Marsh HM. General anesthesia and the lung. Am Rev Respir Dis 1975; 112:541.
44. Mars RL. Chronic renal failure. In: Lubin MF, Walker HK, Smith RB, eds. Medical Management of the Surgical Patient, ed 2. Boston: Butterworths, 1988:343.
45. Anagnostou A, Kurtzman NA. The anemia of chronic renal failure. Semin Nephrol 1985; 5:115.
46. Brenowitz JB, Williams CD, Edwards WS. Major surgery in patients with chronic renal failure. Am J Surg 1977; 134:765.
47. Burke GR, Gulyassy PF. Surgery in the patient with renal disease and related electrolyte disorders. Med Clin North Am 1979; 63:1191.
48. Deutsch S. Anesthetic management of patients with chronic renal disease. South Med J 1975; 68:65.
49. Rowe JW. The influence of age on renal failure. Resid Staff Phys 1978; 24:49.
50. Delcher HK. Diabetes mellitus. In: Lubin MF, Walker HK, Smith RB, eds. Medical Management of the Surgical Patient, ed 2. Boston: Butterworths, 1988:281.
51. Alberti KG, Thomas DJ. The management of diabetes during surgery. Br J Anaesth 1979; 51:693.
52. Bagdade JD, Root RK, Bulger RJ. Impaired leukocyte function in patients with poorly controlled diabetes. Diabetes 1974; 23:9.
53. Fletcher J, Langman MS, Kellock TD. Effect of surgery on blood sugar levels in diabetes mellitus. Lancet 1965; 2:52.
54. Stevens A, Roizen MF. Patients with diabetes mellitus and disorders of glucose metabolism. Anesth Clin North Am 1987; 5:339.
55. Thomas DJ, Platt HS, Alberti KG. Insulin-dependent diabetes: An assessment of continuous glucose-insulin potassium infusion, and traditional treatment. Anaesthesiology 1984; 39:629.
56. Siddiq YK, Gebhart SS. Disorders of the thyroid gland. In: Lubin MF, Walker HK, Smith RB, eds. Medical Management of the Surgical Patient, ed 2. Boston: Butterworths, 1988:292.
57. Utiger RD. Evaluation of abnormal thyroid function tests. In: Kelley WN, ed. Textbook of Internal Medicine. Philadelphia: JB Lippincott, 1989:2293.
58. Utiger RD. Diseases of the thyroid gland. In: Kelley WN, ed. Textbook of Internal Medicine. Philadelphia: JB Lippincott, 1989:2178.
59. Goldmann DR. Surgery in patients with endocrine dysfunction. Med Clin North Am 1987; 71:499.

60. Roizen MT, Hensel P, Lichtor JL, et al. Patients with disorders of thyroid function. Anesth Clin North Am 1987; 5:277.
61. Lampe GH, Roizen MF. Anesthesia for patients with abnormal function at the adrenal cortex. Anesth Clin North Am 1987; 5:245.
62. Siddiq YK, Watts NB. Disorders of the adrenal gland. In: Lubin MF, Walker HK, Smith RB, eds. Medical Management of the Surgical Patient, ed 2. Boston: Butterworths, 1988:301.
63. Gran L, Pahle JA. Rational substitution therapy for steroid-treated patients. Anaesthesiology 1978; 33:59.
64. Morris SJ. Liver disease. In: Lubin MF, Walker HK, Smith RB, eds. Medical Management of the Surgical Patient, ed 2. Boston: Butterworths, 1988:197.
65. Friedman LS, Maddrey WC. Surgery in the patient with liver disease. Med Clin North Am 1987; 71:453.
66. Johnson DA, Cattau EL Jr. Pharmacologic approach to gastrointestinal disease in critical illness. In: Cherrow B, ed. The pharmacologic approach to the critically ill patient. Baltimore: Williams & Wilkins, 1988:322.
67. Conn HO, Blitzer BL. Non-association of adrenocorticoid therapy and peptic ulcer. N Engl J Med 1976; 294:473.
68. Cooke AR. Drugs and gastric damage. Drugs 1976; 11:36.
69. Garner RW, Mowat AG, Hazelman BL. Wound healing after operations on patients with rheumatoid arthritis. J Bone Joint Surg 1973; 55B:134.
70. Schorn D, Mowat AG. Penicillamine in rheumatoid arthritis, wound healing, skin thickness and osteoporosis. Rheumatol Rehab 1977; 16:223.
71. Stark DC, Miller R. Anesthesia for patients with rheumatoid arthritis. Some practical considerations. Orthop Rev 1978; 7:21.
72. Goldman JA. Systemic lupus erythematosus. In: Lubin MF, Walker HK, Smith RB, eds. Medical Management of the Surgical Patient, ed 2. Boston: Butterworths, 1988:257.
73. Hart RG, Easton JD. Management of cervical bruits and carotid stenosis in preoperative patients. Stroke 1983; 14:290.
74. Roedered GO, Langlors YE, Jager KA, et al. The natural history of carotid arterial disease in asymptomatic patients with cervical bruits. Stroke 1984; 15:605.
75. Walker HK. Muscle disease. In: Lubin MF, Walker HK, Smith RB, eds. Medical Management of the Surgical Patient, ed 2. Boston: Butterworths, 1988: 395.
76. Tomarken JL, Britt BA. Malignant hyperthermia. Ann Emerg Med 1987; 16:1253.
77. Eng GD, Epstein BS, Engel WK, et al. Malignant hyperthermia and central core disease in a child with congenital dislocating hips. Arch Neurol 1978; 35:189.
78. Gronert GA. Malignant hyperthermia. Anesthesiology 1980; 53:395.
79. Nelson TE, Flewellen EH. The malignant hyperthermia syndrome. N Engl J Med 1983; 309:416.
80. Wackym PA, Dubrow TJ, Abdul-Rasool IH, et al. Malignant hyperthermia in plastic surgery. Plas Reconstr Surg 1988; 82:878.
81. Bruce DL. Alcoholism and anesthesia. Anesth Analg 1983; 62:84.
82. Putnam L, Jenicek JA, Allen CR, Wilson RO. Anesthesia in the morbidly obese patient. South Med J 1974; 67:1411.
83. Pierce AK, Robertson J. Pulmonary complications of general surgery. Ann Rev Med 1977; 28:211.
84. Watemath CC, Bergman NA. Respiratory compliance in obese patients. Anesthesiology 1974; 41:84.
85. Reisin E, Frohlich ED. Obesity. Arch Intern Med 1981; 141:431.
86. Holm RP. Diagnostic and therapeutic considerations in the obese patient. In: Lubin MF, Walker HK, Smith RB, eds. Medical Management of the Surgical Patient, ed 2. Boston: Butterworths, 1988:271.
87. Boss GR, Seegmiller JE. Age-related physiologic changes and their clinical significance. West J Med 1981; 135:434.
88. Gerstenblith G, Lakatta EG, Weisfeldt ML. Age changes in myocardial function and exercise response. Prog Cardiovasc Dis 1976; 19:1.
89. Weisfeldt ML. Aging of the cardiovascular system. N Engl J Med 1980; 303:1172.
90. Muresan G, Sorbini CA, Grassi V. Respiratory function in the aged. Bull Physiopathol Respir 1971; 7:973.
91. McLachlan MS. The aging kidney. Lancet 1978; 2:143.
92. Greenblatt DJ, Sellers EM, Shader RI. Drug disposition in old age. N Engl J Med 1982; 306:1081.
93. Schumacher GE. Pharmacokinetic factors influencing drug therapy in the aged. Am J Hosp Pharm 1980; 37:559.
94. Berkowitz RJ, Smith RM. Anesthesia for dentistry in children. In: Smith R, ed. Anesthesia for infants and children. St. Louis: CV Mosby, 1980.
95. Campbell RL, Weiner M, Stewart LM. General anesthesia for the pediatric patient. J Oral Maxillofac Surg 1982; 40:497.

3

Immunology and Transmissible Infectious Disease

Peter Quinn

On May 14, 1796, Dr. Edward Jenner, an English country physician, exposed a small scratch on the arm of a young man named James Phipps to infectious material from a cowpox lesion on the hand of another patient, Ms. Sarah Nelmes. Six weeks later, he directly inoculated Mr. Phipps with pus from an intact smallpox pustule. No infection followed. This historic discovery of cross-immunity heralded the beginning of immunology. From Louis Pasteur's rabies immunizations to the current race to develop an HIV vaccine, the field of immunology has undergone incredible growth. There is no area of oral and maxillofacial surgery in which an understanding of the immune mechanism is without benefit. The management of odontogenic infections, hard and soft tissue grafting, proper wound healing, maxillofacial cancer development and treatment, and the use of alloplastic implants all are dependent on the inherent defense mechanisms provided primarily by the immune system. In addition, an understanding of the pathophysiology of communicable disease is paramount to the oral and maxillofacial surgeon and affiliated health care professionals.

THE IMMUNE RESPONSE

General Principles

The primary function of the human immune system is to distinguish self from nonself. Whether protecting itself from internal threats (e.g., malignant cells) or external invaders (bacterial/viral), the system must be able to recognize, process, and respond to antigens. Most antigens are proteins, but other substances like the polysaccharides on bacterial surfaces may provoke the immune response. The majority of antigens have molecular weights of 10,000 or more, but smaller molecules (haptens) can be antigenic if they attach to a body "carrier protein." Whether the antigen is bacterial, viral, food, plant, or tissue (e.g., allogenic bone graft), the basic cellular components of the immune system must be functional for a successful immunologic response to occur.

Pluripotential stem cells differentiate into specific cell lines including lymphocytes, phagocytes, and basophils. Each of these groups of cells has specific functions within cell-mediated immunity (Table 3–1).

Lymphocytes

T-CELLS. The majority of circulating lymphocytes are T-cells (thymus dependent lymphocytes). After maturation in the thymus gland, the cells migrate to peripheral lymphoid tissue, especially the paracortical area of lymph nodes and the periarteriolar portions of the splenic white pulp. T-cells are responsible for host reactions against viruses, fungi, malignancies (tumor antigens), intracellular infections (e.g., tuberculosis, leprosy), and allografted tissue.

T-lymphocytes and the monocyte-macrophage cell

Table 3–1. *Cell Types and Their Function*

Cell Type	Subtype	Function
Lymphocytes	B-lymphocytes	Humoral immunity
	T-lymphocytes	Specific cell-mediated immunity
	Null cells (natural killer cells)	Nonspecific cell-mediated immunity
Phagocytes	Macrophages	Phagocytosis antigen processing
	Polymorphonuclear leukocytes (neutrophils)	Phagocytosis (microbial)
	Eosinophils	Phagocytosis (bacteria, fungi, and immune complexes)
Basophils and mast cells		Immediate hypersensitivity reactions

line function by direct cell-to-cell contact for antigenic destruction or by production of soluble polypeptides that serve specific immune functions such as induction of phagocytosis, or stimulation and proliferation of cell lines (e.g., T-cell growth factor).

The specificity of the immune response is dependent on the development of clones of T-lymphocytes with surface proteins for recognition of specific antigens. An antigen-processing cell (APC macrophage) processes and presents the antigen and links it with a cell surface transplantation antigen (histocompatibility antigen). The combined protein on the surface of the accessory cell is a restriction element. Therefore, T-cells (unlike B-cells) cannot respond to free antigen, but can react to glycoprotein complexes coded for by the major histocompatibility complex on chromosome 6.

There are three types of T-cells: killer, suppressor, and helper. T-killer cells (or cytotoxic cells) are involved in direct cell-to-cell destruction. They are coated with a specific surface protein. Suppressor cells suppress B-cell proliferation for antibody production when appropriate (e.g., after elimination of a viral infection). T-helper cells serve two functions: stimulation of B-lymphocytes for proliferation and production of antibody; and production of interleukin-2 for stimulation and proliferation of T-killer (T8) cells.

Lymphocytes that lack surface antigens (CD4 or CD8) include killer cells and natural killer cells. They cannot specifically recognize antigen but do possess receptors to bind with IgG antibody–coated cells. This antibody-dependent cellular cytotoxicity provides a direct, nonspecific, cell-to-cell surveillance and destruction mechanism for viral and tumor cells that does not require previous exposure.

Another aspect of cell-mediated immunity is the production of cytokines (by macrophages) and lymphokines (by activated lymphocytes). These include interleukins and interferons:

Cytokine/Lymphokine	Function
Interleukin 1	Induces ACTH secretion to stress; stimulates B- and T-cell function; induces neutrophil proliferation
Interleukin 2 (T-cell growth factor)	Stimulates growth of cytotoxic T-cell clones
Interleukin 3	Growth factor for bone marrow; progenitor cell lines and mast cells
Interleukin 4	Stimulates B-cells and enhances major histocompatibility complex (MHC) function
Tumor necrosis factor (TNF)	Direct cytotoxin for some tumor cells; induces fever response
Interferons	Polypeptides that interfere with viral reproduction
Chemotactic factor	Induces chemotaxis in macrophages, eosinophils, and neutrophils (PMN)
Macrophage inhibition factor (MIF)	Aggregates macrophages at site of injury
Blastogenic factor	Proliferates lymphocytes

The mechanisms of cell-mediated immunity are responsible for the following types of clinically relevant reactions:

Immune response to viral and fungal antigens
Contact sensitivity (e.g., poison ivy)
Delayed hypersensitivity reaction (e.g., tine test for tuberculosis)
Immune response to intracellular organisms (e.g., leprosy, brucella)
Host versus graft rejections
Granuloma formation
Immune response to specific tumor cells lines

T-cell–mediated immunity can be assessed in several ways. Delayed hypersensitivity skin tests are used to test immunocompetence. Reactions are induced by intradermal injections of antigens such as tuberculin, candida, mumps, and streptokinase-streptodornase. It is assumed that the patient has had previous exposure to one or more of the antigens. If two or more antigens produce 5 mm or more of induration in 48 hours, one can presume some reasonable level of competence in the cell-mediated response.

Monoclonal antibodies are available for determining the proper ratio of helper (T4) to suppressor (T8) cell populations. The acceptable ratio is approximately 2 to 1. The reversal of this ratio by destruction of the T-helper cell population by CD4-specific HIV viral receptors is the central pathologic process in the acquired immunodeficiency syndrome. Finally, in vitro laboratory testing of T-cell function can be performed with donor cell lines that have been exposed to antigens and are assessed for their ability to proliferate and express T-cell cytotoxic functions in culture.

B-CELLS. Humoral immunity involves the production of immunoglobulins (antibodies) by B-cells. Immunoglobulins can be separated into five distinct classes based on structural differences. The basic structure (Fig. 3–1) is defined by bonded chains of polypeptides with attached carbohydrate molecules. The cavity between the ends of a pair of heavy and light chains (the N portion) forms the *Fab fragment* or the antigen-binding site. This is the variable end and it confers immunologic specificity. The major immunoglobulin classes and their functions appear in Display 3–1.

The *Fc fragment* is the carboxyterminal (constant) region. Its amino-acid sequence is fixed so that this end of the immunoglobulin confers similar biologic properties to this entire class of antibodies. It plays no role in antigen binding but does provide for placental transfer (IgG), passage through mucosal barriers (IgA secretory immunity), intestinal and intravascular transfer (e.g., binding to macrophages, mast cells, platelets), and complement fixation and activation. This interaction between B-cell, precursor T-cells, and antigens accounts for the primary immune response and the secondary (or "amnestic") immune response.

The variable portion of the antibody (Fab) is the amino-acid terminal. Through genetically coded DNA translocations, the amino-acid sequence is specifically engineered to create an antigen-specific antibody. Over a million different "dedicated" pre–B cells can

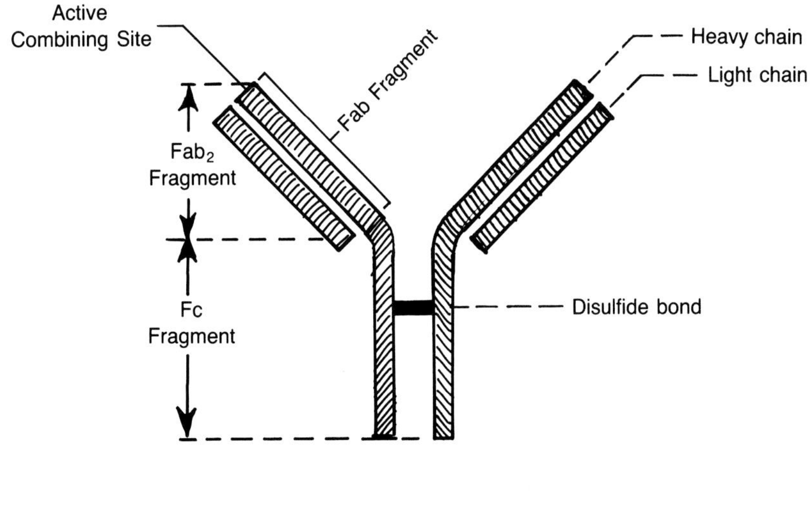

Figure 3-1. *The basic structure of the immunoglobulins (IgG, IgA, IgD, and IgE).*

Display 3–1. Major Immunoglobulins and Functions

IMMUNOGLOBULIN	FUNCTION
IgG	Molecular weight of 150,000; most predominant immunoglobulin (accounts for 75% of circulating immunoglobulin); responsible for the secondary (recall) immune response; easily crosses placenta and diffuses into tissue for efficient antigen interaction. Newborns possess mostly IgG maternal antibodies. Macrophages, neutrophils, and B-cells possess specific IgG-Fc receptors to facilitate opsonization and phagocytosis.
IgM	Large molecular weight (900,000 to 1,000,000) that restricts it to vascular spaces (cannot cross placenta); first immunoglobulin synthesized in the primary immune response, but it is then rapidly replaced by IgG; very efficient for agglutination, opsonization, and bacteriolysis; most efficient Ig for activation of the complement system.
IgA	Primary Ig of all mucosal surfaces and exocrine secretions (e.g., saliva, tears); accounts for 20% of circulating serum immunoglobulin; this secretory immunity is facilitated by production of a glycoprotein (secretory component) to facilitate passage of IgA through mucosal epithelium; IgA functions by forming immune complexes (e.g., IgA–*Streptococcus mutans* binding inhibits the Streptococcus attachment to dental plaque). Some infectious agents (e.g., gonococcus) produce IgA protease to inhibit the Ab-Ag complex formation that normally blocks bacterial entry (immune exclusion).
IgD	Receptor on B-lymphocytes; only trace amounts in serum
IgE	Usually present in small concentrations, but is elevated in immediate hypersensitivity reactions; Fc portions of IgE bind to receptors on mast cells and basophils to release mediators of inflammatory reactions (e.g., histamine, heparin, SRSA). Response is amnestic, so that repeat exposure to antigen causes increasing reaction, possibly resulting in anaphylaxis; also plays a role in reaction to intestinal parasites (helminths).

be produced in the marrow in a single day. After migration to peripheral lymphoid tissue, these precursor cells can be stimulated by antigen binding to their specific immunoglobulin receptor.

Assessment of humoral immune function includes

- Measurement of serum IgA, IgM, and IgG levels (Unless there has been intrauterine infection, there should be no demonstrable levels of IgA or IgM in the neonate.)
- Measurement of naturally occurring antibody levels (e.g., isohemagglutinins to blood group proteins and ubiquitous viral antigens)
- Assessment of current immune response by measuring antibody levels after active vaccination (e.g., pneumococcal, hepatitis B, tetanus)
- In vitro B-cell stimulation with mitogens or drugs in cell culture.

Complement

Another component of the humoral immune system is the complement system. Host defense mechanisms are instituted or amplified by a series of 18 plasma proteins that are sequentially triggered by the complement cascade for several purposes:

- Signal phagocytic cells
- Stimulate chemotaxis
- Mediate immune vascular responses
- Stimulate cytolysis, and
- Facilitate opsonization

The complement system thus serves as a sensing and communication system which facilitates recognition of foreign materials and tissues and then helps other components of the immune system in their defense mission (Fig. 3–2).

A global assessment of the complement system is the CH_{50} test. The test measures the amount of serum needed to lyse 50% of antibody-coated sheep red cells. If a deficiency is suspected, individual assays of C3 and C4 and perhaps other complement components should be ordered.

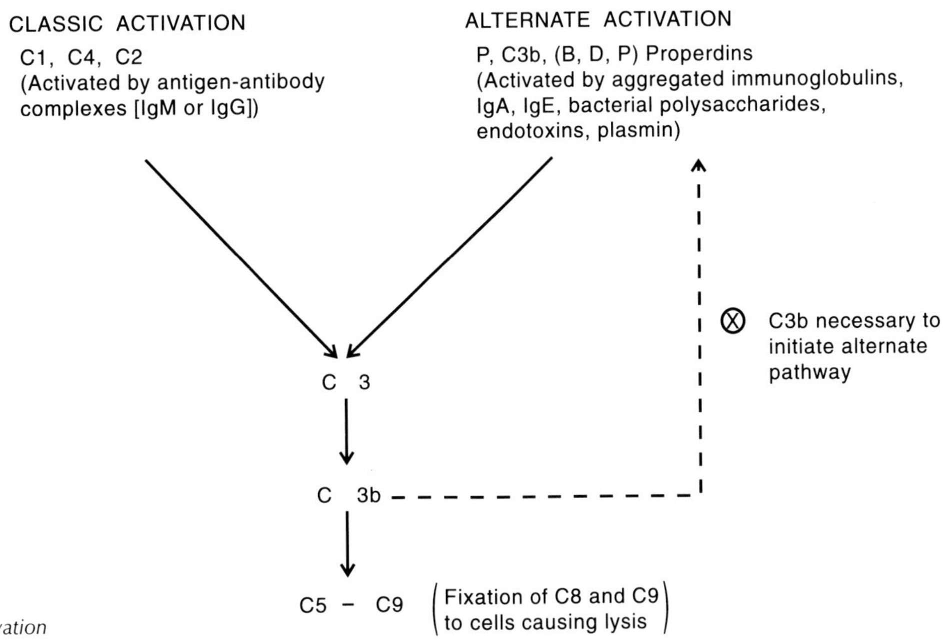

Figure 3-2. *Complement Activation*

Phagocytosis

Lastly, phagocytosis is mediated by circulating and fixed components.

Fixed-tissue phagocytic cells include lymph-node macrophages, microglial brain cells, Kupffer's cells (liver), splenic macrophages, and pulmonary alveolar macrophages.

Circulating phagocytic cells consist of granulocytes, monocytes, and eosinophils.

Bacterial products and complement factors C5a and C3a act as chemoattractants. Polymorphonuclear leukocytes (PMNs) then engulf antibody-coated (opsonized) bacterial cells.

Phagocytosis causes an increase in anaerobic metabolism with a resultant accumulation of lactic acid, thus lowering the pH in the phagocytic vacuole and creating a more bactericidal environ. This mode of metabolism also allows PMNs to be effective in areas of lowered oxygen tension (i.e., abscess cavities). PMN function can be assessed by absolute neutrophil counts, adherence and chemotactic assays, killing assays (*Staphylococcus aureus* and *Candida albicans*), and measurements of oxidative metabolism.

Phagocytosis is bacteria-specific. The toxins produced by invading bacteria (e.g., the erythrotoxin produced by certain streptococci) are highly immunogenic and are neutralized by specific antibodies. These antibodies can also act as opsonins to enhance phagocytosis. Gram-negative organisms such as *Hemophilus influenza* are destroyed by specific antibodies with complement activation. Gram-positive organisms, like streptococci and staphylococci, are resistant to complement-mediated lysis because of their cell wall structure. In this instance, direct phagocytosis is more important. Intracellular bacterial infections with *Mycobacterium* (tuberculosis and leprosy) are resistant to PMN and macrophage phagocytosis. They also elicit poor antibody responses and are associated with T-cell mediated inflammatory responses. Antiviral defense mechanisms are largely antibody mediated. IgA, IgG, or IgM antibodies are involved in the response to more acute extracellular viruses. Acquired immunity to the annual influenza strains is explained on this basis. Chronic viral infections, or "dormant" intracellular viral infections like herpes, can result in both cell-mediated and antibody responses. For example, antibody-dependent cellular cytotoxicity is a unique "combination" mechanism in which antibodies bind to virally infected cells and provide activation of killer T-cells.

Dysfunction of the Immune System

Primary immunodeficiencies are usually genetically inherited recessive disorders. They may affect only B-cells or T-cells, or result in combined-cell deficiencies. Inherited neutrophil and complement disorders are also primary disorders. If only B-cells are affected, measurable immunoglobulin deficiencies result in recurrent bacterial infections with organisms like *Streptococcus pneumoniae*, *S. aureus*, *H. influenzae*, and chronic parasitic infestations (e.g., *Giardia lamblia*). There can be selective deficiencies in specific immunoglobulins (hypogammaglobulinemia), or a total inability to synthesize any Ig (e.g., sex-linked agammaglobulinemia). In this disorder, biopsy reveals hypoplasia of lymph nodes, tonsils, and adenoids. Because T-cell function is intact, the ability to respond to most viral and fungal infections is still present. Malignancies and autoimmune diseases (e.g., rheumatoid arthritis) occur in higher frequencies in agammaglobulinemia. Treatment consists of intermittent injection if immunoglobulin preparations (predominantly IgG, with a trace of IgA and IgM). In spite of this maintenance therapy, infections occur and must be aggressively treated. Secondary B-cell dysfunction can occur with thymoma, transcobalamin deficiency, Epstein-Barr infection, malignancies (e.g., plasma cell transformation to produce myeloma protein), and steroid therapy.

T-cell deficiency is associated with the following:

- Life-threatening opportunistic infections with low-grade pathogens (e.g., fungi, atypical tuberculosis, pneumocystis, measles, herpes, and cytomegalovirus)
- Increased incidence of malignancies
- Chronic diarrhea and wasting
- Exaggerated graft versus host reactions
- Hematologic abnormalities

T-cell absolute counts with T4 to T8 ratios give a quantitative assay, and function can be ascertained by exposing the patient to an allergen (e.g., dinitrochlorobenzene) and then re-exposing 10 to 14 days later to check for specific delayed cutaneous reactivity (i.e., cell-mediated immunity). T-cell deficiency due to a stem-cell defect is best treated by bone marrow transplant from a histocompatible donor. In a thymic defect (e.g., DiGeorge syndrome), the T-cell deficiency may be treated with a thymus transplant. Combined B-cell and T-cell deficiency can be caused by adenosine deaminase deficiency, intrauterine infection (e.g., measles and cytomegalovirus), and also can be induced by pretransplant immunosuppression therapy. The acquired immundeficiency syndrome (AIDS) will be covered separately in this chapter.

Hypersensitivity Reactions

Any immune reaction that results in injury to host tissue is defined as *hypersensitivity*.

Type I: Anaphylaxis (Ab mediated)

Preformed IgE antibodies bind to the surface of target cells (mast cells and basophils) through the Fc region of the immunoglobulin. The cells are now sensitized. On second exposure, the antigen binds to the Fab portion of the IgE, and this Ag-Ab complex causes degranulation. This releases histamine, slow-reacting substance of anaphylaxis (SRS-A), eosinophilic chemotactic factor of anaphylaxis (ECF-A), and leukotrienes.

Manifestations include shock, laryngeal edema, vomiting, diarrhea, vascular permeability, rhinitis, and smooth muscle spasm (bronchoconstriction). Cyclic AMP plays a role in degranulation, because drugs that increase levels of cyclic AMP (theophylline and epinephrine) are therapeutic.

Type II: Cytotoxic Reactions (Ab mediated)

Cell-bound antigens react with either IgG or IgM to trigger the complement cascade. Examples of this complement-dependent cell lysis (mediated by C8 and C9) include idiopathic thrombocytopenic purpura from autoimmune destruction of one's own platelets; autoimmune hemolytic anemia; erythroblastosis fetalis from Rh-negative incompatability (IgG can cross placenta); and Goodpasture's syndrome (autoimmune destruction of the glomerular basement membrane).

Type III: Immune Complex Hypersensitivity Reactions (Ab mediated)

Type III reactions are associated with Ag-Ab complexes (from soluble Ag, not tissue-fixed antigen) that are deposited in tissue and cause complement activation and release of vasoactive amines. Chemoattractants induce PMNs, which phagocytize the Ag-Ab complexes and release lysosomal enzymes. Examples of this type of reaction are serum sickness (Arthus reaction), microbial antigens (e.g., post-streptococcal glomerulonephritis), polyarteritis nodosa, rheumatoid arthritis, and systemic lupus.

Type IV: Delayed Hypersensitivity (cell-mediated)

Delayed hypersensitivity differs from the other three types because it is mediated by T-cells and macrophages. An antigen processing accessory cell presents the Ag to previously sensitized T-cells which release lymphokines. T-cells–activated macrophages are then induced to release lysosomal enzymes, which increase the host tissue damage. Examples of Type IV reactions include autoimmune disease (e.g., Hashimoto's thyroiditis), contact dermatitis (e.g., poison ivy), granulomas from intracellular bacterial infection (tuberculosis and leprosy), and graft versus host disease.

Transplantation

Advances in transplantation immunology have contributed to our understanding of the immune system. Procedures like bone marrow transplantation in hematologic malignancies and cadaveric renal transplants depend on close matching of donor and recipient.

The most important group of antigens to transplantation are the HLA (leukocyte) antigens. These are coded for by a cluster of genes on chromosome 6, the major histocompatibility complex (MHC). There are numerous loci (e.g., HLA-A, HLA-B, HLA-DR, and so forth) with specific alleles at each site. The greater the number of donor-recipient mismatches, the greater the chance of rejection. Autoimmune diseases are also associated with specific phenotypes. For example, HLA-B27 is the antigenic allele that is associated with ankylosing spondylitis, and some insulin diabetics have been linked to DR-3 and DR-4 phenotypes.

Transplants are one of the following:

Xenograft-graft between different species

Allograft-graft between allogenic individuals of the same species, differing in at least one major HLA (e.g., cadaveric renal transplants)

Isograft-graft between syngeneic individuals (e.g., identical twins)

Autograft (self-to-self) tissue graft

The rate of graft rejection differs (acute, hyperacute, or chronic) and depends mainly on the degree of MHC incompatibility. For example, in skin allografts, if there are major MHC differences rejection occurs in 10 to 14 days. Lymphokine-secreting T-cells recruit host macrophages to produce vascular injury, congestion, ischemia, and necrosis. In places where MHC genes are compatible but differences in the minor loci are present, rejection can take months.

The acute rejection reactions involve cytotoxic T-cells and T-cell–secreted lymphokines and usually occur within 2 weeks of transplantation. Hyperacute graft rejection occurs in patients who were presensitized by previous graft and have circulating antigraft serum antibody levels. This immediate reaction is a type II hypersensitivity in which Ag-Ab complexes cause antibody dependent, cell-mediated cytotoxicity (ADCC). The involved antibodies are directed at ABO blood group antigens and MHC antigens. The more common transplant rejection is chronic, secondary to immunosuppressive therapy in the host. Current methods of iatrogenic immunosuppression include the following:

Cytotoxic drugs, such as cyclosporin A, specifically depress activation of T-helper and T-cytotoxic cells while exhibiting little effect on T-suppressor cells.

Steroids cause decrease of leukocyte accumulation at sites of inflammation. This effect is mediated by membrane stabilization and interleukin metabolism.

Anti-lymphocytic sera use specific monoclonal antibodies (e.g., OKT3) to bind host T-cell receptors.

In graft-versus-host reactions, the transplantation of immunocompetent host lymphocytes causes the graft T-cells to react with recipient histocompatibility antigens. This is most likely to occur in patients who are immunosuppressed by drugs or irradiation and is largely a lymphokine induced reaction.

Of particular importance for the oral and maxillofacial surgeon are the potential sources of immunogenicity in osteochondral grafting. The MHC antigens are cell surface antigens associated with osteoid cells and collagen. There is no evidence to suggest that the mineral content of bone (e.g., hydroxyapatite) possesses sensitizing properties. Clearly, the loss of cell viability is related to decreased allograft rejection. Deep-freezing bone (−170° to −20° C) reduces, but does not eliminate, the immune response. Freeze-drying bone bank methods can even further decrease immunogenicity. The ideal method is to increase graft survival without compromising desirable properties like the osteoinduction capabilities of the graft (bone-morphogenic protein or BMP). Heating bone (above 60° C), gamma radiation, and autoclaving may inhibit some rejection mechanisms but they disrupt the basic chemical (e.g., BMP) and structural mechanisms of bone, and can decrease survival on that basis.

COMMUNICABLE DISEASES

Acquired Immunodeficiency Syndrome

Surgeons must be familiar not only with the manifestations of acquired immunodeficiency syndrome (AIDS), but also with the inherent occupational risks of transmission in health care workers. The problem is that asymptomatic carriers (individuals infected with the human immunodeficiency virus [HIV] who do not have AIDS) constitute the majority of infected patients. Asymptomatic patients appear to be more infectious than those with clinically apparent HIV infections.

The human immunodeficiency virus is an oncovirus belonging to the retrovirus family. Retroviruses can produce the enzyme reverse transcriptase. Because this allows the virus to transcribe viral RNA to DNA, HIV can produce double-stranded DNA from single-stranded DNA that has been cleaved from the RNA-DNA hybrid. This new double-stranded DNA inserts itself into the host's nucleus and serves as a template for prolific viral replication. Although multiple cell types have been shown to harbor HIV, the helper T-lymphocyte is most often infected. The implications of this immunity impairment are protean.

"Silent infections" occur with HIV in which antibodies are detectable to the virus, but no clinical or laboratory manifestations are evident. It is theorized that some secondary infection (e.g., hepatitis, syphilis, cytomegalovirus, herpes, and so forth) can activate the virus within the T4 (helper) nucleus and cause viral replication and "budding" of mature virus with dissemination. It is during this process that the T4 cell is destroyed. When sufficient numbers of T-helper-lymphocytes are destroyed, which reverses the normal 2 to 1 ratio of T4 (helper) to T8 (suppressant) cells, the clinical signs of a deficiency in cell-mediated immunity become obvious. Although death occurs approximately 2 years after the diagnosis of AIDS, the incubation period has been reported to be from 6 to 9 years. This figure is lower in risk groups in which multiple concomitant infections cause activation and dissemination of the virus at an earlier stage.

The Centers for Disease Control (CDC) defines four subgroups of HIV infection.

1. Acute. A mononucleosis-like viral illness; because there is a lag in antibody production after HIV exposure for 6 to 8 weeks, a "window" of false negatives can exist.
2. Asymptomatic carriers. No clinical manifestation; majority of HIV infected individuals.
3. Persistent generalized lymphadenopathy (PGL). Previously classified as ARC (AIDS-related complex). Defined as a palpable lymphodenopathy more than 1 cm in diameter in at least two extrainguinal sites, for longer than 3 months. Most patients progress to opportunistic infections (*Pneumocystis carinii* pneumonia, candidiasis, or malignancy [e.g., Kaposi's sarcoma or lymphoma]).
4. Defined HIV Associated Disease States. Patients who have more generalized and serious symptomatology; only those in subgroups C1 and D meet the current strict definition for reporting as AIDS cases according to the CDC.
   a) Subgroup A. Constitutional disease (weight loss more than 10% of baseline; fever or diarrhea for longer than 1 month)
   b) Subgroup B. HIV neurologic disease (dementia, peripheral neuropathy, myelopathy)
   c) Subgroup C. Opportunistic infections indicative of cell-mediated immune deficiency
      C1: Patients with one or more of the following 12 opportunistic infections: *P. carinii* pneumonia (PCP), candidiasis (esophageal, bronchial, or pulmonary), cryptosporidiosis, cryptococcosis, isosporiasis, histoplasmosis, strongyloidiasis (extraintestinal), toxoplasmosis, *Mycobacterium aviarum-intracellulare* (or *M. kansasii*), progressive multifocal leukoencephalopathy, disseminated cytomegalovirus (CMV), disseminated herpes simplex
      C2: Patients with one of the following six secondary infections (not accepted as AIDS under CDC surveillance criteria): salmonella (recurrent), herpes zoster, oral hairy leukoplakia, oral candidiasis, nocardiosis, tuberculosis
   d) Subgroup D. Patients with one or more of three accepted HIV-related malignancies: Kaposi's sarcoma, non-Hodgkin's lymphoma, primary brain lymphoma
   e) Subgroup E. Unclassifiable (as yet) clinical disease states, which could be attributed to defects in cell-

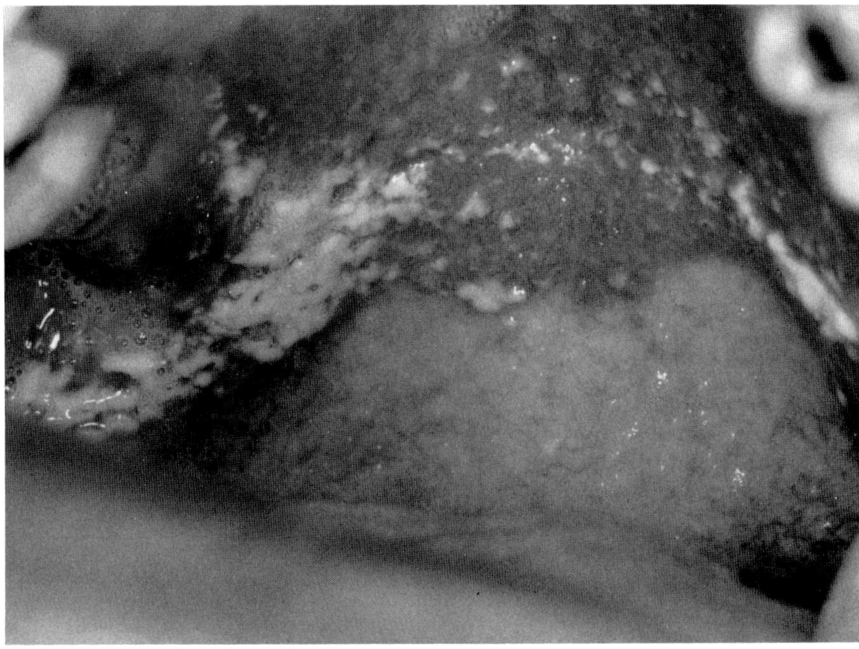

Figure 3–3. *Pseudomembranous candidal infection.*

mediated immunity or nonassociated clinical illnesses complicated by underlying HIV infection

Oral Manifestation of HIV Infection

Oral and maxillofacial surgeons should be particularly aware of the intraoral lesions associated with AIDS. They are generally either fungal/bacterial or viral.

FUNGAL/BACTERIAL. Candidal infection is ubiquitous in HIV infection. It can be limited to the oral cavity or more widely disseminated (e.g., esophageal or gastrointestinal). The four common presentations are erythematous or atrophic; pseudomembranous—the classic "thrush" lesion (Fig. 3–3); hyperplastic (cannot be scraped off mucous membrane, more common in chronic infection); and angular cheilitis.

A potassium hydroxide preparation will show fungal hyphal or a culture can confirm diagnosis. Either nystatin or clotrimazole troches is usually effective therapy. Systemic therapy with ketoconazole may be necessary for persistent lesions. Serious, disseminated candidal infections are treated with amphotericin B for 5 to 10 days.

Cryptococcus neoformans is a nonmycelial budding yeast which has been known to cause mild infections in distinct risk groups like pigeon breeders. It has been reported as the initial manifestation of AIDS and can cause fatal disseminated infection. Histoplasmosis is another fungus carried in bird excretion which can present as intraoral ulceration in immunosuppressed patients. Both require treatment with amphotericin B.

Of particular interest in the bacterial infections are HIV-associated gingivitis (HIV-G) and HIV-associated periodontitis (HIV-P). HIV-G lesions are confined to soft tissues that show a distinct erythema of the free gingiva and attached gingival and alveolar mucosa. In most cases, an intensely red linear band extends 2 to 3 mm apically from the free gingival margins. HIV-P has the features of HIV-G, plus rapid destruction of periodontal attachment and bone loss of 90% in 3 to 6 months has been documented. Uniquely, both HIV-G and HIV-P continue to progress even with removal of plaque and maintenance of good oral hygiene. It does appear that the onset of the disease correlates with a significant drop in the T4 cell count. Reasonably good treatment results have been attained with debridement, surgery when indicated, systemic metronidazole, and topical chlorhexidine therapy.

VIRAL. Intraoral viral infections include herpes simplex and oral hairy leukoplakia. Chronic, nonhealing recurrent herpetic infections are common with HIV

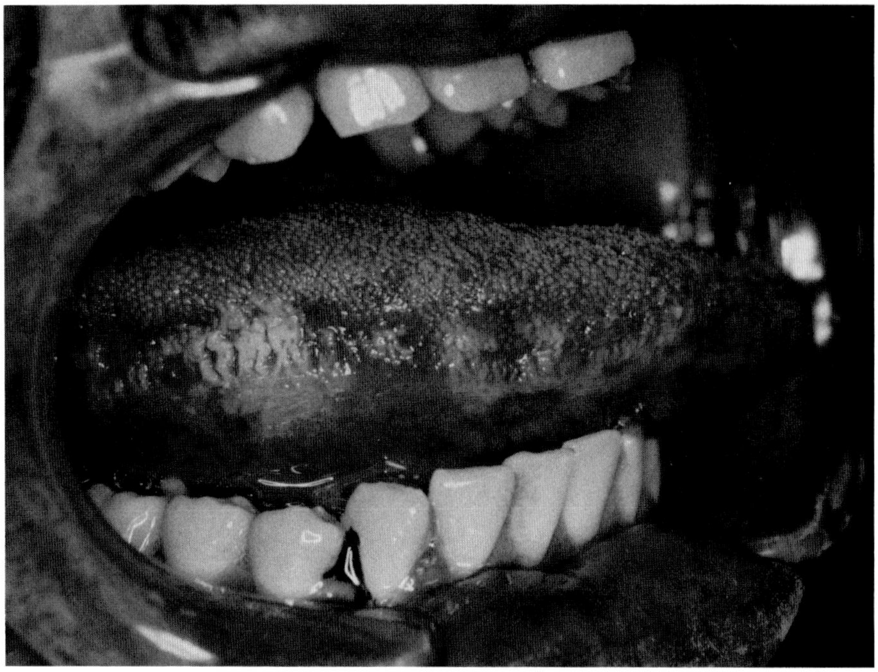

Figure 3–4. *Oral hairy leukoplakia of the lateral border of the tongue.*

infection. Oral acyclovir in doses of 200 to 400 mg five times a day or intravenous acyclovir for persistent or disseminated cases may be effective for severe, chronic, recurrent ulcers.

Oral hairy leukoplaka is an asymptomatic, white plaque that does not rub off, reported predominantly on the lateral border of the tongue or the labial and buccal mucosa. It is a viral-induced hyperplasia caused by the Epstein-Barr virus. Its appearance is now considered pathognomonic for AIDS (Fig. 3–4). Acyclovir has been somewhat effective at a dose of 800 mg four times daily for 2 weeks.

NEOPLASMS. Kaposi's sarcoma is commonly manifest in the oral cavity either as initial lesions or after cutaneous lesions appear; 90% appear on the hard and soft palate. They can present as discreet, flat reddish or purplish discolorations or as macular, ulcerative or hemorrhagic lesions (Fig. 3–5 A, B). Early lesions have been mistaken for pyogenic granuloma both clinically and microscopically. Local treatment includes surgical incision, cryosurgery, intralesional injections of vinblastine, and local radiation therapy. Systemically, tumor regression has been reported with alpha interferon or the combination chemotherapy regimen of ABV (Adriamycin, bleomycin, and vincristine).

Other AIDS-associated malignancies include non-Hodgkin's lymphoma of high-grade histologic type, squamous cell carcinoma of the oral cavity, and basal cell carcinoma.

Detection of HIV Infection

Currently the testing for HIV infection relies on the detection of antibody to the virus. The enzyme-linked immunosorbent assay (ELISA) exposes a patient's serum to plastic wells covered with commercially available HIV antigen. A colorimetric reaction occurs that is directly related to the concentration of HIV antibody in the patient's blood. If the ELISA is positive, it is repeated, and if that is positive, a confirmation Western Blot Assay is performed. In this test electrophoresis is used to identify antigen-antibody complexes which are radio-labeled. There is a high false-positive rate with ELISA and a high false-negative rate with the Western Blot. Also, because both methods detect only antibodies to HIV, an infected patient may go undetected during the "window" period after exposure when antibody levels are not high enough for

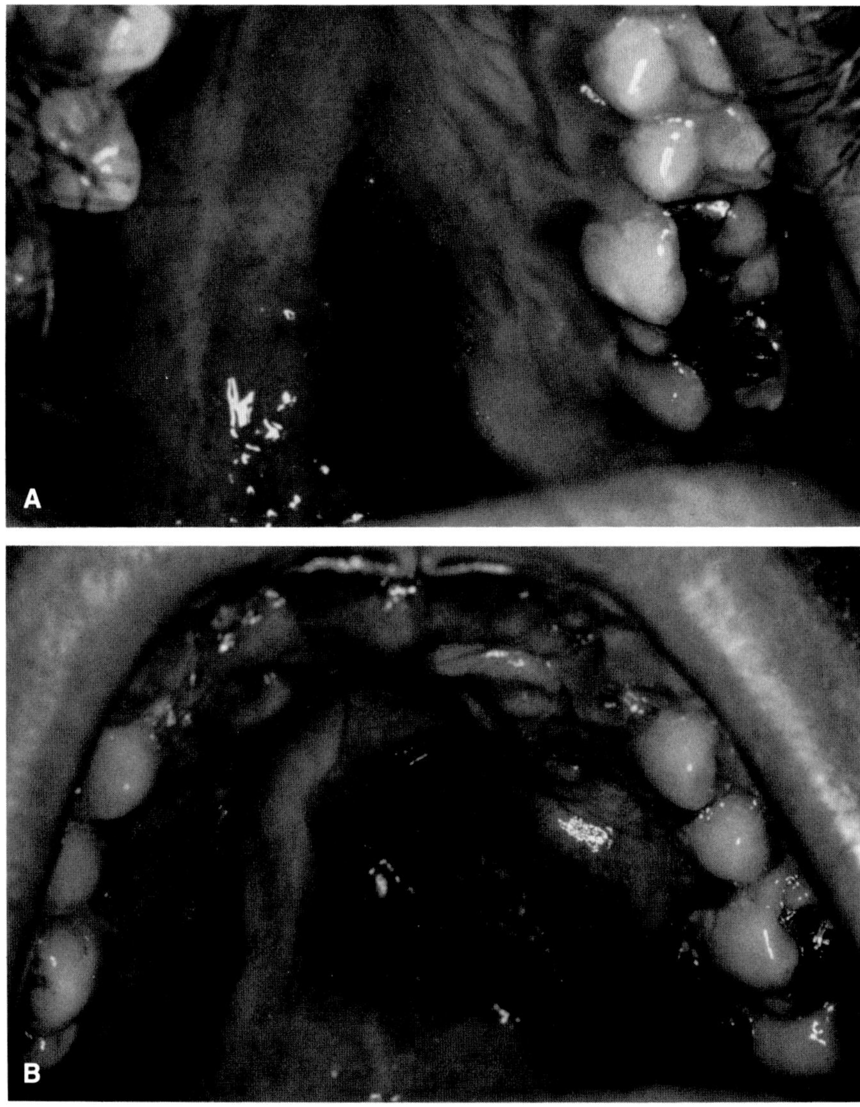

Figure 3–5. *Kaposi's sarcoma. (**A**) Macular intraoral lesion. (**B**) Raised mass lesion of palate.*

detection. Federal law mandates that all blood and plasma be tested for HIV using the ELISA and Western Blot Assays. Yet, cases of HIV transmission have occurred with screened, antibody-negative blood at an estimated rate of twenty-six cases per one million transfusions. Since screening of blood products for HIV has been instituted, the incidence of transfusion-related cases has declined. Current published estimates of the risk are between 1:40,000 and 1:250,000. Likewise, the incidence of infection of hemophiliacs receiving concentrated factor transfusions has also decreased. Although 65% of hemophiliacs in this country are HIV-positive, the majority of these individuals contracted the virus before mid-1985 when suppliers began heat-treating the cryoprecipitates to inactivate the virus.

Risk to Health Care Workers

Prospective studies have shown that occupational transmission of HIV is rare, occurring in approximately 0.4% to 0.5% of significant exposures. Transmission has occurred almost exclusively with blood. Efficiency of transmission by transfusion is 66% to

100%. Percutaneous exposure to HIV-contaminated needles is much less efficient, with a transmission rate of approximately 0.1% to 1%. Exposure of mucous membrane or open wounds to infected blood is thought to be even less efficient, although rare cases have been reported. Because the majority of exposures occur with puncture wounds by surgical instruments and needles, simple measures to decrease "handling" time are recommended. Recapping of needles accounted for one third of all needle-related exposures. Disposable syringes, without any disassembly, had one-fifth the rate of needle-stick injuries as did the older syringes. In addition, the following universal precautions were recommended by the Centers for Disease Control in 1987.

Universal Precautions

- All health care workers routinely should use appropriate barrier precautions to prevent skin and mucous-membrane exposure when contact with blood and the following body fluids is anticipated: semen, vaginal secretions, cerebrospinal fluid, synovial fluid, pleural fluid, peritoneal fluid, pericardial fluid, and amniotic fluid. Universal precautions do not apply to feces, nasal secretions, sputum, sweat, tears, urine, and vomitus unless they contain visible blood.
- Barrier precautions include the following: gloves (vinyl or latex, sterile or nonsterile) for touching blood and body fluids, mucous membranes, or nonintact skin. They should be changed after contact with each patient; masks and protective eyewear should be worn during procedures likely to generate droplets of blood or other body fluids; and gowns or aprons should be worn during procedures likely to generate splashes of blood or other body fluids.
- If contaminated with blood or other body fluids, skin surfaces should be washed immediately. Hands should be washed immediately after gloves are removed.
- Precautions should be taken to prevent injuries caused by needles, scalpels, and other sharp instruments or devices. To prevent needle-stick injuries, disposable needles should not be recapped but disposed of promptly in puncture-resistant containers.
- Although saliva has not been implicated in HIV transmission, in order to minimize the need for emergency mouth-to-mouth resuscitation, appropriate devices (mouthpieces, ventilation bags, etc.) should be available in areas where the need for resuscitation is predictable.
- Health care workers who have exudative lesions or weeping dermatitis should refrain from all direct patient care until the condition resolves.
- Pregnant health care workers are not known to be at a greater risk of contracting HIV infection than health care workers who are not pregnant. However, if HIV infection is contracted during pregnancy, the infant is at risk of infection. Pregnant health care workers should be especially familiar with and strictly adhere to precautions designed to minimize the risk of HIV transmission.

Adapted from Centers for Disease Control publications on universal precautions

Hepatitis

Viral hepatitis is caused by at least six hepatitis viruses: type A; type B; type non-A, non-B (recently identified, also type C); delta hepatitis; hepatitis caused by CMV; and Epstein-Barr virus (EBV). The primary concern for the oral and maxillofacial surgeon is hepatitis B but the surgeon needs to remain cognizant of all forms.

Hepatitis A

Hepatitis A commonly presents as an epidemic from fecal contamination of food and water supplies. The antigen and virus are present in the feces 7 to 10 days before onset of symptoms; but by the time the patient seeks medical attention, both have usually disappeared from the stool.

Hepatitis B

Hepatitis B is an epidemic with an alarming rate of increase. In 1978, the CDC reported 15,000 cases of hepatitis B. Currently that rate has increased 20 times to nearly 300,000 new cases each year. In the United States, serologic evidence of hepatitis B infection occurs at the rate of 30% in the general population. High-risk groups, such as homosexual males, intravenous drug users, mentally retarded individuals in institutions, and hemodialysis patients, may have positive serologic markers in as many as 80% of individuals. Intermediate risk groups include staff of institutions for the mentally retarded and health care workers who have frequent contact with blood. Surgeons have an incidence of positive serologic markers that approaches 30%, ten times that of the general population.

The sequelae of hepatitis B are as follows:

1. Chronic carrier state: Develops in up to 10% of patients; occurs more frequently in anicteric cases. Chronic carriers are usually asymptomatic and thus are "silently" infectious.
2. Chronic persistent hepatitis: Generally benign; progression to cirrhosis or hepatoma is rare.
3. Chronic active hepatitis: Major, late complication in 3% to 5% of cases; can progress to death by cirrhosis.
4. Cirrhosis: Estimated 11% of deaths due to cirrhosis are associated with hepatitis B.
5. Liver cancer (primary hepatoma): Risk of primary liver cancer is 273 times higher for carriers than noncarriers.

The development of anti-HBs, anti-HBc, IgM, and anti-HBe (antibodies to surface antigen, core, and e antigen, respectively), signal the body's full recovery and acquired immunity from hepatitis B infection. Active immunity occurs in approximately 90% of individuals vaccinated with a three-dose regimen of the human plasma–derived Heptavax or the genetically engineered (nonhuman) Recombivax. A booster vaccination is recommended at 5-year intervals.

Hepatitis C (Non A–Non B Hepatitis)

Hepatitis C is largely a diagnosis of exclusion. Transfusion-related hepatitis from blood that has been screened for hepatitis A and B is termed non-A, non-B. It has been renamed hepatitis C for the recently discovered retrovirus thought to be the etiologic agent. FDA approval for a screening test is expected shortly. This should improve the current situation in which 40% of blood carrying hepatitis C escapes the existing two indirect tests.

BIBLIOGRAPHY

Bach MK. Mediators of anaphylaxis and inflammation. Ann Rev Microbiol 1982; ?:371.

Bernier GM. Antibody and immunoglobulins: Structure and function. In: Bellanti JA, ed. Immunology II. Philadelphia: WB Saunders, 1978.

Buckley RH. Immunodeficiency diseases. JAMA 1987; 258: 2844.

Bulloch W. The History of Bacteriology. London: Oxford Press, 1938.

Calvert JE, Maruyama S, Tedder TF, Webb CF, Cooper MD. Cellular events in the differentiation of antibody-secreting cells. Semin Hematol 1984; 21:226.

Centers for Disease Control. AIDS weekly surveillance report—United States. January 18, 1988.

Cohen, S. The role of cell-mediated immunity in the induction of inflammatory responses. Am J Pathol 1977; 88:502.

Coombs RRA, Gell PGH. Classification of allergic reactions responsible for clinical hypersensitivity and disease. In: Coombs RRA, Lachmann PJ, eds. Clinical Aspects of Immunology. London: 1975:761.

Dausset J. The major histocompatibility complex in man. Science 1981; 213:1469.

Fan H, Conner RF, Villarreal LP. The Biology of AIDS. Boston: Jones & Bartlett Publishers, 1989.

Friedman LS, Dienstag JL. Recent developments in viral hepatitis. DM 1986; 32:320.

Gell PGH, Coombs RRA. Clinical Aspects of Immunology, ed 2. Philadelphia: FA Davis, 1968.

Gell PGH, Coombs RRA, Lachman PJ. Clinical Aspects of Immunology, ed 3. Oxford: Blackwell, 1977.

Gerberding JL, Bryant-LeBlanc CE, Nelson K, et al. Risk of transmitting the human immunodeficiency virus, cytomegalovirus, and hepatitis B virus to health care workers exposed to patients with AIDS and AIDS-related conditions. J Infect Dis 1987; 156:1.

Graziano FM, Lemanske RF Jr. Clinical Immunology. Baltimore: Williams & Wilkins, 1989.

Greenspan D, Greenspan JS, Conant M, et al. Oral "hairy" leukoplakia in male homosexuals: Evidence of association with both papillomavirus and a herpes-group virus. Lancet 1984; 2:831.

Greenspan JS, Greenspan D, Schiodt M, Pindborg JJ. AIDS and the Dental Team. Copenhagen: Munksgaard, 1986:96.

Herberman RB. Basic and Clinical Tumor Immunology. Boston: Martinus Nijhoff, 1983.

Howard RJ. Viral infections in surgery. Probl Gen Surg 1984; 1:522.

Klein J. Immunology: The Science of Self-Nonself Discrimination. New York: John Wiley & Sons, 1982.

Lawlor GJ, Fischer TJ. Manual of Allergy and Immunology, ed 2. Boston/Toronto: Little, Brown & Co, 1988.

Newman MG, Nisengard R. Oral Microbiology and Immunology. Philadelphia: WB Saunders, 1988.

Putnam FW, ed. The Plasma Proteins: Structure, Function and Genetic Control, vol 3, ed 2. New York: Academic Press, 1977.

Recommendations of the Immunization Practices Advisory Committee (ACIP). Recommendations for protection against viral hepatitis. Morbidity and Mortality Weekly Report 1985; 34:313.

Redfield RR, Burke DS. HIV infection: The clinical picture. Sci Am 1988; 259 (Oct):90.

Rizzetto M. The delta agent. Hepatology 1983; 3:729.

Robertson PB, Greenspan JS, eds. Oral Manifestations of AIDS. Diagnosis and Management of HIV-Associated Infections. Massachusetts: PSG Publishing, 1988.

Robinson G, Wilson SE, Williams RA. Surgery in patients with acquired immunodeficiency syndrome. Arch Surg 1987; 122:170.

Roger HD, Reinherz EL. Current concepts. T lymphocytes: Ontogeny, function and relevance to clinical disorders. N Engl J Med 1987; 317:1136.

Roitt IM. Essential Immunology, ed 5. Oxford: Blackwell Scientific, 1984.

Rose LF, Kaye D. Internal Medicine for Dentistry, ed 2. St. Louis: CV Mosby, 1990.

Rosina F, Saracco G, Rizzetto M. Risk of post-transfusion infection with hepatitis delta virus: a multicenter study. N Engl J Med 1985; 312:1488.

Rubin RH. Acquired immunodeficiency syndrome. Scientific American, section 7, subsection XI. Rubenstein E, Federman DD, eds. New York: Scientific American, 1990.

Ryan GB, Majno G. Acute inflammation: A review. Am J Pathol 1977; 86:183.

Silverman S Jr, Migliorati CA, Lozada-Nur F, et al. Oral findings in people with or at risk for AIDS: A study of 375 homosexual males. J Am Dent Assoc 1986; 112:187.

Stricof FL, Morse DL. HTLV-III/LAV seroconversion following a deep intramuscular needlestick injury. N Engl J Med 1986; 314:1115.

Trowbridge HO, Emling RC. Inflammation, A Review of the Process, ed 3. Chicago: Quintessence, 1989.

Unanue ER, Benacerraf B. Textbook of Immunology. Baltimore: Williams & Wilkins, 1982.

Update: Acquired immunodeficiency syndrome—United States, 1981–1988. MMWR 1989; 38:229.

Weissmann G. Prostaglandins in acute inflammation. Current Concepts, Upjohn, 1980.

Weissmann G, ed. Mediators of Inflammation. New York: Plenum Publishing, 1974.

Wood MJ, Geddes AM. Antiviral therapy. Lancet 1987; 2:1189.

4

Perioperative Management of the Surgical Patient

Robert Chuong

Comprehensive patient management in the perioperative period requires carefully acquired and maintained skills in the medical management of surgical patients both pre- and postoperatively. This chapter emphasizes concepts of preoperative assessment, fluid and electrolyte balance, surgical nutrition, hematology, general considerations of preparation of the patient for surgery, and general concepts of postoperative management.

PREOPERATIVE ASSESSMENT OF THE SURGICAL PATIENT

The History and Physical Examination

The most fundamental principles of patient assessment are those of attention to detail and employment of a systematic approach to clinical problems. The patient history follows a form beginning with the *chief complaint*. This section states succinctly the patient's description of the problem. As the initial portion of the recorded history it serves to direct the reader's attention toward the problem to be further evaluated. Multiple problems may be included. For example, the patient with an odontogenic infection may present with facial swelling, fever and chills, nausea and vomiting, and syncope. Next is the *history of the present illness*, (*HPI*), in which the specifics of the chief complaint are elaborated. These include alleviating and exacerbating features, associated symptoms, temporal relations to preceding and subsequent events and effects of treatment. This section takes the form of a narrative serving to organize the surgeon's thinking about the problem and documenting the relevant clinical features. Relevant portions of the past medical history, family history, social history, and review of systems should be included.

In the *past medical history* (*PMH*), it is best to describe historical features in the following sequence:

1. Previous hospitalizations and operations with dates, locations, and outcome, if possible.
2. Past and present medical illnesses; the surgeon should specifically ask about rheumatic fever, heart murmurs and other heart problems, asthma and other lung problems, alcoholism, diabetes, hypertension, bleeding disorders, drug abuse, seizures, psychiatric illness, and acquired immunodeficiency syndrome.
3. Medications: It is essential to know the list of agents being used by the patient so that potential drug interactions can be anticipated. Medications should be enumerated including specific doses. Over-the-counter medications such as aspirin or laxatives should be included.
4. Allergies: Any prior adverse drug reactions should be reviewed. If a specific medication is likely to be employed in the perioperative period, such as an anti-

biotic, the patient should be asked specifically about previous experience with that agent. Seasonal allergies may also be included in this section.
5. Health-related Habits: Discussion about alcohol and tobacco consumption previously and presently should be included at this point. Questions should also be directed toward possible use of illicit drugs.

The *review of systems* (*ROS*) is an important part of the comprehensive medical history. Its purpose and design is to prompt patients to recall signs or symptoms of disease in all body systems. As is true for all of clinical practice, the ROS must be reproducibly and efficiently carried through in order to avoid omissions.

The *family history* section should document any systemic or genetically transmitted disease within close family relations. The patient should be asked about previous untoward anesthetic experiences in family members to help identify any potential for malignant hyperthermia. The *social history* should state the patient's occupation, marital status and, possibly, educational background. These variables may be relevant to the determination of disability as well as to planning for postoperative care.

Ambulatory Surgery Consideration

Cost containment in medical care has changed the practice of medicine, particularly the practice of surgery. The surgeon must now be prepared to preoperatively educate patients, initiate all laboratory and medical evaluations on an outpatient basis, and consider alternatives to general anesthesia more frequently. Oral and maxillofacial surgery has been a leader in this manner of clinical practice but, as the complexity of its procedures increases, this speciality must be prepared to adapt to new practice arrangements both in the hospital and in the office.

Informed Consent

Informed consent is a process of patient education about proposed medical or dental treatment given during the period when the patient is deciding among treatment options. The actual form is only a hard copy end-product of the process of patient education.

The informed consent should state the following:

1. Patient's *condition* or problem
2. Proposed treatment and alternatives (including nonsurgical options)
3. Anticipated benefits of that treatment and the possible risks associated with inaction
4. Potential risks associated with the proposed treatment and the probability of such risks
5. *Unpredictability* of treatment outcome and the possible or likely irreversible nature of such treatment
6. Risks associated with anesthesia, particularly if the surgeon administers the anesthetic, such as local or regional blocks (a separate anesthesia consent form may be appropriate)
7. Established familiarity with the verbal or written form of the language in which the informed consent is presented
8. Signature of the patient, his or her guardian if the patient is a minor, one or more witnesses, and the surgeon

Many consent forms will have the patient initial or sign each statement within it, compelling the patient to read and evaluate and presumably understand each item.

The information included in the informed consent must be reviewed personally with the patient by the surgeon. Opportunities must be afforded the patient to ask questions, and second opinions should be encouraged for major elective surgery. The patient should be allowed to take the consent form home for review if desired.

In the emergency setting efforts must be made to elicit informed consent from the patient or from family members. Witnesses to verbal communication should be obtained, preferably from sources outside the surgeon's immediate practice.

FLUID AND ELECTROLYTES

Fluid Compartments

The body maintains a complex balance of fluids and electrolytes, which allows normal cellular function at a variety of levels within various organ systems. The processes of thought, movement, breathing, and all other bodily functions are dependent on movement of ions or limitation of such movement across cell membranes between fluid compartments. It is imperative that the surgeon understands the basic evaluation and management of those processes, typically referred to as "fluid and electrolyte balance," in order to provide optimal patient care.

It is conceptually convenient to consider the body in terms of fluid compartments (Fig. 4–1.). Total body water (TBW) constitutes 50% to 70% of total body weight; the average for young adult males being 60% and for young adult females, 50%. TBW is divided into three compartments: intracellular water (ICF), representing 30% to 40% of body weight; the intravascular or plasma space, representing 5% of TBW; and the extravascular interstitial space, 15% of TBW. The latter two divisions make up the extracellular water (ECF).

Intracellular fluid is primarily within skeletal muscle. The principal cations in this compartment are potassium and magnesium, and the principal anions are phosphates and proteins. Sodium is relatively excluded.

Interstitial fluid is that part of ECF which is extravascular. It includes so-called transcellular fluid such as cerebrospinal and joint fluid. Sodium is the principal cation of ECF, and the major anions are chloride and bicarbonate. Total body sodium regulates ECF volume and it is primarily regulated by aldosterone, which acts at the renal tubules to conserve sodium.

Total body water is regulated by *antidiuretic hormone* (ADH), which is secreted from the posterior pituitary to enhance water retention at the renal tubules. ADH consequently regulates serum osmolarity. Increased levels of ADH occur with trauma, general anesthesia, hypovolemia, or hypertonicity due to water deprivation or any other cause.

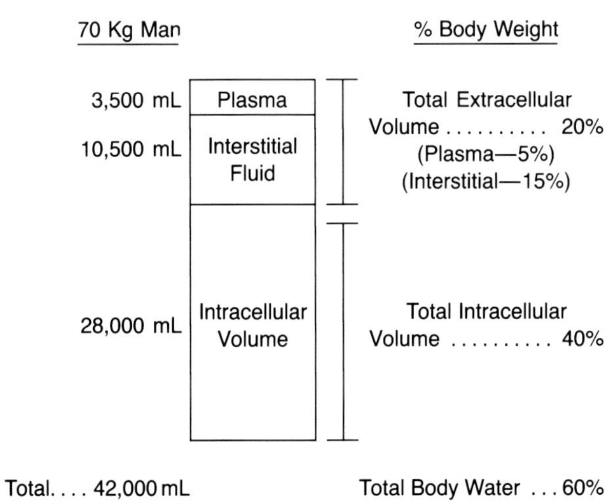

Figure 4–1. *Functional compartments of body fluids.*

"Third space" is a subdivision of the ECF that is inaccessible to the body's normal fluid and electrolyte maintenance mechanisms. It essentially consists of fluids sequestered in a space other than ICF and the typical ECF. For example, fluid within the intestines, although within the body, is not available for rapid fluid and electrolyte shifts; such intraintestinal fluid may be significant with paralytic ileus. Edema from burns or other trauma, as well as ascites due to cirrhotic liver disease are also examples of third space fluid. Significant volumes of "third spacing" can compromise ECF. Surgical management of such circumstances requires an understanding that this fluid can be mobilized eventually (e.g., after resolution of ileus), which can then influence the total effective ECF and possibly cause intravascular volume overload. The normal physiologic response to this process is diuresis.

Fluid and electrolytes tend to equilibrate across the various fluid compartments. Surgery and anesthesia disrupt the normal balance of these variables. The various regulatory mechanisms (renal, ADH, aldosterone) tend to compensate for changes. Surgical management consists of understanding variations in these regulatory mechanisms, the effects of nutrition on fluid and electrolyte parameters, and the potential drug interactions that may influence metabolic changes (e.g., diuretics, hyperalimentation solutions, antibiotics). Surgical management of fluid and electrolytes is based on physical examination, laboratory parameters of blood, urine and sometimes secretions or excretions, and measurement of fluid intake (oral, intravenous, respiratory) and output (urine, stool, wound drainage, gastrointestinal). By its nature, such therapy must be approximate and reliant on the patient's intrinsic capacity to reestablish homeostasis.[1]

Renal Considerations

The kidneys are the major regulators of fluids and electrolytes. The kidneys regulate total body water, acid-base balance in conjunction with the lungs, and serum osmolality. In general, when renal function is adequate, electrolyte and acid-base balance will be normal if sufficient water and electrolytes are provided.

Renal function is best assessed by the specific gravity and pH of the first voided urine. If the specific gravity is 1.016 or greater, is free of glucose and protein, and has a pH of 5.8 or less, renal function is most likely adequate. Serum BUN and creatinine serve as useful screening data to assess renal function. Creatinine clearance is a more direct measure of renal functional capacity. Although a urine collection over longer periods, for example, 12 or 24 hours can be used, it is convenient to calculate a 1-hour creatinine clearance which helps in the estimation of the glomerular filtration rate (GFR). Creatinine is removed from the body only by renal filtration. GFR can thus be calculated:

$$\text{GRF (mL/min)} = UV/P,$$

where U is urine creatinine concentration (mg/dL), V is the urine volume per minute (mL/min), and P is the plasma creatinine concentration (mg/dL). This calculation should be carried out in any patient suspected of early renal compromise by using a 1-hour urine collection from the catheterized bladder. Normal GFR in a young adult is 100 mL/minute or greater. GFR below 30 mL/minute is associated with acute renal failure.

Renal concentrating ability can be evaluated by the ratio U(osm)/P(osm), that is, the ratio between the osmolality of urine to the osmolality of plasma (Table 4–1). In oliguric patients with normal kidneys, U(osm)/P(osm) is greater than 1.3. In acute renal failure, U(osm)/P(osm) is close to 1.0.

Renal tubular function can reliably be evaluated by the urine/plasma creatinine ratio of U (creat)/P (creat). With normal renal function, U(creat/P(creat) is usually about 100, whereas in acute renal failure the value may be 10 or less.

Hormones play a major role in the renal regulation of water and electrolytes. In general, shunting of blood away from the kidneys occurs as a response to trauma and hypovolemia. This results in a decrease in the filtration fraction of blood that perfuses the renal cortex, and increased release of aldosterone with enhancement of sodium conservation. Renal tubular reabsorption of water is enhanced in this setting due to antidiuretic hormones. Decreased flow to the kidneys is perceived by the juxtaglomerular apparatus at the glomerular afferent arteriole, resulting in increased levels of *renin* which, in turn, stimulates release of *angiotensin* and *aldosterone*. The effect of these chemical mediators is to enhance sodium and water retention and to provide a pressor effect through vasoconstriction.

Table 4–1. *Assessment of Volume Status By Urine to Plasma Ratios*

TYPICAL VALUES IN OLIGURIC PATIENTS WITH NORMAL RENAL FUNCTION			
	Urine	***Plasma***	***U/P***
Creatinine (mg/100 mL)	100	1	100
Osmolality (mOsm/L)	400	300	1.3
Sodium (mEq/L)	20	140	0.14
TYPICAL VALUES IN PATIENTS WITH ACUTE RENAL FAILURE			
	Urine	***Plasma***	***U/P***
Creatinine (mg/100 mL)	20	2	10
Osmolality (mOsm/L)	300	290	1.03
Sodium (mEq/L)	110	130	0.9

In the assessment of the surgical patient, basic understanding of the parameters that summarize renal functional capacity as have been discussed above will help determine proper fluid and electrolyte management, specifically water requirements, the need to modify sodium load, and acid-base balance. Drug dosages should be established taking renal function into consideration.[2]

Osmotic Pressure

Osmotic pressure is determined by the number of osmotically active particles or ions per volume measured as milliosmoles (mOsm) per liter. The intracellular and extracellular compartments are separated by the cell membrane, which is effectively a semipermeable membrane. The numbers of osmotically active particles in the two compartments are equal at approximately 300 mOsm/L (serum osmolality). Sodium, being the major cation of ECF, contributes most of the osmotic pressure to this compartment, whereas plasma proteins supply most of the osmotic pressure between plasma and interstitial fluid. Water freely crosses the cell membrane by the influence of osmotic pressure. Any change in osmotic pressure due to changes in electrolyte concentrations will cause a shift in water between the extracellular and intracellular compartments until the osmotic pressure gradient is eliminated.

Alterations of Volume

Volume Excess

Excess body water occurs primarily in three settings: renal failure, hepatic failure, and congestive heart failure. Fluid and electrolyte management must accommodate the inherent decreased fluid output in these disease states. Improper administration of hypotonic solutions can iatrogenically cause a volume excess, or excessive volumes of isotonic fluids can overwhelm the renal capacity for sodium excretion. Excessive ADH secretion, whether due to actual injury to the pituitary gland resulting in inappropriately elevated ADH levels, so called syndrome of inappropriate ADH (SIADH), or due to trauma, pain, anesthesia or anxiety, can cause volume overload.

Management of volume excess is directed towards the cause. Water restriction and judicious use of diuretics are the mainstays of management. Management of pain and anxiety can help to normalize elevated levels of ADH output. Any complicated cases of SIADH require medical consultation. Recognition of the disorder is based on an inappropriately concentrated urine for a given plasma osmolality.

Volume Deficit

Volume deficit, or hypovolemia, is caused by excessive third space fluid sequestration, by external loss of fluid due to bleeding, gastrointestinal output, sweating or other causes, or by failure to supply maintenance fluid replacement. Symptoms are a function of the rapidity of fluid loss and the type of fluid lost. In general, symptoms are most pronounced when isotonic losses occur as compared to loss of water alone, particularly when the loss is rapid.

Urine output is a reflection of the functional ECF, that is, excluding third space fluid. Urine output should be 1 to 2 mL/kg in a child and 0.5 to 1 mL/kg in an adult with normal renal function and adequate perfusion, the latter being a reflection of ECF. Whenever concerns about major alterations in systemic volume exist, a Foley catheter should be placed to accurately monitor output. Fluid replacement must be based on serum osmolality, urine osmolality, serum electrolytes, and clinical signs and symptoms. A central venous catheter, or CVP line, may be appropriate to guide the rate of fluid repletion. A pulmonary artery catheter for pulmonary capillary wedge pressure determination (Swan-Ganz catheter) allows assessment of filling pressures of the left side of the heart and may be extremely important for monitoring fluid administration, particularly in the patient with primary cardiac disease, the goal being to avoid acute pulmonary edema or congestive heart failure.

Fluid replacement can be accomplished using crystalloid or colloid fluid. Each has potential advantages, although among surgeons there is some disagreement as to which is preferred in particular situations. Crystalloids consist of electrolyte and water solutions, which can be administered easily with relatively low cost and without risk of infectious diseases. Colloid preparations contain protein (e.g., albumin preparations) and may better sustain intravascular volume because of their oncotic pressure. When significant blood loss is the cause of hypovolemia, replacement should be blood or blood fractions. When there has been an isotonic fluid depletion, that is, when the entire ECF is deficient, normal saline or lactated Ringer's solution should be employed.[2]

Electrolyte Abnormalities

Calcium

Vitamin D enhances the gastrointestinal absorption and renal conservation of calcium. Calcium metabolism is usually not a consideration in the typical surgical patient, although special circumstances may lead to disturbances of calcium metabolism resulting in relative or absolute hypo- or hypercalcemia.

Hypocalcemia (serum calcium less than 8 mg/dL) may cause perioral and digital paresthesia. Clinical signs and symptoms include muscle cramps, tetany with carpopedal spasm (Trousseau's sign), Chvostek's sign, hyperactive deep tendon reflexes, and prolonged QT interval on the electrocardiogram (ECG). Hypocalcemia may occur transiently owing to hyperventilation, which directly induces a respiratory alkalosis (by decreasing carbon dioxide) which, in turn, increases the amount of calcium bound to serum albumin. This has the effect of transiently decreasing the concentration of free calcium ions, a critical factor in neuromuscular function. Similarly, hypoproteinemia may result in hypocalcemia, although the patient may be completely asymptomatic because the concentration of unbound calcium is normal. In other words, the reported value from the laboratory reflects total extracellular calcium, both protein bound and unbound, and the physiologically active form is the unbound, ionized fraction.

Hypocalcemia may be encountered in settings of hypoparathyroidism, acute pancreatitis, renal failure, fistulas from the small intestine or pancreas, necrotizing fasciitis, or possibly with massive blood transfusion. Serum calcium should be monitored frequently in these settings. Monitoring of the ECG to assess the QT interval is also helpful in more acute circumstances.

Hypercalcemia (serum calcium more than 16 mg/dL) is caused most commonly by hyperparathyroidism or by malignancy with bony metastases. Other causes include sarcoidosis and chronic vitamin D intoxication. Signs and symptoms include weakness, nausea, vomiting, anorexia, weight loss, polyuria, and polydipsia. More severe levels may cause coma. Acute hypercalcemia must be treated emergently by repletion of extracellular volume deficit serving to dilute the calcium, and by the use of drugs such as chelating agents (EDTA), corticosteroids, and mithramycin to decrease the calcium concentration. Hemodialysis may also be employed.

Potassium

Potassium is the primary intracellular cation. Its extracellular, unbound concentration is most critical to cardiac and general neuromuscular function. The ICF contains 98% of the potassium found within the body. The usual dietary intake of potassium is 50 to 100 mEq/day, any excess being excreted in the urine. Because potassium is highly concentrated within cells, any significant tissue injury will release potassium ions into the extracellular fluid compartment or the ECF. Increased extracellular or serum potassium occurs in catabolic states and in states of acidosis, although normal renal function will normalize potassium balance.

Hyperkalemia can be manifested by myocardial irritability as shown electrocardiographically by peaking of T waves, depressed ST segments, and widening of QRS complexes. As hyperkalemia progresses, heart block or cardiac arrest may develop. Gastrointestinal symptoms may develop, including nausea and vomiting, diarrhea, or colic.

Treatment of hyperkalemia consists of measures to counteract the effects of elevated serum potassium and to eliminate potassium from the body. Initially, efforts are made to either sequester potassium intracellularly or to counteract the extracellular effects of potassium. Suppression of a rapid rise in serum potassium can be achieved by intravenous administration of a 10% solution of calcium chloride (10 to 30 mL over 15 min), 50 to 150 mEq of sodium lactate, and 50 to 100 mL of 50% glucose. Sometimes insulin may be given as the glucose is administered. The uptake of glucose promotes cellular uptake of potassium. Sodium lactate raises the pH, which promotes uptake of potassium, essentially exchanging intracellular hydrogen ions for extracellular potassium ions. All of these interventions are ways to reduce serum levels of potassium ions. Absolute elimination of potassium ions may be accomplished by dialysis (peritoneal or hemodialysis) or by use of ion-exchange resins (e.g., Kayexalate) administered per rectum, which allows exchange of sodium for potassium. The potassium-enriched resin is then eliminated per rectum.

Hypokalemia is much more common than hyperkalemia in the surgical patient. The kidneys cannot absolutely conserve potassium even when hypokalemia is present. There is an obligatory renal loss of potassium of roughly 20 mEq/day. Marked hypokalemia may occur secondary to prolonged administration of intravenous fluids with insufficient potassium content. Other causes of hypokalemia include excessive loss of gastrointestinal secretions (e.g., prolonged nasogastric suction, severe diarrhea), use of parenteral hyperalimentation without proper supplementation, or excessive renal excretion of potassium as in patients on chronic non-potassium-sparing diuretic therapy for hypertension or congestive heart failure.

Hypokalemia may be manifested by cardiac irritability, particularly in patients on digoxin. Digoxin toxicity may be enhanced by low serum potassium levels, as indicated by ECG signs of low voltage, ST segment depression, and T-wave flattening.

Hypokalemia is treated by oral or intravenous supplementation. Because the greatest mass of potassium is intracellular, significant hypokalemia as measured by serum potassium (a reflection of extracellular potassium) is difficult to correct quickly. Any potassium administered will equilibrate between ICF and ECF and therefore will typically require large quantities. Potassium is available in 20-mEq and 40-mEq ampules. No more than 40 mEq/hour should be administered intravenously unless ECG monitoring is being performed. In general, if the situation is not pressing, potassium can be administered orally over several days to replete body potassium stores.

Potassium is intimately involved in acid-base regulation. In states of respiratory or metabolic alkalosis, renal excretion of potassium is increased as hydrogen ions are conserved. Hypokalemia itself may produce an alkalotic state, since the renal tubules will tend to preserve potassium ions in exchange for hydrogen ions. Further discussion of acid-base considerations is presented later in this chapter.

Sodium

Sodium is the primary extracellular cation. It is carefully regulated through the kidneys. In states of sodium deficit, unlike the situation for potassium, the kidneys can effectively conserve all sodium. Sodium depletion indicates volume depletion of the ECF compartment. Hyponatremia may be caused by excessive gastrointestinal loss (e.g., vomiting, diarrhea), adrenal insufficiency resulting in inadequate mineralocorticoid function, chronic use of diuretics, chronic nephritis, or restricted dietary intake. Severe losses of ECF externally (e.g., burns, excessive perspiration) or internally by third space sequestration (e.g., ileus) may also deplete the body of sodium. Hyponatremia does not necessarily occur in settings of sodium depletion, particularly when acute changes occur in total body sodium content. Clinical signs of acute sodium depletion are essentially the signs of hypovolemia, including collapsed neck veins, increased hematocrit, tachycardia, furrowing of the tongue, and diminished urine sodium concentration (less than 40 mEq/L). More advanced stages of sodium depletion may be manifested by orthostatic hypotension, oliguria, apathy, and nausea.

Sodium excess is usually caused by renal disease resulting in the inability to excrete sodium properly or by excessive mineralocorticoid (aldosterone) activity. Sodium excess is manifested by the retention of water with edema and associated weight gain. Serum sodium may be normal in this circumstance. Treatment consists of sodium restriction and the use of diuretics. Acute hypernatremia is rare, occurring primarily in settings of administration of hypertonic saline solutions.

Magnesium

Magnesium is the second most common intracellular cation. About one half of total body magnesium is within bone and is slowly exchangeable. The general distribution of magnesium is similar to that of potassium. It plays a vital role in the proper function of many enzyme systems.

Hypomagnesemia occurs in states of poor nutrition as may occur with chronic alcoholism, malabsorption syndromes, starvation, and total parenteral nutrition or prolonged intravenous fluid administration without magnesium repletion. Although the kidneys can conserve magnesium readily, renal excretion of small amounts may continue in severe deficiency states.

Deficiency of magnesium is characterized by neuromuscular irritability with signs and symptoms similar to those of hypocalcemia, including tetany, tremors, hyperactive reflexes, possibly progressing to seizures or coma. Suspicion of this possibility is critical in the surgical patient who exhibits abnormal cerebral function or neuromuscular irritability. Serum magnesium measurements are commonly inaccurate and should be repeated if there is any question about laboratory validity. Even with an apparently normal laboratory value, clinical hypomagnesemia may exist, and administration of magnesium in the form of magnesium chloride or magnesium sulfate may be indicated. Magnesium sulfate 50% may be given intravenously or intramuscularly. Intravenous administration is preferred in states of severe depletion and must be carried out with careful cardiac and clinical monitoring because of potential for magnesium toxicity. Calcium gluconate or calcium chloride should be available to counteract possible toxicity.

Hypermagnesemia is most common with renal failure. Attention should be directed to magnesium-containing medications such as antacids or laxatives (e.g., Maalox, milk of magnesia) in settings of renal compromise. Acute toxicity may occur, manifested by neuromuscular depression (diminished deep tendon reflexes, lethargy, weakness) or cardiac conduction disturbances (prolonged PR, widened QRS, elevated T waves on ECG). Coma may develop. Treatment consists of volume repletion if there is ECF contraction, correction of acidosis which tends to drive magnesium intracellularly, and management of acute symptoms by slow intravenous administration of calcium chloride or calcium gluconate (5 to 10 mEq) or by hemodialysis or peritoneal dialysis.

Management of Fluids

Intraoperative Fluid Management

Fluid must be administered intraoperatively to replace losses. In some cases, such as at the induction of anesthesia, hypotension may be unmasked if there has been a compensated volume deficit preoperatively.

Blood loss should be replaced steadily with crystalloid solution during surgery. In most cases, loss of 500 to 1500 mL of blood is well tolerated without transfusion. Replacement of blood with crystalloid solution at a rate of 3 mL for each 1 mL if blood loss is usually suggested.

Major surgery can cause significant third-spacing of fluid due to edema or transudation of fluid. This volume loss must be replaced intraoperatively. Monitoring of blood pressure, pulse, urine output, and possibly central venous pressure and pulmonary capillary wedge pressure will guide replacement during surgery.

Postoperative Fluid Management

Early after surgery, fluid is administered intravenously to replace any ongoing deficit not replaced intraoperatively, and to supply maintenance fluid. Because fluid requirements are difficult to determine precisely immediately after surgery, frequent reassessment of clinical status, hematocrit, electrolytes, urine output, and wound drainage is essential. Hypotension and tachycardia may indicate hypovolemia. Orthostatic signs should be assessed, as should mental status, skin color and warmth, body temperature, and measurement of fluids administered and fluids lost. Ongoing blood loss should be considered, especially in instances of thoracic, abdominal, or orthopedic surgery in which large volumes may be lost before being clinically obvious.

Maintenance fluid therapy must replace both sensible and insensible fluid loss. Sensible losses are by definition measurable, including urinary, gastrointestinal (e.g., nasogastric suction, colostomy output), surgical drain output, and emesis. Insensible losses must be estimated, although it is relatively constant between 600 mL and 900 mL per day. Insensible losses include water loss through respiration, sweating, and evaporative loss through wounds and may be increased in settings of hyperventilation (e.g., mechanical ventilation), hypermetabolism (e.g., hyperthyroidism, severe burns), and fever. In such settings, insensible loss may exceed 1500 mL/day.

Fluid replacement in the later postoperative period must take into account the diuresis of fluid given during surgery, which was retained due to the inductive effects of surgery and anesthesia on transiently increased levels of aldosterone and ADH. This increased urine output does not need to be replaced. Depending on clinical circumstances, parameters that may help to make a decision about replacement therapy include body weights followed serially, urine and plasma testing for osmolality and sodium concentration, and physical examination.

In general, insensible losses are replaced with 5% dextrose in water (D_5W). Urine losses are usually replaced with salt-containing solution, in spite of the kidneys' capacity to stringently conserve sodium. Tissue catabolism produces water and may, in part, counteract insensible losses.

Serum electrolyte determinations may be helpful in postoperative fluid management, although, in the patient not experiencing extensive sensible losses who is not on diuretics or suffering renal compromise, and who is to be maintained on intravenous fluids for only 2 to 3 days, such determinations are rarely indicated. With more prolonged intravenous fluid therapy, especially without supplementation with oral intake and perhaps metabolic acid-base disturbances, close monitoring of serum and urine electrolytes and osmolality is important. In general, when prolonged intravenous therapy exists, supplemental potassium of at least 40 mEq daily is necessary to account for obligatory renal excretion.

Transfusion Therapy

Transfusion of blood and blood fractions may be necessary preoperatively, intraoperatively, or postoperatively. Patients who demonstrate deficiencies in red cells or platelets may require transfusion in preparation for surgery. Patients with an anemia of chronic disease or a modest anemia of any cause may not require transfusion. In general, the patient with a hematocrit greater than 35% does not warrant preoperative transfusion of blood products. The risks of transfusion must always be considered against the benefits. This is particularly true with respect to the risk of fluid overload, especially in the patient with compromised cardiovascular or renal function, and the risk of transmission of infectious disease such as non-A, non-B hepatitis, human immunodeficiency virus, hepatitis B, and cytomegalovirus (CMV). Transfusion of incompatible blood products is also a potentially fatal problem. In the immunocompromised patient, transfusion of blood products may allow manifestation of graft-versus-host reactions due to transfer of active lymphocytes that may recognize the recipient's cells as foreign. Thus, transfusion is associated with multiple potential risks and must be readily understood in order to appropriately administer or withhold blood products.

Components of Blood

Generally, only that component of blood needed for a given clinical circumstance should be transfused. Put another way, component therapy should be the standard approach to transfusion problems. For example, a patient who is anemic should generally receive packed red cells rather than whole blood to avoid potential fluid overload, especially when the only goal of transfusion in such a setting is to enhance oxygen-carrying capacity. In other settings, anemia of the same degree may best be managed with whole blood, particularly if there is ongoing hemorrhage, a coagulopathy, and hypovolemia. The patient who is thrombocytopenic should receive platelet concentrates. The patient who is deficient in clotting factors manufactured in the liver should receive fresh frozen plasma. Other types of blood components include plasma, leukocyte preparations, cryoprecipitate, and albumin. Each should be used selectively based on carefully considered indications.

WHOLE BLOOD. Whole blood is indicated in settings of acute blood loss of 15% or more of blood volume. Transfusion of whole blood can rapidly restore oxygen-carrying capacity and volume, as well as coagulation factors. Banked whole blood contains essentially no functioning platelets because of their degeneration when stored at room temperatures. Clotting factors V and VIII decrease in biologic activity over 24 hours when blood is stored at 1° to 6° C. Other clotting factors remain relatively stable. Administration of whole blood carries less risk of transmission of infectious disease compared with administration of fresh frozen plasma and packed red blood cells pooled from different donors.

PACKED RED BLOOD CELLS. Packed red blood cells (PRBC) are indicated in situations for which additional oxygen-carrying capacity is required without need for increased intravascular volume. Chronically anemic patients may tolerate hemoglobin concentrations of 7 g/100 mL or less under normal circumstances but may need additional hemoglobin in order to undergo surgery. Transfusion of PRBC would be indicated in such a setting. Each unit of PRBC usually increases the hematocrit by 2% to 3% in an average adult.

DEGLYCEROLIZED RED BLOOD CELLS. Frozen RBC can be stored for years in a glycerol-containing medium at lower than −65° C. Advantages of frozen RBC include long-term preservation; removal of all plasma and isoagglutinins and therefore suitable for patients sensitive to plasma proteins (e.g., IgA-deficient patients who have antibodies to IgA); relatively free of white blood cells; minimal hepatitis risk; rapid infusion possible in patients who are hypervolemic or who have congestive heart failure; storage of rare blood types for later transfusion; and broader use of autologous transfusion.

WASHED RED BLOOD CELLS. RBC washed with saline have less potassium, plasma, and debris from white blood cells and platelets than regular packed RBC. Use of washed RBC may be indicated for patients with a history of febrile reaction to previous transfusion due to leukoagglutinins, and for patients with compromised renal function who are unable to tolerate the potassium present in banked blood.

WHITE BLOOD CELLS. White blood cells (WBC) may be transfused for patients with bone marrow suppression secondary to chemotherapy or massive radiation therapy, or for those with severe neutropenia from sepsis or drug reactions. These life-threatening situations may be helped by WBC transfusion. WBC harvested from many units of compatible blood would be necessary to replace such cells in even one patient; consultations with infectious disease and hematology specialists are therefore indicated.

WBC may induce antibodies, particularly when multiple transfusions are administered. Subsequent transfusions can create anaphylactic reactions and febrile responses. Any patient who is expected to need repeated transfusions should receive WBC-poor blood, as for example, the organ transplant patient.

PLATELET CONCENTRATE. The effectiveness of platelet transfusion is dependent on the time elapsed between drawing of blood from donor to the time of administration. Platelet concentrate should be transfused within 6 hours of phlebotomy. Agitated platelet concentrates kept at room temperature may be used up to 72 hours later.

Platelet transfusion is indicated in the following situations:

Platelet count less than 20,000 if there is any tendency for bleeding
Patients with a platelet count less than 60,000 who are to have extensive or prolonged surgery
Bleeding time greater than 15 minutes in patients who are to have surgery or an invasive procedure such as arteriography
Patients who have experienced severe hemorrhage from trauma or surgery who have received 10 or more units of blood
Patients on cardiopulmonary bypass for 2 hours or longer.

The effectiveness of platelet transfusion is diminished during acute hemorrhage; when its administration is delayed excessively; during a transfusion reaction; in patients with idiopathic thrombocytopenic purpora (ITP), post-transfusion purpura, or thrombocytopenic purpura; in the presence of severe splenomegaly; in the presence of platelet antibodies formed after multiple previous platelet transfusions; and during hyperpyrexia.

As a general guideline, one can expect an increase of 5000 platelets/μL within 1 hour after administration of each unit of random donor platelets. Significantly lower incremental change may indicate an antibody response, which may therefore necessitate HLA tissue histocompatibility matching. When surgery is planned, platelet transfusions should be administered just before and during the time when bleeding will be occurring.

FRESH FROZEN PLASMA. Fresh frozen plasma (FFP) is indicated in settings of coagulopathy due to a deficiency in labile clotting factors. The deficiency is caused by decreased synthesis of such factors due to hepatic dysfunction, congenital deficiency, or transfusion of blood products deficient in these factors.

FFP contains all coagulation factors with minimal cellular debris. It is rich in factors II, V, VII, IX, XII, XIII, and fibrinogen. One unit has a volume of roughly 180 mL to 250 mL.

CRYOPRECIPITATE. Cryoprecipitate is rich in clotting factor VIII. Each unit (5 to 15 mL) contains 80 U of factor VIII, and 200 mg of fibrinogen and is prepared from a single donor. There is no concentration of antibodies in the small volume of a given unit.

Cryoprecipitate may be indicated for management of factor VIII deficiency in hemophilia A and von Willebrand's disease. It may be helpful in the management of hypofibrinogenemia and in the management of uremic bleeding.

NORMAL HUMAN SERUM ALBUMIN. Normal human serum albumin (NHSA) is a sterile preparation of serum albumin obtained by fractionation of blood from multiple donors. It contains at least 96% albumin and is usually prepared as a 25% solution (25 g/100 mL). The primary indication for its use is as a means of increasing serum protein in hypoproteinemia, as in patients with renal or liver disease. NHSA has no hepatitis or HIV risk and can be stored for 3 years at room temperature.

PRETRANSFUSION TESTING. ABO compatibility is the major determinant of transfusion compatibility. Antibodies to the A or B antigens develop in all individuals against those antigens that are intrinsically absent. Type O individuals lack both A and B antigens and therefore have antibodies to both.

The second most important compatibility determination is D antigen testing. The D antigen is part of the Rh group. Anti-D antibodies develop only with previous exposure to D-positive RBC during pregnancy or from transfusion. Routine testing is also done to determine if antibodies exist to other clinically significant RBC antigens through use of the indirect Coombs' test.

Preoperative Transfusion

In general, chronically anemic patients tolerate their condition extremely well and usually tolerate surgery well without first increasing their hemoglobin concentrations into a normal range. For example, patients with chronic renal failure are often severely anemic but usually do not require preoperative transfusion if blood loss is expected to be modest (less than one unit).

To determine if an individual requires preoperative transfusion, the surgeon needs to consider the clinical diagnosis, the amount of bleeding likely during surgery, the presence or absence of symptoms, the level of anemia, and the reticulocyte count, the reticulocyte count being an indicator of the bone marrow's ability to produce RBC.

In general, an anemic patient soon to undergo an operation in which significant blood loss is expected should be transfused preoperatively in a controlled setting. If transfusion occurs 24 hours or more before surgery, the transferred RBC will have regained more physiologic function by the time of surgery.

If blood transfusion is not anticipated during surgery, the surgeon should order a blood clot for "type and screen" preoperatively, which indicates to the blood bank to determine ABO and D types and to determine if there are antibodies to RBC antigens. Blood is not crossmatched. If blood is needed during surgery, an abbreviated crossmatch can be done within a few minutes instead of the three-phase crossmatch which is time-consuming.[3]

Emergency Transfusion

In the emergency setting, a blood sample must be sent as quickly as possible to the blood bank with careful labeling and instructions as to numbers and types of units of blood products necessary initially.

While waiting for blood, large-bore venous access must be established. Large-bore (16 or 14 gauge) peripheral intravenous lines are the first choice for access, being generally preferred over central lines which may have smaller caliber, are associated with more complications, and may be more difficult to insert. Fluid must be administered rapidly as crystalloid (e.g., lactated Ringer's) at a rate of 300 mL to 500 mL per 10 minutes initially, at all times monitoring vital signs and clinical responsiveness of the patient. As blood becomes available, it may be administered even if it is only type-specific (i.e., known to be ABO-compatible) but not completely cross-matched. Cross-matching can be completed even as the transfusion is ongoing. This is generally preferred over administration of uncross-matched type O PRBC. Type O PRBC are indicated in patients needing massive, immediate transfusion. However, generally, circulation can be supported with crystalloid solutions and pressor agents until type-specific blood becomes available a few minutes later.

Autologous Transfusion

For elective surgery in which blood transfusion is required 10% of the time, autologous blood donation is an advisable practice.[4] The potential advantages include avoidance of transmission of infectious agents (hepatitis, HIV) and decreased risk of transfusion reaction and potential for alloimmunization. In addition, there may be advantages to operating on a relatively anemic individual, thereby losing a given volume of relatively dilute blood and subsequently replacing that fluid with red-cell-enriched autologous blood.

As practices vary regionally, the surgeon should be familiar with the protocol of the blood bank support services available in the community. For oral and maxillofacial surgery, autologous donation should be strongly considered before two-jaw orthognathic surgery or other major elective maxillofacial or craniomaxillofacial reconstructive procedures. Patients should receive iron supplementation (e.g., ferrous gluconate 300 mg po tid) and proper nutrition during the donation period.

ACID-BASE BALANCE

Normal cellular function requires a proper environment, one critical component of which is a narrow range of acceptable intracellular and extracellular pH. The human organism tends to produce acids as the byproducts of metabolism so the body must have compensatory systems in place to maintain pH balance. *Acid-base balance* refers to the metabolic and respiratory processes that function to maintain the pH within tolerable ranges (7.40±0.05) when confronted by the production of carbonic acid resulting from the oxidation of foodstuffs and from nonvolatile acids produced by other metabolic processes.

Control of pH is dependent on *buffer systems*, which are physiologic compensations and mechanisms of absolute correction (renal or pulmonary). Buffers consist of a weak acid working with the salt of a strong base with that weak acid, such as sodium bicarbonate (H_2CO_3). Buffers have the capacity to rapidly pick up or release hydrogen ions when confronted with a strong acid or base, which tends to minimize changes in pH.

Buffering is an instantaneous control mechanism. Physiologic compensation for alterations in the concentration of hydrogen ions are slower. This consists of respiratory mechanisms to alter H_2CO_3 concentrations by ventilation, a process that eliminates carbon dioxide through the alveoli, thus tending to decrease H_2CO_3 and therefore to raise pH. The kidneys can control bicarbonate (HCO_3-) and can therefore compensate for changes in hydrogen ion concentration. These compensatory changes can best be understood by understanding the following relationship:

$$H_2O + CO_2 \rightleftarrows H_2CO_3 \rightleftarrows H^+ + HCO_3^-$$

For example, as hydrogen increases, the relation shifts to the left, increasing H_2CO_3, a volatile acid, which can be decreased by increased pulmonary ventilation to eliminate carbon dioxide. Other buffers include phosphate, proteins, and hemoglobin.

Acid-base disturbances are determined by measurement of arterial pH. Venous blood is less reliable since it is more dependent on the state of tissues proximal to the site of venipuncture. In addition to blood pH, the concentration of carbon dioxide in arterial blood (P_{CO_2}) helps to decipher disturbances in acid-base balance. These values are obtained through arterial blood gases (ABGs). ABGs specifically report pH, P_{CO_2}, and P_{O_2}, the latter being a measure of oxygen concentration. The normal value for P_{CO_2} is 40 mm Hg. Increased pulmonary ventilation decreases P_{CO_2} and decreased ventilation increases P_{CO_2}.

The following guidelines will assist the surgeon in using ABGs to evaluate acid-base status[4]:

- A 10 mm Hg shift in the P_{CO_2} accounts for a pH shift of 0.08.
- If the pH is greater than 7.40, alkalosis occurs; if less than 7.40, acidosis.
- If the P_{CO_2} is greater than 40 mm Hg, respiratory acidosis is occurring; if less than or equal to 40 mm Hg the primary derangement is metabolic acidosis.
- For determining the contribution of combined respiratory and metabolic factors to pH alterations, a P_{CO_2} of 60 mm Hg would be expected to lower the pH by 0.16 (0.08 for each 10 mm Hg difference from the normal of 40 mm Hg) to 7.24; if the actual pH is found to be 7.32, then partial metabolic compensation for the respiratory acidosis can be assumed. Similarly, if the P_{CO_2} is 60 mm Hg and the pH is 7.20, then a combined metabolic and respiratory acidosis exists, since the P_{CO_2} alone would be insufficient to account for the observed acidosis.

Metabolic Acidosis

Metabolic acidosis is caused by a decrease in HCO_3^- due to absolute loss, such as through renal mechanisms or through gastrointenstinal fistulae, or due to an increased acid load. Causes of increased acid load include ketosis, such as from diabetic ketoacidosis or from starvation; failure of oxidative metabolism as in shock, resulting in increased lactic acid production; ingestion of large amounts of acidifying salts; and renal failure, both acute and chronic, which can cause decreased ability to excrete hydrogen ions.

When metabolic acidosis occurs, respiratory compensation in the form of increased ventilation tends to occur but may not be effective if there is primary pulmonary pathology (e.g., pneumonia, emphysema) or if other factors are overriding (e.g., anesthesia, mechanical ventilation). Generally treatment is directed towards the primary cause. A pH of less than 7.30 and HCO_3^- less than 15 mEq/L is generally not well tolerated and may require direct intervention with intravenous HCO_3^-. If controllable by pulmonary intervention, as for example an increased ventilatory rate in an individual on mechanical ventilation, such therapy should be instituted first.

Respiratory Acidosis

Respiratory acidosis is due to inadequate pulmonary ventilation and, therefore, inability to adequately eliminate carbon dioxide. Pulmonary insufficiency such as emphysema, pneumonia, adult respiratory distress syndrome, or pulmonary fibrosis can cause respiratory acidosis. Renal compensation is effective only in chronic settings. Acute respiratory acidosis is diagnosed on clinical grounds, as well as by ABGs demonstrating a low pH, elevated P_{CO_2}, and relatively normal serum HCO_3^-. The latter may not be changed due to insufficient time for the renal compensatory mechanisms to have acted to conserve HCO_3^-.

Metabolic Alkalosis

Metabolic alkalosis is usually accompanied by hypokalemia. It is usually caused by loss of acid through the gastrointestinal tract as, for example, following prolonged nasogastric suction with loss of gastric acid. In such settings, hypokalemia occurs secondary to the elevation in pH (decrease in hydrogen ions) in the ECF or excellular compartment. This tends to cause intracellular hydrogen ions to migrate extracellularly, which necessitates a coordinated intracellular shift of potassium thus decreasing extracellular (serum) potassium. In other settings, hypokalemia due to diuretic therapy or hyperaldosteronism may be the primary factor promoting migration of potassium ions from cells into the ECF in exchange across the cell membrane for hydrogen ions, effectively sequestering the latter intracellularly and therefore raising serum or blood pH.

The natural compensation is a decrease in pulmonary ventilation, retention of carbon dioxide, and corresponding increase in H_2CO_3.

Treatment consists of correction of any potassium ion deficit and possible administration of chloride if the alkalosis was caused by loss of gastric acid. Chloride is retained by the renal tubules in exchange for bicarbonate. Potassium ions are exchanged for hydrogen ions in the renal tubules as the kidneys try to preserve hydrogen ions. Consequently, renal excretion of hydrogen ions may increase, necessitating even further potassium replacement. Severe or rapidly developing metabolic alkalosis may require intravenous ammonium chloride.

Respiratory Alkalosis

Hyperventilation with hypocarbia results in respiratory alkalosis. Common causes include general anesthesia, mechanical ventilation, anxiety or hysteria, and some neurologic problems resulting in disturbance of the respiratory center. Respiratory alkalosis is usually short-lived and well tolerated as an isolated disturbance of acid-base balance. It is an important compensatory mechanism for metabolic acidosis, as will be discussed.

Tetany may develop with alkalosis due to pH-dependent binding of calcium ions to serum proteins. As the pH increases, fewer calcium ions may be available, transiently creating a hypocalcemia and therefore a tetanic response.

Respiratory alkalosis is treated by having the patient rebreathe expired gases, or in some settings, breathe a gas mixture that is enriched with carbon dioxide. In settings of mechanical ventilation, the respiratory rate or tidal volume must be decreased to promote retention of carbon dioxide.

Mixed Acid-Base Disturbances

In many instances, acid-base problems are not purely metabolic or purely respiratory in origin, since the human body tends to compensate for any given metabolic disturbance. The rapidity of compensation is dependent on the rate of onset of pH disturbance. Respiratory compensatory mechanisms are much more rapid in onset than metabolic reactions, because the former consists of relatively rapid fluctuations in carbon dioxide, which can be eliminated or retained at the pulmonary alveolar level. The completeness of compensation is dependent not only on the rate of change of the pH but also on the functional capacity of the renal and pulmonary systems to preserve or excrete electrolytes or fixed acids, or to eliminate carbon dioxide in gaseous form (Table 4–2).

As an example, a patient with an arterial pH of 7.60 with a Pco_2 of 33 and total carbon dioxide of 30 has both a respiratory and metabolic alkalosis. One would typically expect an elevation of the Pco_2 to compensate for the alkalosis by respiratory mechanisms, that is, hypoventilation. If the arterial pH was 7.60 and the Pco_2 was 60, the patient has a metabolic alkalosis with incomplete respiratory compensation.

In acidotic states, mixed disturbances may also occur. For example, if the arterial pH is 7.10, the Pco_2 is 50 and the total carbon dioxide is 17, a combined metabolic and respiratory acidosis is present. The normal respiratory response to a decreased pH is hyperventilation to decrease carbon dioxide. If this response is incomplete, as in this example, a diagnosis of respiratory acidosis is established.[5]

HEMATOLOGIC CONSIDERATIONS

Coagulation

Blood coagulation may be initiated by intrinsic or extrinsic pathways (Fig. 4–2). Each consists of a sequence of activation steps, collectively called a cascade, resulting ultimately in the formation of a fibrin clot through the conversion of fibrinogen to fibrin by the proteolytic enzyme thrombin. In this sequence, a small initial stimulus can produce a large effect.

Counteracting the inherent tendency for blood to clot is the fibrinolytic system that is activated by fibrin. The fibrinolytic system consists of the proteolytic enzyme, plasmin, activated from plasminogen. Vascular injury releases plasminogen activators from endothelial cells. Activated factor XII also activates plasmin. The breakdown products, so-called *fibrin split products*, are anticoagulants that tend to engage thrombin with poorly functioning substrates. The longer plasmin reacts with fibrinogen, the smaller the split products, which are less effective in binding with thrombin. In addition, these breakdown products are incorporated into fibrin polymer networks, tending to slow the rate of polymerization and weak-

Table 4–2. *Respiratory and Metabolic Components of Acid-Base Disorders*

	Acute (uncompensated)			Chronic (partially compensated)		
TYPE OF ACID-BASE DISORDER	*pH*	*Pco_2 (respiratory component)*	*Plasma HCO_3^{-*} (metabolic component)*	*pH*	*Pco_2 (respiratory component)*	*Plasma HCO_3^{-*} (metabolic component)*
Respiratory acidosis	↓↓	↑↑	N	↓	↑↑	↑
Respiratory alkalosis	↑↑	↓↓	N	↑	↓↓	↓
Metabolic acidosis	↓↓	N	↓↓	↓	↓	↓
Metabolic alkalosis	↑↑	N	↑↑	↑	↑?	↑

* *Measured as standard bicarbonate, whole blood buffer base, CO_2 content or CO_2 combining power. The base excess value is positive when the standard bicarbonate is above normal and negative when the standard bicarbonate is below normal.*

PHASE I

INTRINSIC

Inactive XII —[Exposed collagen or foreign surface]→ Active XII

Active XII + Inactive XI → Active XI-XII Complex

Active XI-XII Complex + Inactive IX → Active IX

Active IX + VIII + X —[Platelet factors]→ Thromboplastinogen

Autoactivation of Thromboplastinogen + V → Thromboplastin

EXTRINSIC

Tissue Injury → Thromboplastinogen

Thromboplastinogen + VII → Thromboplastinogen-VII Complex

Thromboplastinogen-VII Complex + V + X → Thromboplastin

PHASE II Thromboplastin + Prothrombin —[V and VII]→ Thrombin

PHASE III Thrombin + Fibrinogen + XIII → Fibrin Monomer + Activated XII

Fibrin Monomer + Activated XIII → Fibrin Polymer

Fibrin Polymer —[Activated XIII / Platelets]→ Clot Retraction

Figure 4–2. *Coagulation pathways. Note that Phase I may be activated by either the intrinsic or extrinsic pathways. Phases II and III are common pathways toward the final step of clot formation and clot retraction.*

ening the resulting clot. Interaction between the clotting cascade and the fibrinolytic system is critical to the maintenance of vascular patency following injury.

Laboratory Assessment of Disorders of Coagulation

A wide variety of diseases may predispose to a bleeding disorder. The differential diagnosis is made simpler by a systematic approach. Laboratory testing is a critical element of the diagnostic process, but basic principles must be understood in order to select appropriate screening tests. The surgeon must establish the characteristics of the bleeding disorder. Is the bleeding localized or diffuse? Are there mucosal changes such as petechiae or hematomas? Is the bleeding acute or chronic and are there manifestations of hemodynamic disturbances? Is there a family history of bleeding, drug or alcohol ingestion, or any history of hematologic abnormalities or renal or hepatic disease? Are there any occupational exposures that might predispose to a bleeding disorder? Is there any suggestion of infection, because sepsis may present as a disturbance of coagulation? Once these basic issues have been reviewed, laboratory tests should be ordered.

A complete blood count (CBC) should be obtained to determine the hematocrit and hemoglobin and platelet count. Spontaneous bleeding may occur with platelet counts of less than 50,000. Severe bleeding may occur with platelet counts of less than 20,000. The peripheral blood smear may be helpful for rapid screening purposes; the presence of more than 7 platelets per oil immersion field generally excludes thrombocytopenia as a cause of bleeding. Thrombocytopenia may accompany disseminated intravascular coagulation (DIC), which must be considered in the appropriate clinical circumstances.

The peripheral blood smear showing immature erythrocytes in large numbers may suggest a microangiopathic hemolytic process (as may occur in DIC). Large platelets may be seen if platelet production is increased as a result of premature release of platelets into the peripheral blood (as may occur with idiopathic thrombocytopenia). Bone marrow aspiration or biopsy is indicated if a platelet disorder is suspected. Marrow sampling will yield information helpful to distinguish between increased platelet destruction and decreased platelet production by allowing assessment of the density of megakaryocytes.

Qualitative platelet tests may be necessary should the platelet count be relatively normal with a simultaneous elevated bleeding time. Hematology consultation would be appropriate in this setting.

Coagulation capacity can be screened rapidly by use of the prothrombin time (PT) and the partial thromboplastin time (PTT). *PT* is a measure of the time necessary for fibrin to gel in plasma after calcium and a tissue thromboplastin are added. It reflects the sequential activity of factors VII, X, V, phospholipid, prothrombin, and fibrinogen, that is, the extrinsic pathway. *PTT* measures the activity of the intrinsic pathway of coagulation. In this test, partial thromboplastin (phospholipid) is added instead of tissue thromboplastin. The PTT reflects activation of factor XII and subsequently of factor XI. The PTT is dependent on the activities of all factors except II, VII, and XII.

Bleeding time is a timed measurement of bleeding from a standardized incision of the skin; the Ivy method uses the forearm. Bleeding time may be prolonged with qualitative or quantitative platelet disorders, as well as in disease states characterized by increased capillary fragility.

Normal Red Cell and Hemoglobin Function

Red blood cells carry oxygen from the lungs to various tissues. Although small amounts of oxygen are circulated as a gas in solution within the blood, the overwhelming proportion of oxygen-carrying capacity of blood is within the RBC due to the unique properties of hemoglobin. Hemoglobin has an affinity for oxygen that is altered by a variety of environmental factors including pH, temperature, hypoxia, and anemia. The relation between oxygen content or percent saturation of hemoglobin (% Sat Hb) and the partial pressure of oxygen is described by a sigmoid curve. A "shift to the right" can be caused by a decrease in pH, increase in temperature, or hypoxic conditions such as altitude adaptation or anemia. This rightward shift reflects a decrease in oxygen affinity by hemoglobin, resulting in a greater release of oxygen to hypoxic, acidotic tissues. The shift of the oxygen–hemoglobin dissociation curve in anemia is mediated by the phosphate ester 2, 3,-diphosphoglycerate (2,3-DPG) which binds readily to deoxygenated hemoglobin which, in turn, allows greater production of 2,3-DPG.

Adequate oxygen-carrying capacity of blood is dependent on adequate numbers of RBC in addition to normal concentrations and function of hemoglobin within those cells. Anemia exists when there is inadequate oxygen-transporting material in a given volume of blood. A detailed description and differential diagnosis of anemias is beyond the scope of this chapter. However, general principles of diagnosis based on clinical signs and symptoms will be discussed.

A level of suspicion about possible anemia must be maintained in evaluating any patient who gives a history suggesting chronic blood loss, inadequate diet, use of medications that might suppress bone marrow function (e.g., carbamazepine) or potentiate bleeding (e.g., aspirin), renal or hepatic compromise, and family history positive for anemia (e.g., sickle cell disease or trait, and thalassemia). In addition, physical signs and symptoms must be carefully reviewed on the basis of a thorough medical history and physical examination. Anemia may be suggested by signs and symptoms of myocardial ischemia due to increased myocardial work necessary to satisfy tissue oxygen requirements (tachycardia), fatigue and weakness, which are commonly subtle in onset, shortness of breath, dizziness, or syncope. Other signs may include glossitis of iron deficiency or megaloblastic anemias, ecchymosis or petechiae suggesting an underlying bleeding disorder, abdominal pain with or without melena or hematochezia suggesting gastrointestinal bleeding, or jaundice suggesting hepatic failure with its corresponding dimunition in synthetic capacity.

ROUTINE PREOPERATIVE ORDERS

Written orders before surgery must account for all in-hospital screening and directions for patient preparation in a timely and efficient manner that is clearly interpretable by all persons who may participate in the care of the surgical patient.

A format for preoperative orders is presented in Display 4–1. A logical routine should be established to minimize the likelihood for errors of omission. A

Display 4–1. Preoperative Orders

1. Admit to Dr. ____________________
2. Diagnosis
3. Condition
4. Allergies
5. Vital signs (BP, P, RR, weight)
6. Laboratory Tests (UA, CBC, T&S, etc.)
7. Radiographs
8. Other tests (e.g., ECG, MRI, blood gases)
9. I&O
10. Position (e.g., traction of leg, elevation of head)
11. Wound care (e.g., irrigations, dressings)
12. Activity (e.g., ambulation, bed rest)
13. Diet
14. Operative permit (informed consent)
15. Blood products
16. Consultations
17. Intavenous Fluid
18. Medications
    A. Antibiotics
    B. Analgesic
    C. Antiemetic
    D. Antipyretic
    E. Hypnotic
    F. Sedative
    G. Chronic medications (e.g., digoxin, potassium)
19. Miscellaneous
    A. Transfusion
    B. Respiratory
    C. NPO after midnight
    D. Skin preparation
    E. Voiding

listing of the *diagnosis* is required by most hospitals. This helps the support staff at the hospital to focus on the patient's problem that prompted admission. The *general condition* is indicated next which helps the staff to focus on the patient's systemic status. *Allergies* should be stated; if there are none, that too should be noted. All of these notations are useful reminders to the surgeon as to the patient's status as he or she continues to write orders.

For elective admissions, *vital signs* are typically obtained on a routine basis, usually once per shift. The surgeon may designate other time intervals (e.g., q1h or q4h). A range of acceptable values may be imposed, outside of which the surgeon must be contacted. This is usually more of a consideration in the postoperative period. The range of acceptable monitored values may relate to "neuro vital signs," urine output (UO), central venous pressure (CVP), cerebral spinal fluid pressure, among other vital signs. Serial weights may help in nutritional or fluid management.

Preoperative tests may include radiographs, ECG, and culture and sensitivity studies. Recording of *fluid intake and output*, commonly designated "I & O," may be necessary preoperatively, particularly in trauma patients and those on strict fluid constraints. Patient *position* may be essential to assist in management of related problems such as orthopedic injuries, osteoarthritic cervical spine pathology, or edema due to trauma.

Wounds may require preparation and management prior to surgery. For example, a chronic ulcer of the skin may require debridement for which the surgeon specify "wet to dry dressings with normal saline and fine mesh gauze q4h." *Preparation of the skin* by cleansing or by shaving may be appropriate and should be specified in the preoperative orders.

Patient activity guidelines need to be stated. Bed rest, ambulation, use of walker, bed to chair activity, or any other set of circumstances should be specified. *Respiratory care* such as chest physiotherapy might be included here. *Dietary guidelines* are required, including any special diets. The gastrointestinal tract is route of choice for nutritional supplementation. High-protein, high-calorie foods may be indicated either by oral or by feeding tube administration. Total parenteral hyperalimentation or possibly peripheral intravenous alimentation may be appropriate.

If there is a greater than 10% likelihood of need for *blood products*, these should be ordered preoperatively. If the likelihood of blood products is less than 1%, no blood sample may be necessary preoperatively. If the likelihood of transfusion is somewhat greater, but less than 10%, the surgeon should order a "type and screen" (T & S).

Consultations by other physicians or services may be warranted preoperatively. Anticipation of the need of other types of expertise may be critical at this early stage to optimize subsequent patient care.

Finally, consideration needs to be given to intravenous *fluid* and *medications*. Preoperative medications should be written in a routine sequence, each item being considered for relative or absolute indications. Potential interaction of medications with anesthesia must be considered. In some instances, medications might best be withheld before surgery. For instance, some experts advocate withholding tricyclic antidepressants over a gradually tapering regimen before elective surgery; some advise withholding calcium channel blocking agents before anesthesia because of possible excessive, synergistic myocardial depression when used in conjunction with anesthetic agents. In general, however, chronic medications should be taken by the patient routinely preoperatively with a minimum of water or none at all, including beta-blocking agents. If there is uncertainty about potential drug interaction, discussion with the anesthesiologist, possibly by formal consultation well in advance of surgery, may be appropriate. Potassium supplementation may be necessary before surgery. The first indication of hypokalemia may be from the preoperative laboratory screening data, most likely in the patient on chronic diuretics. Guidelines for potassium ion repletion are presented in the section on fluid and electrolytes. In some cases repletion may not be readily achieved in a short period of time because most of the body's potassium content is intracellular.

Laboratory tests before surgery are routine, but the surgeon must anticipate special needs. For example, the patient on digoxin or anticonvulsants might best be managed with knowledge of blood levels, particularly if there is concern about compliance.

ROUTINE POSTOPERATIVE ORDERS AND DISCHARGE

The principles of writing orders postoperatively are the same as those used before surgery. Orders will usually need to be modified on at least a daily basis to respond to the dynamic changes after surgery and anesthesia. A guideline is presented in Display 4–2.

Special orders relate to maxillofacial surgery. Intermaxillary fixation must be carefully explained to support personnel. Means of rapid and efficient release of fixation should be made obvious by verbal and by written instruction. Oral wound care, nasal care,

Display 4–2. Postoperative Orders

1. Admit to ____________ (e.g., RR, ICU)
2. Operation
3. Condition
4. Allergies
5. Vital signs
6. I&O
7. Position
8. Activity
9. Diet
10. Drains, tubes (NG, Foley, wound, nasal)
11. Voiding (catheter, timing)
12. Respiratory (e.g., turn, cough, ventilate, mechanical ventilation)
13. Laboratory studies (types, frequency)
14. Radiographs (e.g., panoramic, chest)
15. Other studies (e.g., ECG, EEG)
16. Consultations
17. Wound care
18. Blood products
19. Intravenous fluid
20. Medications
    - A. Antibiotics
    - B. Analgesics
    - C. Antiemetic
    - D. Antipyretic
    - E. Hypnotic
    - F. Sedative
    - G. Bowel
    - H. Antiinflammatory (NSAID, steroids)
    - I. Decongestants
    - J. Chronic medications
21. Maxillofacial considerations
    - A. Suction
    - B. Lip care
    - C. Airway
    - D. Sinus precautions
    - E. Scissors, wire cutters
    - F. Mouth rinses, irrigations
    - G. Nasal packing
    - H. Halo
    - I. External fixation pins

external pin site management, and sinus precautions must be specific in detail.

Drains and tubes when used postoperatively require instructions for the nursing staff to follow. Drains may be open or closed. The surgeon must specify dressing care around drains and the nature of suction for the closed systems (wall suction, bulb suction). In certain circumstances, analysis of the chemical composition of drainage is critical to fluid and electrolyte management and even to diagnosis of internal wound problems.

When the patient is deemed to be ready for discharge from the hospital, the patient's family or caretaker must be educated about wound care, fixation, management of emergencies, signs and symptoms of infection, potential effects of medications, restrictions on activities such as driving, sports, and lifting, and the methods of access to the surgeon. Prescriptions should be written in a timely fashion to enhance the transition from hospital to home. Most, if not all, of these considerations can be achieved preoperatively through written materials. However, it is critical to review these with the patient prior to discharge, particularly if unanticipated factors in wound status or type of fixation are present. Follow-up appointments should be clearly established. Special arrangements may be needed before discharge, including those for home therapy and physical therapy. The patient requiring long-term intravenous antibiotic therapy needs coordination with an outpatient intravenous medication service.

NUTRITION OF THE SURGICAL PATIENT

Nutritional Needs

Nutritional considerations in the management of surgical patients are extremely complicated yet critically relevant to patient care. Surgery and anesthesia disrupt the metabolic steady state, initiating a catabolic process which is intensified by periods of limited nutritional intake. Depending on the type of surgical insult and the general metabolic status of the patient preoperatively, periods of relative starvation may be more or less prolonged. Muscle is catabolized for glucose production (gluconeogenesis) early in this phase, with additional protein breakdown from the metabolically active tissues that have been wounded surgically. If prolonged, this process may contribute to problems of wound healing, sepsis, and organ failure, in particular, the renal, hepatic, and pulmonary systems.

The normal adult requires 1800 to 2000 calories per day. Within this requirement is approximately 60g to 70 g of protein, yielding about 10g of nitrogen. This basal caloric expenditure changes very little following minor surgery or minor trauma. Caloric needs increase following more extensive injury, including sepsis. In such circumstances a higher proportion of the caloric requirement is derived from protein because of the relative glucose intolerance that occurs following major injury, including major surgery. This tendency towards hyperglycemia is due partly to catecholamine release, an increased glucagon-to-insulin ratio, and a decreased ability of tissues, especially the liver, to take up glucose. Nutritional therapy in such circumstances is directed towards minimizing catabolism of protein from lean muscle mass by supplying adequate exogenous glucose. In the absence of adequate exogenous glucose, muscle and brain can use ketone bodies for nutrition. Ketone bodies are derived from the breakdown of muscle and specifically from the catabolism of branched-chain amino acids in the liver.

The parenteral requirement for a typical resting young adult is 24 cal/kg/day. A typical 70-kg man would require 1680 calories. The average protein requirement is 0.45 g/kg/day. For protein synthesis a ratio of 200 nonprotein cal/g of nitrogen is necessary. The major limitation of calorie consumption is the rate of glucose use, which is 0.8 to 0.9 g/kg/h, even with exogenous insulin.

Caloric needs may increase perioperatively. Factors that increase caloric requirements include fever, tissue damage resulting in capillary leakage of plasma, the increased metabolic needs necessary for repair of damaged tissues, increased protein loss due to exudation or leakage across renal tubules, and increased respiratory work due to compromise of the airway.

As described by Blackburn et al.,[6] *lean body mass* is defined as body weight minus body fat. Assessment of this compartment is made by measuring the mid-upper arm circumference, the creatinine-height index, and possibly the height-weight index. The latter is least accurate due to the distortion of values one would see in edematous states, as in congestive heart failure. Fat stores are assessed by measurement of the triceps skin fold. Visceral protein is assessed by measuring serum albumin, transferrin, and total iron-binding capacity (TIBC).

Nutritional Support

In general, adequate calories should be supplied as soon as possible following surgery to minimize the mobilization of protein stores within skeletal muscles and the viscera. Those patients in a catabolic state due to stress, injury, or infection should ideally be evaluated nutritionally and have support initiated prior to surgery.

The gastrointestinal tract should be used as the primary pathway for nutrition if it is functional. The goal is to achieve a positive nitrogen balance. Nutritional support may be provided by use of a liquid supplement or use of an elemental diet in addition to the patient's normal preoperative diet. An additional 1000 to 1500 calories per day may be necessary.

An elemental diet consists of amino acids as a source of nitrogen and oligosaccharides as the carbohydrate source. It usually contains little fat and no lactose.[7] Enzymatic breakdown is not required for absorption of these elements from the gastrointestinal tract. In general, blenderized foods or meal-replacement formulas (e.g., Ensure, Isocal) are preferred over elemental diets in patients who have near-normal lipolytic and proteolytic activity in their gastrointestinal tract because they are less costly. These foods consist of high-molecular-weight proteins, fats, and carbohydrates. They can be delivered by feeding tube and should be started slowly by a drip apparatus, starting at about 50 mL of tube feeding and 50 mL of water every 2 hours, working up to 150 mL of each every 3 hours. Gastric retention with potential pulmonary aspiration may cause problems. Frequent assessment of serum electrolytes, glucose, BUN, creatinine, liver function studies, and osmolality is necessary. Hyperosmolar, nonketotic coma with hypernatremia may occur with excessively concentrated feeding solutions.

Parenteral nutrition may be delivered through peripheral veins or through a central vein (internal jugular or subclavian). Peripheral hyperalimentation may be employed when enteral intake is inadequate (less than 1500 Kcal per day). Typically a solution of 3% to 4% amino acids (e.g., Aminosyn, Freamine) can be mixed with 5% to 10% dextrose and be administered by peripheral vein. A fat emulsion (e.g., Intralipid or Liposyn) can be administered simultaneously. Such peripheral hyperalimentation can supply up to 1800 Kcal and 1 gram of amino acids per kilogram of body weight per day. If greater caloric requirements exist (greater than 2000 Kcal daily) for more than 2 weeks, a central venous catheter should be placed for total parenteral nutrition (TPN). Use of a large central vein allows use of hypertonic solutions containing up to 5% amino acids and 25% dextrose. Electrolytes, vitamins, and trace elements can be added. When TPN is employed for periods of months, care must be taken to provide adequate B-complex vitamins, ascorbic acid, folic acid, and the fat-soluble vitamins A, D, and E. Intramuscular administration of vitamin K and vitamin B_{12} must be provided.

Complications associated with TPN include catheter-related sepsis due to seeding of bacteria from distant sites, such as from the urinary tract, the lungs, or the wound, or from local violation of the sterile port. Strict catheter management techniques are essential to minimize the incidence of infection. Each hospital employs its particular protocol for such circumstances, which must be understood by all health care personnel. In general, central catheters should not be violated for administration of drugs or for blood sampling for laboratory tests.

In the setting of prolonged nutritional support, especially with TPN, particular attention should be directed to certain electrolytes and vitamin needs. Magnesium is necessary for normal neurologic function. Hypomagnesemia is manifested by perioral and extremity tingling or by agitation. The recommended daily intake of magnesium is 25 mEq of which approximately 8 mEq is absorbed; more is necessary when there is severe diarrhea or liver disease. Hypomagnesemia should be considered in any unexplained neurologic abnormality.

Hypophosphatemia can cause coma. The normal daily requirement for phosphate is 90 mEq, which may not be provided in prolonged states of poor nutrition. Trace elements such as iodine, copper, zinc, chromium, manganese, and fluoride can be provided by giving a unit of plasma protein every week or two during TPN support. Calcium is necessary daily for proper neurologic function and maintenance of bone. Adults require 200 to 400 mg of calcium daily which should, if possible, be administered by the gastrointestinal tract.

Water-soluble vitamins B and C are essential to wound healing, with vitamin C being essential for collagen cross-linking. They have no significant toxic effect in physiologic amounts. The commercial vitamin preparation MVI can be administered in one bottle of hyperalimentation fluid daily along with 1 mg of folic acid. Fat-soluble vitamins (A, D, E, K) can cause toxicity with overdosage. Vitamin K (10 mg) should be administered twice weekly. It is absorbed only in the presence of bile salts. Vitamin K deficiency, resulting in inadequate levels of the vitamin K–dependent coagulation factors VII, IX, X, and prothrombin, can develop due to biliary tract obstruction or malabsorption states (e.g., sprue, celiac disease). Gut bacteria are responsible for the synthesis of vitamin K and, therefore, sterilization of the gut due to prolonged use of broad-spectrum antibiotics may lead to deficiency of this vitamin.[8]

SPECIAL CONSIDERATIONS

Postoperative Urinary Retention

Urinary retention after surgery is common, occurring more frequently in the bedridden patient and in elderly males with prostate disease. Excessive fluid administration without bladder decompression may cause loss of bladder tone and retention of urine. Narcotic analgesics and anesthetic agents in general may interfere with bladder function.

The normal capacity of the bladder is 500 mL. If greater than this volume is sustained over a period of hours, permanent damage may result. Urine output must be monitored postoperatively and, for operations that are either prolonged (greater than 3 hours) or involve significant disturbance of fluid and electrolyte balance, intraoperative monitoring of urine output is necessary using a urinary catheter. The patient should be encouraged to get out of bed to void. If there is concern about urine retention, physical examination consisting of palpation and percussion of the suprapubic and lower abdominal areas should be performed. An urge to urinate in response to manual pressure is consistent with bladder distension (Crede sign). Percussion to establish the superior extent of the bladder should begin at or above the umbilicus so as to avoid overlooking a markedly distended bladder. This is particularly important in the comatose or otherwise uncooperative patient.

Hemodynamic instability, particularly tachy- and bradydysrhythmias, should prompt consideration of urine retention within the differential diagnosis while ruling out primary cardiovascular or metabolic etiologies. Relief of bladder distension may diminish excessive sympathetic or cholinergic activity.

If the bladder is distended and the patient is unable to void, the bladder should be catheterized. If less than 300 mL of urine are produced, the catheter is generally removed. If 500 mL or more are released, consideration should be given to leaving the catheter in to gravity drain for 24 hours, or more. Rapid drainage of extremely large volumes of urine should be interrupted by periodic clamping of the catheter to avoid precipitous hypotension due to altered autonomic tone.

Aspiration Pneumonitis

Aspiration of oral secretions and small amounts of blood is common after surgery during the emergence from general anesthesia and during the early postanesthesia period when protective pharyngeal reflexes are depressed. Small amounts of such secretions and blood may produce a mild pneumonitis, which usually resolves with increasing patient activity, deep breathing, turning, and coughing.

More significant aspiration pneumonitis may result from vomiting and aspiration of gastric contents or large volumes of blood. Gastric contents can cause a severe chemical pneumonitis due to its acidic nature. Once diagnosed, immediate access to the tracheobronchial system must be established through endotracheal intubation or bronchoscopy to allow suctioning and saline irrigation to dilute the concentration of the aspirated materials. Antibiotics should be instituted on a prophylactic basis due to the high likelihood for mucosal disruption and secondary bacterial pneumonitis. The use of systemic steroids is controversial. Consultation with a pulmonary specialist should be initiated after stabilization of the airway.

Postoperative Developments

Fever

Fever in the postoperative period is common. Early after surgery and anesthesia low-grade temperature elevations in the range of 100° to 101°F rectally are common. Atelectasis and aspiration of small amounts of blood or oral secretions probably accounts for most of these situations during the first 48 hours postoperatively. General anesthesia itself may contribute to a temporary disruption of central temperature regulation. Breakdown of blood products within the tissues may also contribute to early postoperative fever.

Beyond the first 48 hours, persistent postoperative fever is usually due to bacterial infections of the lungs, urinary tract, or surgical wound. Other areas of infection may include catheter sites from peripheral intravenous lines, arterial lines, or central venous lines. Adverse drug reactions should be considered in the differential diagnosis of both early and late postoperative fever, even when there has been no new agent introduced. The manifestations of drug intolerance may be subtle. An elevated eosinophilic cell count may be suggestive. In the absence of rash, pruritis, or other signs of an allergic phenomenon, altered drug therapy or elimination of medications may be necessary after infectious etiologies have been ruled out.

Altered Mental Status

In the postoperative period, altered states of mentation and consciousness may be encountered, much more commonly in the elderly individual. In general, consideration should be directed toward two factors, namely the cause or causes of such changes and the effects of such lack of cooperation upon surgical healing and general recuperation.

In some instances the diminished consciousness may be due to delayed metabolism of anesthetic agents caused by hepatic or renal insufficiency. The duration of action of anesthetic agents varies widely according to the general body habitus of the patient. Some anesthetic agents dissolve preferentially in fat deposits; particularly in obese individuals, after a long period of anesthesia, the emergence from anesthesia can be slow as the agent is gradually released from those fat stores.

Greatly prolonged states of depressed consciousness should prompt further investigation. The surgeon and anesthesiologist must evaluate for possible cerebral hypoxia, possibly on the basis of a primary cerebrovascular event, whether embolic or hemorrhagic, or whether due to inadequate ventilation and oxygenation during the anesthesia or early postoperative period. Cerebral hypoxia may occur due to inadequate RBC replacement, perhaps in conjunction with compromised cardiac output due to hypovolemia, myocardial ischemia, or cardiac dysrhythmias. Elderly individuals are often affected by vascular compromise within the cerebral and cardiac tissues. Such individuals may not tolerate even modest compromises in cerebral perfusion. Depending on the type of surgery, embolic phenomena should be considered, including emboli of fat, air, or atherosclerotic plaque.

Altered mental status may be caused by metabolic disturbances postoperatively. Profound hypoglycemia during anesthesia may have occurred in the insulin-dependent diabetic and gone undetected. Severe disturbances in acid-base and electrolyte balance may cause alterations in mental status, an example being hypomagnesemia. Septicemia should be considered in the appropriate setting within the differential diagnosis of altered mental status after surgery, particularly in the immunocompromised host who may not be able to demonstrate the expected febrile response.

Some individuals display signs of organic brain syndrome during the postoperative period, which is often triggered by the unfamiliar hospital environment, including unfamiliar noises from monitoring devices, sleep disturbance, loss of sense of time, and possibly prolonged sensory deprivation, particularly in the intensive care unit setting. Consultation with a neurologist is helpful. The surgeon must first perform a basic neurologic examination to rule out focal deficits.

Workup of the altered mental status postoperatively should include a basic neurologic examination. This should include assessment of orientation to time, place, and identity, and of strength, coordination, cranial nerve function, and deep tendon reflexes. The laboratory workup should include arterial blood gases to rule out hypoxia and hypercarbia, and screening chemistry parameters including sodium, potassium, magnesium, and glucose. Renal and hepatic function should be assessed by BUN, creatinine, SGPT, SGOT, LDH, direct and indirect bilirubin, and alkaline phosphatase. Urine specific gravity and electrolytes may be helpful. In certain settings a drug screen for sedatives and hypnotics may be appropriate. If narcotics have been employed, reversal with naloxone may be attempted. Lethargy associated with dystonic reactions should prompt the surgeon to consider an extrapyramidal reaction to antidepressant medications; intravenous diphenhydramine might be considered.

Tubes and Drains

Various tubes and drains are used during surgery and in the postoperative period to facilitate removal of body fluids. In general, tubes and drains are used for obliteration of dead space in a surgical wound and removal of materials or fluids that are harmful to the site in which it is placed, including blood, purulence, and gastrointestinal secretions.

In the maxillofacial region, drains are commonly employed after incision and drainage of infections. Minor oral abscesses may not require drain placement, because incision and drainage and the use of appropriate antibiotics may be sufficient. Infections involving the deep fascial spaces of the head and neck usually require drain placement. In general, drains should be placed in the most dependent location to facilitate drainage with the help of gravity. In the maxillofacial region this is often best achieved through extraoral incision and drainage.

Chest tubes are used in a variety of settings and, in general, are employed to evacuate air (e.g. pneumothorax) or to evacuate fluid (e.g. hemothorax; malignant pleural effusions). Hemothorax may be secondary to chest trauma often in conjunction with pneumothorax, or it may be secondary to surgical insult as with pulmonary segment or lobar resection. The maxillofacial surgeon encounters chest tubes most commonly in the setting of traumatic pneumothorax in the multiply injured patient or after the procurement of rib grafts used for maxillofacial reconstruction. In general, chest tubes may be placed to suction if there is a persistent air leak until the pleura becomes adherent to the chest wall, thus sealing the leak. If there is no persistent air leak but there continues to be a small pneumothorax as determined by serial chest radiographs and clinical examination, the tube should be placed to "underwater drainage," so-called water seal. This allows the egress of air but prevents inflow of air.

REFERENCES

1. Schrier RW, Berl T. Disorders of water metabolism. In: Schrier RW, ed. Renal and Electrolyte Disorders. Boston: Little, Brown, 1976:1.
2. Schrier RW. Renal sodium excretion, edematous disorders, and diuretic use. In: Schrier, RW, ed. Renal and Electrolyte Disorders. Boston: Little, Brown, 1976:45.
3. The Use of Blood. North Chicago, IL: Abbott Laboratories, 1971:21.
4. Postoperative care. In: Donoff RG, ed. Manual of Oral and Maxillofacial Surgery, chap. 6. St. Louis: CV Mosby, 1987:139.
5. Davenport, HW. The ABC of Acid-Base Chemistry, ed. 5. Chicago: University of Chicago Press, 1969.
6. Blackburn GL, Bistrian BR, Maini BS, Schlamm HT, Smith MF. Nutritional and metabolic assessment of the hospitalized patient. J Parenteral Enterol Nutrition 1977; 1:11.
7. Michel L, Serrano A, Malt RA. Current concepts: Nutritional support of hospitalized patients. N Engl J Med 1981; 304:1147.
8. Blackburn GL, Maini BS, Pierce EC. Nutrition in the critically ill patient. Anesthesiology 1977; 47:181.

II

PRINCIPLES OF DENTOALVEOLAR SURGERY

5

Basic Principles of Dentoalveolar Surgery

Stanley A. Berman

Although the scope of oral and maxillofacial surgery has expanded in many directions, the mainstay of most practices remains dentoalveolar surgery. It is imperative that surgeons possess extensive knowledge and use sound surgical skills in this fundamental aspect of the profession. These basics provide for the most efficient and effective delivery of care and also provide the opportunity to develop new procedures and techniques in the ever-expanding realm of oral and maxillofacial surgery.

THE INTRAORAL FLAP

The intraoral flap is an incision in soft tissue designed to allow access to the underlying area and follows the basic parameter of all surgical flaps. There are a variety of different types of intraoral flaps, each of which has been designed to solve a particular problem. These include the envelope flap, the envelope flap with relieving incision, the semilunar flap, and the palatal flap. In any intraoral flap, the tissue is retracted from the surgical site, the procedure is performed, and the flap is replaced to cover and protect the site so healing can occur.

Basic Intraoral Flap Design

Proper flap design can mean the difference between atraumatic surgery and prolonged postoperative healing. In designing a functional intraoral flap it is essential to make the base wide enough to ensure an uninterrupted flow of blood to the margins of the flap. It is also important to make the flap as thick as possible for the same reason. If the blood supply is compromised, all or part of the flap can become necrotic, causing dehiscence and thus delayed healing. Another cause of dehiscence is inadequate flap size. The flap should be large enough to expose the entire surgical site and extend over intact bone. When the flap is too small, the sutured incision will rest over a surgical void rather than intact bone, causing the incision to dehisce. Whenever dehiscence occurs, the wound must heal by secondary intention.

The design of the flap should take into consideration certain vital structures. Those in the maxilla are found on the palate. These are the neurovascular bundles exiting through the greater palatine and the nasopalatine foramina. The vital structures in the mandible are the lingual and mental nerves and those found in the floor of the mouth. The lingual nerve becomes very superficial at the distal lingual aspect of the third molars. The mental nerve exits the bone of the mandible in the bicuspid region.

One of the most important aspects of a successful flap is proper retraction. Although the commonly accepted method of retracting is to use a round-ended retractor to hold back the flap, this can result in some undesirable consequences. When attention is focused on the surgery, the tendency is to put unnecessary pressure on the flap, occasionally causing the flap to tear. Torn flaps heal more slowly than sharply in-

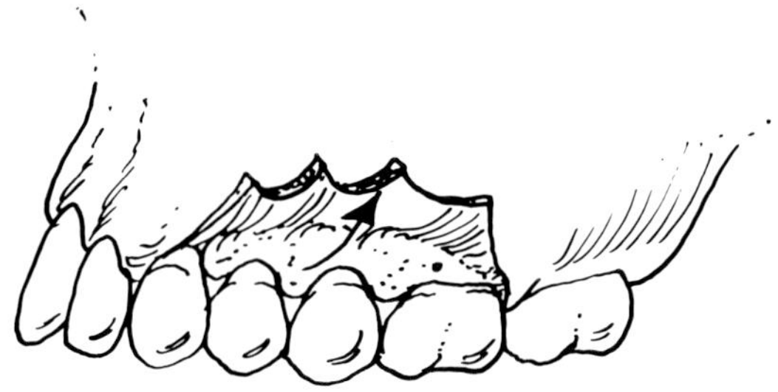

Figure 5–1. *An envelope flap is made by incising in the gingival sulcus and reflecting tissue to expose underlying structures.*

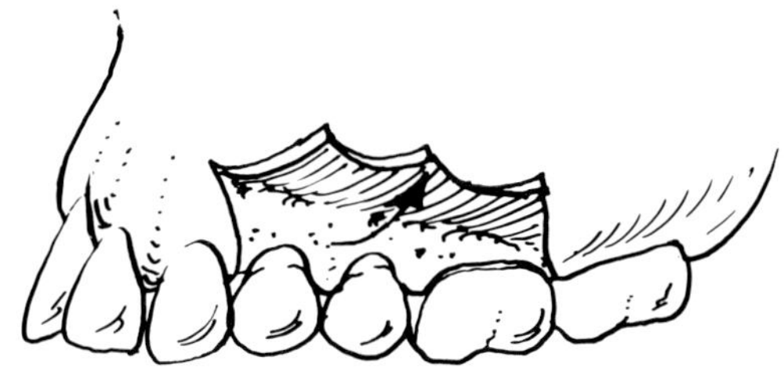

Figure 5–2. *The envelope flap is converted to a three-corner flap by making a release incision at the anterior end of the incision.*

cised flaps, thus resulting in prolonged healing and excess pain.

The Envelope Flap

The envelope flap is the simplest type of flap, as there are no releasing incisions. It is commonly used when limited access is needed for the removal of roots or to perform a surgical extraction. If the patient is dentulous, the incision is made in the gingival sulcus; if the patient is edentulous, the incision is usually made at the crest of the ridge (Fig. 5–1). There is no optimum length for an envelope flap. It is made the size necessary to allow for proper access. Because incisions heal across and not along their length, the length of an incision does not affect the healing time. It is not advisable to attempt an envelope flap around a curved structure, like the cuspid eminence, because these flaps are difficult to reflect and tend to tear easily.

Envelope Flap With Vertical Release Incisions

When vision or access is not sufficient, an envelope flap may need a release incision. This incision can be made on either end of the envelope flap, but is usually made at the anterior end as it provides the best visibility and access (Fig. 5–2). Another criteria would be to avoid vital structures. The vertical release incision should be made on an oblique angle, which allows the base to be wider than the free margin. For best results, a vertical release incision should not be made through the papilla or directly on the facial surface of the attached gingiva because both predispose the surgical site to periodontal compromise. The release incision allows for superior apical access; however, a contraindication for the use of a vertical relieving incision is that it requires an extended period of healing compared with the simpler flap design.

Semilunar Flap

The semilunar flap is a form of envelope flap basically used for apical exposure. Unlike an envelope flap, the incision is not at the crest of the ridge, but is made completely in unattached gingiva. The flap needs an adequate margin of bone beyond the surgical site, and a good margin of unattached gingiva (Fig. 5–3).

A potential problem in semilunar flap design is that the incision may be made too close to the gingival sulcus, disrupting the blood supply to the tissue, causing necrosis and poor healing. It is also possible to underestimate the size of the pathology underneath the tissue and design the flap too small. This compromises the principle of extending the incision over good bone and leads to dehiscence and slow healing.

Palatal Flap

The palatal flap is primarily designed for the removal of palatal tori. The palatal blood supply, except for minor anastomoses, does not cross the midline. Flaps designed to cross the midline without incorporating adequate blood supply from the lateral can cause complete or partial necrosis of the flap. The easiest in-

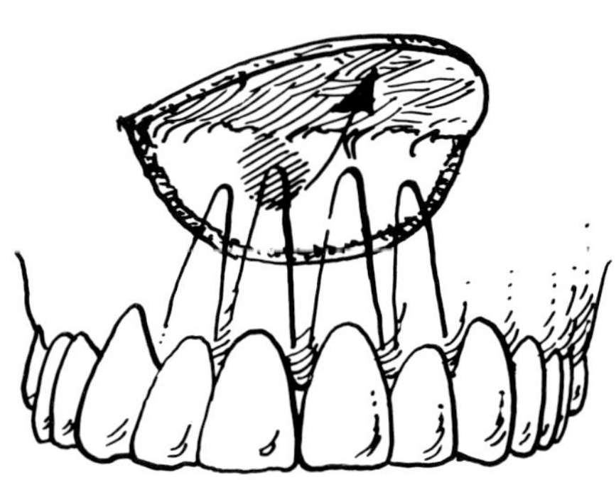

Figure 5–3. *The semilunar flap is used most commonly to expose periapical pathology.*

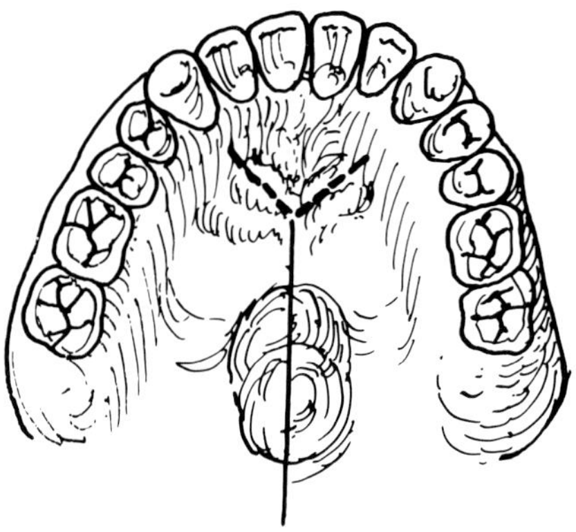

Figure 5–4. *A midline palatal incision with* Y*-shaped releasing incisions at the anterior end provides excellent access for removal of palatal torus.*

cision to expose palatal tori is the straight midline anteroposterior incision. If access with the incision is not adequate, the anterior end can be extended by Y-sloped incisions (Fig. 5–4). The center of this Y incision frequently becomes slightly necrotic and has to heal by secondary intention. In general, the mucosa over the dense cortical bone of the torus is very thin; therefore, flap necrosis is most prevalent after removal of a torus. For the removal of impacted cuspids or supernumerary teeth in the anterior maxilla, a standard envelope flap is used. The only vital structures involved in reflecting the anterior flap are the nasopalatine vessels and nerve. These rarely cause a problem with operative bleeding and tend to heal well. Occasionally the patient experiences some numbness of the anterior palate but is seldom bothered by it. In most cases, the anesthesia resolves itself quickly.

In using palatal flaps, caution needs to be observed to prevent overextension of the anteroposterior incision into the soft palate. This can cause unnecessary bleeding, which can be difficult to control. Another potential bleeding problem can occur if a branch of the greater palatine artery or vein is severed when the anteroposterior flap is torn or reflected aggressively.

Torn Flaps

To avoid torn flaps, the flap should be well designed to provide adequate access, employing releasing incisions where necessary. In preparation for the incision, it is important that the surgical blade be sharp. Extensive procedures or multiple extractions may necessitate a second or third blade.

SURGICAL EXTRACTIONS

A surgical extraction needs to have a flap for access and may require the tooth to be sectioned and removed in sections. Anatomic abnormalities, such as accessory roots, hypercementosis, root curvatures, dilacerations, or a span of roots that is larger than the neck of the tooth, can be diagnosed by x-ray film and can often indicate a surgical extraction. There are also instances in which crowns or other existing restorations impinge on the tooth to be extracted, and if a surgical extraction is not performed, damage to the restoration may occur.

Technique for Minimal Flap Extractions

When a root is fractured at the gingival margin and there is no crown left to grasp with a forcep, the tooth can still be delivered without a major flap or surgical sectioning. An incision is made to free the papilla on both sides of the tooth, providing room to seat a narrow-beaked forcep. The forcep is manipulated up under the slightly loosened flap until the beaks are over the lip of alveolar bone so tooth and bone are firmly grasped (Fig. 5–5). The root is then delivered in the usual fashion.

Techniques for Removal of Single-Rooted Teeth

For the removal of a single-rooted tooth fractured below the bone level or near the apex, the basic principles include good lighting and good suction of the socket. Sometimes the root tip will come out after brisk suctioning. Root tip picks can be used, but care should be taken, since they are very delicate instruments and can break with overzealous use (Fig. 5–6). If immediate results are not obtained with the root tip pick, the effort should be discontinued, and a purchase point should be made in the periodontal ligament space. This will allow for the use of a larger elevator.

Another option for the removal of a root tip is the use of an endodontic file. The file can be used whenever a canal is visualized. The point should be screwed into the canal as far as possible. With fingers or a hemostat clamped to the file, the root can be removed slowly (Fig. 5–7).

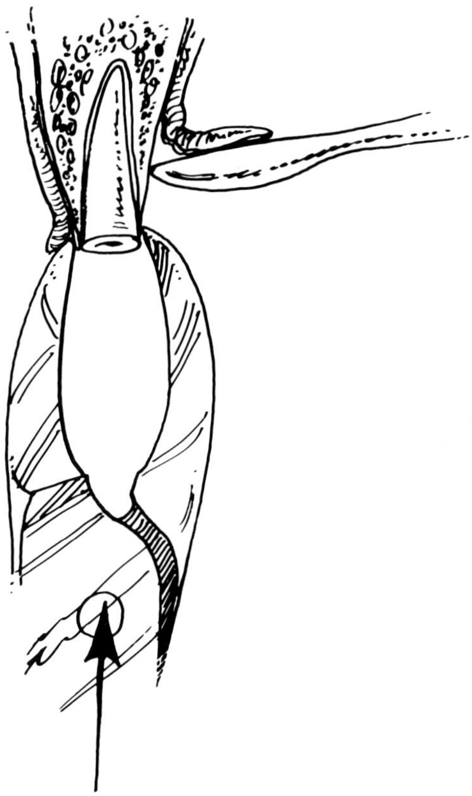

Figure 5–5. *To deliver a root fractured at the gingival margin, the buccal tissue is minimally reflected so that a bit of bone can be grasped along with the root.*

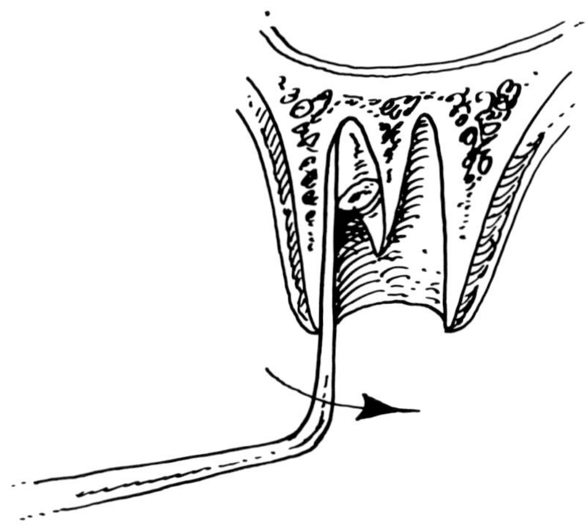

Figure 5–6. *A root tip pick is used to tease the apical 2 to 3 mm of root from the socket.*

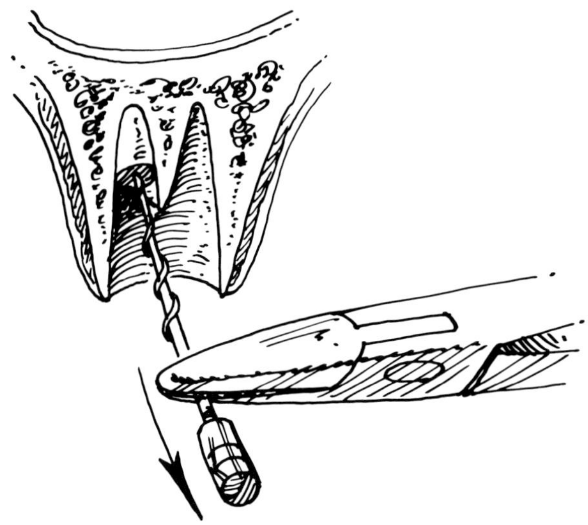

Figure 5–7. *An endodontic file can be used to engage the root tip and elevate it from the socket.*

Techniques for Removal of Multi-Rooted Teeth

Multirooted teeth present different surgical problems from single-rooted teeth. The roots usually have to be removed separately, which necessitates sectioning of the tooth. The objective is to convert a two- or three-rooted molar into single-rooted sections. In the removal of mandibular molars, the tooth is sectioned buccolingually (Fig. 5–8). Using a straight elevator, the tooth is split into two single-rooted teeth with crowns, which are removed with a forcep.

A variation of this technique requires formation of an envelope flap and removal of enough buccal bone to visualize the bifurcation. This enables the surgeon to horizontally section one root away from the crown and second root (Fig. 5–9). Using a lower molar forcep, this crown and second root can be removed in one piece. After the remaining root is removed, the socket needs to be debrided, the flap coapted back into place, and sutured.

The procedure for removing maxillary molars is the same as that used for mandibular molars, except that the maxillary molars have three roots instead of two. An envelope flap should be used and buccal bone removed to expose the trifurcation. A horizontal cut is made through the two buccal roots, leaving the palatal root attached to the crown. With a maxillary molar forcep, the crown and palatal roots can be removed in one piece, leaving the two buccal roots.

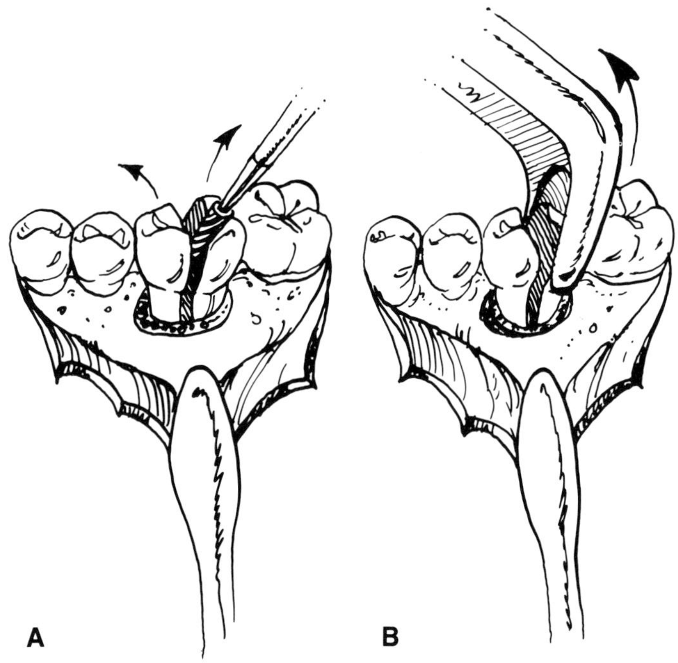

Figure 5–8. *(**A**) Lower molar is sectioned buccolingually, separating it into a mesial and a distal single-rooted tooth. (**B**) The two "teeth" are delivered with a forcep.*

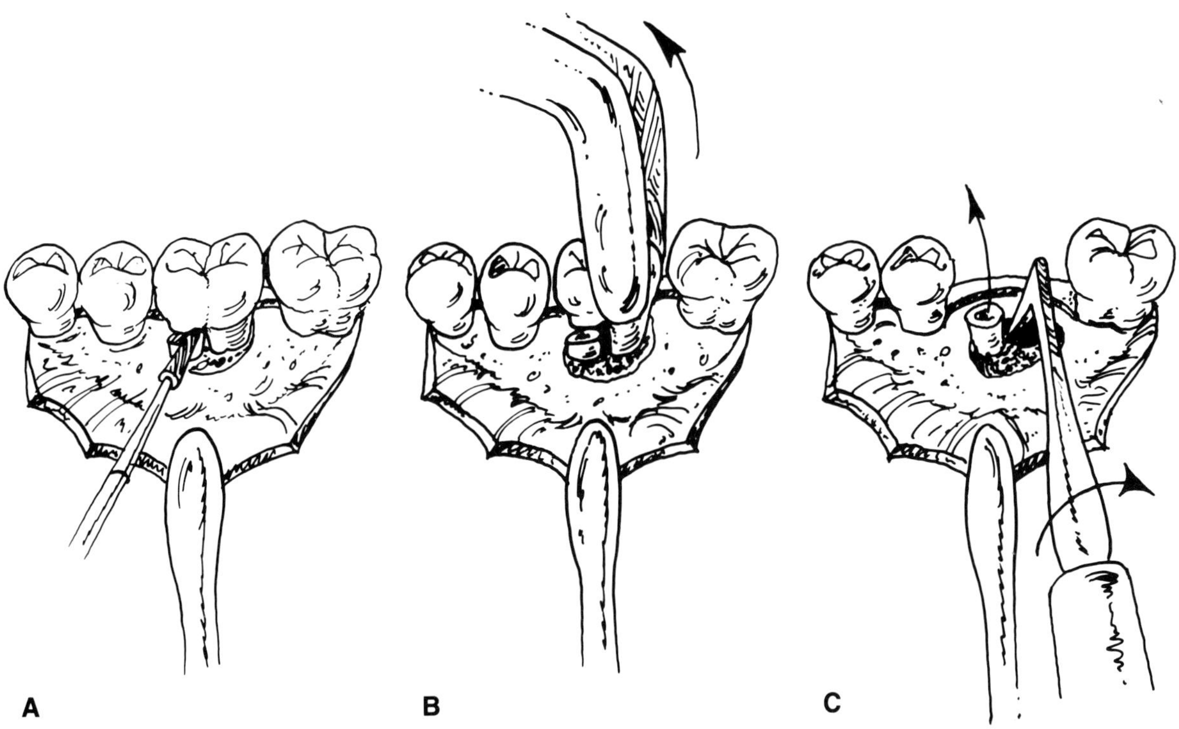

Figure 5–9. *Mandibular molar removal. (**A**) An envelope flap is reflected, a small amount of buccal bone is removed, and the mesial root is sectioned. (**B**) The crown and distal root are removed with a forcep. (**C**) The mesial root is removed with a triangular elevator.*

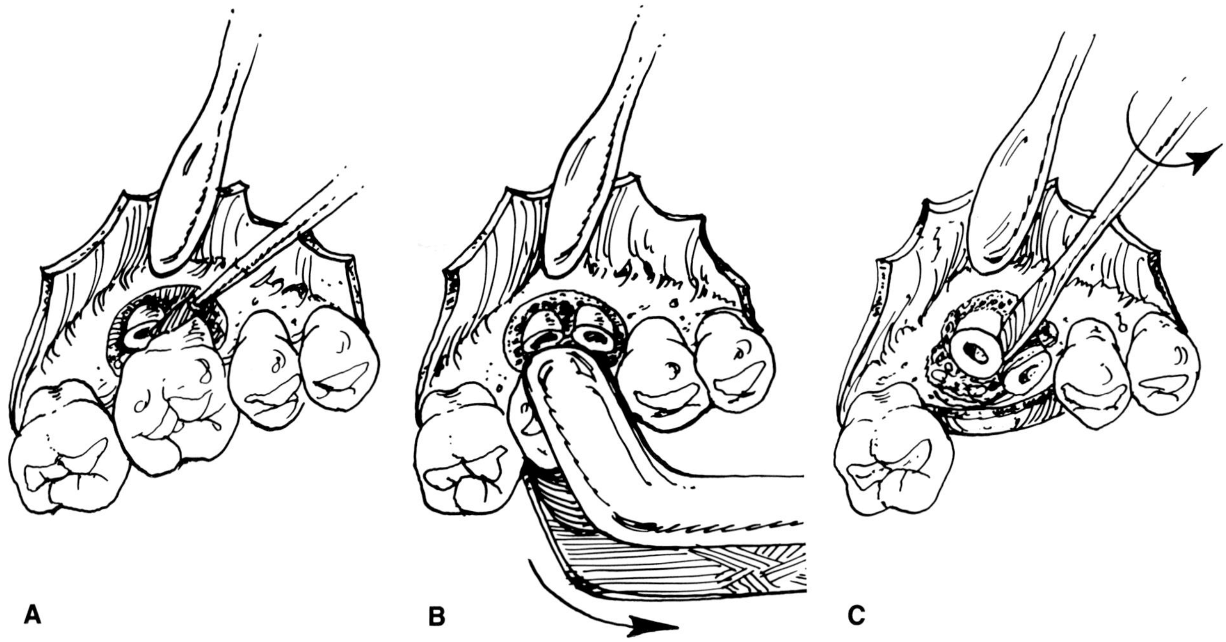

Figure 5–10. *Maxillary molar removal. (**A**) An envelope flap is reflected, buccal bone is removed, and the two buccal roots are sectioned. (**B**) The crown and palatal roots are removed with a forcep. (**C**) The two buccal roots are delivered with a straight elevator.*

These can then be removed with an elevator or a narrow-beaked forcep (Fig. 5–10). It is not always necessary to section maxillary molars that are firmly embedded in excessive bone; rather, an envelope flap can be reflected, buccal bone removed to expose the trifurcation, and the tooth can be removed in one piece using a forcep.

Proximity to the sinus is a major concern when dealing with fractured or decayed roots in maxillary molars. It is inadvisable to exert apical pressure in an attempt to loosen these roots. In these cases, root tip picks should be used to tease loose root tips only. The proper approach for firmly embedded root tips is an envelope flap, buccal bone removal sufficient to visualize the root, and elevation from the apex away from the sinus towards the crest of the ridge (Fig. 5–11). If the palatal root tip is large enough to see the nerve canal, an endodontic file is a useful instrument.

When to Leave Root Tips

The criteria for root tips that need removal are well defined and include roots that have an apical lesion on x-ray film, or those with visible pathology or infection. However, there are instances in which it is better to leave root tips in place. If the root is near a vital structure which may be injured during extraction, has the potential to be displaced into the sinus, inferior alveolar canal, or submandibular space, or would require the destruction of excess bone, the root should be left in place. It is rare to have postoperative sequelae. When a root tip is left, the patient should be informed of the circumstances and understand the decision. Films should be taken, and full documentation on the patient's chart is mandatory. Followup films should be repeated at 6 and 12 months to ensure uneventful healing.

Alveoloplasty

Alveolectomy is indicated when many teeth adjacent to each other are removed. The ability to wear a prosthesis successfully may hinge on performing a proper alveolectomy. Undercuts and sharp spicules need to be revised, as well as irregularities caused by extractions performed at different times. The bone that would normally resorb away naturally can be trimmed and smoothed at this time without any long-term loss.

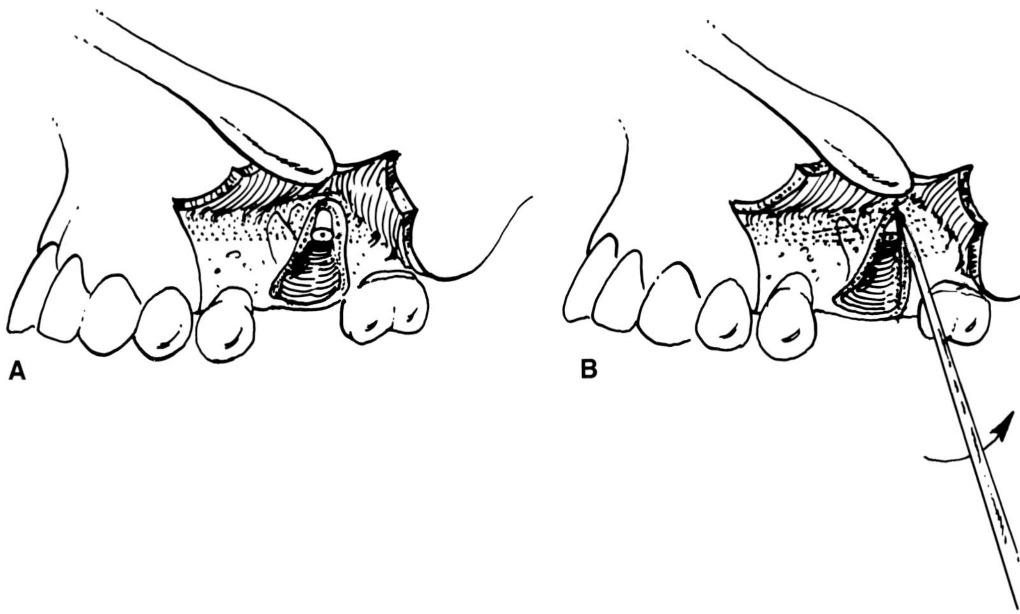

Figure 5–11. *To avoid displacing a fractured root into the sinus, apical pressure should be avoided. (**A**) A three-corner flap is reflected and buccal bone is removed to expose the entire root. (**B**) A straight elevator is then used to deliver the root to the occlusal.*

In smoothing and preparing the ridge, it is important to remove as little bone as possible. The standard alveolectomy, in conjunction with extraction, should be performed by a crestal incision, reflection of the flap, trimming of undercuts, and removal of spicules and sharp bony projections using rongeurs and bone files. The tissue should be trimmed, removing all torn papillae and granulation tissue. Following this, the area should be well irrigated, the gingiva coapted back into place, and sutured.

Interseptal Bone Removal

When teeth are removed in the maxilla and the patient has a protruded buccolabial plate of bone, a form of alveoloplasty in which the interseptal bone is removed is indicated. It usually necessitates the removal of four to six teeth to be successful. A minimal gingival flap is reflected. The interseptal bone is removed with a rongeur and the bone plate compressed and fractured inward. The tissue is then sutured. This technique allows for a reasonable reduction in the thickness of the ridge and provides a smooth base on which to construct a proper prosthesis.

COMPLICATIONS OF EXODONTIA

The elevator and the forcep are the two basic instruments in the armamentarium, and of the two, the elevator is more likely to be misused. To use the elevator properly, it should be wedged between tooth and alveolar bone. Although this is basic procedure, the adjacent tooth is often improperly used as a fulcrum. Fractured crowns, fractured restorations, and loosened and traumatized adjacent teeth are the inevitable results. Teeth with conical roots, if used as a fulcrum, can be avulsed. In addition, second molars can be loosened if the elevator is used improperly on mesioangled third molars, which are hooked under the marginal ridge. A tooth which has been avulsed while extracting another tooth should be treated immediately. This tooth should receive the same treatment as any other traumatically avulsed tooth. The tooth needs to be replaced immediately and stabilized with splints or bonding materials. A root canal is usually needed at a later date.

Forceps also can cause trauma when not handled correctly. There is a great deal of pressure exerted with the use of forceps. If the forcep is not protected by the surgeon's other hand acting as a buffer, damage can occur to surrounding tissue.

Fracture of Alveolar Bone

Alveolar bone usually fractures from overzealous buccal or lingual luxation. There is always some expansion of bone during an extraction. Sometimes this expansion of bone goes beyond the socket and involves the adjacent teeth. If there is extensive expansion, there will be tearing and bleeding into the periodontal space of the adjacent teeth. This can result in these teeth becoming sensitive and loose. Upon examination, these teeth will show no etiology for the pain being experienced. Consequently, the only treatment for this problem is routine bone compression after each extraction.

Because the buccolabial plate of bone is sometimes thin and fragile, it is possible for small pieces of bone to be broken off as a result of the trauma from the extraction. These pieces of bony alveolus often come out attached to the tooth. In other instances, they may be obviously displaced in the socket and therefore be easily removed. Furthermore, they may be fractured and still attached to the periosteum. The fractured piece of bone retains its blood supply if it is still attached to soft tissue, or it can become avascular and die. Unfortunately, if these pieces of alveolar bone go undetected, they act as foreign bodies, causing low-grade discomfort and the formation of granulation tissue.

There are instances in which large pieces of alveolar bone are fractured during an extraction. Because these pieces still maintain a viable blood supply, the treatment of choice is to attempt to save them.

Fracture of the Tuberosity

The same basic principles for alveolar bone fractures also apply to fractures of the tuberosity. Because the tuberosity is the end of the alveolar arch, the distal side has no support. The sinus can fill the majority of the tuberosity, leaving only an eggshell-thin plate, which can fracture when a molar with widely divergent roots is extracted. It is important when extracting posterior teeth to evaluate the x-ray films for sinus size and bone thickness. If in the course of removing a tooth the tuberosity becomes loosened, several options are available. If the tooth is being removed because of overeruption or malposition, or is decayed but not symptomatic, the extraction can be discontinued. This permits the surgeon to stabilize the tuberosity with an arch bar and allow sufficient time (6 weeks) to elapse for it to heal (Fig. 5–12). If the tuberosity is only slightly loose, discontinuing surgery may be the only treatment needed. If the tooth is infected or painful, extraction must be continued. The gingiva around the tooth should be loosened, and an attempt to remove some bone initiated. This bone removal can make the extraction easier. It is imperative not to compromise the blood supply to the bone by separating the bone from the periosteum. If after the tooth is removed the tuberosity is still attached at the periosteum, the bone and soft tissue are stabilized with sutures. The gingival flap should be repaired with a watertight closure, using horizontal mattress sutures and a running suture line. Sound surgical practice dictates that the opposite hand should always be positioned on the tooth, as well as on the alveolus or tuberosity. This allows the surgeon to feel the first signs of movement and hopefully prevent the fracture from occurring.

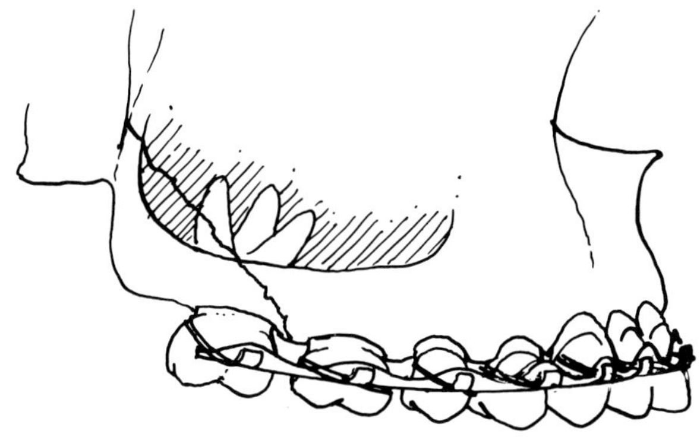

Figure 5–12. *When a tuberosity is fractured, the tooth should be wired to an arch bar and allowed to heal for 6 weeks. A surgical extraction with sectioning of the roots is carried out at the second operation.*

Maxillary Sinus Perforation

A perforation of the sinus can occur in the course of removing teeth in the maxilla. The severity of perforation can range from a slight opening at the apex of a root socket to a large bony defect which requires major repairs. Existing conditions can precipitate a perforation; for instance, when the alveolar bone surrounding the tooth is extremely thin and the majority of the tooth structure lies within the sinus, a traumatic routine extraction can cause a perforation. Also, chronic or acute infection, cysts, periapical granulomas, tumors, and extruded root canal material can cause destruction of alveolar bone, leading to sinus perforation when an extraction is performed. If the sinus is healthy, small perforations (2 to 4 mm) at the apex of the socket will be protected by the clot and will heal without complications. When dealing with a moderate-size perforation (more than 5 mm) an attempt should be made to close the mucosa over the extraction site. If there is sufficient tissue, placement of sutures is all that is required. Sometimes, however, buccal bone needs to be removed in order to approximate the tissue. If the opening is large, a buccal flap procedure is necessary to make a watertight closure over the defect.

The objective in performing a buccal flap procedure is to release enough tissue to make a watertight closure over an extraction site (Fig. 5–13). An incision is made along the crest of the ridge and through the extraction site. Release incisions are made on both sides of the incision, extending lateral at an angle to make the base wider than at the crest. The periosteum is reflected into the buccal vestibule, exposing the socket and the buccal bone. With the flap reflected, the periosteum is incised horizontally to provide relaxation of the flap. The palatal mucosal edges of the socket are reflected slightly and freshened, allowing better union of tissue. Horizontal mattress sutures are then placed over the socket to suture the flap to the palatal mucosa. A running suture is then placed along the length of the flap that lies directly over the socket. This produces a two-layer closure. Because the release incisions are over bone, interrupted sutures can be used. The patient should be placed on antibiotics, antihistamines, and a nasal spray.

It is important to inform patients about postoperative care so they do not inadvertently prolong the healing process. They need to understand the importance of sneezing with their mouth open, wiping their nose instead of blowing it, avoiding mechanical cleaning devices such as Water Piks, and keeping foreign objects out of the healing socket.

Root Tip in Sinus

If a root tip is pushed into the sinus, the surgeon should carefully weigh whether it should be removed. It is advisable when dealing with a small 2- to 3-mm root that is not infected or has no visible pathology to allow it to remain in place. The patient should be apprised of the situation and be allowed to take an active part in the decision process.

A root that is larger than 2 to 3 mm or has some visible pathology should be removed. If the root can be delivered through the existing defect without enlarging it, a major procedure can be avoided. There are some root removal techniques designed to achieve

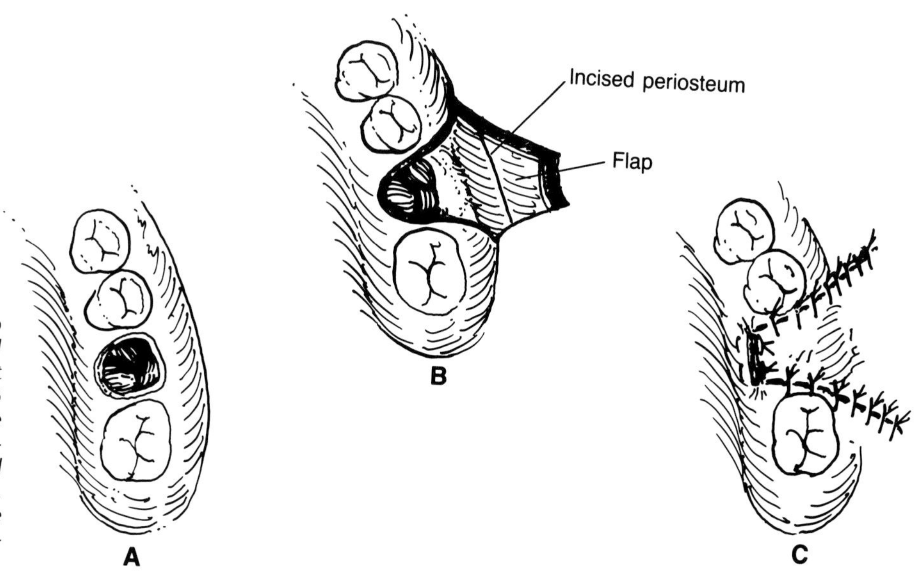

Figure 5–13. *The buccal flap technique for closure of an oral antral communication. (**A**) A defect in the sinus floor larger than 5 or 6 mm. (**B**) Buccal oblique release incisions are made, the flap reflected, and the periosteum incised horizontally to provide relaxation. (**C**) The flap is sutured into place with horizontal mattress and simple sutures.*

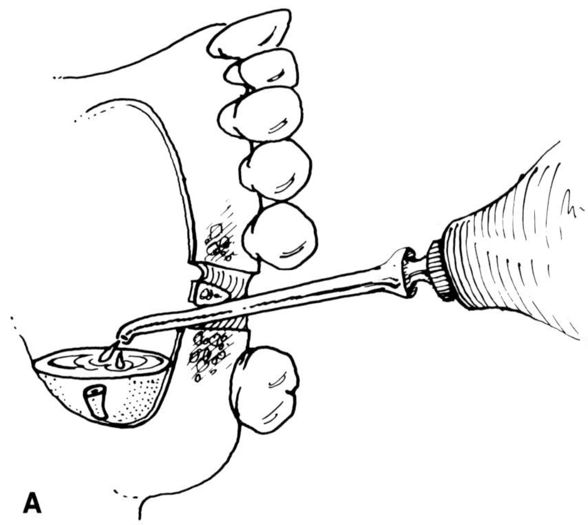

A

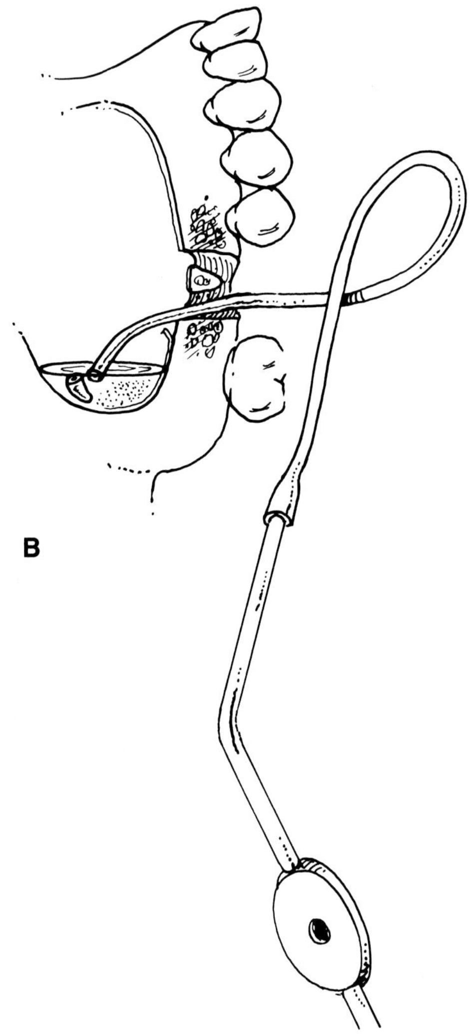

B

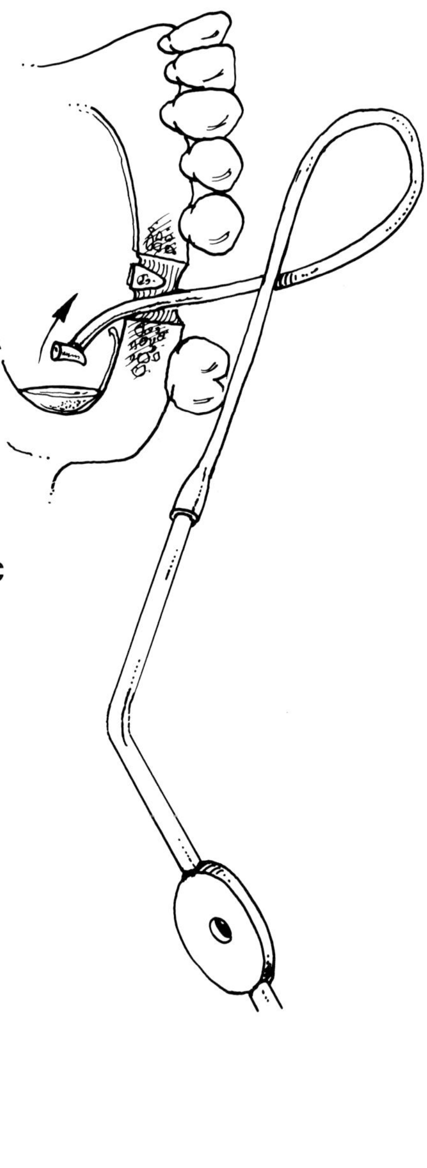

C

Figure 5–14. *Retrieval of a small root tip may be accomplished with a suction catheter. (**A**) With the patient in a horizontal position, sterile water (5–10 mL) is injected into the sinus by way of the perforation. (**B**) A catheter the same size as the perforation is manipulated into the water, and the suction is attached. (**C**) The root tip will be caught against the catheter tip and removed with the catheter.*

this outcome. One approach is to place the patient in a horizontal position in the chair. Using a bulb syringe, sterile water is injected through the perforation into the sinus. The root tip will fall back to the posterior aspect of the sinus. A flexible catheter is inserted into the perforation, and the other end should be attached to a suction tip. The catheter should be manipulated to the posterior aspect of the sinus. As the water is suctioned into the catheter, the root tip may also be suctioned up and will occlude the cut end of the catheter. Frequently a change in sound can be heard when the root tip attaches to the catheter and blocks the opening. The catheter should then be carefully withdrawn with the root tip attached (Fig. 5–14). Sometimes this procedure needs to be repeated because the root tip adheres to the mucosa and does not drop to the posterior of the sinus when irrigated. When the root is removed, the socket should be sutured closed with a figure-eight suture. The standard regimen of antibiotics, antihistamines, and nasal sprays should be instituted.

For the removal of large roots or roots with pathology, the Caldwell-Luc procedure is used (Fig. 5–15). An incision is made in the canine fossa above the roots of the teeth. The flap should be reflected upward, and the infraorbital nerve located. A hole is then made through the bone into the sinus and enlarged with a Kerrison rongeur. The sinus is irrigated in order to re-

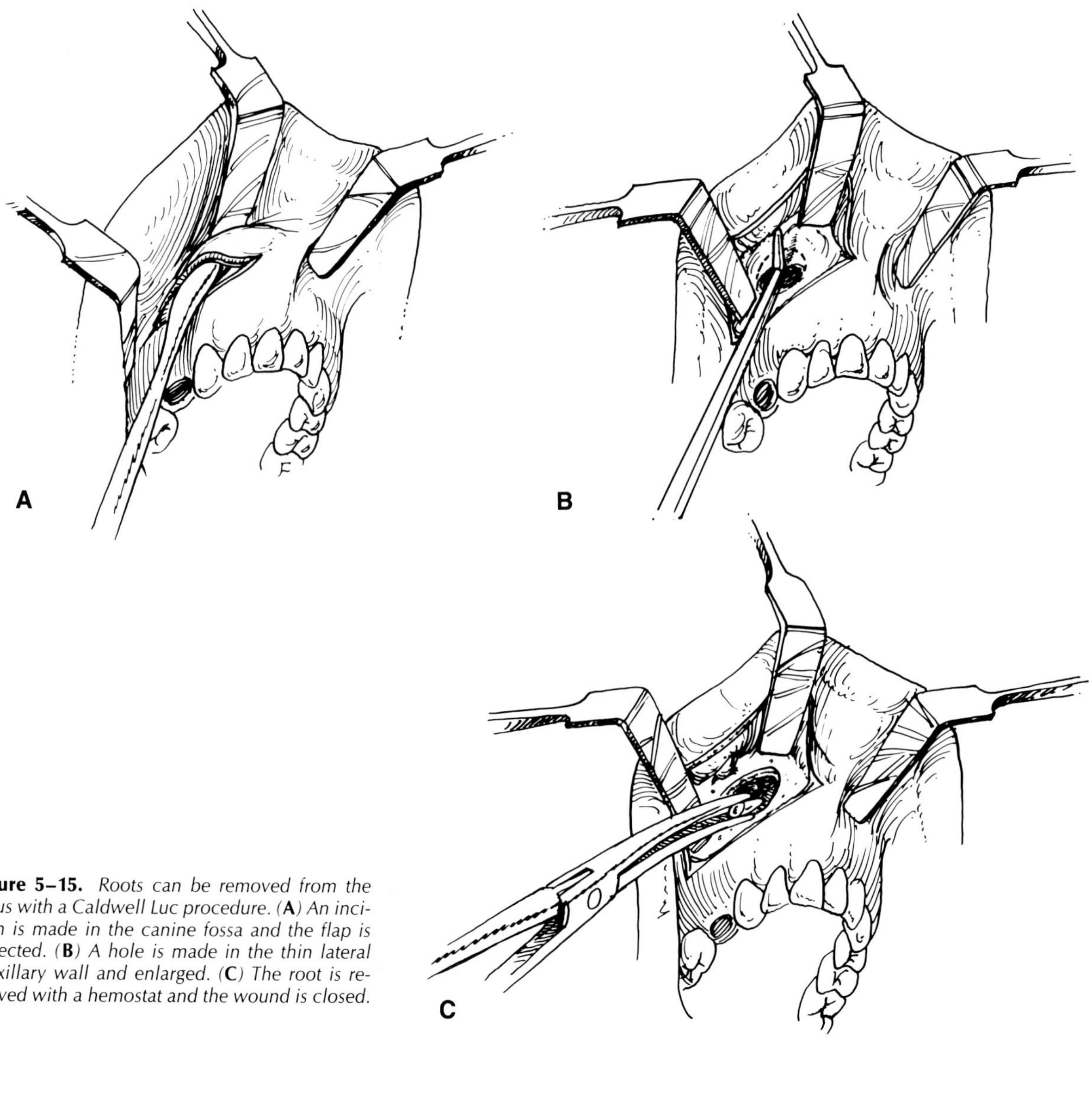

Figure 5–15. *Roots can be removed from the sinus with a Caldwell Luc procedure. (**A**) An incision is made in the canine fossa and the flap is reflected. (**B**) A hole is made in the thin lateral maxillary wall and enlarged. (**C**) The root is retrieved with a hemostat and the wound is closed.*

move blood clots and debris. The root is retrieved and the flap replaced.

Root in the Submandibular Space

Because of the anatomy of the lingual aspect of the mandible, some roots of third molars are not covered with bone and extend into the submandibular space. Fracture of such a root may result in its displacement into the submandibular space.

If the root is displaced through the socket and into the space, a flap approach is needed to remove it. Films should be taken, both lateral and anteroposterior views, to locate the root in the space. Because of the location of the lingual nerve, flap design should be approached cautiously. A lingual envelope flap, reflected carefully, may give sufficient access. With slow dissection and good light, the root tip may be visualized. Because the root tip has a tendency to slide away and elude retrieval, an attempt should be made to stabilize it with a finger or an instrument. If after a reasonable effort the root cannot be removed, the site should be sutured closed and the patient placed on antibiotics. It is advisable to wait 10 days to 2 weeks before making another attempt at removal. During this time, the root will become fibrosed in place and thus easier to remove.

Roots in Infratemporal Fossae

Displacement of maxillary third molars into the infratemporal fossa is an uncommon complication of third molar removal, which happens most commonly with distoangular impactions. When excessive force is used in removing maxillary third molars, the tooth or root can be pushed easily through the thin wall of bone surrounding it and disappear from view. If this occurs, the surgical procedure should be suspended and x-ray films taken. Lateral skull and anteroposterior views are needed to determine whether the tooth has been displaced into the infratemporal fossa or the maxillary sinus. If the films confirm the tooth is in the fossa, the incision should be enlarged and retracted. Once the tooth is visualized, a curet should be positioned behind the tooth to prevent it from being displaced further into the fossa. The tooth should be grasped cautiously with a hemostat or Russian forceps. If the tooth slips from the grasp and is lost, or if the tooth is not easily located, surgery should stop and the incision closed. Radiographs are taken and the patient is observed on a weekly basis for 3–4 weeks. At that time, two options exist: remove the tooth which now is less likely to be elusive due to fibrosis, or continue careful follow-up. If the patient has a restricted range of motion or has pain the tooth should be removed. If the patient is without symptoms, it may be best to leave the tooth alone. If surgery is chosen, immediate preoperative radiographs should be made to aid in localization.

Usually, proper instrumentation can prevent a tooth or root entering the infratemporal fossa. When the flap is retracted and the tooth visualized, the elevator should be placed on the mesiobuccal surface to elevate downward and backward. At this time, the retractor should be removed and placed posterior to the tooth. This will guide the tooth downward into the mouth and block the path to the infratemporal fossa.

Nerve Damage

In the mandible, the inferior alveolar and the lingual nerves are the most likely to sustain injury during routine dentoalveolar surgery. The long buccal nerve is rarely damaged. The inferior alveolar nerve is vulnerable in the third molar socket area and where the branches lying in soft tissue emanate from the mental foramen. The inferior alveolar nerve lies adjacent to the roots of the third molar, sometimes entwining between or through the roots. Because x-ray films are only two-dimensional, they cannot determine the relation between the root and the nerve; therefore, even in the most skilled hands, there are instances when the nerve will be compromised, regardless of what approach is attempted. This possible complication should be discussed thoroughly with the patient prior to surgery. If the root of the third molar breaks and the use of an elevator becomes necessary, care should be taken to avoid forcing the root into the nerve canal. To prevent this from occurring, proper visualization is necessary before any attempt is made to remove the root. Interseptal bone can also be dislodged from the socket and pushed into the nerve canal, blocking it off. This blockage will prevent future nerve regeneration.

At the point where the nerve loses its bony protection at the mental foramen and branches into soft tissue, surgical damage may also occur. Lacerations and torn flaps are the most common cause of nerve damage. When surgery is performed in this area, the nerves should be identified by blunt dissection and retracted out of the surgical field. If this is not possible, the retractor should be positioned to protect the nerve, especially from rotary instruments. In designing a flap in this area, release incisions should be made cautiously.

If the nerve is damaged anywhere along its course, varying degrees of paresthesia or anesthesia can occur. This could involve the lip, chin, and labial mucosa. Since the condition can be temporary, careful documentation of its extent should be kept and compared on each subsequent visit. If it appears to be diminishing over the course of a few months, no further treatment is needed; however, if the paresthesia does not appear to be resolving on its own, an evaluation for microsurgery should be initiated.

Another nerve that is vulnerable is the lingual branch of the fifth nerve. This nerve frequently passes through the tissue lingual to the third molar and superior to the crest of the ridge. It often lies precariously close to the site of lower third molar surgery, and may in some cases actually lie within the tissue covering the buried molar.

One of the primary causes of lingual paresthesia is nerve damage, as a result of tearing the lingual tissue during removal of third molars. Another cause of paresthesia is fracture of the lingual bone plate. If the lingual nerve is not superior to the crest of the ridge, it invariably lies against the lingual bone plate. If the plate is fractured during surgery, it is preferable to leave it in place. Attempts at removal can precipitate damage to the nerve. In removing buried third molars, surgeons do not reflect the lingual portion of the lower flap. As a consequence, when they elevate the tooth upward, they inadvertently tear the unreflected flap. This can be avoided if the lingual aspect of the flap is loosened very carefully so that the tissue is not bound to the buried crown. The nerve that crosses the distal lingual cusp may be manipulated during the loosening process, but should not sustain any permanent damage.

BIBLIOGRAPHY

Kohn MW, Chase DC, and Marciani RD. Surgical misadventures. Dent Clin North Am 1973; 17:533.

Laskin DM. Extraction of teeth—exodontia. In Laskin DM, ed. Oral and Maxillofacial Surgery, Vol. II. St. Louis: CV Mosby, 1985:3.

Meyer, RA Complications of exodontia. In: Waite DE, ed. Textbook of Practical Oral and Maxillofacial Surgery, ed 3. Philadelphia: Lea & Febiger, 1987:145.

Peterson LJ. Prevention and management of surgical complications. In: Peterson LJ, ed. Contemporary Oral and Maxillofacial Surgery. St. Louis: CV Mosby, 1988:265.

Peterson LJ. Principles of complicated exodontia In: Peterson LJ, ed. Contemporary Oral and Maxillofacial Surgery. St. Louis: CV Mosby, 1988:185.

Peterson LJ. Principles of uncomplicated exodontia. In: Peterson LJ, ed. Contemporary Oral and Maxillofacial Surgery. St. Louis: CV Mosby, 1988:133.

6

Principles of Management of Impacted Teeth

Larry J. Peterson

The atraumatic removal of impacted teeth is one of the most commonly performed surgical procedures by the oral and maxillofacial surgeon. Removal of the impacted tooth is usually considered to be an office procedure, but extensive training, skill, and experience are necessary to perform this procedure in an atraumatic fashion. When the surgeon is untrained and inexperienced, the incidence of complications rises significantly.[62] Not only must the surgeon who performs third molar surgery be well trained and experienced in this procedure but also he or she must be able to decide whether asymptomatic impacted teeth need removal. In many situations, this decision will be made based on clinical experience and professional judgment; in others the decision will be clear cut and easy to make. In an era of skyrocketing medical expenses and concerns with cost containment, the surgeon will be called upon more and more frequently to justify surgical procedures, including removal of third molars.

The purposes of this chapter are to review and discuss the indications and contraindications for the removal of impacted teeth, to discuss the classification and determination of the degree of difficulty of the surgery, to discuss the parameters of perioperative patient care, to discuss the likely complications and their management following third molar surgery, and to review the controversies surrounding the removal of asymptomatic impacted teeth.

DEVELOPMENT OF THE MANDIBULAR THIRD MOLAR

The mandibular third molar is the most commonly impacted tooth. It also presents the greatest surgical challenge and invites the greatest controversy when indications for removal are considered. When the surgeon is determining whether a specific third molar will become impacted and whether it should be removed, he or she needs to have a clear understanding of the development and movement of the third molar between the ages of 7 and 25. Although an individual tooth may not follow the usual trends, the majority will, and therefore the surgeon will need to understand these movements for the decision-making process.

A number of longitudinal studies have been performed that have clearly defined the development and eruption pattern of the third molar.[3–6] The mandibular third molar tooth germ is usually radiographically visible by age 9 (Table 6–1), and cusp mineralization is completed approximately 2 years later. At this point the location of the tooth is the anterior border of the ramus with the occlusal surface facing nearly directly anteriorly. The level of the tooth germ is approximately at the occlusal plane of the erupted dentition. Crown formation is usually complete by age 14, and the roots are approximately 50% formed by age 16. During this time, the body of the mandible grows in length at the expense of resorption of the anterior

Table 6–1. *Development of Lower Third Molar*

	Average Age (years)	*Range (years)*
Tooth germ visible	9.8	7.5–12.1
Cusp mineralization complete	11.9	8.8–14.7
Crown formation complete	14.1	10.5–18.1
Roots, one-half formed	16.3	12.6–20.2
Roots, formed; apex open	18.2	14.4–22.1

border of the ramus. During this process the relative position of the third molar to the adjacent teeth changes, with the third molar assuming a position at approximately the root level of the adjacent second molar. The angulation of the surface of the crown becomes more horizontal also. The roots are completely formed with an open apex by age 18. By age 24, 95% of all the molars which will erupt have completed their eruption.

The change in orientation of the occlusal surface from facing straight anteriorly to straight horizontally occurs primarily during root formation. During this time the tooth rotates from being horizontal to mesial to vertical. Therefore, the normal development and eruption pattern, assuming the tooth has sufficient room to erupt, brings the tooth into its final position by age 20.

Most third molars do not follow this typical sequence, and instead become impacted teeth. Approximately half do not assume the vertical position and remain as mesioangular impactions. There are several possible explanations for this. The Belfast Study Group[6,7] claims that there may be differential root growth between the mesial and distal roots, which causes the tooth to either remain mesially inclined or to rotate to a vertical position depending on the amount of root development. In their studies, they have found that underdevelopment of the mesial root will result in a mesioangular impaction. Overdevelopment of the same root will result in overrotation of the third molar into a distoangular impaction. Overdevelopment of the distal root, commonly with a mesial curve, is responsible for the severe mesioangular or horizontal impaction. The Belfast Group has noted that, whereas the expected normal rotation is from horizontal to mesioangular to vertical, failure of rotation from the mesioangular to the vertical position is also very common and, to a lesser extent, worsening of the angulation from a mesioangular to a horizontal impaction and overrotation from mesioangular to distoangular. These overrotations from mesioangular to horizontal and from mesioangular to distoangular occur during the terminal portion of root development.

A second major reason for the failure of the third molar to rotate into a vertical position and erupt into position has to do with the relation of the bony arch length to the sum of the mesiodistal widths of the teeth in the arch. Several studies[5,8,9] have demonstrated that when there is inadequate bony length there is a higher proportion of impacted teeth. In general, patients with impacted teeth almost invariably have larger teeth than those with normal teeth.[9] Even when the tooth-bone relation is favorable, a lower third molar that is positioned laterally to the normal position will almost always fail to erupt.[5] This may be the result of the dense bone present in the external oblique ridge.

A final factor that seems to be associated with an increased incidence of impaction is retarded maturation of the third molar. When dental development of the tooth lags behind the skeletal growth and maturation of the jaws, there is an increased incidence of impaction. This is most likely a result of a decreased influence of the tooth on the growth pattern and resorption of the mandible.

The number of impacted teeth observed in the population appears to be increasing. The probable explanation for this is the fact that a large percentage of the population now lives in communities where the water is fluoridated, and there is a consequent lack of severe dental disease. The result is that fewer permanent premolars and molars are being extracted during the teenage years. Whereas the early loss of teeth allowed more room for the erupting third molar, the current trend to retain all 28 teeth results in a greater incidence of impacted third molars.[6]

INDICATIONS FOR REMOVAL OF IMPACTED TEETH

An impacted tooth can cause the patient mild to serious problems if it remains in the unerupted state. Not every impacted tooth actually causes a problem of clinical significance, but each does have that potential. A body of information has been collected based on extensive clinical experience and clinical studies from which indications for removal of impacted teeth have been developed. For some indications, there is lack of hard data gained from long-term prospective longitudinal studies.

Pericoronitis Prevention or Treatment

When a third molar, usually the mandibular third molar, partially erupts through the mucosa, the potential for the establishment of a mild to moderate inflammatory response similar to gingivitis and periodontitis exists. In certain situations, the patient may actually experience a severe infection, which may require vigorous medical and surgical treatment. The bacteria that are most commonly associated with pericoronitis are *Peptostreptococcus*, *Fusobacterium*, and *Bacteroides*.[10–12] Initial treatment of pericoronitis is usually aimed at debridement of the periodontal pocket by irrigation or by mechanical means, disinfection of the pocket with an irrigation solution such as hydrogen peroxide or chlorhexidine, surgical management by extraction of the opposing maxillary third molar and occasionally of the offending mandibular third molar, and systemic antibiotic therapy in severe cases.

Prevention of recurrent pericoronitis is usually achieved by removal of the involved mandibular third molar. Although operculectomy has been recommended for management of this problem, the soft tissue redundancy usually recurs due to the relationship between the anterior border of the ramus and the fully or partially erupted mandibular third molar. Pericoronitis can occur whenever the involved tooth is partially exposed through the mucosa, but most commonly occurs around mandibular third molars that have soft or hard tissue over the posterior aspect.[13]

Approximately 25% to 30% of impacted mandibular third molars are extracted because of pericoronitis or recurrent pericoronitis.[14–18] Pericoronitis is the most common reason for removal of impacted third molars after age 20. With increasing age, the incidence of pericoronitis as an indication for removal of impacted teeth also increases.

Prevention of Dental Disease

Dental caries can occur in the mandibular third molar or in the adjacent second molar, most commonly at the cervical line. Due to the patient's inability to effectively clean this area, and because the third molar is inaccessible to the restorative dentist, caries in the second and third molar are responsible for extraction of impacted third molars in approximately 15% of the patients.[14–18] As with pericoronitis, the presence of caries and eventual pulpal necrosis are responsible for an increasing percentage of extractions with increasing age.

The presence of the partially impacted third molar and the patient's inability to clean the area thoroughly may result in early advanced periodontal disease. This is the primary reason for removal of approximately 5% of impacted third molars.[14–18] In patients whose dental health is poor and who have partially erupted third molars, the periodontal condition around the second molar and partially erupted third molar can become extremely severe at an early age.

Orthodontic Considerations

The presence of the impacted third molar, especially the mandibular third molar, has been felt for many years to be responsible for a variety of orthodontic problems. These problems fall into three general areas.

Crowding of Mandibular Incisors

Perhaps one of the most controversial issues regarding mandibular third molars has been the issue of their influence on crowding of mandibular incisor teeth, especially after orthodontic therapy. A variety of studies have been reported that support both sides of the controversy. Many of these studies have been reviews of small numbers of patients[19] or have been reviews of anecdotal information.[20] The Belfast third molar study has been a long-term longitudinal study which has carefully followed a large number of patients in a variety of clinical situations to determine whether or not the presence of the lower third molar has an influence on mandibular anterior crowding.[6,8,21] The Belfast study has documented that one of the most important, if not the most important, factor in late crowding of the lower incisor teeth is the presence of impacted third molars. The study also points out that there may be other factors involved, but probably none are as important as the impacted third molar. Therefore, it would appear prudent to consider removal of impacted third molars in patients who are undergoing orthodontic treatment for crowded mandibular incisors or in whom a tight anterior occlusion will exist in the postorthodontic state.

Obstruction of Orthodontic Treatment

In some situations, the orthodontist will attempt to distalize the molar teeth because the presence of an impacted third molar may inhibit or even prevent this procedure. Therefore, if the orthodontist is attempting to move the buccal segments posteriorally, removal of the impacted third molar will facilitate treatment and allow it to be achieved more predictably.

Obstruction of Orthognathic Surgery

When LeFort I osteotomies or sagittal split osteotomies are planned, presurgical removal of the impacted teeth may be extremely helpful in the surgical procedure. This is especially true if rigid fixation with screw fixation is to be employed in the mandible. Most surgeons recommend that the impacted third molars be removed at least 9 to 12 months before sagittal split osteotomy of the mandible. Although this involves a very small percent of all impacted third molars, it is a critical issue for those patients who are to undergo these procedures.

Prevention of Odontogenic Cysts and Tumors

In the impacted third molar that is left intact in the jaw, the follicular sac which was responsible for the formation of the crown may undergo cystic degeneration and form a dentigerous cyst. The follicular sac could also develop into odontogenic tumors. These sequences of events have frequently been cited as a reason for removal of asymptomatic teeth, and although it remains a very potential problem, in terms of percentages it is a very rare occurrence. In retrospective surveys of large numbers of patients,[14–18] between 1% and 2% of all third molars which are removed are removed because of the presence of odontogenic cysts and tumors. Of additional importance, is that when these pathologic entities are seen, they usually occur in patients under age 40.

Management of Unexplained Pain

Occasionally patients will complain of jaw pain in the area of an impacted third molar, which has neither clinical nor radiographic signs of pathology. In these situations, removal of the impacted third molar frequently results in resolution of this pain. At this time, there is no plausible explanation as to why this relief of pain occurs. Approximately 1% to 2% of mandibular third molars that are removed are removed for this reason.[14–18]

When a patient presents with this type of complaint, the surgeon must make sure that all other sources of pain are ruled out before suggesting surgical removal of the third molar. In addition, the patient needs to be informed that removal of the third molar may not necessarily relieve the pain completely.

Root Resorption of Adjacent Teeth

Third molars in the process of eruption may cause root resorption of adjacent teeth. The general view is that malaligned erupting teeth may restore the roots of adjacent teeth, just as succedaneous teeth resorb the roots of primary teeth during their normal eruption sequence. The actual occurrence of significant root resorption of adjacent teeth is not clear, although it may be as high as 7%.[22] If root resorption is noted on adjacent teeth, the surgeon should consider removing the tooth as soon as is convenient. In most cases the tooth will repair itself with the deposition of a layer of cementum over the resorbed area. However, if resorption is severe, and the mandibular third molars displace significantly into the roots of the second molar, both teeth will probably have to be removed.

Teeth Under Dental Prosthesis

Before construction of a removable or fixed prosthesis, the dentist should make sure that there are no impacted teeth in the edentulous area which is being restored. If such teeth are present, the general recommendation is that they be removed before the final placement of the prosthesis. Teeth which are completely covered with bone, which show no pathologic changes, and which are in patients who are over age 40 are unlikely to develop problems. However, if a removable tissue-borne prosthesis is to be constructed on a ridge where an impacted tooth is covered by a millimeter or two of bone, it is highly likely that the overlying bone will be resorbed, perforation of the mucosa will occur, and the area will become painful and often infected. After the infection is resolved by surgical and medical treatment, the tooth will need to be removed and the dental prosthesis either dramatically altered or a new one made in its place.

Each individual situation must be viewed separately, and the risks and benefits of removal of the impacted tooth must be given careful consideration. In older patients with tooth- or implant-borne fixed prosthesis, asymptomatic deeply impacted teeth can be left in place. However, if a removable prosthesis is used and the overlying bone around the impacted tooth is thin, the teeth should generally be removed before the final prosthesis is constructed.

Prevention of Jaw Fracture

Patients who engage in contact sports, such as football, the martial arts, and some so-called noncontact sports such as basketball, should consider having their impacted third molars removed to prevent jaw fracture during competition. An impacted third molar presents an area of lowered resistance to fracture in the mandible and, therefore, is a common site for fracture. Additionally, the presence of an impacted third molar in the line of fracture may cause increased complications in the treatment of the fracture.

SUMMARY

The preceding discussion has dealt with the indications for removal of symptomatic impacted third molars. Most clinicians agree that should a patient present with one or more of the above pathologic problems or symptoms, the involved teeth should be removed. It is much less clear as to what should be done with teeth that are impacted before they cause these problems. Most of the symptomatic, pathologic problems that result from third molars occur as a result of a partially erupted tooth. There is a lower incidence of problems associated with a complete bony impaction.

Therefore, in making the decision as to whether or not a third molar should be removed, it is important to take into consideration a variety of factors. First, the available room in the arch into which the tooth can erupt: if such room exists, then the clinician may choose to defer the extraction until eruption is complete. The next consideration is the status of the impacted tooth and the age of the patient. It is important to remember that the average age of complete eruption is age 20, but that eruption can occur up to age 24. Teeth that appear to be mesioangular impactions at age 17 may eventually become more vertical in their angulation as they erupt into the mouth. If insufficient room exists to accommodate the tooth, and a soft tissue operculum exists over the posterior aspect of the tooth, then the sequelae discussed above are likely to occur. It is fairly well established at this point that the position of retained third molars will not change after age 25, and the incidence of symptomatic problems will be related primarily to whether or not they perforate the soft tissue.[14]

CONTRAINDICATIONS FOR REMOVAL OF IMPACTED TEETH

The decision to remove a given impacted tooth must be based on a careful evaluation of the potential benefits versus the potential risks. In situations in which pathology exists the decision to remove the tooth is uncomplicated, because it is necessary to remove the tooth to treat the disease process. Likewise, there are situations in which removal of impacted teeth will be contraindicated because the surgical complications and sequelae outweigh the potential benefits. The general contraindications for removal of impacted teeth can be grouped into three primary areas: patient's age and poor health and surgical damage to adjacent structure.[23]

Extremes of Age

Healing generally occurs more rapidly and more completely in younger patients; however, surgical removal of unerupted third molars in the very young is contraindicated. Although some clinicians report[77] that removal of the tooth bud of the developing third molar at age 8 or 9 can be accomplished with minimal surgical morbidity, the general consensus is that this is not a prudent procedure. The original view was based on the belief that accurate growth predictions could be made and, therefore, an accurate determination could be made of whether a given tooth would be impacted. If such a determination were to be the case, then the tooth bud could be removed relatively atraumatically in the very young patient. The evidence at this time, however, is contradictory to that opinion, and the general consensus is that removal of the tooth bud at this stage may, in fact, be unnecessary because the involved third molar may erupt into proper position.

As a patient becomes older, there is decreased healing response,[24] which may result in a greater bony defect postoperatively than was present because of the impacted tooth. Additionally, the surgical procedure grows more and more difficult as the patient ages owing to a more densely calcified bone, which is less flexible and more likely to fracture. As a patient ages, the response to the surgical insult is tolerated less easily, and the recuperation period increases in length. There is overwhelming clinical evidence to support the fact that the number of days missed from work and other normal activity following third molar extraction is much higher in the patient who is over age 40 as compared with patients under age 18.

As a general rule, if a patient has a fully impacted third molar, which is completely covered with bone, has no obvious potential source of communication with the oral cavity, and has no signs of pathology such as enlarged follicular sac, and if the patient is over age 40, the tooth probably should not be removed. Long-term follow-up by the patient's dentist should be performed periodically with a radiograph every several years to ensure that no adverse sequelae occur. If there are signs of pathology, or if the overlying bone is very thin and a removable denture is to be placed over that tooth, the tooth probably should be removed before the final prosthesis is constructed.

Compromised Medical Status

Patients who have impacted teeth may have some compromise in their health status, especially if they are older. As age increases, so does the incidence of moderate to severe cardiovascular disease, pulmonary disease, and other health problems. Thus, the combination of advanced age and compromised health status may contraindicate the removal of impacted teeth which have no pathologic processes.

Other factors may compromise the health status of younger people, such as congenital coagulopathies, asthma, and epilepsy. In this group of patients, it may be necessary to remove impacted teeth before the incipient pathologic process becomes fulminate. Thus, not only in the older compromised patient but also the younger compomised patient, the surgeon will occasionally need to remove symptomatic as well as asymptomatic third molars. The compromised medical status becomes a relative contraindication and may require the surgeon to work closely with the patient's physician to manage the patient's medical problems.

Surgical Damage to Adjacent Structures

Occasionally an impacted tooth is positioned such that its removal may seriously compromise adjacent nerves, teeth, and other vital structures, making it prudent to leave the impacted tooth in situ. The potential complications must be weighed against potential benefits of surgical removal of the tooth. When fully developed, totally bone-impacted third molars are present around the inferior alveolar nerve, it may be best to leave that impacted tooth in place and not risk permanent anesthesia of the alveolar nerve. In such situations, the potential risk of development of pathologic problems would be relatively small and, therefore, the advantage of removal of such a tooth would not outweigh the potential risks. Surgical extraction of impacted third molars that results in significant bony defects may not heal adequately in older patients and, in fact, may result in loss of adjacent teeth rather than improvement or preservation of periodontal health. This also would be viewed as a contraindiction to removal of the impacted tooth.

SURGERY AND PERIOPERATIVE CARE

Determining Surgical Difficulty

Preoperative evaluation of the third molar, both clinically and radiographically, is a critical step in the surgical procedure for removal of impacted teeth. The surgeon pays particular attention to the variety of factors known to make the impaction surgery more or less difficult.

A variety of classification systems have been developed to aid in the determination of difficulty. The three most widely used are angulation of the impacted tooth, the relationship of the impacted tooth to the anterior border of the ramus, and the depth of the impaction and the type of tissue overlying the impacted tooth. It is generally acknowledged that the mesioangular impaction, which accounts for approximately 45% of all impacted mandibular third molars, is the least difficult to remove. The vertical impaction (40% of all impactions) and the horizontal impaction (10%) are intermediate in difficulty, whereas the distoangular (5%) is the most difficult.

The relationship of the impacted tooth to the anterior border of the ramus is a reflection of the amount of room available for the tooth eruption as well as the extraction. If the length of the alveolar process anterior to the anterior border of the ramus is sufficient to allow tooth eruption, the tooth is generally less difficult to remove. Conversely, teeth that are essentially buried in the ramus of the mandible are more difficult to remove. The depth of the impaction under the hard and soft tissue is likewise felt to be an important consideration in determining degree of difficulty. This is the most commonly used factor in determining difficulty; that is, soft tissue, partial bony, and complete bony impaction.

In a recent study to determine which of the three classification systems has the greatest impact upon the degree of difficulty[25] found that the third system, depth of the impaction and type of overlying tissue, was the most predictable in determining the length of time for impaction surgery when timed by a stopwatch. Factors such as angulation of the impaction, relationship of the tooth to the anterior border of the ramus, and root morphology had little influence on the time that surgery would require.

Other factors have been implicated in making the extraction process more difficult. Root morphology can be either conical fused roots, or separate and divergent, with the latter being the more difficult. A large follicular sac around the crown of the tooth provides more room for access to the tooth, making it less difficult to extract than one with essentially no space around the crown of the tooth.

An overall important determinant of difficulty of extraction is the age of the patient. When impacted teeth are removed before age 20, the surgery is almost always less difficult to perform. The roots are usually incompletely formed, thus requiring less bone removal to remove them. There is usually a broader pericoronal space formed by the follicle of the tooth, thereby providing additional access for tooth extraction without bone removal. Because the roots of the impacted teeth are incompletely formed, they are usually separated from the inferior alveolar nerve. In contradistinction, removal of impacted teeth in patients of older age groups is almost always more difficult. The roots are usually completely formed and thus longer, which requires more bone removal, and closer to the inferior alveolar canal, which increases the risk of postsurgical anesthesia and paresthesia. The follicular sac with age almost always degenerates, which makes the pericoronal space thinner; as a result more bone must be removed for access to the crown of the tooth. Finally, there is increasing density and decreasing elasticity in the bone, thus requiring greater bone removal to deliver the tooth from its socket.

In summary, the degree of difficulty of the surgery to remove an impacted tooth is determined primarily by two major factors:

Depth of impaction and type of overlying tissue
Age of the patient

Full bony impactions are always more difficult to remove than soft tissue impactions and, given two impactions of the same depth, the impaction in the older patient would always be more difficult than the one in the younger patient.

A corollary of surgical difficulty is one of difficulty of recovery from the surgery. As a general rule, the more difficult and time-consuming the surgical procedure is, the more difficult and prolonged the postoperative recovery period. It is more difficult to perform surgery in the older individual, and it is more difficult for these patients to recover from the surgical procedure.

Technique of Surgery

The technique for removal of impacted third molars is one that must be learned on a theoretical basis and then performed repeatedly to gain adequate experience. There is more variety in presentation of the surgical situation of impacted third molars than in any other surgical procedure. Therefore, extensive experience is required to master the procedure of their removal. A large number of textbooks is available which describe the technique for removal of the different types of impactions.

In general, the approach must be one in which the surgeon gains adequate access to the underlying bone and tooth through a properly designed and reflected soft tissue flap. Bone must be removed in an atraumatic, aseptic, non-heat-producing technique, and as little bone removed and damaged as possible. The tooth is then divided into sections and delivered with elevators, using judicious amounts of force in order to prevent complications. Finally, the wound must be thoroughly debrided mechanically and by irrigation so as to provide the best possible healing environment in the postoperative period.

The initial step in removing impacted teeth is to reflect a mucoperiostal flap, which is adequate in size to permit access. The most commonly used flap is the envelope flap, which extends from just posterior to the position of the impacted tooth anteriorly to approximately the level of the first molar (Fig. 6–1A,B). If the surgeon requires greater access to remove a deeply impacted tooth, the envelope flap may not

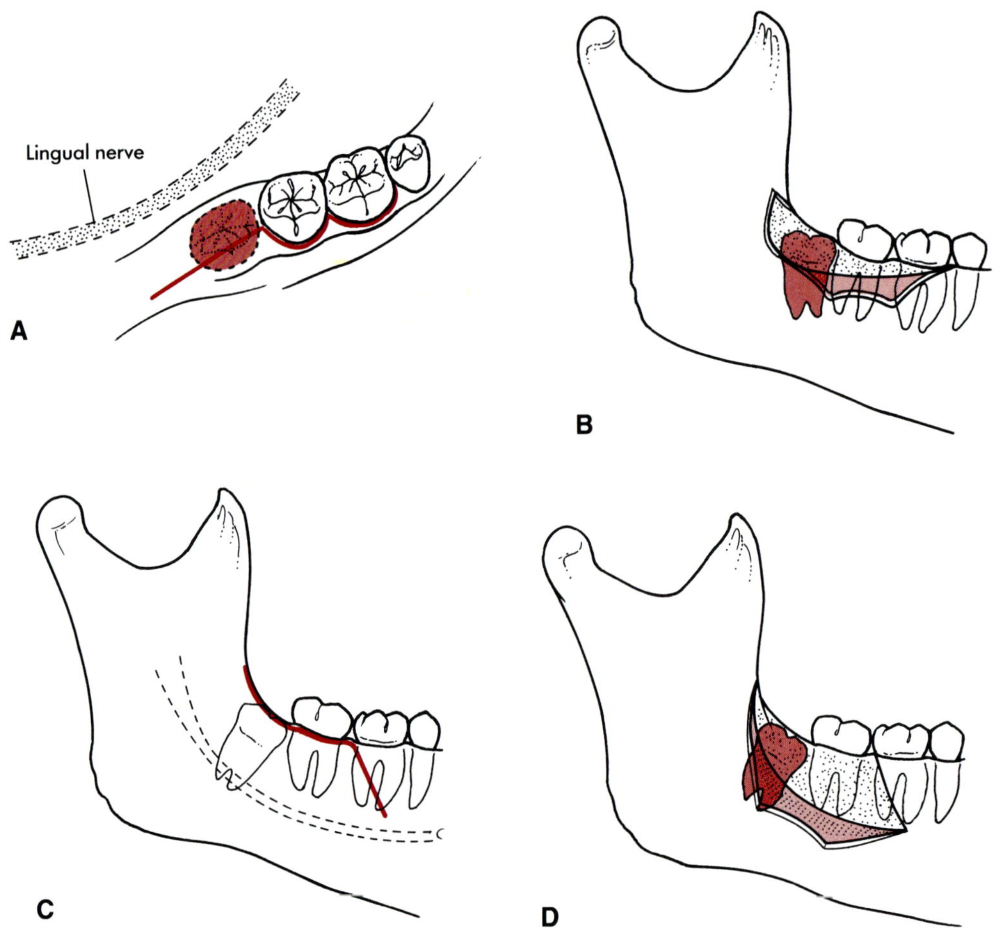

Figure 6–1. **(A)** *Envelope incision is most commonly used to reflect soft tissue of mandible for removal of impacted third molar. Posterior extension of incision should diverge laterally to avoid injury to lingual nerve.* **(B)** *Envelope incision is reflected laterally to expose bone overlying impacted tooth.* **(C)** *When three-cornered flap is made, release incision is made at mesial aspect of second molar.* **(D)** *When soft tissue flap is reflected by means of release incision, greater visibility is possible, especially at apical aspect of surgical field. (Peterson LJ, Ellis E III, Hupp JR, Tucker MR: Contemporary Oral and Maxillofacial Surgery. St. Louis, CV Mosby, 1988)*

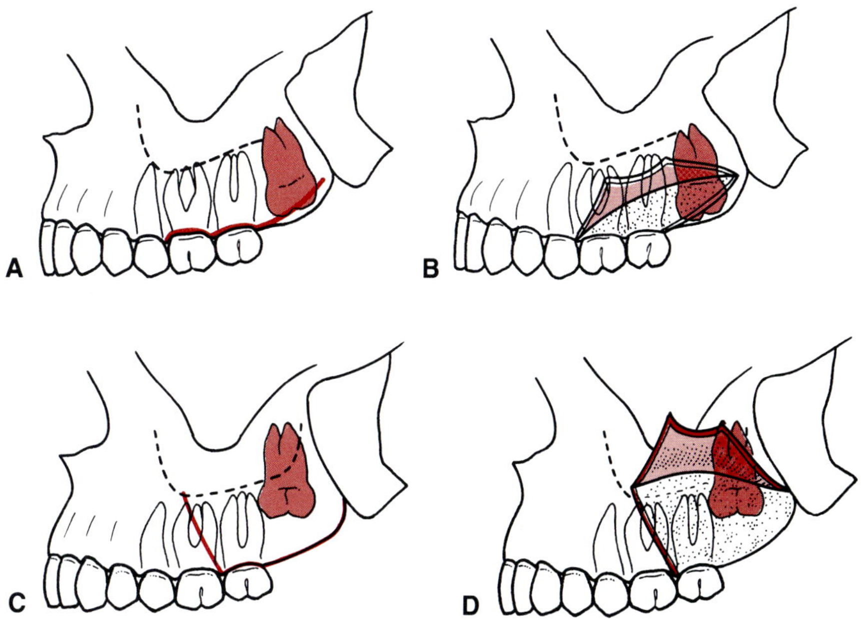

Figure 6–2. **(A)** *Envelope flap is the most commonly used flap for removal of maxillary impacted teeth.* **(B)** *When soft tissue is reflected, bone overlying third molar is easily visualized.* **(C)** *If tooth is deeply impacted, release incision can be used to gain greater access.* **(D)** *When three-cornered flap is reflected, there is greater visibility of bone's more apical portions. (Peterson LJ, Ellis E III, Hupp JR, Tucker MR: Contemporary Oral and Maxillofacial Surgery. St. Louis, CV Mosby, 1988)*

provide enough access. In that case, a release incision is done on the anterior aspect of the incision, creating a three-cornered flap (Fig. 6–1C,D). The envelope incision is usually associated with fewer complications and tends to heal more rapidly and with less pain than the three-cornered flap. A small artery, the buccal artery, is sometimes encountered when creating the releasing incision, and this may be mildly bothersome during the early portion of the surgery.

The posterior extension of the incision must extend to the lateral and up the anterior border of the mandible. The incision should not continue posteriorly in a straight line, because the mandible diverges laterally. If the incision were to be extended straight, the knife would enter the sublingual space and likely damage the lingual nerve. The mucoperiosteal flap is reflected laterally to the external oblique ridge with a periosteal elevator and held in this position with a retractor such as an Austin or Minnesota.

The most commonly used incision used for the maxillary third molar is also an envelope incision (Fig. 6–2A,B). It extends posteriorally from the distal buccal line angle of the second molar and anteriorally to the first molar. A releasing incision is rarely necessary for the maxillary third molar (Fig. 6–2C,D).

The second major step is to remove the bone from around the impacted tooth. Most surgeons use a high-speed, low-torque, air-driven handpiece, although a few surgeons still choose to use a chisel for bone removal. The most recent advance is the relatively high-speed, high-torque electric drill, which has some significant advantages in reducing the time required for bone removal and tooth sectioning. It is essential that the handpiece exhausts the air out of the surgical site to prevent emphysema or air embolism, and that the handpiece can be sterilized completely, usually in a steam autoclave.

The bone on the occlusal, buccal, and distal aspects of the impacted tooth is removed down to the cervical line. The amount of bone that needs to be removed will vary with the depth of the impaction. It is almost never necessary and is, in fact, advisable not to remove any bone on the lingual aspect because of the likelihood of damage to the lingual nerve (Fig. 6–3). A variety of burs can be used to remove bone, but the most commonly used are the number-8 round bur, and a 703 Fisher bur.

For maxillary teeth, bone removal is done primarily on the lateral aspect of the tooth down to the cervical line to expose the entire clinical crown. Frequently the bone on the buccal aspect is thin enough that it can be removed with a periosteal elevator or a chisel using hand pressure.

Once the tooth has been sufficiently exposed, it is sectioned into appropriate pieces so that it can be delivered from the socket. The direction in which the

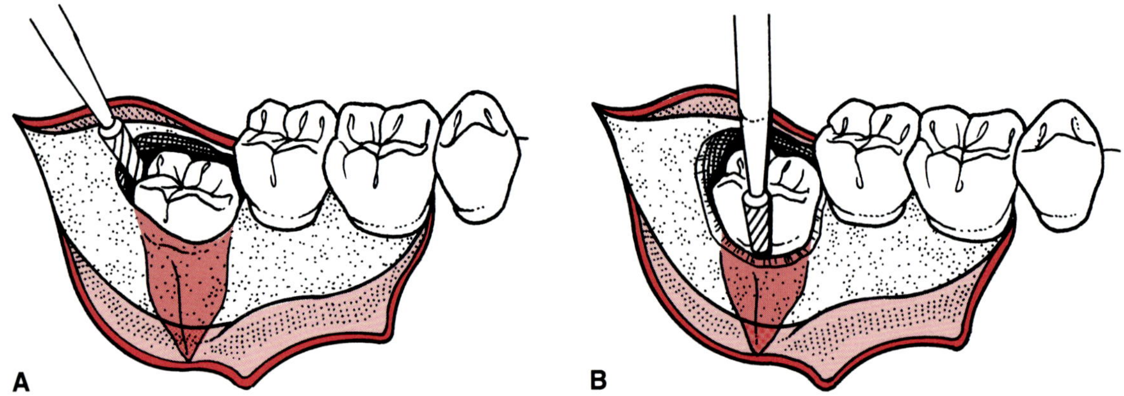

Figure 6–3. **(A)** *After soft tissue has been reflected, bone overlying occlusal surface of tooth is removed with a fissure bur.* **(B)** *Bone on buccal and distal aspect of impacted tooth is then removed with bur. (Peterson LJ, Ellis E III, Hupp JR, Tucker MR: Contemporary Oral and Maxillofacial Surgery. St. Louis, CV Mosby, 1988)*

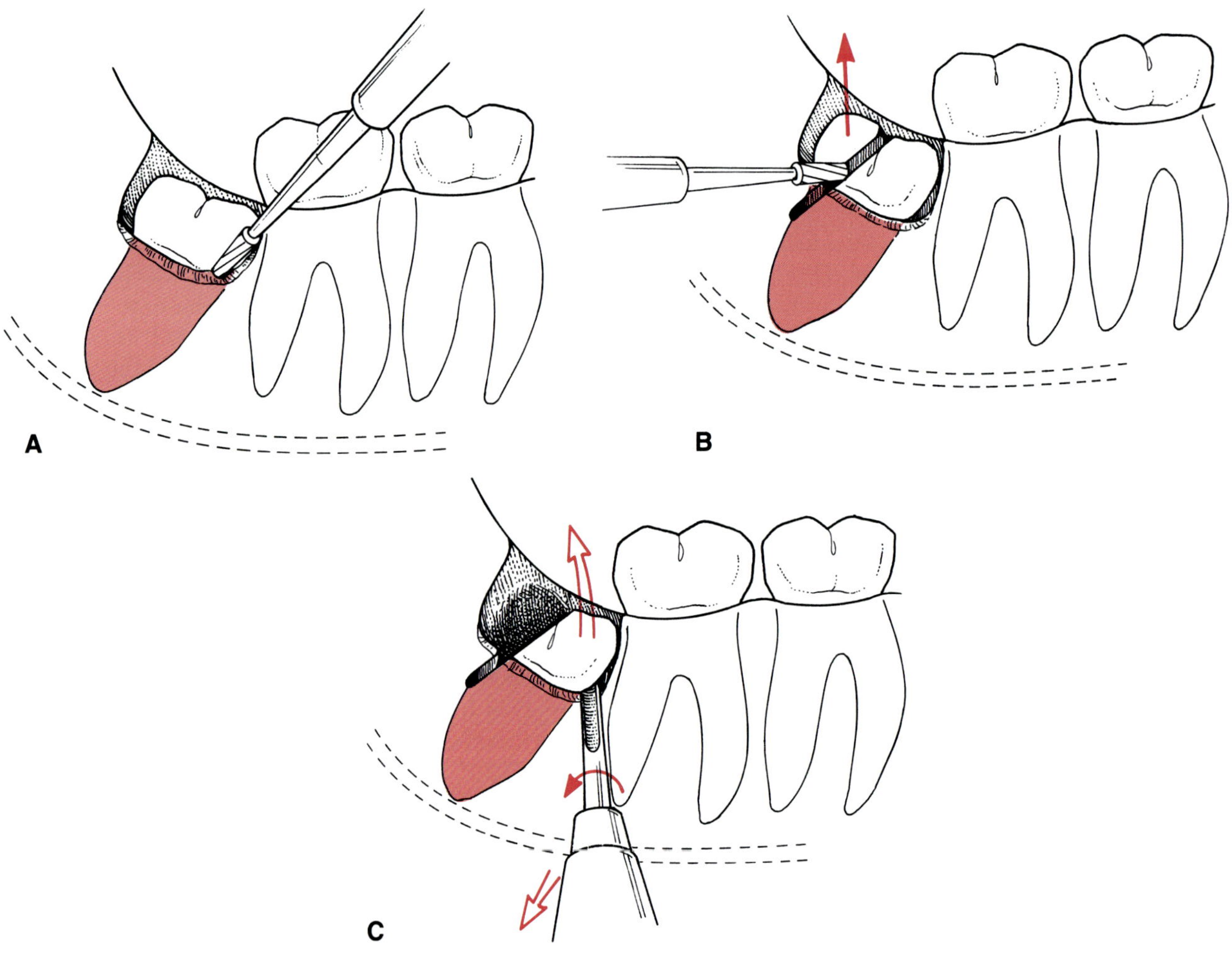

Figure 6–4. **(A)** *When removing mesioangular impaction, buccal and distal bone are removed to expose crown of tooth to cervical line.* **(B)** *Distal aspect of crown is then sectioned from tooth. Occasionally it is necessary to section entire tooth into two portions rather than to section distal portion of crown only.* **(C)** *After distal portion of crown has been delivered, small straight elevator is inserted into purchase point on mesial aspect of third molar, and tooth is delivered with rotational and lever motion of elevator. (Peterson LJ, Ellis E III, Hupp JR, Tucker MR. Contemporary Oral and Maxillofacial Surgery. St. Louis, CV Mosby, 1988)*

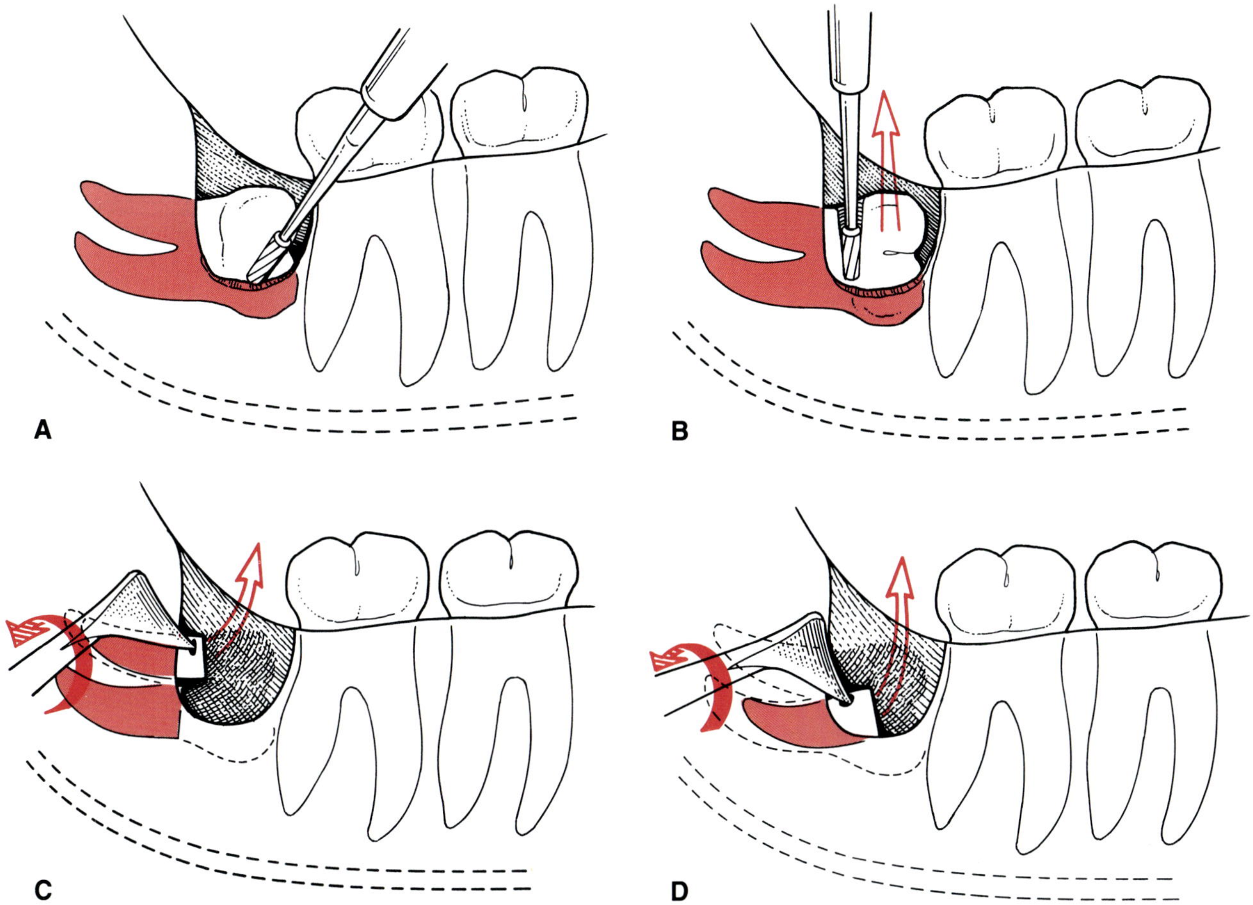

Figure 6–5. **(A)** *During removal of horizontal impaction, bone overlying tooth—that is, bone on distal and buccal aspect of tooth—is removed with bur.* **(B)** *Crown is sectioned from roots of tooth and delivered from socket.* **(C)** *Roots are delivered together or independently by Cryer's elevator used with rotational motion. Roots may need to be separated into two separate parts; occasionally, purchase point is made in root to allow Cryer's elevator to engage it.* **(D)** *Mesial root of tooth is elevated in similar fashion. (Peterson LJ, Ellis E III, Hupp JR, Tucker MR: Contemporary Oral and Maxillofacial Surgery. St. Louis, CV Mosby, 1988)*

impacted tooth is divided is dependent upon the angulation of the impaction. Tooth sectioning is performed either with a bur or chisel, but since the advent of high-speed drills, the bur is most commonly used because it provides a more predictable sectioning. The tooth is usually divided three quarters of the way through to the lingual aspect, and then split the remainder of the way with a straight elevator or similar instrument. This prevents injury to the lingual cortical plate and reduces the possibility of damage to the lingual nerve.

The mesioangular impaction is usually the least difficult to remove. After sufficient bone has been removed, the distal half of the crown is sectioned off from the buccal groove to just below the cervical line on the distal aspect of the tooth. This portion of the tooth is delivered, and the remainder of the tooth is delivered with a small straight elevator placed at a purchase point on the mesial aspect of the cervical line. An alternative is to prepare a purchase point in the tooth with the drill and use a crane pick or Cryer's elevator in the purchase point to deliver the tooth (Fig. 6–4).

The horizontal impaction usually requires removal of more bone than the mesioangular impaction. The crown of the tooth is usually sectioned from the roots and delivered with a Cryer's elevator. The roots are then displaced into the socket, which was previously occupied by the crown, and delivered into the mouth.

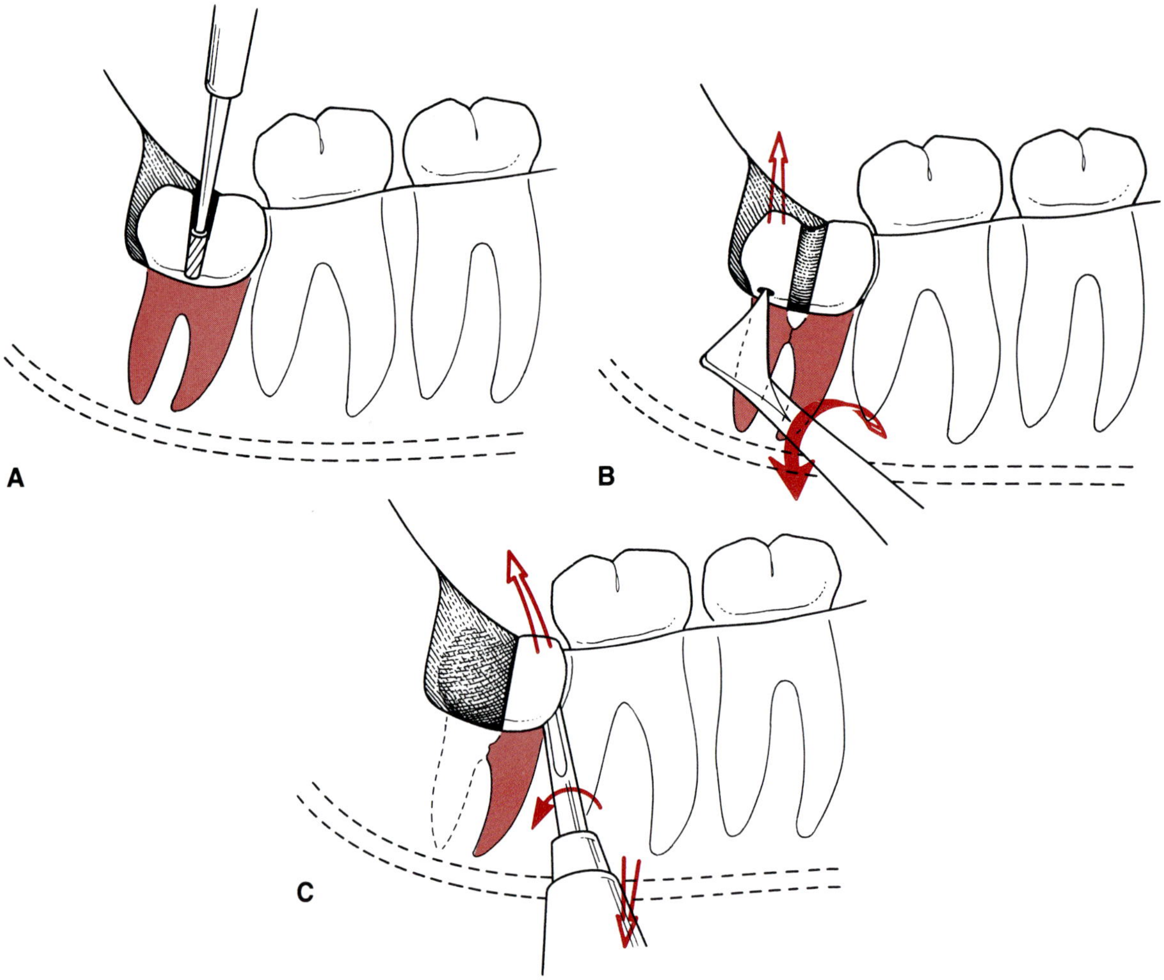

Figure 6–6. **(A)** *When removing vertical impaction, bone on occlusal, buccal, and distal aspects of crown is removed, and tooth is sectioned into mesial and distal sections. If tooth has a fused single root, distal portion of crown is sectioned off in manner similar to that depicted for mesioangular impaction.* **(B)** *Posterior aspect of crown is elevated first with a Cryer's elevator inserted into small purchase point in distal portion of tooth.* **(C)** *Small, straight number-301 elevator is then used to elevate mesial aspect of tooth by rotary and levering motion. (Peterson LJ, Ellis E III, Hupp JR, Tucker MR: Contemporary Oral and Maxillofacial Surgery. St. Louis, CV Mosby, 1988)*

Occasionally they may need to be sectioned into separate portions and delivered independently (Fig. 6–5).

The vertical impaction is one of the more difficult ones to remove if it is impacted very deeply. The procedure for bone removal and sectioning is similar to the mesioangular impaction in that occlusal, buccal, and distal bone are removed first. The distal half of the crown is sectioned and removed, and the tooth is elevated by applying a small straight elevator at the mesial aspect of the cervical line. The option of preparing a purchase point in the tooth is also frequently used, same as for the mesioangular impaction (Fig. 6–6).

The most difficult tooth to remove is the distoangular impaction. After removal of bone, the crown is usually sectioned from the roots just above the cervical line and delivered with a Cryer's elevator. A purchase point is then prepared in the tooth and the roots delivered together or sectioned and delivered independently with a Cryer's elevator (Fig. 6–7). Extraction of this impaction is more difficult than the others because more distal bone must be removed, and the

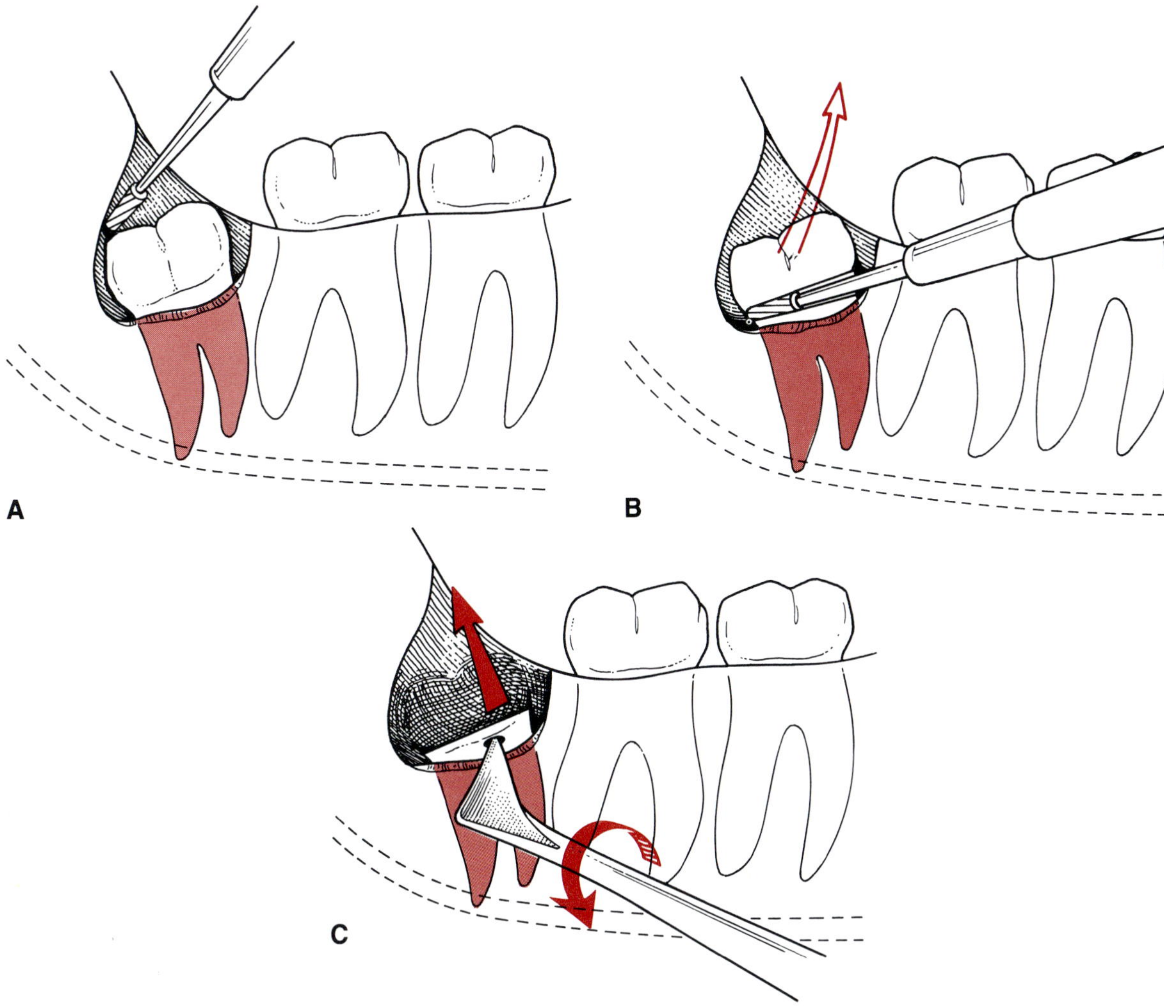

Figure 6–7. **(A)** *For distoangular impaction the occlusal, buccal, and distal bone is removed with a bur. It is important to remember that more distal bone must be taken off than for vertical or mesioangular impaction.* **(B)** *Crown of tooth is sectioned off with bur, and crown is delivered with straight elevator.* **(C)** *Purchase point is put into remaining root portion of tooth, and roots are delivered by Cryer's elevator with wheel-and-axle motion. If roots diverge, it may be necessary in some cases to split them into independent portions. (Peterson LJ, Ellis E III, Hupp JR, Tucker MR: Contemporary Oral and Maxillofacial Surgery. St. Louis, CV Mosby, 1988)*

tooth tends to be elevated posteriorally into the ramus portion of the mandible.

Impacted maxillary third molars are rarely sectioned because the overlying bone is thin and relatively elastic. In patients with thicker bone, the extraction is usually accomplished by removing additional bone rather than by sectioning the tooth. The tooth should never be sectioned with a chisel, because the tooth may be displaced into the maxillary sinus or infratemporal fossa when it is struck with the chisel (Fig. 6–8).

Once the impacted tooth is delivered from the alveolar process, the surgeon must pay strict attention to debriding the wound of all particular bone chips and other debris. The best way to accomplish this is to mechanically debride the socket and the area under the flap with a periapical curet. A bone file should be used to smooth any rough, sharp edges of the bone. A mosquito hemostat is usually used to remove any remnant of the dental follicle. Finally, the socket and wound should be thoroughly irrigated with saline or sterile water (30 to 50 mL is optimal).[26] Within certain

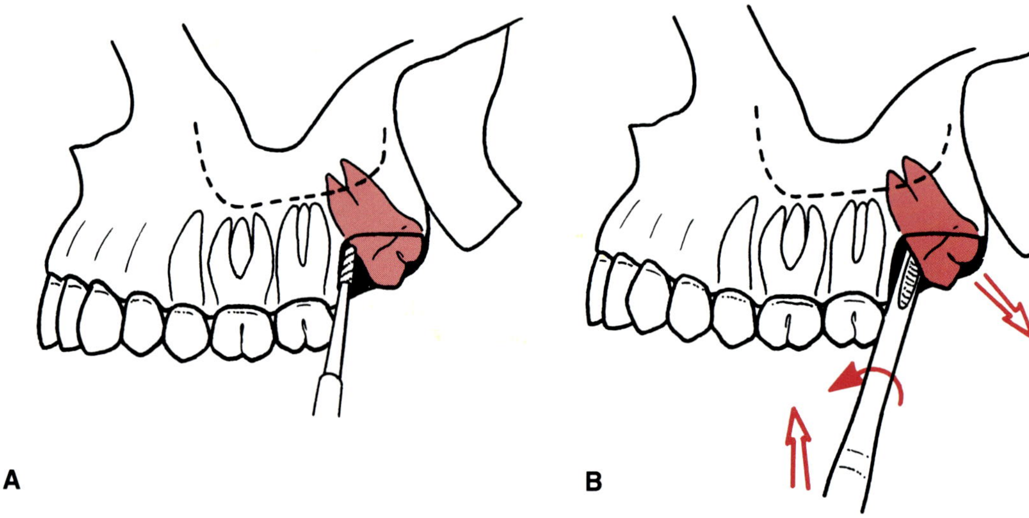

Figure 6–8. *Delivery of impacted maxillary third molar.* **(A)** *Once soft tissue has been reflected, a small amount of buccal bone is removed with a bur or a hand chisel.* **(B)** *Tooth is then delivered by a small straight elevator with rotational and lever types of motion. Tooth is delivered in the distobuccal and occlusal direction. (Peterson LJ, Ellis E III, Hupp JR, Tucker MR: Contemporary Oral and Maxillofacial Surgery. St. Louis, CV Mosby, 1988)*

limitations, the more irrigation that is used, the less likely the patient is to have a dry socket, delayed healing, or other complications.

The incision should usually be closed by primary intention. The flap is returned to its original position and the initial suture placed at the posterior aspect of the second molar. Additional sutures are placed as necessary.

Use of Perioperative Systemic Antibiotics

One of the primary goals of the surgeon in performing any surgical procedure is to prevent postoperative infection as a result of surgery. To achieve this goal, prophylactic antibiotics are necessary in some surgical procedures. Most of these procedures fall into the clean/contaminated, or contaminated categories of surgery. The incidence of postoperative infections in a clean surgery is related more to operator technique than to the use of prophylactic antibiotics.

Surgery for the removal of impacted third molars clearly fits into the category of clean/contaminated surgery; however, the exact incidence of postoperative infection is unknown. In the usual sense of the word, infection probably is a rare occurrence following third molar surgery. This means that it would be unusual to see pain, swelling, and pus production, which requires incision and drainage or antibiotic therapy to treat. The incidence of such infections is probably less than 2% for most surgeons. In general, an excellent surgeon would expect to have an infection rate in the range of 2% to 3%. It is difficult, and probably impossible, to reduce infection rates below 3% with the use of prophylactic antibiotics. Therefore, it is unnecessary to use prophylactic antibiotics in third molar surgery to prevent postoperative infections in the normal healthy patient. Although the literature contains many papers that discuss the use of prophylactic perioperative antibiotics, there is essentially no report of their usefulness in prevention of infection following third molar surgery.[27,28]

A more subtle type of wound healing problem that occurs after the surgical removal of the impacted mandibular third molar is so-called alveolar osteitis or dry socket. This disturbance in wound healing is most likely caused by the combination of saliva and anaerobic bacteria. The use of prophylactic antibiotics in third molar surgery does, in fact, reduce the incidence of dry socket. Other techniques that reduce bacterial contamination of the socket, such as copious irrigation, preoperative rinses with chlorhexidine, and placement of antibiotics in the extraction socket, are also effective.[28–36] Once again, the issue of risks versus benefits becomes important. Although systemic antibiotics are effective in the reduction of postoperative dry socket, they are no more effective than local nonsystemic measures. The increase of antibiotic-related complications such as allergy, resistant bacteria, gastrointestinal side effects, and secondary infections are not outweighed by the benefits. Therefore, the use of perioperative systemic antibiotic administration does not seem to be valid.

Use of Perioperative Steroids

Just as the oral and maxillofacial surgeon desires to minimize the use of infection following third molar surgery, he or she also has a major interest in reducing the perioperative morbidity. The use of corticosteroids to help minimize swellng, trismus, and pain has gained wide acceptance in the oral and maxillofacial surgery community. The method of usage, however, is extremely variable, and which is most effective has yet to be clearly delineated.

There is little doubt that an initial intravenous dose of steroid at the time of surgery has a major clinical impact on swelling and trismus in the early postoperative period. However, if the initial intravenous dose is not followed up with additional doses of steroids, this early advantage disappears by the second or third postoperative day. Maximum control of swelling requires that additional steroids be given for 1 or 2 days following surgery. The two most widely used steroids are dexamethasone and methylprednisolone. Both of these are almost pure glucocorticoids, with little mineralocorticoid effect. Additionally, these two appear to have the least depressing effect on leukocyte chemotaxis. Common dosages of dexamethasone are 4 to 12 mg given intravenously at the time of surgery. Additional oral dosages of 4 to 8 mg twice a day for the day of surgery and two days afterwards leads to the maximum relief of swelling, trismus, and pain. Methylprednisolone is most commonly given intravenously 125 mg at the time of surgery followed by significantly lower doses, usually 40 mg three or four times daily taken orally for the day of surgery and for two days after surgery.

High-dose, short-term steroid usage is associated with minimal side effects. They are contraindicated in the patient with gastric ulcer disease, active infection, and certain types of psychosis. The administration of perioperative steroids may increase the incidence of alveolar osteitis after the third molar surgery, but the data is lacking as to the precise degree of increase.[37–41]

COMPLICATIONS OF IMPACTION SURGERY

Surgical removal of impacted third molars is associated with a moderate incidence of complications, around 10%.[42,43] These complications range from the expected and predictable ones such as swelling, pain, trismus, and mild bleeding to more severe and permanent complications such as inferior alveolar nerve anesthesia and fracture of the mandible. The overall incidence of complication and the severity of these complications are associated most directly with the depth of impaction, that is, whether it is a complete bony impaction or not, and to the age of the patient.[44–46] Because of factors already discussed, removal of impacted teeth in the older patient is associated with a higher incidence of postoperative complications, especially alveolar osteitis, infections, and inferior alveolar nerve anesthesia. The removal of complete bony impactions is likewise associated with increased postoperative pain and morbidity and an increase in the incidence of inferior alveolar nerve anesthesia.

Another determinant of the incidence of complications of third molar surgery is the relative experience and training of the surgeon. The less experienced surgeon will have significantly higher incidence of complications than the trained, experienced surgeon.[1,2]

Common Postsurgical Sequelae

After the surgical removal of an impacted third molar, certain normal physiologic responses will occur. These include such things as mild bleeding, swelling, trismus, and pain. All of these are interpreted by the patient as being unpleasant and, therefore, they should be minimized as much as possible.

Bleeding can be minimized by using good surgical technique and by avoiding tearing of flaps or excessive trauma to the overlying soft tissue. When a vessel is cut the bleeding should be stopped in order to prevent secondary hemorrhage after the patient leaves the office. The most effective way to achieve hemostasis following surgery is the application of a moist gauze pack directly over the site of the surgery with adequate pressure. This is usually done by having the patient bite down on a moist gauze pad. In some patients, immediate postoperative hemostasis is difficult. In situations such as this, a variety of techniques can be employed to help secure hemostasis, including oversuturing and application of topical thrombin on a small piece of absorbable gelatin sponge (Gelfoam) into the extraction socket. The socket can also be packed with oxidized cellulose (Oxycel or Surgicel). Unlike the gelatin sponge, oxidized cellulose can be packed into the socket under pressure. In some situations, microfibriller collagen (Avitene) can be used to promote platelet plug formation. Patients who have known acquired or congenital coagulopathies will require extensive preparation and preoperative planning before third molars are removed surgically.

Postsurgical edema or swelling is an expected sequela of third molar surgery. As discussed earlier, the parenteral administration of corticosteroids is frequently employed to help minimize the swelling which occurs. The application of ice packs to the face may make the patient feel more comfortable but has no effect on the size of swelling.[47] The swelling usually reaches its maximum by the end of the second postoperative day and is usually resolved by the fifth to seventh day.

Trismus, or inability to open the mouth the normal amount, is also a normal and expected morbidity of third molar surgery. Patients who are given steroids for the control of edema, also tend to have less trismus.[38–40] Trismus usually reaches its maximum on the second day and resolves by the end of the first week.

Another postsurgical morbidity expected with third molar surgery is pain. The postsurgical pain begins when the effects of the local anesthesia subside and reaches its maximum intensity during the first 12 hours postoperatively.[48] Pain which requires analgesics for control rarely extends beyond 48 hours.[49] A large variety of analgesics is available for management of postsurgical pain. The most common ones are combinations of aspirin or acetaminophen with codeine and its congeners, and the nonsteroidal antiinflammatory analgesics. Women appear to be more sensitive to postoperative pain than men,[49,50] and will generally require more analgesics than men. Analgesics should be given before the effect of the local anesthesia subsides. That way the pain is usually easier to control, requires less drug, and may require a less potent analgesic. Administration of nonsteroidal analgesics before surgery may be beneficial in aiding in the control of postoperative pain.

The most important determinant of the amount of postoperative pain that will occur is the length of the operation,[51] but neither swelling nor trismus correlates with the length of time of the surgery. There is a strong correlation between postoperative pain and trismus, indicating that pain may be one of the principle reasons for limitation of opening after the removal of impacted third molars.[51]

A common postsurgical complication related to the surgical removal of impacted third molars is infection. The incidence of infection following the removal of third molars is very low, ranging from 1.7% to 2.7%.[52] Infections after removal of mandibular third molars is almost always a minor complication. About 50% of them are the localized, subperiosteal abscess type infections, which occur 2 to 4 weeks after a previously uneventful postoperative course. These are usually attributed to debris which is left under the mucoperiosteal flap, and are easily treated by surgical drainage. Of the remaining 50%, rarely is the postoperative infection sufficient to warrant surgery, antibiotics, and hospitalization. Infections occur in the first postoperative week after third molar surgery approximately 0.5% to 1% of the time. This is a very desirable infection rate, and cannot be lowered by the administration of prophylactic antibiotics.

One of the most frequent problems encountered in removing third molars is fracture of a portion of the root, which may be difficult to retrieve. In these situations, the root fragment may be displaced into the submandibular space, into the inferior alveolar canal, or into the maxillary sinus. Uninfected roots left within the alveolar bone have been shown to remain in place without postoperative complications.[53] The pulpal tissues undergo fibrosis, and the root becomes totally incorporated within the alveolar bone. Aggressive and destructive attempts to remove portions of roots that are in precarious positions seem to be unwarranted and may cause more damage than benefit.

Alveolar Osteitis

The incidence of alveolar osteitis or dry socket following the removal of impacted mandibular third molars varies between 3% and 25%. Most of the variation is most likely a result of the definition of the syndrome.

When dry socket is defined in terms of pain that requires the patient to return to the office, the incidence is probably in the range of 20% to 25%.

The pathogenesis of alveolar osteitis has not been absolutely defined but is most likely the result of lysis of a fully formed blood clot before the clot is replaced with granulation tissue. This fibrinolysis occurs during the third and fourth day and results in symptoms of pain and malodor after the third day or so following extraction. The source of the fibrinolytic agents may be from tissue, saliva, or bacteria.[54] The role of bacteria in this process can be confirmed empirically based on the fact that systemic and topical antibiotic prophylaxis reduces the incidence of dry socket by approximately 50% to 75%.

The incidence of dry socket seems to be higher in patients who smoke cigarettes[55,56] and in female patients who take oral contraceptives.[52] Its occurrence can be reduced by several techniques, most of which are aimed at reducing the bacterial contamination of the surgical site. Presurgical irrigation with antimicrobial agents, such as chlorhexadine, reduces the incidence of dry socket by up to 50%.[2] Copious irrigation of the surgical site with large volumes of saline is also effective in reducing dry socket.[26] Placing small amounts of antibiotics such as tetracycline or lincomycin also curbs the incidence of alveolar osteitis.[57–60]

The goal of treatment of dry socket is to relieve the patient's pain during the delayed healing process. This is usually accomplished by irrigation of the socket which is involved, very gentle mechanical debridement, and placement of an obtundent dressing, which usually contains eugenol. The dressing may need to be changed on a daily basis for several days and then less frequently after that. The pain syndrome usually resolves within 3 to 5 days, although it may take as long as 10 to 14 days in some patients. There is some evidence that topical antibiotics, such as metronidazole, may hasten resolution of the dry socket.[61]

In summary, alveolar osteitis is a disturbance in healing that occurs after the formation of a mature blood clot but before the blood clot is replaced with granulation tissue. The primary etiology appears to be one of excess fibrinolysis, with bacteria playing an important but yet ill-defined role. Antimicrobial agents delivered by perioperative mouth rinses, topically placed in the socket, or administered systemically all help to reduce the incidence of dry socket. Mechanical debridement and copious saline irrigation of the surgical wound also are effective in reducing the incidence of dry socket. A rational approach may be to provide preoperative chlorhexadine rinses for approximately 1 week before surgery, irrigate the wound thoroughly with normal saline at the conclusion of surgery, place a small square of gelatin sponge saturated in tetracycline in the socket, and continue chlorhexidine rinses for 1 additional week. This combination approach would reduce the incidence of dry socket to a level of 1% to 2%.

Nerve Disturbances

Surgical removal of mandibular third molars places both the lingual and inferior alveolar branches of the third division of the trigeminal nerve at risk for injury. The lingual nerve is most often injured during soft tissue flap reflection, whereas the inferior alveolar nerve is injured when the roots of the teeth are manipulated and elevated from the socket. The generally accepted incidence of injury to the inferior alveolar and lingual nerve following third molar surgery is about 3%, although it has been reported as high as 11.5% for the lingual nerve.[42–45,62–64] Only a small proportion of these anesthesia and paraesthesia problems remain permanent. However, there is a significant incidence of some minor alterations and sensation after injury caused by third molar surgery. As many as 45% of nerve compression injuries, which are typical in third molar surgery, result in a permanent sensory abnormality.[65]

Inferior alveolar nerve injury is most likely to occur in specific situations. The first and most commonly reported predisposing factor is complete bony impaction of mandibular third molars. The angulation classification most commonly involved is usually mesioangular or vertical impaction. Radiographic signs that indicate that the involved third molar is intimately associated with the canal are diversion of the path of the canal by the tooth, darkening of the apical end of the root indicating that it is included within the canal, and interruption of the radiopaque white line of the canal.[66] When these signs are noted on preoperative evaluation of the radiograph, the surgeon should take extraordinary precautions, such as extra bone removal or sectioning the tooth into extra pieces, to avoid injury to the nerve. Special efforts should be made to ensure that patient education is in order and that informed consent is obtained.

When an injury to the lingual or inferior alveolar

nerve is diagnosed in the postoperative period, the surgeon should begin long-term planning for its management. These issues are dealt with elsewhere in this book.

Miscellaneous Complications

The complications already discussed are the common ones, which account for more than 90% of the complications in surgery to remove impacted third molars. Several additional complications occur only very rarely, and will be mentioned only in passing.

Maxillary third molars that are highly positioned may have only thin layers of bone posteriorly separating them from the infratemporal fossa, or anteriorly separating them from the maxillary sinus. Small amounts of pressure in slightly wrong directions can result in displacement of maxillary third molars into these spaces. When a maxillary third molar is displaced posteriorly into the intratemporal fossa, the surgeon should try to manipulate the tooth back into the socket with finger pressure placed high in the buccal vestibule near the pterygoid plates. If this is unsuccessful, the surgeon can attempt to recover the tooth by placing the suction tip into the socket and towards the posterior. If both of these maneuvers are unsuccessful in recovering the tooth, the most effective technique is to allow the tooth to undergo fibrosis and to return 2 to 4 weeks later to remove it. If the tooth is totally asymptomatic, is not causing any restriction in jaw movement, and is not causing pain, the surgeon should consider leaving the tooth in place. If the decision is made to remove the tooth, three-dimensional localization of the tooth should be made before surgery is initiated. If the tooth is displaced into the maxillary sinus, retrieval is usually done by a Caldwell-Luc procedure at the same appointment. The surgeon should localize the tooth with at least a one-dimensional and preferably a three-dimensional radiograph before performing the retrieval surgery.[67]

Fracture of the mandible during removal of impacted mandibular third molars is a rare occurrence. The typical situation is a deeply impacted third molar, most commonly in an older individual with dense bone. The surgeon places excessive pressure on the tooth with an elevator in an attempt to deliver the tooth or tooth section into the mouth; fracture occurs, and the remaining portion of the tooth is easily retrieved. The surgeon then should perform an immediate reduction and fixation of the fracture. If the surgeon has the experience and the armamentarium available, rigid internal fixation with miniplates is an excellent choice in this unfortunate situation. Wire fixation and application of intermaxillary fixation is an acceptable alternative.

PERIODONTAL HEALING AFTER THIRD MOLAR SURGERY

One of the important reasons for removing impacted third molars is to preserve periodontal health, or in some situations to treat a periodontitis which is already in existence.[13] A relative contraindication to the removal of impacted third molars is a situation in which there is good periodontal health and a complete bony impaction in an older patient. Removal would be contraindicated because the healing response in older patients would most likely result in a postsurgical defect that was greater than the presurgical one.

Much attention has been given to the two parameters of periodontal health following third molar surgery, those of bone height on the distal aspect of the second molar, and attachment level and pocket depth also on the distal aspect of the second molar. In applying these two parameters to the example given, several important factors must be taken into consideration. First is whether the impacted third molar is a complete bony impaction or a partial impaction. In partial impaction, there are already a periodontal pocket on the distal aspect of the third molar and an osteal defect in the bone on the distal root of the second molar. Potentially rapid periodontal destruction is risked by retention of the third molar. The postoperative measurement of the bone will show both lower bone level and deeper pocket depths than would be desirable. Therefore, careful comparisons of preoperative measurements with postoperative measurements are essential in determining the effect of the removal of the impacted tooth.

Also of importance is the separation of patients into groups by ages. Patients age 19 and younger are usually grouped together, as are ages 20 to 35 and older than 35. Because the healing response is potentially different for these age groups[24] it is important that their individual responses to surgery be noted.

The bone height after third molar surgery in most situations remains at the preoperative level,[68–70] although some studies have indicated net gain in bone level after surgery.[71] If the bone level on the distal aspect of the mandibular second molar is compromised by the presence of the third molar, it will usually remain at that level following healing of the bone. There is universal agreement that bone healing will be better if surgery is done before the third molar resorbs the bone on the distal aspect of the second molar and while the patient is young.[70–75] The greatest bony defect will occur in situations in which the third molar has resorbed extensive amounts of bone from the second molar, in an older patient, which compromises bony repair and bone healing.

The other periodontal parameter of importance is attachment level or, less accurately, sulcus or pocket depth. As with bone levels, if the preoperative pocket depth is great, the postoperative pocket depth is also likely to be deep. In most studies, the attachment level has been found to be at essentially the same level as preoperatively.[68,74,75] In older patients with complete bony impactions, pocket depth and attachment levels may be significantly poorer than preoperatively. However, in patients younger than age 19 even removal of complete bony impactions results in no compromise in attachment level or pocket depth. Initial healing after third molar surgery usually results in reduction in pocket depth in young patients.[70] The long-term healing in this group continues for up to 4 years after surgery, with continuing reduction in probable pocket depths.[73] However, long-term follow-up of older patients clearly demonstrates that this long-term healing does not occur.[71,73]

Periodontal healing following third molar surgery is clearly best when the impacted tooth is removed before it becomes exposed in the mouth, before it resorbs bone on the distal aspect of the second molar, and when the patient is as young as possible.[68–75] If the third molar is partially impacted and is partially exposed in the mouth, it should be removed as soon as possible. The reason for this is that there is already a deep and potentially destructive periodontal lesion which is impossible for the patient to clean. Even if the patient is asymptomatic, the impacted tooth should be removed as soon as possible to allow the best periodontal healing after surgery as possible. In these situations the periodontal healing will be compromised because of the fact that there was already a destructive lesion caused by the presence of the partially impacted third molar.

The completely impacted third molar in a patient older than age 35 should probably be left intact unless some pathology develops. Removal of asymptomatic, completely impacted third molars in these older patients will result in pocket depths that are significantly greater and potential loss of alveolar bone on the posterior aspect of the second molar.

SUMMARY

The issue of whether to remove impacted third molars has generated much controversy over the last two decades. The reason for this controversy has been the lack of long-term prospective studies which have followed large groups of patients with impacted teeth to determine the eventual outcome of leaving impactions in situ. During the 1980s, a large number of papers appeared that have helped to clarify some of the issues concerning third molars. For example, only an extremely small percentage of third molars that are left in place actually form cysts or tumors. Therefore, prevention of cysts and tumors becomes almost a nonreason for removal of asymptomatic third molars.

It is also clear that mandibular third molars will continue to erupt beyond age 18 or 20, frequently continuing in their migration until age 24 or 25. However, in the vast majority of these situations there will be a soft tissue or bone tissue flap over the distal aspect of the erupted third molar, which has the great potential to cause pericoronitis. In fact, the tooth which is most likely to be involved in pericoronitis is the erupted, vertically positioned third molar with a soft tissue flap over the posterior. Although most attempts at very early prediction of impaction and removal of tooth buds at age 8 or 9 have now been generally abandoned, it is reasonably possible that by age 17 or 18 the dentist and surgeon can reasonably predict whether there will be adequate room for the tooth to erupt with sufficient clearance of the anterior ramus to prevent soft tissue overhangs (as in patients with large jaws and relatively small teeth). Likewise, patients who have had premolar extractions for orthodontics may also have sufficient room for the third molars to erupt into a functional occlusion without distal soft tissue excess.[6]

Soft tissue and bone tissue healing will occur at its

maximum level if the surgery to remove impacted third molars is done as early possible. By age 17, if the diagnosis of inadequate room for functional eruption can be made, then the asymptomatic third molar should be removed. Even though the tooth may be completely covered with soft and hard tissue, the periodontal health of the second molar will be maximized by removing the third molar at that time. The application of the principle of decision analysis to the extraction of asymptomatic third molars has been attempted.[76] Early efforts have been interesting, but the data are insufficient to provide accurate values for the various branches of the algorithm. As more and more information is gathered through intermediate and long-term studies, decision analysis concepts will undoubtedly play a role in formulating the best treatments for asymptomatic molars.

REFERENCES

1. Sisk AL, Hammer WB, Shelton DW, Joy ED Jr. Complications following removal of impacted third molars: the role of the experience of the surgeon. J Oral Maxillofac Surg 1986; 44(11): 855.
2. Larsen PE. The effect of a 0.12% chlorhexidine rinse on the incident of alveolar osteitis following the surgical removal of impacted mandibular third molars. J Oral Maxillofac Surg (in press).
3. Rantanen AV. The age of eruption of the third molar teeth. Acta Odontol Scand 1967; 25(Suppl): 48.
4. Engstrom C, Engstrom H, Sagne S. Lower third molar development in relation to skeletal maturity and chronological age. Angle Orthod 1983; 53(2): 97.
5. Richardson ER, Malhotra SK, Semenya K. Longitudinal study of three views of mandibular third molar eruption in males. Am J Orthod 1984; 86(2): 119.
6. Richardson ME. The effect of mandibular first premolar extraction on third molar space. Angle Orthod 1989; 59(4): 291.
7. Richardson ME. Pre-eruptive movements of the mandibular third molar. Angle Orthod 1978; 48(3): 187.
8. Ng F, Burns M, Kerr WJS. The impacted lower third molar and its relationship to tooth size and arch form. Eur J Orthod 1986; 8:254.
9. Forsberg CM. Tooth size, spacing, and crowding in relation to eruption or impaction of third molars. Am J Orthod Dentofacial Orthop 1988; 94(1): 57.
10. Heimdahl A, Nord CE. Treatment of orofacial infections of odontogenic origin. Scand J Infect Dis 1985; 46(Suppl): 101.
11. Van Winkelhoff AJ, Carlee AW, deGraaff J. Bacteroides endodontalis and other black-pigmented bacteroides species in odontogenic abscesses. Infect Immun 1985; 49:494.
12. Mombelli A, Buser D, Lang NP, Berthold H. Suspected periodontopathogens in erupting third molar sites of periodontally healthy individuals. J Clin Periodontol 1990; 17:48.
13. Leone SA, Edenfield MJ, Cohen ME. Correlation of acute pericoronitis and the position of the mandibular third molar. Oral Surg 1986; 62(3): 245.
14. Lysell L, Rohlin M. A study of indications used for removal of the mandibular third molar. Int J Oral Maxillofac Surg 1988; 17:161.
15. Nordenram A, Hultin M, Kjellman O, Ramstrom G. Indications for surgical removal of the mandibular third molar. Swed Dent J 1987; 2:23.
16. Stanley HR, Alattar M, Collett WE, Stringfellow HR Jr, Spiegel EH. Pathological sequelae of "neglected" impacted third molars. J Oral Pathol 1988; 17:113.
17. von Wowern N, Nielsen HO. The fate of impacted lower third molars after the age of 20. Int J Oral Maxillofac Surg 1989; 18:277.
18. Schroeder DC, Cecil JC III, Cohen ME. Retention and extraction of third molars in naval personnel. Milit Med 1983; 148(1): 50.
19. Ades AG, Joondeph DR, Little RM, Chapko MK. A long-term study of the relationship of third molars to changes in the mandibular dental arch. Am J Orthod Dentofac Orthop 1990; 97(4): 323.
20. Bishara SE, Andreasen G. Third molars: a review. Am J Orthod 1983; 83(2): 131.
21. Richardson ME. The role of the third molar in the cause of late lower arch crowding: a review. Am J Orthod Dentofac Orthop 1989; 95:79.
22. Nitzan D, Keren T, Marmary Y. Does an impacted tooth cause root resorption of the adjacent one? Oral Surg 1981; 51(3): 221.
23. Peterson LJ. Principles of management of impacted teeth. In: Peterson LJ, ed. Contemporary Oral and Maxillofacial Surgery. St Louis: CV Mosby, 1988:223.
24. Amler MH. The age factor in human extraction wound healing. J Oral Surg 1977; 35:193.
25. Larsen PE, Mesieha ZS, Peterson LJ, Beck FM. Impacted third molars: radiographic features used to predict extraction difficulty. J Dent Res 1991; 70:551.
26. Sweet JB, Butler DP, Drager JL. Effects of lavage techniques with third molar surgery. Oral Surg 1976; 42(2): 152.
27. Happonen RP, Backstrom AC, Ylipaavalniemi P. Prophylactic use of phenoxymethylpenicillin and tinidazole in mandibular third molar surgery, a comparative placebo controlled clinical trial. Br J Oral Maxillofac Surg 1990; 28:12.
28. Bystedt H, Nord CE. Effect of antibiotic treatment on postoperative infections after surgical removal of mandibular third molars. Swed Dent J 1980; 4:27.
29. Bystedt H, von Konow L, Nord CE. Effect of tinidazole on postoperative complications after surgical removal of impacted mandibular third molars. Scand J Infect Dis 1981; 26(suppl): 135.
30. Hellem S, Nordenra A. Prevention of postoperative symptoms by general antibiotic treatment and local

bandage in removal of mandibular third molars. Int J Oral Surg 1973; 2:273.
31. Kaziro GSN. Metronidazole (flagyl) and arnica montana in the prevention of post-surgical complications, a comparative placebo controlled clinical trial. Br J Oral Maxillofac Surg 1984; 22:42.
32. Krekmanov L, Nordenram A. Postoperative complications after surgical removal of mandibular third molars. Int J Oral Maxillofac Surg 1986; 15:25.
33. Krekmanov L, Hallander HO. Relationship between bacterial contamination and alveolitis after third molar surgery. Int J Oral Surg 1980; 9:274.
34. Krekmanov L. Alveolitis after operative removal of third molars in the mandible. Int J Oral Surg 1981; 10:173.
35. Macgregor AJ, Addy A. Value of penicillin in the prevention of pain, swelling and trismus following the removal of ectopic mandibular third molars. Int J Oral Surg 1980; 9:166.
36. Rood JP, Murgatroyd JM. Metronidazole in the prevention of "dry socket." Br J Oral Surg 1979–80; 17:62.
37. Hooley JR, Francis FH. Betamethasone in traumatic oral surgery. J Oral Surg 1969; 27:398.
38. Huffman GG. Use of methylprednisolone sodium succinate to reduce postoperative edema after removal of impacted third molars. J Oral Surg 1977; 35:198.
39. Pedersen A. Decadronphosphate in the relief of complaints after third molar surgery. Int J Oral Surg 1985; 14:235.
40. Beirne OR, Hollander B. The effect of methylprednisolone on pain, trismus, and swelling after removal of third molars. Oral Surg 1986; 61:134.
41. Bystedt H, Nordenram A. Effect of methylprednisolone on complications after removal of impacted mandibular third molars. Swed Dent J 1985; 9:65.
42. Nordenram A. Postoperative complications in oral surgery. Swed Dent J 1983; 7:109.
43. Goldberg MH, Nemarich AN, Marco WP. Complications after mandibular third molar surgery: a statistical analysis of 500 consecutive procedures in private practice. J Am Dent Assoc 1985; 111:277–279.
44. Bruce RA, Frederickson GC, Small GS: Age of patients and morbidity associated with mandibular third molar surgery. J Am Dent Assoc 1980; 101:240.
45. Osborn TP, Frederickson G, Small IA, Torgerson TS. A prospective study of complications related to mandibular third molar surgery. J Oral Maxillofac Surg 1985; 43:767.
46. Hinds EC, Frey KF. Hazards of retained third molars in older persons: Report of 15 cases. J Am Dent Assoc 1980; 101:246.
47. Forsgren H, Heimdahl AN, Johansson B, Krekmanov L. Effect of application of cold dressings on the postoperative course in oral surgery. Int J Oral Surg 1985; 14:223.
48. Seymour RA, Blair GS, Wyatt FAR. Post-operative dental pain and analgesic efficacy. Br J Oral Surg 1983; 23:290.
49. Seymour RA, Walton JG. Pain control after third molar surgery. Int J Oral Surg 1984; 13:457.
50. Seymour RA, Meechan JG, Blair GS. An investigation into post-operative pain after third molar surgery under local analgesia. Br J Oral Maxillofac Surg 1985; 23:410.
51. Pedersen A. Interrelation of complaints after removal of impacted mandibular third molars. Int J Oral Surg 1985; 14:241.
52. Nordenram A, Grave S. Alveolitis sicca dolorosa after removal of impacted mandibular third molars. Int J Oral Surg 1983; 12:226.
53. Knutsson K, Lysell L, Rohlin M. Postoperative status after partial removal of the mandibular third molar. Swed Dent J 1989; 13:15.
54. Nitzan, DW. On the genesis of "dry socket." J Oral Maxillofac Surg 1983; 41:706.
55. Sweet JB, Butler DP. The relationship of smoking to localized osteitis. J Oral Surg 1979; 37:732.
56. Meechan JG, MacGregor IDM, Rogers SN, Hobson RS, Bate JPC, Dennison M. The effect of smoking on immediate post-extraction socket filling with blood and the incidence of painful socket. Br J Oral Maxillofac Surg 1988; 26:402.
57. Swanson AE. A double-blind study on the effectiveness of tetracycline in reducing the incidence of fibrinolytic alveolitis. J Oral Maxillofac Surg 1989; 47:165.
58. Nordenram A, Sydens G, Odegaard J. Neomycin-bacitracin cones in impacted third molar sockets. Int J Oral Surg 1973; 2:279.
59. Goldman DR, Kilgore DS, Panzer JD, Atkinson WH. Prevention of dry socket by local application of lincomycin in Gelfoam. Oral Surg 1973; 35:472.
60. Hall HD, Bildman BS, Hand CD. Prevention of dry socket with local application of tetracycline. J Oral Surg 1971; 29:35.
61. Mitchell L. Topical metronidazole in the treatment of "dry socket." Br Dent J 1984; 156:132.
62. Kipp DP, Goldstein BH, Weiss WW Jr. Dysesthesia after mandibular third molar surgery: a retrospective study and analysis of 1,377 surgical procedures. J Am Dent Assoc 1980; 100:185.
63. Wofford DT, Miller RI. Prospective study of dysesthesia following odontectomy of impacted mandibular third molars. J Oral Maxillofac Surg 1987; 45:15.
64. Mason DA. Lingual nerve damage following lower third molar surgery. Int J Oral Maxillofac Surg 1988; 17:290.
65. Robinson PP. Observations on the recovery of sensation following inferior alveolar nerve injuries. Br J Oral Maxillofac Surg 1988; 26:177.
66. Rood JP. The radiological prediction of inferior alveolar nerve injury during third molar surgery. Br J Oral Maxillofac Surg 1990; 28:20.
67. Oberman M, Horowitz I, Ramon Y. Accidental displacement of impacted maxillary third molars. Int J Oral Maxillofac Surg 1986; 15:756.
68. Osborne WH, Snyder AJ, Tempel TR. Attachment levels and crevicular depths at the distal of mandibular second molars following removal of adjacent third molars. J Periodontol 1982; 53:93.

69. Meister F Jr, Nery EB, Angell DM, Meister RC. Periodontal assessment following surgical removal of mandibular third molars. Gen Dent 1986 (Mar-Apr); 120–123.
70. Kugelberg CF, Ahlstrom U, Ericson S, Hugoson A. Periodontal healing after impacted lower third molar surgery. Int J Oral Surg 1985; 14:29.
71. Marmary Y, Brayer L, Tzukert A, Feller L. Alveolar bone repair following extraction of impacted mandibular third molars. Oral Surg 1985; 60:324.
72. Ash MM Jr, Costich ER, Hayward JR. A study of periodontal hazards of third molars. J Periodontol 1962; 33:209.
73. Kugelberg CF. Periodontal healing two and four years after impacted lower third molar surgery. Int J Oral Maxillofac Surg 1990; 19:341.
74. Grondahl HG, Lekholm U. Influence of mandibular third molars on related supporting tissues. Int J Oral Surg 1973; 2:137.
75. Chin Quee TA, Gosselin D, Miller EP, Stamm JW. Surgical removal of the fully impacted mandibular third molar. J Periodontol 1985; 56:625.
76. Tulloch JFC, Antczak AA, Wilkes JW. The application of decision analysis to evaluate the need for extraction of asymptomatic third molars. J Oral Maxillofac Surg 1987; 45:855.
77. Ricketts RM. Studies leading to the practice of abortion of lower third molars. Dent Clin NA 1979; 23(3): 393.

7

Management of Pain and Anxiety

Joel Weaver

Since the discovery of general anesthesia nearly a century and a half ago by the dentists Horace Wells and William T. G. Morton, the successful management of pain and anxiety has played a key role in the advancement of the specialty of oral and maxillofacial surgery. As new sedatives, analgesics, anxiolytics, and local and general anesthetic drugs have been discovered, doctors have used them to develop newer and safer techniques to control pain and anxiety in the ambulatory patient. Formalized anesthesia training in both the inpatient and outpatient settings provides a solid foundation on which the surgeon can build and refine these techniques.

The 1985 National Institutes of Health Consensus Conference on Sedation and Anesthesia in the Dental Office reaffirmed the necessity, as well as the safety, of in-office pain and anxiety control.[1] The American Dental Association's policy statement on sedation, deep sedation, and general anesthesia in 1986 recognizes the right of qualified dentists to provide such methods within the office.[2] Most states have implemented dental board laws or regulations governing the administration of sedation and ambulatory general anesthesia by dentists. In order to better organize and prepare the office for potential emergencies, the American Association of Oral and Maxillofacial Surgeons publishes the *Office Anesthesia Evaluation Manual*.[3] Guidelines for sedation and anesthesia in the dental office have been developed by a number of dental organizations.[1,4,5] From these official documents are the following definitions.

- *Sedation:* A depressed level of consciousness which may vary from light to deep.
- *Conscious sedation:* A minimally depressed level of consciousness that retains the patient's ability to independently and continuously maintain the airway and to respond appropriately to physical stimulation and verbal command at any time, produced by a pharmacologic or nonpharmacologic method or a combination thereof. The loss of consciousness should be unlikely and the drugs and techniques used should carry a margin of safety wide enough to render the unintended loss of consciousness unlikely.
- *Deep sedation:* A controlled state of depressed consciousness or unconsciousness from which the patient is not easily aroused, which may be accompanied by a partial or complete loss of protective reflexes including the inability to independently maintain a patent airway and respond purposefully to physical stimulation or verbal command, produced by a pharmacologic or nonpharmacologic method or a combination thereof.
- *General anesthesia:* A controlled state of unconsciousness accompanied by a partial or complete loss of protective reflexes, including the inability to independently maintain a patent airway and respond purposefully to physical stimulation or verbal command, produced by a pharmacologic method, or a combination thereof.

These definitions must be kept in mind, because the intended depth of central nervous system depression and the likelihood of unintended additional depression determines to a great extent the need for additional monitors, equipment, and auxiliary personnel.

For conscious sedation, the recommended minimum number of office personnel is two, the anesthesia-trained surgeon and an auxiliary. In addition to continuous visual monitoring (including the level of consciousness, color, and the rate and depth of respirations) patients under conscious sedation must have their blood pressure and heart rate recorded pre- and postoperatively and at a minimum of 15-minute intervals. Continuous monitoring of the cardiovascular and respiratory systems is a necessity and is most efficiently accomplished with a precordial stethoscope and a pulse oximeter. Extremely light, single-drug conscious sedation techniques (such as N_2O-O_2) require only continuous visual monitoring.

The recommendations for deep sedation and general anesthesia are essentially identical to each other, since deeply sedated patients may have periods of unconsciousness. The minimum number of office personnel is three: the anesthesia-trained surgeon who directs the anesthesia, a trained auxiliary who continuously monitors the patient's vital signs and adjunctive monitors, and the surgical assistant. Vital signs must be recorded at 5-minute intervals. In addition to those monitors used for conscious sedation (precordial stethoscope, pulse oximeter, and blood pressure cuff) a cardioscope is essential to more readily detect anesthetic emergencies.

Measurement of end-tidal carbon dioxide (capnography) can detect carbon dioxide retention due to decreased rate or depth of respirations as well as respiratory obstruction or apnea. Capnography is the most accurate monitor to verify proper endotracheal tube placement, and as technologic advances occur and acceptance increases, it is likely that capnographs with apnea alarms will be an emerging standard of care for intubated and probably for non-intubated patients as well.

The office where ambulatory sedation or general anesthesia is performed must be properly equipped to assure the highest margin of safety for the patient. Such equipment and drugs must be well-organized, routinely checked for proper function, and readily available, preferably at an arm's reach. Back-up systems for oxygen delivery, suction, and light must be available.

PREOPERATIVE PATIENT EVALUATION

The old adage "never treat a stranger" is never more important than in the oral and maxillofacial surgeon's office. Preoperative evaluation of the oral surgical patient consists of four major parts:

1. Complete past medical history
2. Physical examination
3. Psychologic evaluation
4. Determination of American Society of Anesthesiologists (ASA) physical status

The past medical history includes a thorough review of systems. Special emphasis is placed on the cardiovascular and respiratory systems, previous illnesses and hospitalizations, previous anesthetics, allergies, exercise tolerance, and current medications which the patient takes or is supposed to take.

The emphasis for the physical examination of the ambulatory patient is placed on inspection and auscultation. The surgeon observes the patient for cyanosis, clubbing, dyspnea, hyperpnea, body build, and airway obstruction. A difficult airway may be anticipated for patients with protruding maxillary incisors, a short muscular neck, retrognathia, micrognathia, poor mobility of the mandible and neck,[6] a large tongue, and a distance from the symphysis to the thyroid cartilage of less than 6.5 cm (approximately the width of 3 fingers) (Fig. 7–1).

The outpatient oral surgical patient is frequently anxious about the proposed surgical-anesthetic experience. Additionally, long-standing emotional and psychological problems may add to the stress of the experience. These factors must be weighed by the surgeon and consideration given to them in developing an acceptable pain and anxiety control plan.

The American Society of Anesthesiologists developed the ASA Physical Status Classification System to estimate the medical risk for a patient undergoing a surgical procedure. Although it was designed primarily for patients who were to receive a general anesthetic, the system is presently used for all patients, even those requiring only local anesthesia. The system as described by Schneider[7] has six risk categories:

ASA I: A patient without systemic disease; a normal healthy patient
ASA II: A patient with mild systemic disease, no functional limitation
ASA III: A patient with severe systemic disease, definite functional limitation
ASA IV: A patient with severe systemic disease that is a constant threat to life
ASA V: A moribund patient unlikely to survive 24 hours with or without operation
ASA E: Emergency operation of any variety; the "E" precedes the patient's physical status

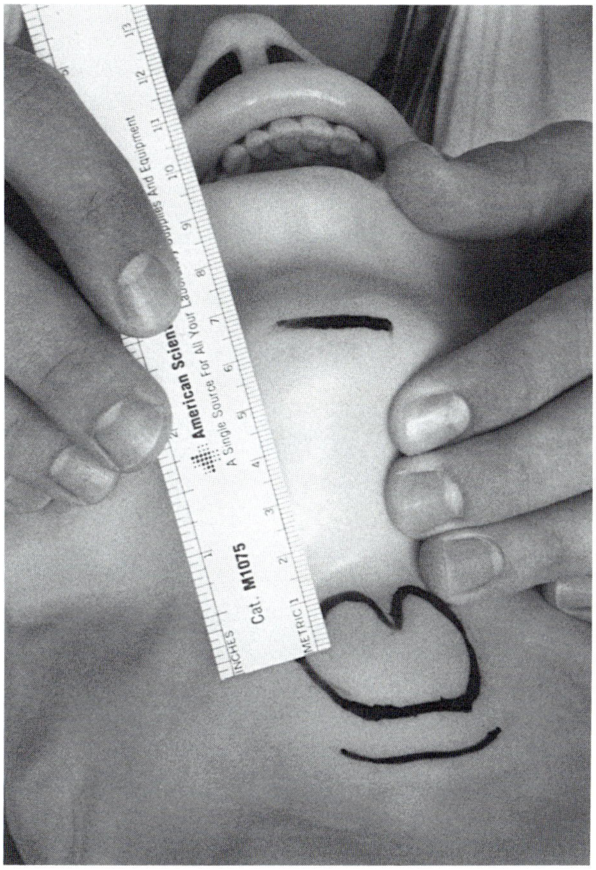

Figure 7–1. *In an adult a space of 6.5 cm. (approximately 3 fingers) from mandible (menton) to the thyroid notch with the head extended suggests that endotracheal intubation via direct laryngoscopy in the adult is attainable.*

Generally only healthy patients (ASA I) or those with mild systemic disease (ASA II) are candidates for deep sedation or general anesthesia in the dental office. ASA III patients may be candidates for conscious sedation and may be at less overall risk when pain and anxiety are controlled in this manner. ASA IV patients are usually treated for only brief appointments and with complete adjunctive monitoring, usually with profound local anesthesia alone or with the lightest levels of conscious sedation. ASA V patients are obviously never treated in the dental office. True unscheduled emergency patients are generally considered to have a full stomach and are definitely not candidates for deep sedation or general anesthesia in the office.

Once all of the pertinent patient information is gathered, the surgical and anesthetic plans may then be developed. It is absolutely essential that each plan be developed individually depending on the patient's needs and desires, physical status, and the surgical considerations. The benefit-risk ratio of each alternative is carefully weighed and the patient is eventually advised accordingly. Written, informed consent including alternative methods is strongly encouraged.

CLINICALLY SIGNIFICANT PHARMACOLOGIC ASPECTS OF ANESTHETIC AND ADJUNCTIVE DRUGS

Local Anesthetics and Vasoconstrictors

Lidocaine and mepivacaine have been long regarded as the standard local anesthetic drugs for modern dentistry. Their somewhat short duration is enhanced by the addition of the vasoconstrictors epinephrine and levonordefrin. Because mepivacaine causes somewhat less vasodilation than lidocaine, a 3% solution of mepivacaine is more effective when vasoconstrictors are unwanted or a relatively short anesthetic is desired.

Bupivacaine and etidocaine are long-acting anesthetics which significantly postpone the onset of postoperative pain in the mandible. Contemporary practice among many oral and maxillofacial surgeons is to use lidocaine or mepivacaine for a rapid onset of anesthesia and to inject bupivacaine for a prolonged effect postsurgically. The additive effects of each component toward the maximum recommended local anesthetic and vasoconstrictor doses must be borne in mind. Alternatively, etidocaine may be used since it has rapid onset and prolonged anesthetic effects. The maximum recommended doses and the expected duration of soft tissue anesthesia for the most commonly used local anesthetics are listed in Table 7–1.

The American Dental Association has long recommended a maximum dose of 200 μg of epinephrine for patients with heart disease.[8,9] A reduction in this amount may be necessary for some medically compromised patients, since circulating levels of epinephrine from infiltration with large doses of local anesthetics are greater than those produced by vigorous exercise or pheochromocytoma.[10,11] Clinical research indicates that 1 μg/kg of epinephrine during halothane anesthesia is unlikely to increase the incidence of cardiac dysrhythmias.[12] In the absence of specific epinephrine dosage guidelines for specific medical conditions,

Table 7–1. *Local Anesthetics: Dosages and Duration*

Trade Name	Contents	Maximum Doses: Children, in mg/kg	Maximum Doses: Healthy Adults, in mg (No. cartridges)	Duration of Anesthesia: (soft tissue) Maxillary Infiltration (min)	Duration of Anesthesia: Inferior Alveolar Block (min)
Xylocaine with epinephrine	2% lidocaine hydrochloride; 1:100,000 epinephrine	7	500 (14)	170	190
Carbocaine with neo-cobefrin	2% mepivacaine hydrochloride; 1:20,000 levonordefrin	6	400 (11)	130	185
Carbocaine	3% mepivacaine hydrochloride	6	400 (7.5)	90	165
Citanest Forte	4% prilocaine hydrochloride; 1:200,000 epinephrine	8	600 (8.25)	140	220
Citanest	4% prilocaine hydrochloride	8	600 (8.25)	105	190
Marcaine with epinephrine	0.5% bupivacaine hydrochloride; 1:200,000 epinephrine	3	225 (25)	340	440
Duranest with epinephrine	1.5% etidocaine hydrochloride; 1:200,000 epinephrine	6	400 (15)	280	470

(Data from Neidle EA, Yagiela JA. Pharmacology and Therapeutics for Dentistry, ed 3. St. Louis: CV Mosby, 1989:244)

such a dose (1 μg/kg) would also seem to be reasonable for medically compromised patients. This roughly translates into four cartridges of 1:100,000 epinephrine for a 70-kg patient.

Benzodiazepines

The benzodiazepines are by far the most widely used anxiolytics in oral surgery. They cause less cardiorespiratory depression than the barbiturates and produce excellent anterograde amnesia, even in the consciously sedated patient. Diazepam, the prototypic drug in this class, produces a dose-dependent clinically effective sedation for approximately 30 to 45 minutes, but its slow terminal elimination half-life (T 1/2 beta) and active metabolites prolong complete recovery. Midazolam is a water-soluble benzodiazepine which causes less venous irritation than diazepam. Like diazepam it produces suitable sedation and amnesia for similar periods of time. Its terminal elimination half-life (2 to 4 hours) is considerably shorter than diazepam, an important factor after the patient is escorted home. Compared to diazepam, midazolam is two to four times as potent as a sedative.[13]

Early reports of significant respiratory depression and apnea with midazolam have been attributed to rapid administration of relatively large incremental doses, co-administration of other depressant drugs, particularly narcotics, and increased sensitivity in aged or debilitated patients.[14] Significant arterial oxygen desaturation has been observed in healthy oral surgery outpatients undergoing intravenous sedation with a combination of midazolam and fentanyl.[15] Midazolam must be used in a setting fully equipped for monitoring and treating the unconscious patient.

The dose for intravenous, conscious sedation with midazolam alone in the average, healthy adult ranges from 0.1 to 0.15 mg/kg. When combined with typical analgesic doses of narcotics, the suggested dose of midazolam is decreased approximately 25%. Slow titration of 1-mg increments of midazolam is necessary, particularly when deep sedation or unconsciousness are to be avoided.

For deep sedation or general anesthesia the dose of midazolam may be increased up to 0.3 mg/kg, but prolonged amnesia and recovery may occur.[16,17] A more practical approach for ambulatory patients is to give usual sedative doses of midazolam or midazolam-narcotic, followed by combinations of nitrous oxide–oxygen and 10- to 20-mg increments of methohexital to achieve the desired sedative-anesthetic state and an acceptably short recovery time.

Flumazenil, a specific benzodiazepine antagonist,

is an excellent agent for the rapid reversal of all benzodiazepines.[18,19] It has been shown to reverse all of the effects of benzodiazepines such as respiratory depression, apnea, unconsciousness, slow recovery, and paradoxical reactions, as well as sedation, anxiolysis, muscle relaxation, and amnesia. The onset time of titrated intravenous doses of flumazenil is generally 1 to 2 minutes and somewhat longer (1 to 5 min) for benzodiazepine-induced coma. The intravenous dose range is 0.1 to 10 mg with the expected minimum effective dose being 0.4 mg. Although flumazenil alone has very limited agonistic effects (mild anxiolysis and anticonvulsant) it may cause seizures in benzodiazepine-controlled epileptics and anxiety and symptoms of acute withdrawal in patients with benzodiazepine dependency.

The terminal elimination half-life of flumazenil is 0.83 to 1.5 hours, considerably shorter than most benzodiazepine agonists. Because of the relatively short duration of its competitive mechanism of action at benzodiazepine receptor sites, flumazenil may permit the effects of the agonist to reappear.[20] The "overdose patient" may revert to coma, and the sedated outpatient who may feel completely normal after flumazenil reversal may later become resedated, a particular hazard if postoperative instructions against driving a car are not followed. Whether or not this drug becomes popular in everyday clinical practice, it does offer the surgeon increased flexibility in safely managing patient anxiety.

Narcotic Analgesics

Narcotic analgesics are frequently administered parenterally with sedatives for conscious sedation, deep sedation, and general anesthesia. Since they are well-known respiratory depressants, relatively small doses of narcotics are used to produce sedation and euphoria and to reduce the total doses of other sedative drugs administered. The analgesic component provided by a low-dose narcotic appears to reduce the patient's reaction to the local anesthetic injection and to provide a smoother sedative/anesthetic course.

Meperidine, a synthetic narcotic, has been used for many years in ambulatory sedation and anesthesia. It provides sedation, euphoria, analgesia, and mild anticholinergic activity, particularly xerostomia. It is intermediate in duration of action, only mildly releases histamine, and is cost-effective.

Fentanyl, another synthetic narcotic, is also widely used by oral and maxillofacial surgeons. Its short duration of action is more consistent with most office procedures, although the respiratory depressant effects appear to outlast its analgesia. Fentanyl causes virtually no histamine release. A disadvantage however, is fentanyl's initiation of truncal or chest wall muscle rigidity, a condition in which positive pressure ventilation of the patient is difficult or impossible. Truncal rigidity usually occurs with large doses of fentanyl (50 to 100 μg/kg) for cardiac surgery, but also has been reported by dentists using small doses (100 μg) for sedation.[21,22] Potentiation of the respiratory depressant effects of sedative and anxiolytic drugs is well known.[16] Fentanyl, therefore, is most safely used for a continuously well-monitored patient breathing supplemental oxygen for whom there are drugs (naloxone, succinylcholine) and resuscitation equipment standing by.

Sufentanil, a derivative of fentanyl, is approximately ten times more potent but offers essentially no therapeutic advantage over the parent drug for the oral and maxillofacial surgeon. Alfentanil, another fentanyl derivative, is considerably less potent but has a much shorter redistribution half-life (T 1/2 alpha) than fentanyl. This drug is frequently administered by continuous intravenous infusion with nitrous oxide–oxygen and muscle relaxants for inpatient general anesthesia. Whether it is useful for nonintubated outpatient oral surgery patients remains to be seen.

The agonist-antagonist narcotics, such as pentazocine, butorphanol, and nalbuphine, are also useful in outpatient sedative-anesthetic procedures. Like pure agonist narcotics, analgesic effects and respiratory depression both increase with the dose administered. However, at high doses, there appears to be a ceiling effect for the respiratory depression, and thus the antagonistic effects of these drugs are revealed. Moreover, their antagonistic effects may precipitate abstinence syndrome (narcotic withdrawal) if inadvertently administered to a narcotic-dependent patient. These drugs are known to increase the incidence of dysphoric reactions postoperatively.[23] The federal government has classified butorphanol and nalbuphine as prescription-only items but not as controlled substances, apparently because of the lack of substantial evidence of abuse potential. This classification does not require the practitioner at this time to maintain special drug purchase, inventory, or administration records.

The pure narcotic antagonist naloxone possesses great affinity for narcotic receptors but has essentially no agonist activity. It readily reverses the sedative, analgesic, and respiratory depression associated with narcotic agonist and agonist-antagonist drugs. Naloxone is not routinely used to hasten recovery in ambulatory dental patients because of increased costs, the potential for the return of narcotic depression, and the sudden onset of pain and sympathetic stimulation; the precipitation of abstinence syndrome in the narcotic-dependent patient is also possible. Following initial positive pressure ventilation with 100% oxygen, naloxone is the drug of choice for the immediate reversal of narcotic-induced respiratory depression.

Barbiturates

Among the many barbiturates available for sedation or the induction of general anesthesia, three are selected for their use for the oral and maxillofacial surgeon. Pentobarbital, classified as a short-acting barbiturate derivative, provides a smooth intravenous conscious sedation for office procedures of intermediate duration. Amnesia and significant respiratory depression are usually not noted with intravenous conscious sedation with pentobarbital. Combinations of pentobarbital with other sedatives, analgesics, or anxiolytic drugs may produce deep sedation with accompanying amnesia and respiratory depression.

Thiopental and methohexital, ultrashort-acting barbiturates, are highly lipid soluble and cross the blood-brain barrier rapidly. They produce profound sedation in relatively small intravenous doses (10 to 50 mg). Amnesia and respiratory depression are common. Obtunded protective airway reflexes, laryngospasm, and apnea can occur during deep sedation with these agents. Their greatest advantage is a smooth, pleasant induction (1 to 3 mg/kg methohexital or 3 to 5 mg/kg thiopental) and a rapid recovery due to redistribution from the brain to other body storage sites. Cumulative effects of multiple, small doses may prolong recovery as these sites become saturated. However, for short procedures, no other drugs have yet successfully replaced the ultrashort-acting barbiturates for rapid onset, profound sedation with accompanying amnesia, and rapid recovery. Methohexital has a significantly higher clearance rate compared to thiopental and its terminal elimination half-life (1.5 to 4 hours) is considerably shorter than thiopental (10 to 12 hours). Methohexital may provide a more rapid recovery compared to thiopental, but at the expense of occasional hiccups and involuntary movements.

Nonbarbiturate Sedative-Hypnotics

Etomidate and propofol are two relatively new drugs which may replace the ultrashort-acting barbiturates in anesthesiology. Etomidate produces less cardiovascular depression than the barbiturates, but unfortunately it also produces involuntary body movements and has been implicated in depressing adrenal cortical function.

Propofol, a poorly water-soluble compound, is formulated in a white, milky, oil-egg phosphosphatide glycerol emulsion. Following an intravenous bolus, two redistribution phases are noted. The first redistribution half-life (T 1/2α) is 1.8 to 8 minutes and the second slower phase is 34 to 64 minutes. The terminal elimination half-life (T 1/2β) is 300 to 700 minutes.

Propofol is an ultrashort-acting agent which provides a smooth, pleasant, rapid induction of anesthesia, similar to methohexital but with significantly faster recovery.[24] Compared to anesthesia with midazolam, recovery from propofol is significantly more rapid.[25] Recovery time and costs are significantly reduced with propofol compared to thiopental-isoflurane.[26]

Induction boluses of propofol decrease mean arterial pressure, systemic vascular resistance, and cardiac index without a change in heart rate.[27] Pain on injection has been reported and is dependent on the site of the injection. It can be minimized if large veins such as on the forearm are used.[28]

Induction doses of 2.5 mg/kg of intravenously administered propofol with or without 1 or 2 μg/kg of fentanyl are used commonly. Such doses are frequently associated with apnea. Nitrous oxide–oxygen and either intermittent boluses of propofol (30 to 50 mg) or a continuous infusion of propofol (100 to 200 μg/kg/min) are used for anesthetic maintenance. Continuous infusions of 70 to 100 μg/kg/min of propofol after initial sedation with small boluses of propofol have also been reported as highly satisfactory for sedation.[29-31]

Propofol has the potential for altering existing outpatient anesthetic practice. Despite its greater cost compared with methohexital, propofol can provide the benefits of enhanced patient acceptance and increased office efficiency with decreased chair-time recovery time, and associated expenses. Likewise, the use of the continuous infusion pump provides a smoother anesthetic course and reduces the total amount of drug administered.

Dissociative Anesthetics

Ketamine is a valuable agent for unmanageable pediatric and mentally handicapped patients in ambulatory anesthesia. Intramuscular ketamine in a dose of 1 to 4 mg/kg produces within a few minutes a markedly sedated patient for 15 to 30 minutes. Although depression of protective reflexes and respiration are not remarkable, enhanced salivary secretions and laryngospasm are potential problems. Supplementation with nitrous oxide–oxygen, local anesthetics, and titrated intravenous small boluses of ketamine (0.25 to 0.5 mg/kg) will prolong this deep sedation state. Larger doses of up to 10 mg/kg for general anesthesia induction are likely to prolong recovery. Ketamine causes bronchodilation which may be beneficial, particularly for the asthmatic. Bizarre dreams and hallucinations are associated with ketamine and must be considered when analyzing the risk-benefit ratio of ketamine. However, they are less likely to occur in children and when smaller sedative doses are given. Benzodiazepines may be given with ketamine to promote a smooth sedation and emergence. Midazolam 0.07 to 0.15 mg/kg followed by 0.25 to 0.5 mg/kg of intravenous ketamine has produced excellent sedation, amnesia, and analgesia for the injection of local anesthetics without producing significant cardiorespiratory depression.[32]

Inhalation Anesthetics

Nitrous oxide, the first recognized anesthetic agent, still plays a prominent role in modern anesthesiology. Although it lacks potency, nitrous oxide adds to the sedative, analgesic, and amnesic effects of other anesthetic agents. Its rapid elimination is particularly suitable for ambulatory patients, whether used alone for conscious sedation or in combination with intravenous drugs for deep sedation or general anesthesia.

The potent inhalation agents currently in common use are halothane, enflurane, and isoflurane. Of these three, halothane is the preferred induction agent for children. It has the least pungent odor, providing a smooth anesthetic course and rapid recovery. Halothane is the most dysrhythmogenic, particularly during light anesthesia or in the presence of hypercarbia and exogenously administered epinephrine. A limitation of 1 μg/kg of epinephrine infiltrated in the oral region during halothane anesthesia is suggested.[12] The existence of halothane-induced hepatotoxicity has been debated for decades without resolution. As with the other potent inhalation anesthetics, halothane can trigger malignant hyperthermia.

Enflurane and isoflurane are significantly less dysrhythmogenic than halothane. The safety of infiltration of the surgical site with epinephrine during anesthesia with enflurane (2 μg/kg of epinephrine) or isoflurane (3 μg/kg of epinephrine) is enhanced compared to halothane.[12] However, when used as the sole induction agents their relatively unpleasant odor produces a slow, often stormy, induction.

Two new, potent inhalation agents on the horizon may offer significant advantages for outpatient anesthesia. Desflurane (I-653) has a very low blood–gas solubility coefficient (0.42), which is similar to nitrous oxide (0.47), and thus it produces a rapid onset of anesthesia and rapid recovery.[33,34] Compared with similar agents used today, it is less potent (MAC equals 5%–7%) but undergoes little or no metabolism. It has a somewhat pungent odor and may cause a stormy induction similar to isoflurane.

Sevoflurane also has a low blood-gas solubility coefficient (0.6–0.7) and has a potency (MAC = 1.7%) similar to enflurane. Its lack of pungency permits a smooth induction, and it does not appear to sensitize the myocardium to epinephrine. About 2% of sevoflurane that is administered is metabolized. These agents of the future may eventually improve the safety and convenience of inhalation ambulatory anesthesia.

TECHNIQUES FOR CONTROL OF PAIN AND ANXIETY

Local Anesthesia

Profound local anesthesia is the foundation on which nearly all sedative-anesthetic techniques are based. Standard infiltration and nerve block techniques are most often used. The Akinosi inferior alveolar nerve block is frequently performed for mandibular anesthesia in patients with limited opening,[35] whereas the Gow-Gates mandibular nerve block may be chosen as an alternative to the standard inferior alveolar nerve block when the patient can open widely.[36] An intraoral maxillary nerve block through the greater palatine canal is an acceptable alternative for the more traditional techniques of maxillary anesthesia.[37]

The periodontal ligament injection is recommended as a supplement to any other local anesthetic technique which is not entirely successful. The small amount of drug injected under significant pressure into the periodontal ligament apparently produces its effect as an intraosseous infiltration. Usually placed on the distal aspect of single-rooted teeth and on the mesial and distal aspects of multi-rooted teeth, the periodontal ligament injection produces profound anesthesia of relatively short duration.[38]

Conscious Sedation

Conscious sedation as previously defined may be attained by many routes with a variety of agents. For the anesthesia-trained oral and maxillofacial surgeon, the drugs and techniques chosen will, in part, depend upon whether deep sedation is also an acceptable alternative. For instance, although small doses of methohexital may provide conscious sedation, it is not a drug recommended for a patient who is not a candidate for deep sedation, because that might inadvertently occur. Other sedatives for such a patient should be chosen that are less likely to produce deep sedation or unconsciousness.

Oral Conscious Sedation

Among a variety of oral drugs available for conscious sedation, diazepam (5 to 20 mg) has a long history of usage as an oral preoperative sedative. However, its prolonged elimination half life and active metabolites make it less desirable in ambulatory patients. Triazolam is rapidly absorbed orally and appears to be acceptable for the ambulatory patient. Adult doses of 0.25 to 0.5 mg of triazolam produce significant sedation and amnesia. Because profound sedation may occur, patients should be orally sedated in the office after the presence of an escort is assured.

Inhalation Conscious Sedation

Nitrous oxide–oxygen conscious sedation offers several advantages compared with other techniques. It has a rapid onset, short recovery, and is not a significant cardiovascular nor respiratory depressant. However, this sedation alone is infrequently used by oral and maxillofacial surgeons because profound sedation and amnesia rarely occur in the absence of excitation, agitation, and other side effects associated with high concentrations of nitrous oxide. The additional oxygen inhaled may be beneficial for some medically compromised patients. When used in combination with other central nervous system depressants, it tends to increase the depth and duration of their effects, including respiratory depression. However, it reduces the dosages of these other agents and makes other sedative techniques more controllable.

Intramuscular Conscious Sedation

The intramuscular route for conscious sedation in the oral and maxillofacial surgeon's practice is usually limited to patients with poor venous access and those who will not or cannot cooperate for successful venipuncture. Midazolam may be used alone (0.08 mg/kg) or in reduced dosage when administered with a narcotic. Midazolam is considerably better absorbed and is less painful compared to an intramuscular injection of diazepam. The peak effect occurs in 30 to 45 minutes. Supplemental oxygen is advisable, because the calculated dose may produce excessive central nervous system depression. Low-dose ketamine (up to 1 mg/kg) may be an alternative. Intrabuccal, submucosal, or subcutaneous routes offer no advantage over the intramuscular route for these agents.

Intravenous Conscious Sedation

Titration of small doses of sedative, analgesic, or anxiolytic drugs to a conscious endpoint for each individual patient is the great advantage of the intravenous route of drug administration. Midazolam alone or in combination with a narcotic, with or without nitrous oxide–oxygen supplementation, is widely used for modern intravenous conscious sedation. Pentobarbital alone or in combination with meperidine and scopolamine (Jorgenson technique) may be an acceptable alternative. Intravenous diazepam alone may provide conscious sedation with less risk of inadvertent deep sedation, apnea, or other serious complications, particularly for the elderly or debilitated patient.

Deep Sedation

Deep sedation may result from the use of larger doses of the same drugs or drug combinations used for conscious sedation or the addition of certain agents such as methohexital. The combination of intravenous midazolam, fentanyl, nitrous oxide–oxygen, and small increments of methohexital is widely used for deep sedation. For very brief procedures, methohexital alone provides an acceptable deep sedative effect. Propofol may be substituted for methohexital. Effective local anesthesia is, of course, the foundation on which all of these techniques are based.

Intramuscular ketamine (2 to 4 mg/kg) produces excellent deep sedation for approximately 30 minutes. An anticholinergic such as atropine should be included (often mixed in the same syringe) to reduce the enhanced salivation caused by ketamine. Nitrous oxide–oxygen by nasal hood or small intravenous increments of ketamine prolong the deep sedation. A benzodiazepine may be beneficial in reducing the incidence of ketamine-induced hallucinations.

General Anesthesia

General anesthesia may result from the use of larger doses of the same drug or drug combinations used for deep sedation or the use of potent inhalation agents. Baseline sedation is typically attained with benzodiazepines, narcotics, or nitrous oxide, followed by induction doses of methohexital (1 to 3 mg/kg) or propofol (1 to 3 mg/kg). Local anesthetics are then administered. The airway is usually maintained with proper head and mandibular position. A nasal hood permits inhalation of nitrous oxide–oxygen, and a gauze screen is placed to prevent aspiration of secretions, blood, or surgical fragments. A nasopharyngeal tube may be placed to aid in maintenance of the airway.

Induction of general anesthesia with a potent volatile anesthetic such as halothane is the best alternative to the parenteral route, especially for children. The volatile potent anesthetic agents may also be selected to maintain general anesthesia after intravenous induction with methohexital or propofol. A nasal hood, a nasopharyngeal tube, or an oral or nasal endotracheal tube may be used to facilitate gas delivery.

OUTPATIENT RECOVERY AND CRITERIA FOR DISCHARGE

Most oral surgical procedures are of short duration and, therefore, clinical recovery is also short. Complete recovery may be difficult to determine and may take hours to days to occur. There are several different stages of recovery, namely home readiness, street fitness, and complete recovery.[39]

The *home-ready* patient is oriented to person, place, and time, can ambulate unassisted (although an escort must be present), and has stable vital signs. A *street-fit* patient has recovered enough psychomotor skills to walk alone on a street, but not enough to operate heavy machinery. The surgeon must strongly consider the effects on the duration of recovery for all sedative-anesthetics used in ambulatory patients. A recovery level of home-readiness is acceptable provided the escort is present. Other than with nitrous oxygen conscious sedation, no sedated patient must ever leave the office unescorted. Because recurrence of sedation may happen when the specific antagonists for benzodiazepines and narcotics are no longer effective, reversal with these drugs does not eliminate the need for an escort.

Although assessment of the patient's home-readiness is mostly subjective, future quality assurance issues may require more objective criteria. In addition to stable vital signs, patients may need to demonstrate their return to near baseline scores on psychomotor tests such as the Trieger test or driving simulators.

PREVENTION, RECOGNITION, AND MANAGEMENT OF COMMON ANESTHETIC EMERGENCIES

A thoroughly reviewed past medical history and a careful physical examination are the two most useful methods to prevent anesthetic emergencies. Anesthetic equipment and drugs must be organized and readily available. The staff must be prepared to anticipate untoward events and manage them appropriately. Patients must be observed and monitored carefully to facilitate recognition of adverse events, hopefully before they become medical emergencies.

Problems with the airway or ventilation are traditionally the most likely causes of anesthetic mishaps. Unfortunately, the adequacy of ventilation has been difficult to access. Observations of chest movements, the reservoir bag, and patient color and ausculation of breath sounds are very crude estimations of proper ventilation. The pulse oximeter and the capnograph have markedly improved our ability to monitor respiratory function. Technologic advances in transcutaneous oxygen and carbon dioxide monitors may further enhance respiratory monitoring in the future.

Mechanical obstruction of the airway by the tongue is very common and easily managed if recognized. Other causes include enlarged tonsils, edema, infection, pharyngeal gauze partition, and foreign bodies. The practitioner must be immediately capable of providing proper care by repositioning the head, inserting an oral or nasopharyngeal airway, and by performing direct laryngoscopy or cricothyroidotomy, if necessary.

Secretions, irrigation solution, blood, and surgical debris may precipitate laryngospasm. High-pitched "crowing" sounds are produced on inspiration during partial spasms, whereas no sounds are produced during a complete or total laryngospasm. Suctioning deeply into the laryngopharynx and then application of positive pressure oxygen usually resolves this problem. The depth of anesthesia may also be increased to decrease laryngeal irritability. If oxygen saturation drops significantly, a small intravenous dose of succinylcholine (5 to 10 mg) may be given to relax the laryngeal muscles to permit positive pressure ventilation. This low dose may not resolve the spasm nor permit predictable relaxation for direct laryngoscopy should that become necessary. Less time will be lost if a full dose of succinylcholine (1 mg/kg) is initially administered.

Bronchospasm must be included in a differential diagnosis whenever ventilatory difficulties develop. Whether the consequence of asthma, histamine release, anaphylaxis, airway manipulation and stimulation, or aspiration, it must be recognized early and vigorously treated in a timely fashion. Increased airway pressure and significant wheezing during bronchospasm may be associated with severe hypoxemia and hypercarbia.

Aspiration of foreign bodies such as teeth, bone, blood, and irrigation solution is a recognized danger during oral and maxillofacial surgery, particularly for those patients who are deeply sedated or under general anesthesia. A properly positioned pharyngeal gauze partition and the availability of a high-volume evacuation system are necessary to decrease this risk.

The aspiration of gastric contents is also a significant risk, especially during nonintubated, outpatient general anesthesia. Risk factors for aspiration in ambulatory patients include obesity, diabetes, hiatal hernia, advanced pregnancy, and recent consumption of food or beverage. Aspiration of at least 25 mL of gastric contents of a low pH (2 to 2.5) is likely to produce serious morbidity. Management of aspiration includes suctioning the pharynx and administration of 100% oxygen. The lung fields are auscultated and bronchospasm is managed. Endotracheal intubation for oxygenation with positive end-expiratory pressure (PEEP) and direct tracheal suctioning may be necessary. Pulmonary lavage, prophylactic antibiotics, and glucocorticosteroids are generally not indicated. Transportation to the emergency room is recommended whenever aspiration is suspected.

Malignant hyperthermia is likely to occur only in those settings where known triggering agents such as volatile inhalation anesthetics and succinylcholine are frequently used. The vast majority of intravenous sedative-anesthetic drugs used in the office are considered to be nontriggering agents. Malignant hyperthermia is usually first manifested as an unexplained tachycardia and elevated end-tidal carbon dioxide level. Muscle rigidity, cyanosis, dysrhythmias, and elevated temperature are also noted. Intravenous dantrolene (1–10 mg/kg), oxygen, and cooling the patient are important initial treatment steps. Stabilization of serum potassium, acid-base balance, and kidney function are also therapeutic goals.

Ambulatory sedative and anesthetic techniques administered in the office of oral and maxillofacial surgeons have a long history of safety and cost effectiveness. For such procedures to remain viable in the future, anesthesia training opportunities must be continually upgraded and expanded in both the inpatient and outpatient areas. Research in anesthetic drug development and use must also remain in the forefront of oral and maxillofacial surgery if the specialty is to retain this privilege.

REFERENCES

1. National Institutes of Health. Consensus development conference statement on Anesthesia and Sedation in the Dental Office. JADA 1985; 111:90.
2. DeForest A. Dental anesthesiology: The policies of the American Dental Association in the past and its plans for the future. Anesth Prog 1986; 33:206.
3. Office Anesthesia Evaluation Manual, ed 3. American Association of Oral and Maxillofacial Surgeons, 1986.
4. Rosenberg, MB, Campbell RL. Guidelines for intraoperative monitoring of dental patients undergoing conscious sedation, deep sedation, and general anesthesia. Oral Surg Oral Med Oral Pathol 1991; 71(1):2.
5. American Academy of Pediatric Dentistry. Guidelines for the elective use of conscious sedation, deep sedation, and general anesthesia in pediatric patients. Pediatr Dent 1985; 7(4): 224.
6. Cass NM, James NR, Lines V. Difficult direct laryngoscopy complicating intubation for anesthesia. Br Med J 1956; 1:488.
7. Schneider AJL. Assessment of risk factors and surgical outcome. Surg Clin North Am 1983; 63:1113.
8. Report of the special committee of the New York Heart Association, Inc, on the use of epinephrine in connection with procaine in dental procedures. J Am Dent Assoc 1955; 50:108.
9. Vasoconstrictors. In: Accepted Dental Therapeutics, ed 40. Chicago: American Dental Association, 1984:205.
10. Cotton BR, Henderson HP, Achola KJ, Smith G. Changes in plasma catecholamine concentration following infiltrations of large volumes of local anesthetic solutions containing adrenaline. Br J Anaesth 1986; 58:593.
11. Cryer PE. Physiology and pathophysiology of the human sympathoadrenal neuroendocrine system. N Engl J Med 1980; 303:436.
12. Johnston RR, Eger EI, Wilson C. Comparative interaction of epinephrine with enflurane, isoflurane and halothane in man. Anesth Analg 1976; 55(5):709.
13. White PF, Vasconez LO, Mathes SA, et al. Comparison of midazolam and diazepam for sedation during plastic surgery. J Plast Reconstr Surg 1988; 81:703.
14. Food and Drug Administration. Drug Bulletin 1987; 17:5.
15. Tucker MR, Och MW, White RP. Arterial blood gas levels after midazolam or diazepam administered with and without fentanyl as an intravenous sedative for outpatient surgical procedures. J Oral Maxillofac Surg 1986; 44:688.
16. Berggren L, Eriksson I. Midazolam for induction of anaesthesia in outpatients—a comparison with thiopentone. Acta Anaesthesiol Scand 1981; 25:492.
17. Verma R, Ramasubramanian R, Sachar RM. Anesthesia for termination of pregnancy: Midazolam compared with methohexital. Anesth Analg 1985; 63:792.
18. Forster A, Juge O, Louis M, Nahory A. Effects of a specific benzodiazepine antagonist (RO-15-1788) on cerebral blood flow. Anesth Analg 1987; 66:309.
19. White PF, Shafer A, Boyle WA, et al. Benzodiazepine antagonism does not provoke stress response. Anesthesiology 1989; 70:636.
20. Darragh A. Antagonism of the central effects of 3-methylclonazepam. Br J Clin Pharmacol 1982; 14:871.
21. Vaughn RL, Bennett CR. Fentanyl chest wall rigidity syndrome—a case report. Anes Prog 1981; 28(2): 50.
22. Rosenberg M. Muscle rigidity—a case report. Anesth Prog 1977; 24(2): 50.
23. Garfield JM, Garfield FB, Philip BK, et al. A comparison of clinical and psychologic effects of fentanyl and nalbuphine in ambulatory gynecologic patients. Anesth Analg 1987; 66:1303.
24. Doze VA, Westphal LM, White PF. Comparison of propofol with methohexital for outpatient anesthesia. Anesth Analg 1986; 65:1189.
25. Forrest P, Galletly DC. Comparison of propofol and antagonized midazolam anaesthesia for day-case surgery. Anaesth Intensive Care 1987; 15:394.
26. Marias ML, Maher MW, Wetchler BV, Korttila K, Apfelbaum J. Reduced demands on recovery room resources with propofol (Diprivan) compared to thiopental-isoflurane. Anesth Rev 1989; 16:29.
27. Grounds RM, Twigley AJ, Carli F. The haemodynamic effects of intravenous induction: Comparison of the effects of thiopentone and propofol. Anaesthesia 1985; 40:735.
28. MacKenzie N, Grant IS. Comparison of the new emulsion formulation of propofol with methohexitone and thiopentone for induction of anesthesia in day cases. Br J Anaesth 1985; 57:725.
29. Valtonen M, Salonen M, Foressell H, Scheinin M, Viinarnaki O. Propofol infusion for sedation in outpatient oral surgery—a comparison with diazepam. Anaesthesia 1989; 44:730.
30. Rodrigo MRC, Jonsson E. Conscious sedation with propofol. Br Dent J 1989; 166:75.
31. MacKenzie N, Grant IS. Propofol for intravenous sedation. Anaesthesia 1987; 42:3.
32. White PF, Vasconez LO, Mathes SA, et al. Comparison of midazolam and diazepam for sedation during plastic surgery. J Plast Reconstr Surg 1988; 81:703.
33. Yasuda N, Targ AG, Eger EI II. Solubility of I-653, sevoflurane, isoflurane and halothane in human tissues. Anesthesiology 1988; 69:A615.
34. Eger EI II, Johnson BH. Rates of awakening from anesthesia with I-653, halothane, isoflurane and sevoflurane: A test of the effect of anesthetic concentration and duration in rats. Anesth Analg 1987; 66:977.

35. Akinosi JO. A new approach to the mandibular nerve block. Br J Oral Surg 1977; 15:83.
36. Gow Gates, GAE. Mandibular conduction anesthesia: A new technique using extra-oral landmarks. Oral Surg 1973; 36:321.
37. Mercuri LG. Intraoral second division nerve block. Oral Surg 1979; 47:109.
38. Moore KD, Reader A, Meyers WJ, Beck M, Weaver J. A comparison of the periodontal ligament injection using 2% lidocaine with 1:100,000 epinephrine and saline in human mandibular premolars. Anesth Prog 1987; 34:181.
39. Korttila K. Postanesthetic cognitive and psychomotor impairment. Int Anesthesiol Clin 1986; 24:59.

8

Risk Management in Oral and Maxillofacial Surgery

Arthur W. Curley
Ronald B. Marks

Recent statistics indicate that as many as one out of every ten dentists may be sued each year. In many states, this statistic, although alarming, does not reveal the severity of the problem. For example, in California, nearly all of the oral surgeons can anticipate being sued at least once in their career, and some statistics indicate that as many as 50% of the oral surgeons will be sued a second time.

Basically three reasons account for the increase in the number of suits against dentists: the current legal system, the public's changing attitude toward dentistry, and increasing competition in the dental community. When looking at the current state of the legal system one must remember that most state legislatures are composed of attorneys. After the laws are written they are subject to interpretation by judges, most all of whom are attorneys. The United States is one of the only countries that allows contingency fees and does not require plaintiffs to post bonds to provide some compensation to successful defendants. The politics of the system encourages the expansion of the tort liability system, changes the nature of the evidence necessary to prove a case, and increases the amount and nature of damages that may be awarded.

The general public's attitude toward dentistry has changed significantly in recent years. In the past, although no one liked going to a dentist, doctors were usually given the benefit of the doubt in cases of unsuccessful treatment. However, in this era of consumerism, dentistry is often viewed in the same light as a nonprofessional service.[1] The public often believes that when a product does not work, it is somehow inherently defective or was negligently manufactured.[2] This new attitude has been spawned in part by competitiveness within the profession, as well as aggressive marketing in the dental industry.

In many situations a patient may seek the advice of another practitioner, who, not meaning to be critical, may refer to a different method of treatment that would have been preferable. The patient then concludes that he or she received improper treatment. Thus, the doctor must be particularly aware of the pitfalls of casual remarks concerning the patient's prior treatment plan or the results of previous care.

Dentistry is a significant part of the change in the health care industry in America. There is growing competition for the millions of dollars spent on dental care. In order to attract these dollars, many practitioners will attempt to induce patients to seek treatment because they offer either a new treatment method or offer a special discount for treatments. This type of competitive marketing often breeds discontent within the profession and draws quick criticism.

Armed with an understanding of these problems,

the provider of dental healthcare must prepare a simple risk management program to provide the necessary defense against claims of dental malpractice. Dentistry is a target for attorneys, not because there is more malpractice but because dentists are simply easier targets.

THE AMERICAN LEGAL SYSTEM

In order to carefully manage one's practice, a minimal understanding of the legal system is essential. This understanding, along with good office risk management, will help the practitioner minimize exposure to claims of malpractice.

The state legislature essentially writes the fundamental rules for the regulation of the practice of dentistry. However, with rare exceptions, these laws do not specifically control the quality of dentistry. The legislature merely sets forth what types of health care may be provided by dentists and what aspect of dental treatment may be provided by nonlicensed individuals. The state legislature has a significant role in the determination of the type of malpractice suit a patient may file, the ease with which such claims can be prosecuted, and the amount of damages that may be awarded to a plaintiff.

Terminology

A *crime* is defined as a prescribed unlawful action against a person known as a victim. A criminal case is prosecuted by a district attorney who represents the State. A criminal proceeding is initiated by the filing of a complaint on behalf of the people of the State. In criminal cases, the State seeks imprisonment of the defendant or the payment of a fine. A criminal complaint against a dentist could involve actions such as insurance fraud, unlicensed personnel providing dental treatment, or drug abuse.

A *civil claim* (or *tort*) is one in which the harm is to an individual. The claim is made by that same individual. In civil cases, the individual harmed (the plaintiff) seeks monetary damages. Such damages are designed to repay the patient for lost expenses and pain and suffering, without necessarily intending to punish the dentist. However, some cases allow the recovery of punitive damages, which are designed to punish the dentist. These are distinguished from a fine because payment is made directly to the patient rather than to a governmental agency.

Malpractice is defined in most states as the failure to meet the standard of care or negligence.[3] This is generally not the subject of statutory regulation. In other words, the state legislature does not set forth rules as to how a specific procedure should be performed; that is determined by the standard of care, as judged by other doctors. However, there are exceptions. For example, some states regulate the administration of anesthesia. Violation of such regulations that cause harm to a patient may be grounds for a malpractice claim.

Court System

The role of the courts in our system is to interpret the laws written by the legislature. The court system has various levels.

Small claims courts have some unusual distinctions. First, attorneys are not allowed to present cases on behalf of clients, there are no juries, and the money that can be discussed in the case is limited to a maximum specific amount, such as \$1000 or \$1500. Dentists frequently use this arena to compel patients to pay past fees owed.

The municipal courts, or city courts, are the next highest authority after small claims courts. However, here also there are limitations as to the damages that may be sought. Many jurisdictions do not allow for claims in excess of \$25,000. At this level the parties may be represented by attorneys, and in many circumstances juries will hear the evidence and decide the "issue of fact."

The superior, district, or circuit court is the next highest and the most common arena for most dental malpractice claims. Claims in excess of the municipal or city jurisdiction limits are heard in this court. There is generally no limit on the amount of damages that may be awarded. Parties in this situation are almost always represented by attorneys, and most trials are heard by a jury composed of anywhere from six to twelve members of the community.

Parties who are unhappy with the results at the trial level may appeal the decisions to the appellate court, a panel of judges (no juries). The cases are argued exclusively by attorneys. Most states have two levels of appellate courts: district courts of appeal and the state supreme court. On rare occasions, a claimant may find a federal or national issue involved in the trial, and appeal the decision of the state supreme court to the federal appellate system. Here again, the claim is heard only through the arguments of attorneys, without juries. Appellate courts may only rule as to the correctness of the trial judges' decisions.

THE LAW AND THE HEALTH PROFESSIONS

As a general rule, civil liability against a doctor may be labeled one of two basic categories: negligence or intentional conduct. Negligence may be divided further into negligent commission or performance of an act and the negligent omission, or failure to perform a required act.

In order to prevail in an action against a doctor, a plaintiff must establish a doctor-patient relationship, and that a breach of the duty established by that relationship proximately or legally caused damages and injuries. Traditionally, acceptance of the duty is implied once the doctor and patient begin interaction. A *breach* is defined as a doctor's failure to adhere to the standard of care i.e., malpractice.

Also, ordinary negligence of the office staff is imputed to the doctor, and it is no defense that staff failed to follow procedure unless their conduct was well beyond the scope and course of employment.

Standard of Care

Standard of care is determined not by statute nor by the decision of judges. Rather, this standard is defined and determined by the testimony of experts at trial or deposition (sworn testimony given outside the courtroom). The law with regard to the standard of care is extremely vague and subject to the interpretation of expert witnesses. Normally the only guideline is a statement read to a jury that it is the doctor's "duty to use the care and skill ordinarily exercised in like cases by reputable members of the profession practicing in the same or similar locality and under similar circumstances."

Traditionally, this rule has held that if a doctor followed the practices of his local community he or she was not negligent. However, doctors belong to national associations and frequently attend national conferences. Because of these national educational efforts and a modern medical practice, the locality rule has, for the most part, been abandoned. Most courts now consider the locality rule extinct and accept a national standard of care.

Expert Witnesses

The standard of care requires a doctor to exercise prudent practice, as testified to by reputable members of his profession. It is important to recognize that the law does not require expert witnesses to be exclusively trained in oral and maxillofacial surgery. Other healthcare providers frequently testify as experts (e.g., plastic surgeons, neurologists, anesthesiologists, and otolaryngologists) in malpractice cases. Thus, a careful practitioner must consider the possibility that his or her work will fall under the scrutiny of other doctors not necessarily trained as oral and maxillofacial surgeons. The law also places no special requirements on the training of a doctor in order for them to testify as an expert. The courts do not require the expert witness to have any special credentials or training in the procedure that is the subject matter of the litigation. Instead, the judge will indicate that it is a matter of witness credibility and that the jury should consider the witness's training only in determining what weight to give the testimony, as compared with other experts.

The prudent practitioner must carefully present and document alternative forms of treatment discussed with the patient, particularly when using relatively new techniques, medications, or instruments.

Abandonment

Abandonment is a legal concept and a violation of the standard of care. Put simply, once a doctor begins a specific treatment on a patient, that procedure must be completed regardless of whether the doctor is receiving payment. This rule of law applies to all treatment including implants, restorations, appliances, and completion of orthodontic therapy. Once a patient's condition is altered by treatment, the doctor must complete therapy until the patient's condition is returned to a stable situation.[4]

At this time, the issue of a dental practitioner's

rights of refusal of treatment of patients suffering from acquired immunodeficiency syndrome (AIDS) or those who test positive for the human immunodeficiency virus (HIV) is not resolved. Most states and federal law now classify an AIDS patient in the same category as a handicapped individual, and thus a health care provider may not legally refuse to give treatment.[5] This is a form of abandonment. Even if there is no physical injury to the patient, such individuals may bring a suit against the doctor for refusing treatment and for causing emotional distress. Also, it is no defense that staff refused to treat an AIDS patient. The doctor is the employer and should educate or replace staff who refuse to follow the law.

Statute of Limitations

The law does not favor stale claims. Typically, most jurisdictions require that an action be brought within 1 to 3 years after the time the patient knew or should have known of the injury *and* its negligent cause. However, the courts are very liberal as to when the patient should have obtained this knowledge. Judges are adverse to throwing out a claim based on a circumstantial understanding of the patient.

Some states, by way of tort reform, have put an absolute limit on the statute of limitations. Typically, they require a patient to bring an action to trial within 3 years from the time of the injury, regardless of knowledge as to the negligent cause. However, courts frequently find exceptions to this rule, and thus the careful doctor must recognize that claims may be brought anywhere from 3 to 5 years after the last treatment. The time is tolled in cases of undiscovered nontherapeutic retained instruments or fraud by the doctor.

The Burden of Proof

The standard of care must be proved by a preponderance of evidence and not beyond a reasonable doubt as required in a criminal action. This is an important distinction. Typically, a jury is told they may have 49.9 % doubt as to the defendant's liability. Yet, if they have 50.1% belief in liability, they must award the full measure of damages. If the jury believes the evidence is fifty-fifty, they must find for the defendant.

In the event a jury finds that a doctor failed to meet the standard of care, they must then find that the negligence was the proximate or legal cause of some injury. The typical standard is the "but for" rule; for example, but for the negligence of the doctor's failure to prescribe antibiotics, the patient would not have suffered a severe infection. Legal cause is used when there are multiple concurrent causes. The rule in such cases is that the jury must find that the defendant's negligence was a substantial, although not an exclusive, factor in causing the injury.

Damages

In the event the jury finds there was a breach of the standard of care proximately causing injury, they are then told to decide what damages will make the plaintiff whole. Damages are divided into three categories: general damages, special damages, and punitive damages. The jury may not speculate as to the amount of these damages.

General damages are defined as the pain and suffering (physical and emotional) that has been or will be experienced by a patient. In most states this award has no limitation and is left to the discretion of the jury or judge. Dental verdicts for general damages have ranged from a few thousand dollars to amounts as high as two million dollars. Typically, a jury makes a decision as to general damages by analyzing whether the injury is permanent or temporary and the age, occupation, and preexisting health of the patient. Also, spouses may sue for loss of comfort, support, and society of the patient.

Special damages are defined as monetary losses suffered or to be suffered by the patient. Typical damages have been awarded for dental treatment, psychologic counseling, hospitalization for infection, transportation costs to and from treatment centers, housekeepers' fees, wage loss due to incapacitation, future wage loss, future hospitalization and treatment, and even wardrobe considerations when patients have lost or gained considerable weight.

Punitive exemplary damages are defined as an award designed to punish or make an example of the defendant. This doctrine is not designed to repay the patient for past suffering or expenses. Initially this was designed to punish intentional conduct (e.g., striking someone without his or her permission). This was usually quasi-criminal conduct and required intentional actions on behalf of the defendant. Where it is found that the defendant's conduct was performed in a conscious disregard for the rights and safety of others, many states allow the award of punitive damages. The Conscious Disregard rule applied to the dental profession includes conduct in which the doctor knew that a certain test should have been performed but consciously chose to not use that test. This rule has been used in periodontal cases in which the doctor knew about periodontal probes but chose not to use the instruments. While inconceivable that a doctor would intend to harm the patient, this is in effect the allegation by way of this unusual doctrine.

It is extremely important to note that punitive damages are based on a percentage of the defendant's net worth and is not related to the injury caused to the plaintiff. The wealthier the defendant, the more damages that may be awarded to the patient, irrespective of the harm suffered.

Legal Forms

A *request for records* is usually the first document formally announcing a claim. This is normally a written authorization from an attorney for release of records. This demand letter is usually accompanied by a release from the patient. When both of these items are present, the dentist must, in most states, release copies of the records, x-ray films, models, or any other items requested regardless of whether the patient owes any money or has yet to complete treatment. At this point, no efforts should be made to contact the patient or the attorney.

The *complaint* is the first legal document filed with the court stating the lawsuit. Today's dental practitioner should not be alarmed if there are rather gross and confusing allegations. Complaints routinely allege that the doctor had inadequate training, intended to harm the patient, used unproven techniques, and defrauded the patient. The courts allow a plaintiff to allege anything, although proving it is another matter. It is important for today's practitioner to note that the law takes quite seriously time limits set in responding to certain documents. Typically, a complaint must be answered within 30 days or the doctor is deemed to have admitted everything set forth in the complaint, and then the court need only decide the amount of damages to award the patient. Upon receipt, the doctor should immediately advise his or her insurance company or attorney.

The *answer* is the formal response to the complaint. If filed on time, it negates the possibility of a default judgment for failure to respond. A typical answer will deny all of the allegations and set forth claims that the patient was responsible for his or her own injuries. In most cases these documents are filed by attorneys.

Discovery is that process by which both sides to a litigation obtain evidence. Discovery includes subpoena of records, written questions submitted to each side (known as interrogatories), and depositions (sworn oral testimony). A doctor should never release original records without first consulting his or her counsel. Any notices received from the plaintiff or the plaintiff's attorney should be immediately forwarded to the doctor's insurance company, or once counsel is appointed, sent to the assigned attorney.

INFORMED CONSENT

Legal Requirements

The doctrine of informed consent has its roots in the legal principle known as "battery." *Battery* is defined as the touching of a person without the consent of that person. Traditionally, to be a battery, treatment must have been an intentional, unlawful, and offensive contact by a health care provider and without the consent of the patient. In such situations, a doctor would be held liable for any negative effects of the treatment, successful or not, regardless of the standard of care.[6] To defend these claims, the doctor had to show evidence of consent, which is implied in most healthcare settings. As the delivery of healthcare became more complicated, it became necessary to establish a standard as to the information to be given to a patient before surgery. Thus, the original doctrine of implied consent was replaced by "informed" consent. A healthcare provider must disclose such additional information as a skilled practitioner of good standing would provide under the same or similar circumstances. This provider-based doctrine remained in force until the early 1970s. Today, informed consent is a legal rather than medical doctrine. A doctor must advise a patient of the reasonable alternatives and the known risks of serious bodily injury inherent in a proposed procedure. The discussion must be in lay terms so the reasonable patient may make an informed decision.

The doctrine of informed consent has been further extended to include the requirement that doctors advise patients of the risk of *not* having treatment. This has been extended to cases such as a patient's refusal to have x-ray films, periodontal surgery, biopsies, and laboratory tests.

The law does not require that every known risk be discussed. Indeed, it has been frequently ruled that there is no duty to discuss minor risks inherent in common procedures when such procedures very seldom result in serious ill effects. Examples include the fact that some patients have been known on very rare occasions to die from the effects of local anesthetic or to sustain serious infections as a result of giving blood. There is also no duty to make disclosure of risks when the procedure is simple and the danger remote and commonly understood to be remote.

The mere consent of the patient without the disclosure of the risks of the treatment renders the doctor subject to liability for any injury if a reasonably prudent person in the patient's position would not have consented to the treatment if he or she had known the risks. This part of the consent law, known as the reasonable person standard, is perhaps the most significant tool for the defense of the doctor. The jury is to judge a patient not by twenty-twenty hindsight; rather, the measuring stick is what a reasonable person would have done had he or she known of the risks and alternatives of treatment and refusal of treatment.

The most important aspect of informed consent is documentation. Many studies have shown that patients do not remember much of what they have been told by their physician or dentist. Patients who have undergone open heart surgery have had their informed consents tape-recorded in detail. Postoperatively, these patients could recall no more than about 40% of the information provided. The studies indicate retrograde amnesia from the effects of the anesthetic, the stress of the surgery, and the human tendency to simply want to block out unpleasant experiences. The conclusion of these studies is to "get the consent in writing."[7]

Charting

Before using an informed consent document, the dental practitioner must first chart the necessity of the treatment. This includes the diagnosis of the problem, the recommendations and alternatives discussed with the patient, and some documentation of the discussion of the risks of the procedure. Typically, this is done by way of a written consent form after the doctor makes the appropriate chart entries. Some practitioners have resorted to audio or video recordings of the consultation during which the risks are discussed. These are acceptable methods if the patient consents to the recording.

At a minimum any consent form should include the following:

Name of the doctor who will perform the treatment (in some jurisdictions a patient cannot consent to treatment by a clinic or dental group)
In lay terms a description of the proposed treatment
Brief description of what the treatment is expected to accomplish
General and specific indication of the risks associated with the treatment
Brief indication of reasonable alternatives to the procedure
Provision for acknowledgment by the patient after being given an opportunity to ask questions of the doctor

It is recommended that any consent form be fashioned so that it can be tailored to the specific procedure for a specific patient. The document should have alternative paragraphs which may be checked or deleted where applicable. The forms must always provide for the patient's dated signature, witnessed by a staff member and signed and dated by the doctor. The staff member's signature allows for the identification of an important lay witness in the event there is a dispute.

Specific Procedures

Because of the complexities associated with most oral surgery procedures, it is recommended that written informed consent be obtained for most procedures. Specifically, and at a minimum, a patient should be warned of the following procedures and risks:

Molar exodontia and apical surgery: Permanent numbness, partial loss of taste, sinus communication, and subsequent repair, serious postoperative infection, limited jaw opening or temporomandibular joint (TMJ) dysfunction requiring physical therapy, jaw fracture necessitating repair surgery

Intravenous anesthesia (conscious and general): Intravenous irritation, allergic response, cardiac arrest and death

Implant surgery: Failure necessitating removal, permanent numbness, sinus communication, infection, and TMJ dysfunction

Orthognathic surgery: Failure or relapse requiring additional surgery, cosmetic failure, serious infection, permanent numbness, loss of taste or smell, speech and hearing changes, TMJ dysfunction

RECORDKEEPING

Today's practitioner has one major defense against litigation: good records. The law sees recordkeeping differently from perhaps the average doctor. The records are any tangible evidence of the conduct, activity, communication and interactions between the doctor, staff, and patient. Thus, in attempting to create and maintain good records the doctor should be aware that records include: the chart and insurance billings, health history questionnaires,[8] office pamphlets, letters regarding billing inquiries, models, photographs, letters received and sent, referral slips, laboratory reports, specialist reports, telephone logs and records, and prescription or medications slips.

Due to the extended statutes of limitation, it is recommended that the prudent practitioner maintain all of the office records for at least 10 years. Ideally, charts should be preserved for the entirety of the practice. After 10 years they can be stored at another location. Models and photographs should be maintained at least 8 to 10 years.

Another important consideration is that too often the practitioner, because of the press of time or a busy schedule, does not note "normal" conditions. One should consider a dental chart very much like a hospital chart which contains the history and physical and notes about the normal as well as abnormal findings.

A recognized set of abbreviations should be developed for the office, kept on file, and used by all staff members.

A major source of litigation and the unfavorable resolution of claims is altered records. Never, under any circumstances, attempt to change or alter the records. If for some reason one is compelled to make additions, the additions should always be put in the records in the normal sequence, not squeezed between other dates. The addition should be dated the date it is actually made. If it refers to another entry in the chart the doctor should simply note within the body of the entry that it is referring to some other date no matter how old the other entry.

LITIGATION

Pretrial Discovery

Perhaps the single most important aspect of litigation is the process known as discovery. This process allows each party to request and observe all of the evidence and legal theories that will be offered by the opponent. Put simply, the courts do not favor surprise at the time of trial. Part of the intent of the discovery system is to provide each party a clear understanding of the issues so that an out-of-court resolution is more likely.

Of all the tools available in discovery the deposition is probably the most important single item. Ninety to 95% of all dental malpractice suits never reach the actual trial stage of litigation. A few cases are dismissed on technicalities such as running of the statute of limitations, or because of the failure of the plaintiff to show any issue for the jury to decide. However, most cases resolve as a result of a payment by the doctor or insurance company to the plaintiff. Almost all evidence is introduced by way of testimony in the depositions of the parties and witnesses. Thus, in cases where the defendant does well in deposition the resolution may often be favorable for that defendant.

A deposition is very much like being a witness before a judge and jury. The primary difference is that testimony is given outside of a courtroom. Traditionally, most depositions are taken at the offices of the doctor giving the deposition or at the office of the attorney asking the questions. During the deposition both parties are always allowed to be present. Thus, a defendant may anticipate that the plaintiff/patient may be present during testimony. The defendant doctor is encouraged to attend the testimony of the plaintiff. Other individuals present would include the court reporter and the attorneys for all other parties.

Traditionally, the testimony is taken down by a court reporter who then transcribes it into a question and answer form. A copy is then provided to the defendant for correction of any transcription errors. Many states allow videotaping of the deposition and subsequent viewing by the jury at trial. Typically, a defendant should anticipate being deposed for at least 2 to 4 hours, and often the deposition may last more than an entire day.

Every party to a lawsuit must give their deposition on notice issued by an opposing party. Other witnesses in the case must be subpoenaed.

The Trial Process

Typically, a dental malpractice claim does not come to trial until 3 to 5 years after the last dental visit, and it is not unusual for a doctor to be in court 8 to 10 years after the patient was last seen. Because of the shrinking tax dollars available to many state governments the current civil court system is very crowded. Often there will be many false starts in which a doctor and his attorney are called down to trial only to be told that there are no available courtrooms and that the matter will be scheduled for a new court date 3 to 4 months in the future. In some situations this continuance may occur two or three times before the action is ever finally brought to trial.

The defendant doctor should be present throughout all phases of the trial, which typically lasts from 5 to 10 days. After completion of the pretrial motions the attorneys begin jury selection. The jury is composed of a random sample of members of the community. Typically, the courts rely on voter registration and driver's licenses to identify prospective jurors.

Many potential jurors ignore the court's request for their attendance. Others are excused because of their occupation. In many states professionals are automatically eliminated from juries. Next, individuals who would experience extreme financial hardships by being required to sit as a juror are dismissed. Thus, when a jury pool is finally called to a courtroom it is often composed of 30 or 40 individuals who are retired, housewives, unemployed, or students, or who are in occupations that may not require their services for lengthy periods of time. Next, the attorneys may challenge and exclude a limited number of jurors believed not favorable to one party. Although it has often been said that it is everyone's civic duty to act as a juror it is also true that many find a way to get off a jury. In the final analysis a doctor must recognize that the jury will be composed of individuals who lack the sophistication and education to understand complex healthcare issues and who may decide the case sympathetically. (It is very rare that a doctor is left on the jury.)

All evidence in a case comes in by way of verbal testimony. Even physical evidence such as films, records, models, and so forth must be authenticated by verbal testimony. Most jurisdictions allow the defendant to be called as the first witness on behalf of the plaintiff's case. After direct testimony each witness is then cross-examined by the opposing attorney. In dental malpractice cases it usually takes about a half day for each expert witness. At the conclusion of all testimony the attorneys are allowed to give closing statements and argument. Plaintiff's attorney will start, followed by the defense attorney and then finally the plaintiff's attorney will conclude with rebuttal. Typically, this is a no-holds-barred presentation by counsel. The court specifically indicates to the jury that the statements of counsel are not evidence and thus some rather dramatic interpretations are presented by counsel. The evidence may be reread to the jury, exhibits may be demonstrated, and counsel may often engage in borderline theatrics.

At the conclusion of the closing remarks the court will then read instructions to the panel. These instructions advise the jury as to the law they should use in deciding the standard of care, proximate cause, and damages.

In the event either party is unhappy with the verdict they may appeal the jury's decision to the trial court. The complaining party will ask the judge of the trial court to rule that there was misconduct by the jury, or an error of law made by the court. Seldom are such motions successful. With few exceptions, verdicts against dentists are usually either paid or settled for a lesser amount. In general, appellate courts are very hesitant to upset a jury award.

Alternative Dispute Resolution Procedures

Arbitration

A frequently used alternative to the expensive and time-consuming trial process is arbitration. This form of dispute resolution has been shown to effectively reduce the cost and time of litigation by as much as 60%. Such savings translate into reduced premiums and costs to the defendant doctor. Several states have passed binding arbitration statutes. The patient, before treatment, must sign a very specific binding arbitration form, waiving the right to trial by jury.

The majority of states have legislation that allows for court-ordered nonbinding arbitration. Such legislation provides for a damage threshold which is used to determine the eligibility of a given case for arbitration. A determination of the amount of any potential award of damages is made by the court, and cases in which the likely verdict does not exceed the statutory damage threshold are assigned to nonbinding arbitration. The parties do not give up their right to trial by jury, and the results of arbitration are not admissible at trial. Additionally, the time required to bring the case to trial is tolled until the conclusion of nonbinding arbitration. Either party may reject the arbitration award. However, certain sanctions in the form of monetary penalties are assessed against the party requesting a new trial, if the trial does not result in a verdict greater than the arbitration award.

The discovery process in arbitration cases is identical to normal litigation. The only difference is the presentation of the evidence at the time of arbitration as compared with a formal trial. The parties will still have depositions taken, records subpoenaed, independent medical examinations performed, and interrogatories propounded and answered. However, in arbitration, evidence is admissible without the necessity of personal testimony. In a typical arbitration, only the plaintiff, defendant, and their respective attorneys will be present. A court-appointed or agreed panel of arbitrators will hear the evidence. The arbitrator, usually an attorney, will review all the depositions, records, and other evidence, in addition to hearing from the parties. The appearance of the defendant at the arbitration proceeding is just as important as at deposition or trial. The arbitrator serves as both the judge and the jury. A defendant doctor should prepare for arbitration in the same fashion as would be expected for a deposition or trial testimony. A formal courtroom proceeding lasts anywhere from 7 to 10 days, whereas an arbitration rarely lasts more than one day due to the informality of the proceedings and the ability to use discovery items in place of live witnesses.

Statistics indicate that a significant number of cases are resolved following arbitration, either by settlement or acceptance of the decision of the arbitrator.

Peer Review Committees

The traditional alternative dispute resolution method has been the use of peer review committees. A patient with a complaint has the matter reviewed by local members of a dental society or a state-appointed board of quality assurance. However, few states have allowed the findings of peer review committees to be binding on the patient. The only sanction afforded the committee is the authority to discipline a member doctor who refuses to abide by a decision. In most cases disciplinary action is limited to dismissal from the society. Peer review societies cannot award general damages, and awards of specific damages are limited to the amount of the charges paid to the defendant and, in some cases, the cost of obtaining of the dental treatment in question elsewhere.

Most states encourage peer review without fear of undue scrutiny. Therefore, the internal workings of a peer review committee are generally not subject to discovery and are inadmissible at trial.[9] This protective limitation on access to the use of peer findings is designed to promote the viability and effectiveness of the review process by discouraging second guessing and removing the fear of litigation challenging the findings of a reviewing panel. Unfortunately, many patients simply use peer review as a testing ground for possible malpractice actions. Also, expert witnesses testifying on behalf of the plaintiff are afforded the opportunity to study the peer review findings and incorporate favorable aspects into their testimony. However, many disputes are successfully resolved by peer review decisions.

LIABILITY INSURANCE

Until the early 1980s most dentists were able to obtain occurrence liability insurance to protect them against claims of dental malpractice. This type of coverage can be defined as an insurance policy in which all treatment occurring during the policy period is covered regardless of when the actual claim is made (i.e., year of treatment must equal year of insurance, no matter when the suit is brought). Because of wide fluctuations in the claims experience many insurance carriers have abandoned this type of coverage and have moved to "claims-made" coverage.

Claims-made insurance policies cover claims made while the policy is in effect (i.e., year of coverage must equal year of suit). Claims-made policies afford the insurance carrier more predictability as to current claims experience, and rates are more reflective of the current trends. Claims-made policies are less expensive in the first year and then increase in price until maturity in approximately the fifth year, at which time the premium is about equal to an occurrence liability policy.

A retiring or disabled practitioner must purchase a "prior acts" policy rather than continuing to purchase annual claims-made coverage. The cost of such a policy is usually one-and-one-half times the annual premium. Many companies provide that if the insured has been with the company for a specified number of years or has passed a specific age, then prior acts coverage is included and no further premium need be paid. (Caveat: When terminating or changing insurance, a doctor must be careful to either have had an occurrence policy or purchase prior acts coverage if insured under claims-made policies.)

REFERENCES

1. Time Magazine, March 24, 1986.
2. Gwilliam G. Esq. Dental malpractice: Who cares? CTLA Form April 1985.
3. Restatement of Torts, 2nd ed. §245A, *Katz v Hebbing*, 205 Cal 629, 271 P. 1062 (1928).
4. *McNamara v Emmons*, 36 C.A. 2d 199, 97 P. 2d 503 (1039).
5. *Doe v Centinela Hospital*, 57 USLW 2034 (CD Cal 1988), Federal Rehabilitation Act of 1973, §504.
6. California Book of Approved Jury Instructions §6.11, *Cobbs v Grant*, 1972, 8 Cal. 3d 229, 104 Cal Rptr 505, 502 P. 2d 1.
7. Robinson G. Ann Thorac Surg 1976; 22(3):9.
8. McCarthy FM. A new patient-administered medical history developed for dentistry. J Am Dent Assoc 1985; 111:595.
9. California Code of Evidence §1157, §1157.5.

BIBLIOGRAPHY

Howard WW, Parks AL. The Dentist and the Law, ed 3. St. Louis: CV Mosby, 1973.

Morris WO. Dental Litigation, ed 2. Charlottesville, VA: Michie, 1977.

Schafler NL. Medical Malpractice: Handling Dental Cases. Colorado Springs: Shepard's/McGraw-Hill, 1985.

Schroeder OC Jr, Gardner AF. Dental Jurisprudence: A Handbook of Practical Law. MA: PSG Publishing, 1980.

Woodall IR, Bentley JM. Legal, Ethical, and Management Aspects of the Dental Care System, ed 2. St. Louis: CV Mosby, 1983.

III

MANAGEMENT OF INFECTIONS OF THE JAWS

9

Odontogenic Infections: Anatomic and Microbiologic Considerations

Robert D. Marciani

Odontogenic infection has been a part of human existence since prerecorded history. When early man experienced a toothache, his clinical course was most certainly painful and very likely, occasionally lethal. He relied on his own natural defenses and eventual loss of the tooth for a cure. As the human species evolved and diets became more refined, dental disease became more common. Cro-Magnon humans lived 25,000 years ago and showed evidence of destructive tooth attrition.[1] Dental caries and periapical and periodontal abscesses occurred in all periods of recorded Egyptian history.[2] Skulls of pre-Columbian Peruvians show evidence of both caries and periodontitis.[3] Hippocrates described an Athenian boy with decayed teeth, jaw pain, and facial swelling. The pain ceased when spontaneous suppuration occurred in the right ear.[4] Hippocrates related human illness in part to "peccant humors" which must be evacuated to achieve resolution of diseases.

The greatest doctors of antiquity practiced medicine by observation, knowledge of anatomy, and fundamental physical examination. They recognized odontogenic infection and applied principles of care that are relevant centuries later.

The fundamentals of infection management that were practiced by the great masters of ancient civilizations are as important today as they were in early times. The successful treatment of the infected patient begins with the application of these fundamentals. A broad understanding of odontogenic infections is achievable when the principles of care are mastered.

PRINCIPLES OF INFECTION MANAGEMENT

Consistent therapeutic results is the goal of every treatment regimen, irrespective of the disease process. Odontogenic infections generally respond in a predictable manner to four principles of care: removal of cause, incision and drainage, appropriate antibiotic care, and supportive care.

Removal of Cause of Infection

Identifying the source of an infection is the first step in the development of a treatment plan to control inflammatory diseases of the head and neck. Acute infections of the perioral region are commonly associated with periapical, periodontal, subperiosteal, sinus, pericoronal, or salivary gland disease. The early resolution of odontogenic infections is strongly influenced by the timing of surgical intervention.

When is surgical intervention to remove the cause of the pain and swelling indicated? Delaying the extraction of a tooth, for example, until the cellulitis was "walled off" by the host's specific and nonspecific defense mechanisms was a common practice in the preantibiotic era. Prompt surgical intervention is the recommended treatment for odontogenic infections in concert with antibiotics and suitable supportive care. Surgical care should only be delayed when intercurrent systemic illness must be corrected to permit a safer operative course. The practice of placing the patient on antibiotics and waiting for spontaneous drainage and decreased swelling is usually inappropriate.

Incision and Drainage

The importance of abscesses draining did not escape the attention of the masters of antiquity. Hippocrates, in his fourth book on epidemics noted, "Egesistratus had a suppuration near the 'eye.' An abscess manifested itself near the last tooth; the eye directly got quite well; there was a dense discharge from the gums. It seemed as though a suppuration at the third tooth were going to take place, but it went back and suddenly the jaw and the eye swelled up."[4] The experience of contemporary clinical practice endorses the importance of draining the abscess. The practitioner treating orofacial infections must know the anatomy of head and neck spaces, microbiologic considerations, the indigenous oral flora, pathogenic mechanisms, surgical techniques of incision and drainage, culture and sensitivity techniques, and have the ability to interpret the results of all pertinent laboratory tests.

Antibiotics

Antibiotic agents produced by microganisms occur naturally and continuously in soil, sewage, water, and other natural habitats. Mankind has benefitted immeasurably from the substances derived from one living organism to kill another organism.[5] To be of practical value in the treatment of infection, an antibiotic must exert its effects on the invading microorganisms without seriously damaging the cells of the host. It is remarkable that so many compounds with such selective activity have been developed. As far as is known, all antimicrobial agents are effective because they enhance the natural defense mechanisms of the host.

The principal result of antibiotic activity is retardation of organism growth. When present in sufficiently high concentrations, some drugs kill bacteria in vivo as well as in vitro. The importance of the patient's immune and inflammatory defense mechanisms cannot be overstated. Antimicrobial agents, even the most potent ones, do not (except in uncommon instances) cure infection simply by virtue of their activity against the responsible organism. The high percentage of therapeutic failures of infected patients with impaired immune reactions is testimony to the importance of the host's response. The use of antibiotics is a vital, if not absolutely essential, step in the management of orofacial infections. An in-depth understanding of the history, mechanisms of action, spectrums of activity, and reactions to antibiotics is essential to the care of the infected patient.

Supportive Care

An important adjunct to infection treatment is the fulfillment of the patient's nutritional, fluid and electrolytes, analgesic, and anesthetic needs. The debilitated patient is less capable of resisting the spread of infection than one who is otherwise healthy. Intercurrent disease may interfere with the speedy resolution of infection or encourage such life-threatening complications as mediastinal or intracranial extension, retropharyngeal spread and airway obstruction, pleuropulmonary suppuration, and hematogenous dissemination to heart valves. Maintenance and replacement fluids must be infused to achieve correct fluid and electrolyte balance. Drug interactions and untoward antibiotic events must be anticipated and prevented. Pain and suffering must be alleviated with suitable analgesics. The psychosocial and economic impact on the patient's life must be considered.

OROFACIAL ODONTOGENIC INFECTIONS

Microbiologic Considerations

The microflora associated with odontogenic infections is complex and generally reflect the indigenous oral flora. Odontogenic infections are usually polymicrobial and involve four to six organisms. Each organism in this complex flora does not have equal pathogenic potential. The numerically predominant, cultivable microflora are not necessarily the most important organisms cultured. It also may not be necessary to eradicate the complete microflora for effective therapy.[6]

Understanding the microbiology of odontogenic infections begins with a review of the indigenous oral flora, the environment of the oral cavity, and the attributes of microorganisms overall.

The mouth is a warm moist environment that provides a variety of surfaces for bacterial colonization. Moist surfaces are freely exposed to the cleansing action of saliva. Protected crypts are found in the occlusal surfaces of teeth, between the teeth, and along the gingival margin. Large bacterial masses develop on the teeth; epithelial cell desquamation prevents the accumulation of comparable masses on mucosal surfaces. The largest biomass of bacteria is found on the surfaces of the teeth and on the dorsum of the tongue.

Oral Flora

The oral cavity contains an estimated 200 microbial species.[7] Many of these organisms are anaerobic bacteria that can be shown with quantitative cultures to dominate the flora of the oral cavity. Most anaerobic infections involve bacteria that are normal inhabitants of the adjacent oral structure.

Saliva contains 10^8 to 10^9 bacteria, which are continuously being shed from the tongue surface.[8] Veillonella and various types of streptococci predominate, in a ratio of 3 to 10 anaerobes for each aerobe. The tooth surface harbors large numbers of *Actinomyces viscosus, Streptococcus mutans, Streptococcus miteor,* and *Streptococcus sanquis*. The largest bacterial concentrations are found in the gingival sulcus. A lush anaerobic flora which includes *Bacteroides melaninogenicus, Fusobacterium nucleatum,* and anaerobic streptococci inhabit the sulcus.[9] These organisms are the predominant identifiable pathogens in odontogenic abscesses, aspiration pneumonia, and lung abscess.

Bartlett and Gorbach[7] described flora studies showing that populations of bacteria form distinctive ecosystems within the oropharynx. Different bacteria are found in the nose, pharynx, tongue, buccal mucosa, tooth surface, and gingival crevice. Four factors are considered important in colonization patterns: bacterial adherence, IgA, bacterial antagonism, and environmental conditions. Different bacteria have the propensity to adhere to certain cell types. Adherence also appears to play a role in certain pathologic conditions; an extraneous organism must attach to cells before it can invade the host. Gibbons and vanHoute[10] described the ability of *S. pyogenes* to adhere to normal pharyngeal cells but not bladder epithelial cells; the opposite relationship applies to common urinary tract pathogens such as *Escherichia coli.*[11] *S. pyogenes* has a greater affinity for pharyngeal cells from patients with rheumatic fever.[12] Selective adherence of this type may explain the pathophysiology of bacterial endocarditis, pharyngitis, urinary tract infections, and a variety of enteric diseases.[13]

Johanson et al.[14] and Laforce et al.[15] have shown that the normal cell-microbe relation is disrupted in the presence of serious illness. Pharyngeal and buccal epithelial cells from healthy persons have little affinity for coliform bacteria. These organisms appear to attach well to cells from patients who are ill. The extent of the attachment correlates with the severity of the disease. This mechanism may explain why coliforms are seldom found in the oropharynx of healthy persons but are relatively common in patients who are seriously ill. Normal flora is reestablished following recovery from the illness.

Bartlett and Gorbach[7] established bacterial antagonism as an important factor in determining colonization patterns. They suggested that bacteria compete for receptor sites or nutrients and that elimination of the normal flora promotes ingrowth by extraneous forms to "fill the void." Other investigators have observed that antimicrobial administration to even healthy persons is commonly associated with unusual colonization patterns in the oropharynx.[16,17]

Onishi et al.[18] reported the oxidation-reduction potential (E_h) obtained on gingival, tongue, and interdental spaces. E_h values for periodontal pockets, plaque, and the gingival crevice are -5 mV, -200 mV, and -300 mV, respectively. An E_h of -300 mV simulates the environment in the colon, which is sufficiently low in atmospheric oxygen to support the growth of fastidious anaerobes. The predominance of anaerobes in the normal oral flora is not paradoxical if one does not assume that atmospheric oxygen has easy access to the oral cavity. Eskow and Loesche[19] have studied oxygen tensions in the human oral cavity. Gas analysis of the buccal fold indicates a PO_2 of less than 1%, suggesting minimal gas exchange where the cheek approximates gingival and tooth surfaces.

Attributes of Microorganisms

There are countless numbers of microorganisms but only a small number are capable of causing disease in humans.[20] Microorganisms that are pathogenic for humans are placed in groups arranged in a sequence of increasing complexity of organization. Viruses are classified as either DNA or RNA, with RNA viruses more commonly pathogenic for humans. Energy-generating and biosynthetic mechanisms are absent in viruses; viral replication requires the active participation of the host cells. Viruses replicate by attaching to host cells, penetrating, uncoating, replicating and translating viral nucleic acid, maturing, and releasing to infect other cells. Chlamydias are susceptible to antimicrobials such as sulfanilamide, chloramphenicol, and tetracycline. In humans, chlamydia causes trachoma, inclusion blennorreah, lymphogranuloma venereum, psittacosis, and possibly nonspecific urethritis. Mycoplasmas are not susceptible to antimicrobials that interfere with cell wall synthesis. Only one species of *Mycoplasma*, *M. pneumonia*, the etiologic agent of primary atypical pneumonia, is pathogenic for humans. Rickettsias have a cell membrane that is usually permeable and require an arthropod vector for perpetuation in nature and for transmission to the human host. They lose viability rapidly in most extracellular environments and generally produce severe infections with exanthemata (e.g., Rocky Mountain spotted fever) in humans. Bacteria are the predominant organisms in orofacial infections. A more detailed review of the structure, classification, staining reactions and oxygen tolerance qualities of bacteria will be discussed subsequently.

Spirochetes are not important pathogens in orofacial infections. Three genera are pathogenic for humans and are susceptible to penicillin G in low doses. Fungi differ from human cells in size, morphology, complexity of cellular organization, modes of reproduction, and cellular differentiation. The rigid fungal cell wall differs chemically from the bacterial cell; the synthesis of fungal cell walls is not blocked by the penicillins or other agents that interfere with the synthesis of bacterial cell walls. The cell membranes of fungi are unlike those of bacteria in that they are rich in sterols, particularly ergosterol. Amphotericin B has a high affinity for sterols and is, therefore, an excellent antimicrobial for fungal infections. Protozoa are medically important organisms that infect the intestines (*Entamoeba histolytica*), blood and hematopoietic system (*Plasmodium*), genital tract (*Trichomonas*), and parenchymal cells and cells of the endoreticular system.

Bacteria

Orofacial infections are managed successfully when the principles of infection management are implemented. These principles are few and relatively easily applied. It is important for the surgeon to approach the care of the infected patient with a biologic basis for his treatment. Bacteria are the common pathogens of orofacial infections and much is known about bacterial cells. An in-depth understanding of the fundamental characteristics of the bacteria and their relation to the human cell will help the surgeon make enlightened patient care decisions. A schematic representation of a prototype bacterial cell is shown in Figure 9–1.

The cell wall is a structure found in bacterial but not in human cells. The cell wall imparts mechanical strength to bacteria, thus permitting the organism to survive in a wide range of environmental conditions. Salts and metabolites have a much higher concentration inside the bacterial cell than outside; osmotic rupture is prevented by the rigid cell wall. In gram-positive bacteria, the cell wall is 20 to 80 nm thick and constitutes 20% to 40% of the dry weight of the cell. The cell wall of gram-negative bacteria is less than 10 nm thick and constitutes about 15% of the dry cell weight.

The basic structure of the bacterial cell wall is a peptidoglycan layer made up of polysaccharide chains cross-linked by oligopeptides, resulting in one huge, complex molecule. The polysaccharide chain contains alternating units of N-acetylglucosamine and N-acetylmuramic acid. The latter is a compound unique to bacterial cell walls. The proteinaceous compounds of the gram-positive cocci and the lipopolysaccharides of gram-negative bacteria form the part of the cell wall external to the basal peptidoglygan layer. A capsular layer may be found in some strains external to the cell wall.

Walls and capsules are exceedingly important structures. Capsules probably interfere with phagocytosis

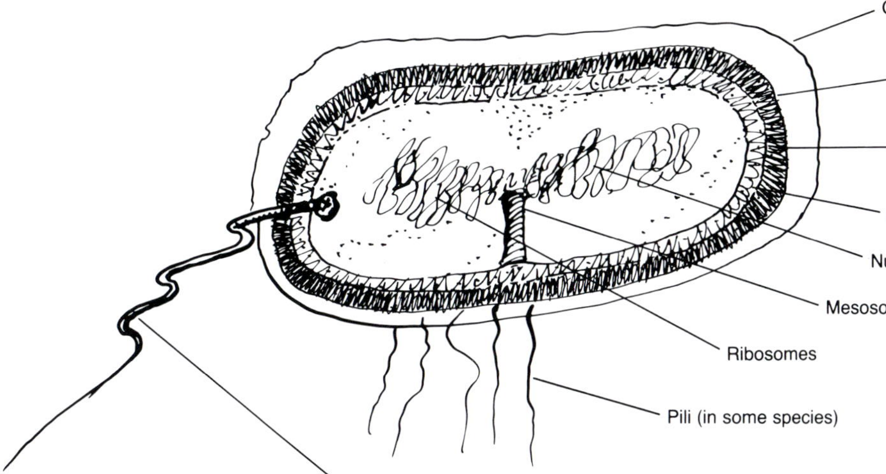

Figure 9–1. *Schematic drawing of a typical bacterium.*

and thereby increase their pathogenicity. Antimicrobials may be rendered ineffective by the structure of the cell wall. The lipopolysaccharide layer can impair or prevent the entry of some antimicrobial molecules.

Antibiotics such as penicillin that interfere specifically with cell wall synthesis are effective antibacterial agents because they attack a structure that is not present in the human cell. Penicillin is the principal antibiotic used to treat odontogenic infections. The chemical composition of the bacterial cell wall makes it vulnerable to the action of penicillin, which interferes with cell wall synthesis.

Morphologically, chemically, and functionally the bacterial cell membrane resembles the human cell. There are several important differences including the absence of sterols in bacteria. (Sterols are compounds that are credited with conferring toughness on membranes.) Also absent in bacteria are an internal membrane system of structures similar to the endoplasmic reticulum, Golgi complex, and nuclear membrane of the human cell.

The bacterial cytoplasm contains ribosomes, the only organelles found in the cytoplasm. The ribosomes of bacteria and human cells are similar in general structure but differ significantly in size, weight percentage of RNA subunits, and number of protein subunits. These structural differences account for the effectiveness of selected antimicrobials that inhibit the protein synthesis of bacteria without appreciably disrupting this same function in the human cell.

Nucleus and nucleolus as distinct, identifiable structures are not found in bacterial cells. Bacterial cells contain regions where DNA aggregates but it is not separated from the cytoplasm by nuclear membranes. As a result, the genetic material of bacteria is more accessible to antimicrobial agents than the coding material of human cells.

Bacterial shape (coccal, bacillary, curved), staining reaction (gram stain, acid fast), and oxygen tolerance (aerobic, anaerobic, facultative) are the most useful identifying characteristics of bacteria to the clinician. Gram stain is particularly useful to establish the presence of organisms within minutes of obtaining a specimen for culture and antibiotic sensitivity. A positive gram stain implies retention of a gentian violet stain which is associated with some bacteria and all fungi. A negative reaction, failure of retention of a gentian violet stain, is generally associated with organisms that have physical-chemical properties that are the reverse of gram-positive species. In addition to establishing the shapes of the organisms present, that gram stain provides information that is useful in selecting an antibiotic and indirectly may suggest the presence of anaerobic organisms when cultures are reported as having no growth. An example of a gram stain is shown in Figure 9–2.

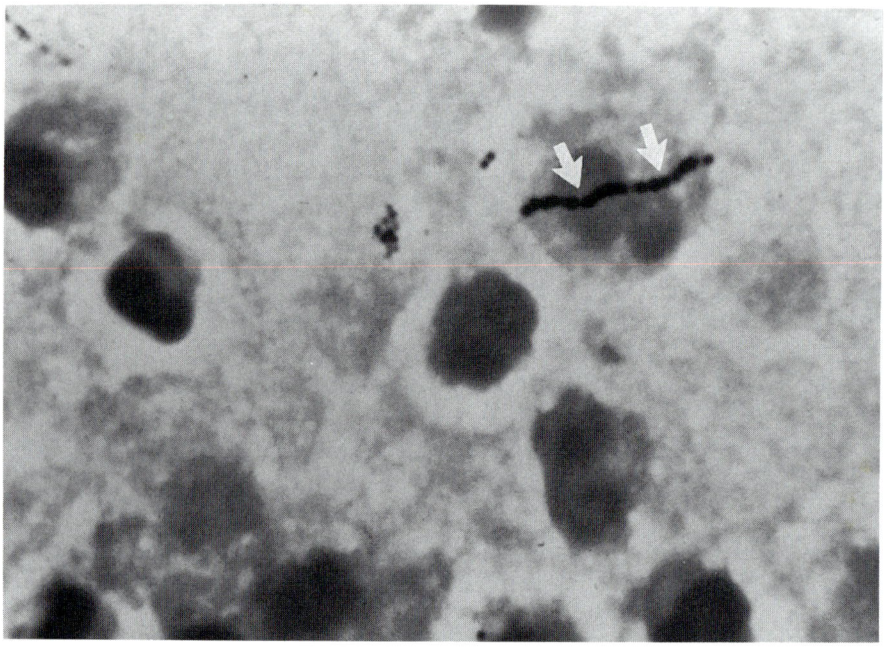

Figure 9–2. *Example of a gram stain. These gram-positive cocci are arranged in a chain.*

Medically Important Bacteria

Most medically important bacteria fall into one of five major groups: gram-positive cocci, gram-negative cocci, gram-positive bacilli, gram-negative bacilli, and acid-fast bacteria. Gram-positive streptococcus is the most common organism in odontogenic infections and is frequently seen in specimens taken from dental abscesses. Gram-negative cocci are represented by *Veillonella* (anaerobe) and *Neisseria* species, organisms that are not major pathogens in odontogenic infections but are often reported as growing in the infected tissue specimen. Actinomyces is an important gram-positive bacilli which is a common inhabitant of the oral cavity and usually only becomes pathogenic when tissue is damaged. Actinomyces is a fastidious anaerobe that should always be suspected when odontogenic infections become chronic and gram-positive rods are found. *Corynebacterium diphtheriae* is a facultative gram-positive rod that frequently is found in cultures obtained from the head and neck, but is of no clinical significance. The gram-negative bacilli are common pathogens in dental infections. *F. nucleatum* and *B. melaningenicus* are important anaerobic gram-negative rods that frequently are grown from oral pus. The Enterobacteriaceae and other facultative gram-negative rods are uncommon in oral infections in healthy adults, but may be opportunistic pathogens in the elderly or debilitated patient.

GRAM-POSITIVE COCCI. Streptococci are gram-positive cocci that occur in pairs or chains. They may exhibit gram variability with increasing age of culture. Streptococci may be further grouped by blood hemolysis or antigenic structure (Lancefield groups). Alpha hemolysis appears as small colonies surrounded by a greenish zone of hemolysis; β-hemolysis by a clear zone of hemolysis; and gamma hemolysis with no changes in the blood agar. *S. pyogenes*, a common pathogen responsible for upper respiratory infections and post-streptococcal sequelae such as rheumatic fever, rheumatic heart disease, and glomerulonephritis is usually beta hemolytic. Enterococci are usually nonhemolytic, but may exhibit α- or β-hemolysis. Differential media allow selective morphologic identification of certain microbial colonies. The colony morphology and type of hemolysis are initial screening tests to determine further steps in identification of an isolate. Lancefield grouping may be clinically important in odontogenic infections when the serologic type (e.g., group D enterococci) helps to identify an organism resistant to penicillin.

S. pyogenes usually inhabit the nasopharynx and skin. They seldom cause oral infection and are usually penicillin sensitive. The enterococci, such as *S. faecalis*, usually inhabit the gastrointestinal tract, vagina, and pharynx. These organisms may comprise up to 10% of cultivable organisms of the gingival sulcus and exhibit resistance to penicillin and other antibiotics. *S. sanguis* usually inhabits the throat, gut, and nasopharynx. Fifteen percent of cultivable organisms of coronal plaque, 8% of sulcus organisms and a significant percentage of organisms on the dorsum of the tongue are *S. sanguis*. These organisms are usually sensitive to penicillin.[8] *S. salivarius* usually inhabits the mouth and throat and is also sensitive to penicillin.

Anaerobic gram-positive cocci are divided into several genera including peptococci (anaerobic staphylococci) and peptostreptococci (anaerobic streptococci). These organisms can be very difficult to isolate and grow because they are often accompanied by other bacteria in an infection. Most perimandibular space infections involve a polymicrobial flora in which anaerobic bacteria are the dominant isolates.[21–24]

The genus *Staphylococcus* contains the important pathogen *S. aureus*, and the less virulent *S. epidermidis*. Both are common resident flora of the skin and nasal mucosa. These gram-positive cocci occur singly, in pairs, or in clusters. They may be pigmented white, beige, or gold. Usually a coagulase test is used to differentiate the more pathogenic *S. aureus* (coagulase positive) from the usually benign *S. epidermidis* (coagulase negative). The majority of strains of *S. aureus* and *S. epidermis* currently isolated in the United States produce penicillinase, an enzyme that destroys the β-lactam ring of penicillin.

Pneumococci are important pathogens in the lungs, meninges, paranasal sinuses, and the middle ear. *S. pneumoniae* frequently is cultured in meningitis related to basalar skull fractures associated with midface fractures.[25]

GRAM-NEGATIVE COCCI. *Neisseria* are small gram-negative cocci typically arranged in pairs with adjacent sides flattened. They are common throat flora and are often found in cultures of the head and neck. They are usually nonpathogenic in the oral cavity.

Veillonella are small anaerobic gram-negative cocci that are common in the oral cavity and are rarely considered pathogens.

GRAM-POSITIVE RODS. *Corynebacterium diphtheriae* are small, nonsporulating gram-positive bacilli. They are part of the normal oral flora and generally are not pathogenic there.

Nocardia (aerobic) and *Actinomyces* (anaerobic) are closely related bacilli that appear as small, branching gram-positive or gram-variable rods which may form filaments or tangled mats. They may form small, yellowish flecks or balls composed of delicate, branching gram-positive bacilli. These flecks or sulfur granules may be more evident to the naked eye in the threads of gauze or a cotton swab.

Clostridium is a large, anaerobic, sporulating gram-positive bacillus that produces gas and a foul odor in both the specimen and the culture. *C. perfringens* (*welchii*) is the species most commonly associated with gas gangrene, a disease rarely found in the head and neck.

C. tetani are obligate anaerobes. They have been cultured from soil, house and operating room dust, fresh and salt water, and gun wads. Tetanus is a disease manifested primarily by neuromuscular dysfunction. It is caused by tetanal toxin, an extremely potent exotoxin produced by *C. tetani*.[26]

GRAM-NEGATIVE RODS. *Haemophilus influenzae* are aerobic, pleomorphic, nonacid-fast, nonmotile, nonsporulating, and usually capsulated organisms that are important pathogens in children under 5 years of age. Since 1974, strains of ampicillin-resistant *H. influenzae* have been isolated from CSF and blood in children with meningitis or bacteremia.[27]

Enterobacteriaceae (e.g., *E. coli*, *Klebsiella*, *Proteus mirabilis*) are gram-negative enteric bacilli that inhabit the gastrointestinal tract and are the major pathogens of the abdominal viscera and urinary tract. They are facultative organisms and are uncommon pathogens in odontogenic infections in healthy adults.

P. aeruginosa is an important pathogen in the leukopenic, burned, immunosuppressed, or debilitated hospitalized patient. It has a sweet, fruity odor and is usually identified by its characteristic yellowish green pigment.

Bacteroides, *Fusobacterium*, and *Leptothrix* are anaerobic gram-negative rods. *Bacteroides* and *Fusobacterium* species are obligate anaerobes that are important pathogens in odontogenic infections.

ORAL MICROFLORA AND THE BACTERIOLOGY OF ORAL INFECTIONS

The microbial specificity in odontogenic infections was more clearly delineated when technologic advances in sampling and anaerobic culturing became available. Improved methods for species identification and taxonomy facilitated differentiating bacterial compositions for dental caries, gingivitis, and different forms of periodontitis compared with cultures from healthy tissues.[28-30] The microbial specificity in orofacial infections arising from odontogenic sources reflects the combined influence of the indigenous oral flora and the unique microbiota of the underlying conditions. *Bacteroides*, *Peptostreptococcus*, and *Streptococcus* are the most prevalent isolates.[6] When anaerobic culture techniques were not used, only streptococci were recovered. Staphylococci and aerobic gram-negative rods are not commonly associated with odontogenic infections. Gram-negative rods may become important pathogens in selected patients with serious underlying disease.[31]

These findings serve to further emphasize the importance of anaerobic culture and rapid transport of specimens to establish accurately the organisms present in odontogenic infections. Appropriate specimen collection is ideally obtained extraorally or by direct needle aspiration of fluids from the infected site to avoid contamination by the surrounding oral flora.

The bacteriology of 21 permandibular closed-space infections was studied prospectively using optimal bacteriologic techniques to collect, transport, and process specimens.[32] There was an average of six microbial species per specimen, including approximately four anaerobes and two aerobes. The predominant aerobes were α-hemolytic and non-hemolytic streptococci; the predominant anaerobes were peptostreptococci, *B. melaninogenicus*, and *F. nucleatum* infections. Fourteen of these patients had x-ray film evidence of a periapical abscess or an oral examination which showed gingivitis. Specimens were obtained by percutaneous needle aspiration or through a percutaneous surgical incision to avoid contamination by bacteria on mucosal surfaces. Anaerobic bacteria were recovered in every specimen, usually as part of a complex flora, which included a total of 123 isolates with 39 strains of aerobes and 84 strains of anaerobes.

Assessment of the records of 173 pyogenic dental infections revealed a predominance of facultative anaerobic streptococci and gram-negative bacteria.[22]

These and other bacteriologic findings[23,24] indicate that most perimandibular space infections involve a polymicrobial flora in which anaerobic bacteria are the dominant isolates. The choice of antibiotics should be heavily influenced by these findings when culture data is unavailable, anaerobic cultures are suspect, or the patient's clinical course is unfavorable.

ROUTES OF TRANSMISSION

The role of surgical intervention in the treatment of orofacial infections can not be overemphasized. Prompt and appropriate surgical intervention is the most important step in the management of odontogenic infections. Other orofacial infections, such as sialadenitis and sinusitis, may require nonsurgical therapy alone or surgical manipulation only after a reasonable course of conservative therapy has been tried. The surgeon must have an in-depth knowledge of the fascia and fascial spaces of the head and neck and the relation of these spaces to each other. Accurate knowledge of the anatomy of these spaces and the surgical approaches for drainage of pus is an absolute requirement for surgeons treating head and neck infections. The reader is encouraged to make a detailed review of this subject in a suitable anatomy textbook.[33]

Superficial Fascia

The subcutaneous tissue of the head and neck compose the superficial fascia. The superficial fascia contains a variable amount of fat and generally encloses voluntary muscles in its deep portion. This attachment to the muscles of facial expression translates into the ability of the human face to communicate effectively without speaking. Rarely do infections of the head and neck involve the muscles of the face and their tight fascial attachments. The subcutaneous tissue of the face is also tightly attached to the underlying bone. Exceptions include the subcutaneous tissue of the eyelids, the subgaleal space, and the buccal space occupied by the buccal fat pad. The buccal space and the superficial orbital space are common sites for the spread of odontogenic infection. Involvement of the superficial tissues of the eye should alert the surgeon to the potential of orbital cellulitis, vision impairment, and intracranial infection.

Deep Fascia

Hollinshead[33] described the cervical fascia as having several more or less distinct layers (Fig. 9–3). The layers in the front of the neck continue around the posterior aspect of the neck. Thus, the anterior cervical fascial layer also has a posterior segment. To avoid confusing the various layers of the deep cervical fascia, the surgeon should recall the individual levels and compartments, from the most superficial to the deepest, and further consider the location of the space above and below the hyoid bone. Hollinshead proposes a simple concept of the superficial deep cervical fascia encircling the entire neck deep to the subcutaneous tissue while other layers by their dispositions and fusions form two unpaired and one paired compartment within the superficial fascia. The layer surrounding the entire neck is the superficial (anterior) layer. It surrounds the trapezius, omohyoid, sternocleidomastoid, and infrahyoid muscles. Superiorly the superficial layer attaches to the hyoid bone and inferiorly is split to form the suprasternal space of Burns. The prevertebral (posterior, deep) layer encloses the neck and attaches again at its point of origin.

The pretracheal or middle layer of fascia passes behind the strap or infrahyoid muscles and blends with the superficial fascia at the lateral edges of these muscles. The pretracheal layer extends into the superior mediastinum and can be involved by odontogenic infection through its retrovisceral portion. The retrovisceral-retropharyngeal space extends behind the pharynx to the base of the skull. It is through this pathway that infections in the head and neck reach the mediastinum.

The prevertebral layer of fascia attaches to the transverse process laterally and divides into two layers anteriorly called the *alar fascia* (Fig. 9–4). The anterior layer of the alar fascia forms the posterior boundary of the retrovisceral space. The posterior layer is made up of the prevertebral fascia, which consists of the connective tissue immediately against the anterior surfaces of the prevertebral muscles and the vertebral bodies. The danger space lies between the layers of the

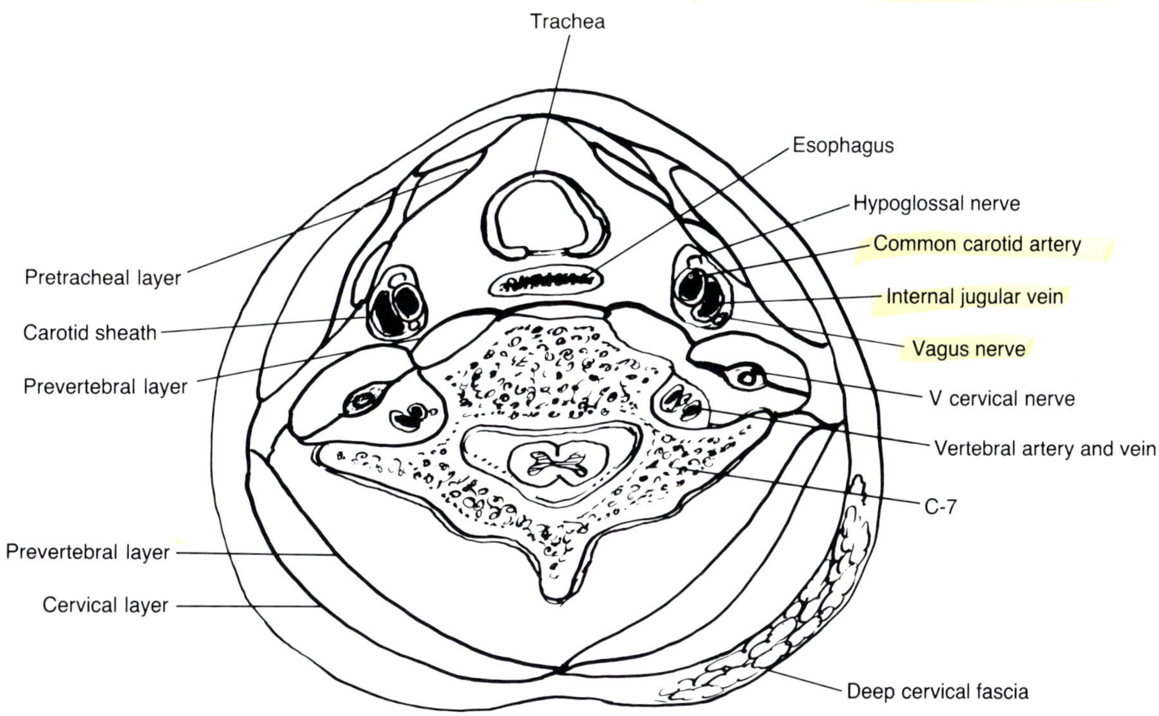

Figure 9–3. *Chief cervical fascial layers (*heavy lines*) below the hyoid. Note the relation of the superficial and deep layers.*

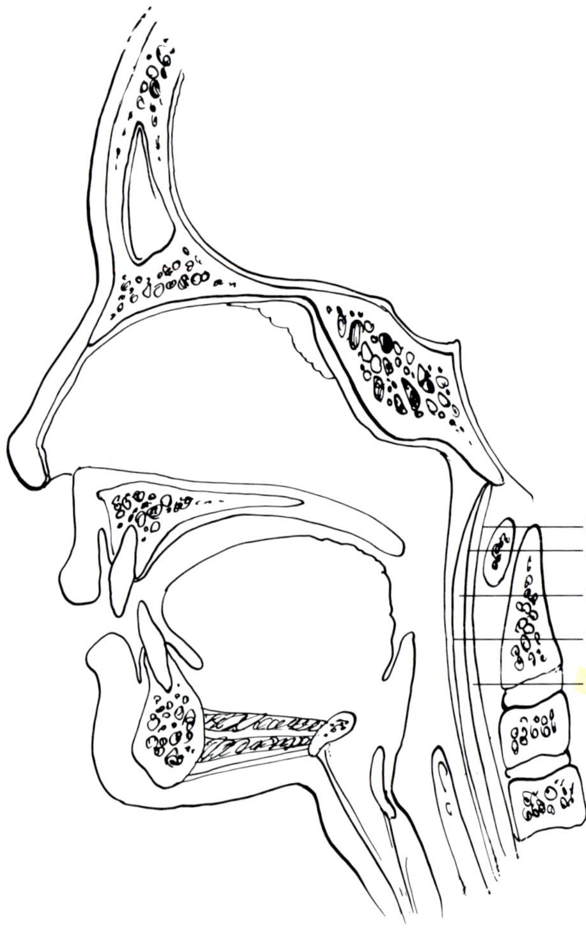

Figure 9–4. *Deep cervical fascial layers and spaces below the cranial base and above the hyoid. Note the continuation of the spaces below the hyoid bone.*

alar fascia. It extends upward as far as the base of the skull and downward as far as the diaphragm. Grodinsky and Holyoke[34] theorized that infections of the danger space most commonly arise from infections of the retrovisceral-retropharyngeal space. The carotid sheath, surrounding the internal jugular, common carotid artery, and vagus nerve, is interposed between the superficial and pretracheal layers anteromedially and the prevertebral layer posteriorly.

Fascia and Spaces Above the Hyoid Bone

The spaces of the head and neck that are of importance to the clinician are formed by the superficial layer of the deep cervical fascia extending upward from the hyoid bone and the anterior border of the sternocleidomastoid to the mandible and the zygomatic arch. The superficial fascia splits around the structures of the mouth floor, the mandible and the muscles of mastication, and the parotid gland. The fascial layers and spaces above the hyoid bone are shown in the sagittal section in Figure 9-4. The danger space and the retrovisceral space show no interruption, but are continuous with the danger space and the retropharyngeal space above the level of the hyoid bone.

The space of the body of the mandible is shown in Figure 9–5. The split of the fascia around the mandible creates a space that surrounds the periapical

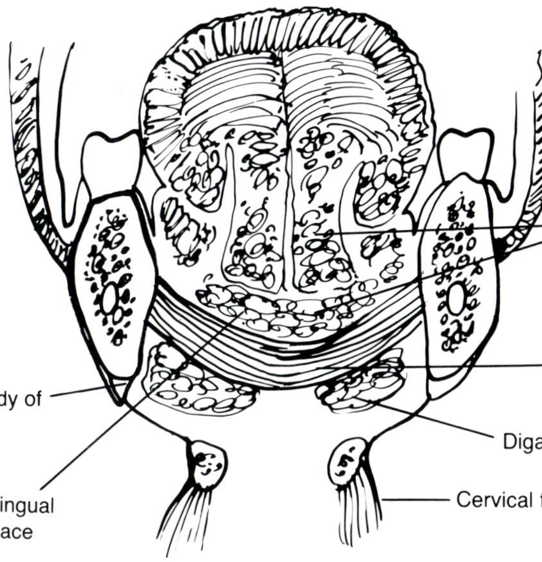

Figure 9–5. *Space of the body of the mandible. Note the relation of the submandibular and the sublingual spaces to the mandible.*

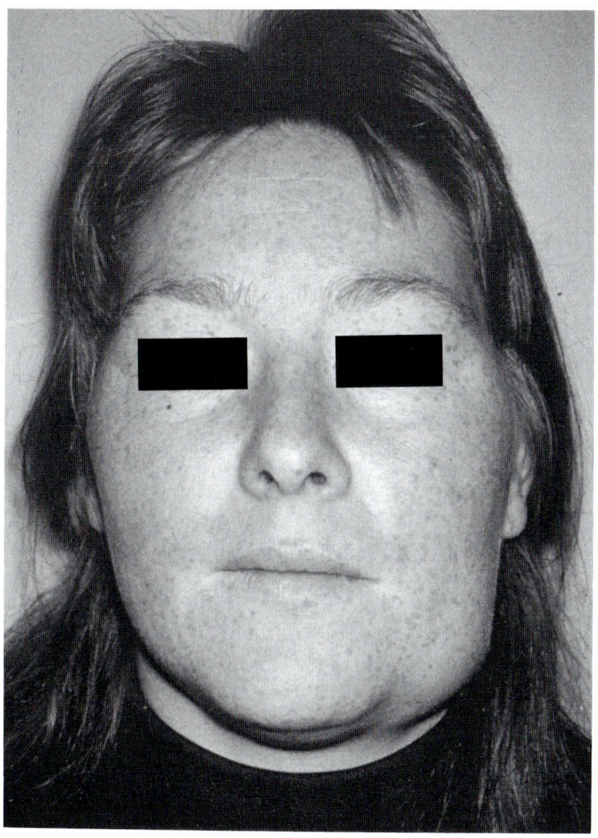

Figure 9–6. *Paramandibular and submandibular space swelling is characteristic of odontogenic infections originating from posterior mandibular teeth.*

area of the teeth and provides a route for the spread of periapical infection away from bone. It is limited anteriorly by the attachment of the anterior belly of the digastric muscle and posteriorly by the attachment of the medial pterygoid muscle to the mandible.

The paramandibular and submandibular spaces form the fascial compartments above and below the mylohyoid muscle and are continuous with the lateral pharyngeal space (Fig. 9–6). Posterior to these spaces the superficial layer of cervical fascia splits to enclose the ramus of the mandible, the masseter, the medial pterygoid, and the lower portion of the temporal muscle (Fig. 9–7).

The space of the parotid gland encloses the parotid gland and its associated lymph nodes, the facial nerve, and the great vessels which pass through it (Fig. 9–8). Infections of the parotid gland are usually confined to the duct and acinar system of the gland and rarely penetrate through the fascia surrounding the gland.

IDENTIFICATION OF BACTERIA

The organisms responsible for infection are usually identifiable. To aid in identifying them, a representative specimen must be collected, examined grossly, and then submitted for culture and sensitivity testing. When collecting specimens from the infected site certain steps should be followed.

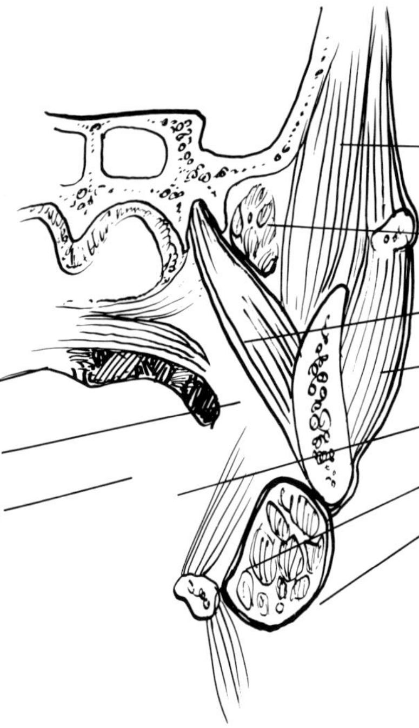

Figure 9–7. *Masticator space encloses the medial and lateral ramus of the mandible, the masseter, the medial pterygoid, and the temporal muscle.*

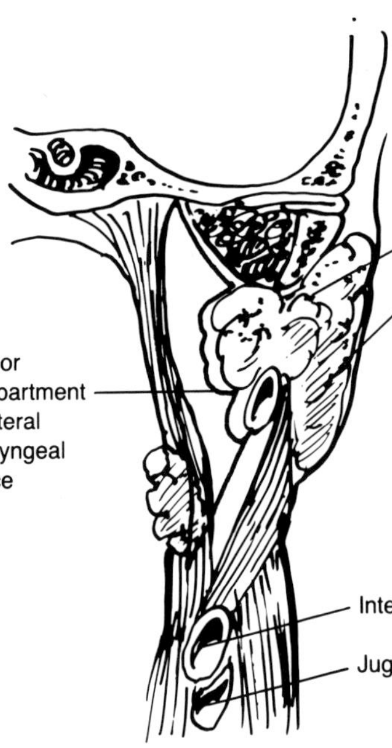

Figure 9–8. *Space of the parotid gland.*

1. Choose the material most likely to reflect the disease process.
2. Obtain the specimen in a manner that avoids contamination by the patient's own flora (Fig. 9–9).
3. Collect a specimen of sufficient volume for microbiologic examination and culture.
4. If possible, obtain specimens before initiating antimicrobial therapy.
5. Use an appropriate container and transport system.
6. Deliver the specimen promptly to the lab.

The infected tissue sample should be grossly examined for characteristic odors, cellular and bacterial debris, and the presence of normal body fluids. The following are examples of gross examination findings:

- Anaerobic infections frequently produce a foul-smelling pus.
- Characteristic odors are associated with certain microorganisms (*S. faecalis*, feces; *Pseudomonas aeruginosa*, fruity).
- Yellowish flecks or balls (sulfur granules) visible to the naked eye may be formed by actinomyces and identified in the drainage material.

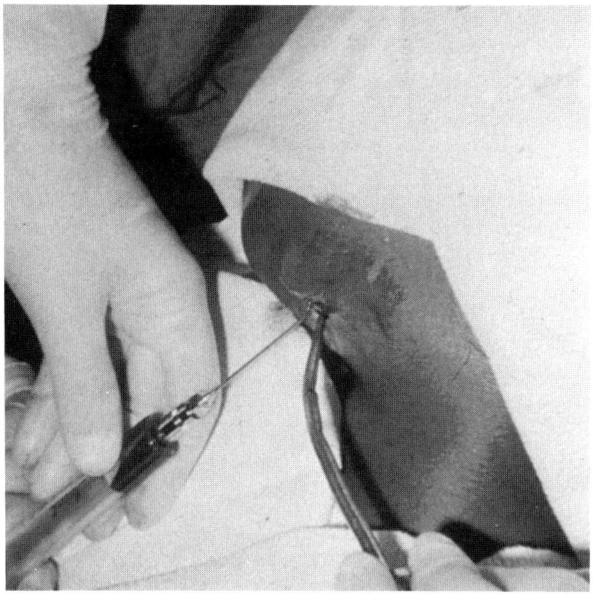

Figure 9–9. *Extraoral aspiration of pus from the submandibular space.*

- In patients with meningitis, the cloudy appearance of CSF is often the first confirmation of the diagnosis.
- Sputum can often be differentiated from saliva on the basis of color, consistency, and odor.
- Thin, "dish-water" drainage may indicate necrotic fascia.
- Stringy, thin secretions from a drainage site involving salivary glands may indicate a salivary gland fistula.

REFERENCES

1. Lufkin AW. A History of Dentistry, ed 2. Philadelphia: Lea & Febiger, 1948.
2. Ruffer, A. Studies in the Paleopathology of Egypt. Chicago: University of Chicago Press, 1921:315.
3. Studies in Paleo-Odontology. Pacific Dent Gaz, 1929–1930.
4. Guerini V. History of Dentistry. Philadelphia: Lea & Febiger, 1909:53.
5. Sande MA, Mandell GL. Antimicrobial agents. General considerations. In: Goodman LS, Gilman A. Pharmacological Basis of Therapeutics, ed 7. New York: Macmillian, 1985:1066.
6. Chow AW, Roser SM, Brady FA. Orofacial odontogenic infections. Ann Intern Med 1978; 88:392.
7. Bartlett JG, Gorbach SL. Anaerobic infections of the head and neck. In: Roth GI, Calmes R. Oral Biology. St. Louis: CV Mosby, 1981:401.
8. Loesche WJ. Ecology of the oral flora. In: Newman MG, Nisengard R. Oral Microbiology and Immunology. Philadelphia: WB Saunders, 1988:351.
9. Sanz M, Newman MG. Dental plaque and calculus. In: Newman MG, Nisengard R. Oral Microbiology and Immunology. Philadelphia: WB Saunders, 1988:367.
10. Gibbons RJ, vanHoute J. Bacterial adherence in oral microbial ecology. Annu Rev Microbiol 1975; 29:19.
11. Ellen RP, Gibbons, RJ. Virulent surfaces; removal of this protein impairs adherence. Parameters affecting the adherence and tissue tropisms of *Streptococcus pyogenes*. Infect Immun 1974; 9:85.
12. Selinger DS, Julie N, Reed WP, et al. Adherence of Group A streptococci to pharyngeal cells: A role in the pathogenesis of rheumatic fever. Science 1978; 201:455.
13. Reed WP, William RC Jr. Bacterial adherence: First step in pathogenesis of certain infections. J Chronic Dis 1978; 67:72.
14. Johanson WG, Pierce AK, Sanford JP. Changing pharyngeal bacteria flora of hospitalized patients. N Engl J Med 1969; 21:1137.
15. Laforce FM, Hopkins J, Trow R, et al. Human and oral defenses against gram-negative rods. Am Rev Respir Dis 1976; 114:929.
16. Sprunt K, Redman W. Evidence suggesting importance of the role of inter-bacterial inhibition in maintaining balance of normal flora. Ann Intern Med 1968; 68:579.
17. Thonard JC. Host defense mechanisms in the oral mucosa. Oral Med Oral Path 1976; 42:234.
18. Onishi J, Kondo W, Uchiyama Y. Preliminary report on the oxidation-reduction potential obtained on surfaces of gingiva and tongue and in interdental space. Bull Tokyo Med Dent Univ 1960; 7:161.
19. Eskow RN, Loesche WJ. Oxygen tensions in the human oral cavity. Arch Oral Biol 1971; 16:1127.
20. Chang RS, Beaman BL, Rinaldi MG, et al. Attributes of infectious agents. In: Hoeprich PD, Jordan MC, eds. Philadelphia: JB Lippincott, 1989:2.
21. Bartlett JG, O'Keefe P. The bacteriology of perimandibular space infections. J Oral Surg 1979; 37:407.
22. Morey EF, Moule AJ, Higgins TJ. Pyogenic dental infections—a retrospective analysis. Aust Dent J 1984; 29:150.
23. Young EW, Johnson WT, Lundin R, et al. Evaluation of treatment provided patients hospitalized with orofacial odontogenic infections: A retrospective study. Oral Surg 1985; 59:28.
24. Johnson WT. Managing odontogenic infections. AFP 1984; 29:167.
25. Overturf GD. Bacterial meningitis. In: Hoeprich PD, Jordan MC, eds. Infectious Diseases, ed 4. Philadelphia: JB Lippincott, 1989:1114.
26. Orenstein WA, Wassilah SG, Hinman AR. Tetanus. In: Hoeprich PD, Jordan MC, eds. Infections Diseases, ed 4. Philadelphia: JB Lippincott, 1989:1173.
27. Liu C. Epiglottitis, laryngitis, and laryngotracheo-

bronchitis. In: Hoeprich PD, Jordan MC, eds. Infectious Diseases, ed 4. Philadelphia: JB Lippincott, 1989:328.

28. Schachtele CF. Dental caries. In: Schuster GS, ed. Oral Microbiology and Infectious Disease. Baltimore: Williams & Wilkins, 1983:197.
29. Patters MR. Periodontal disease. In: Schuster GS, ed. Oral Microbiology and Infectious Disease. Baltimore: Williams & Wilkins, 1983:234.
30. Van Palenstein, Helderman WH. Microbial etiology of periodontal disease. J Clin Periodontal 1981; 8:261.
31. Valenti WM, Trudell RB, Bentley DW. Factors predisposing to oropharyngeal colonization with gram-negative bacilli in the aged. N Engl J Med 1978; 298:1108.
32. Bartlett JG, O'Keefe P. The bacteriology of perimandibular space infections. J Oral Surg 1979; 37:404.
33. Hollinshead WH. Anatomy for Surgeons: The Head and Neck, ed 2. New York: Harper & Row, 1968:306.
34. Grodinsky M, Holyoke EA. The fasciae and fascial spaces of the head and adjacent regions. Am J Anat 1938; 63:367.

10

Clinical Considerations in Head and Neck Infections

Robert D. Marciani

EVALUATION OF THE PATIENT

Physical Examination

Patients with odontogenic and other head and neck infections present with signs and symptoms that generally are strongly suggestive of the underlying disease process. Typically the patient complains of pain, loss of function, and swelling; signs of systemic involvement may also be apparent. The clinician must accurately assess the severity of the infection, establish the patient's general condition, and institute immediate therapy if the patient is seriously ill. Pertinent details concerning the location of the infection, duration of the problem, and etiologic factors should be established. Associated systemic diseases that may be contributing to the infection must be identified by a precise review of systems and the patient's past medical history. Of particular importance is the management of concurrent diseases such as diabetes, malnutrition, and the effects of immunosuppressive drugs.[1]

Physical examination of the head and neck must establish the etiology of the infection and which anatomic sites are involved adjacent or distant from the central focus of the infection. A screening neurologic examination should be done on every patient to establish a baseline level of consciousness, eye signs, respiratory patterns, and generalized motor responses. Visual acuity changes and evidence of extraocular muscle impairment must be noted in the patient's record. The clinician must further demonstrate his appreciation for the potential of head and neck infections to spread to other vital organs by clearly recording positive and negative findings in the patient record. Subsequent new historical and physical examination findings must also be annotated. Patients with serious head and neck infections must have a complete history and physical review with particular attention paid to the neurologic, ophthalmologic, cardiovascular, and respiratory systems.

Physical examination findings of head and neck infections are presented in Table 10–1. The cardinal signs of inflammation—rubor, tumor, calor, and dolor—usually are evident.[2] The redness occurs secondary to local vasodilation and the swelling from the accumulation of tissue fluid or pus. Heat also results from the vasodilation and an increased blood flow to the area. Dolor, or pain, is caused by pressure on nerve endings from tissue distention. Fever and tachycardia are the most common systemic signs of a severe infection. Intraoral examination immediately establishes the degree of mandibular opening. Trismus may be related to the spread of infection to the muscles of mastication and suggests deep space involvement. Lateral pharyngeal space infection, for ex-

Table 10–1. *Physical Examination Findings in Head and Neck Infections*

ODONTOGENIC		
Large carious lesion	Thermal response changes	Percussion sensitivity
Parulis	Sinus tracts	Pus
Dentoalveolar swelling		Space swelling
Trismus		
SALIVARY GLAND		
Swelling (persistent)	Tenderness	Decreased salivary flow
Swelling (intermittent)	Purulence	Sialoliths
SINUSES		
Swelling (antral wall)	Nasal discharge	Epiphora
Swelling (orbit)	Quadrant tooth sensitivity	Disconjugate eye movements
Swelling (nasal)		
ORBIT		
Lid edema	Ptosis	Proptosis
Chemosis	Ophthalmoplegia	Optic neuritis
Blindness	Sensory changes V2, V3	

ample, can cause trismus, dysphagia, swelling, and displacement of the uvula and mandibular angle swelling. Frank abscess or cellulitis of this space can be easily overlooked when an intraoral examination is curtailed because of decreased jaw opening. The lateral pharyngeal space must always be evaluated when peripharyngeal space involvement is suspected. Teeth are evaluated visually, by percussion, and by hot and cold and electrical stimulation. Large carious lesions and poorly repaired teeth are strongly suggestive of sources of infection. Periodontal pockets should be probed for periodontal defects and abscess formation. Oral and circumoral foreign bodies should be ruled out. Salivary glands are palpated for tenderness and massaged to observe for the quantity and quality of secretions at the duct orifices.

The anatomic relation of the structures of the head and neck encourage substantial overlap of clinical findings, which may confuse the diagnostician. An infected upper first molar, for example, may present with the same physical examination findings as acute maxillary sinusitis. An inflamed submandibular gland might be misdiagnosed as a submandibular space infection of odontogenic origin.

Laboratory and Radiographic Evaluation

Preoperative laboratory testing of the infected patient should include those studies pertinent to the appropriate preparation of the patient for surgery; other laboratory tests necessary to diagnose intercurrent disease are also indicated. Routine laboratory tests such as CBC, differential white blood cell (WBC) count, and sedimentation rate are necessary for serious infections and may be the only evidence of an occult head and neck infection. Dental infections, otitis media, or sinusitis may present as a fever of unknown origin without clinically apparent signs and symptoms. Naschitz and Yeshurun[3] reported five cases (14%) in a series of immunocompetent patients with fever of undetermined origin with occult infection in the facial area. In most of these patients local signs were absent, laboratory investigations were noncontributory, and antibiotic treatment was ineffective. Surgical drainage of pus was followed a few days later by defervescence.

Elevated white blood cell counts with increased percentages of immature WBC will occur variably depending on the severity of the infection. Patients with local signs and symptoms of head and neck infection will usually have associated minor WBC changes.

Radiographic and diagnostic imaging of the head and neck to establish the presence of infection in deep spaces or to corroborate clinical findings of the cause of the infection is an essential step in the patient's evaluation. Panographic and periapical dental radiographs are generally adequate to diagnose the etiology of odontogenic infections. Computed tomography (CT) and magnetic resonance imaging (MRI) are useful in locating infection in the lateral pharyngeal space, orbit, brain, neck, and mediastinum. The ability of modern diagnostic imaging techniques to distinguish tissue and fluid densities, establish mass contours, and delineate the extent of infiltration into adjacent tissues is extremely helpful in planning surgical approaches.[4–6]

ODONTOGENIC INFECTIONS: CLINICAL PRESENTATIONS

Odontogenic infections originate in the dental pulp or the periodontal or pericoronal tissues. The dental pulp most commonly is the source of dentoalveolar abscesses.

Pulpal Infection

Necrosis of the pulp can be caused by physical and chemical injury and infection resulting from carious exposure of the contents of the pulp chamber. Invasion of the pulp produces either a localized or generalized pulpal infection.[7] The subjective and objective findings of pulpal necrosis depend on the portal of entry to the pulp permitting spontaneous drainage. If the infected tooth is spontaneously draining through a sinus tract or through a tooth, the patient may be asymptomatic. If drainage is obstructed, rapid involvement of the entire pulp results in pulpal necrosis. The subsequent clinical course of the pathologic pulp depends on many factors. If drainage is established through the coronal portion of the tooth before the inflammatory products irritate periapical alveolar bone, a periapical granuloma may develop. This process is asymptomatic and will persist as long as drainage through the tooth continues.

Acute dentoalveolar infections are managed by removing the infected pulp and obliterating the pulp chamber with root canal therapy, or extracting the infected tooth and draining the periapical infection. Three treatment options have been advocated when a diagnosis of acute alveolar abscess is made[8]: incision and drainage, extraction as the primary treatment, and intensive medical care, with surgical intervention postponed. The immediate aim in treating infection using the preceding options is to create drainage, which in turn prevents the spread of infection, relieves pain, and starts the resolution of the condition. If there is a well localized accumulation of pus, an incision into the abscess cavity will create drainage in the simplest manner possible. Continuous drainage must then be established with a suitable drain. With drainage established, the patient will be relieved of discomfort almost immediately and extraction of the tooth can be deferred. Extraction is next in the order of preference and should be done, in many cases of acute infection, when fluctuance is not present and when the removal of the tooth will produce drainage. Secondly, extraction can be the primary treatment if the offending tooth can be removed atraumatically.

An alternative, if not similar, approach to the management of acute dentoalveolar abscesses is to extract the involved tooth and incise and drain the abscess at the same time irrespective of tooth mobility. This approach offers several advantages over sequential treatment of infection:

- The removal of the etiology of the infection is the most important step in the treatment of infection.
- The time necessary to resolve the infection will be shortened.
- Multiple procedures can be avoided resulting in health care cost reduction.
- The patient may return to gainful activity sooner.

The perils of tooth extraction in the presence of swelling is a myth that has been passed from one generation of dentists to another.[8] In 1951 Krogh[9] showed a 3% complication rate when 2626 teeth were removed at the time of initial examination. Martis and Karakasis[10] completed a similar study in which they treated 1376 acute dentoalveolar abscesses by immediate extraction; a 3% complication rate was also reported. Hall et al.[11] randomly divided 350 patients with odontogenic cellulitis into two groups. The first group had extractions performed on the day of initial presentation. Treatment of the second group was delayed until the fourth day to allow for localization of the infection to occur. In neither group did extractions appear to have an effect on the spread of infection. The patients who received the early treatment recovered more rapidly and required subsequent incision and drainage less frequently than in those patients in whom the treatment was delayed. In addition, those with later extractions had a greatly increased incidence of extraoral drainage.

Extraction of teeth, incision and drainage, and antibiotic care can be accomplished concurrently almost without exception. Delaying full treatment of the infection may be necessary because of the patient's general health, or because of operating room availability. Under these conditions incision and drainage using local anesthesia may reduce pain, decrease the potential for the infection to spread, and begin the resolution of the condition.

Periodontal Infection

Periodontal disease is a chronic and progressively destructive bacterial process involving the supporting structures of the teeth. Unlike the symptoms associated with infected pulp tissue, inflammatory products produced in periodontal infection usually drain freely, and the patient experiences little, if any, discomfort.[12] An acute process similar to that of pulpal involvement will develop when drainage from the infected area is interrupted. The diagnosis of periodontal abscess is entertained when there is no obvious carious lesion and periodontal probing and radiographic findings suggest this disease. In most cases acute periodontal infections are confined to the local dentoalveolar tissues and do not spread to the deep spaces of the head, jaws, and neck. The clinician, however, should recognize the potential for these infections to spread to distant sites when patient factors and local conditions such as the failure to drain are present.

Treatment of periodontal infections includes curettage and debridement of inflammatory gingival sulcus material, drainage of pus, or removal of the involved tooth. Antibiotic therapy should be initiated when drainage cannot be achieved or when the infection has spread to distant tissues or the patient shows systemic signs of infection.

Pericoronal Infection

Pericoronitis occurs when debris and microorganisms located under a soft tissue operculum overlying a partially erupted tooth (usually an erupting or partially impacted third molar) provoke an inflammation. The tissue operculum is often traumatized by the opposing tooth, which either precipitates the infection or contributes to its progression by persistently traumatizing the operculum. Usually the pericoronal inflammation remains localized and is easily managed initially by irrigating under the operculum and extracting the opposing third molar. Antibiotics are indicated when lymphadenopathy is present or the patient demonstrates constitutional symptoms. If drainage is interrupted or systemic factors enhance the virulence of the infection, the entrapped exudate will extend to the deep spaces of the jaws. Radiographically the underlying bone may not be involved. Frequently the bone distal to the partially erupted lower third molar will be destroyed; it presents as a radiographic radiolucency (Fig. 10–1).

Removal of impacted lower third molars with pericoronitis should be delayed when the surgeon judges the operative procedure to be complex, the tooth is severely impacted, bone removal will be necessary, or a prolonged surgical procedure is anticipated. The pericoronitis should be resolved or substantially reduced in its intensity by the conservative measures previously outlined.

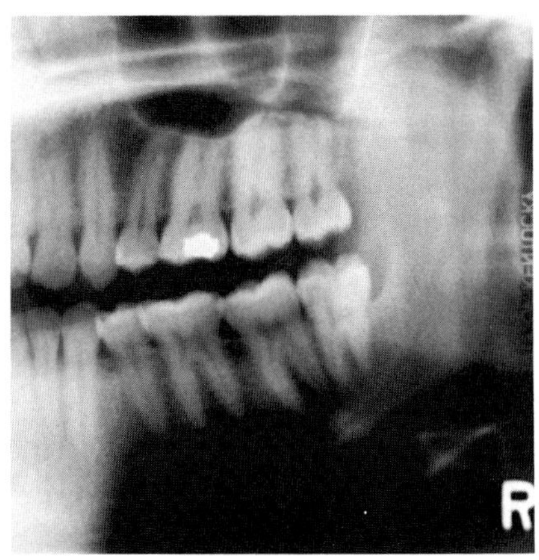

Figure 10–1. *Partially erupted right mandibular third molar appears on radiographs as a radiolucency distal to the crown.*

Table 10–2. *Potential Sites of Drainage of Head and Neck Space Infections*

Space	Site of Incision and Drainage
Masticator	Inferior border of the mandible
Temporal	Above the zygomatic arch (both superficial and deep spaces)
Submandibular	Below the inferior border of the mandible in the submandibular triangle
Lateral pharyngeal	Intraorally along the pterygomandibular raphe
	Extraorally at the angle of the mandible
Buccal	Intraorally in the mandibular mucobuccal fold
Paramandibular	Intraorally in the buccal sulcus
Infratemporal	Above and lateral to the maxillary tuberosity

ODONTOGENIC INFECTIONS: SURGICAL MANAGEMENT

General Techniques

The surgical techniques necessary to manage localized and spreading odontogenic infections are basically simple once the cause of infection is removed. The location of the infection in fascial spaces must be established and the appropriate surgical openings made for drainage (Table 10–2). The sites of drainage of the spaces of the head and neck are generally positioned to achieve dependent drainage, avoid important anatomical structures, minimize undesirable cosmetic sequelae, and allow further surgical manipulation of the drainage site. Extraoral incisions should, whenever possible, be placed in healthy skin to avoid extensive scarring resulting from drains placed directly into areas of fluctuation. The clinician may be tempted to use the existing point of spontaneous drainage for an incision and drainage (I & D) location to avoid a second scar. Often this location is not dependent and the poor quality of the compromised tissue predisposes this site to greater scarring.

The technique of I & D seldom varies irrespective of the space requiring surgical entrance. A 1- to 2-cm incision is made through skin and subcutaneous tissue. A hemostat is then used to bluntly dissect through the intervening tissues until the involved space is entered. Before the I & D, the surgically prepared surface tissue should be penetrated with an 18-gauge needle and an aspirate of pus obtained. The aspirate should be of a sufficient quantity to allow aerobic, anaerobic, gram-stain, and other indicated cultures to be obtained. When pus or serosanguineous fluid are not withdrawn, sterile saline can be injected into the infected space and retrieved for submission to the microbiology laboratory.

The location and the number of drains necessary to treat a circumoral and deep space infection are determined by the route the hemostat must be directed to enter the space and the likelihood that drainage will flow unimpeded to the incision opening. The lateral pharyngeal, masticator, temporal, sublingual, and submandibular spaces can be entered through one incision site in the midline of the submental area. From this location the base of the skull can be reached (Fig. 10–2). A single opening, however, to manage multiple deep spaces is ill-advised and should be discouraged. Establishing an opening into the infected space is a preliminary step; maintaining patency of the opening and the subsequent continuous flow of pus is of equal importance. Long routes of drainage should be avoided. The lateral pharyngeal space, for example, may be more effectively drained intraorally than from a submandibular or submental location. The shortest and most direct route to the pus consistent with the preservation of important anatomic structures and cosmetic considerations should determine the I & D site. Drains must be placed into the depths of the infected spaces and periodically observed for patency and effectiveness.

Rubber drains are very useful and inexpensive. Idoform and Selfedge gauze strips can be used as a

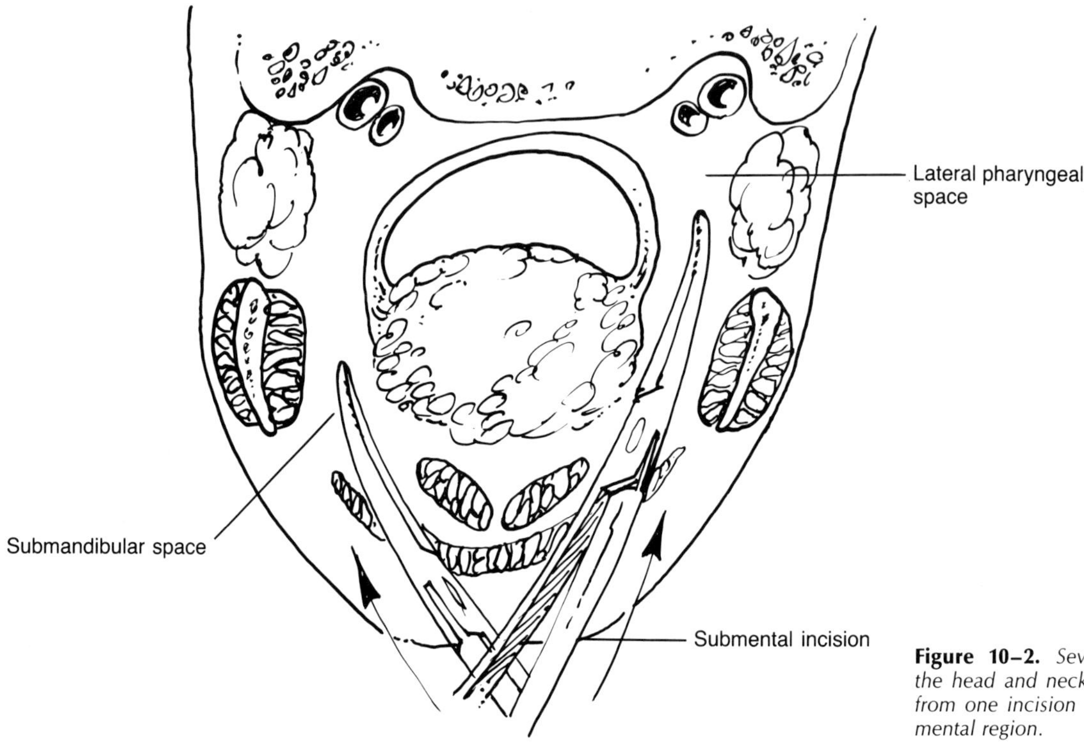

Figure 10–2. *Several spaces of the head and neck are accessible from one incision site in the submental region.*

substitute for rubber drains or to pack an infected wound open. Jackson Pratt drains allow drainage and irrigation of the infected site. This drainage system is effective but more expensive than rubber drains.

Drains should be left in place until the wound stops draining. Care must be taken to identify normal oral secretions and to avoid prolonged drainage. Salivary gland fistulas can develop from drains placed extraorally. The sublingual gland acinir are easily penetrated during the course of draining the sublingual space. Once leakage of saliva commences into the drain site it will persist uninterrupted until the drain is removed. A mixture of saliva and pus can be mistaken for copious amounts of inflammatory debris and result in prolonging antibiotic and general patient care. The clinician should suspect salivary secretions when the drainage is watery and stringy, the patient is subjectively improved, and WBC counts have returned to normal levels.

In general, cellulitis from odontogenic infections will spread along tissue planes to adjacent spaces. Infections arising from the maxillary teeth will result in swelling of the upper half of the face, whereas cellulitis initiated by lower teeth will involve the lower half of the face and neck. Ultimately the entire side of the face and the contralateral spaces may be involved regardless of the origin of the infection. In the nondebilitated host, most untreated odontogenic infections will tend to localize and drain spontaneously. If an unusual combination of microorganisms is involved or host defenses are compromised, odontogenic infections will spread rapidly.[12]

Maxillary Odontogenic Infections

Infection spreading from maxillary teeth commonly involves the buccal and canine spaces. Less commonly the infratemporal and temporal spaces may be involved. As with all odontogenic infections, the lateral and retropharyngeal spaces can also be involved.

Canine Space Infections

The anterior maxillary teeth are anterior to the insertion of the buccinator muscle. Cellulitis initially

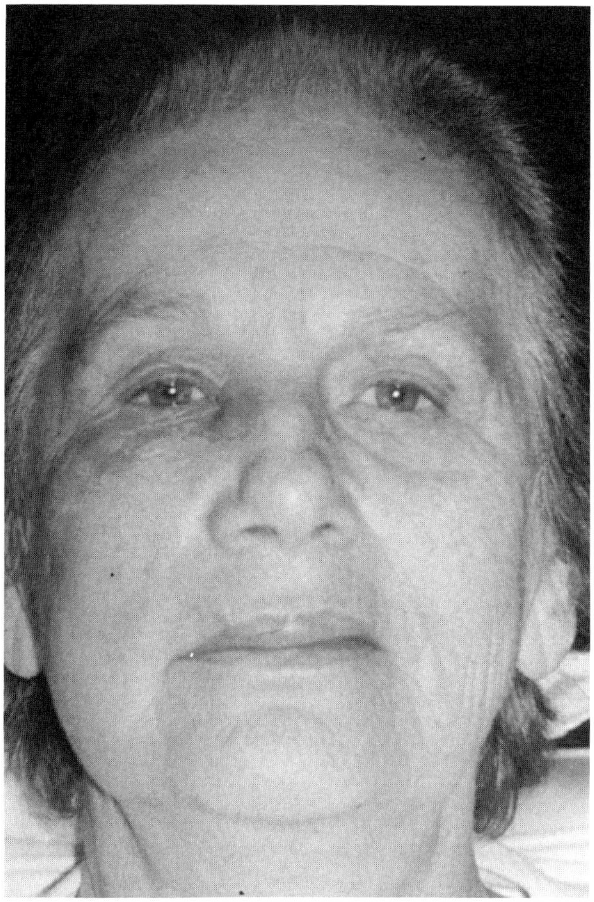

Figure 10–3. *Canine space infection has caused periorbital edema.*

spreads to the upper lip and canine fossa; frequently the superficial periorbital space is involved. The clinical appearance is that of a sick patient with a swollen upper lip and edematous periorbital tissue (Fig. 10–3). Treatment consists of pulp canal therapy or extraction, surgical drainage, and antibiotics. The canine space is directly drained in the mucobuccal fold adjacent to the canine fossa.

Infratemporal Space Infections

Infection in the infratemporal space can be indolent and difficult to diagnose using clinical parameters alone. Trismus, persistent pain, and failure of an odontogenic infection to improve following surgical intervention and antibiotics should alert the clinician to the possibility of involvement of this space. The infratemporal space is bounded medially by the lateral plate of the pterygoid process and the pharynx, posteriorly by the parotid gland, anteriorly by the maxilla, and superiorly by the roof of the infratemporal fossa. The relation of the fossa to the orbit and the potential direct communication of infection through the inferior orbital fissure into the eye is of vital importance.

Infections of the infratemporal space are commonly associated with other deep space infections, usually the buccal and temporal spaces. Isolated infections of the infratemporal space are rare but can be the initial site of inflammation originating from involvement of the posterior maxillary teeth. The maxillary third molar is often the source of the infection, and the infratemporal space should be studied by CT scanning or MRI when clinically marked trismus and pain are present following maxillary third molar surgery or associated with periapical pathology of teeth in the posterior maxilla (Fig. 10–4A,B). Further signs of infection such as external swelling or redness in the preauricular area and inferior to the zygomatic arch may be minimal. The infection may proceed to involve the entire cheek (buccal space) and eyelids (superficial orbital space) and proceed to the deep spaces of the pharynx and mandible. When the pharynx is involved dysphagia is a common finding. Infection that does extend into the orbit penetrating the orbital septum will produce proptosis, optic neuritis, vision loss, and ophthalmoplegia.

Temporal Space Infections

The superficial temporal space is bounded by the temporalis fascia and the temporalis muscle. The deep temporal space is limited deep to the temporalis muscle by its origin from the skull. Involvement of the deep and superficial temporal spaces can be secondary to infections of the infratemporal and masseteric spaces. Patients complain of trismus, pain, and headaches. Persistent diffuse headache, chills, and fever may be early signs of intracranial involvement. No other clinical signs of meningitis or encephalitis may be evident. The presentation of this infection is similar to that of the infratemporal space (Fig. 10–5). Swallowing complaints are not usually a feature of temporal space cellulitis.

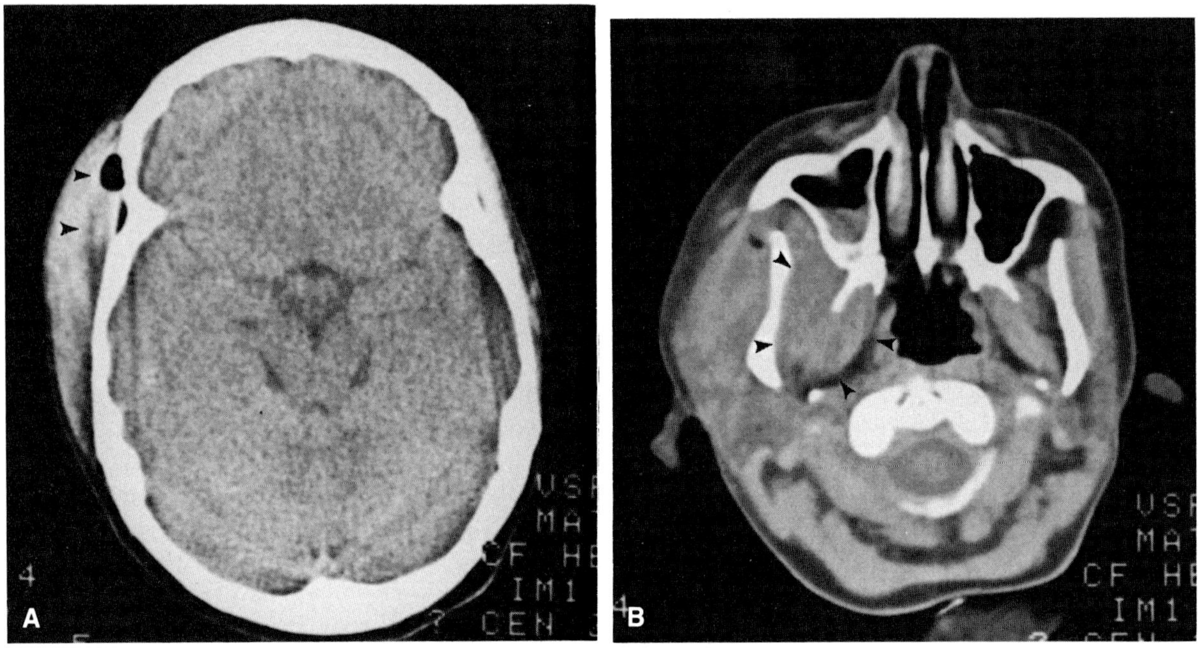

Figure 10–4. *(**A**) CT scan of a temporal space infection. Note the air fluid level in the superior deep temporal space (arrows). (**B**) Infratemporal and temporal spaces show swelling (arrows).*

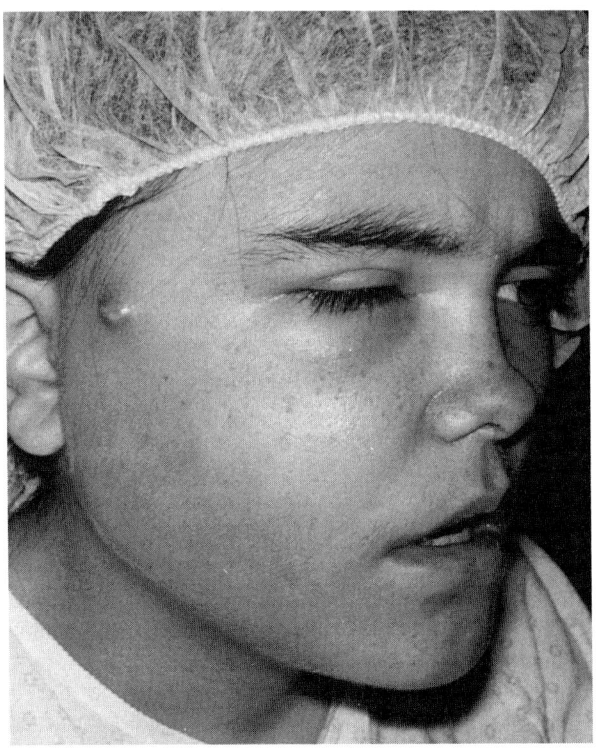

Figure 10–5. *Temporal space infection with involvement of the superficial periorbital space.*

Temporal space infections are unlike other deep space infections. Swelling may be minimal, fluctuance is usually not appreciated, and spontaneous external drainage rarely occurs. Drainage can be obtained through an intraoral incision under the zygomatic arch (Fig. 10–6) or extraorally in the temple area (Fig. 10–7). When drainage persists and the soft tissues overlying the temple appear "boggy" and "ballooned" away from the skull, the temporal fascia under the swollen area has necrosed. Drainage will persist until the necrotic fascia has been removed. The surgeon may successfully remove the dead fascia by simply irrigating through the I & D openings (Fig. 10–8) and blindly exploring the temporal space with a hemostat (Fig. 10–9). Occasionally, it may be necessary to extend the extraoral I & D opening 2 to 3 cm to facilitate direct access to the necrotic fascia (Fig. 10–10). Supplemental incisions are incorporated when debridement can not be completed through the original drainage incision. Use of through-and-through drains, packing of the temporal space, and frequent irrigation are not acceptable alternative therapies to the removal of the necrotic fascia.

Scarring and persistent trismus is minimized by physiotherapy to reestablish interincisal opening and excursive movements. The potential for loss of jaw

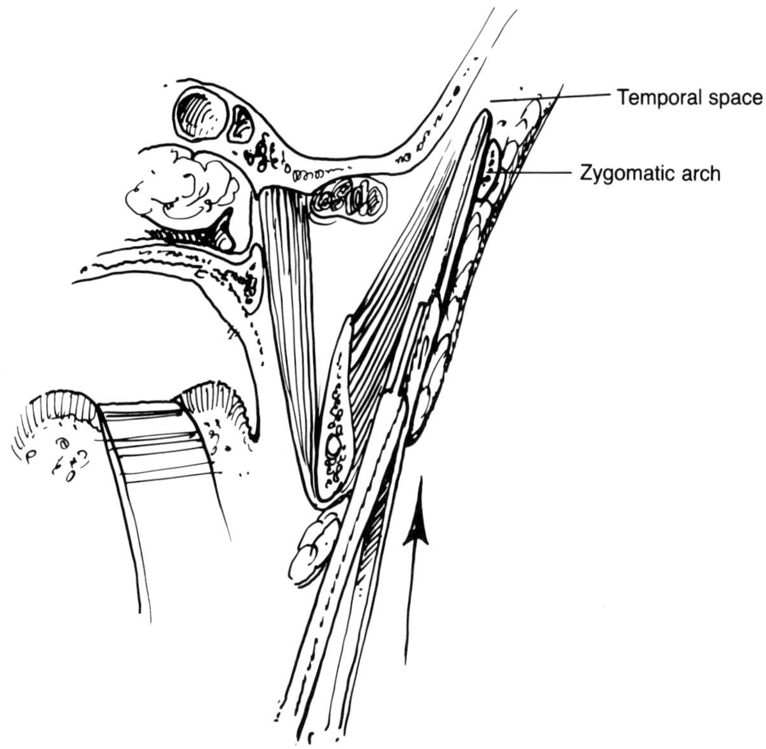

Figure 10–6. *Intraoral drainage of the temporal space. The zygoma buttress is palpated with the cheek extended. An incision is made posterior to the buttress in the midportion of the maxillary mucobuccal fold and a closed hemostat is thrust through the opening and directed under the zygomatic arch superiorly (arrow). Both the superfacial and deep temporal spaces must be entered.*

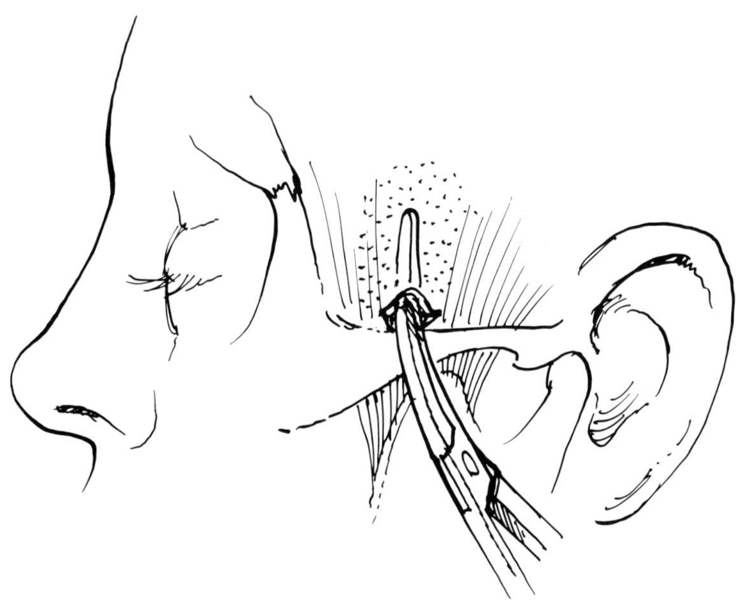

Figure 10–7. *Extraoral drainage of the temporal space. The tip of the hemostat must contact the temporal bone to establish drainage in the deep temporal space.*

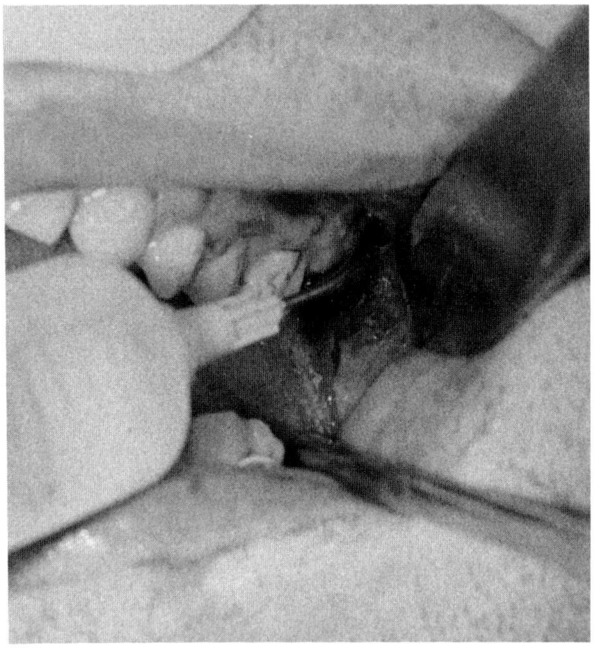

Figure 10–8. *Brisk irrigation will facilitate disruption of poorly attached, necrotic temporal fascia.*

function must be explained to the patient during the earliest stages of treatment so that patient cooperation may be established.

Buccal Space Infections

The buccal space lies between the buccinator and superficial fascia anterior to the superficial and deep temporal spaces. Infections limited to this space are generally not severe; the cheek is swollen, trismus is usually not apparent, and the patient generally has few constitutional symptoms. Untreated infections will eventually spread to other spaces and behave in a much more threatening fashion or will drain spontaneously. It is often difficult to determine the character of buccal swellings and their relation to potential sites of odontogenic infections. The buccal space can be involved from both maxillary and mandibular infections. Surgical access to the buccal space is placed in the superior portion of the mandibular buccal sulcus (Fig. 10–11). An opening at the inferior margin of the buccal space facilitates dependent drainage.

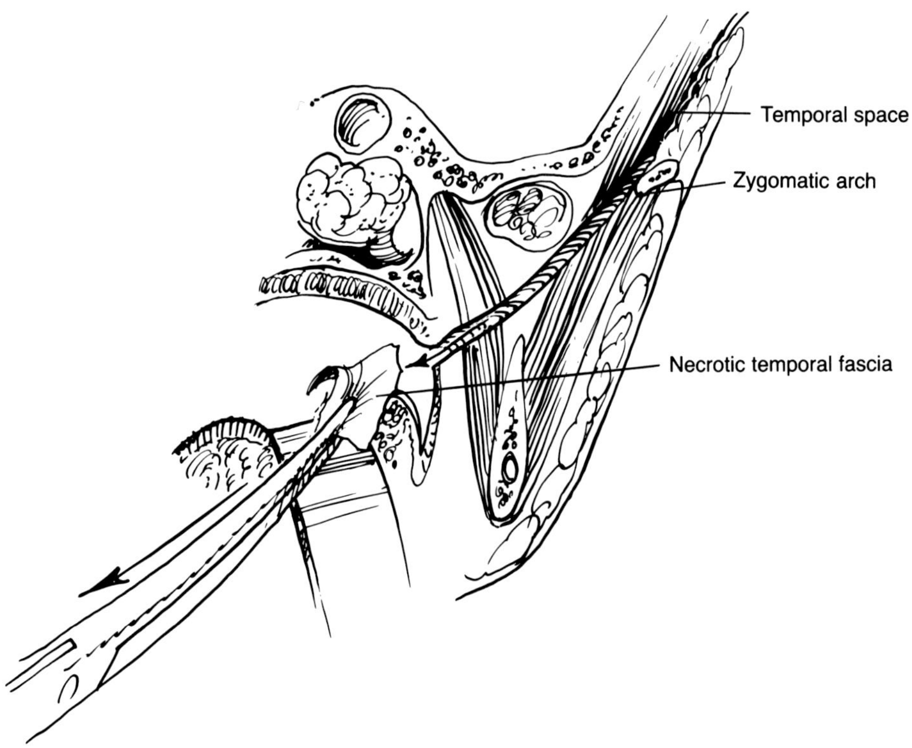

Figure 10–9. *Necrotic temporal fascia is removed through the intraoral drainage site. The distended temporal soft tissue is explored with the hemostat after briskly irrigating the deep temporal tissues.*

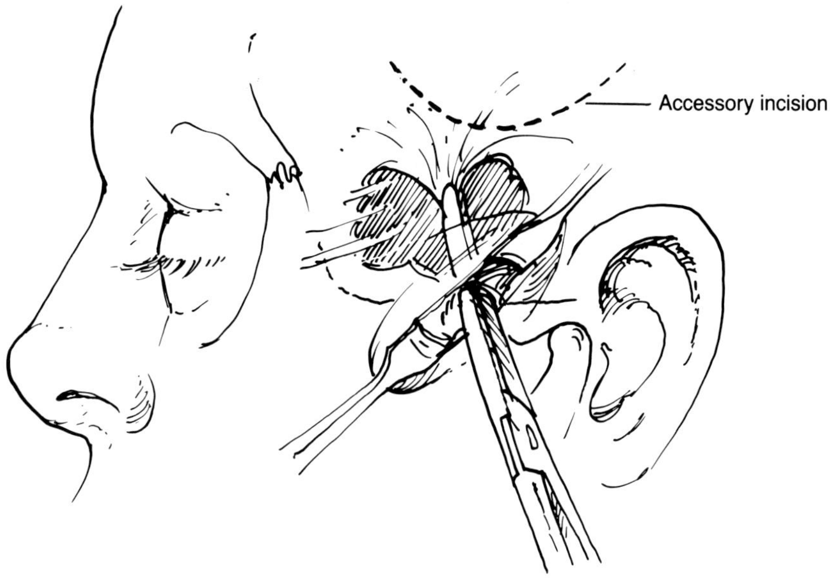

Figure 10–10. *Extraoral approach to remove necrotic temporal fascia. The extraoral drainage site may be extended posterior to the temporal branch of the facial nerve. Additional incisions through skin and subcutaneous tissue are added superiorly to facilitate wider debridement.*

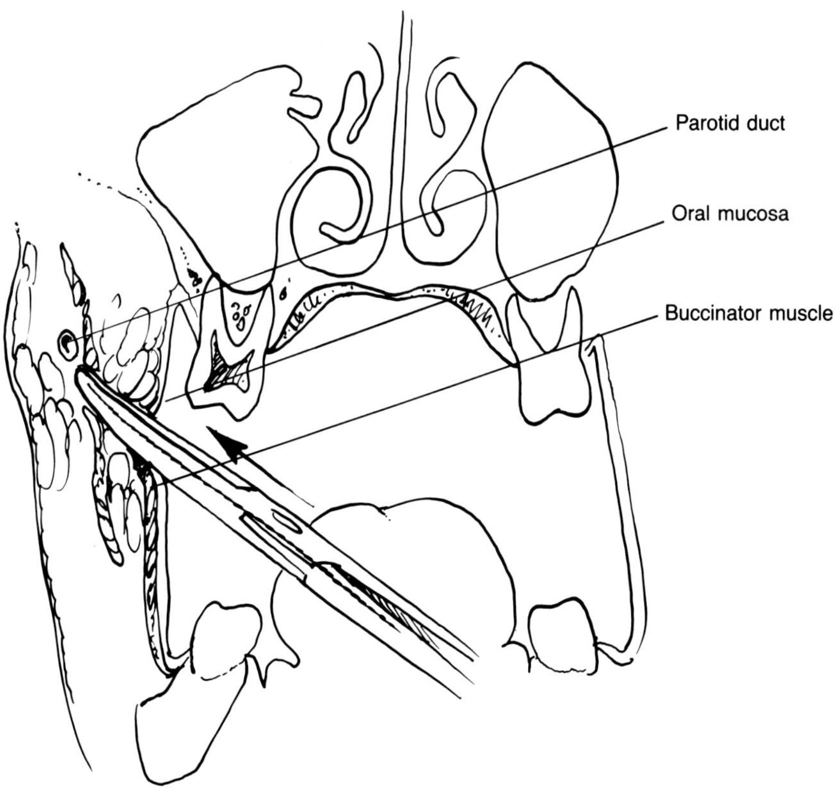

Figure 10–11. *Access for intraoral drainage of the buccal space is made through the cheek.*

Mandibular Odontogenic Infections

Infections originating in mandibular incisors and canines may spread either labially or lingually. If the root apices are above the insertion of the mentalis muscle and the infection perforates buccally, the cellulitis and pus formation will remain intraorally. When mandibular infection spreads lingually, either the sublingual space or the submandibular triangle will be involved, depending on the relation of the apices of the teeth above or below the mylohyoid muscle. Premolars and first molars vary in their apical relation to the mylohyoid. The apices of the second and third molars are generally below the mylohyoid; the submandibular space will most likely be involved and extraoral localization apparent.

Sublingual Space Infections

The sublingual space occupies the floor of the mouth between the mucosa and mylohyoid muscle. Involvement of this space results in swelling of the mouth floor, pain, difficulty in swallowing, and a decrease in tongue mobility. Spread of infection into the submandibular space is highly likely when floor-of-the-mouth infections are inadequately treated. Large accumulations of pus invariably are accompanied by submandibular swelling. I & D of the sublingual space should be done from an extraoral approach when submandibular space involvement is assumed (Fig. 10–12). Isolated sublingual space infection may be drained intraorally and nondependent drainage established.

Damage to the capsule of the sublingual gland is often a sequela of infection in the mouth floor. Persistent drainage following I & D placement may represent sublingual gland secretions.

Submandibular Space Infections

Submandibular space infections are characterized by firm swellings, pain, tenderness to palpation, and limited trismus compared to masseteric space involvement (Fig. 10–13).

Swellings in the submandibular space not related to odontogenic infection can be mistaken for a cellulitis of dental etiology. Inflammatory conditions, neoplasms, and obstructive disorders of the submandibular gland can cause a tender swelling below the mandible. Metastatic and primary neoplastic diseases involving the submandibular node can also present as submandibular triangle enlargements and be incorrectly diagnosed as spreading odontogenic infection.

The submandibular space includes the sublingual space and is limited superiorly by oral mucous membrane and the tongue. The superficial layer of cervical fascia forms the inferior boundary as it extends from the hyoid bone to the mandible. The space below the mylohyoid muscle is divided by the anterior belly of the digastric muscle into the submental and submaxillary spaces. The submental space lies medial to the anterior belly of the digastric; the submaxillary space is formed by the anterior and posterior bellies of the digastric muscle and the hyglossus muscle medially.

I & D of the submental and submandibular spaces should be done from an extraoral approach. Surgical sites placed in healthy tissue below the inferior border of the mandible at the midline and the midbody region provide adequate access (Fig. 10–14A–D).

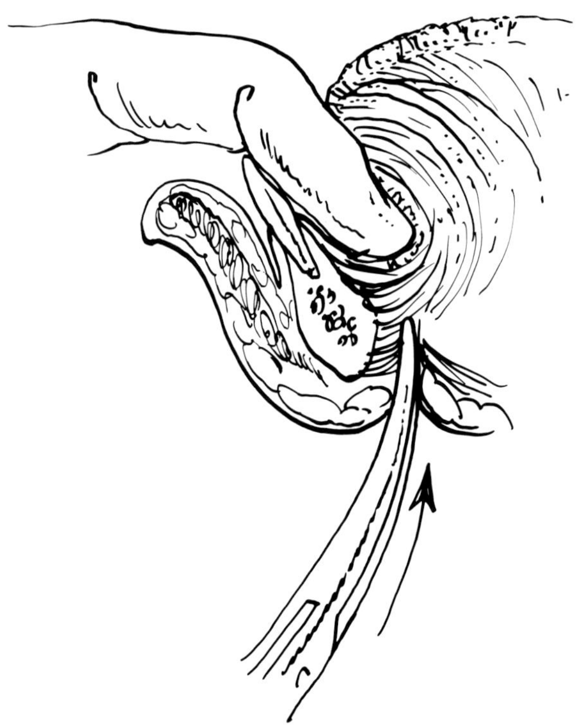

Figure 10–12. *The sublingual space drained extraorally. The surgeon places the fingers of one hand intraorally to palpate and direct the extraorally placed hemostat into the sublingual space. The oral mucosa should not be perforated.*

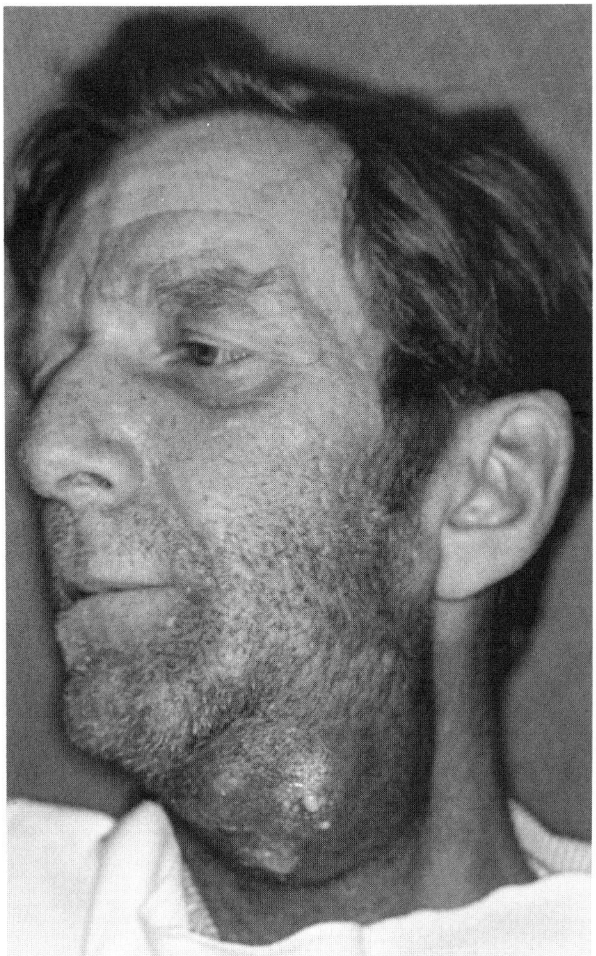

Figure 10–13. *Submandibular space infection. The skin of the submandibular triangle is thin and necrotic. Spontaneous drainage is present.*

The surgical management of diffuse floor-of-mouth and submandibular space infections must include provisions for airway management. The airway is best protected by preventing respiratory obstruction with prompt, aggressive surgical intervention and high doses of intravenous antibiotics. If the circumstances are those of impending or progressing airway embarrassment, endotracheal intubation by a skilled clinician should be done immediately. Tracheostomy should only be considered when more conservative measures are ineffective or unavailable. Fiberoptic intubation is of particular value when conditions of severe trismus and swelling exist.

If bilateral involvement of the sublingual and submandibular spaces occurs, severe dysphagia and respiratory obstruction may ensue. The clinical significance and morbid potential of bilateral deep infections in the mouth floor, submandibular triangle, and neck have been recognized for hundreds of years. Ludwig described such an infection in 1836, a condition that still bears his name.[13]

The original clinical description of Ludwig's angina was that of a "woody" edema of the submental tissue, a firm swelling sublingually, a well-defined border of neck edema, and the absence of infection in regional lymph nodes. Thoma[14] further described the widespread cellulitis in the mouth floor as originating in the submandibular space. He regarded the origin to be almost exclusively from abscesses of mandibular molars, because the roots of these teeth extend below the attachment of the mylohyoid muscle. The classic description of Ludwig's infection is that of a brawny induration without fluctuation in the early stages of the disease, and frequently purulence is not identified.

In 1943, Williams and Guralnick[15] reported their findings in 51 cases and with a mortality rate exceeding 54%. The early reports of Ludwig's angina described hemolytic streptococci and staphylococci as the most frequent causative organisms.

Ludwig's angina, when critically reviewed using modern diagnostic imaging techniques, anaerobic cultures, and contemporary patient management protocols, is not a unique infection separate and distinct from other space infections. It is, in fact, an extensive spread of infection throughout the mouth floor and neck caused by the same organisms responsible for less morbid head and neck infections. Reports of anaerobic organisms as pathogens in complicated oral facial cellulitis became more common in the 1970s. The emergence of anaerobic organisms should not be construed as a change in the pathogenic flora responsible for the infection but, rather, a refinement in culture techniques required to grow these organisms.[16, 17]

Masticator Space Infections

The masticator space includes all of the muscles of mastication, the mandibular ramus, the zygomatic arch, and the temporal bone. Swellings of this space are commonly associated with mandibular third molar infections or spread of infection from the contiguous

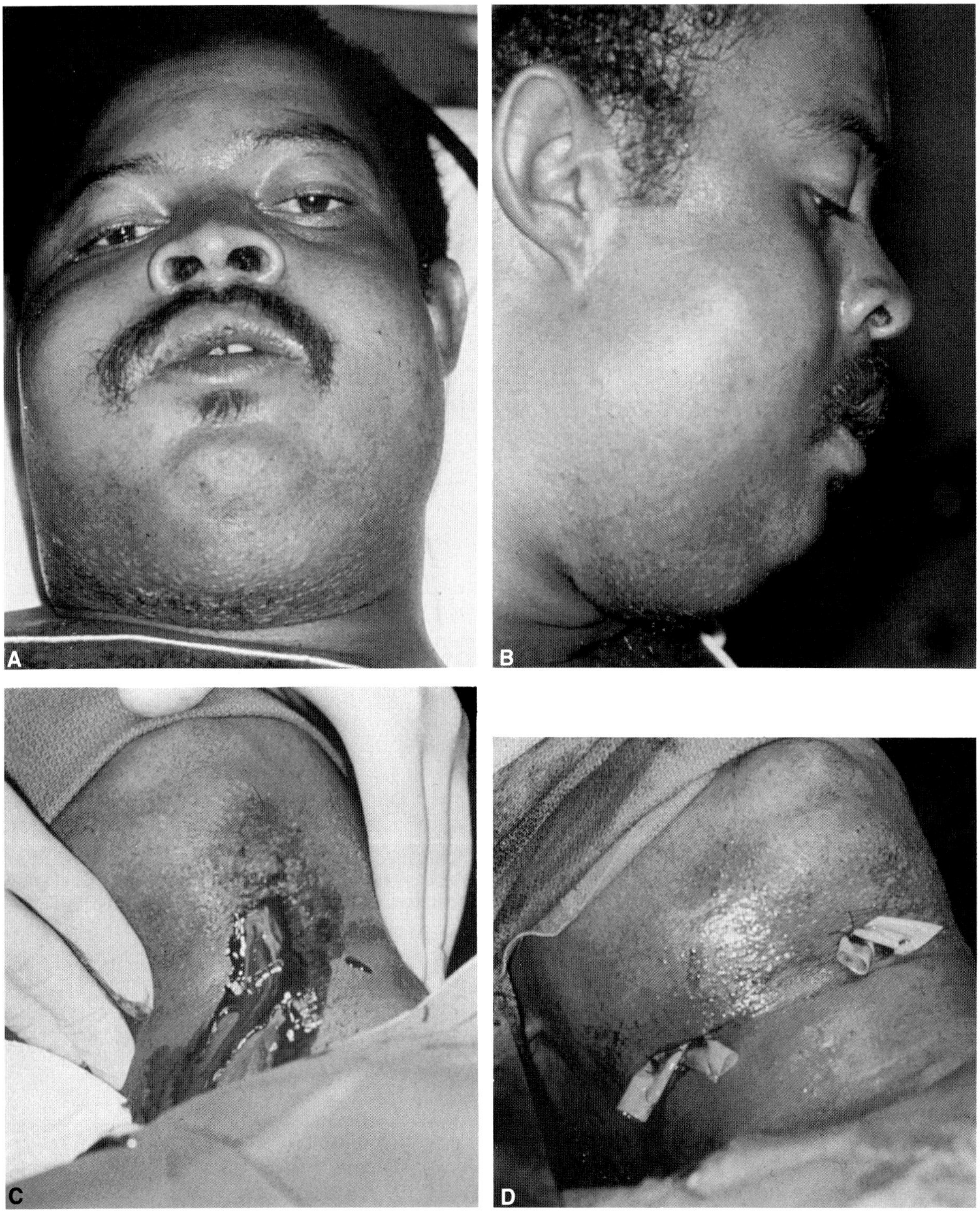

Figure 10–14. *Bilateral submandibular, sublingual space, and parapharyngeal space involvement. (**A, B**) Diffuse face and neck edema. (**C**) Drainage from an incision site at the submental midline. (**D**) Multiple incision sites and drains ensure direct access to the involved space and the shortest route for drainage.*

submandibular space and the lateral pharyngeal compartment. The clinical characteristics of masseteric space infections are trismus, pain, and swelling in the area of the body and angle of the mandible (Fig. 10–15). The patient is usually febrile and complains of difficulty swallowing. Swelling may also be evident on the medial side of the mandible in the retromolar region. Involvement of the medial compartment of the masticator space may be less apparent, however, and may be overlooked if not carefully examined. I & D is directly achieved below the angle of the mandible, preferably in a skin fold (Fig. 10–16).

Lateral and Retropharyngeal Space Infections

Mandibular and maxillary odontogenic infections may involve the lateral or retropharyngeal spaces. The medial wall of the lateral pharyngeal space is continuous with the fascia forming the carotid sheath. The retropharyngeal space provides a direct route into the mediastinum. Lateral pharyngeal space infections are characterized by displacement of the lateral wall toward the midline (Fig. 10–17). Isolated masticator space involvement will not produce distortion of the palate or the uvula. Trismus and difficulty swallowing are prominent features of lateral pharyngeal space infection. Examination of the posterior and lateral pharynx may be difficult as a result of reduced mouth opening; the presence of infection may, therefore, not be clinically observable. The clinician must maintain a high level of suspicion of pharyngeal space involvement and purposely observe for its characteristic signs in every patient irrespective of the cause or primary location of a head and neck infection.

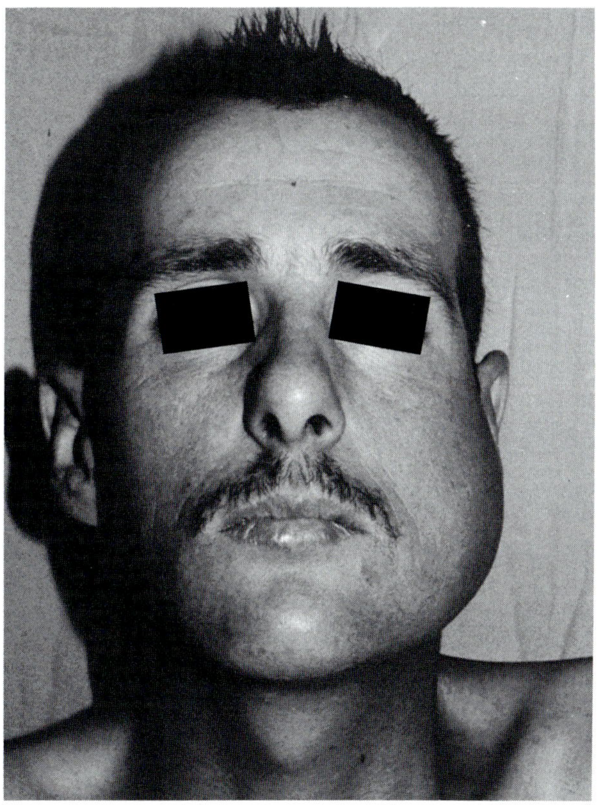

Figure 10–15. *Masticator space infection has produced left ramus and angle of mandible swelling. Trismus is a common finding.*

The symptoms of lateral pharyngeal infections will vary according to the location of the infection in either the anterior or posterior, or both compartments. Dzyak and Zide[18] described the four cardinal signs of anterior compartment involvement: trismus, induration and swelling at the angle of the jaw, fever, and pharyngeal bulging. Involvement of the medial pterygoid muscle accounts for the trismus. The anterior compartment ends at the level of the angle of the jaw. Swelling in this area may only be apparent in the late stages of the infection, if felt at all.

Posterior compartment infection is characterized by septicemia with little pain or trismus. Acute mediastinitis can ensue, because this space communicates with the retropharyngeal space. Swelling is usually internal and deep and can often be missed because it is behind the palatopharyngeal arch. Chow et al.[7] described serious complications when the posterior compartment is involved, including respiratory obstruction from edema of the larynx, thrombosis of the jugular vein, and erosion of the internal carotid artery. Neurologic involvement of cranial nerves IX and XII and of the cervical sympathetic chain with ipsilateral Horner's syndrome have been reported.[19]

The retropharyngeal space usually becomes infected from medial extension of the lateral pharyngeal space. Trauma to the retropharyngeal space from foreign bodies or from traumatic nasoendotracheal intubation can rarely cause a primary infection.

In addition to odontogenic infections other common sites of origin of parapharyngeal infection include the tonsils, adenoids, parotid gland, and lymph nodes draining the nose, pharynx, and teeth.[20]

The potential for perforation of a lateral space abscess at the time of intubation is a possibility, but the

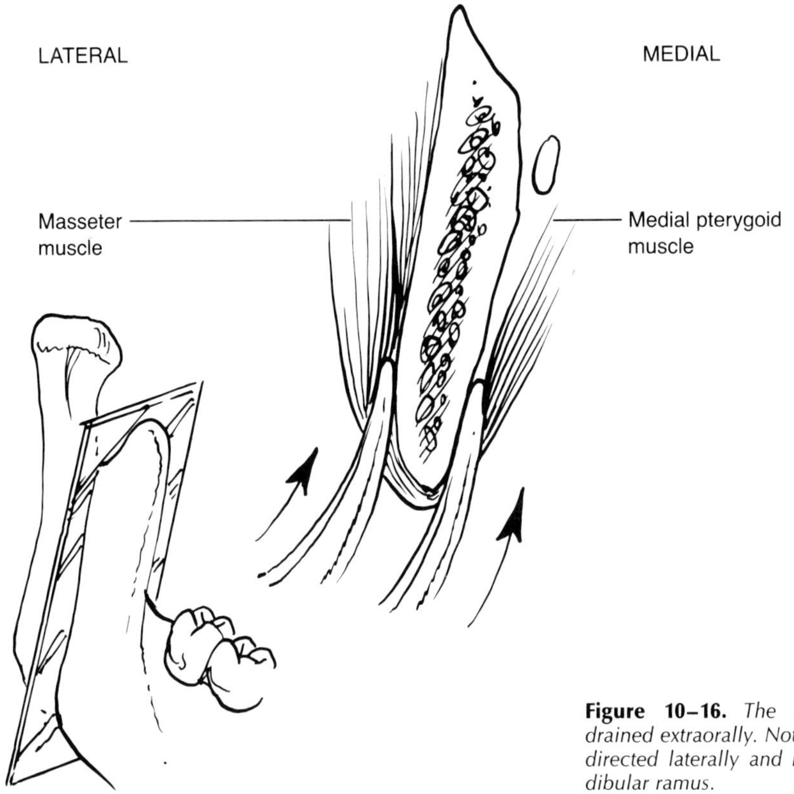

Figure 10–16. *The masticator space is drained extraorally. Note that the hemostat is directed laterally and medially to the mandibular ramus.*

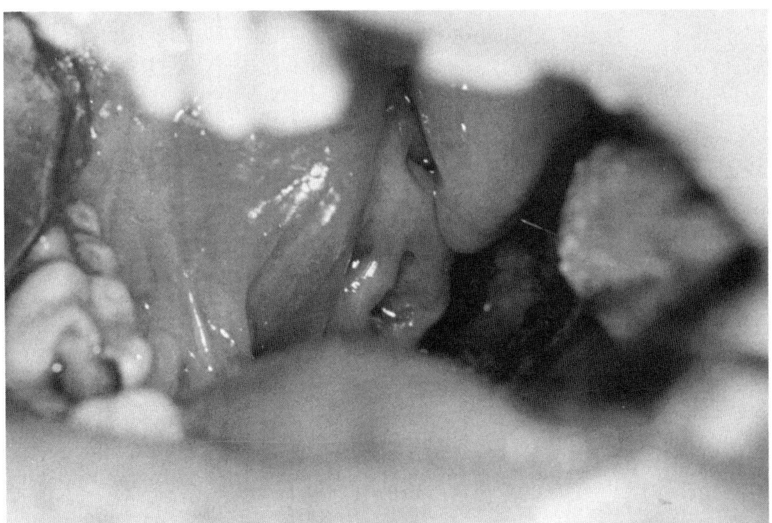

Figure 10–17. *Lateral pharyngeal space infection. The uvula is deviated to the unaffected side. The peritonsillar and adjacent soft palate areas are swollen.*

resultant sequela of seeding the lungs with pathogens and pus should not prevent a well planned and controlled intubation.

The lateral pharyngeal space can be drained extraorally from a location at the angle of the mandible identical to that of the masticator space opening. An intraoral incision over the pterygomandibular raphe allows direct access medial to the lateral pharyngeal space and laterally to the medial compartment of the masticator space (Fig. 10–18). An incision directly

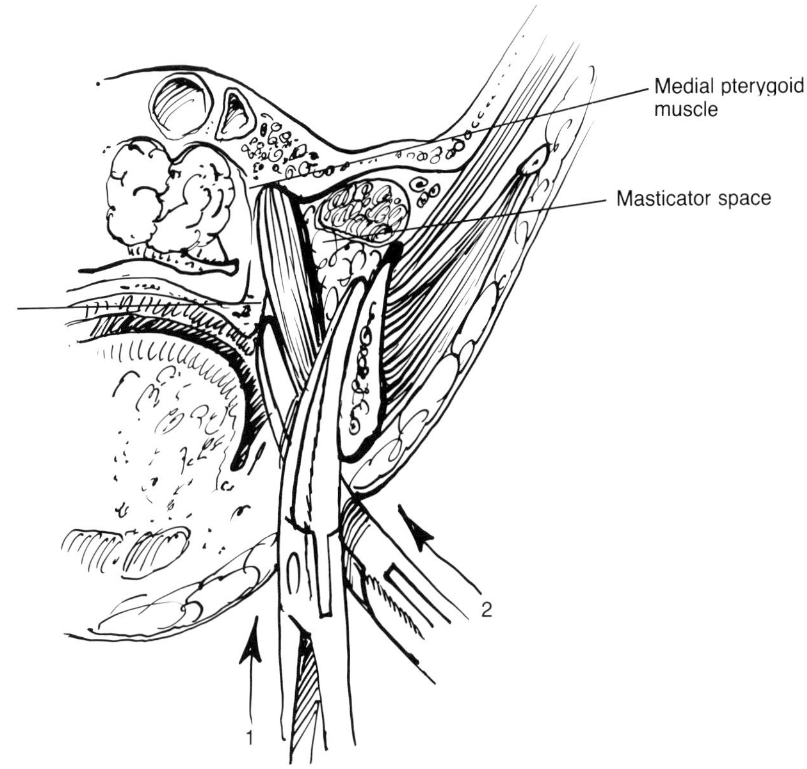

Figure 10–18. *The lateral pharyngeal space is entered through an incision along the pterygomandibular raphe. The hemostat is directed medially into the lateral pharyngeal space or laterally into the medial portion of the masticator space.*

over the superior margin of the lateral pharyngeal space will cause brisk hemorrhage and, therefore, should be avoided. After the mucosa overlying the pterygomandibular raphe is incised, blunt dissection medially and laterally will allow entrance into the adjacent spaces.

HEAD AND NECK INFECTIONS

Peritonsillar Abscess

Peritonsillar abscess (PTA) was a life-threatening disease before the advent of antibiotics. Yung and Cantrell[21] described the reports of an estimated 226 deaths in England in 1875. PTA is a very common deep infection of the head and neck which, if left untreated, may rupture spontaneously or progress to a parapharyngeal space infection. Modern therapies for peritonsillar abscess have included I & D and immediate tonsillectomy.[22] More recently Spires et al.[23] reported the results of a prospective clinical study of aspiration of peritonsillar abscess as opposed to I & D. The 62 patients were treated with either I & D or needle aspiration alone. The recovery period was similar in both groups, but 2 of the 41 patients treated with aspiration had an immediate recurrence. Both patients were successfully treated with subsequent I & D.

In a review of 50 cases of quinsy tonsillectomy, Yung and Cantrell[22] found the abscess was localized to the upper pole of the tonsil in only 38 patients. In 12 patients, the abscess was in the midportion or lower pole and would not have been drained by the standard I & D. Contralateral abscesses were present in four cases, suggesting that approximately 20% of PTA cannot be adequately drained by standard I & D.

The indications for tonsillectomy including PTA remain controversial. Herbild and Bonding[24] found that the probability of late recurrence of PTA was affected by the patient's age and medical history. Fifty percent of patients with no prior throat symptoms remained asymptomatic following I & D, and in patients over 40 years old the chance of recurrence was low.

The clinician who routinely treats odontogenic infections must consider the diagnosis of PTA when patients present with complaints of dysphagia and trismus. The most common physical findings are an asymptomaic tonsillar swelling, deviation of the uvula, and trismus. These findings are consistent with those of lateral pharyngeal space abscess of odontogenic origin. A differential diagnosis of isolated pharyngitis and associated PTA can be made by ruling out an odontogenic etiology for these findings.

There is ample clinical evidence to support aspiration of PTA as the initial procedure of choice.[25–27] Needle aspiration should be performed sequentially, as described by Spires et al.[23] at three different points with an 18-gauge needle. The area lateral to the superior tonsillar pole should be aspirated initially with two additional aspirations 1- and 2-cm inferior to the initial point (Fig. 10–19). If only the most superior point is aspirated, then 33% of the abscesses may be missed.

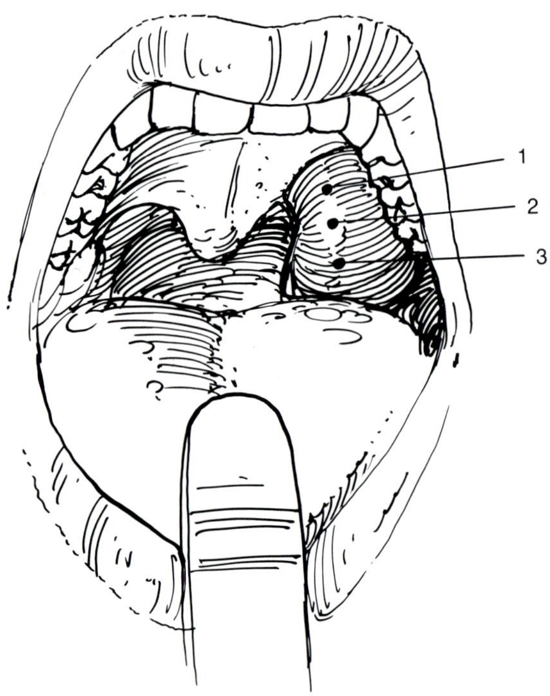

Figure 10–19. *Three levels of needle aspiration are recommended to evacuate the pus from peritonsillar abscesses.*

Anaerobic and aerobic cultures should be obtained in all patients. Patients should receive appropriate antibiotic therapy. A 10-day course of phenoxymethyl penicillin (2 g/day) or, if a penicillin allergy exists, erythromycin (1 g/day) should be initiated. Brook[28] reported that anaerobes were found in all cases of PTA. Spires et al.[23] recommend that antimicrobials, such as clavulanic acid derivatives, be used if the initial response is unsatisfactory.

Acute Orbital Cellulitis

Etiology and Presentation

Acute orbital cellulitis is an uncommon but serious complication arising from a midface infection. It usually occurs in acute sinusitis mainly in adolescents and children without previous sinus problems, but also frequently from dental infections[29] (Fig. 10–20A,B). Orbital cellulitis originates from neighboring sinuses in 70% to 80% of cases. In the adult, bacterial frontal sinusitis is the most frequent cause. In children, spread from ethmoidal sinuses is more common. Other causes include scarlet fever, trauma to neighboring tissues, odontogenic abscesses, middle ear infections, and intracranial infections.[31] Still other less common infectious causes have been reported by Stone and Stratigos[32] in their literature review of multiple reports of orbital cellulitis. They cite a variety of etiologies including cellulitis of the skin of the face and nose, blepharitis, dacryocystitis, dacryoadenitis, hordeolum, erysipelas, herpes simplex stomatitis, varicella, and mumps.[33–36] Traumatic causes include blunt trauma leading to fracture of the nose or zygoma. Preexisting chronic maxillary sinusitis from a deep periodontal pocket leading to orbital cellulitis as a complication of a zygoma fracture has also been reported.[37] Penetrating injuries of the orbit have resulted in serious intraglobular infection.[33]

Neoplasms in or near the orbit or paranasal sinuses can create orbital swelling by blocking venous drainage. Orbital rhabdomyosarcomas must be considered, especially in children.[38] Orbital cellulitis comprises diffuse edema of the orbital contents with infiltration of the globe and the adipose tissue of the orbit with inflammatory cells and bacteria.[31]

Odontogenic infections of maxillary and mandibular teeth can give rise to orbital cellulitis and all of the attendant sequela of orbital abscess, optic neuritis,

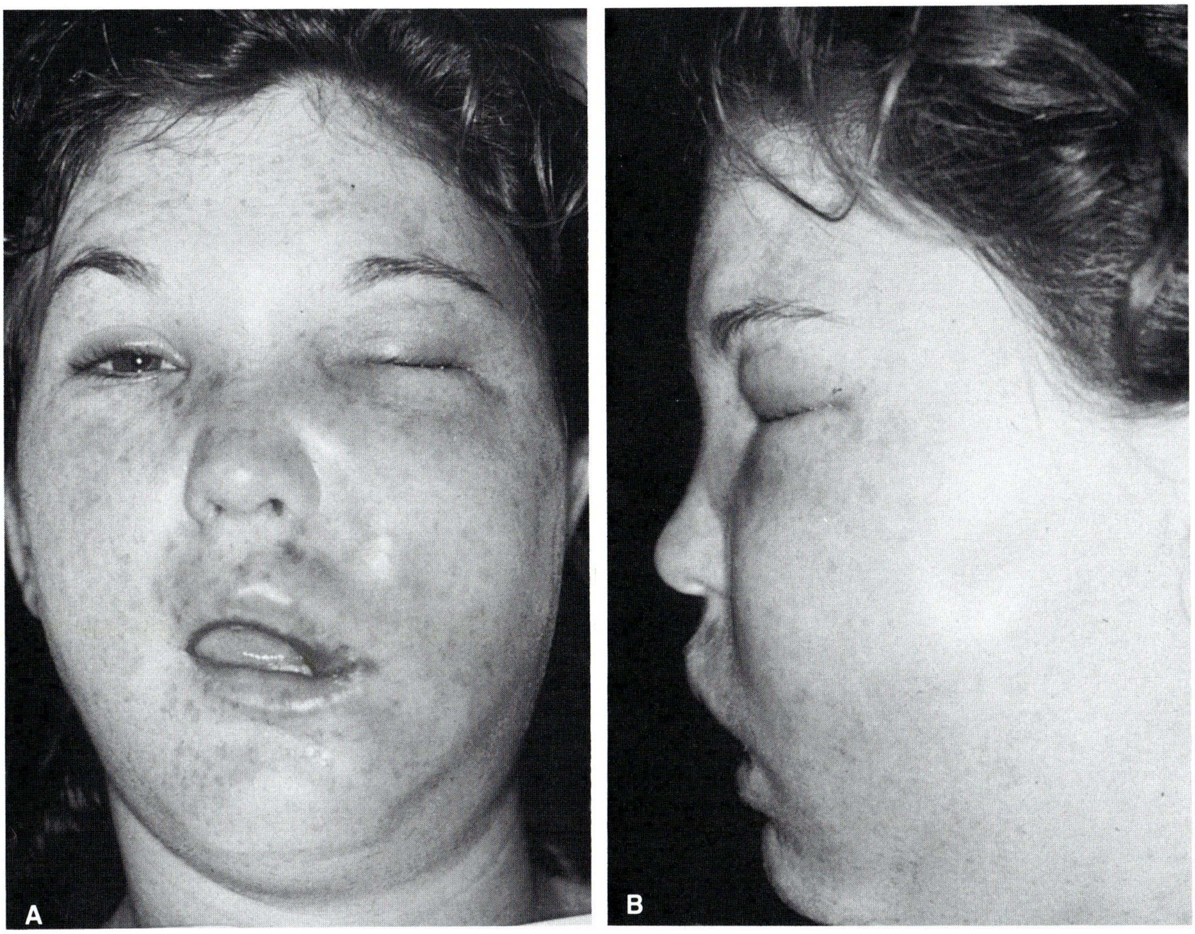

Figure 10–20. *(A,B) Orbital cellulitis following maxillary third molar extraction. The superficial periorbital, temporal, and buccal spaces are also involved.*

cavernous sinus thrombosis, blindness, and death (Fig. 10–21). In one reported series 10 of 190 cases of orbital cellulitis were caused by dental infections. Of the entire group studied, 15 patients suffered partial or total vision loss and two were left with abducent nerve paralysis. Orbital cellulitis of dental origin constitutes a small percentage of the total cases of globe involvement, usually from maxillary teeth, although infection in the mandible can spread through the paranasal sinuses, deep facial circulation, and orbital tissues, resulting in the expected morbid sequela.[32]

Early signs of orbital involvement must be identified and vigorous antibiotic and surgical therapy initiated. The appearance of orbital cellulitis has been generally classified using clinical criteria. Swelling and redness of the eyelids, chemosis, exophthalmos, and dull pain are usually present. Chandler et al.[39] classified cases into five groups by increasing severity of infection. Obstructive nontender edema, contrasted with inflammation and cellulitis, is seen in groups I and II (inflammatory edema and orbital cellulitis). The presence and location of pus determines the next two groups (subperiosteally in group III; within orbital tissues, group IV). Cases which progress to cavernous sinus thrombosis are placed in group V.

Management

Once the early signs of orbital cellulitis become evident (eye pain, chemosis, proptosis, and subjective vision changes) the patient should be hospitalized and

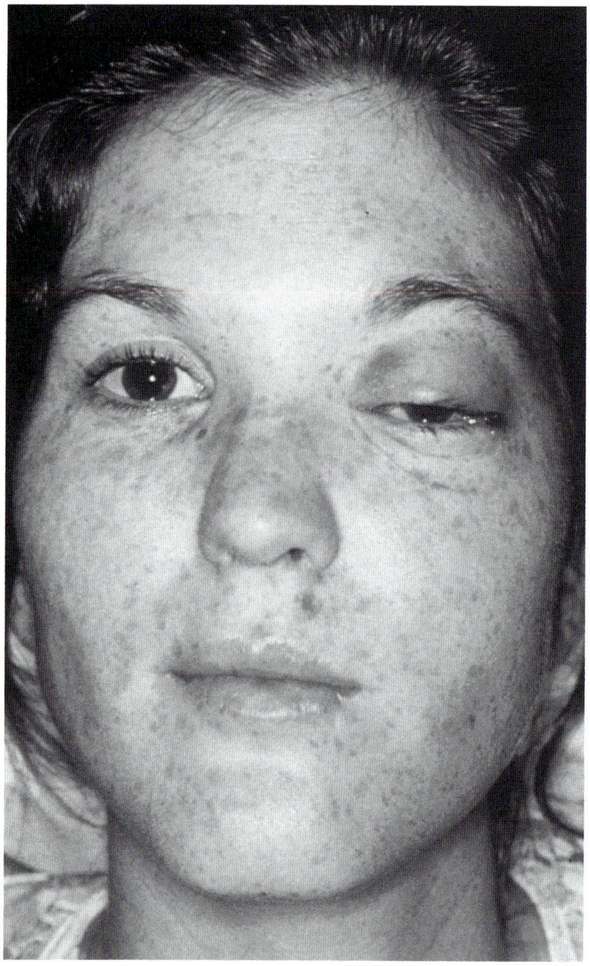

Figure 10–21. *Orbital cellulitis. Marked ptosis and proptosis are results of involvement of the occulomotor nerve and the extrinsic muscles of the eye.*

broad coverage antimicrobial therapy administered intravenously. The choice of antibiotics in the early stages of evaluation depends on the suspected etiology and the patient's general condition. Early diagnosis and the immediate institution of appropriate medical and surgical therapy are imperative. Bullock and Fleishman[42] recommend a multiple drug regimen of agents administered intravenously and in high doses. In general, when gram-staining and cultures of the infecting organisms are unavailable, initial therapy should include a penicillinase-resistant penicillin. Ampicillin should be included for patients who are under age 4 to provide coverage against *Haemophilus influenzae*.[43] Bullock and Fleishman[42] warn that a patient with orbital cellulitis may respond dramatically to initial antimicrobial therapy, only to relapse several days later after an orbital abscess has formed.

Surgical management depends on the circumstances of the individual case. In all cases the precipitating etiology must be removed and the appropriate incision and drainage established. If the paranasal sinuses are the source of infection, then an operation suitable for the pathology present should be done (e.g., ethmoidectomy, Caldwell-Luc operation, or frontal sinus trephination).

Odontogenic infections should be managed in a manner previously described. The orbit may require surgical drainage, the timing of which depends on surgical judgment. Duke-Elder[44] and Dingman[45] have stressed the difficulties inherent in deciding when to drain the orbit. If drainage is attempted prematurely, a localized infection may be disseminated throughout the orbital tissues. Delaying drainage of an orbital abscess, on the other hand, may result in loss of vision, cavernous sinus thrombosis, meningitis, subdural empyema, or brain abscess.

Bullock and Fleishman[42] advocate large incisions made over the region of a suspected abscess or in the supranasal quadrant of the orbit (Lynch incision) (Fig. 10–22). Additional incisions can be made if needed. Drains should be placed in the wounds and advanced a small distance each day.

Local measures to complement surgical intervention and antibiotic treatment should be an integral part of the treatment. Care should be taken to prevent exposure keratitis which, in itself, can cause the loss of an eye.[46] The general well-being of the patient including vital signs and WBC count should be measured daily.[32] The earliest changes in eye signs should signal the initiation of frequent daily testing of visual acuity, occular motility, exophthalmos, and visual fields.

Intracranial Infection

Neurologic complications of odontogenic infections may become manifest as a cavernous sinus thrombosis, a brain abscess, or a meningitis. Cavernous sinus thrombosis has been reported as a more frequent neurologic complication of dental infection than brain abscesses and subdural empyema.[47] The classic neurologic clinical signs of acute cavernous sinus thrombosis are proptosis with periorbital edema, thrombosis of the retinal vein, supraorbital sensory

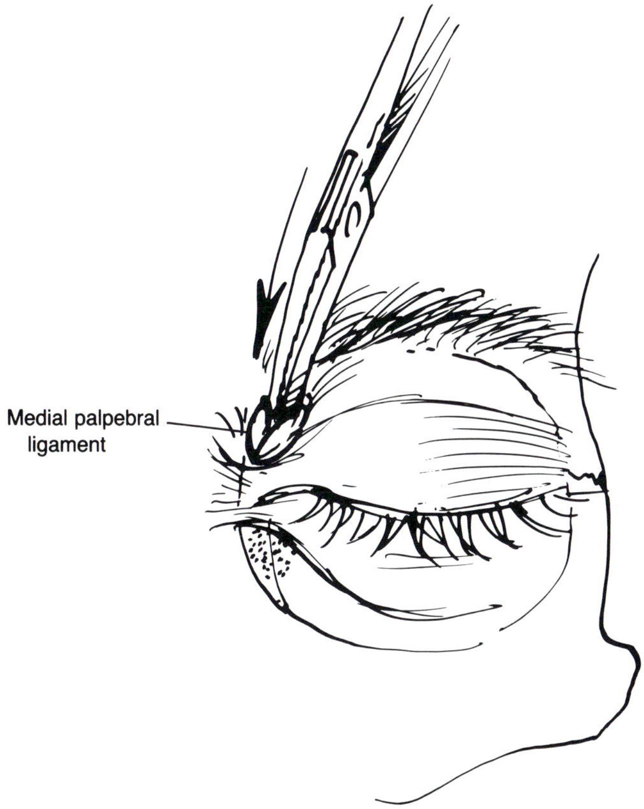

Figure 10–22. *Lynch incision is used to drain an orbital abscess. The anterior ethmoid artery should be identified on the medial wall of the orbit. The periorbita is penetrated in order to open into the internal eye.*

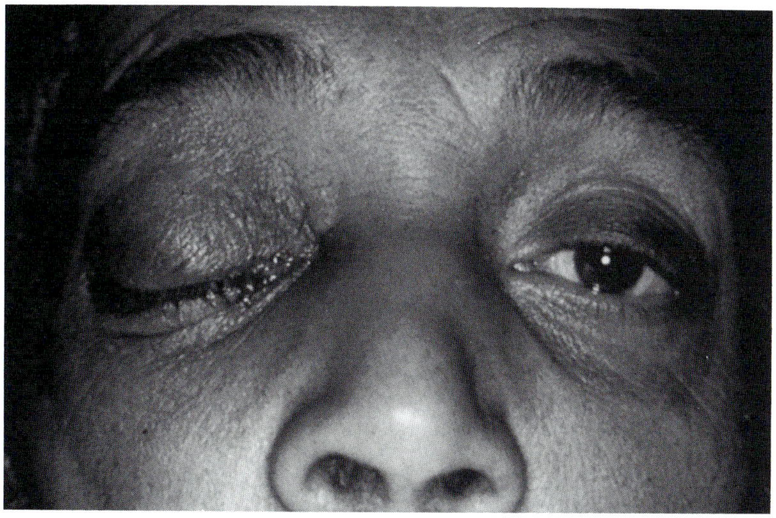

Figure 10–23. *Cavernous sinus thrombosis. Patient exhibits marked proptosis and ptosis.*

changes, ophthalmoplegia, ptosis, dilated pupils, and abolishment of corenal reflexes[48] (Fig. 10–23). Associated findings directly related to the orofacial infection are often found. Dental infections of either jaw can be the nidus for brain infection by way of the facial, angular, inferior, and superior ophthalmic veins, or by a direct route through openings in the temporal bone.[49]

Brain abscesses associated with dental infection have an extremely high mortality rate compared with other foci and are difficult to control with antibiotics alone. Clinically, there may be a latent period of several days or weeks before the appearance of symptoms of intracranial involvement. Initial complaints may be mild, consisting mostly of headaches, malaise, and apathy. Neurologic signs may appear later, depending on the location of the lesion. When intracranial infection is suspected, the appropriate neurologic studies including CT scan and MRI should be done immediately.

Chronic meningitis has been reported in patients with dental infections.[50–52] Four patients with a history of initial fever for 2 to 4 weeks followed by fever peaks every third to sixth day with afebrile intervals for months were described. Three of them had presumed foci of infection in maxillary teeth. The findings of *Streptococcus milleri* antigen in cerebrospinal fluid in one patient in this group inspired a search for other organisms commonly associated with odontogenic infection.

Facial and Cervical Infections Associated With Gas-Producing Bacteria

Gas-producing infections in the head and neck region are rarely reported. Gonty and Costich[53] described two cases of severe facial and cervical infections caused by gas-producing organisms. Altemeier and Culbertson,[54] in 1948, classified gas-producing conditions and evinced the ways that gas may be introduced into the tissue by extrinsic factors such as severe trauma, improper irrigation of wounds, and injury of the respiratory organs or intrinsic factors, such as infection caused by gas-producing organisms. Crepitant cellulitis and gas gangrene can occur spontaneously, without previous trauma or surgery.

Drake et al.[55] stated that gas gangrene or myonecrosis may be caused by clostridial or nonclostridial organisms, and that the two groups of organisms are indistinguishable on clinical grounds. The characteristics of gangrene are as follows:

Severe pain in the wound
Toxemia
Drowsiness, fever, tachycardia
Intensely tender edematous wound
Sweet- or foul-smelling discharge
Dead muscle
Gas formation with or without crepitus
Overlying skin that is gangrenous or erythematous; occasionally with a coppery hue and bullous formation

Gas formation, if not evident by the presence of crepitus, may be apparent by radiographic examination (Fig. 10–24). Both anaerobic and aerobic bacteria of nonclostridial crepitant cellulitis have been cultured in gas-producing infections.

It is important to note that the anaerobes found commonly in odontogenic infections may produce gas in individual tissues. The most likely cause of gas in tissue in infections associated with odontogenic etiology is nonclostridial but nevertheless indicative of serious infection.

Anaerobic	***Aerobic***
Bacteroides fragilis	Pyogenic cocci
Bacteroides melaninogenicus	*Streptococcus*
Peptostreptococcus	*Enterococcus*
	Staphylococcus
	Coliform bacteria
	Escherichia
	Proteus
	Klebsiella
	Enterobacter
	Serratia
	Pseudomonas
	Herelle
	Diphtheroids

Clostridial cellulitis is more common than true clostridial myonecrosis and represents a mild form of the disease.[55] Clostridial infections localized to the subcutaneous tissue (clostridial crepitant cellulitis) are serious, but early adequate treatment usually resolves the infection.[56]

Crepitant nonclostridial cellulitis of the head and neck occurs infrequently, and, although the potential morbidity and mortality associated with these infections is increased compared to other head and neck infections, early diagnosis and aggressive treatment can minimize the untoward sequela.[53]

Necrotizing Fasciitis

Necrotizing fasciitis is a relatively rare acute infectious process that is characterized by rapidly progressive necrosis of subcutaneous tissue and fascia (Figs.

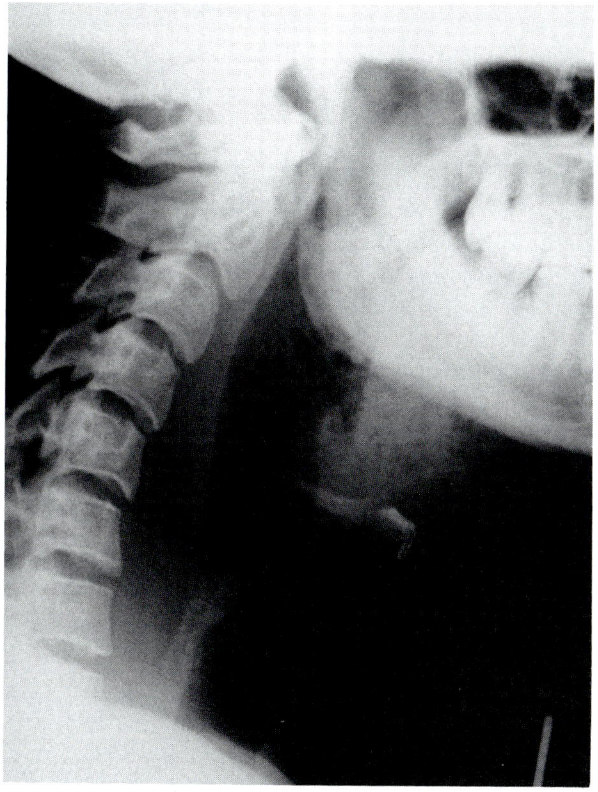

Figure 10–24. *Lateral cervical radiograph. Air is present in the retropharyngeal tissues.*

10–25 and 10–26). Rea and Wyrick[57] described this clinical entity and identified it as synonymous with such destructive lesions reported in the older literature as acute streptococcal gangrene, gangrenous erysipelas, necrotizing erysipelas, and hospital gangrene. Accompanying the widespread necrosis of the superficial fascial is extensive undermining of the surrounding tissue and the possibility of systemic toxicity. Necrotizing fasciitis must be differentiated from erysipelas, progressive bacterial synergistic gangrene, anaerobic streptococcal gangrene, and gas gangrene. Erysipelas is a spreading cellulitis and lymphangitis with raised, slightly defined, irregular reddish borders. In necrotizing fasciitis the involved skin is pale red without distinct borders and with blisters or bullae (see Fig. 10–25). Pale red areas progress to a distinct purple color. Progressive bacterial synergistic gangrene usually develops more slowly, with fewer signs of toxicity. The gangrene frequently involves the edges of previous wounds. Anaerobic streptococcal gangrene develops rapidly and the affected skin is hot, red, swollen, and painful. Rea and Wyrick[57] distinguished this entity from necrotizing fasciitis by the tissues involved. If the fascia is primarily infected, the diagnosis is necrotizing fasciitis; if the muscle is principally infected a diagnosis of streptococcal myositis or clostridial myositis (gas gangrene) should be considered.

Cervicofacial necrotizing fasciitis is a much less common condition than fasciitis of the abdomen, perineum, or extremities. Spankus et al.[58] identified 29 cases in the world literature and added 3 new cases. The mortality rate in their series was 22% with an increase in the death rate of males over age 40. Sperry and McFeeley[59] reported five cases of necrotizing fasciitis and presented a review of the causative factors and the medicolegal implications. The risk of devel-

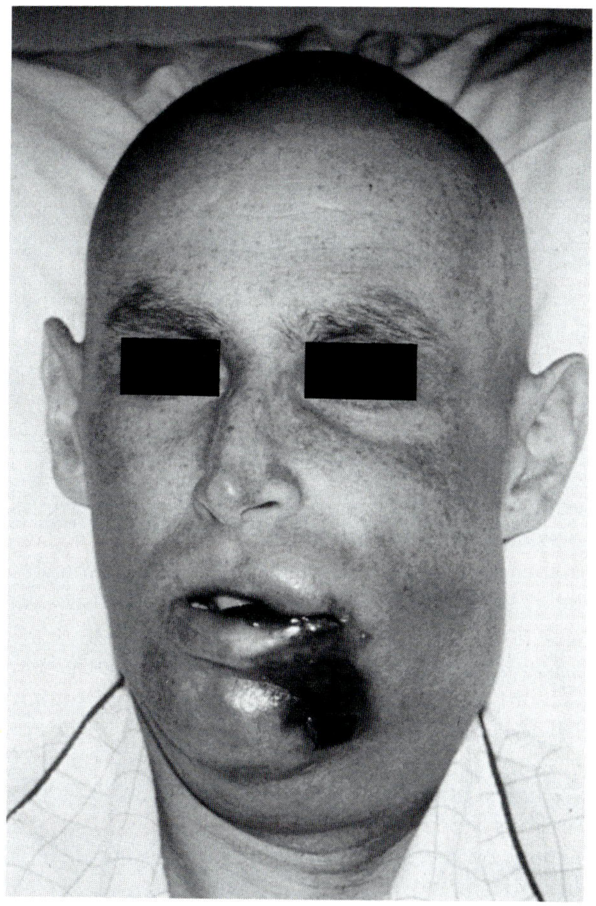

Figure 10–25. *Necrotizing fasciitis is seen in a terminally ill leukemia patient 18 hours after gentle scaling of a lower left bicuspid periodontal defect. Diffuse necrosis of the left lower lip is present.*

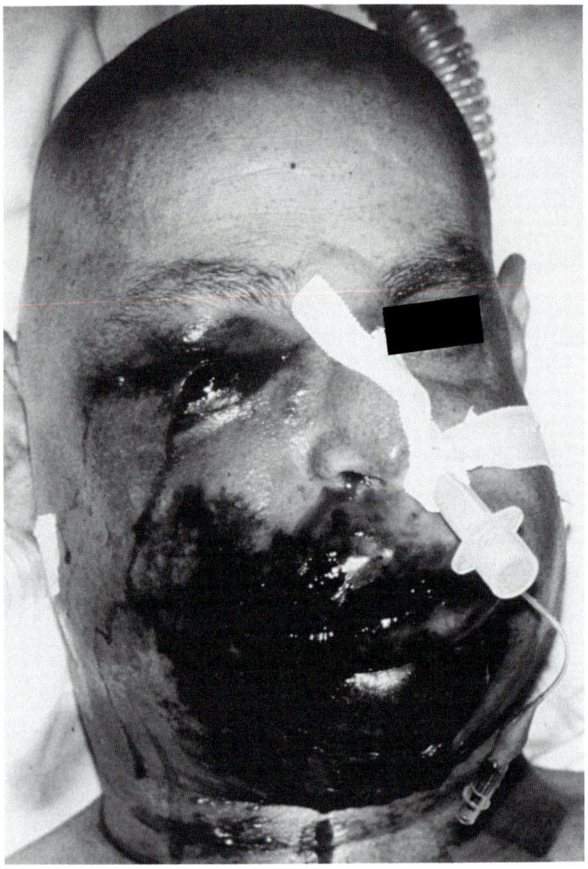

Figure 10–26. *Necrotizing fasciitis in the patient shown in Figure 10–25 48 hours after tooth scaling. The necrosis had spread throughout the face and neck; death ensued.*

oping this destructive disease is exacerbated by the presence of predisposing conditions (50% of cases demonstrate intercurrent diseases) including diabetes mellitus, atherosclerotic coronary vascular disease, and alcoholism.

Because necrotizing fasciitis was often mistaken for cellulitis or erysipelas in the past, it was initially treated conservatively with extremely morbid results.[60] The disease would continue to progress along the fascia and ultimately involve the skin. The gangrenous appearance of the skin would encourage a diagnosis of "wet gangrene" and radical excision would be performed without the true disease process recognized.[61] In its early stages, the disease process can present with a deceptively benign superficial appearance that may persist as chronic drainage and a resistant infection. A clinically troublesome but initially benign course may develop in an otherwise relatively healthy patient. Klabacha et al.[62] proposed a classification of soft tissue infections based on tissue plane involvement. They considered necrotizing fasciitis a type III infection by virtue of the superficial fascia being the major tissue plane involved.

Aerobes and obligate anaerobes have been cultured in synergistic combination, thus dispelling the earlier belief that the infection was caused by streptococci and staphylococci.[63] Giuliano et al.[64] completed a microbial study of 16 patients with necrotizing fasciitis that revealed two distinctive types of bacterial findings. Anaerobic and facultative anaerobic bacteria, such as enterobacteriaciae and streptococci other than group A (at least one anaerobe in combination with facultative anaerobic bacteria) were cultured from type I patients. Type II patients (3 of 16) had group-A streptococci (pyogene) alone, or in combination with staphylococci (*epidermidis* and *aureus*), without the occurrence of anaerobic bacteria. Group-A streptococci and staphylococci were not isolated from type I patients. In all cases, the clinical findings and the progression of the disease were closely identical.

Type I or type II organisms may be introduced into the tissues by a variety of means including trauma from surgery, insect bite,[65] hypodermic needle injection,[66] intravenous needle placement,[67] burns, cuts, abrasions, contusions,[57] peritonsillar infections,[68] boils, or any type of penetrating trauma.[69] Inevitably, as previously described, patients affected generally have a concomitant systemic condition.

Balcerak et al.[60] reviewed the literature and incorporated their own clinical findings to describe the classic infectious process which usually begins 2 to 4 days after the initial insult. The skin becomes smooth, tense, and shiny; no sharp demarcation may be seen between normal and affected skin. The disease process can progress extremely rapidly when serious intercurrent disease exists. The dusky discoloration of the skin appearing as small purplish patches with ill-defined borders is the pathognomonic sign of necrotizing fasciitis. Blisters or bullae a few millimeters in diameter will appear in the skin of the involved areas. The tissue beneath the blisters becomes necrotic and blue in color. Thrombosis of the nutrient vessels that pass through the zone of involved fascia causes the localized necrosis of skin. If treatment is delayed or inadequate the disease progresses to frank cutaneous gangrene that forms a superficial slough, beneath which can be seen the liquefaction of fat and necrosis of the fascia.[69] Mitz and Peyronie[70] described the fascial plane involved in cervicofacial necrotizing fasciitis and the superficial musculoaponeurotic system (SMAS). The longitudinal sheath attaches to the parotid sheath in the parotomasseteric area and is part of the cervicocephalic fascia investing the muscles of expression and is continuous from the head to the neck. The SMAS is continuous with the posterior part of the frontalis muscle in the upper face and with the platysma in the lower face and neck. Infection may spread along this plane along the investing fascia of the temporalis and frontalis muscles to eventually reach the galea aponeurotica. In isolated necrotizing fasciitis, bone and muscle are not initially involved unless they are part of the original trauma.[71] Ladingham and Tehrani[72] postulated that the fascia alone is primarily involved and muscle tissue initially spared because the avascularity of the fascial planes favors subcutaneous spread by anaerobic organisms.

Balcerak et al.[60] described the elements of successful treatment of necrotizing fasciitis: early recognition of the infection process, aggressive surgical intervention, systemic medical and supportive therapy, intensive antibiotic therapy, and aggressive early surgical care.

Diagnosis of soft tissue destruction and gas can be helped by radiographs and CT scans.[73, 74] Frozen section biopsy[75] and digital dermofluorometry[76] can be employed as aids to diagnose and to evaluate vascular viability in exploratory flap design.

The initial surgical approach to necrotizing fasciitis is wide, extensive fasciotomy incisions with exposure and exploration of all involved fascia and gross debridement of necrotic tissue.[60] Clinically, the extent of the destructive lesion is diagnosed by passing a blunt instrument through an existing traumatic skin break, or an incision made down to fascia, in which the probe can be easily passed in all directions along the fascial sheath.[67] The extent of fascial involvement cannot be determined by the overlying skin. The surgeon must anticipate much wider actual fascial necrosis than is superficially apparent.[72]

Fasciotomy incisions in the skin are made over existing necrotic areas or in the skin creases, when possible (Fig. 10–27). Balcerak et al.[60] advise this technique:

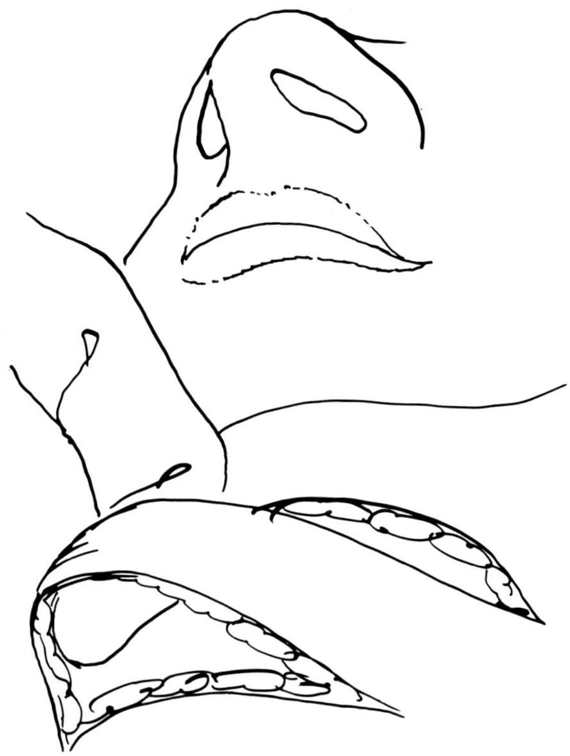

Figure 10–27. *Surgical approach to necrotizing fasciitis in the neck. An incision is made in a skin fold down to fascia. The extent of dissection is determined by blunt finger dissection.*

- Fasciotomy incisions should parallel major blood vessels, and the vascular supply to the tissue flaps created must be maintained.
- It is not necessary to excise all of the overlying skin, only that which is definitely necrotic.
- The extent of dissection is determined by using a gloved finger to undermine the infected tissue until the finger cannot pass further with a reasonable amount of manual pressure.

The skin is hyperesthetic or anesthetic to pinprick in the area of necrosis; these neurologic findings strongly suggest the likelihood of an underlying fasciitis.[77] Presumably, the cutaneous nerves in the subcutaneous tissue are destroyed by the necrotizing process.[61] A thin, gray, serosanguineous "dishwater fluid" exudate which may be foul smelling can be encountered along with a dull gray necrotic fascia during the debridement procedure.[78]

Following the extensive fasciotomy incisions, the wounds should be irrigated and dressed with packs impregnated with standard medicaments such as zinc peroxide, hydrogen peroxide,[79] normal saline solution,[78] and 0.5% silver nitrate. Once the infectious process is arrested, the wound can be treated as an extensive burn.[66] The necrotic area should be dressed several times daily and the wound reexplored to identify additional necrotic areas requiring debridement.

Antibiotic coverage must be broad and administered intravenously. High doses of penicillin, an aminoglycoside, a penicillinase-resistant antibiotic, and an anaerobic antimicrobial agent should be instituted immediately when necrotizing fasciitis is suspected. Once suitable cultures have been obtained and the infecting organisms identified, the antibiotic regimen can be adjusted to suit the organisms grown.

Important local and systemic findings may be associated with cervicofacial necrotizing fasciitis. The patient may feel very ill, report weakness, and appear apathetic.[69] Tachycardia, a slight temperature elevation, leukocytosis or leukopenia, and transient bone marrow inhibition are common findings.[79] Fulminant, advanced cases may show severe anemia secondary to bacterial hemolysins. Serum calcium levels may be low.[81]

Supportive care and management of intercurrent disease are critically necessary to limit and cure the infection process. Fluid and electrolyte balance, including restoration of calcium intravenously and transfusons to correct anemia, is essential to limiting local and systemic complications.[81]

Serious local complications of cervicofacial necrotizing fasciitis include extension to cervical viscera, mediastinal pneumonia, lung abscesses, arterial erosion, internal jugular venous thrombosis, and cranial neuropathies.[82] Death, directly related to necrotizing fasciitis, is most often a result of overwhelming sepsis, respiratory failure, renal failure, or multiorgan system failure.[83]

Mediastinitis

Mediastinitis caused by a descending head and neck infection occurs rarely. Suppurative mediastinitis is most commonly the result of esophageal perforation, either secondary to esophagoscopy or tumor erosion.[84]

Pearse[85] reported 110 patients with suppurative mediastinitis. Sixty-four were the result of esophageal perforation; suppurative lymphadenitis and retropharyngeal abscesses were next in frequency with 13 and 11 patients, respectively. Other etiologies accounted for the remaining 22 cases. Levine et al.[84] presented five cases of mediastinitis secondary to odontogenic infection and described a technique for transcervical drainage of the anterior and posterior mediastinum. Although the incidence of intrathoracic complications from odontogenic infections is low, the morbidity and mortality associated with intrathoracic infection is high. Two patients died in Levine's series because of a delay in diagnosis and the fulminant nature of the disease. Steiner et al.[86] reported one case of odontogenic infection leading to cervical emphysema and fatal mediastinitis. Other cases of fatal mediastinitis secondary to odontogenic infection can be found in the literature.[87, 88] Pearse[85] further reported a mortality rate over 50% when patients with esophageal perforations were excluded from the series. Estrera et al.[89] reviewed the literature and found 21 patients with mediastinitis reported between 1966 and 1983 and added ten additional cases. Of these 31 patients, odontogenic infections were the etiology in 17 and retropharyngeal abscesses in ten patients. The mortality rate of these patients was 42% (13 of 31).

The route of infection between the fascial spaces of the head and neck and the mediastinum has been previously discussed. A detailed account of the anatomy of the mediastinum and its interrelation with the spaces above the clavicle can be found in other written descriptions.[90, 91] Levin et al.[84] emphasized several key anatomic considerations. There are three primary routes that an infection can take to spread from the neck to the mediastinum. The pretracheal space descends into the anterior mediastinum where, at the level of the carina, its fascia fuses with the pericardium and the adventitia of the great vessels, and also becomes adherent to the parietal pleura. These connections account for the frequent association of empyema and pericardial effusions with anterior mediastinal abscesses. The viscerovascular space includes the carotid sheath and its neural and vascular structures. Mosher,[92] in 1929, called this route the "Lincoln's Highway" for extension of pus. Major vessel ruptures and cranial nerve deficits can occur when this space is involved. More commonly infections from the retropharyngeal and retrovisceral spaces extend into the mediastinum. The retropharyngeal space becomes the retrovisceral space at the level of the esophagus and trachea. This space extends from the skull base inferiorly into the posterior mediastinum. The "danger space" of the neck formed by the alar fascia does not have the clinical significance as a route of infection that its name would imply. Infection of this space is rare and almost always secondary to vertebral osteomyelitis.[93]

The clinical history and physical examination findings generally include complaints of a sore throat, difficulty swallowing, fever, chills, productive cough that may be foul smelling and bitter tasting,[88] shortness of breath, and pleuritic chest pain. Adventitious lung sounds may be present, and the lung may be tympanic to percussion.

CT scanning or MRI, if obtainable, are extremely useful in diagnosing mediastinitis. Levine et al.[84] effectively used CT scanning if the patient could tolerate the positioning involved in obtaining an accurate scan. They recommended relying on conventional radiographs to disclose neck swellings and gas dissecting into the mediastinum. The x-ray film findings must be interpreted to account for previous drainage procedures in the neck. A widened mediastinum, suggestive of mediastinal involvement, must also be cautiously interpreted to account for the position of the patient during the exposure of the film. The presence of brawny edema extending from the neck onto the chest wall, especially if associated with crepitance, is highly suggestive of severe cervical-mediastinal infection.[84]

The treatment of suppurative mediastinitis parallels that of all infections. The etiology of the infection must be managed (if odontogenic, the indicated teeth must be removed), an aggressive broad coverage antibiotic regimen initiated, and surgical drainage established from all the spaces involved above and below the clavicle. Levine et al.[84] favor a transcervical approach for most descending infections. The neck is approached through an incision anterior to the sternocleidomastoid muscle and extended across the midline inferiorly (Fig. 10–28). If the neck is involved bilaterally, a circumferential, apron-type incision is preferred. All the involved spaces in the neck are opened, drained, and debrided of necrotic tissue. The anterior mediastinum is entered through the pretracheal space and the mediastinum opened to the level of the tracheal bifurcation using blunt finger dissection (Fig. 10–29). Blunt dissection reduces the risk of damage to vascular structures. The posterior mediastinum is entered by extending the dissection of the retrovisceral space inferiorly.

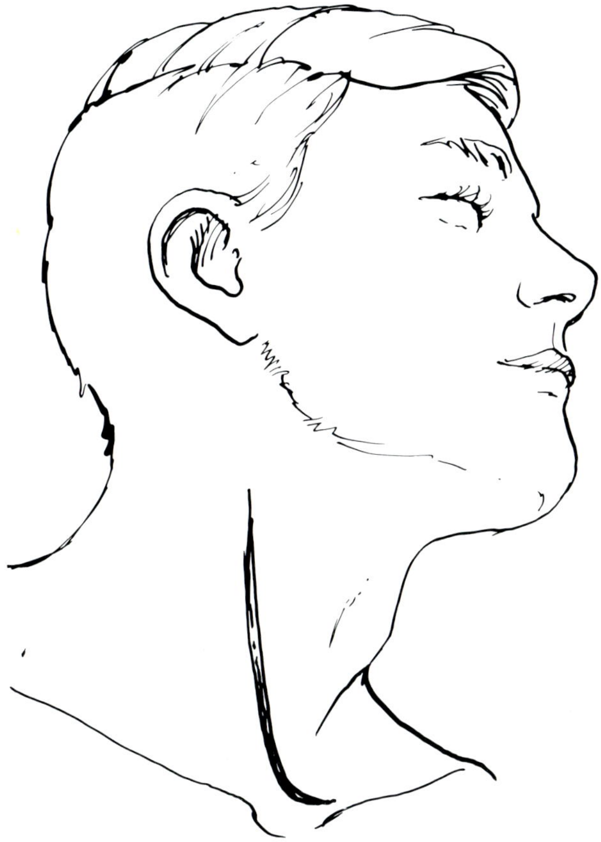

Figure 10–28. *Surgical approach to suppurative mediastinitis. Transcervical incision is made anterior to the sternocleidomastoid muscle and extends across the midline inferiorly.*

The involved spaces are copiously irrigated and soft suction drains placed to provide continuous drainage of the mediastinum to minimize the risk of erosion into major vessels (Fig. 10–30). Levine et al.[84] further recommended insertion of a chest tube to rule out the presence of an empyema, even if there are no radiologic signs preoperatively. An early decision to perform a tracheostomy must be made. If the patient has not previously received a tracheostomy, serious consideration must be given to establishing a controlled surgical airway at the inferior portion of the neck incision. Accidental dislodgment of an endotracheal tube in a patient with massive upper airway edema could be fatal.

Postoperatively, the patient is maintained in the Trendelenberg position to facilitate drainage from the mediastinum. Three of Levine's patients required secondary drainage procedures in spite of meticulous

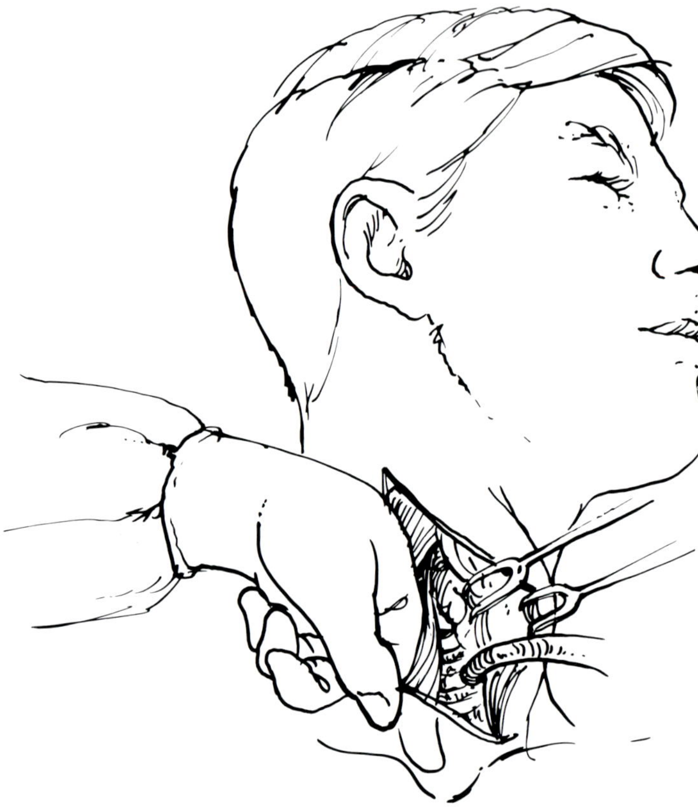

Figure 10–29. *Suppurative mediastinitis. The mediastinum is entered and opened to the level of the tracheal bifurcation using blunt finger dissection.*

wound care and frequent irrigations to break up any remaining loculations. Additional surgical procedures are not uncommon.

Pediatric Infections

Abscesses of the head, jaws, and neck in children parallel similar adult conditions and the same general principles of management apply for effective treatment. The frequency of acute odontogenic infections has declined and the need for emergency care concomitantly reduced. Brook[94, 95] studied the microbiology of abscesses of the head and neck in children to establish further the polymicrobial anaerobic and aerobic nature of these infections. The factors predisposing the children to infection were trauma (13 patients), dental infection (nine), tonsillitis (six), fetal monitoring (five) and congenital cyst (three). Correlation between the predisposing conditions and the bacteria recovered from the infected tissue demonstrated a high frequency of anaerobic bacteria in patients with dental infections, tonsillitis, or after fetal monitoring. Aerobic bacteria, primarily *S. aureus*, were recovered from patients with trauma or in patients with no predisposing conditions.

The management of head, perioral, and neck infections in children is influenced by the patient's ability to cooperate, the extent and location of the infection, and the child's general systemic condition. Chronic odontogenic infections associated with unrestorable deciduous teeth in an otherwise asymptomatic patient may be observed when space maintenance is desired and a dentoalveolar parulis is present. Acute conditions are treated using the same principles applied to adults. Patient management requirements may preclude treatment under a local anesthetic and general anesthesia may be necessary. Inpatient care should be extended to patients who show signs of systemic involvement, have deep space infection, or require general anesthesia. Laboratory tests may not be of value until dental infections reach the stage of acute

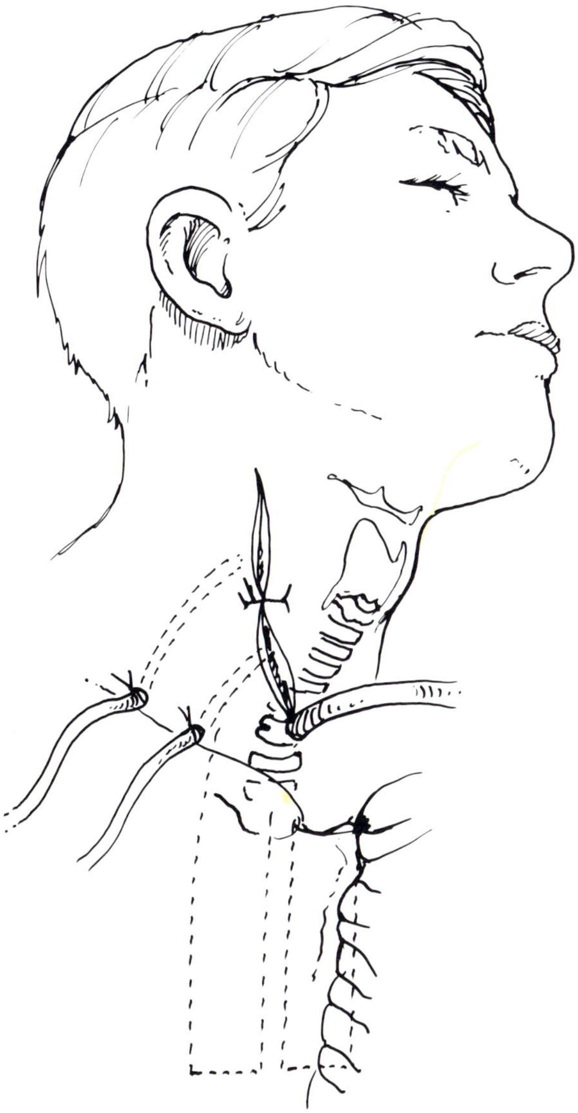

Figure 10–30. *Suppurative mediastinitis. Suction drains are placed into the mediastinum to maintain drainage.*

cellulitis.[96] The patient often will be afebrile until the dental infection has progressed beyond the periradicular area.

Actinomycosis of the Jaws

"Lumpy jaws" was the sobriquet used to describe actinomycosis in cattle and in humans. Lebert reported actinomycosis in humans in 1857; Israel, in 1878, saw granules similar to those described in cattle, and in 1891 he and Wolff cultured anaerobic filamentous organisms from human clinical material.[97] *Actinomyces israeli* was thought to be the same agent as that infecting cattle. *A. bovis*, as currently classified, has never been isolated from man, although both *A. israeli* and *A. bovis* have been found in cattle.[98]

The historical description of actinomycosis is that of an acute or chronic swelling of the involved cervicofacial area with multiple sinuses developing in the skin overlying the abscess, through which pus drains[99] (Fig. 10–31). *A. israeli* is part of the normal oral flora inhabiting dental plaque, dental caries, calculus, and particularly the tonsillar crypts.[100] Trauma to the soft tissues, including surgical manipulation, is thought to facilitate the penetration of the *Actinomyces* organism into tissues with reduced oxygenation, which creates

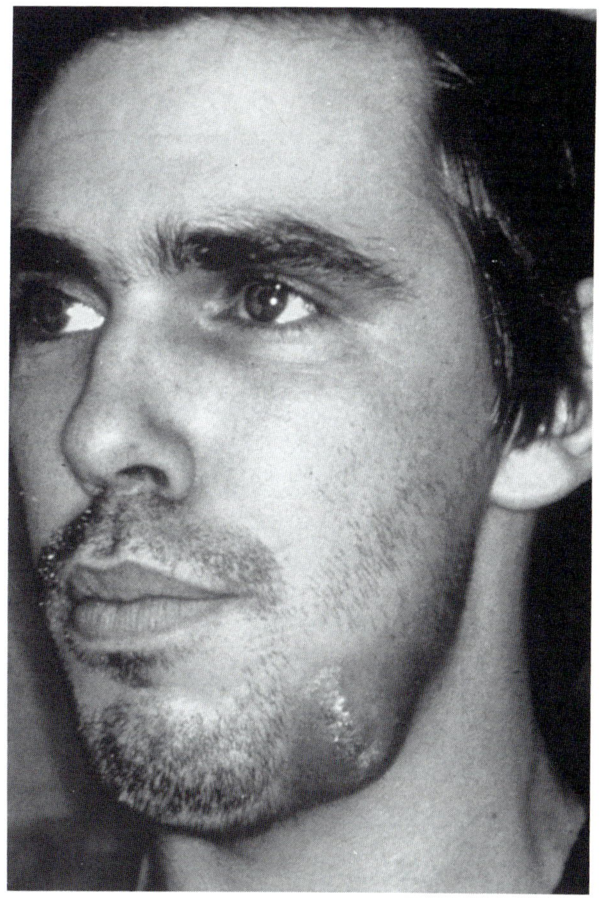

Figure 10–31. *Actinomycosis. Note the necrotic skin and the multiple draining fistulas (courtesy of Dr. Richard C. Ziegler).*

a favorable environment for growth of actinomycotic organisms displaced from the normal oral flora.[101] Actinomycosis is similar to other infections of the jaws in that the synergistic activity of other organisms contributes to the pathogenicity of a mixed infection. Culturing of *Actinomyces* is often difficult because of the mixed nature of the infection and the anaerobic qualities of the organism. The need for a reduced oxygen environment may account for the greater prevalence of actinomycotic infections in the mandible compared with the maxilla, which has a better blood supply providing more oxygen and better circulation.[102]

Actinomycotic osteomyelitis of the facial bones, maxilla, and mandible is best treated by high doses of intravenous antibiotics and prolonged oral antibiotic therapy, together with surgical management of necrotic bone and sinus tracts. Aqueous penicillin G is the drug of choice in the nonallergic patient and is administered intravenously every 3 hours in doses of 1 to 3 million units for 3 to 6 weeks or until draining sinus tracts have resolved, followed by oral penicillin, 2 g/day for at least 3 additional months after all evidence of infection has subsided. Surgical debridement of dead bone, granulation tissue, and necrotic debris to create an environment less favorable to anaerobes is an essential step in achieving successful management of actinomycotic infections. Peabody and Seabury[103] reported cures with sulfa drugs, streptomycin, erythromycin, chloramphenicol, and tetracycline, alone or in combination. Tetracycline is recommended as a second-choice drug.

Soft tissue actinomycosis may respond to routine oral antibiotic therapy and not require intravenous antibiotics or extensive surgical intervention. A unique feature of actinomycotic infection is the dense fibrous connective tissue reaction peculiar to the organism. This reaction may prevent the penetration of therapeutic doses of the antibiotic into the infected tissue, thereby necessitating extensive surgical intervention and the high-dose penicillin regimen.[104]

Osteomyelitis of the Jaws

Osteomyelitis is an inflammatory condition of bone involving the medullary cavity, the haversian systems, and the adjacent cortex. The mandible is more commonly involved than the maxilla, although a high incidence of the disease in the maxilla was reported by Adekeye and Cornah.[105] Osteomyelitis may be classified as follows[106]:

Acute suppurative osteomyelitis
Chronic suppurative osteomyelitis
Chronic sclerosing osteomyelitis
—diffuse
—focal
Chronic osteomyelitis with proliferative periostitis (Garre's chronic nonsuppurative sclerosing osteomyelitis)

The incidence of osteomyelitis of the jaws has been greatly reduced in developed countries since the advent of antibiotics.[107] The causes of osteomyelitis may be clinically apparent when the historical and physical examination findings reveal a traumatic episode, a chronically inflamed carious tooth, an infection in an adjacent anatomical structure (e.g., otitis media), a metastatic septic focus releasing septic thrombi, or advanced chronic periodontitis.[108] Other cases of osteomyelitis occur in medically compromised patients with altered resistance to infection because

Display 10–1. Acute Suppurative Osteomyelitis: Clinical and Laboratory Features

History	Pain; carious or periodontally involved tooth; recent tooth extraction; infection of adjacent anatomic site; debilitating disease; malaise
Clinical	Diffuse swelling; pus discharge; acute or chronic pulpitis; periodontal abscess; fever; trismus
Laboratory	Elevated WBC count; elevated ESR. Histopathology: medullary spaces filled with inflammatory cells which are mainly polymorphonuclear leukocytes; lacuna may be devoid of osteocytes.
X-ray films	Often no x-ray findings or localized periapical radiolucencies

Display 10–2. Chronic Suppurative Osteomyelitis: Clinical and Laboratory Features

History	Previous episode of odontogenic infection or acute suppurative osteomyelitis; debilitating disease; infection of adjacent anatomic site; lip anesthesia or paresthesia; chronic jaw pain; malaise is unlikely.
Laboratory	Elevated ESR and a low-grade leukocytosis may be present. Histopathology: fibrous scar with attempts at osteogenesis characterized by osteoblastic rimming around new bone, together with multiple sequestra with evacuated lacuna.
X-ray films	Patchy areas of radiolucency and radiopacity suggesting bone destruction and sequestrum formation

of neoplasia, drug therapy, tuberculosis,[109] blood dyscrasias,[110] syphilis,[111] malnutrition, and metabolic diseases such as osteopetrosis.[112]

The elements of successful treatment of osteomyelitis of the jaws are strongly dependent on the accurate diagnosis and classification of the disease. The salient historical, clinical, and radiographic features are contained in Displays 10–1 through 10–5.

Acute Suppurative Osteomyelitis

Acute osteomyelitis remains an important infection because chronic osteomyelitis may develop if the primary infection is not eliminated by proper treatment. The designation of acute versus chronic osteomyelitis is somewhat arbitrary; acute osteomyelitis is characterized by those features contained in Display 10–1.

Polymicrobial bacteriologic findings are common to both acute and chronic osteomyelitis. Organisms isolated are *Streptococcus* species, *Bacteroides* species, *Lactobacillus* species, *Eubacterium* species, and *Klebsiella* species. Other frequently cultured organisms include *S. aureus*, *Escherichia coli*, *Veillonella parvula*, *Fusobacterium nucleatum*, and *Peptostreptococcus magnus*.[113] Anaerobic organisms are frequently isolated in equal numbers from all stages of osteomyelitis of the jaws. However, it remains an important infection because chronic osteomyelitis may develop if the primary infection is not eliminated by proper treatment.

The principles of infection management previously discussed for odontogenic infections are similarly applied in the treatment of osteomyelitis of the jaws. Careful clinical and radiographic evaluation to establish undiagnosed foci of infection (teeth, foreign bodies, dead or necrotic bone) will reduce the opportunity for microorganisms to become ensconced in environments favorable to their growth. Aggressive surgical debridement and removal of the cause, intravenous antibiotics, and prolonged oral antibiotic therapy based on culture and sensitivity information are critical elements of successful therapy. Once the

Display 10–3. Chronic Sclerosing Osteomyelitis—Focal: Clinical and Laboratory Features

History	Previous history of odontalgia; patients are younger than age 20.
Clinical	Decreased sensation in the tooth related to the radiopacity; no other specific clinical findings
Laboratory	No distinguishing laboratory findings
X-ray films	A well circumscribed radiopaque mass of sclerotic bone often related to a tooth root; localized radiopacity in an edentulous area of the jaw

Display 10–4. Chronic Sclerosing Osteomyelitis—Diffuse: Clinical and Laboratory Features

History	Pain and local swelling often in cyclic exacerbations; previous tooth extractions; short term antibiotic therapy; more common in young female adults
Clinical	Swelling along the inferior border of the mandible; facial asymmetry; trismus; teeth and gingiva usually normal; lymphadenopathy is infrequent; fistulation to the mouth or skin surface does not occur.
Laboratory	Elevation of temperature and ESR associated with exacerbations of the disease; normal WBC count; normal phosphate activity; and normal routine tests of humoral and cellular immunity. Histopathology: most characteristic changes are coarse, irregular bone trabeculae in fibrotic, partly calcified, or amorphous marrow spaces. Small infiltrates of mononuclear cells, mainly plasma cells and lymphocytes; single multinucleated osteocytes in lacunae along the borders of trabeculae.
X-ray films	The radiographic appearance varies considerably with the stage of the disease and age of the patient. Discreet thin zones with increased density to the lower border of the mandible indicating periosteal hyperactivity and disposition of bone (early finding) Osteolytic areas as well as zones of sclerotic bone appearing early after the onset of symptoms A local cortical bone deficit often at the mandibular angle Children and young adults with increased mandibular volume in width and superior-inferior dimensions Adults with tendency toward reduction of mandibular volume, especially in the angle region Shortening of tooth roots a frequent finding, may be of diagnostic value since it is not seen in fibrous dysplasia of the jaws.

Display 10–5. Chronic Osteomyelitis With Proliferative Periostitis: Clinical and Laboratory Features

History	Young persons are most often affected; asymptomatic, mandibular infection in permanent first molars with necrotic pulps or other deciduous or succedaneous teeth.
Clinical	Afebrile, bone hard swelling on the lateral aspect of the mandible with the overlying mucosa appearing normal; moderate facial asymmetry
Laboratory	Normal WBC, ESR, and alkaline phosphatase. Histopathology: vascular fibrous marrow with new reactive bone and osteoid tissue with osteoblasts bordering many of the trabeculae; inflammatory cells are usually not evident.[126]
X-ray films	A focal overgrowth of bone of the lateral surface of the mandible cortex described as cortical "onion skinning." Radiographs of the involved medullary areas often show mixed radiolucent-radiopaque areas and a carious tooth with a periapical radiolucent area.[127]

acute episode has subsided, clinical and radiographic follow-up should continue for months or longer to observe for early recurrence and retreatment.

Chronic Suppurative Osteomyelitis

Chronic osteomyelitis of the jaws has a varied clinical appearance and an uncertain origin because the original cause of the acute problem may no longer be present. Wannfors and Hammarstrom[114] reported a retrospective study of 24 cases of chronic osteomyelitis based on histories and historic material. No specific correlation could be found between clinical symptoms and morphologic changes in bone. In certain patients, bacteria were found in foci such as osteolytic lacunae of necrotic bone and dentinal tubules of embedded tooth fragments. In these foci, the bacteria could maintain an inflammatory reaction in bone by escaping the immunologic defenses of the host and avoiding the effects of antibiotics. The mandibular canal may be a pathway for the spread of infection.

Treatment of chronic osteomyelitis of the jaws involves removal of all the suspected causes and wide surgical debridement of dead bone, granulation tissue, and chronic exudate (Fig. 10–32). Removal of the buccal plate of the mandible at the infection site when the lower jaw is involved usually eliminates a source of infection and increases antibiotic levels through the blood supply of the buccal tissues. Intravenous antibiotics selected from the results of culture and sensitivity provided by the incubation of granulation tissue and infected bone should be maintained at high levels for several weeks, followed by long-term oral antibiotics. Signs of recurrence should be evaluated for undetected nidus of infection, and immediate aggressive surgical and antibiotic retreatment should be initiated. Intercurrent disease must be considered and general reevaluation of the patient is always indicated.

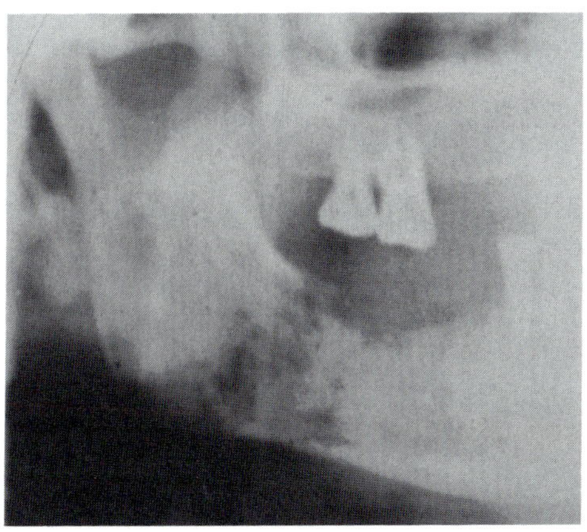

Figure 10–32. *Chronic suppurative osteomyelitis is viewed by panographic radiograph. Advanced destruction of the right body of the mandible occurred while patient endured one year of pain and discomfort.*

Chronic Sclerosing Osteomyelitis

Sclerosing osteomyelitis of the jaws is usually divided into focal and diffuse types.[115] The focal type, also known as condensing osteites, has a pathognomonic radiographic appearance (Fig. 10–33). It is of little clinical significance and generally requires no treatment. The diffuse type (DSO), is primarily confined to the mandible and may prove to be a diagnostic and therapeutic dilemma (Fig. 10–34).

The cause of DSO is thought to be a low-grade medullary infection which causes endosteal and periosteal reactions.[116] Differences of opinion regarding

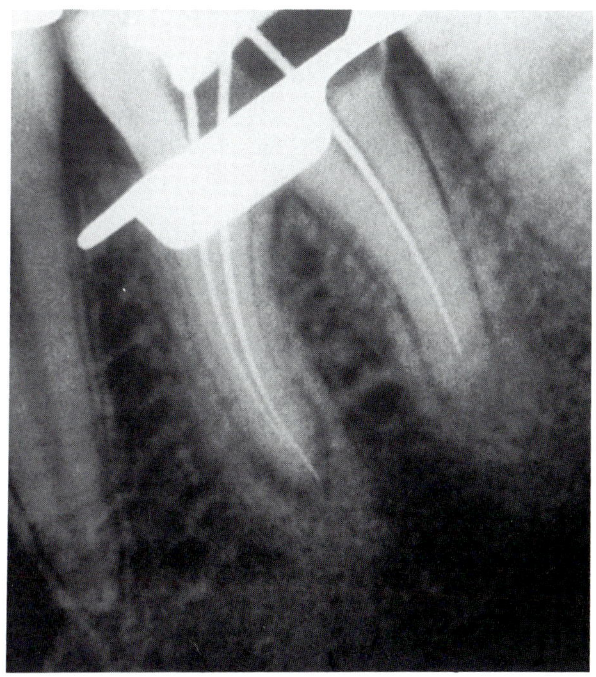

Figure 10–33. *Focal-type chronic sclerosing osteomyelitis (periapical radiograph). Note the radiopacity at the apex of the endodontically treated molar (courtesy of Dr. Doug Damm).*

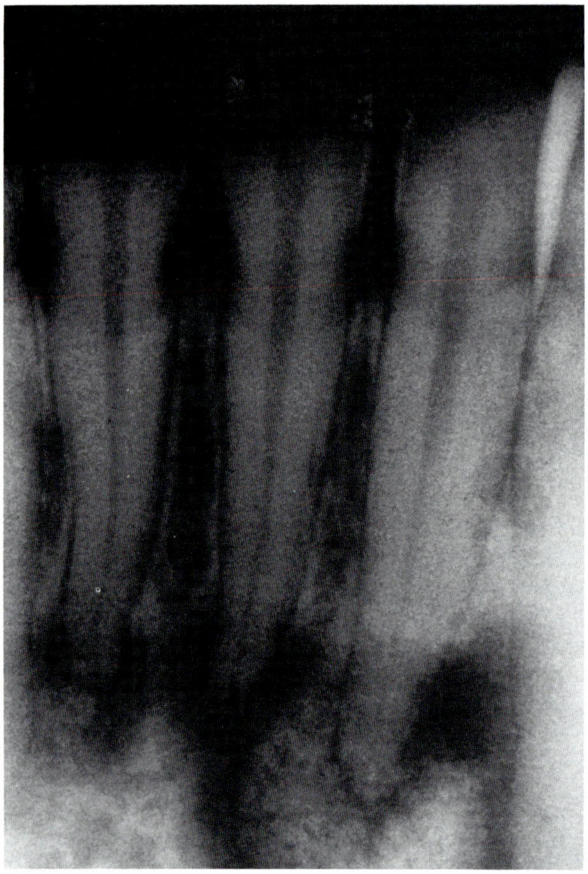

Figure 10–34. *Diffuse-type chronic sclerosing osteomyelitis (periapical radiograph) (courtesy of Dr. Doug Damm).*

the pathogens involved in this disease have been reported. Turlington[117] stated that pathogens are routinely found. Other investigators[118] claim that bacteria usually cannot be grown. Jacobsson and Hollender[119] reported their long-term follow-up of 21 patients with DSO of the mandible treated in Göteborg, Sweden. Despite great efforts to isolate pathogenic organisms, they found only "normal flora" dominated by *Propionibacterium acnes* or *S. epidermidis*. Jacobsson and Hollander[119] hypothesized that an endogenic infection colonized by normal inhabitants of the mucosa or skin preceded by a hematogenous or local dental infection accounted for the scarcity of true pathogens. They further theorized that an earlier infection led to the formation of thrombophlebitis, which may cause a reduction of normal phagocyte function in the sinusoids of bone. A reduction in local circulation may additionally contribute to the creation of an environment conducive to the growth of endogenic anaerobic organisms.

Jacobsson and Hollender[119] recommended that early diagnosis and antibiotic treatment should be initiated as part of a treatment plan, as follows:

1. Treatment should be initiated with penicillin, even if cultures are negative, and continued for at least 3 months unless a culture or sensitivity test shows that another type of antibiotic would be more favorable.
2. If nonsteroidal antiinflammatory agents are unable to suppress the pain and swelling, cortisone therapy should be given.
3. The patient should be kept under observation for several years.
4. Stretch exercises in patients with trismus should be avoided, and tooth extractions should be performed only when there are rigorous indications and only under antibiotic coverage.
5. If the initial therapy fails and the clinical symptoms and radiographic change progress, decortication should be done. Decortication is most successful when the osteomyelitis does not extend too far into the mandibular ramus.
6. Cortisone is a valuable aid in the therapy and is strongly advocated in late chronic stages after antibiotics have failed.

Patients enrolled in the Göteborg study who were treated elsewhere for their trismus by stretch exercises generally were not helped. On the contrary, stretch exercises seemed to accelerate the progression of the disease. An acute exacerbation of symptoms was also frequently recorded following tooth extractions.

Chronic Osteomyelitis With Proliferative Periostitis

In cases in which a carious tooth is the causative factor, extracting the involved tooth and antibiotic therapy are recommended. Treatment should be individualized to the needs of each patient, but there is little evidence to suggest reduction of the periosteal mass is necessary (Fig. 10–35). Physiologic remodeling usually occurs in almost all patients, providing that the causative tooth is removed and sequestrectomy of dead bone is performed.[120]

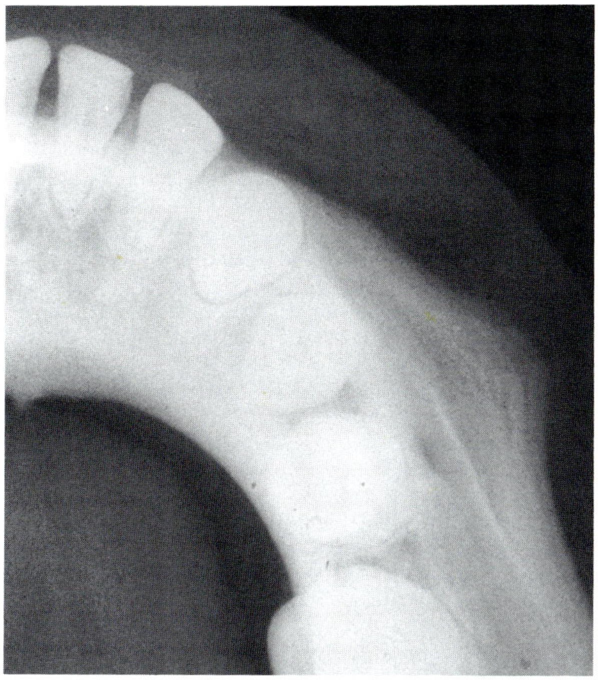

Figure 10–35. *Chronic osteomyelitis with proliferative periostitis is evident on occlusal radiograph. Note the focal overgrowth of cortical bone on the buccal surface of the mandible (courtesy of Dr. Doug Damm).*

Pediatric Infections

Inflammation of the bone marrow in children may be classified in a manner identical to the descriptions used for adults. Osteomyelitis in infants is reported to occur more commonly in the maxilla, because the maxillary sinus in the new bone is still developing and immature.[121] Statistical analysis of osteomyelitis cases in young people show a greater incidence of osteomyelitis in adults (older than 10 years) than children.[122] Osteomyelitis in children can be more aggressive than the adult variety because the immature root apices of the molar region are close to the mandibular canal, which is extremely porous and incomplete.[123] Inflammation can extend along the canal and reach the ascending ramus. Resistance against disease may also contribute to the seriousness of the infection.

Treatment of osteomyelitis of the jaws in children should include all the therapeutic recommendations that apply to the adult patient. Surgical treatment, however, must be tempered for infants and children to address the forming dentition and maxillofacial growth and development.

Hyperbaric Oxygen Treatment

Hyperbaric oxygen therapy has been considered as a useful adjunct in treatment of chronic osteomyelitis, but its true value has not been conclusively demonstrated.[124] In chronic diffuse sclerosing osteomyelitis and in patients in whom decortication and antibiotic therapy have failed, hyperbaric oxygen treatment in combination with antibiotics and surgery may be indicated.[125]

REFERENCES

1. Piecuch JF. Odontogenic infections. In: Symposium on medical emergencies in the dental office. Dent Clin North Am 1982; 26:129.
2. Goldberg MH, Topazian RG. Odontogenic infection and deep fascial space infection of dental origin. In: Topazian RG, Goldberg MH, eds. Management of infections of the oral and maxillofacial regions. Philadelphia: WB Saunders, 1981:156–203.
3. Naschitz JE, Yeshurun D. Occult infection in the facial area presenting as fever of unknown origin. Isr J Med Sci 1985:995.
4. Eames FA, Peters JC. CT findings in lingual abscess. J Comput Assist Tomogr 1983; 7(3):544.
5. Flood TP, Laurence BS, Lee JM, et al. Computed tomography in the management of oribital infections associated with dental disease. Br J Ophthalmol 1982; 66:269.
6. Unger JM, Chintapalli KN. Computed tomography of the parapharyngeal space. J Comput Assist Tomogr 1983; 7:605.
7. Chow AW, Roser SM, Brady FA. Orofacial odontogenic infections. Ann Intern Med 1978; 88:392.
8. Guralnick W. Odontogenic infections. Br Dent J 1984; 156:440.
9. Krogh HW. Extraction of teeth in the presence of acute infections. J Oral Surg 1951; 9:136.
10. Martis CS, Karakasis DT. Extractions in the presence of acute infections. J Dent Res 1975; 54:59.
11. Hall HD, Gunter JW, Jamison HC, et al. Effect of time of extraction on resolution of odontogenic cellulitis. J Am Dent Assoc 1968; 77:626.
12. Chow AW, et al. Orofacial odontogenic infections. Ann Intern Med 1978; 88:392.
13. Grodinsky M. Ludwig's angina: Anatomical and clinical study with review of literature. Surgery 1939; 5:678.
14. Thoma KH. Oral Surgery, ed 3. St Louis: CV Mosby, 1958:937.

15. Williams AC, Guralnick WC. Diagnosis and treatment of Ludwig's angina: Report of 20 cases. N Engl J Med 1943; 228:443.
16. Quayle AA. Bacteroides infection in oral surgery. J Oral Surg 1974; 32:91.
17. Gross BD, Roark DT, Meador RC, et al. Ludwig's angina due to bacteroides. J Oral Surg 1976; 34:456.
18. Dzyak WR, Zide MF. Diagnosis and treatment of lateral pharyngeal space infections. J Oral Maxillofac Surg 1984; 42:243.
19. Zangenbrunner DJ, Dajani S. Pharyngomaxillary space abscess with carotid artery erosion. Arch Otolaryngol 1971; 94:447.
20. Schwartz HC, Bauer RA, Davis NJ, et al. Ludwig's angina: Use of fiberoptic laryngoscope to avoid tracheostomy. J Oral Surg 1974; 32F:608.
21. Yung AK, Cantrell RW. Quinsy tonsillectomy. Laryngoscope 1976; 86:1714.
22. Yung AK, Cantrell RW, Bonding P. Tonsillectomy a chaud. J Laryngol Oto 1973; 87:1171.
23. Spires JR, Owens JJ, Woodson GE, et al. Treatment of peritonsillar abscess: A prospective study of aspiration vs incision and drainage. Arch Otolaryngol Head Neck Surg 1987; 113:984.
24. Herbild D, Bonding P. Peritonsillar abscess. Arch Otolaryngol Head Neck Surg 1981; 107:540.
25. Herzon FS, Aldridge JH. Peritonsillar abscess needle aspiration. Arch Otolaryngol Head Neck Surg 1981; 89:910.
26. Herzon FS. Permucosal needle drainage of peritonsillar abscess. Arch Otolaryngol Head Neck Surg 1984; 10:104.
27. Schechter GL, Sly DE, Roper AL, et al. Changing face of treatment of periotonsillar abscess. Laryngoscope 1982; 92:657.
28. Brook I. Aerobic and anaerobic bacteriology of peritonsillar abscess in children. Acta Paediatr Scand 1981; 70:831.
29. Guindi GM. Acute orbital cellulitis: A multidisciplinary emergency. Br J Oral Surg 1983; 21:201.
30. Sorsby A. Modern Ophthalmology, vol. 2. London: Butterworths, 1963:598.
31. Janakarajah N, Sukumaran K. Orbital cellulitis of dental origin: Case report and review of the literature. Br J Oral Maxillofac Surg 1985; 23:140.
32. Stone A, Stratigos GT. Mandibular odontogenic infection with serious complications. Oral Surg 1979; 47:395.
33. Gans H, et al. Treatment of acute orbital complications. Arch Otolaryngol 1974; 100:329.
34. Aries DR. Orbital cellulitis. J Laryngol Otol 1974; 88:559.
35. Healy GB. Acute periorbital swelling. Laryngoscope 1972; 82:1491.
36. Walters FC, et al. Acute orbital cellulitis. Arch Ophthalmol 1976; 94:785.
37. Hovinga J, Christiaans BJ. Odontogenic infection leading to orbital cellulitis as a complication of fracture of the zygomatic bone. J Cranio Maxillo Fac Surg 1987; 15:254.
38. Vaughan D, Asbury T. General Ophthalmology, ed 8. Los Altos: Lange Medical, 1977:159.
39. Chandler JR, et al. Pathogenesis of orbital complications in acute sinusitis. Laryngoscope 1970; 80:144.
40. Smith AT, Spence JT. Orbital complications resulting from lesions of the sinuses. Ann Otol Rhinol Laryngol 1948; 57:5.
41. Welsh LW, Welsh JJ. Orbital complications of sinus disease. Laryngoscope 1974; 84:88.
42. Bullock JD, Fleishman JA. The spread of odontogenic infections to the orbit: Diagnosis and management. J Oral Maxillofac Surg 1985; 43:749.
43. Watters EC, Waller PH, Hiles DA, et al. Acute orbital cellulitis. Arch Ophthalmol 1976; 6:426.
44. Duke-Elder S. The occular adnexa, part 2. In: System of Ophthalmology, vol 13. St Louis: CV Mosby, 1974:859.
45. Dingman RO. The management of acute infections of the face and jaws. Am J Orthod 1939; 25:780.
46. Jarret WH, et al. Occular complications of infection in paranasal sinuses. Arch Ophthalmol 1969; 81:683.
47. Shaw RE. Cavernous sinus thrombophlebitis. Br J Surg 1952; 40:40.
48. Mehrotra MC. Cavernous sinus thrombosis with generalized septicemia. Oral Surg 1965; 19:715.
49. Tatoian JA, LaDow SC, Disque F, et al. Meningitis and temporal lobe abscess of dental origin: Report of a case. J Oral Surg 1972; 30:423.
50. Hollin SA, Hayashi H, Gross SW. Intracranial abscesses of odontogenic origin. Oral Surg 1967; 23(3): 227.
51. Valachovic R, Hargreaves JA. Dental implications of brain abscess in children with congenital heart disease. Oral Surg 1979; 48(6): 459.
52. Hedstrom SA, Nord CE, Ursing B. Chronic meningitis in patients with dental infections. Scand J Infect Dis 1980; 12:117.
53. Gonty AA, Costich ER. Severe facial and cervical infections associated with gas-producing bacteria: Report of two cases. J Oral Surg 1981; 39:702.
54. Altemeier WA, Culbertson WR. Acute non-clostridial crepitant cellulitis. Surg Gynecol Obstet 1948; 87:206.
55. Drake SG, King AM, Slack WK. Gas gangrene and related infection: Classification, clinical features, and aetiology, management and mortality: A report of 88 cases. Br J Surg 1977; 64:104.
56. Nichols RL, Smith JW. Gas in the wound: What does it mean? Surg Clin North Am 1975; 55:1289.
57. Rea WJ, Wyrick WJ. Necrotizing fasciitis. Ann Surg 1970; a72:957.
58. Spankus EM, Flint PW, Smith RJ, et al. Craniocervical necrotizing fasciitis. Otolaryngol Head Neck Surg 1984; 92:261.
59. Sperry K, McFeely PJ. Medicolegal aspects of necrotizing fasciitis of the neck. J Forensic Sci 1987; 32:273.
60. Balcerak RJ, Sisto JM, Bosack RC. Cervicofacial ne-

crotizing fasciitis: Report of three cases and literature review. J Oral Maxillofac Surg 1988; 46:450.

61. Wilson B. Necrotizing fasciitis. Am Surg 1952; 19:416.
62. Klabacha ME, Stankiowicz JA, Cleft SE. Severe soft tissue infection of the face and neck: A classification. Laryngoscope 1982; 92:1135.
63. Gallia LJ, Johnson JT. Cervical necrotizing fasciitis. Otolaryngol Head Neck Surg 1981; 89:935.
64. Giuliano A, Lewis F, Hadley K, et al. Bacteriology of necrotizing fasciitis. Am J Surg 1977; 134:52.
65. Bahna M, Canalis RF. Necrotizing fasciitis (streptococcal gangrene) of the face. Arch Otolaryngol 1980; 106:648.
66. Wilson B. Necrotizing fasciitis. Am Surg 1952; 18:416.
67. Gibboney W, Lemons JA. Necrotizing fasciitis of the scalp in neonates. Am J Perinatol 1986; 3:58.
68. Wenig BL, Shikowitz MJ, Abramson AL. Necrotizing fasciitis as a lethal complication of peritonsillar abscess. Laryngoscope 1984; 94:1576.
69. Crosthwaite RW, Crosthwaite SR, Jorgan JL, et al. Necrotizing fasciitis. J Trauma 1964; 4:149.
70. Mitz V, Peyronie M. The superficial musculoaponeurotic system (SMAS) in the parotid and cheek area. Plast Reconstr Surg 1976; 58:80.
71. Andrews EC, Cruz AB. Necrotizing fasciitis. Diagnosis and treatment. Tex Med 1969; 65:50.
72. Ladingham IM, Tehrani MA. Diagnosis, clinical course and treatment of acute dermal gangrene. Br J Surg 1972; 62:364.
73. Fisher JR, Conway MJ, Takeshita RT, et al. Necrotizing fasciitis. Importance of roentgenographic studies for soft tissue gas. JAMA 1979; 241:803.
74. Rogers JM, Gibson JV, Farrar WE, et al. Usefulness of computerized tomography in evaluating fasciitis. South Med J 1984; 77:782.
75. Stamenkovic I, Lew PD. Early recognition of potentially fatal necrotizing fasciitis, the use of frozen section biopsy. N Engl J Med 1984; 310:1689.
76. Bongard FS, Elings VB, Markinson RE. New uses of fluorescence in the surgical management of necrotizing soft tissue infection. Am J Surg 1985; 150:281.
77. Svensson LG, Brookstone AJ, Willstead MB, et al. Necrotizing fasciitis in contused areas. J Trauma 1985; 25:260.
78. Javenicus RV, Hann SF, Batt MD. Necrotizing fasciitis. Surg Gynecol Obstet 1982; 154:97.
79. Crewson WN. Fatal necrotizing fasciitis developing after tooth extraction. Am Surg 1973; 39:525.
80. Wilson B, Crosswaite, Drake-Lee AB, Broughton SJ, Rampling A, et al. Necrotizing fasciitis. J Laryngol Otol 1983; 97:193.
81. Gallia LJ, Johnson JT. Cervical necrotizing fasciitis. Otolaryngol Head Neck Surg 1981; 89:935.
82. Gehna M, Canalis RF, Alexander DW, Leonard JR, Trail ML. Vascular complications of deep neck abscesses. Laryngoscope 1967; 77:364.
83. Majeski JA, Alexander JW. Early diagnosis, nutritional support and immediate extensive debridement improve survival in necrotizing fasciitis. Am J Surg 1983; 145:784.
84. Levine TM, Wurster CF, Krespi YP. Mediastinitis occurring as a complication of odontogenic infections. Laryngoscope 1986; 96:747.
85. Pearse HF. Mediastinitis following cervical suppuration. Ann Surg 1938; 108:588.
86. Steiner M, Grau MJ, Wilson DL, et al. J Oral Maxillofac Surg 1982; 40:600.
87. McCurdy JA, MacInnis FL, Hays LL. Fatal mediastinitis after a dental infection. J Oral Surg 1977; 35:726.
88. Hendler BH, Quinn PD. Fatal mediastinitis secondary to odontogenic infection. J Oral Surg 1978; 36:308.
89. Estrera AS, Landay MJ, Grisham JM, et al. Descending necrotizing mediastinitis. Surg Gynecol Obstet 1983; 157:545.
90. Pearse HE, Beck AL. Deep neck infection. Ann Otol Rhinol Laryngol 1939; 48:940.
91. Spilka CJ. Pathways of dental infections. J Oral Surg 1966; 24:111.
92. Mosher HP. The submandibular fossa approach to deep pus in the neck. Trans Am Acad Ophthalmol Otolaryngol 1929; 34:19.
93. Bryan CS, King BG, Bryant RE. Retropharyngeal infection in adults. Arch Intern Med 1974; 134:127.
94. Brook I. Microbiology of abscesses of the head and neck in children. Ann Otol Rhinol Laryngol 1987; 96:429.
95. Brook I, Finegold SM. Aerobic and anaerobic bacteriology of cutaneous abscesses in children. Pediatrics 1981; 67:891.
96. Travis RT, Steinle CJ. The effects of odontogenic infection on the complete blood count in children and adolescents. Pediatr Dent 1984; 6:214.
97. Yenson A, Defries HO, Deeb ZE. Actinomycotic osteomyelitis of the facial bones and mandible. Otolaryngol Head Neck Surg 1983; 91:173.
98. Mandell G, Douglas RG, Bennett JE. Principles and practice of infectious diseases. New York: John Wiley & Sons, 1979.
99. Steinhouse D, MacDonald DG. Low grade osteomyelitis of the jaws with actinomycosis. Int J Oral Surg 1974; 3:60.
100. Steinhouse D. Intraoral actinomycosis: Report of five cases. Oral Surg 1975; 39:547.
101. Hirsch SA. Cervicofacial actinomycosis following surgical trauma in rats. Oral Surg 1978; 46:827.
102. Hamner JE, Schaefer ME. Anterior maxillary actinomycosis: Report of a case. J Oral Surg 1965; 23:60.
103. Peabody JW, Seabury JH. Actinomycosis and nocardiosis. Am J Med 1960; 28:99.
104. Peabody JW, Seabury JH, Estridge CE, Prather R, Hughes FA Jr, et al. Actinomycosis: A 24-year-old experience. South Med J 1972; 65:839.
105. Adekeye, Cornah J. Osteomyelitis of the jaws: A review of 141 cases. Br J Oral Maxillofac Surg 1985; 23:24.

106. Ord RA, El-Attar A. Osteomyelitis of the mandible in children. Clinical presentations and review of management. Br J Oral Surg 1987; 25:204.
107. Shakenovsky BN, Ripamonti U, Lownie JF. Chronic osteomyelitis of the jaws. Int J Oral Maxillofac Surg 1986; 15:352.
108. Daramola JD, Ajabe HA. Chronic osteomyelitis of the mandible in adults: A clinical study of 34 cases. Br J Surg 1982; 20:58.
109. Sepheriadou T, Yannoulopoulos A. Tuberculosis of the jaws. J Oral Maxillofac Surg 1986; 44:158.
110. Daramola JO. Massive osteomyelitis of the mandible complicating sickle cell disease: Report of case. J Oral Surg 1981; 39:144.
111. Yusuf H, Ballacharaya MN. Syphilitic osteomyelitis of the mandible. Br J Oral Surg 1982; 20:122.
112. Albers-Schonberg H. Roentgenbilder einer selten knochenerkrankung. MMW 1904; 51:365.
113. Calhoun KH, Shapiro RD, Stiernberg CM, et al. Osteomyelitis of the mandible. Arch Otolaryngol Head Neck Surg 1988; 114:1157.
114. Wannfors K, Hammarstrom L. Infections foci in chronic osteomyelitis of the jaws. Int J Oral Surg 1985; 14:493.
115. Shafer WG. Chronic sclerosing osteomyelitis. Oral Surg 1957; 15:138.
116. Shafer WG, Hine MK, Levy BM. A Textbook of Oral Pathology, ed 3. Philadelphia: WB Saunders, 1974:455.
117. Turlington EG. Chronic sclerosing nonsuppurative osteomyelitis. In: Kay LW, ed. Oral Surgery. Copenhagen: Munksgaards Forlag, 1973:120.
118. Panders AK, Hadders HN. Chronic sclerosing inflammations of the jaw. Oral Surgery 1970; 30:396.
119. Jacobsson S, Hollender L. Treatment and prognosis of diffuse sclerosing osteomyelitis (DSO) of the mandible. Oral Surg 1980; 49:7.
120. Nortja CJ, Wood RE, Grotepass F. Periostitis ossificans versus Garre's osteomyelitis II. Radiographic analysis of 93 cases in the jaws. Oral Surg 1988; 66:249.
121. Gorlin RJ, Goldman HM. Thoma's oral pathology I. St Louis: CV Mosby, 1970:368.
122. Gunge M, Yamamoto H, Katch T, et al. Suppurative osteomyelitis of the mandible in a child. Int J Oral Maxillofac Surg 1987; 16:99.
123. Kamijoh Y. Oral Anatomy I. Osteology. Tokyo: Anatom, 1978:217.
124. Strauss MB. Chronic refractory osteomyelitis: Review and role of hyperbaric oxygen. Hyperbaric Oxygen Rev 1980; 1:231.
125. Van Merkesteyn JPR, Bakker DJ, Van Der Waal I, et al. Hyperbaric oxygen treatment of chronic osteomyelitis of the jaws. Int J Oral Surg 1984; 13:386.
126. Eversole LR et al. Proliferation periostitis of Garre: Its differentiation from other neoperostosis. J Oral Surg 1979; 37:725.
127. Lichty G, Langlais RP, Aufdemorte T. Garre's osteomyelitis. Oral Surg 1980; 50:309.

11

Antibiotics for Head and Neck Infections

Robert D. Marciani

SELECTION OF ANTIMICROBIAL DRUGS

Selecting the appropriate antibiotic regimen for a patient with an odontogenic infection or other head and neck infection of nonodontogenic etiology does not usually require the expertise of a clinician with special training in infectious disease. Adequately trained surgeons can select and implement acceptable antibiotic protocols when the cause of the infection is identifiable and the response of the organisms to antimicrobial drugs is understood. Consultation with infectious disease experts should be considered when patients have severe intercurrent disease that may alter their response to therapy, when there is eminent danger of major morbidity or mortality, when the responsible surgeon is unfamiliar with the organisms isolated, or in other circumstances that would indicate that multidisciplinary care is necessary.

In the initial therapy of life-threatening infections in which a bacterial cause is suspected, the emphasis should be on extended-spectrum antibiotic coverage. Initial therapy is based on clinical assessment and diagnosis. Definitive antibiotic coverage should be initiated after organisms are isolated, identified and, when indicated, in vitro susceptibility tests are obtained.

In severe infections, antimicrobial agents should be given parenterally initially to ensure the maximum effect of the drug. Optimal dosage must be established for those antimicrobial agents that have frequent side effects. Combinations of antibiotics are indicated in infections caused by *Pseudomonas aeruginosa*, Enterococcal group-D streptococci, resistant pathogens, and life-threatening infections.

Laboratory examination of pus and inflammatory debris is very important but not always necessary. Localized dentoalveolar abscesses in patients who do not show any signs of systemic involvement do not require culture and sensitivity testing. Odontogenic infections confined to the periradicular area of the alveolus may, under certain circumstances, not require any antibiotics when definitive surgical therapy can be delivered. Laboratory aid for the selection of antimicrobial therapy is always indicated in severe head and neck infections when the causative organisms are unclear or the patient's condition fails to improve. By contrast, certain organisms have stable, predictable susceptibilities that can be relied on to respond uniformly to the appropriate antibiotic therapy. The organisms frequently responsible for odontogenic infections, for example, have been consistently sensitive to penicillin, a fact that allows the clinician to empirically select this drug for initial therapy with a high likelihood of success.

Antimicrobial selection is influenced by the basic characteristics of antibiotics susceptibility tests, logistical considerations, and patient factors:

Activity of the antibiotic against the pathogenic organism
The least toxic alternative
The site of infection

Renal and hepatic function
Allergy and pregnancy
Cost

Susceptibility testing is essential when organisms vary in susceptibility. An active drug may be ineffective because of route of administration, inadequate dosage, infected foreign body, abscesses, inadequate drainage, or inability of the drug to reach the site of infection. Intravenous antimicrobial therapy may be necessary because of the seriousness of the infection, the site of the infection, or diminished host resistance.

Initial Therapy versus Definitive Therapy

The initial treatment of suspected or proved bacterial infections is influenced by the patient's condition, the progress of the infection, and initial Gram-stain results. Ideally, clinical samples of pus should be obtained from the infected site. Gram-stain results can be available within minutes of obtaining the sample and, when considered in conjunction with the patient's clinical condition, can contribute to the choice of antimicrobial therapy. Antibiotic therapy based on definitive bacteriologic information is unavailable for a period of 24 hours after the culture material has been submitted. Preliminary anaerobic culture results are not generally reported until 48 hours following the onset of incubation.

During the period of 48 hours or longer when only incomplete bacteriologic information is available, treatment is based entirely on clinical information obtained by history, physical examination, white blood cell (WBC) differential counts, radiographic findings, and the skills and experience of the surgeon.

Unlike infections in other anatomical regions, odontogenic infections usually are clinically apparent, the causative organisms are generally predictable, bacteremia is seldom a complication, and surgical intervention has a significant curative effect on the course of the infection. When the site of the primary infection and the circumstances under which it developed are known, a reasonable prediction of the pathogens present can be made.[1]

The choice of antibiotics should be based on the probable source of infection, on Gram-stained smears of appropriate clinical specimens, and on the immune status of the patient. Current patterns of bacterial resistance in the hospital and the community should also be considered.

Choices in Drug Administration

Route of Administration

Most of odontogenic infections can be managed with oral antibiotics. In severe infections or in milder infections occurring in immunologically compromised patients, antimicrobial agents should be given parenterally. Intravenous administration can give more rapid and higher blood levels and ultimately higher tissue levels. Intramuscular administration is painful and inconvenient if repeated injections are necessary, but it may be useful when more predictable blood levels are desirable without relying on direct intravenous medication. The absorption of orally administered antimicrobial agents is too variable from patient to patient to be reliable in severe infections. Patient compliance with oral medications must always be considered when deciding on the route of administration.

The merits of intravenous administration of antibiotics must be balanced against the need for hospitalization and the obvious increased costs to the patient for this therapy. Home health care providers may administer intravenous antibiotics to outpatients. The increased costs and risks of toxic and untoward sequela when the intravenous route is used must be justified by the dangers of the infection. In general, each intravenous dose should be administered over a relatively short period of time to achieve peak blood levels when conditions such as endocarditis, osteomyelitis, actinomycosis infections, and severe infections caused by gram-negative bacilli are being treated.

Dosage of Antimicrobial Agents

Antimicrobial agents with a wide margin between therapeutic and toxic blood levels (therapeutic index) such as the penicillins, can be administered in dosages that are relatively imprecise compared to more toxic drugs like the aminoglycosides. In essence, the same dosage amount of penicillin can be dispensed to most adults who have good liver and kidney function. For antimicrobial agents in which the margin between therapeutic and toxic levels is narrow (low therapeutic index), the dosage must be precisely calculated based on the patient's lean body weight.

Care must be taken not to underdose the patient when aminoglycosides are used. Therapeutic blood levels must be achieved if the antibiotic is to be effective and if the hazard of creating resistant strains by underdosing is to be avoided. In severe infections maximal doses should be administered to patients with normal kidney function. The correct dose should be calculated in milligrams per kilogram, based on the specific recommendations for the individual aminoglycoside and divided into three equal doses given every 8 hours. Peak and trough blood levels should be obtained 30 minutes before and after the drug is administered. Serum and urine creatinine levels should be continually determined.

Combinations of Antimicrobial Agents

Most odontogenic infections can be treated using a single penicillin in one of its preparations. Infections, in general, can be treated with a single antibiotic agent when the pathogens are known and the pattern of antimicrobial susceptibility established.

Overall, combination therapy is desirable when synergism occurs and the microorganism is more readily destroyed or neutralized.[1] Certain organisms (*Pseudomonas* and enterococcal group-D streptococci) are well known for their resistance to single drug therapy and are, therefore, routinely treated with combination agents.

Combination initial therapy is also indicated in the presence of severe infection of uncertain etiology or when an antibiotic with a specific but otherwise limited effectiveness is used to treat a polymicrobial infection. Metronidazole is a useful antianaerobic drug with little activity against aerobic gram-positive cocci or rods. It is an effective antibiotic when combined with other agents to treat odontogenic infections. It should not be used, however, as the sole agent when oral organisms are the suspected or known pathogens.

Multiple antimicrobial agents increase the risk of superinfections, encourage adverse side effects, and may substantially elevate the cost of therapy.[1] When multiple agents are used, it is wise to avoid the simultaneous use of agents that have similar toxic side effects.

Recurrence or Persistence of Fever During Therapy

Several possibilities should be considered when a patient shows an initial favorable response to therapy but fever returns: the presence of an abscess that requires drainage; drug fever related to one of the antimicrobial agents (most commonly seen with the penicillins and cephalosporins but not limited to them); a clinical laboratory error leading to inadequate therapy; superinfection; the wrong antibiotic is being administered or the dose is inadequate; and patient noncompliance.

Patients with drug fever often look relatively well, their fever is low grade and continuous, and is the only "sign" of infection. Pulse rate during the febrile periods is usually normal. Laboratory studies may show a normal WBC count with the exception of an eosinophilia. A drug rash may also suggest the possibility of a drug fever. A drug fever will resolve when the antibiotic is discontinued.

Laboratory Tests Used to Guide Antimicrobial Therapy

Laboratory tests are helpful in guiding antimicrobial therapy. There are many factors that contribute to the clinical response of an infected patient. Among these, the susceptibility of the infecting organism to antimicrobial agents and the adequacy of antimicrobial dosage and diffusion into the infected site can be measured. The clinician, however, should not rely on in vitro tests as the only means of determining the patient's response to treatment.

Many bacteria have predictable antimicrobial susceptibility patterns. It may not be necessary to routinely test these organisms. Organisms, such as pneumococci, group A β-hemolytic streptococci, and most gonococci (penicillin-resistant strains of *Neisseria gonorrheae* have been isolated) are routinely susceptible to penicillin G.

In Vitro Susceptibility Test

Tests of microbial susceptibility in vitro are indicated when the susceptibility of an organism is not completely predictable or to determine whether resistance has developed during the course of therapy.[2] An organism is generally considered susceptible if the concentration of antimicrobial agent necessary to inhibit its growth in vitro is lower than that usually attainable in blood. The results of laboratory tests must be interpreted cautiously. They can vary depending on the preparation of antimicrobials, inoculum size of the organism, duration, and temperature of incubation, definition of inhibitory end points, and the cation content and pH of the specific medium.

Anaerobes are not routinely tested for susceptibility. Testing procedures are more complex than for aerobic and facultative organisms, and anaerobic susceptibility must be specially requested from the laboratory.

Determination of Bacterial β-Lactamase Activity

A number of bacterial isolates are resistant to penicillin, ampicillin and, to a lesser degree, the cephalosporins because they produce a β-lactamase that inactivates the antimicrobial agent.[3] Rapid methods for detection of β-lactamase allows testing as soon as colonies are isolated, often 12 to 24 hours before susceptibility tests are available.

Serum Bactericidal Activity

Serum bactericidal activity of an antibacterial is established by incubating the serum of treated patients with the infecting organism to determine the highest dilution of the serum that is bactericidal. Serum levels can be obtained at peak and trough levels. This method has been used for many years (Schlichter test) to establish bactericidal titers.[4]

Assay of Antimicrobial Activity in Serum

Serum concentrations of antimicrobial agents must be tested when the toxicity level of the agent is close to the therapeutic range. Accurate measurement of serum concentrations is necessary when an aminoglycoside, for example, is the agent of choice, or in patients with renal failure who are receiving drugs excreted by the kidney. Pretreatment conditions, such as hearing loss, renal damage, blood dyscrasias, and liver disease, can modify the dosage administered or exclude an antibiotic from the therapeutic regimen.

Serum concentrations can be correlated with minimum inhibitory concentration (MIC) values to verify the adequacy of treatment; organisms that are marginally susceptible require a more precise estimation of antimicrobial serum activity and should be tested accordingly.

Antimicrobial Agents

The choice of an antimicrobial agent to treat odontogenic infection or other infections of the head and neck must be made rationally using the basic characteristics and properties of individual agents as a guide for selection.

Classification and Mechanism of Action

The chemical structure of an antibiotic is the most common basis for its classification. It is a distinguishing characteristic that facilitates recognition of drugs with like structures and very similar activities that may have different pharmacodynamics.[5]

The antibiotics presently available may also be classified into several groups on the basis of their mechanism of action[6] (Table 11–1): agents acting on the cell walls, agents interfering with protein synthesis, agents affecting the cell membrane by exerting a detergent effect, agents affecting nucleic acid metabolism, and drugs affecting intermediary metabolism.

A classification of antibiotics based on their clinical effectiveness is related to the spectrum or microorganisms that they inhibit (i.e., narrow, extended, or broad spectrum agents). Penicillin G is considered a

Table 11–1. *Antibiotics and Their Mechanism of Action*

Mechanism of Action	Antibiotic Examples
Cell wall action	Penicillin, cephalosporins, vancomycin
Protein synthesis interference	Erythromycin, chloramphenicol, tetracycline
Detergent effect	Polymyxin, nystatin, amphotericin
Nucleic acid metabolism interference	Ciprofloxacin, metronidazole
Intermediary metabolism	Trimethoprim, sulfonamides

narrow-spectrum antibiotic because it is primarily effective against gram-positive cocci and rods. The tetracyclines and chloramphenicol are examples of extended-spectrum agents because they suppress multiplication of both gram-positive and gram-negative bacteria.

For an antibiotic to be of value as part of infection management, it must exert its effects on the invading organism without seriously damaging the cells of the host.[7] The patient's immune defenses must be functioning to ultimately overcome the infection. The principal result of antibiotic activity is retardation of the rate of bacterial growth. When present in sufficiently high concentrations, some drugs kill bacteria in vivo and in vitro. The effectiveness of an agent, even the most potent, does not cure infections simply by virtue of its activity against the responsible organism. The bactericidal compounds may, in certain infections, be more effective agents compared with bacteriostatic drugs, but they also require the effective intervention of various humoral and cellular defense mechanisms of the host.

Resistance of Organisms to Antibiotics

Each antibiotic agent has a spectrum of activity that determines its effectiveness. There are many determining factors, the principal one being whether the antibacterial effect suppresses an essential life process in the microorganism. β-lactamase and other substances can be produced by the organism that will inactivate the antibacterial agent. Bacteria, particularly staphylococci, produce β-lactamase enzymes that inactivate the penicillins by cleavage of the 6-aminopenicillanic acid nucleus to yield penicillic acid derivatives.

Bacterial resistance occurs as the result of genetic alterations of the bacterial cell. These alterations are transferred from generation to generation. Bacterial resistance may be natural or acquired. Natural resistance implies that a fundamental, inherent resistance occurs as a consequence of antibiotic therapy.

Chromosomal resistance normally occurs in a stepwise fashion. Succeeding exposures to the antibiotic initiate further genetic changes, which result in a greater degree of resistance to the antimicrobial agent. The antibiotic acts to select each increasingly resistant mutant, allowing it to multiply and exhibit more mutational changes in its progeny. Low doses of antibiotics can contribute to this selection process. Higher concentrations may inhibit the still susceptible first- and second-step mutants before they can grow and produce progeny containing additional mutations.[7]

Acquired drug resistance may develop in bacteria growing in the presence of antibiotics in vivo and in vitro. Antibiotics differ in their propensity to develop acquired resistance. Penicillin resistance develops in a slow stepwise manner, whereas resistance to erythromycin occurs rapidly with only a few steps or spontaneous mutations required before resistance develops. Streptomycin very commonly induces bacterial resistance in a single step.

Hospital-acquired methicillin-resistant *Staphylococcus aureus* has become a serious clinical problem. As the growth of drug resistance organisms multiplies they eventually outnumber the sensitive microbes; at this stage the antibiotic as a single agent is no longer useful for infected patients. Organisms that become insensitive to one antibiotic may simultaneously become resistant to another to which it is chemically related. Concurrent drug therapy may prevent the emergence of resistance organisms or diminish the speed in which they develop.

Inherent to the selection of the appropriate antibiotic regimen is a fundamental understanding of the basic properties of the pathogens commonly involved in head and neck infections. In many instances bacteriologic testing will not be essential to the outcome of treatment. Delaying the administration of an antibiotic until culture and sensitivity reports are available is inappropriate, although obtaining a pus specimen before treatment may be advisable. In odontogenic infections, the well-informed clinician can make a reasonable early choice of antibiotics based on knowing the etiology of the disease, the pathogens commonly implicated as the infecting organisms, the patient's clinical condition, and the established effectiveness of the available antimicrobials for dental infections. There are, however, infections in which careful bacteriologic studies are essential to proper treatment.

Determining the etiology of an infection is helpful in the selection of the most effective drug. There may, however, be a wide variation in the susceptibility to antimicrobial agents of different strains of certain species of organisms.[7] Knowledge of the sensitivity pattern of a pathogen will aid in the choice of a drug. Although the ability to inhibit growth of the causative organism is an important factor in selecting an antibiotic, other factors must also be considered, such as the nature of the illness, a history of hypersensitivity, and the cost of the drug. A patient who cannot swallow pills or is vomiting would be a poor choice for an orally administered agent. A patient with a history of a hypersensitivity reaction or organ damage that would be placed at further risk of untoward sequela by receiving the antibiotic, must not be reexposed to the same agent. In rare circumstances, a specific infection may require using an antibiotic under these conditions. If such is the case, every effort must be made to establish the risk-benefit ratio to the patient and to scrupulously monitor the patient for the earliest signs of allergic or toxic reactions.

The cost of different antibiotics with a similar spectrum of antimicrobial and mechanism of action can vary greatly. Penicillin continues to be an attractive drug for odontogenic infections because it is effective, has a low incidence of toxicity, and in its penicillin G and V preparations, is relatively inexpensive. The cephalosporins, by contrast, generally are not indicated as the drug of initial choice for dental infections and are substantially more expensive. The same or better clinical results are achievable with penicillin at a dramatically lower cost.

Concentrations and Distributions

Blood is the transport medium for drugs and is the most accessible tissue to measure the concentration of an antibiotic in vivo. The value of this measurement must be viewed from the perspective that the infectious process is not actually intravascular; accurate data identifying the concentrations of antibiotics at the actual site of infection is not obtainable by simple clinical and laboratory means.

The concentration and distribution of antibiotics is influenced by absorption from the site of administration; elimination usually in the urine or in other secretions; catabolism primarily by the liver, but also by the kidneys and other organs with some drugs; and passage into tissues and body fluids, with or without fixation by specific tissues and microorganisms. Hoeprich[5] recommends antibiotic concentrations in the blood four or five times greater than the MIC of the infecting organism. In the final analysis, empiric interpolation, clinical experience, the severity of the illness, and the location of the infection will determine the antibiotic regimen.

The location of the infection may present special problems to the delivery of antiinfective agents. The blood-brain barrier must be penetrated by the antibiotic if infections of the central nervous system are to be successfully managed. The penetration of drugs into tissues, secretions, and compartments of the body is affected by factors other than the concentrations attained in blood. Passage from the blood is favored by small molecular size, lack of electrical charge at pH 7.4, solubility in lipids, and little or loose binding by plasma proteins.[5]

Antimicrobial Prophylaxis in Surgery

Antimicrobial prophylaxis regimens recommended by the American Heart Association to prevent bacterial endocarditis should be followed when patients with heart valves, rheumatic heart diseases or other cardiac abnormalities undergo oral surgical procedures. The indications for antimicrobial prophylaxis for patients with prosthetic joints, vascular grafts, transplants, and other allografts in oral surgery patients is not clearly defined. Prophylaxis is generally recommended.

Antimicrobial prophylaxis for "clean surgery" is usually not indicated unless it involves implantation of prosthetic material such as an artificial joint.[8] If indicated, a single dose of a parenteral antimicrobial given within 30 minutes of an operation usually provides adequate tissue concentrations throughout the procedure.[9] When surgery is delayed or prolonged, a second, intraoperative dose is advisable, unless the prophylactic agent has an extended serum half-life. Postoperative doses of prophylactic drugs are generally unnecessary and potentially harmful.

Use of prophylactic antimicrobial drugs for routine oral surgical procedures in a noninfected patient is not necessary and contraindicated. Although considered clean-contaminated from the standpoint that the mouth is teeming with organisms, the microbiota of the oral cavity should not be considered a threat to the healthy patient in the same manner as "dirty-surgery" at other sites. A perforated abdominal viscus, a compound fracture, or a laceration due to an animal or human bite is often followed by infection; this is not the case with exodontia or routine soft tissue or preprosthetic procedures.

Prophylaxis with cefazolin or other antimicrobial drugs decreases the incidence of wound infections after head and neck operations that involve an incision through the oral and pharyngeal mucosa. Infection rates in uncontaminated head and neck surgery are too low to justify prophylaxis.[10] Cefazolin has the advantage of a longer serum half-life and causes less pain with intramuscular injection. Single-dose prophylaxis with second-generation cephalosporins that have extended serum half-lives (cefotetan, ceforanide, cefonicid) has no advantage over single-dose cefazolin or cefoxitin prophylaxis unless the surgery is protracted, in which case the injection of cefazolin or cefoxitin can be repeated. Third-generation cephalosporins should not be used for surgical prophylaxis.[8]

ANTIMICROBIAL AGENTS USEFUL FOR OROFACIAL INFECTIONS

The Penicillins

The penicillin derivatives have consistently remained the drug choice for most orofacial infections. As a group, the penicillins are the most frequently and widely used of the antimicrobial agents because they are effective, rarely toxic, and relatively inexpensive. They are bactericidal, are well distributed throughout the body spaces and, in certain derivatives, have an extended spectrum of activity. Allergenicity is the most common and serious problem associated with the use of penicillins. Toxicity does occur with individual penicillin drugs, although it is rare compared with that with aminoglycosides. The older penicillins, such as penicillin G and V, have the decided advantage of extremely low cost compared to the newer penicillins and the cephalosporins.[11]

The mode of action and the main pharmacologic properties of penicillin interfere with the production of an effective cell wall, resulting in the rupture of the cell by osmotic lysis. The β-lactam antibiotics will all have a similar mechanism of action.

Chemically, all of the penicillin derivatives are similar in that they contain the same basic nucleus, 6-aminopenicillanic acid. The pharmacologic properties of the basic nucleus can be altered by adding various sidechains to the nucleus which will result in a change in the chemical properties of the compound. Important new penicillin compounds with properties such as acid stability, resistance to the penicillinases, or increased antibacterial spectrum of activity have been developed.[12] Many of the penicillin compounds are destroyed by gastric acid and cannot be used as oral agents. Those penicillins not destroyed in the stomach are absorbed in the duodenum and give peak levels in the serum within 1 hour. Absorption from injection is also rapid unless the compound is combined with a salt that slows its absorption, such as procaine.[13]

Penicillin G and V

The narrow spectrum penicillins are generally effective against gram-positive cocci and rods, spirochetes, and most of the anaerobes associated with orodental infections. Penicillin G is effective against most strains of *Neisseria*, but relatively large parenteral doses are required for treatment of infections caused by this gram-negative cocci.[12]

The half-life is normally 30 minutes in a patient with healthy kidneys, but can be increased to 10 hours in the anuric patient. If hepatic disease is coincident with renal insufficiency, the rate of clearance of penicillin from the blood decreases almost to zero. The inability of the body to clear the penicillin under these conditions indicates that the liver is the major site of extrarenal handling of the drug. Much of the administered dose of penicillin is bound to plasma proteins.

Aqueous crystallin penicillin G (potassium or sodium penicillin G) is used when a rapid effect or a high serum concentration of the drug is required or when the drug is given intravenously.[14] Because of its acid liability, penicillin G is usually administered parenterally. When given orally, the blood levels will be lower than those obtained with penicillin V. When injected intramuscularly, maximal plasma concentrations are reached within 30 to 60 minutes; the drug disappears from the plasma in 3 to 6 hours, depending on the size of dose given.[11]

Aqueous penicillin G should be administered intramuscularly or by intravenous injections in divided 3-hour doses. In severe odontogenic or other head and neck infections, the intravenous route is preferred (2 to 3 million units every 3 hours). The responsible clinician must monitor the patient's fluid and electrolyte balance whenever large doses of aqueous penicillin are administered. Sodium penicillin G contains approximately 100 mg of sodium in each 1 million units. Potassium penicillin G contains 1.7 mEq, or 65 mg of potassium in each 1 million units. Hyperkalemia may result from the injudicious administration of additional potassium under these circumstances and precipitate cardiac complications.

Penicillin V is acid stable and is the preferred derivative for oral administration when this route is suitable for the infection present. It is the agent of first choice for orally administered treatment of the usual odontogenic infections.[12] Absorption of potassium penicillin V from the gastrointestinal tract may produce peak serum concentrations within 30 minutes; detectable levels of the drug are maintained for 4 hours. Oral forms of penicillin should not, however, be the preparation of choice when parenteral penicillin G is needed. Penicillin V should be given in doses of 125 to 500 mg four times daily.

Procaine Penicillin G

Procaine penicillin G is indicated when a longer acting preparation is desired and high blood levels are not required. It can be given intramuscularly one to three times daily in amounts of 300,000 to 1.2 million units. Precautions must be taken to observe for allergic reactions following injections with this preparation, because it is more likely to produce an adverse immune response than is aqueous crystalline penicillin G. Procaine penicillin G is absorbed comparatively slowly after intramuscular injection, a characteristic that should be considered advantageous when treatment is combined with the faster acting aqueous preparations. Maximal plasma concentrations occur within 1 to 2 hours and detectable concentrations in the blood may be present for 24 hours.[11]

Penicillinase-Resistant Penicillins

After oral administration, 30% to 40% of penicillin G and 60% of penicillin V is absorbed from the small intestine. Once absorbed from the gastrointestinal tract or intramuscular site, penicillin enters all body fluids except the cerebral spinal fluid. Inflammation of the meninges or administration of massive doses of intravenous penicillin facilitates passage of the antibiotic in the central nervous system. Both penicillin G and V are well distributed into most soft tissue sites; the amount of penicillin found in bone is a fraction of the plasma concentration. Osteomyelitis of the jaws requires combined surgical debridement and high-dose antibiotic therapy to allow the agent to achieve sufficiently elevated bone levels.[15]

After parenteral administration of penicillin G, 90% to 100% of the dose is excreted in the urine within several hours. Urinary excretion mechanisms consist of active renal tubular secretion (90%) and glomerular filtration (10%). Metabolism and excretion by the liver is the major route of elimination when rapid tubular excretion is reduced by renal disease or drugs such as probenecid. The major excretory route following oral administration is from the intestine, with 20% of the dose appearing in the urine.

Bacterial resistance to penicillin G and V develops in a slow stepwise fashion and usually is caused by the selection of mutants that elaborate β-lactamases (penicillinases). Although most of the organisms commonly involved in odontogenic infections remain susceptible to penicillin, some anaerobes are resistant and exhibit increased resistance. Resistance to the penicillins results from the production of penicillinase. This enzyme is properly called a β-lactamase because it cleaves the four-membered β-lactam ring of the molecule, thereby inactivating the drug.

In certain mixed infections, penicillinase produced by staphylococci or gram-negative organisms constituting a minor component of the infection may protect a major pathogen, which is sensitive to penicillin. Thus, a normally effective dosage regimen may be rendered inadequate in the area of the infection because of penicillinase secreted into the immediate environment.

The emergence of penicillinase-producing strains of *S. aureus* prompted the development of the parenteral and oral semisynthetic penicillinase-resistant penicillins. The mechanism of resistance to the action of penicillinase by these compounds is thought to be steric hindrance conveyed to the drug by the acyl side chain, which prevents opening of the β-lactam ring. The activity of the penicillinase-resistant penicillins against streptococci is less than that of penicillin G. A majority (60% to 80%) of the *S. aureus* strains found in hospitalized patients are resistant to penicillin G and other nonpenicillinase-resistant derivatives.[12]

Methicillin was the first of the semisynthetic penicillinase-resistant penicillins.[17] It is rarely used currently because of the high incidence of interstitial nephritis. For oral use against penicillinase-producing strains of staphylococci, cloxacillin and dicloxacillin are preferred. Cloxacillin or dicloxacillin are the agents of choice for oral administration because they are absorbed well from the gastrointestinal tract. For severe infections, a parenteral formulation of nafcillin or oxacillin should be considered.[18] Occasional strains of coagulase-positive staphylococci and many strains of coagulase-negative staphylococci are resistant to penicillinase-resistant penicillins, and are usually known as methicillin-resistant staphylococci. These strains are also resistant to cephalosporins and to imipenem. Vancomycin, with or without rifampin or gentamicin may be used for these resistant strains.[18] The role of the penicillinase-resistant derivatives is insignificant for the majority of dental infections. When *S. aureus* is suspected as the etiologic agent, initial therapy with a suitable penicillinase-resistant derivative should be instituted until the results of bacteriologic culturing are obtained.[12]

Extended-Spectrum Penicillin Derivatives

The extended-spectrum penicillins provide increased activity against some gram-negative bacilli. They do not resist the action of penicillinase unless combined with clavulanic acid or sulbactam. Generally, the antibacterial spectrum of the ampicillin-like antibiotics includes gram-positive aerobes, but they are less active than is penicillin G against such organisms.[12] Based on their therapeutic use, three groups of extended-spectrum penicillins are currently available:

1. Ampicillin-like derivatives: ampicillin, amoxicillin, cyclacillin, hetacillin, and bacampicillin
2. Carbenicillin-like derivatives: carbenicillin, ticarcillin, piperacillin, mezlocillin
3. Azlocillin

The combination of extended-spectrum penicillins with clavulanic acid (Augmentin [Beecham], Timentin [Beechum]), and sulbactam (Unasyn [Roerig]) are β-lactamase sensitive antibiotics and β-lactamase inhibitor combinations now available in the United States.

When ampicillin was originally introduced for clinical use, it was effective against a number of gram-negative aerobes including *Haemophilus influenzae*, enterococci, *E. coli*, *Proteus mirabilis*, salmonella, and shigella. A number of strains of these organisms have now become resistant and the ampicillin-like agents are no longer effective. The usefulness of ampicillin has been limited by increasing bacterial resistance produced by bacterial β-lactamases that enzymatically inactivate the drug.[19] All of the extended-spectrum penicillins are inactivated by penicillinase.

The ampicillin-like antibiotics are well absorbed following oral administration. Amoxicillin, bacampicillin, and cyclacillin demonstrate increased absorption over ampicillin even in the presence of food.[20] Metabolism of these antibiotics is similar to that described for penicillin G and V.

Ampicillin and ampicillin-like antibiotics are useful agents when treating mixed infections or certain gram-negative infections. Ampicillin alone is active against a broad range of pathogenic bacteria including group A and group B streptococci, pneumococci, enterococci, many strains of *E. coli* and *P. mirabilis*, gonococci, and *H. influenzae*, and many beta-lactamase–negative anaerobes.[19] They are less effective against the gram-positive organisms than is penicillin G and should not be used as a substitute for penicillin G and V. Amoxicillin is well absorbed from the gastrointestinal system so that t.i.d. dosing is feasible. It is the preferred agent for oral administration.[12]

The carbenicillin-like agents and azlocillin have an antibacterial range similar to that of ampicillin but are especially useful for their important added activity against gram-negative bacilli such as *Pseudomonas* and indole-positive *Proteus* species.[21] Since they are only given parenterally their use is properly limited to hospitalized patients with serious gram-negative infections.

Combinations of Extended-Spectrum Penicillins and β-Lactamase Inhibitor

Amoxicillin and ticarcillin in fixed ratio combinations with the β-lactamase inhibitor clavulanic acid have been marketed under the trade names Augmentin (Beecham) and Timentin (Beecham), respectively. Clavulanic acid is a β-lactam derivative which exhibits slight intrinsic antibacterial activity. However, its major use is in its ability to competitively and irreversibly bind bacterial β-lactamase enzymes and therefore extend the spectrum of the previously susceptible β-lactam antibiotics to include β-lactamase–producing strains. Clavulanic acid does not extend the spectrum of activity to bacteria that do not produce β-lactamase and are intrinsically resistant.

Augmentin is a fixed ratio combination of amoxicillin trihydrate and potassium clavulanate. It is recommended for the oral treatment of otitis media, sinusitis, human and animal bite infections caused by susceptible organisms, and other gram-negative and mixed infections. Important pathogenic bacteria that are not vulnerable to amoxicillin alone such as *H. influenzae*, *Brahamella catarrhalis*, and *S. aureus* are susceptible to the combination. The usual adult dose is one Augmentin tablet every 8 hours. Clavulanic acid does not affect the pharmacokinetics of amoxicillin. Tablets of Augmentin contain 250 mg or 500 mg of amoxicillin and 125 mg of clavulanic acid. Two 250-mg tablets (2:1 amoxicillin to clavulanic acid ratio) are not equivalent to one 500-mg tablet (4:1 ratio). Higher doses of clavulanic acid may lead to a greater incidence of diarrhea. Both amoxicillin and clavulanic acid are acid stable, rapidly absorbed, and widely distributed following oral administration.

Timentin is a fixed ratio combination of ticarcillin disodium, a β-lactam antibiotic, and clavulanic acid. It is used parenterally to treat penicillinase-producing strains of bacteria which are otherwise susceptible to ticarcillin alone, particularly *P. aeruginosa*.

Ampicillin sodium with sulbactam (Unasyn [Roerig]) is the third β-lactam antibiotic and β-lactamase inhibitor combination to become available in the United States. Sulbactam, a penicillanic acid sulfone, is a semisynthetic β-lactamase inhibitor with limited antibacterial activity of its own. The addition of sulbactam to ampicillin extends the in vitro activity of ampicillin to include β-lactamase–producing strains of *H. influenzae*, *Neisseria*, *S. aureus*, and other pathogenic bacteria. Many anaerobes, including *Bacteroides fragilis* are susceptible to this drug combination.[22–24] The indications for Unisyn are the same as for Augmentin.

Adverse Reactions to Penicillins

Allergic reactions are the chief side effects encountered with the use of penicillins.[25] Cross-allergenicity among the semisynthetic and natural penicillins is high; the common 6-aminopenicillanic acid nucleus apparently providing the target area for the adverse immune response. The incidence of allergic reactions to penicillin varies between the oral and parenteral derivatives of the drug. The intensity of the reaction is less with the oral form of the drug than with aqueous penicillin G given by injection. Procaine penicillin administered intramuscularly and penicillin applied locally have a distinctly higher incidence of allergic reaction due to the procaine salt, not to the penicillin. Allergy to the penicillins occurs in 3% to 5% of the population and in approximately 10% of people who have previously received the drug. An immune response is more likely to occur with larger doses and prolonged administration of the agent. Life-threatening anaphylactoid reactions occur in 0.02% of the patients given a penicillin derivative, and 10% of these are fatal.[26]

Penicillins have a large therapeutic index, which is a decided advantage of the drug. Side effects include nausea, vomiting, and diarrhea. These reactions are dose related and usually are caused by the irritative properties of the penicillins. Superinfections may result when the normal oral, genitourinary, or gastrointestinal microflora are altered (e.g., thrush, vulvovaginitis secondary to Candida). Ampicillin has been identified as one of the antimicrobial drugs causing *Clostridium difficile*, a toxin-associated diarrhea of colitis (pseudomembranous ulcerative colitis).[27] Massive doses of penicillin administered to patients with impaired renal function may result in visual and auditory hallucinations, generalized convulsions, and coma. Occasionally residual brain damage can occur. In rare cases the penicillins may cause blood dyscrasias. Granulocytopenia and anemia have occurred after the administration of methicillin and oxacillin.[10]

Interstitial nephritis is a serious, but rare complication of penicillin therapy. This reaction has been reported more frequently with methicillin and large doses of penicillin G. Fever, eosinophilia, hematuria, proteinuria, and pyuria are findings associated with interstitial renal changes.[28] Patients receiving large doses of penicillin or other prolonged antimicrobial therapy should be monitored frequently for red blood cells in the urine and incipient eosinophilia, early findings suggestive of renal changes. Table 11–2 contains an overview of the adverse reactions reported with the penicillins.

The Cephalosporins

First and Second Generation

Cephalosporins have been grouped into generations on the basis of their spectrum of activity against gram-negative rods. All first-generation drugs have a similar spectrum and include many gram-positive cocci (but not enterococci or methicillin-resistant staphylococcus), *E. coli*, *Klebsiella pneumoniae*, *P. mirabilis*, and oral anaerobes. First-generation cephalosporins,

Table 11–2. *Adverse Ractions to Penicillins*

Penicillins	*Reaction*
ALL PENICILLINS	Allergic reactions which can be anaphylactic Skin rashes, drug fever, diarrhea, neuromuscular irritability Nephropathy
INDIVIDUAL DRUGS	
Ampicillin, amoxicillin	Skin rash, diarrhea, pseudomembranous colitis
Carbenicillin	Hypokalemic alkalosis, sodium overload, platelet dysfunction
Methicillin	Interstitial nephritis, anemia, neutropenia, granulocytopenia
Nafcillin	Thrombophlebitis, elevated SGOT
Oxacillin	Elevated SGOT, granulocytopenia
Augmentin	Diarrhea
Timentin	Pain at the injection site
Unasyn	Pain at the injection site

such as the parenteral drugs cephalothin (Keflin, Seffin) and cefazolin (Ancef, Kefzol) and the oral agent cephalexin (Keflex), are the most active of all cephalosporins against staphylococci and nonenterococcal streptococci.[29]

Second-generation cephalosporins include the parenteral agents cefamandole (Mandol), cefuroxime (Zinacef, Kefurox), Cefonicid (Monocid), cefoxitin (Mefoxin), and cefotetan (Cefotan), and the oral agents cefaclor (Ceclor) and cefuroxime axetil (Ceftin). In vitro, these agents are more effective than first-generation agents against *E. coli*, *Klebsiella* species, and *P. mirabilis*.[30] Many strains of enterobacter, *Serratia*, indole-positive proteus, *H. influenzae*, *Neisseria gonorrhea*, *N. meningitidis*, and anaerobes are covered by selected agents in this group.[31] β-lactamase–producing strains of ampicillin-resistant *H. influenzae* are inactivated by cefuroxime and, to a lesser extent, cefamandole.[32] Cefoxitin is of special interest to the clinician treating head and neck infections because of its marked activity against anaerobes including *B. fragilis*.

ACTIVITY, ABSORPTION, AND EXCRETION. The cephalosporins differ chemically from the penicillins only in that the β-lactam ring is fused to a six-member ring rather than a five-member ring. The mechanism of action of the cephalosporins is very similar to that of the penicillins. They interfere with the terminal step in bacterial cell wall synthesis and may also cause an increase in cell wall breakdown. Generally, their action is bactericidal. The cephalosporins have a relatively broad spectrum of activity that includes both gram-positive and gram-negative aerobes.[12]

The use of the cephalosporins was identified in the late 1960s as antibiotics that resisted the β-lactamases and, therefore, could be considered as substitutes for penicillin. The early aspirations for drugs capable of resisting the penicillinases were lost with the emergence of cephalosporinases that imparted an enzymatic resistance to the cephalosporins. The continued search for newer cephalosporins is driven by the need for agents with broader spectrums, that is, activity against gram-negative and anerobic organisms, greater resistance to beta-lactamase enzymes, and improved pharmocokinetics for passage into certain fluid spaces and extending the duration of action.

Many of the cephalosporins are poorly absorbed from the gastrointestinal tract because of their acid liability. Cephalexin, cefadroxil, cefaclor, cefuroxime, and cephradine are resistant to acids and are available for oral use.

The ability of an antibiotic to enter a variety of body fluids is of special importance in head and neck infections because of the potential for eye and intracranial involvement. The cephalosporins penetrate most body fluids but do not enter the aqueous humor of the eye and the cerebrospinal fluid (CSF). Ceftriaxone and moxalactam can provide therapeutic levels in the CSF. The cephalosporins generally have short half-lives of under 2 hours, with many of the agents having values of less than 1 hour. Ceftriaxone and cefadroxil may be given twice daily because of their 9-hour half-life.[12]

As with the penicillins, the kidney excretes most of the cephalosporins intact by glomerular filtration and proximal tubular secretion. Tubular excretion can be inhibited by probenecid. Patients with reduced creatinine clearance must have their dose reduced consistent with their kidney function to avoid toxicity from high serum concentrations.

CLINICAL USE. First-generation cephalosporins are effective alternatives to penicillins in treating staphylococcal and nonenterococcal streptococcal infections in patients who are allergic to penicillin.[33] Care must be taken to avoid cross-reactions. The cephalosporins should be avoided when the patient presents with a history of a substantial allergic reaction to a penicillin derivative. The cephalosporins may be used to treat odontogenic and orofacial infections when penicillin and erythromycin are contraindicated or when the causative organism is especially sensitive to the cephalosporins. Generally, for most oral infections, the cephalosporins are not recommended because of the predictable effectiveness of the penicillins and the considerably higher costs of the cephalosporins.[12]

The first-generation cephalosporins are the agents of choice for prophylaxis in cardiovascular, orthopedic, biliary, pelvic, and intraabdominal surgery because they cost less and have an effective and narrow range of activity.[34] Cefazolin is particularly useful as a prophylactic antibiotic because of its longer half-life than other first-generation agents.[30] Cefoxitin has been used with an aminoglycoside to treat mixed aerobic-anaerobic infections below the clavicle.[35] Cefonicid, because of its long half-life of 4.5 hours, may be administered once a day to treat less severe infections.[36] Several studies have concluded that infections caused by gram-negative bacilli susceptible to the cephalosporins should be treated with an aminoglycoside as well. The use of the cephalosporins as single agents for gram-negative organisms is unpredictable and, therefore, requires combination therapy.[37,38]

Third-Generation Cephalosporins

The third-generation cephalosporins are less active than the older cephalosporins against gram-positive cocci but more active against enteric gram-negative bacilli, including nosocomially acquired strains resistant to multiple antibiotics and moderately active against *P. aeruginosa.* These agents can be divided into two groups based on their activity against *P. aeruginosa* (Table 11–3).

Cefotaxime has been the most used third-generation cephalosporin and can serve as a comparison drug. It does not improve the coverage provided by first-generation cephalosporins against gram-positive cocci (a characteristic that decreases its usability in odontogenic infections). The resistance that cefotaxime demonstrates to the β-lactamases permits this drug to provide a potent broad spectrum of activity against the aerobic gram-negative bacteria that is markedly greater than that provided by first- and second-generation agents.[39,40] Cefotaxime has only moderate activity against anaerobes compared to cefoxitin. It should not be considered as the first drug of choice for odontogenic infections.

Cefoperazone is more active against *Pseudomonas* species than other third-generation cephalosporins but less active against many gram-negative bacilli.[41]

ACTIVITY, ABSORPTION AND EXCRETION. The kidneys are the principal route of excretion of most of the first-, second- and third-generation agents. Hepatic elimination predominates for cefoperazone and ceftriaxone, for which 40% of their elimination is hepatic.[30] Third-generation cephalosporins do penetrate through inflamed meninges to attain effective drug concentrations in the CSF. Cefoperazone is an exception to this activity.

CLINICAL USE. Third-generation cephalosporins are not indicated for treatment of gram-positive infections

Table 11–3. *Third-Generation Cephalosporin Activity Against* Pseudomonas aeruginosa

Cephalosporin	*Active*	*Not Active*
Cefotaxime (Claforan)		X
Ceftriaxone (Rocephin)		X
Ceftizoxime (Cefizox)		X
Moxalactam (Moxam)		X
Ceftazidime (Fortez, Tazidime)	X	
Cefoperazone (Cefobid)	X	

commonly found in head and neck infections. Moxalactam and ceftazidime, particularly, do not demonstrate consistent activity against these organisms and generally should not be used.[30]

Adverse Effects of the Cephalosporins

The chemical similarity of the cephalosporins to the penicillins has resulted in cross-sensitivity which must be considered when these agents are used in patients with severe penicillin allergies. If the reaction to penicillin was of the acute, immediate type supported by the findings of angioedema, urticaria, or anaphylactic shock, then cephalosporins should be given only as a last resort. The practitioner must be prepared to manage severe allergic emergencies prospectively by taking every precaution before administering the drug.

Cephalosporins are fairly safe antibiotics. Adverse reactions, which are uncommon and usually reversible, include thrombophlebitis, pain at the injection site, diarrhea, pseudomembranous colitis, and transient disturbances in hepatic, renal, or hematologic function. Gastrointestinal symptoms may result more frequently from cefoperazone than from the other agents.[42]

Bleeding problems of clinical significance have been associated with moxalactam more often than the other drugs in this group.[43] Impairment in normal hemostasis may result from hypoprothrombinemia and abnormalities in platelet aggregation.[44]

Erythromycin

Erythromycin has been the second choice antibiotic for odontogenic infections. It was particularly useful for patients who are allergic to penicillin and was thought to have a reasonable spectrum of activity against the organisms commonly cultured primarily by aerobic techniques. The widespread use of anaerobic cultures has demonstrated the polymicrobial nature of odontogenic infections and the predominance of anaerobes, a few of which are resistant to erythromycin.

ACTIVITY, ABSORPTION, AND EXCRETION. Erythromycin acts by inhibiting protein synthesis in susceptible microorganisms by binding to bacterial ribosomes to competitively inhibit access of transfer RNA-amino acid complexes to the messenger RNA-ribosome complex.[45] Its binding site on the bacterial ribosome is identical to that of clindamycin, lincomycin, and chloramphenicol. The antibacterial spectrum of erythromycin is similar to that of penicillin G but also includes *Staphylococcus*, *Haemophilus* species, *Mycoplasma*, *Rickettsia*, and *Chlamydia*. This spectrum of activity includes most of the oropharyngeal anaerobes commonly grown from dental infections. Fifty percent of the strains of *S. aureus* isolated from hospital patients are resistant to erythromycin. Resistance of other organisms involved in head and neck infections also has emerged. Strains of *S. pneumoniae*, viridans group of streptococci, enterococci, *H. influenzae*, and *S. pyogenes* are unaffected by erythromycin.[46]

Erythromycin is well absorbed from the gastrointestinal tract, but the base agent must be protected from stomach acid by the formation of acid-insoluble salts (stearate) or esters (estolate) or by coating with acid-insoluble films (enteric coating). Food in the stomach reduces the absorption of this drug except with the estolate and an enteric-coated formulation E-Mycin (Upjohn, Kalamazoo, MI).[47, 48] The enteric-coated preparation is preferred because of the cholestatic hepatitis associated with the estolate formulation.

Erythromycin is excreted primarily in the bile; only 2% to 5% is excreted in the urine. Concentrations in the bile may exceed ten times those in plasma. Erythromycin diffuses readily into tissues; CSF levels are approximately 20% of corresponding plasma levels.[49]

CLINICAL USE. The primary indication for erythromycin is in out-patients allergic to penicillin, with mild infections, who do not suffer from gastrointestinal diseases. Most of the gram-positive aerobic microorganisms and oral anaerobes are susceptible to erythromycin. An inherent disadvantage of erythromycin is the rapid development of resistance among certain microorganisms, which will be encouraged if the patient is not compliant with the dosing schedule and the duration of therapy. Effective inhibitory concentrations must be maintained with this bacteriostatic drug or resistance will be further encouraged. The bacteriostatic activity of the drug, the tendency for organisms to develop resistance, and the overall decreased effectiveness of erythromycin compared to penicillin makes it a secondary drug for the treatment of odontogenic infections.

ADVERSE EFFECTS. The most commonly encountered problem is gastrointestinal disturbances in the form of nausea, epigastric distress, vomiting, and diarrhea. These adverse effects may encourage patients to reduce their adherence to the dose schedule or the amount of drug taken per dose. The irritative properties of the drug are dose related, and care should be taken not to give unnecessarily high quantities of the agent. The enteric coating of erythromycin appears to reduce the gastrointestinal disturbance.

Allergic reactions to erythromycin occur relatively infrequently compared to the penicillins and present as a rash, pruritis, fever, and eosinophilia.[12] Intravenous erythromycin burns and is irritating to the venopuncture site. The cholestatic hepatitis reported with erythromycin estolate, and rarely with erythromycin ethylsuccinate, appears to be a unique form of drug allergy to the ester moiety rather than to the erythromycin base.[50, 51]

Clindamycin and Lincomycin

Lincomycin is obtained from *Streptomyces lincolnesis*, so named because it was isolated from soil near Lincoln, Nebraska. Clindamycin, the deoxy, chloro derivative of lincomycin can be given orally as well as parenterally and is the more active of the two agents. Clindamycin has unique characteristics that make it very useful in the management of odontogenic infections caused by a polymicrobial flora with multiple anaerobes which may be resistant to penicillin or for patients who are allergic to penicillin. In fact, the proportion of penicillin-resistant *Bacteroides* species from the oropharynx has been on the increase.[52] When patients are seriously ill with orofacial infections that may be due to these organisms, or when the response to penicillin is delayed, clindamycin treatment should be considered.

ACTIVITY, ABSORPTION, AND EXCRETION. Clindamycin acts by inhibition of protein synthesis in a manner similar to that previously described for erythromycin. Low concentrations are bacteriostatic; bactericidal activity can be achieved in vivo with usual clinical doses. Clindamycin is active against gram-positive aerobes including staphylococci but not to the extent of the penicillin G preparations. Its activity against most anaerobes is superior to that of any other antibiotic. This agent should be held in reserve to treat those orofacial infections caused by anaerobes resistant to other antibiotics. *B. fragilis* should be treated with clindamycin when this organism is cultured and the patient appears refractory to other antibiotic regimens.

Clindamycin is well absorbed from the gastrointestinal tract. The presence of food in the stomach does not appreciably impair absorption (95% of the agent will enter the body), but peak serum levels may be delayed. Peak serum levels are achieved 1 hour after a 600-mg intravenous dose.[53]

With the exception of the CSF, clindamycin penetrates body tissues well. Even when the meninges are inflamed, only small concentrations of clindamycin are found in the CSF.[54]

The distribution of clindamycin into bone is excellent, with active concentrations equaling or exceeding the plasma concentration.[55] The affinity of clindamycin for bone does not necessarily result in superior treatment results of osteomyelitis of the jaws.

Clindamycin is metabolized by the liver and excreted in inactive form in the urine. With impaired renal function, excretion in the feces is increased. Adjustments of dosage may be required in patients with hepatic dysfunction. The presence of active drug in the intestine can produce significant alterations of the microflora, resulting in superinfections.

CLINICAL USE. Clindamycin is indicated for the treatment of serious orofacial infections caused by anaerobes resistant to penicillin. Clindamycin should not be used as a substitute for penicillin or other drugs that are effective against orofacial and odontogenic infections.

ADVERSE EFFECTS. The gastrointestinal disturbances associated with clindamycin have been well publicized; antibiotic-associated colitis (AAC) occurs in some patients receiving this agent.[56] Animal studies showed that clindamycin suppresses the growth of some normal bowel flora while permitting the overgrowth of certain clindamycin-resistant strains of *C. difficile*. Diarrhea is the most common adverse effect associated with clindamycin and occurs in approximately 20% of patients (10% secondary to changes in bowel flora and up to 10% secondary to AAC).[57] This may occur after either oral or parenteral administration. The frequency of AAC has been reviewed with clindamycin as well as other agents. A study of such cases revealed that 31% of the patients had been given a cephalosporin, 27% were given ampicillin, and 11% received clindamycin; the remaining percentage involved most of the other antibiotics.[58] Diarrhea (more than five loose stools daily) should immediately prompt the agents to be discontinued and the diarrhea treated with absorbents (Kaopectate [Upjohn]) or resins (cholestyramine). Narcotic antidiarrheal agents such as Lomotil are contraindicated because they encourage intestinal spasms resulting in retention of the cytotoxins in the colon.[12] Proctoscopy may be indicated when diarrhea persists. Severe cases are treated with vancomycin. If recognized early and use of the drug is discontinued, clindamycin-associated colitis is usually self-limiting; however, fatalities have occurred. The drug should not be readministered. AAC has occasionally appeared after use of clindamycin has been discontinued. The clinician must be alert to this possibility and be sensitive to patients' complaints of changes in bowel habits that continue for a considerable time following administration of clindamycin and other agents.

Blood dyscrasias including neutropenia, thrombocytopenia, and agranulocytosis have been associated with prolonged therapy with clindamycin and lincomycin.[12]

Tetracyclines

Tetracyclines are closely congeneric derivatives of the polycyclic substance naphthacenecarboxamide. They are active in vitro against many urinary tract pathogens, are safe, and inexpensive. Tetracyclines should not be used for the treatment of infections in pregnant women or children who are younger than age 12, since staining of developing dentition can occur. Although the tetracyclines are frequently used to treat specific gram-negative bacilli and *Chlamydia* infections, they are rarely the first choice agent for orofacial infections.

Tetracycline is effective as adjunctive therapy for refractory cases of adult periodontitis and juvenile periodontosis unsuccessfully managed by conventional periodontal therapy.[12]

ACTIVITY, ABSORPTION, AND EXCRETION. The tetracyclines act by inhibiting protein synthesis and are bacteriostatic only. They are considered a broad-spectrum antibiotic with activity against many aerobic gram-positive cocci, gram-negative bacteria (both aerobes and anaerobes), spirochetes, *Actinobacillus actinomycetemcomitans*, *Chlamydia*, *Rickettsia*, and *Mycoplasma*.[12] Much resistance to the tetracyclines now exists due to extensive use and their "static" mechanism of action. Tetracyclines should not be used to treat staphylococcal, group A β-hemolytic streptococcal, or *S. pneumoniae* infections because of the occurrence of resistant strains.[53]

Tetracyclines are usually administered orally, and care must be taken to avoid certain food groups such as milk and other dairy products. Absorption from the gastrointestinal tract is incomplete and is influenced by the derivative, individual patient, presence of food, and concomitant administration of products containing certain cations such as aluminum-hydroxide gels, sodium bicarbonate, calcium and magnesium salts, and iron preparations.[59] Absorption is probably decreased by chelation and an increase in gastric pH. Minocycline and doxycycline are more effectively absorbed than the other tetracyclines, have longer half-lives, and are administered in lower, less frequent doses. Peak serum levels occur at 2 hours after oral administration (500 mg tetracycline or 200 mg doxycycline or minocycline).[53]

Tetracycline's affinity for bone is well known to researchers studying this tissue. Unfortunately, the agent partitions in bone to form complexes with hydroxyapatite that are biologically inactive.[60] It penetrates well into other body tissues. Spinal fluid levels are approximately one fourth those in plasma, and inflammation of the meninges is not a prerequisite for penetration of tetracyclines into the CSF.[53]

Tetracyclines are metabolized by the liver and concentrated in the bile. Excretion takes place primarily in the urine for most of the tetracyclines with less elimination through the feces. An exception is doxycycline, which may be useful in patients with impaired renal function because of its extrarenal mode of excretion.[53]

CLINICAL USE. Tetracyclines have a limited usefulness in orofacial infections. With the exception of treating refractory periodontitis, juvenile periodontosis, and a susceptible odontogenic infection that is resistant to penicillin and erythromycin, they are rarely first-choice antibiotics.

ADVERSE EFFECTS. Allergic reactions are infrequent and usually appear as skin rashes. Anaphylactic reactions have occurred after both oral and parenteral administration.[61] Oral symptoms of allergy include cheilosis, brown and black coating of the tongue, and soreness of the oral mucosa.[12]

Adverse effects involving multiple organ systems have been produced by the tetracyclines. Generally they may be grouped into those reactions caused directly by the irritating qualities of the drug such as gastrointestinal disturbances, superinfections, and direct toxicity. The tetracyclines are the most likely of all the antibiotics to cause superinfections with bacteria, fungi, and yeast. Antibiotic-associated colitis should be investigated whenever severe diarrhea is reported.

Chloramphenicol

Chloramphenicol inhibits protein synthesis by blocking polypeptide linkage on the messenger RNA-ribosome complex.[62] Chloramphenicol possesses a wide spectrum of activity; it is primarily bacteriostatic, although it may be bactericidal to certain species under some conditions. Its use in orofacial cellulitis is generally limited to severe odontogenic infections that are threatening the orbital contents or the brain. The emergence of newer drugs with less toxicity than chloramphenicol but equally effective against anaerobes has lessened the need for this historical drug.

ACTIVITY, ABSORPTION, AND EXCRETION. Chloramphenical penetrates well into all tissues, including the brain and CSF and is effective treatment for brain abscesses and bacterial meningitis caused by susceptible organisms. As previously stated, chloramphenicol is highly active in vitro against anaerobic organisms, including *B. fragilis*, an organism of special interest in odontogenic infections.

Chloramphenicol is rapidly and completely absorbed from the gastrointestinal tract, and absorption is not impaired by the simultaneous administration of food or antacids. Peak serum levels are achieved 1 to 2 hours after an oral or intravenous dose of 1 g of chloramphenicol. It is inactivated in the liver by glucuronyl transferase and excreted in the urine.

CLINICAL USE. Chloramphenicol is the drug of choice for the treatment of typhoid fever and other systemic *Salmonella* infections.[52] Because of its toxicity, chloramphenicol is not a first-choice antibiotic for orofacial infections. It has a primary role in the treatment of infectious diseases normally unrelated to the head and neck. When serious head and neck infections are encountered that are a threat to the eye or brain, chloramphenicol can be a useful agent.

ADVERSE EFFECTS. Hypersensitivity reactions to chloramphenicol are uncommon. The most common toxic effect is bone-marrow suppression. Chloramphenicol-associated pancytopenia occurs correlated with dose and idiosyncratically. Complete blood and platelet counts should be obtained at least three times a week for patients who are receiving chloramphenicol.[53]

Vancomycin

Vancomycin is a narrow-spectrum bactericidal antibiotic that was introduced in 1956. Its primary use has been as a substitute for penicillin in the prophylaxis of the heart valve patient and as a methicillin-resistant staphylococcal agent.[63]

Vancomycin hydrochloride is not effective by the oral route for the treatment of systemic infections. The drug may be given orally for the treatment of antibiotic-associated pseudomembranous colitis produced by *C. difficile* in combination with parenteral vancomycin.

ACTIVITY, ABSORPTION, AND EXCRETION. Vancomycin is effective against gram-positive organisms, cocci, and bacteria; most oral anaerobes; and against gram-negative cocci such as *Neisseria*. It is bactericidal to susceptible organisms, having an action on both the cell wall and the cell membrane.[64] Vancomycin does not traverse the uninflamed meninges.

Vancomycin is not absorbed from the gastrointestinal tract and must be given intravenously for the therapy of systemic infections. Excretion is by the kidneys as the active drug. In patients with impaired renal function, dose or frequency of administration must be modified to prevent toxic side effects.

CLINICAL USE. Indications for vancomycin therapy include serious methicillin-resistant staphylococcal infections, antibiotic-induced enterocolitis, and antibiotic prophylaxis for the penicillin-allergic patient with prosthetic heart valves. Vancomycin is used for patients with prosthetic heart valves because they are at increased risk of developing endocarditis from dentally caused bacteremia. The organisms commonly implicated in endocarditis usually are susceptible to vancomycin. In addition, the presence of nonhemolytic streptococci (enterococci) in the oral cavity that are resistant to other antibiotics can cause endocarditis. A further advantage of vancomycin is the lack of cross-allergenicity with penicillin. The chief disadvantage of this agent is the limitations of intravenous administration.[12]

ADVERSE EFFECTS. Among the allergic reactions that have been produced by vancomycin are macular skin rashes and anaphylaxis.

The major adverse effect of vancomycin is neurotoxicity; only the auditory nerve is involved. Kidney damage also occurs following prolonged administration. Thrombophlebitis is a common problem, but the incidence can be reduced by slow infusion. Intramuscular injections are contraindicated because of severe tissue necrosis at the injection site.

Too rapid intravenous administration of vancomycin can cause a sudden decrease in blood pressure frequently referred to as the "red man syndrome" or "red-neck syndrome." The sudden drop in blood pressure can be severe and may be accompanied by flushing a maculopapular or erythematous rash, urticaria, angioedema, wheezing, dyspnea, and pruritis. Histamine release causing a negative inotropic and vasodilating action appears to be partly responsible for the vancomycin-induced hypotension. The release of histamine also appears to cause the erythema and rash of the face, neck, chest, and upper extremities. The hypotension reaction is related to the rate of infusion of vancomycin; rapid infusion (10 min or less) has most often been associated with decreases in blood pressure. The hypotension reaction has been reported in patients who were infused with the drug over periods of an hour or more.

Hypotensive reactions to vancomycin can be minimized by administering the antibiotic over a period of one hour or longer. Blood pressure should be monitored before, during, and after the infusion. If a hypotensive reaction or other findings suggestive of the red man syndrome develop, antihistamines, intravenous fluids, and corticosteroids should be administered. Vasoactive reactions usually resolve spontaneously within hours after the drug has been discontinued.

Patients receiving intravenous vancomycin may also complain of severe throbbing pain in the muscles of the back and neck. This commonly occurring, but unexplained, adverse effect can also be minimized by slow administration of the antibiotic.

Metronidazole

The antianaerobic activity of metronidazole (Flagyl) was discovered in 1962 when Shinn[65] observed that a patient afflicted simultaneously with a trichomonal infection and Vincent's gingivitis was cured of both conditions after receiving metronidazole for the trichomonal infection. Before Shinn's observation, metronidazole virtually was used exclusively as an antiparasitic agent. The clinical implications of the potential role of the agent in the management of anaerobic infections remained obscure for more than a decade until the development of a relatively simple, reliable, and inexpensive method of detection of these organisms became available.[66]

Before the introduction of Flagyl IV (Searle) the primary antibiotics used to treat anaerobic odontogenic infections were penicillin G, clindamycin, and chloramphenicol. Penicillin G is not effective against *B. fragilis*, and other resistant oropharyngeal strains of anaerobes are now emerging. Clindamycin does not cross the blood-brain barrier, and therefore it is not indicated for the treatment of central nervous system infections. Chloramphenicol is a highly effective anti-anaerobic drug that has serious toxic side effects which can be fatal.

Metronidazole is a consistently bactericidal drug against obligate anaerobes at readily achievable serum levels. It is distributed rapidly throughout nearly all the tissues of the body, readily crosses the blood-brain barrier, and attains therapeutic concentrations in brain abscesses. Metronidazole cannot be depended on as a single-drug therapy for odontogenic infections because it does not appear to possess any clinically relevant activity against facultative anaerobes or obligate aerobes.[67]

ACTIVITY, ABSORPTION, AND EXCRETION. Muller[66] described the action of metronidazole on anaerobic organisms as a function of the interaction of this agent with electron-transporting proteins, similar to ferredoxin, a low-redox-potential electron-transporting protein. The change in the metronidazole molecule produced by this interaction inside the anerobic cell produces cytotoxic products that kill the cell. The intracellular activation of metronidazole to a bactericidal metabolite occurs whether or not the cells are dividing, because it depends on an active metabolic process. Metronidazole hydrochloride (Flagyl IV) is indicated in the treatment of serious infections caused by susceptible anaerobic bacteria. In a mixed aerobic and facultative anaerobic infection, antibiotics appropriate for the treatment of the nonanaerobic organisms should be used in addition to metronidazole.

Within an hour of administration, at least 80% of the oral dose of metronidazole is usually absorbed.[68] Food intake does not significantly influence the bioavailability of the drug.[69]

Metronidazole is metabolized by hydroxylation, oxidation, and glucuronide formation. Sixteen percent of a dose is excreted in the urine as unaltered metronidazole, 25% as the major metabolite, and 14% as conjugates of both. The major pathway of elimination of metronidazole is in the urine (60% to 80% of an administered dose); fecal excretion accounts for 6% to 15%.

CLINICAL USE. Metronidazole has been found to be effective in anaerobic infections including those caused by *B. fragilis* infections resistant to clindamycin, chloramphenicol, and penicillin.[70] It is an extremely useful agent for odontogenic infections involving *Bacteroides* species when it is used in combination with β-lactam antibiotics to control the aerobic and facultative bacteria. Metronidazole's ability to penetrate into the central nervous system provides additional merit to its use when the eye and the brain are threatened by infection.

ADVERSE EFFECTS. The two most serious adverse reactions reported in patients treated with metronidazole have been convulsive seizures and peripheral neuropathy, the latter characterized mainly by numbness or paresthesia of an extremity. Adverse reactions reported during treatment with oral metronidazole include nausea, sometimes accompanied by headache, anorexia, and occasionally vomiting, diarrhea, epigastric distress, abdominal cramping, and constipation. If patients receiving metronidazole drink alcoholic beverages, they may experience abdominal distress, nausea, vomiting, flushing, headache, and modification of the taste of alcoholic beverages has also been reported.[71]

The Aminoglycosides

Aminoglycoside antibiotics have a molecular structure consisting of amino sugars in glycosidic linkage. By convention, those agents originating from the genus *Streptomyces* are labeled "mycins" (e.g., kanamycin), and those originating from the genus *Micromonospora* are labeled "micins" (gentamicin).[72] They are useful in head and neck infections when enteric gram-negative bacteria are cultured (usually in patients over age 60 or those who have a compromised immune response).

Aminoglycosides have little or no activity against anaerobic organisms, are poorly absorbed from the gastrointestinal tract, and do not penetrate well into the CSF. These pharmacologic considerations alone make the aminoglycosides poor agents for the usual odontogenic infection.

ACTIVITY, ABSORPTION, AND EXCRETION. The aminoglycoside antibiotics penetrate the cell wall and cytoplasmic membrane of susceptible organisms and act on the bacterial ribosomes. They are bound to the ribosomes and cause misreading of the genetic code; thus, incorrect amino acids are inserted into the peptide chain and faulty proteins produced (i.e., interfere with protein synthesis).[72] The aminoglycoside antibiotics are generally clinically ineffective against *S. pyogenes*, *S. pneumoniae*, meningococcus, and anaerobic organisms. They are active against *S. aureus* but are less effective than the penicillins or the cephalosporins. Gentamicin, tobramycin, and amikacin are equally useful against most aerobic gram-negative rods. *Pseudomonas* strains resistant to gentamicin may sometimes be susceptible to tobramycin or netilmicin and often are susceptible to amikacin, ceftazidime, imipenem, aztreonam, and ciprofloxacin.

The aminoglycosides are excreted primarily by the kidneys and undergo no detectable metabolic change.

Numerous nomograms and formulas have been reported for the estimation of aminoglycoside dosage in patients with renal failure.[74] These aids can be helpful in planning initial treatment and establishing the ideal therapeutic concentrations of the aminoglycoside without reaching toxic levels.

CLINICAL USE. Aminoglycosides have a role in the treatment of aerobic gram-negative rods, although with decreasing indications. Combinations of an aminoglycoside and a penicillin or cephalosporin frequently achieve a greater effect than either agent alone. This effect has clear clinical benefit in enterococcal and in serious *Pseudomonas* infections.[73]

ADVERSE EFFECTS. The major adverse effect of the aminoglycosides is damage to the kidney and the eighth cranial nerve. Nephrotoxic effects are related to longer durations of therapy and are almost always reversible. The ototoxicity may involve either auditory or vestibular function, frequently is permanent, and is caused by excess peak plasma levels.

Newer Beta-Lactam Antibiotics

Carbapenems

Carbapenems are β-lactam antibiotics with an exceptionally broad spectrum. Imipenem is the carbapenem antibiotic currently available. It is used in combination with cilastatin sodium, a compound that inhibits the metabolism of imipenem by renal dipeptidases and thereby increases urinary concentrations of the drug.[75] Imipenem has the broadest antimicrobial spectrum of activity of any antibiotic. It is the most active of the newer agents against gram-positive cocci, approaching the level of penicillin.[76]

ACTIVITY, ABSORPTION, AND EXCRETION. More than 90% of most species of gram-negative organisms are susceptible to imipenem including those resistant to other β-lactam agents and aminoglycosides.[77] The activity of imipenem against *P. aeruginosa* compares favorably with ceftazidime, and its anaerobic activity is comparable to that of metronidazole and clindamycin.[78] Neither imipenem nor cilastatin sodium is absorbed appreciably from the gastrointestinal tract and, therefore, the drugs must be given parenterally.

Only low concentrations of imipenem enter the CSF following intravenous administration. The antibiotic is distributed to saliva, wound fluids, and bone.

If imipenem is administered without cilastatin sodium, the kidneys partially hydrolyze the drug to a microbiologically inactive metabolite, and only 5% to 43% of the dose is excreted unchanged in urine. With cilastatin sodium, approximately 70% of the imipenem dose is excreted unchanged in urine within 10 hours.

CLINICAL USE. Imipenem has been used for a variety of both community-acquired and nosocomial infections when multiply resistant gram-negative bacilli or mixed aerobic and anaerobic organisms are suspected.[30] Its high anaerobic activity and action against gram-positive cocci make it an attractive drug for odontogenic infections. Imipenem's broad spectrum, however, may invite unwanted resistance and superinfections. Imipenem may be useful in head and neck infections when the patient is immunocompromised, is allergic to other more commonly used antibiotics, or has a life-threatening infection.

ADVERSE EFFECTS. Gastrointestinal upset is the most common side effect of imipenem. Hypersensitivity reactions occur in about 3% of patients. Seizures have been reported in 1.5% of patients receiving imipenem and cilastatin sodium.[30]

Monobactams

Aztreonam (Azactam) is a β-lactam antibiotic that is a synthetic analogue of an antibiotic initially isolated from solid bacteria.[79] It is resistant to hydrolysis by most β-lactamases and does not induce production of β-lactamases.[80]

ACTIVITY, ABSORPTION, AND EXCRETION. Aztreonam has a spectrum of activity that resembles the aminoglycosides. Aerobic gram-negative bacilli are particularly susceptible. Most of the Enterobacteriaceae, for example, are susceptible to aztreonam comparable to the extent they are to third-generation cephalosporins and the extended-spectrum penicillins.

The usual dosages of aztreonam are eliminated primarily unchanged in the kidneys.[81]

CLINICAL USE. Aztreonam is contraindicated as a single drug for odontogenic infections. The narrow spectrum of activity of the monobactams precludes their use for mixed infections that contain anaerobic organisms. Aztreonam is a potential replacement for aminoglycosides in head and neck infections requiring combination therapy.

ADVERSE EFFECTS. Aztreonam has minimal cross-allergenicity with other β-lactam drugs and, therefore, can be used in patients allergic to penicillins or cephalosporins.[82] The monobactams have the same toxicity profile as most of the other β-lactam antibiotics.[83]

Quinolones

Ciprofloxacin is a synthetic quinolone that is representative of this group of antiinfective agents. It is usually bactericidal in action inhibiting DNA-gyrase in susceptible organisms.

ACTIVITY, ABSORPTION, AND EXCRETION. The newer quinolones possess an expanded spectrum of antibacterial activity. Most of the fluorinated compounds are moderately active against gram-positive bacteria, including methicillin-resistant *S. aureus*, *E. coli*, *Klebsiella*, *Enterobacter*, and *Proteus*. Ciprofloxacin has minimal activity against many streptococci and essentially no activity against anaerobes, two activity deficiencies that limit its use in odontogenic infections.

The clinical pharmacology of the fluoroquinolones is generally characterized by rapid oral absorption; urinary drug concentrations that markedly exceed the MIC for all common bacterial pathogens; wide distribution into body tissues; and half-lives sufficiently long to allow dosing every 12 to 24 hours.[84]

Quinolones undergo both renal and hepatic elimination. The kidneys excrete metabolites and the parent drug by way of glomerular filtration and tubular secretion.

CLINICAL USE. Norfloxacin and ciprofloxacin have established roles in treating urinary tract, lower respiratory tract, infectious diarrhea, skin and skin structure, and bone and joint infections. Barrier[85] reported preliminary clinical data suggesting that the oral quinolones will allow cost-effective, outpatient therapy for gram-negative and bacterial infections that previously required parenteral antiinfectives and hospitalization.

ADVERSE EFFECTS. Serious adverse drug reactions were reported in less than 1% of patients. The most frequently reported symptoms included nausea (1.9%); headache (1.8%); dizziness (1.2%); and abdominal pain, upset stomach, constipation, and flatulence (0.3% each). Patient gastrointestinal complaints were comparable with those found in the study by Corrado et al.[86] Many patients (3.3%) reported central nervous system symptoms (dizziness, headache, tremors, and restlessness) that, in many cases, were associated with concomitant theophylline therapy. The fluoroquinolones significantly increase peak and trough serum theophylline concentrations.[87] Theophylline concentrations were measured in the toxic range in 30% of patients experiencing increases.

REFERENCES

1. Hermans PE. General principles of antimicrobial therapy. Mayo Clin Proc 1977; 52:603.
2. Rosenblatt JE. Laboratory tests used to guide antimicrobial therapy. Mayo Clin Proc 1977; 52:611.
3. Thornsberry C, Baker, CN, Kirven LA, et al. Susceptibility of ampicillin-resistant *Haemophilus influenzae* to seven penicillins. Antimicrob Agents Chemother 1976; 9:70.
4. Schlichter JG, Maclean H. A method of determining the effective therapeutic level in the treatment of subacute bacterial endocarditis with penicillin: a preliminary report. Am Heart J 1947; 34:209.
5. Hoeprich PD. Antimicrobics and antihelminthics for systemic therapy. In: Hoeprich PD, ed. Infectious Diseases, ed 2. Hagerstown: Harper & Row, 1977:152.
6. Gale EF. Mechanisms of antibiotic action. Pharmacol Rev 1963; 15:481.
7. Montgomery EH. Principles and mechanisms of antibiotic therapy. In: Neidle EA, Yagiela JA, eds. Pharmacology and Therapeutics for Dentistry, ed 3. St Louis: CV Mosby, 1989:493.
8. Antimicrobial prophylaxis in surgery. Med Lett Drugs Ther 1987(Oct 9); 29(750): 91.
9. DePiro JT, et al. Single dose systemic antibiotic prophylaxis of surgical wound infections. Am J Surg 1986; 152:552.
10. Johnson JT, Wagner RL. Infection following uncon-

taminated head and neck surgery. Arch Otolarngol 1987(April); 113:368.
11. Wilkowske KG. The penicillins. Mayo Clin Proc 1977; 52:616.
12. Montgomery EH, Kroeger DC. Use of antibiotics in dental practice. Dent Clin North Am 1984; 28:433.
13. Weinstein L. The penicillins. In: Goodman LS, Gilman A, eds. The Pharmaceutical Basis of Therapeutics, ed 4. Philadelphia: Macmillan, 1970:1204.
14. Wormer DC, Martin WJ, Nichols DR, et al. Concentrations in serum of procaine and crystalline penicillin G administered orally or parenterally. Antibiot Med 1955; 1:589.
15. Smilack JD, Filitte, WH, Williams TW Jr. Bone concentrations of antimicrobial agents after parenteral administration. Antimicrob Agents Chemother 1976; 9:169.
16. Drucker DB, Jolly M. Sensitivity of oral organisms to antibiotics. Br Dent J 1971; 131:442.
17. Gilbert DN, Sanford JP. Methicillin: critical appraisal after a decade of experience. Med Clin North Am 1970; 54:1113.
18. The choice of antimicrobial drugs. Med Lett Drugs Ther 1986(March 28); 28(710): 36.
19. Ampicillin/Subactam (Unasyn). Med Lett Drugs Ther 1987(Aug 28); 29(747): 79.
20. Sutherland R, Croydon EAP, Rolinson GN. Amoxicillin: A new semisynthetic penicillin. R Med J 1972; 3:13.
21. Bodey GP, Whitcar JP Jr., Middleman E, et al. Carbenicillin therapy for pseudomonas infections. JAMA 1971; 218:62.
22. Wexler M et al. Antimicrobial Agents Chemother 1985; 27:876.
23. JA Retsema, et al. Sulbactam/ampicillin vitro spectrum, potency and activity in models of acute infection. Rev Infect Dis 1986; 8:s528.
24. Jones, et al. Susceptibility of *Haemophilus ducreyi* to ampicillin and sulbactam in vitro. Antimicrob Agents Chemother 1986; 29:1110.
25. Corr DJ, Wellman WE. Reactions to penicillin. I. Review of the literature concerning severe reactions (English and North America). Minn Med 1956; 39:599.
26. Rudolph AH, Price EV. Penicillin reactions among patients in venereal disease clinics: a national survey. JAMA 1973; 223:499.
27. Bartlett JG. Antimicrobial agents implicated in Clostridium difficile toxin-associated diarrhea of colitis. Johns Hopkins Med J 1981; 149:6.
28. Appel GB, Neu HC. The nephrotoxicity of antimicrobial agents. N Engl J Med 1977; 296:663.
29. Moellering RC Jr, Swartz MN. The newer cephalosporins. N Engl J Med 1976; 294:24.
30. Donowitz GR, Mandell GL. Beta-lactam antibiotics (second of two parts). N Engl J Med 1988; 318:490.
31. Sanders CV, Greenberg RN, Marier RL. Cefamandole and cefoxitin. Ann Intern Med 1985; 103:70.
32. Eykn S, Jenkins C, King A, Phillips I. Antibacterial activity of cefuroxims, a new cephalosporin antibiotic, compared with that of cephaloridine, cephalothin, and cefamandole. Antimicrob Agents Chemother 1976; 9:690.
33. Stillerman M, Isenberg HD, Moody M. Streptococcal pharyngitis therapy: comparison of cephalexin, phenoxymethyl penicillin, and ampicillin. Am J Dis Child 1972; 123:457.
34. DiPiro JT, Bowden TA Jr, Hooks VH III. Prophylactic parenteral cephalosporins in surgery: Are the newer agents better? JAMA 1984; 252:3277.
35. Drusano GL, Warren JW, Saah JA, et al. A prospective randomized controlled trial of cefoxitin versus clindamycin-aminoglygoside in mixed anaerobic-aerobic infections. Surg Gynecol Obstet 1982; 154:715.
36. Wallace RJ Jr, Niefield SL, Waters S, et al. Comparative trial of cefonicid and cefamandole in the therapy of community-acquired pneumonia. Antimicrob Agents Chemother 1982; 21:321.
37. Glew RH, Pavick RA. Early synergistic interactions between amikacin and sit beta-lactam antibiotics against multiple resistant members of the Enterobacteriaceae. Antimicrob Agents Chemother 1984; 26:378.
38. Giamarellou H. Aminoglygoside plus beta-lactams against gram-negative organisms: Evaluation of in vitro synergy and chemical interactions. Am J Med 1986; 80 (Suppl 6B): 126.
39. Richmond MH. Beta-lactamase stability of cefotaxime. J Antimicrob Chemother 1980; 6(Suppl A): 13.
40. Schrinner E, Limbert M, Penasse L, et al. Antibacterial activity øf cefotaxime and other newer cephalosporins (in vivo and in vitro). J Antimicrob Chemother 1980; 6(Suppl A): 25.
41. Kayser FH. Microbiological studies of cefoperazone. Clin Ther 1980; 3(Special Issue): 24.
42. Platt R. Adverse effects of third-generation cephalosporins. J Antimicrob Chemother 1982; 10(Suppl C): 135.
43. Weitekamp MR, Aber RC. Prolonged bleeding times and bleeding diathesis associated with moxalactam administration. JAMA 1983; 249:69.
44. Satter FR, Weitkemp MR, Ballard JO. Potential for bleeding with the new beta-lactam antibiotics. Ann Intern Med 1986; 105:924.
45. Lorian V. The mode of action of antibiotics on gram-negative bacilli. Arch Intern Med 1971; 128:623.
46. Sprunt K, Leidy G, Redmon W. Cross resistance between lincomycin and erythromycin in viridans streptococci. Pediatrics 1970; 46:84.
47. Griffith RS, Black HR. Comparison of the blood levels obtained after single and multiple doses of erythromycin estolate and erythromycin stearate. Am J Med Sci 1964; 247:69.
48. Fraser DG. Selection of an oral erythromycin product. Am J Hosp Pharm 1980; 37:1199.
49. Weinstein L. Antimicrobial agents. In: Goodman LS, Gilman A, eds. The pharmacological basis of therapeutics, ed 5. New York: Macmillan, 1975:1124.
50. Sullivan D, Csuka ME, Blanchard B. Erythromycin ethylsuccinate hepatotoxicity. JAMA 1980; 243:1047.
51. Tolman KG, Sannella JJ, Freston JW. Chemical struc-

ture of erythromycin and hepatotoxicity. Ann Intern Med 1974; 81:58.
52. The choice of antimicrobial drugs. Med Lett Drugs Ther 1988 (Mar 25); 30(762): 33.
53. Wilson WR. Tetracyclines, chloramphenicol, erythromycin, and clindamycin. Mayo Clin Proc 1977; 52:635.
54. Panzer JD, Brown DC, Epstein WL, et al. Clindamycin levels in various body tissues and fluids. J Clin Pharmacol 1972; 12:259.
55. Bystedt H, Dahlback A, Dornbusch K, et al. Concentrations of azidocillin, erythromycin, doxycycline and clindamycin in human mandibular bone. Int J Oral Surg 1978; 7:442.
56. Swartzberg JE, Maresca RM, Remington JS. Clinical study of gastrointestinal complications associated with clindamycin therapy. J Infect Dis 1977; 135 (Suppl):99.
57. Tedesco FJ, Barton RW, Alpers DH. Clindamycin-associated colitis: a prospective study. Ann Intern Med 1974; 81:429.
58. Bartlett JG. Antimicrobial agents implicated in *Clostridium difficile* toxin-associated diarrhea of colitis. Johns Hopkins Med J 1981; 149:6.
59. Neuvonen PJ, Gothoni G, Hackman R, et al. Interface of iron with the absorption of tetracyclines in man. Br Med J 1970; 4:532.
60. Smilack JD, Flittie WH, Williams TW Jr. Bone concentrations of antimicrobial agents after parenteral administration. Antimicrob Agents Chemother 1976; 9:169.
61. Furey DG, Tan C. Anaphylactic shock due to oral demethylchlortetracycline. Ann Intern Med 1969; 70:357.
62. Lorian V. The mode of action of antibiotics on gram-negative bacilli. Arch Intern Med 1971; 128:623.
63. Geraci JE, Heilman FR, Nichols DR, et al. Some laboratory and clinical experiences with a new antibiotic, vancomycin. Proc Staff Meet Mayo Clin 1956; 31:564.
64. Geraci JE. Vancomycin. Mayo Clin Proc 1977; 52:631.
65. Shinn DL. Vincent's disease and its treatment. Amsterdam: Excerpta Medica 1977; 438:334.
66. Muller M. Metronidazole: Its action on anaerobes. J Infect Dis 1979; 9:4.
67. Sutter VL, Finegold SM. In vitro studies with metronidazole against anaerobic bacteria. Metronidazole. Proceedings of the International Metronidazole Conference. Excerpta Medica 1977:279.
68. McGilveray IJ, Midha KK, Loo JCK, et al. The bioavailability of commercial metronidazole formulations. Int J Clin Pharmacol 1978; 16:110.
69. Melander A, Kahlmeter G, Kamme C, et al. Bioavailability of metronidazole in fasting and nonfasting healthy subjects and in patients with Crohn's disease. Eur J Clin Pharmacol 1977; 12:69.
70. Finegold SM. Antimicrobial therapy of anaerobic infections: A status report. Hosp Pract 1979; 14:71.
71. Flagyl IV. A clinical and laboratory profile. Searle Pharmaceuticals, Inc. Chicago, Illinois, 1980.
72. Brewer JS. Antimicrobial agents II. The aminoglycosides. Mayo Clin Proc 1977; 52:675.
73. Gregaory D, Hirschman JV. Prudent use of the aminoglycosides. Postgrad Med 1978; 64:97.
74. McHenry MC, Gavan L, Gifford RW Jr, et al. Gentamicin dosage for renal insufficiency: Adjustments based on endogenous creatinine clearance and serum creatinine concentration. Ann Intern Med 1971; 74:192.
75. Oates JA, Alastair JJ, Wood MD. Beta-lactam antibiotics. N Engl J Med 1988; 318:490.
76. Kropp H, Gerckens L, Sundelof JG, et al. Antibacterial activity of imipenem: The first thienamycin antibiotic. Rev Infect Dis 1985; 7(Suppl 3): S389.
77. Jones RN. Review of the in vitro spectrum of activity of imipenem. Am J Med 1985; 78(Suppl 16A): 22.
78. Braveny I. In vitro activity of imipenem—a review. Eur J Clin Microbiol 1984; 3:456.
79. Sykes RB, Cimarusti CM, Bonner DP, et al. Monocyclic beta-lactam antibiotics produced by bacteria. Nature 1981; 291:489.
80. Bush K, Freudenberger JS, Sykes RB. Interaction of aztreonam and related monobactams with beta-lactamases from gram-negative bacteria. Antimicrob Agents Chemother 1982; 22:414.
81. Swabb EA. Review of the clinical pharmacology of the monobactam antibiotic aztreonam. Am J Med 1985; 78 (Suppl 2A):11.
82. Saxon A, Hassner A, Swabb EA, et al. Lack of cross-reactivity between aztreonam, a monobactam antibiotic, and penicillin in penicillin–allergic subjects. J Infect Dis 1984; 149.
83. Newman TJ, Dreslinki GR, Tadrus SS. Safety profile of aztreonam in clinical trials. Rev Infect Dis 1985; 7 (Suppl 4):S648.
84. Norris S, Mandell GL. The quinolones: History and overview. In: Andriole VT, ed. The Quinolones. London: Academic Press, 1988:1.
85. Barrier SL. Economic impact of oral ciprofloxacin: A pharmacist's perspective. Am J Med 1987; 82(Suppl 4A): 387.
86. Corrado ML, Struble WE, Peter C, et al. Norfloxacin: Review of safety studies. Am J Med 1987; 82(Suppl 6B): 22–6.
87. Wijnands WJ, Vree TB, Herwaarden CL. Enoxacin decreases the clearance of theophylline in man. Br J Clin Pharmacol 1985; 20(6):538.

IV

PRINCIPLES OF MANAGEMENT OF SINUS DISEASE

12

Diagnosis and Management of Sinus Disease

Arthur A. Gonty

It is important to have a sound understanding of the anatomy and pathophysiology of the paranasal sinuses. Swelling of the nasal mucosa caused by allergy or infection can result in obstruction of the ostia of the major sinuses and lead to sinusitis. Injury to the sinuses may lead to infection. Injury to the maxillary sinus mucosa by odontogenic infection, pathologic conditions, or surgery may lead to sinusitis or oroantral fistula formation. Knowledge of the microbiologic characteristics of acute and chronic sinusitis aids in the medical and surgical management of acute and chronic sinusitis.

This chapter describes the anatomy, radiology, pathophysiology, and microbiology of sinus disease. Major emphasis is placed on the maxillary sinus, but the other sinuses are included for completeness. Medical and surgical management of sinus disease, including complications resulting from sinus disease, are presented.

ANATOMY OF THE PARANASAL SINUSES

The Maxillary Sinus

The maxillary sinus begins to develop in early fetal life. An evagination burrows from the middle meatus of the nasal cavity into the maxilla. At birth the maxillary sinus is present but small. It continues to increase in size until the permanent teeth have erupted. The average size of the maxillary sinus is 34 mm anteroposteriorly, 33 mm in height, and 23 mm in width.[1] The capacity of the sinus varies from 9.5 to 20 mL with an average capacity of 15 mL.

Drainage of the maxillary sinus occurs through its ostium. The ostium is located on the highest part of the medial wall of the antrum. It is variable in its size, position, and efficacy in draining the sinus.[2] The structure of the nasal cavity and the position of the nasal septum may cause anatomic obstruction and limit access to the ostium. These anatomic abnormalities can contribute to the development of maxillary sinusitis.

The ethmoid bulla lies above the uncinate process of the ethmoid bone. Lying between these two structures is the hiatus semilunaris (Fig. 12–1). The channel leading from the nasal frontal recess to the hiatus semilunaris is called the infundibulum (Fig. 12–2). The location of the maxillary ostium is variable in the course of the infundibulum. This area, the middle meatus and the anterior and middle ethmoid air cells, is called the ostiomeatal complex and is thought to be crucial in the health of the maxillary and frontal sinuses. It is the area currently drawing considerable attention in intranasal sinus endoscopy.

The roof of the maxillary sinus is the floor of the orbit. The infraorbital nerve runs through the infraorbital canal at the rim of the orbit. The bone is rela-

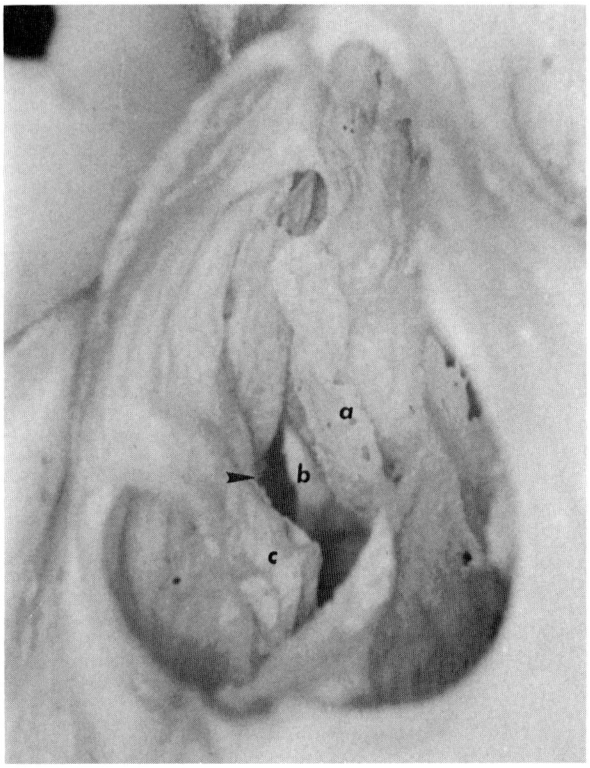

Figure 12–1. *The bony landmarks of the infundibular area of the lateral nasal wall are shown. a indicates middle turbinate;* b, *ethmoid bulla;* c, *the inferior turbinate obstructs the view of the uncinate process, and hiatus semilunaris* (arrow).

tively thin at the roof of the sinus and can be easily fractured with a blow to the globe, producing an orbital blowout fracture. The floor may also be thin enough to have a dehiscence, which may allow passage of infection from the antrum to the orbit.

The antral mucosa is composed of a single layer of pseudostratified, ciliated, columnar epithelium. The tunica propria is very thin and is composed of a superficial loose connective tissue layer and a deep compact layer, which fuses with the periosteum to form the mucoperiosteum.[3] The tunica propria contains goblet cells and mucosal glands. The mucociliary apparatus protects the sinuses against infection by removing the organisms trapped in the mucus through the ostium.

Acute infections such as those caused by the common cold virus result in a completely reversible inflammatory process of the nasal and sinus mucosa.[3] If a secondary bacterial infection occurs, secretions can become mucopurulent and occasionally flecked with blood. As long as drainage of the ostium is maintained, normal mucosa and function will return. Chronic sinusitis results from either a persistent acute inflammatory process or by repeated bouts of acute sinusitis. Squamous metaplasia of the antral mucosa ultimately occurs and is irreversible. Chronic sinusitis may be classified pathologically into two major types: hypertrophic (polypoid) and atrophic (sclerosing).

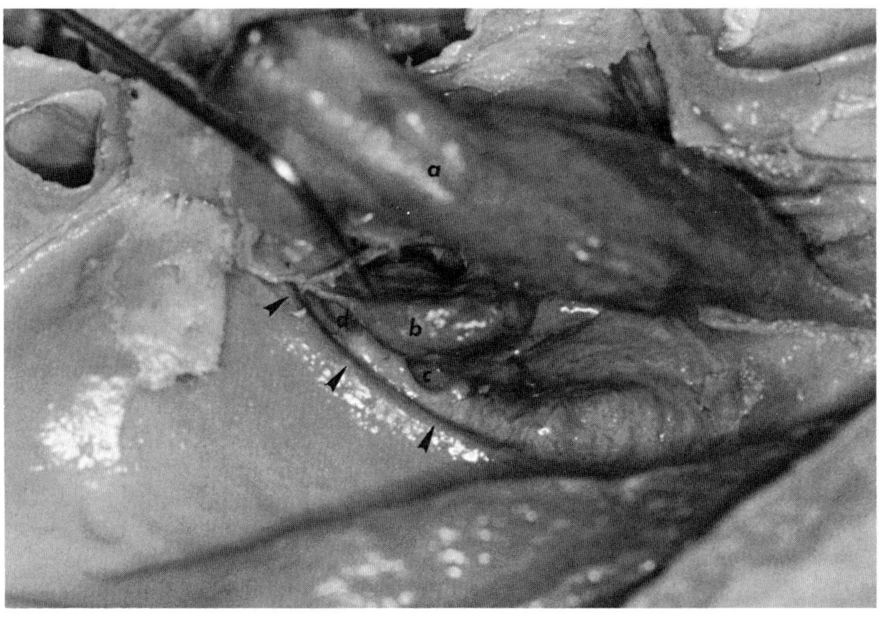

Figure 12–2. *A cadaver view of the lateral nasal wall. a indicates the middle turbinate that is elevated;* b, *the ethmoid bulla;* c, *the ostium of the maxillary sinus;* d, *the ostium of the nasal frontal duct, and infundibular area* (arrow).

The Ethmoid Sinus

The ethmoid bone is shaped like a cross. The crista galli forms the superior extension of the cross, and it extends into the anterior cranial fossa. The inferior extension forms the perpendicular plate of the nasal septum. The horizontal projections form the cribriform plate to which are attached, bilaterally, a body of air cells called the ethmoid labyrinth (Fig. 12–3). The average adult dimensions of the ethmoid labyrinth is 4 to 5 cm in length, 2.5 to 3 cm in height, and 0.5 cm in width anteriorly and 1.5 cm in width posteriorly.[4]

The ethmoid air cells begin their development during the fifth month in utero. The cells that develop in the ethmoid bone itself are called intramural cells, and those that invade other bones such as the frontal, sphenoid, and maxilla are called extramural air cells.

A thin plate of bone forms the medial wall of the orbit. This plate is called the lamina papyracea. There can be dehiscences in the bone that may provide a direct passage for infection from the air cells into the orbit. The ethmoid air cells are divided into anterior and posterior air cells. The anterior cells can invade the frontal bone and supraorbital rim. These air cells have their own ostia and drain into the frontal recess and infundibular region of the middle meatus of the nose. The posterior air cells drain through their own ostia in the the superior meatus. They can grow and expand into the sphenoid sinus area (Fig. 12–4).

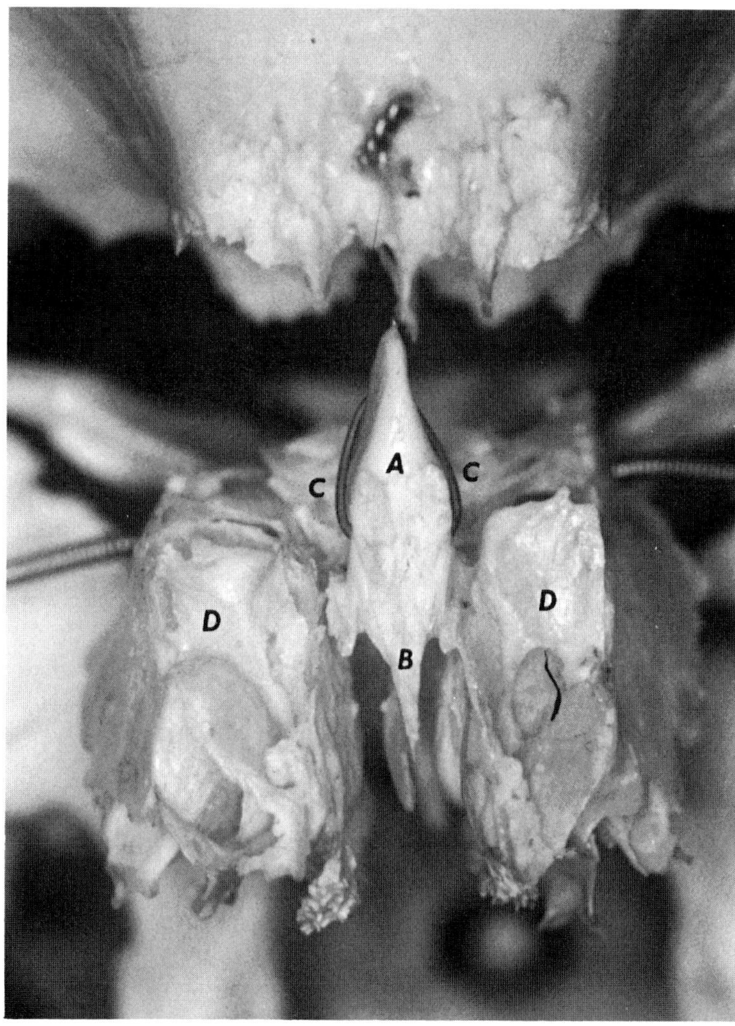

Figure 12–3. *The ethmoid bone. A indicates the crista galli; B, the perpendicular plate; C, the cribiform plate; D, the ethmoid labyrinth.*

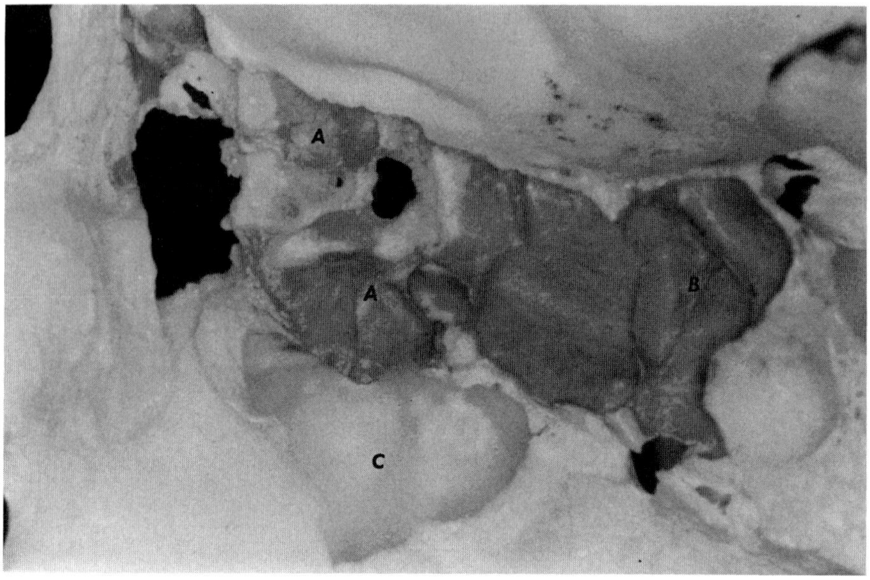

Figure 12–4. *The lateral wall of the nasal cavity. A indicates anterior ethmoid air cells; B, posterior ethmoid air cells; C, superior portion of the maxillary sinus.*

The Frontal Sinus

The frontal sinus develops from an evagination in the frontal recess of the nasal cavity into the frontal bone at 3 to 4 months during fetal life. Anterior ethmoid air cells may also be responsible for the formation of the frontal sinus by invading the frontal bone. About the age of 6 years, the frontal sinus becomes radiographically evident. The average adult frontal sinus is 28 mm in height, 27 mm in width, and 17 mm in depth.[1] The frontal sinus is divided into two sinuses by a variably positioned septum, making the sinuses asymmetrical. The frontal sinus drains through the nasal frontal duct or occasionally through an ostium directly into the nasal cavity (Fig. 12–5). The nasal frontal duct can be serpentine in its pathway to the nasal cavity—the result of growth and expansion of the anterior ethmoidal air cells.[5] The nasal frontal opening is located in the middle meatus (Fig. 12–6). The posterior table of the frontal sinus can be thin, which may allow for erosion of the bone and spread of infection from the sinus intracranially.

The Sphenoid Sinus

The sphenoid sinus is a paired sinus separated by a complete bony septum and is located in the center of the skull (Fig. 12–7). The sphenoid sinus drains through an ostium located high above the floor of the sinus, which drains into sphenoethmoidal recess in the superior nasal meatus. The sphenoid sinus is almost round in shape. The average adult cavity is 14 × 14 × 12 mm with the anteroposterior dimension being the shortest.[1]

The sphenoid sinus is surrounded by many important structures, including the cavernous sinus, pituitary gland, optic nerves, and frontal lobes of the brain (Fig. 12–8).

RADIOLOGY OF THE PARANASAL SINUSES

Conventional Radiology

The use of conventional radiography for the evaluation of uncomplicated sinus disease and facial trauma is still useful today. Clinical evaluation plus conventional radiography provide the information necessary to make the diagnosis of sinus disease in most conditions. When clinical evaluation and conventional radiography are unable to correlate and confirm the diagnosis of sinus disease, when the clinical findings indicate the spread of infection beyond the paranasal sinuses, or when the plain radiographs reveal a mass that is expanding or destroying bone, computed tomography (CT) is indicated.[6]

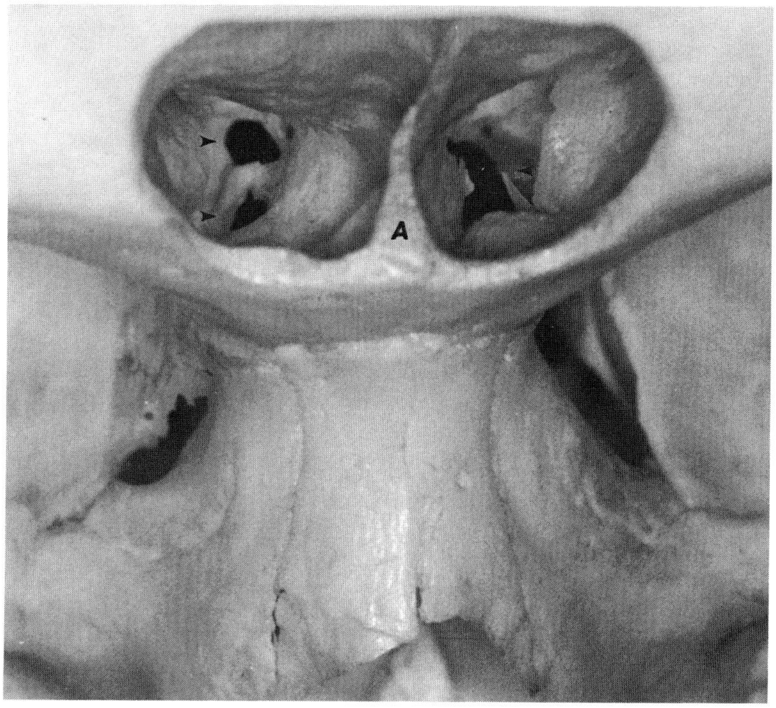

Figure 12–5. *Axial view of the frontal sinuses. A indicates septum, and the arrow indicates the nasal frontal ostia.*

The Waters' radiograph is the single most important view for evaluating sinus disease and facial trauma. The technique gives an unobstructed view of the maxillary sinuses by positioning the patient's head so the petrous ridges of the temporal bones are not superimposed over the sinuses (Fig. 12–9).

The Caldwell[7] view is designed to provide a clear view of the frontal and ethmoid sinuses without superimposition of portions of the sphenoid bone, and it differs from the Waters' radiograph by obstructing the maxillary sinuses from view by superimposition of the petrous ridges of the temporal bone (Fig. 12–10).

The lateral view of the head is particularly good for evaluating the frontal and sphenoid sinuses. The lateral view provides information about the anteroposterior (AP) depth of the frontal sinuses, fractures of the outer table of the frontal sinuses, and the degree of pneumatization of the sphenoid sinuses. In the lateral projection, shadows of opposing sinuses and other bony and soft tissue structures are superimposed, making diagnosis of unilateral sinus disease difficult (Fig. 12–7).[8]

The submentovertex radiograph is made to evaluate the sphenoid sinuses and the foramina of the base of the skull (Fig. 12–11). A modified submentovertex view that is underexposed is the best view for evaluation of fractures of the zygomatic arches.

The panoramic radiograph is particularly useful for evaluation of the degree of pneumatization of the maxillary sinuses and its relationship to the maxillary teeth (Fig. 12–12). The panoramic radiograph adequately shows mucus retention cysts, odontogenic cysts, and fibroosseous lesions. The panoramic view, however, is not as useful a diagnostic tool of maxillary sinusitis as is the Waters' view.

Computed Tomography

Computed tomography offers improvement in contrast resolution over conventional radiography and pluridirectional tomography.[9] CT scans give a simultaneous display of air, bone, and soft tissues with high-spatial resolution, making it superior to conventional tomography.[10] This makes it ideal for evaluating the paranasal sinuses. CT scanning is performed on the axial, coronal, and sagittal planes. The axial plane is the easiest to obtain. The coronal plane requires the patient to hyperextend the neck. This scan may be

Text Continued on Page 232

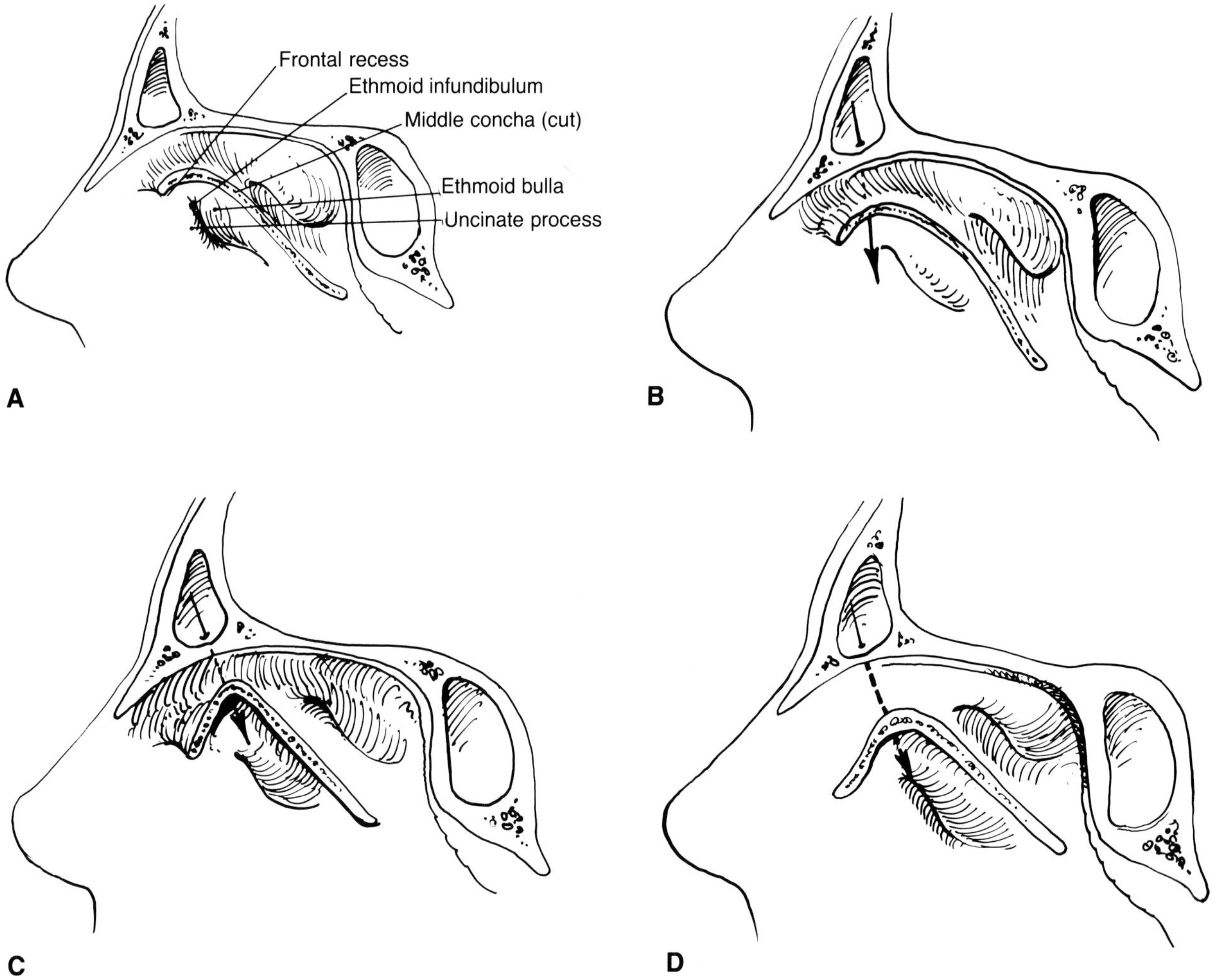

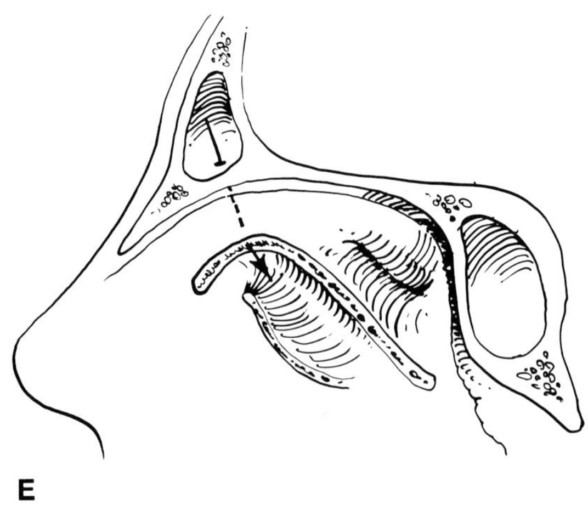

Figure 12–6. *Variations in the location of the opening of the frontal sinus.* **A** *shows the general anatomy depicted in these diagrams. The remainder of the diagrams show the approximate percentages and variation in drainage of the frontal sinuses.* **B** *shows drainage into the frontal recess anterior to the infundibulum;* **C**, *drainage above but not into the infundibulum;* **D**, *drainage into the infundibulum;* **E**, *drainage above the bulla. (Adapted from Hollinshead HW. Anatomy for surgeons: the head and neck, vol. 1 ed 2. p. 286. New York: Harper & Row, 1968)*

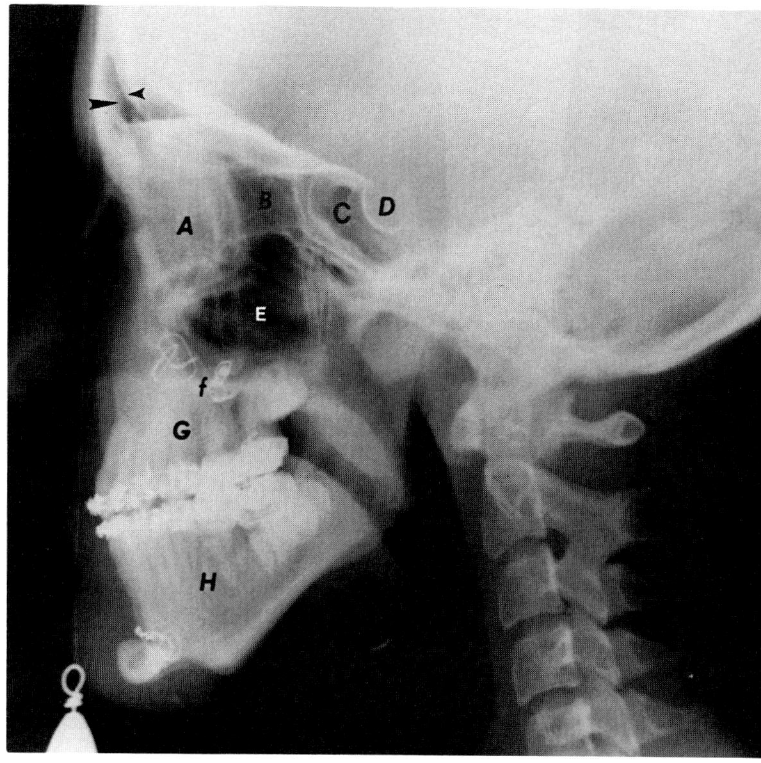

Figure 12–7. *Structures viewed in lateral view: frontal sinuses* (large arrow) *and inner table of frontal sinus* (small arrow). *A indicates orbits; B, ethmoid sinuses; C, sphenoid sinuses; D, sella tursica; E, maxillary sinuses; F, palate; G, maxilla; H, mandible.*

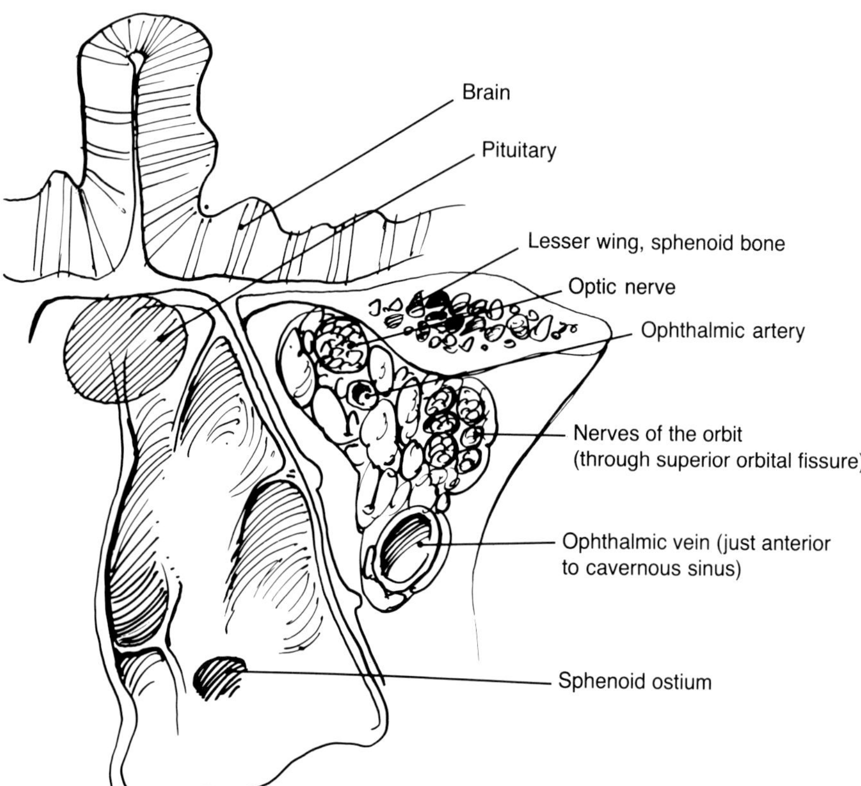

Figure 12–8. *The sphenoid sinus cut coronally at the apex of the orbit. Note the close approximation of the sphenoid to the optic nerve and ophthalmic artery, the ophthalmic vein just anterior to the cavernous sinus, the brain, and the pituitary gland, which sits in the sella tursica superior to the sphenoid sinus and is depicted by the circular broken line.*

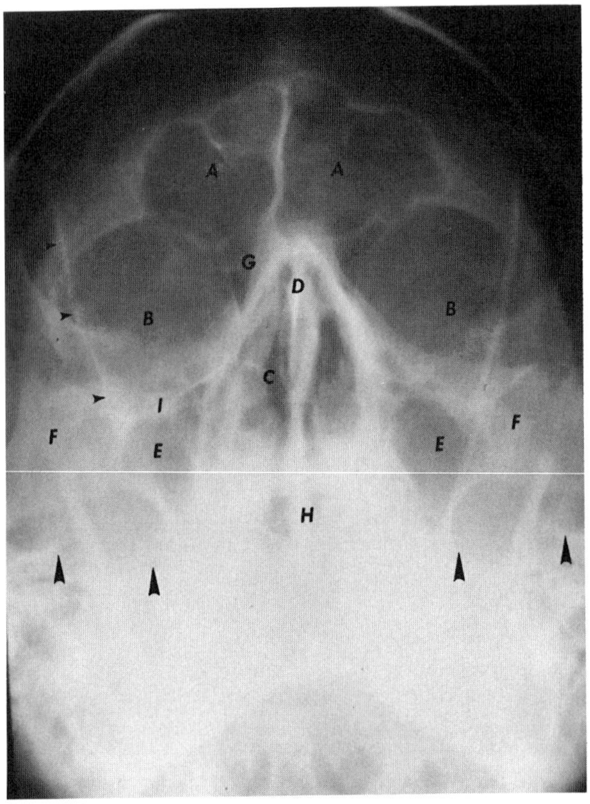

Figure 12–9. *Structures viewed in Waters' view. A indicates frontal sinuses; B, orbits; C, nasal cavity; D, nasal septum; E, maxillary sinuses; F, zygomas; G, ethmoid sinuses; H, sphenoid sinuses; I, infraorbital foramen; small arrows, temporal line (linea innominata); large arrows, petrous ridge.*

difficult to obtain on the patient who has a fractured neck or severe arthritis. The sagittal view requires a large gantry and special set-up.[11] The combination of axial and coronal views gives excellent details of the paranasal sinuses. Reconstructed CT images provide less than optimal delineation of facial structure, but they can be used for patients who are unable to hyperextend their neck for a coronal view and when sagittal views are technically not possible.

Contrast enhancement is often used with CT, but it is not particularly helpful in the evaluation of the paranasal sinuses because there is equal enhancement of tumor and normal soft tissue. When intracranial extension of a lesion is suspected, clinically or by plain CT scans, contrast increases the identification of the interface between the tumor and normal brain tissue.[12] The use of fast scanners and contrast may be useful in identifying vascular lesions. Other advantages of con-

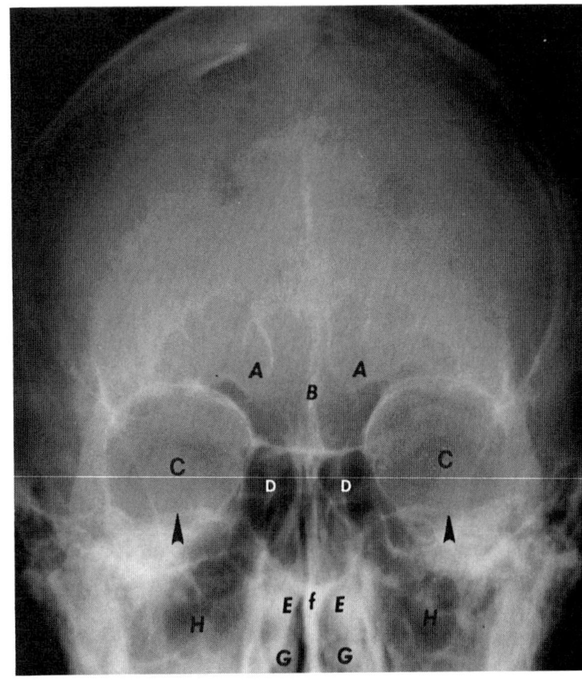

Figure 12–10. *Structures viewed in a Caldwell view. A indicates frontal sinuses; B, frontal septum; C, orbits; D, ethmoid sinuses; E, nasal cavity; F, nasal septum; G, turbinates; H, maxillary sinuses obstructed by petrous ridge (arrows).*

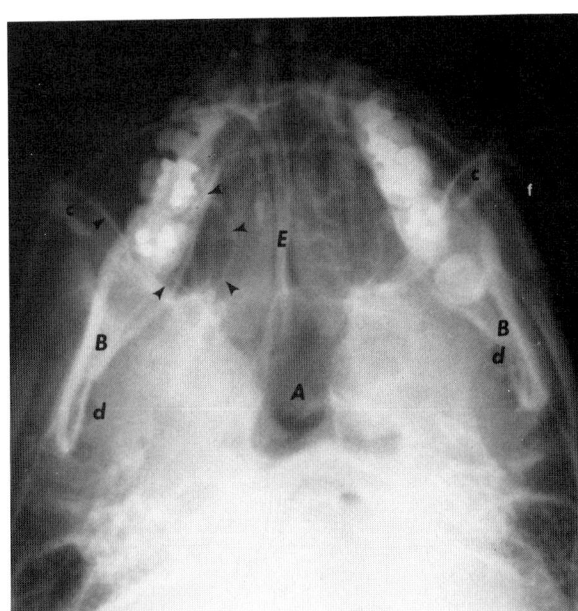

Figure 12–11. *Structures viewed in a submentovertex projection. A indicates sphenoid sinus; B, rami of mandible; c, buttress of zygoma; d, foramen ovale; E, nasal septum; f, zygomatic arch; small arrows, outline of orbit.*

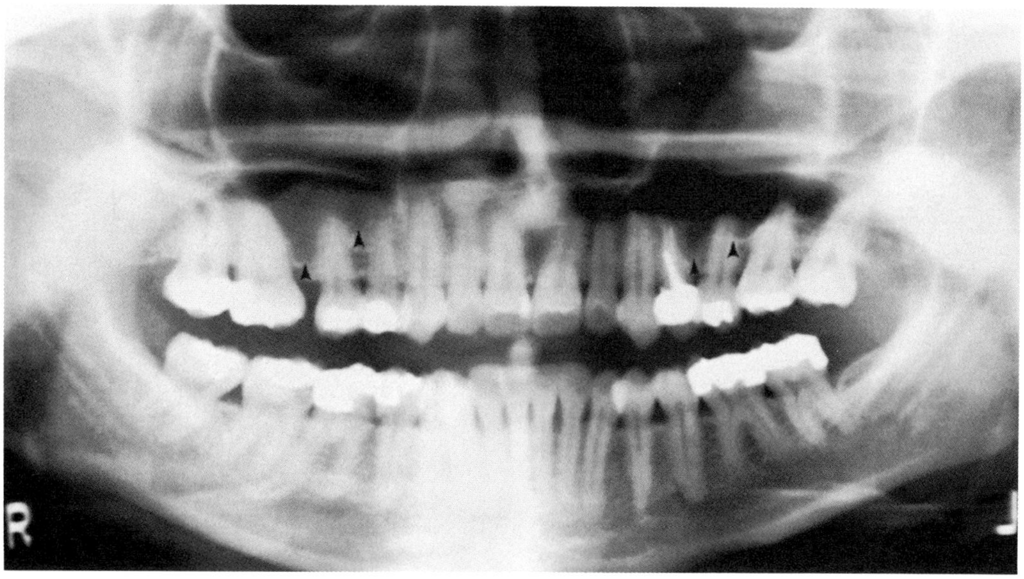

Figure 12–12. *A panoramic view shows bilateral pneumatized maxillary sinuses, especially in the bicuspid region where the sinus reaches the crest of the alveolar ridge* (small arrows). *A pseudocyst can be seen in the right maxillary premolar region.*

gic pansinusitis, whereas bacterial sinusitis is more trast administration include differentiation of fluid from solid tissue within the sinus, demonstration of inhomogeneity of a mass resulting from necrosis or formation of a cyst or abscess, and improved delineation of normal orbital structures when they are displaced.[6]

The mucosa of the sinuses is in such close approximation to the bone that the mucosa cannot be seen on CT scans. Any bulge of soft tissue seen in the sinus is abnormal and may represent mucosal inflammation, hematoma, cysts, polyps, or tumors.[13] Figures 12–13 and 12–14 represent normal axial and coronal CT scans of the paranasal sinuses and associated landmarks.

Radiographic Survey Of Pathology Of The Paranasal Sinuses

Allergy in the form of hay fever may result in rhinitis and lead to secondary changes in the maxillary sinuses as a result of obstruction of their ostia.[3] Swelling of the nasal turbinates may be seen radiographically in allergic rhinitis. Allergic sinusitis is more likely to cause bilateral sinusitis (especially maxillary) or even aller-likely to be unilateral. Allergy may cause polyp formation in the antral mucosa. These polyps can develop to such a large size that they extend through the ostia into the nasal cavity. Because the ostium is far back in the hiatus semilunaris, the polyps fall back through the posterior choana, producing antrochoanal polyps.[14] Air fluid levels are rarely seen in allergic disease,[15] whereas they are more commonly seen in bacterial sinusitis and trauma (Fig. 12–15). Mucosal thickening is also seen in bacterial sinusitis. Simple antral sinusitis almost never results in an airless sinus.[15] When this is seen, some other cause should be suspected, such as mucocele, a large polyp, fungal infection, or a tumor (Fig. 12–16). Chronic sinusitis often is first seen radiographically with thickened or sclerotic bone (Fig. 12–17). A long history of sinusitis, chronic pain, and exacerbations of subacute sinusitis may help to determine if the chronic sinusitis is active.

Cysts and cyst-like processes arising from the sinus mucosa may be classified as pseudocysts, retention cysts, and mucoceles.[16] Pseudocysts are formed by the accumulation of fluid beneath the mucoperiosteum, which lifts off the bone and floor of the sinus to form the characteristic dome-shaped structure that is commonly seen on panographic radiographs (Fig. 12–18).

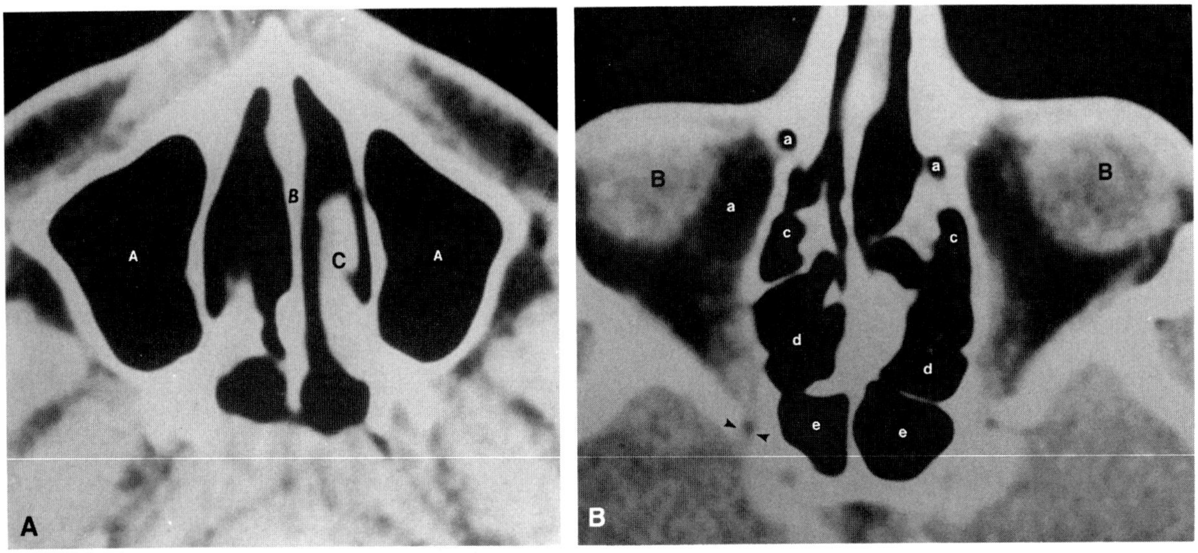

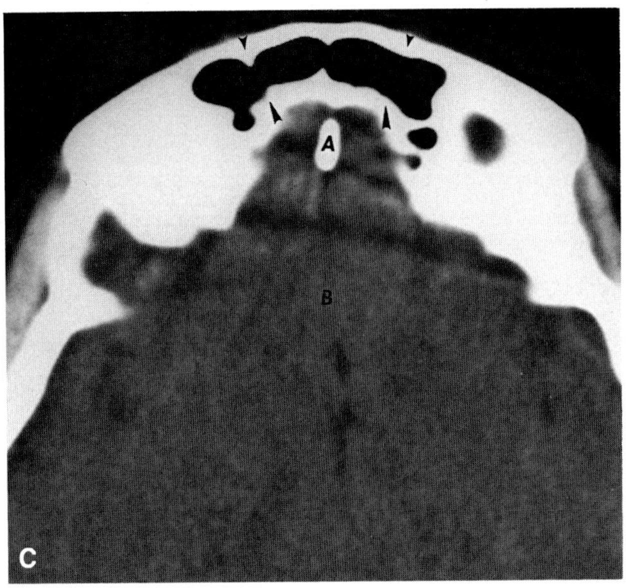

Figure 12–13. (**A**) *Axial computed tomographic (CT) view of the maxillary sinuses.* a *indicates maxillary sinus;* B, *nasal septum;* C, *turbinate (soft tissue window).* (**B**) *Axial view of the ethmoid and sphenoid sinuses.* a *indicates nasolacrimal canal;* b, *globes;* c, *anterior ethmoid air cells;* d, *posterior ethmoid air cells;* e, *sphenoid sinuses with septum; small arrows, optic canal (soft tissue window).* (**C**) *Axial view of the frontal sinuses.* A *indicates crista galli;* B, *brain; small arrows, anterior table; medium arrows, posterior table of frontal sinuses (soft tissue window).*

The histologic appearance of the wall of a pseudocyst is that of normal or inflamed antral lining. The pathogenesis of polyps of the sinonasal tract is probably similar. Polyps form by accumulation of fluid in the loose connective tissue of the lamina propria. The clinical difference between the two lesions is that the sinus mucosa associated with the polyp is thickened by edema and is not in a pseudocyst. Pseudocysts are typically dome-shaped, whereas polyps are often pendulous or irregular in shape. Polyps can be surgically removed intact, whereas pseudocysts burst. Polyps are often multiple, whereas pseudocysts are usually solitary but can be bilateral. Pseudocysts are harmless and generally require no treatment. Periapical and periodontal disease may play a significant role in the origin of maxillary pseudocysts.[17] If there is suspicion that odontogenic disease may be the cause of a pseudocyst, vitality testing of the suspected teeth should be performed. Elimination of the dental disease may result in resolution of the pseudocyst.

Retention cysts are caused by blockage and subsequent dilation of ducts of the seromucinous glands of

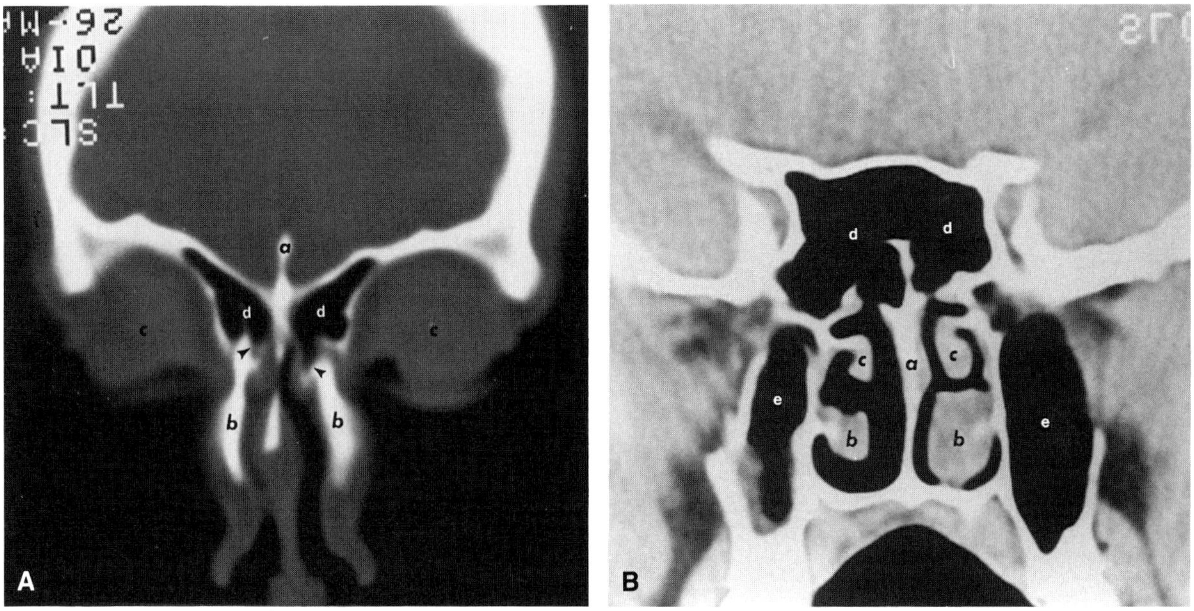

Figure 12–14. *(**A**) Coronal (CT) view of the frontal sinuses. A indicates crista galli; b, frontal processes of the maxilla; c, globes; d, frontal sinuses; small arrows, nasofrontal ostia (bone window). (**B**) Coronal CT view of the sphenoid sinuses. a indicates vomer; b, inferior turbinates; c, middle turbinates; d, sphenoid sinuses; e, posterior portion of the maxillary sinuses (soft tissue window).*

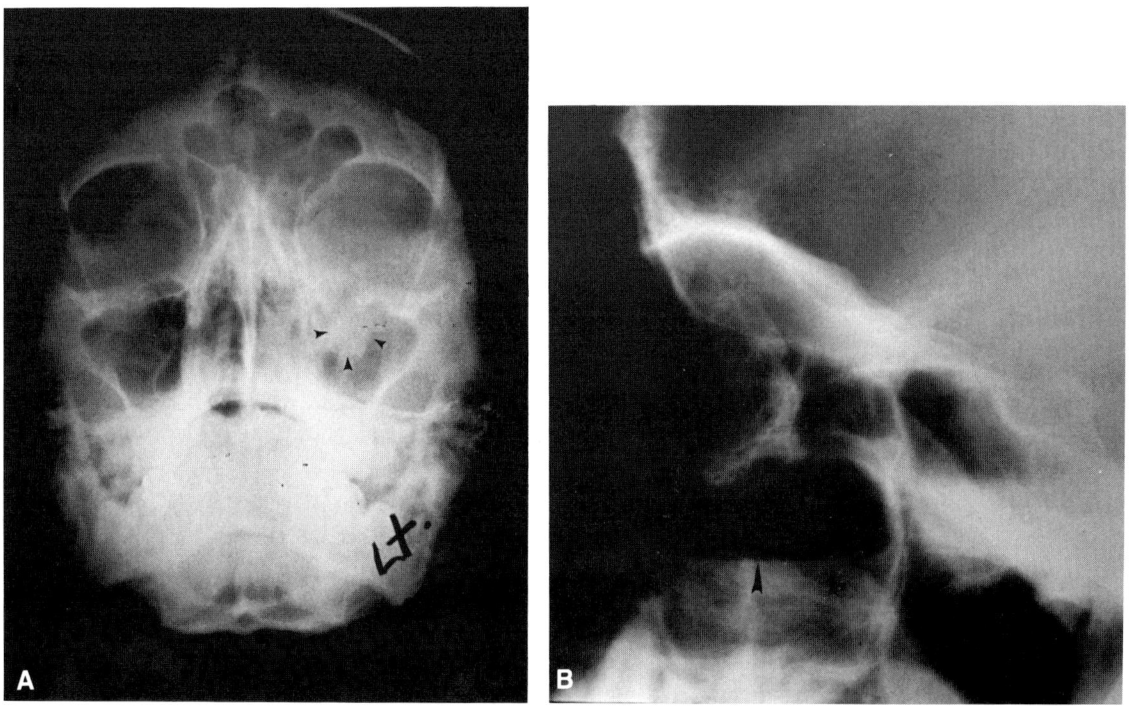

Figure 12–15. *(**A**) Cloudy left maxillary antrum as a result of an orbital blow-out fracture. Small arrows outline orbital contents hanging into the sinus. (**B**) Lateral view showing air-fluid level of the maxillary sinuses. Arrows mark the height of the fluid level.*

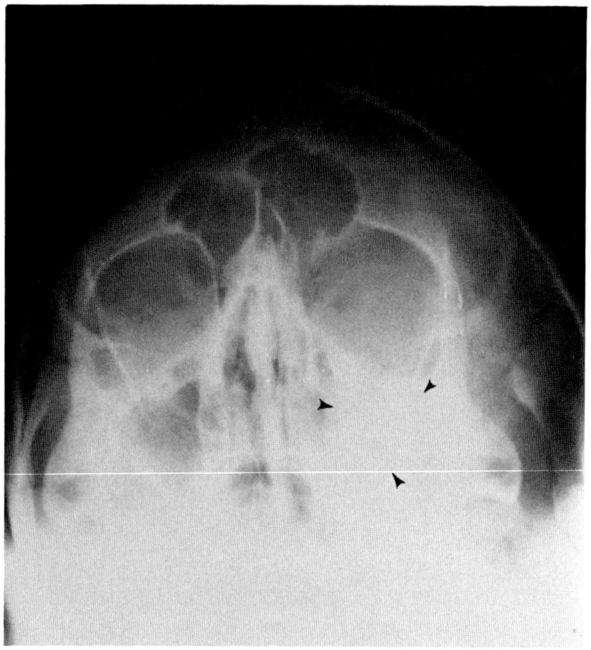

Figure 12–16. *Waters' view showing complete opacification of the left maxillary sinus as a result of aspergillosis. The patient sustained a left zygoma fracture that was repaired by open reduction and internal fixation 1 year prior to developing aspergillosis.*

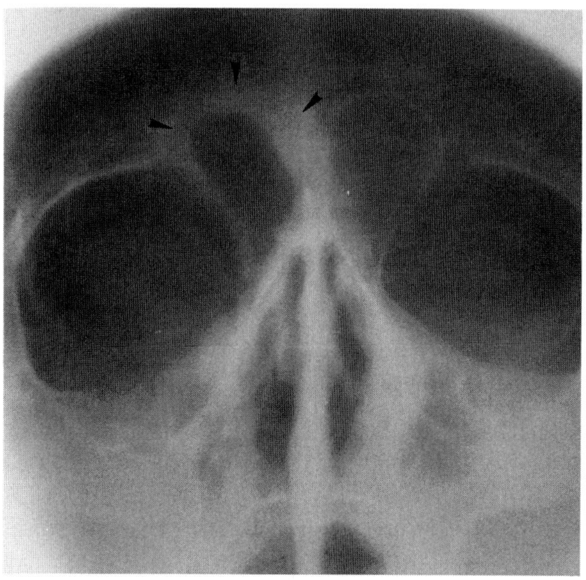

Figure 12–17. *Waters' view showing chronic sinusitis of the maxillary sinuses and the right frontal sinus. Note the sclerotic bony margin of the right frontal sinus indicative of chronic sinusitis.*

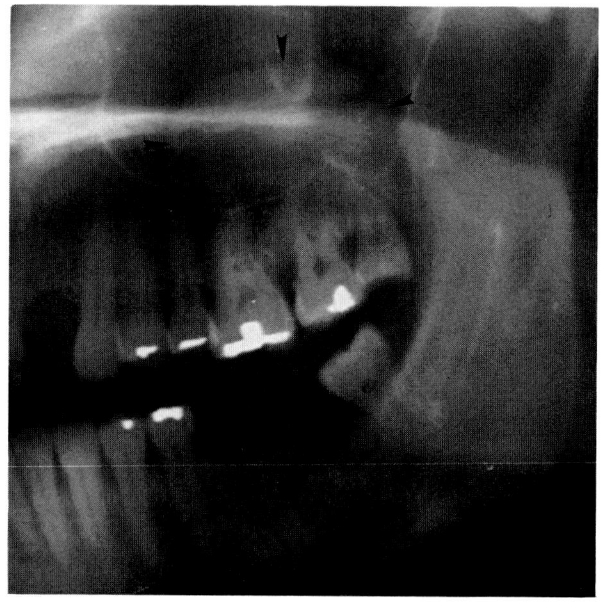

Figure 12–18. *A panoramic view showing a pseudocyst of the maxillary antrum.*

the sinus and are consequently lined with epithelium.[16] The cysts are small, occur in inflamed mucosa, and may be found with antral polyps. They are seldom seen on radiographs.

Mucoceles of the paranasal sinuses are well-recognized lesions that most commonly occur in the frontal sinuses, less frequently in the ethmoid sinuses, and rarely in the maxillary sinuses.[18] Som and Shugar[19] reported that 10% of the mucoceles in their study occurred in the maxillary sinus. Mucoceles are expansive and potentially destructive lesions, which differentiates them from pseudocysts. They form when the sinus ostium is obstructed. However, the majority of antral mucoceles are of the primary type of mucocele—resulting from inflammation, allergy, or malignant disease. A postoperative mucocele that only partially fills the antrum and has a different appearance can occur after a Caldwell-Luc operation. Radiographically, in its initial stages of development, an antral mucocele appears as a completely clouded, airless sinus with normal sinus walls (Fig. 12–19). As a mucocele expands, it can cause bony erosion and destruction. CT enhancement can be used to differentiate a mucocele from a slowly growing tumor. Most tumors are enhanced to a variable degree, whereas mucoceles are

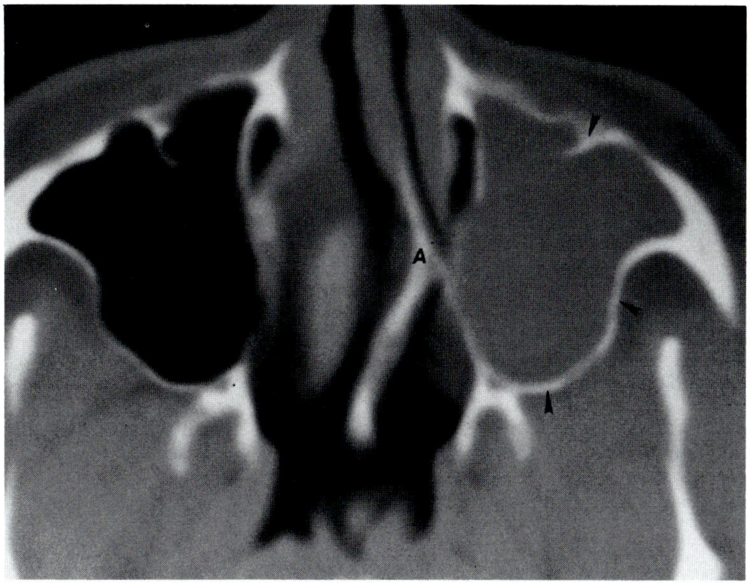

Figure 12–19. *CT scan showing complete obstruction of the maxillary antrum by a mucocele (arrows). Note the deviated nasal septum (A) obstructing the region of the sinus ostium. The patient complained of severe headaches, which resolved immediately after surgical removal of the mucocele.*

not. A pyocele, an infected mucocele, is enhanced at its periphery, giving a rim effect to the mass.[19]

ACUTE SINUSITIS

Maxillary

Etiology

The single most common cause of maxillary sinusitis is a viral upper respiratory tract infection. The viruses responsible for the common cold are the rhinoviruses (30%) and the coronavirus (20%).[20] Approximately 0.5% of common colds are complicated by sinus infection.[21] Rhinitis results in nasal congestion leading to narrowing or obstruction of the sinus ostium. Viral infection can also lead to sinus epithelial injury and alteration of mucociliary action. As a result of these changes, bacterial invasion occurs, resulting in sinusitis. Allergic rhinitis can also lead to similar changes, causing bacterial sinusitis.

Maxillary sinusitis can occur when the sinus membrane is violated following extraction of teeth, facial trauma, and maxillary osteotomies. Odontogenic infections of the maxillary teeth can also lead to maxillary sinusitis; the incidence of this is much lower than when the sinus is invaded by surgery or trauma. The signs and symptoms of acute maxillary sinusitis are listed in Display 12–1.

Display 12–1. Signs and Symptoms of Acute Maxillary Sinusitis

SIGNS

1. Pain on pressure over the anterior maxillary sinus wall
2. Purulent discharge over the inferior nasal turbinate
3. Fever
4. Malaise
5. Inability to work

SYMPTOMS

1. Cheek pain with referral to the frontal region
2. Increased pain on bending
3. Maxillary posterior teeth feel like "pegs"
4. Hyposomia

Patients with head injuries or who are critically ill may develop sinusitis when nasally intubated for prolonged periods.[22–24] Many of these patients may have facial fractures involving the sinuses, which may compound the problem of extended nasal intubation. The exact length of time before sinusitis develops is not specified but 1 week seems critical. The diagnosis of sinusitis is difficult because of the lack of clinical signs. Evidence of mucopurulent drainage from the nose may help diagnose sinusitis, but by the time this appears, seeding of bacteria to other areas may have occurred. Septic shock, meningitis, and intracranial infection can result from the sinusitis. Isolated maxillary sinusitis may occur, but pansinusitis may also develop. Obstruction of the sinus ostium by a large bore nasotracheal tube is thought to be the cause. Oral intubation prevents this occurrence, and tracheostomy is indicated when prolonged airway management is necessary. Early diagnosis, removal of the nasal tube, and medical treatment corrects the sinusitis.

Systemic disorders such as allergy, Kartagener's syndrome, cystic fibrosis, and immunodeficiency may lead to sinusitis. Kartagener's syndrome consists of situs inversus, bronchietasis, and sinusitis. It appears to result from a structural defect of the cilia. Other causes of ciliary structural abnormality are primary ciliary dyskinesia, immotile cilia syndrome,[20,25] and retinitis pigmentosa.[26] Nasal and bronchial biopsy are performed to confirm these diseases. Cystic fibrosis with its highly viscous mucus secretion and development of nasal polyps may lead to sinusitis, particularly in children.[27] Immunocompromised patients have a quantitative deficit of neutrophils. The more profound the neutropenia, the greater the incidence of bacterial and fungal infections.[28]

Microbiology

The pathogens commonly isolated from the antrum in acute sinusitis are *Haemophilus influenza* and *Streptococcus pneumoniae*.[29–31] One study states that these two bacteria account for over half the cases of maxillary sinusitis.[32] *Haemophilus influenzae*, *Streptococcus pneumoniae*, and *Branhamella catarrhalis* are commonly isolated in children with acute maxillary sinusitis.[27,33,34] *Streptococcus pyogenes* is occasionally found in acute maxillary sinusitis. The incidence of anaerobes cultured in acute maxillary sinusitis varies greatly, being present in none to 23% of cases.[30]

The role of *Staphylococcus aureus* in sinusitis is now considered to be much less significant than in the past. In one study[35] *Staphylococcus aureus* was found in the nasal cavities of approximately one third of the subjects. Earlier studies that used the nasal swab technique for culturing purposes in acute sinusitis resulted in a higher percentage of staphylococcus isolates. Recent studies that use needle-aspirate techniques for culturing sinuses show that the incidence of staphylococcus as a major pathogen in sinusitis has diminished.

Anaerobic and facultative bacteria are commonly isolated in chronic sinusitis or in sinusitis resulting from dental infections.[36,37] The lowering of the oxygen content and pH of the sinus cavity supports the growth of anaerobic organisms by providing them with optimal oxidative-reduction potential as a result of ostial obstruction.[38] The common anaerobic bacteria, listed in their order of frequency, are: anaerobic cocci, *Bacteroides* species (including *B. melaninogenicus* and *B. fragilis*), *Propionibacterium acnes*, and *Fusobacterium* species. Common facultative bacteria are: α-hemolytic streptococci, *Staphylococcus aureus*, and *Streptococcus pyogenes*.[37] These findings also apply to children with chronic maxillary sinusitis. Antibiotic management must be directed at this variety of bacteria. The increasing emergence of β-lactamase–producing *Bacteroides* species (other than *Bacteroides fragilis*) and the presence of resistant *Staphylococcus aureus* requires that alternatives to penicillin be used.

Ethmoid Sinusitis

Acute ethmoid sinusitis is seen more commonly in children than adults. The microbiologic characteristics are similar to that found in maxillary sinusitis. *Haemophilus influenzae* and *Branhamella catarrhalis* should be suspected in children under the age of 6 years. Fever and irritability are often associated with ethmoiditis in children. Blood cultures appear to be more accurate in identifying the offending microorganisms associated with ethmoiditis in children than in adults. The most common cause of orbital cellulitis in children is acute ethmoiditis. Orbital complications are usually unilateral but may be bilateral.[39] Extraocular motility may be somewhat limited. Mucopurulent discharge may be present intranasally. Orbital cellulitis occurs more commonly in children under the age of 6 years, but more severe orbital involvement, although less common, occurs in older children and young adults.

Frontal Sinusitis

Acute frontal sinusitis can be a serious condition. The clinical signs of acute frontal sinusitis may be severe frontal pain, tenderness, or pain during palpation over the frontal bone; redness, swelling, or fluctuation of the soft tissue over the frontal bone; and purulent exudate in the nasal cavity. Radiographic evidence of cloudiness, thickened sinus membranes, and air fluid levels help confirm the diagnosis of frontal sinusitis. The microorganisms of acute frontal sinusitis are similar to the other paranasal sinus infections. Extension of frontal sinus infections can lead to orbital cellulitis and abscess, cavernous sinus thrombosis, subdural and brain abscess, meningitis, and osteomyelitis. These complications are discussed later.

Sphenoid Sinusitis

Lew reported that headache is the most common initial symptom of acute sphenoid sinusitis.[40] The headache is usually unilateral and involves the frontal, temporal, or occipital region. Lew stresses that severe headache that interferes with sleep and is not relieved by aspirin may be an early diagnostic sign. Pain or paresthesia over one of the branches of the trigeminal nerve may occur. Fever is often present. A purulent discharge is frequently found in the middle and superior tubinate region. Patients may be lethargic or comatose. The changes in neurologic status or pain or paresthesia of the trigeminal pathways indicate extension of infection beyond the sphenoid sinus into the brain or cavernous sinus. CT scanning is the most useful tool in the diagnosis of sphenoid sinusitis. *Streptococcus pneumoniae* combined with other streptococcal species is the most common microorganism isolated. *Staphylococcus aureus* is also frequently cultured.

Management of Acute Sinusitis

Medical therapy is the primary treatment for acute sinusitis in children and adults. Antibiotic therapy appears to be the most important ingredient for successful management of acute sinusitis. Systemic and topical decongestants are administered in the management of sinusitis to shrink the boggy nasal and sinus mucosa and, in doing so, to increase the patency of the ostia of the sinuses. Pain control may be required. In the patient with atopic conditions, management of rhinitis by an allergist may be necessary to help prevent or contain the development of sinusitis.

The aminopenicillins are effective against many of the organisms commonly isolated in acute and chronic sinusitis, including *Haemophilus* organisms, *Branhamella* organisms, *Streptococcus pneumoniae*, α- and β-hemolytic streptococci, and *Peptostreptococcus*, *Peptococcus*, *Fusobacterium*, and *Bacteroides* species. The aminopenicillins ampicillin and amoxicillin are not effective against most *Staphylococcus* organisms. Additionally, many strains of *H. influenzae* are also resistant. The addition of β-lactamase inhibitors increases the activity of ampicillin and amoxicillin against these two bacteria. Amoxicillin with clavulanate (Augmentin) is the drug of choice for oral use and ampicillin with sulbactam (Unasyn) is the drug of choice for parenteral use.

In patients who are allergic to penicillin, alternative choices for acute sinusitis treatment include trimethoprim-sulfamethoxazole (Bactrim and Septra), and cefaclor (Ceclor). Trimethoprim-sulfamethoxazole and cefaclor are effective against *Haemophilus influenzae* and *Streptococcus pneumonia*. The response of acute sinusitis to ampicillin, amoxicillin, cefaclor, and trimethoprim-sulfamethoxazole is similar.[32,41] The length of time for the administration of antibiotics in acute sinusitis is controversial, but most clinicians suggest a minimum of 10 days of antibiotic therapy is necessary. All patients should undergo radiographic follow-up to evaluate the efficacy of therapy. The patient must be clinically asymptomatic despite the persistence of high titers of bacteria in the sinus.[31]

Systemic decongestants reduce the edema of the nasal mucosa in the acute stages of rhinitis secondary to a cold or allergy. They are commonly prescribed in combination with an antibiotic to help maintain the patency of the sinus ostium when the sinus membrane

Display 12–2. Medical Management of Acute Sinusitis

ANTIBIOTIC	SYSTEMIC DECONGESTANT	TOPICAL DECONGESTANT
Amoxicillin	Dimetapp Extendtabs	Afrin
Augmentin®	Entex L A	Otrivin
Bactrim or Septra®		
Ceclor®		

has been violated during the extraction of teeth. This may prevent the development of an oral-antral fistula. Dimetapp Extendtabs (brompheniramine, phenylephrine, and phenylpropanolamine) and Entex L A (phenylpropanolamine and guaifenesin) are typical systemic decongestants. Dimetapp produces a drying effect on secretions, whereas Entex produces a thinning effect on secretions. Both have their advocates. Most decongestants contain an antihistaminic that produces varying degrees of sedation, and the sympathomimetic may elevate the blood pressure further in hypertensive patients. Systemic decongestants should be used prudently.

Topical decongestants such as Neo-Synephrine (phenylephrine), Afrin (oxymetazoline), and Otrivin (zylometazoline) are commonly used. Neo-Synephrine's duration of action is approximately 1 hour, whereas Afrin and Otrivin last approximately 6 hours. Topical decongestants should be used for approximately 3 days and then discontinued. Overuse can result in rebound nasal congestion or rhinitis medicamentosa with extensive use (Display 12–2).

Steam inhalation may also be effective in the management of sinusitis. The steam helps liquefy and mobilize tenacious nasal mucus, and the heat helps cause vasoconstriction.[20]

If there is no evidence of improvement of sinusitis, needle aspiration of the sinus through the lateral wall of the nose under the inferior turbinate or through the canine fossa is indicated to obtain material for culture. When culture and sensitivity results become available, an appropriate antibiotic can be selected. Antral lavage may be performed at the same time as aspiration. If signs of worsening or extension of the infection beyond the antrum or other sinuses is evident, surgical intervention is indicated. A transnasal antral window or a Caldwell-Luc procedure with a nasal antral window in maxillary sinusitis is indicated. Frontal sinus trephination (Fig. 12–20) is indicated in nonresponsive or worsening frontal sinusitis. External ethmoidectomy (Fig. 12–21) and transnasal sphenoidectomy is indicated when those sinuses do not respond to medical therapy or there is evidence of extension of the infection.

CHRONIC MAXILLARY SINUSITIS

Etiology

The most common cause of chronic maxillary sinusitis is the persistence of acute sinusitis or repeated bouts of acute sinusitis. Melen[42] proposed the following criteria to define chronic sinusitis:

1. Facial pain, nasal congestion, or abnormal secretions remain or reappear during a period of at least 3 months
2. Sinus radiography or sinus endoscopy reveals persistent localized or generalized mucosal swelling with or without secretion
3. Chronic maxillary sinusitis of rhinogenous origin that does not heal after conservative treatment consisting of one or more courses of antibiotics of 10 days duration, nose drops or oral decongestants, and antral lavage
4. Chronic maxillary sinusitis of dental origin that existed when oral antral fistula was present or when radiographs or examination showed an indistinct border or close connection between the diseased maxillary sinus mucosa and the apex of nonvital teeth, an inflammatory periodontal or periapical lesion, or the follicle of an impacted tooth in connection with a periodontal or periapical lesion

Cystic fibrosis, Kartagener's syndrome, large adenoids, and cleft palate may lead to chronic sinusitis in children.[43]

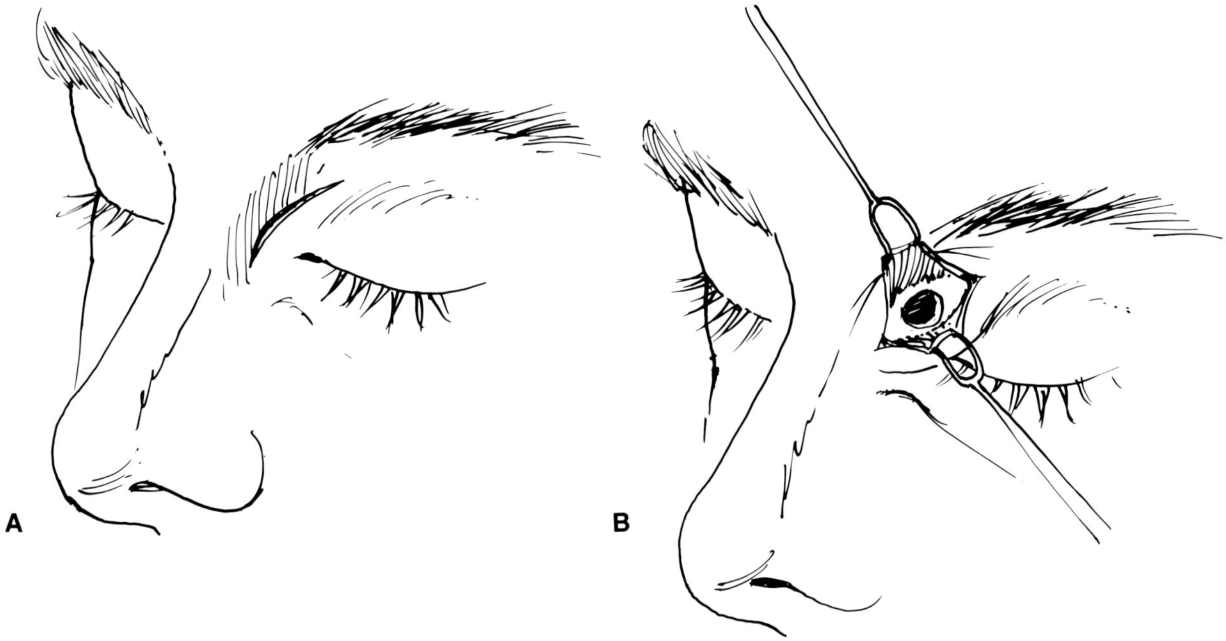

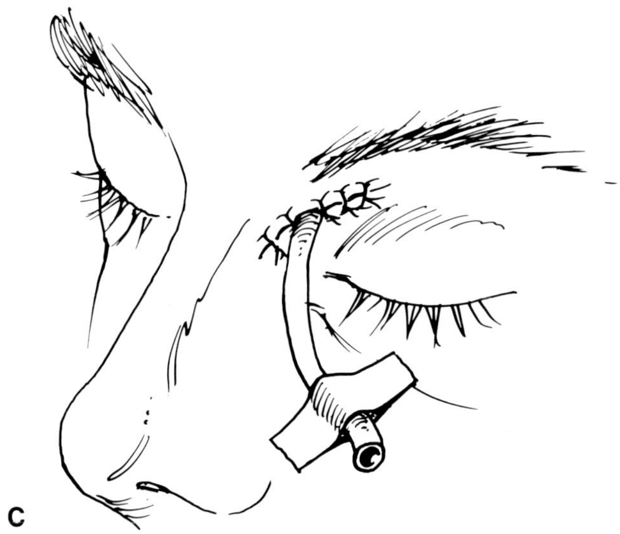

Figure 12–20. *(**A**) The incision for a frontal sinus trephination is made in the superomedial orbital rim. (**B**) A periosteal flap is reflected, and a hole is drilled at the medial supraorbital rim into the floor of the frontal sinus. (**C**) A small drain is inserted into the sinus for drainage and the incision is closed. The drain is usually removed in 2 to 3 days.*

Signs and Symptoms of Chronic Maxillary Sinusitis

In adults, chronic sinusitis may first be seen clinically with a foul nasal or postnasal discharge. Pain and pressure in the maxillary dentition and over the affected antrum may be present. Pain is not always a consistent finding in chronic maxillary sinusitis, however. If the patient has an exacerbation of acute or subacute sinusitis superimposed over chronic sinusitis, pain may be the chief complaint. Nasal stuffiness and hyposmia may be a feature of chronic sinusitis. Day and night cough may be a complaint. Dental pain may be co-existent (Display 12–3).

Children are first seen clinically with a chronic nasal discharge and nasal obstruction.[43] Young chil-

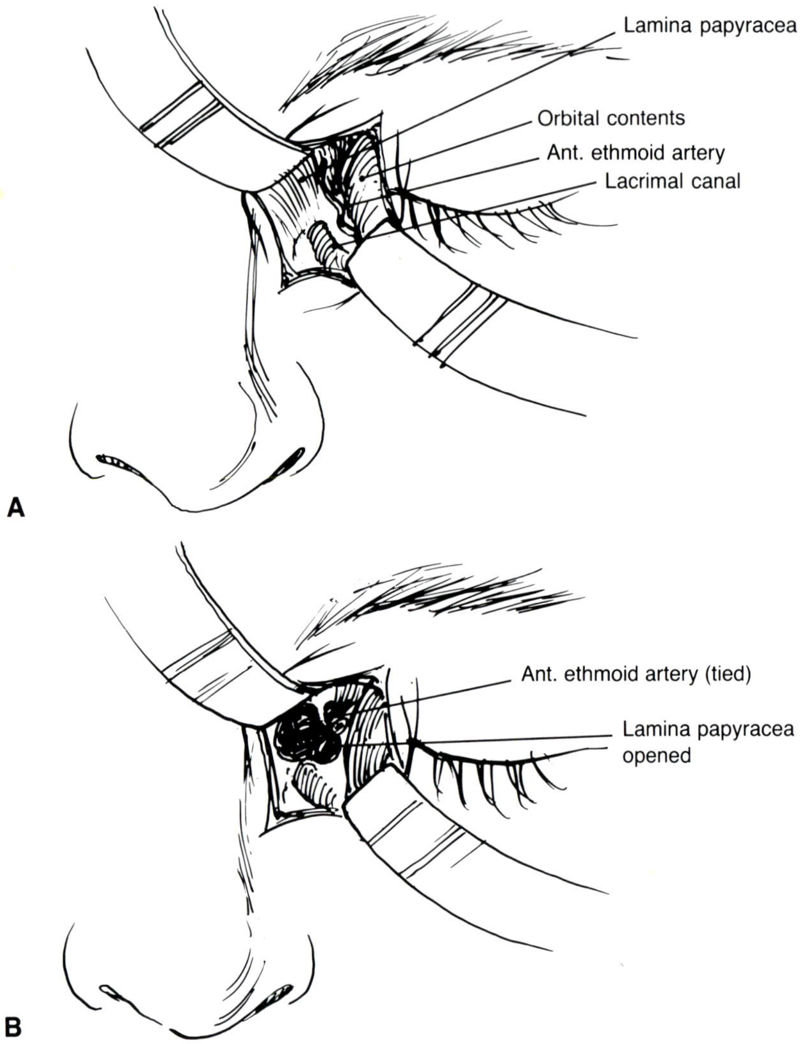

Figure 12–21. *(**A**) When performing an external ethmoidectomy, a periosteal flap is reflected posteriorly along the medial wall of the orbit while retracting the globe laterally until the anterior ethmoid artery is exposed. It is ligated and the medial wall of the ethmoid bone is exposed to the posterior ethmoid artery. (**B**) The lamina papyracea is removed and the ethmoid air cells are eradicated.*

Display 12–3. Signs and Symptoms of Chronic Maxillary Sinusitis

SIGNS	***SYMPTOMS***
Rhinorrhea	May be pain free
Postnasal drip	Pressure headaches
Day or night cough	Hyposomia
Nasal stuffiness or obstruction	Dental pain

dren rarely verbalize discomfort or pain, whereas older children may. Infection may spread to the nasolacrimal duct causing chronic dacrocystitis, and involvement of the auditory tube may induce serous or suppurative otitis media. Irritability and fatigue occur, and lymphadenopathy may be present.

Microbiology

The microorganisms found in chronic sinusitis are predominantly anaerobic.[36,37,44] The poor drainage and increased intrasinus pressure during inflammation reduces oxygen tension and provides an optimum oxidation-reduction potential for anaerobic bacteria growth.[38] In the past it was thought that the sinuses were sterile.[45] Brook, however, studied the bacterial flora in noninflamed maxillary sinuses in 12 adults.[46] He administered aseptic aspiration of the sinuses under general anesthesia. Anaerobes were isolated in all 12 patients. Of these, 42% were anaerobes and 58% were mixed flora. The mechanism by which pathologic bacteria reach the sinus is not clear. One hypothesis is that the anaerobic bacteria reach the sealed off sinus by the lymphatic or venous systems. Aerobic and anaerobic bacteria in the normal sinuses may become pathogenic when the sinus drainage is obstructed. Suppressed local host resistance as a result of low-oxygen tension leads to acute infection with aerobic bacteria such as *H. influenzae* and *S. pneumoniae* predominating. Complete lack of oxygen in the purulent stage supports the growth of anaerobes.

Sinusitis occurs secondary to dental origin in 10% of patients.[32] In these patients, mixed anaerobic infections is common. This is not surprising because odontogenic infections of periapical or periodontal origin are often of mixed aerobic and anaerobic flora. The anaerobic organisms commonly found in chronic maxillary sinusitis include microaerophilic bacteria and anaerobic *Streptococcus, Bacteroides, Viellonella, Corynebacterium,* and *Fusobacterium* species.

Actinomyces and *Nocardia* organisms are two other bacteria that may rarely infect the sinuses.[47] *Actinomyces* organisms appear to affect the maxillary sinus more often than do *Nocardia* organisms. Histologically, actinomycotic infections are granulomas of confluent nodules, in the center of which are colonies of *Actinomyces* organisms surrounded by polymorphic leukocytes, granulation tissue, and fibrous connective tissue.[44] Clinically, actinomycotic sinus infections are usually unilateral and may occur following injury or trauma to the sinuses. The patient may complain of pain or pressure over the affected sinus as in chronic sinusitis. Surgical management with a Caldwell-Luc operation and antibiotic therapy with penicillin is recommended.

Aspergillus organisms are the most common fungus found in sinus infections (Fig. 12–22).[48–52] The species involved in aspergillosis are generally *A. fumigatus* or *A. flavus.* They can be recognized histologically by their septated hyphae. They can invade the sinuses without predisposing factors such as immunosuppressive therapy. After aspergillosis, infection by *Phycomycetes* organisms, commonly *Mucor* species or *Rhizopus* species, are the next most frequent fungi to invade the sinuses. Mucormycosis is more commonly found in patients with debilitating diseases, diabetes mellitus, and other metabolic disturbances.

Mild fungal infections are treated by surgical inter-

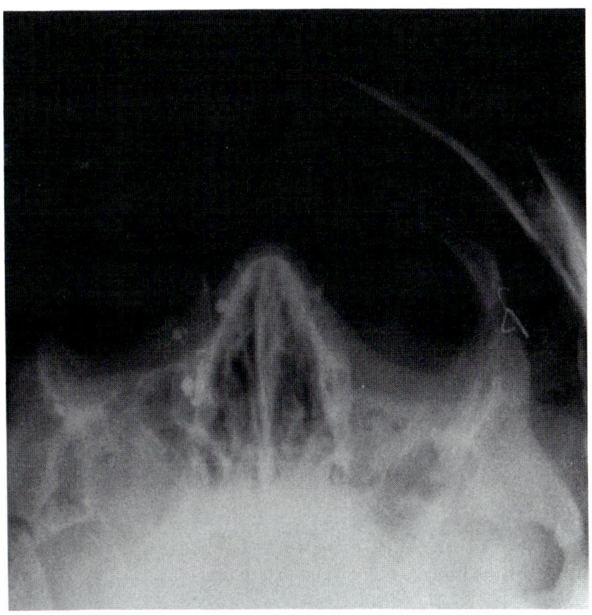

Figure 12–22. *The Waters' view shows bilateral cloudy maxillary sinuses. The right sinus had an aspergillus fungal ball removed from it at the time of surgery. The patient complained of chronic pain from the right sinus before surgery. The radiopaque material is dye from a previous dacrocytogram and the wire ligature from a previous reduction of a zygoma fracture.*

vention with the Caldwell-Luc operation. The progressively destructive and the fulminant infections require aggressive surgical management, in addition to antifungal antibiotic therapy with amphotericin B. Management of concurrent disease is absolutely necessary.

Mucormycosis occurs in many forms: pulmonary, disseminated, soft tissue, paranasal, rhinoorbital, and rhinocerebral. The latter, which is also referred to as rhinocerebral phycomycosis, includes infections of the nasal and paranasal sinuses with extension to the brain.[44] It is rarely seen in healthy individuals, but it occurs more commonly in uncontrolled diabetes mellitus, in persons undergoing immunosuppression therapy for lymphoma or leukemia, and in prolonged corticosteroid use. It is a severe illness with fever and mental deterioration. A black crusting of the nasal septum and turbinates may be seen. Weakness of the third, fourth, and sixth cranial nerves may be a feature if cavernous sinus thrombosis develops. Loss of vision can occur with extension into the orbit.

Mucomycosis is frequently fatal. However, Parfrey reported that there was a 73% survival rate of patients since 1970 as compared with 7% before 1970.[53] He attributed this to early diagnosis. Biopsy is needed to make the diagnosis, and culture is necessary to identify the species. Histologically, broad, nonseptate hyphae with right-angle branching are seen. Aggressive surgical management to remove dead and devitalized tissue is required. Amphotericin B is given intravenously, and the underlying disease process must be controlled.

Management of Chronic Maxillary Sinusitis

As previously defined, chronic sinusitis is a persistent infection that has been present for at least 3 months. It has resisted conservative and medical therapy or has gone undiagnosed for some time. It is imperative that surgical drainage be established either by intranasal antrostomy or by the Caldwell-Luc operation with the creation of a nasal antral window. In sinusitis of dental origin, dental treatment combined with local sinus surgery is necessary. Patients with chronic maxillary sinusitis must be followed over a long period. Sinus radiograph or sinoscopy should be performed annually, even if the patient is asymptomatic.

Endoscopic Paranasal Sinus Surgery

The Europeans were the first to report the advantages of endoscopic sinus surgery. It was not until Messerklinger[55] documented his findings in English in 1978 that U.S. otolaryngologists became interested in sinus endoscopy. He described the anatomy and pathology of the middle meatus and anterior and middle ethmoid air cells of the nose. Whenever two mucosal layers come into contact, there is a disruption of mucociliary clearance, resulting in an increased potential for infection even in the presence of a patent maxillary or frontal ostium. This area of the nasal cavity is called the ostiomeatal unit[56] and is the focus of endoscopic surgery (Fig. 12–23).

Modern paranasal endoscopic surgery may be divided into two approaches, the Messerklinger or Wigand.[57] Both techniques use a rigid endoscope through the nasal route. Using the Messerklinger approach, the surgeon enters the ethmoid bulla and then works forward to the frontal recess, removing diseased sinus tissue. The maxillary and frontal ostium can be enlarged by this approach. A total sphenoethmoidectomy and supramiddle turbinate antrostomy are performed in the frontal recess in the Wigand approach. The advocates of the nasal endoscopic sinus surgery believe that eradication of disease from the ostiomeatal area will allow adequate drainage of the maxillary and frontal sinuses and that the diseased sinus mucosa will return to normal.

A well-documented history, physical examination, fiberoptic rhinoscopy, and CT scanning are imperative before endoscopic sinus surgery. Routine radiography does not show the anterior ethmoid region well. CT scanning is an important and necessary part of the planning and execution of endoscopic surgery.

Endoscopic paranasal sinus surgery is recommended as a superb diagnostic tool and can achieve excellent functional results with low morbidity in certain diseases, but standard techniques also have unsurpassed functional results with low morbidity. The removal of a benign maxillary sinus tumor is an absolute indication for a Caldwell-Luc operation. Simple retention cysts (if they become symptomatic), mucoceles, pyoceles, dental cysts and tumors of dental origin, antrochoanal polyps, inverted papillomas, mesenchymal tumors, and fibroosseous lesions require a Caldwell-Luc operation.[58]

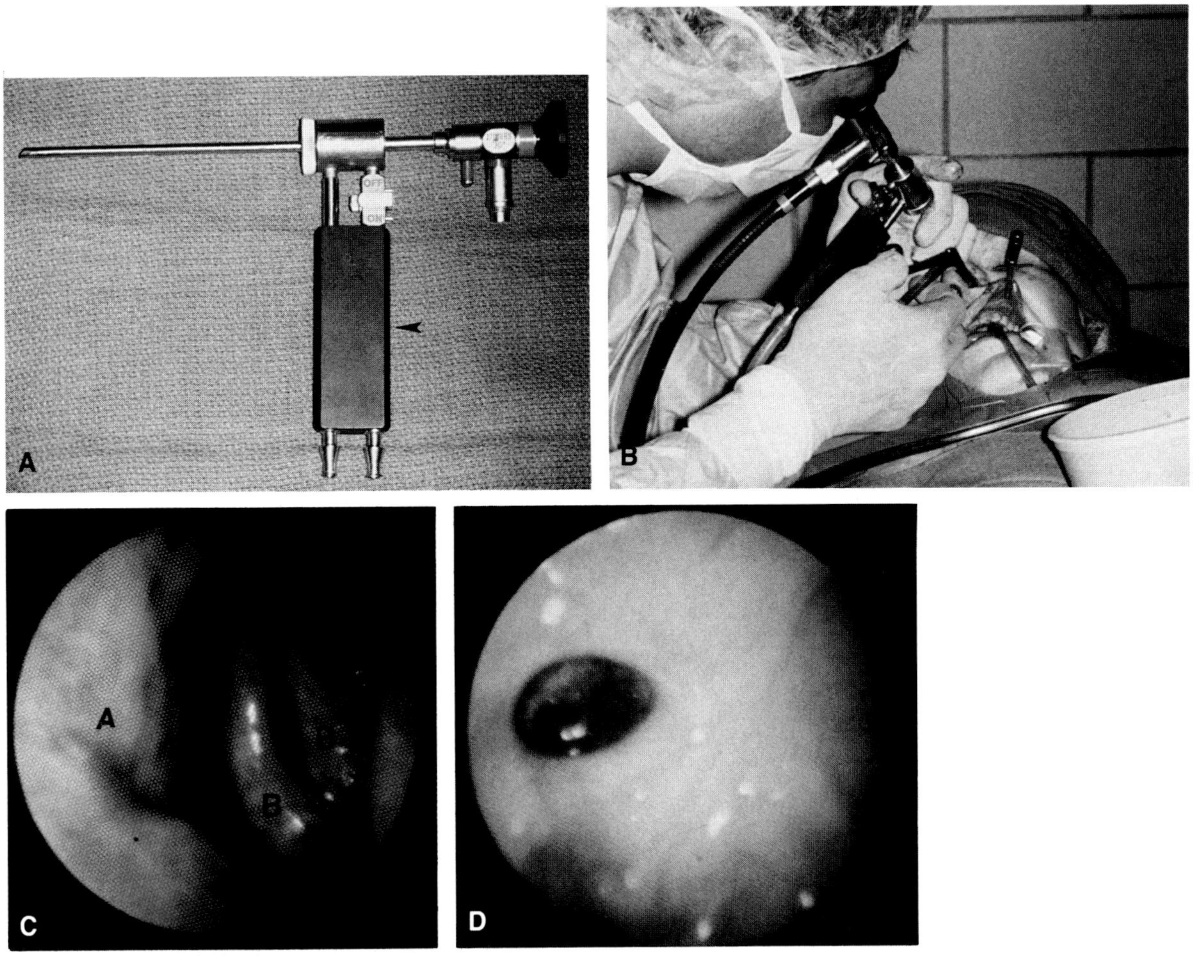

Figure 12–23. *(**A**) A picture of a 30°-wide angle nasal endoscopy telescope with suction irrigator control (arrow). (**B**) Nasal endoscopy with telescope and suction irrigator in the nose. Rongeur used to remove the pathologic condition in the osteameatal area and irrigator probe placed through the canine fossa into the maxillary sinus to assist with visualization. (**C**) Endoscopic view. A indicates nasal septum; B, double process middle turbinate. (**D**) Nasal endoscopic view of a patent maxillary sinus ostium surrounded by white scar tissue. The patient had complaints of chronic maxillary sinusitis following closure of an oroantral fistula several years earlier. (Contributed by Sanford Archer, MD, Division of Otolaryngology, University of Kentucky Medical Center)*

There is a "learning curve" associated with paranasal endoscopic sinus surgery. The complication rate decreases with experience. Significant complications associated with endoscopic surgery include: hemorrhage, cerebrospinal leak, blindness, orbital hematoma, diplopia, and subcutaneous orbital emphysema. Postoperative complications include: synechia, antrostomy closure, nasolacrimal duct injury, and recurrent disease.

The Caldwell-Luc Operation

Henri Luc was born in France in 1855, and George Caldwell was born in the United States in 1866. Both men were interested in rhinology and independently developed a surgical technique for the treatment of maxillary sinusitis. Their initial treatment was of maxillary sinusitis of dental origins. Caldwell published a brief paper on the operation in 1893 in the New York

Display 12–4. Indications for the Caldwell-Luc Operation

1. Retrieval of a root or tooth from the sinus
2. Enucleation of odontogenic cysts or mucoceles from the sinus
3. Removal of odontogenic tumors from the sinus
4. Treatment of acute maxillary sinusitis resistant to medical therapy or showing evidence of extending beyond the boundaries of the sinus
5. Treatment of chronic sinusitis
6. Management of oroantral fistula
7. Repair of fractures of the antrum or zygoma

Medical Journal. Luc gave Caldwell credit for describing an operation very similar to his own. It is highly unlikely that either man was aware of the other's work. The indications for the Caldwell-Luc operation are described in Display 12–4.

The Caldwell-Luc operation is best performed with the patient under general anesthesia. It requires that the surgeon wear a headlight for good visualization. The incision is made either around the necks of the teeth or approximately 2 mm above the mucogingival junction (Fig. 12–24). A releasing incision is carried anteriorly over the canine eminence and a posterior releasing incision is positioned according to the pathologic conditions present in the antrum. A full-thickness mucoperiosteal flap is elevated to expose the canine fossa region of the lateral maxillary wall. Care is taken to protect the infraorbital nerve from injury when elevating the flap.

An opening is created in the canine fossa area above the roots of the maxillary teeth, or it may be made further posteriorly, depending on the location of the pathologic condition (Fig. 12–25). A rotating bur or back-biting rongeur is used to create the opening (Fig. 12–26). The opening created is approximately 2.5 cm in diameter. The diseased material is removed from the sinus. If the sinus mucosa is healthy and the ostium patent, the sinus mucosa does not need to be removed or a nasal antral window created. This may be done, for example, if a root or tooth is removed from the sinus immediately after being displaced into the antrum. If the antral mucosa is generally diseased, it is removed with antral curettes; if only a small area of

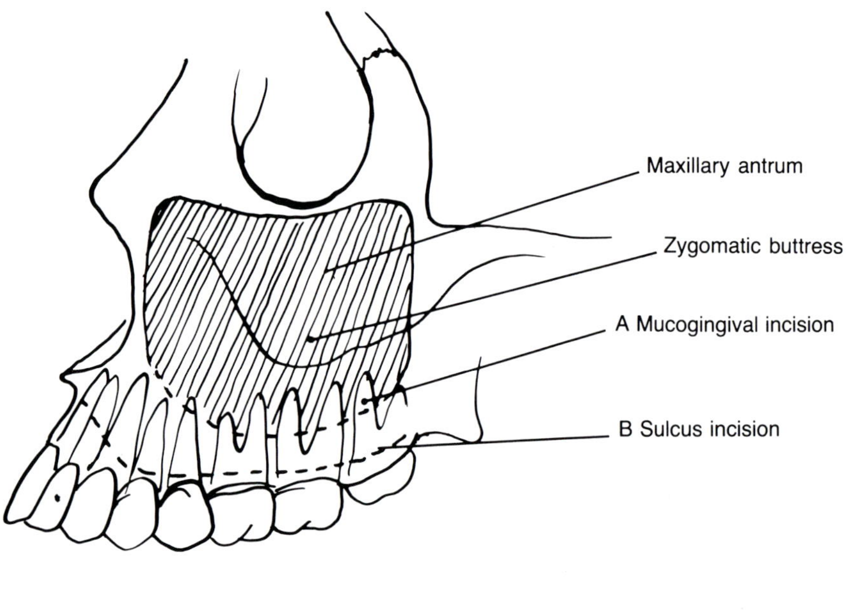

Figure 12–24. *A indicates the standard incision for the Caldwell-Luc operation; B, the sulcular incision is used for instances where using the standard incision might result in closure of the incision line over a bony opening.*

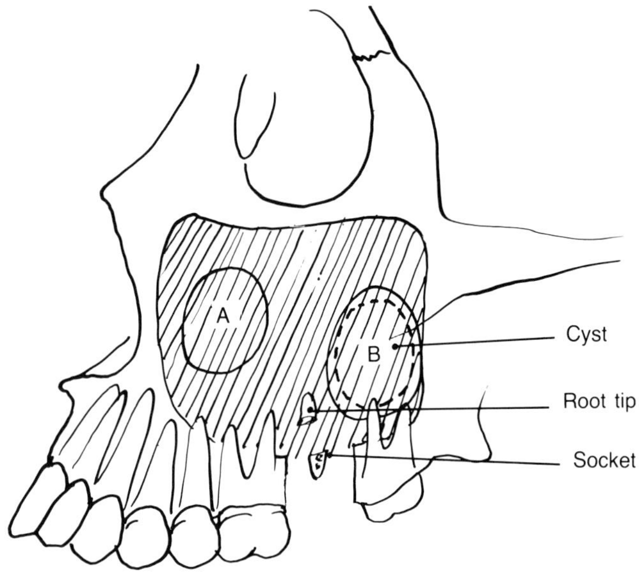

Figure 12–25. *A indicates the standard Caldwell-Luc opening into the maxillary sinus for retrieval of a root or tooth; B, a modified opening at the posterior maxilla for removal of lesions that arise in the posterior maxillary sinus.*

the mucosa is diseased, the healthy mucosa should not be removed. The contents of the sinus are sent to a pathology laboratory for histologic examination. Swabs of purulent material or tissue specimens are subjected to aerobic, anaerobic, acid fast, and fungal cultures and antibiotic sensitivity tests.

A nasal antral window is created transantrally into the inferior meatus to establish dependent drainage. The window must be large enough to prevent spontaneous closure. It should be at least 2 cm in length and 1 cm in height (Fig 12–27). The nasal mucosa is incised transantrally through the nasal antral window

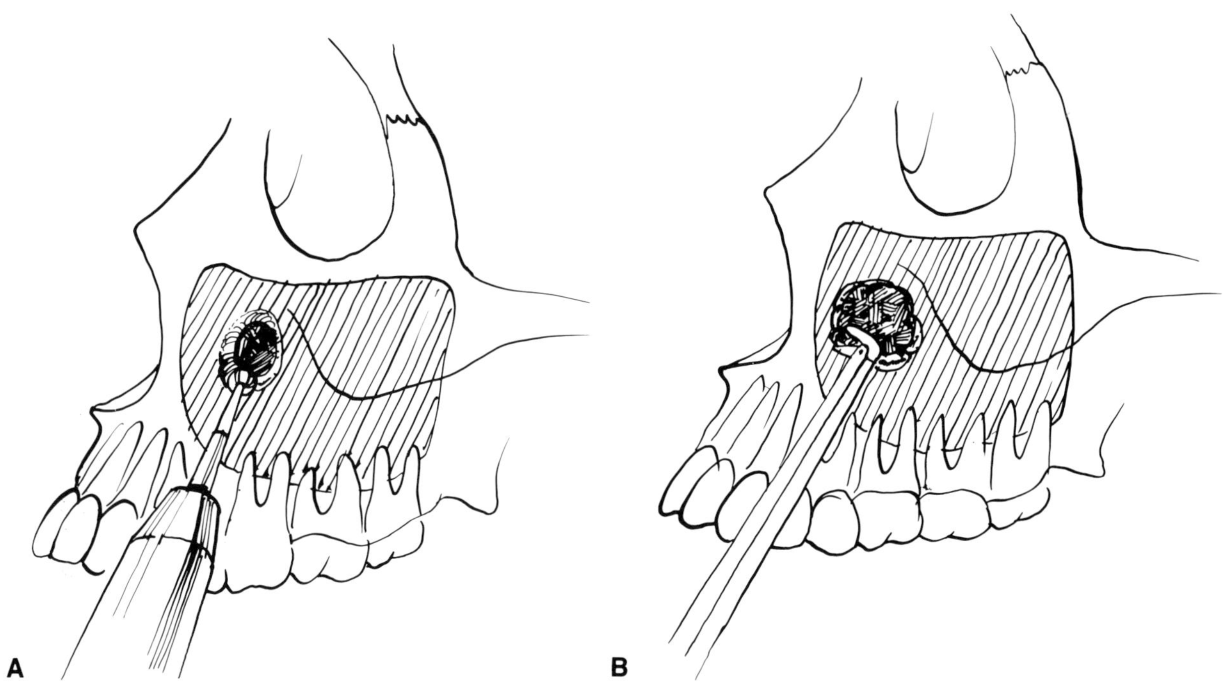

Figure 12–26. *The opening into the antrum can be created by (**A**) a bur and drill and (**B**) a back-biting rongeur.*

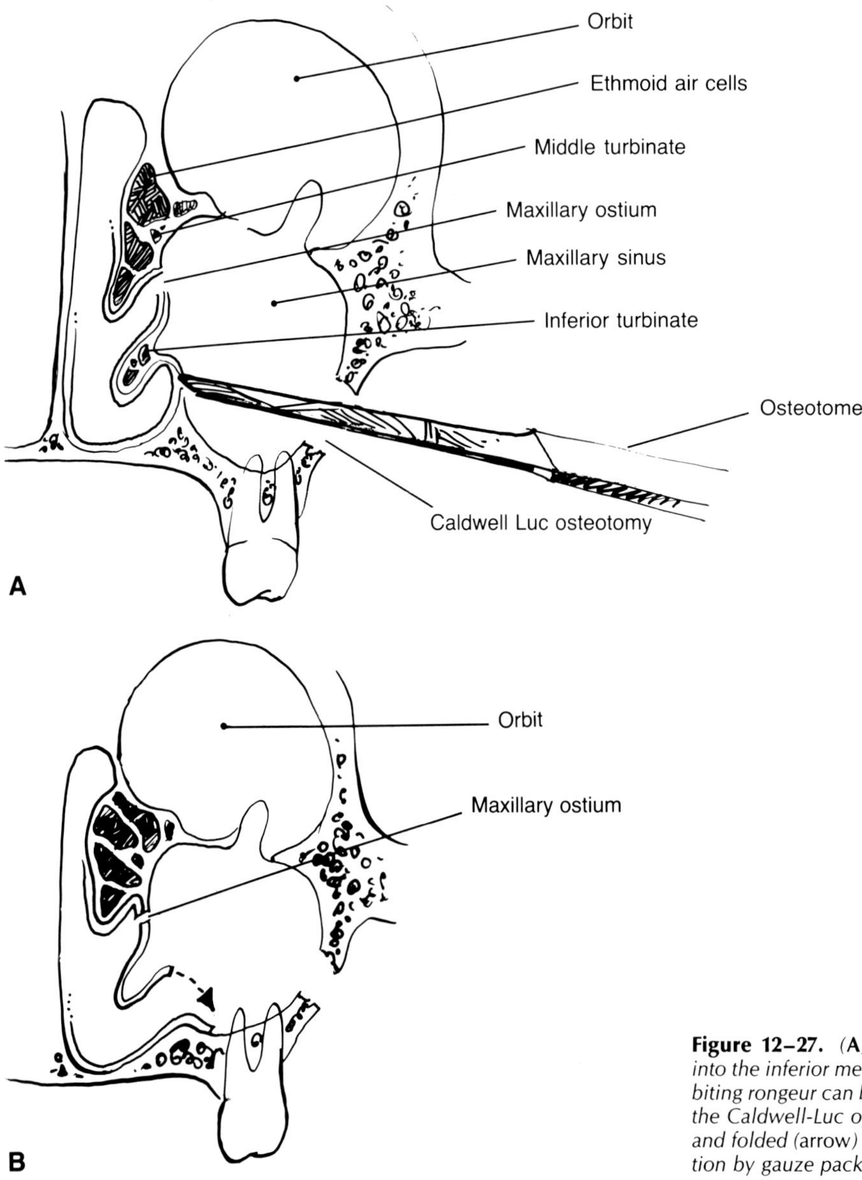

Figure 12–27. (**A**) *A nasal antral window being created into the inferior meatus of the nasal cavity. A chisel or back-biting rongeur can be used to remove the bony wall through the Caldwell-Luc opening.* (**B**) *The nasal mucosa is incised and folded* (arrow) *into the antrum, where it is held in position by gauze packing.*

and then folded into the antrum. The folded nasal tissue is held in place with antral packing. Iodoform gauze impregnated with topical antibiotic is passed through the window into the nose and sutured to the ala of the nose. The sinus is packed loosely with the end of the gauze extending from the window into the antrum (Fig. 12–28). The gauze pack is not placed when the antral mucosa is healthy. In some instances the gauze may be used to control hemorrhage or to prevent potential infection in healthy mucosa. In these instances it may be packed into the sinus through the Caldwell-Luc opening, tunneled under the oral mucosa some distance from the Caldwell-Luc incision, and then punctured through into the oral cavity. It is then sutured to the maxillary vestibule. The oral mucoperiosteal flap is sutured into its original position or is stretched to cover a bony defect such as an oral antral fistula. The antral packing is normally left in place for 4 to 7 days, but when intended as a fracture stabilization, it may be left in place for 2 weeks.

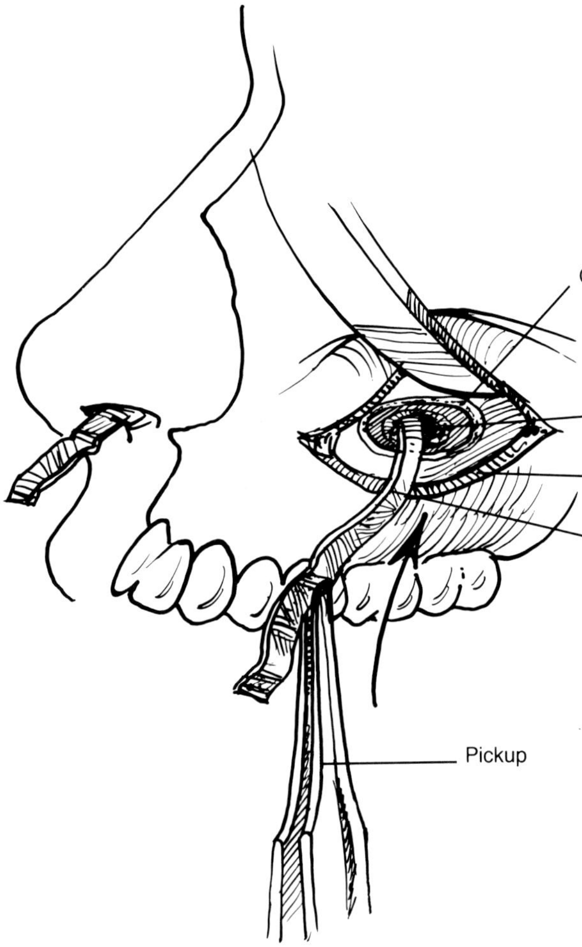

Figure 12–28. *Iodoform gauze impregnated with a topical antibiotic is passed through the antral window and pulled to the nares where it is sutured. The antrum is then packed lightly for infection and hemostatic control with the remaining gauze. It is later removed from the sinus by pulling it through the nose.*

Some patients with significant inflammatory sinus disease may have increased vascularity resulting in significant intraoperative bleeding. It is prudent to perform the Caldwell-Luc operation on these types of patients in the hospital.

The postoperative complications associated with the Caldwell-Luc operation are usually minor in nature. Murray reviewed 45 patients undergoing 60 Caldwell-Luc operations.[59] The majority of the procedures were performed for chronic sinusitis. Recurrent sinusitis was the most common complication. Protracted numbness of the teeth, gingiva, and lip caused by injury to the infraorbital or anterior superior alveolar nerves occurred to a minor degree. Persistent cheek swelling, oral antral fistula, and dental complications also occurred.

SURGICAL PROCEDURES INVOLVING THE MAXILLARY SINUS

Sinus Complications during Tooth Extraction

The maxillary molar teeth are normally in close proximity to the antrum. If the sinus is pneumatized, roots of the premolar and molar teeth may extend well into the antrum. These teeth must be removed cautiously, especially if they have divergent or dilacerated roots. Surgical sectioning (Fig. 12–29) of the roots from the crown and from each other, in addition to judicious apical force, may prevent the fracturing of alveolar bone, resulting in the exposure of the sinus (Fig. 12–30), or the forcing of a root into the sinus. Care

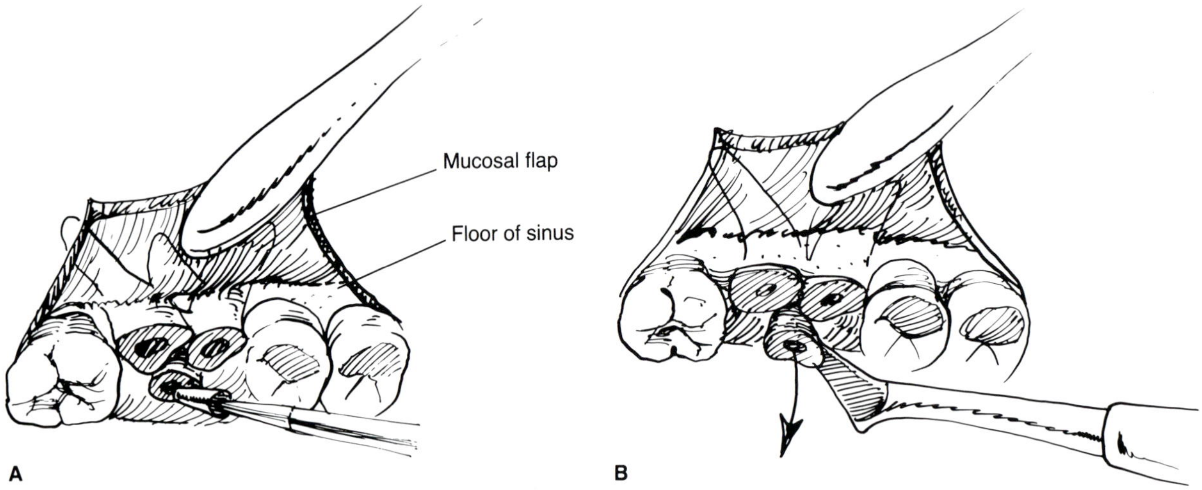

Figure 12–29. *(**A**) A tooth with divergent roots in a pneumatized sinus has a mucoperiosteal flap reflected. The crown of the tooth is cut off. Individual roots are separated from one another. (**B**) Judicious force is required when a straight elevator is used to elevate the roots, while the pendant shaped elevator is used to apply occlusally directed force.*

must be taken not to cut too deep into the frucation of the tooth and not to remove too much buccal bone because the bur can cut a hole into the pneumatized sinus.

If exposure of the sinus is suspected when removing a tooth, examination of the socket for a perforation with a good light, irrigation, and suctioning is necessary. Having the patient hold his or her nose and gently blow while examining the area of suspected perforation will demonstrate the opening. Questioning the patient about a history of sinusitis is important because an already diseased sinus tolerates the violation to a lesser extent. In addition, if the tooth has a periapical infection, the chance of antral infection is greater.

If the patient has a healthy sinus, an oroantral communication of under 4 to 5 mm will most likely heal spontaneously.[60–62] Precautions after sinus surgery, including sneezing with the mouth open, refraining from blowing the nose or sucking through a straw, and smoking cessation, must be emphasized to the patient to help the healing process. Prescribing an antibiotic and systemic and topical decongestants is imperative at the time of acute injury.

Maxillary sinusitis is present when an untreated oroantral communication has persisted for more than 48 hours.[63] Surgical closure of an antral communication is indicated if the opening is over 4 to 5 mm in size at the time of injury. If the patient has a history of sinus disease, closure of the perforation is indicated even if the opening is less than 4 mm.[64]

The most common surgical technique for the closure of an acute oroantral perforation is the buccal flap procedure described by Rehrmann.[65] Careful planning must be done in the design of the buccal flap so that it can be used to close the communication. If a root tip is pushed into the sinus and a flap must be elevated, it should be designed so that it can be used to close a bony alveolar defect after root retrieval. Great care must be given to developing the flap with proper undermining and horizontal periosteal releasing incisions to create a water-tight closure without tension (Fig. 12–31). Standard precautions after sinus surgery, an amoxicillin, and systemic and topical decongestants are recommended after the operation. The advantage of the buccal flap procedure is that it allows the Caldwell-Luc operation and the closure of the oroantral fistula to be performed simultaneously if sinus disease is present. The disadvantage of the buccal flap procedure is that 50% of patients experience permanent reduction of vestibular height.[63] This could pose a problem for the edentulous patient requiring a prosthesis.

The buccal trapezoidal flap described by Moczair[66] is slid distally a distance of one tooth for closure of an oroantral fistula (Fig. 12–32). The advantage is no loss

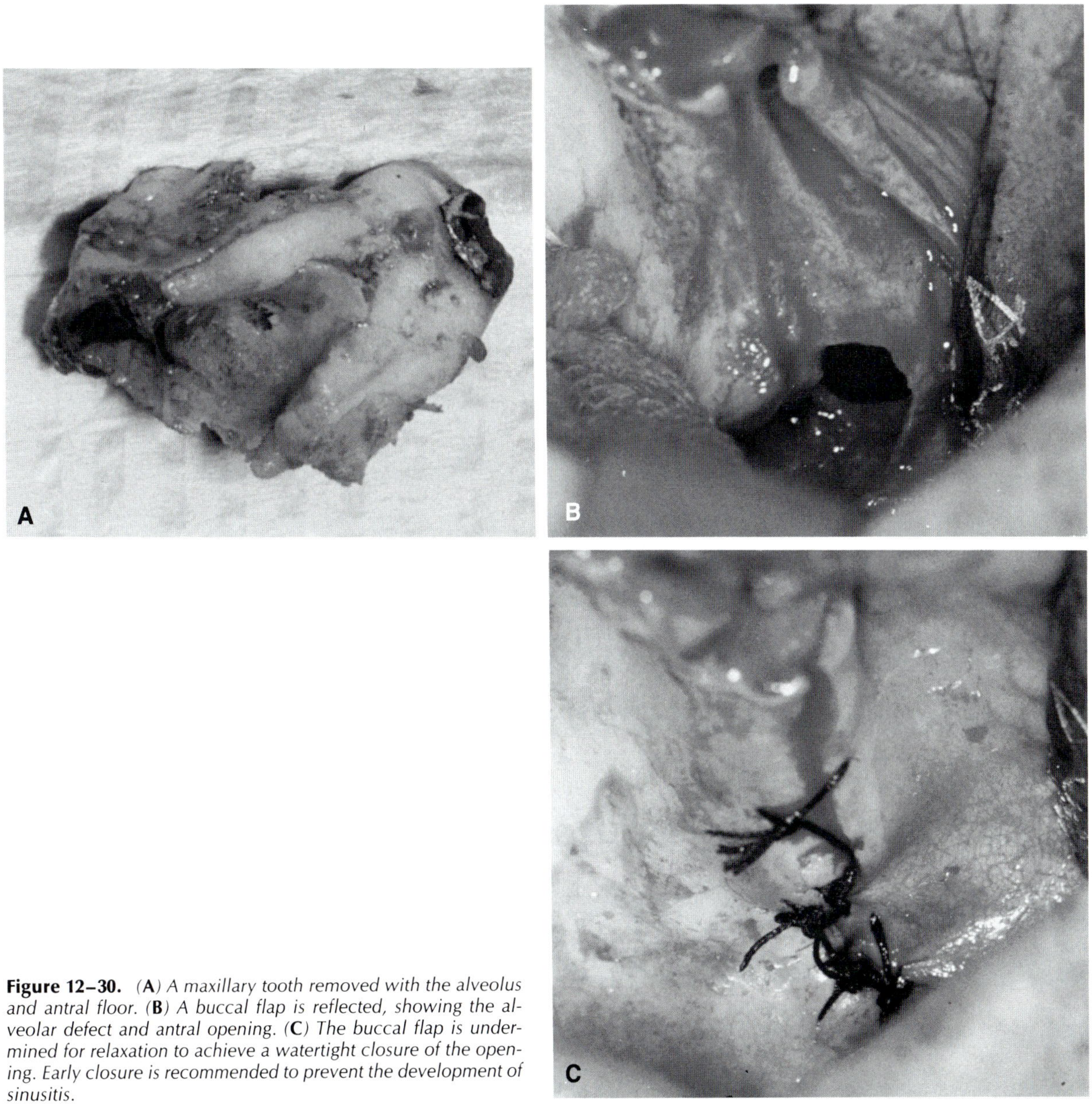

Figure 12–30. *(**A**) A maxillary tooth removed with the alveolus and antral floor. (**B**) A buccal flap is reflected, showing the alveolar defect and antral opening. (**C**) The buccal flap is undermined for relaxation to achieve a watertight closure of the opening. Early closure is recommended to prevent the development of sinusitis.*

of buccal vestibular height; however, the disadvantage is scarring of the anterior releasing incision.[63] This flap is recommended for use in the edentulous patient. It is also a useful flap for closure of a fistula in the hard to reach location distal to the maxillary molars in the tuberosity area.

If a small, uninfected root tip (2 to 3 mm) is pushed through the floor of the antrum, it may lie between the sinus membrane and the floor or may perforate the membrane. No attempt to retrieve the root tip should be made.[64] The root tip will fibrose and generally cause no problem. The patient should be informed of the occurrence, and a radiograph should be taken to document the root tip position. Closure of the perforation should be performed with a figure-of-8 suture over the socket to hold the blood clot.

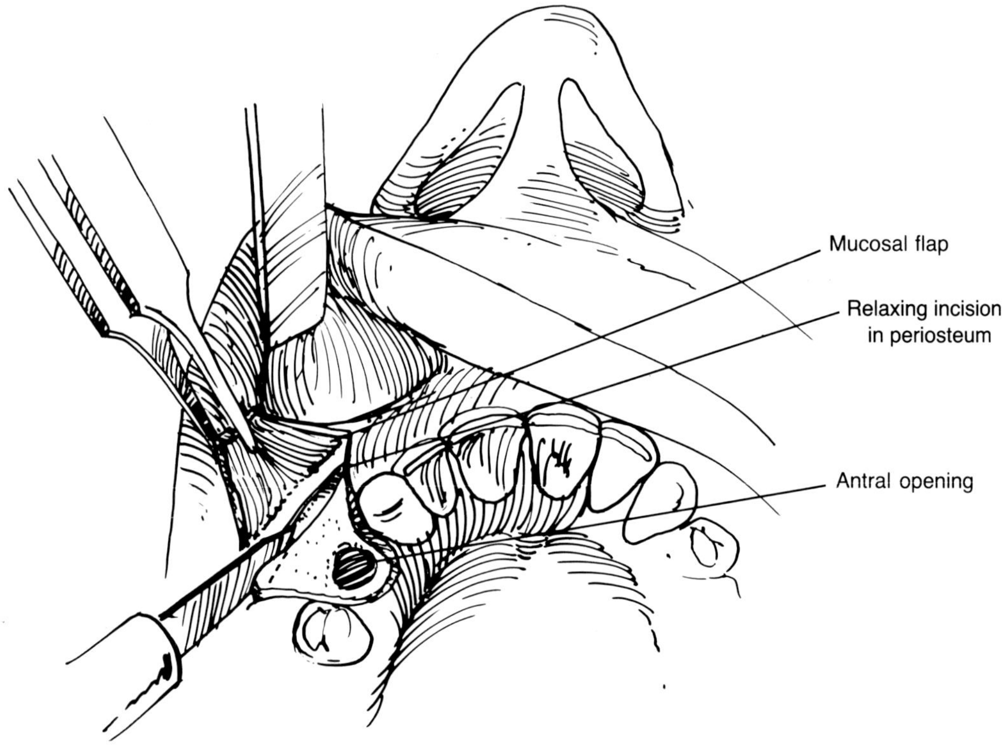

Figure 12–31. *A buccal flap is elevated and a horizontal periosteal relaxing incision is made to increase the mobility of the flap to close the oroantral fistula or opening.*

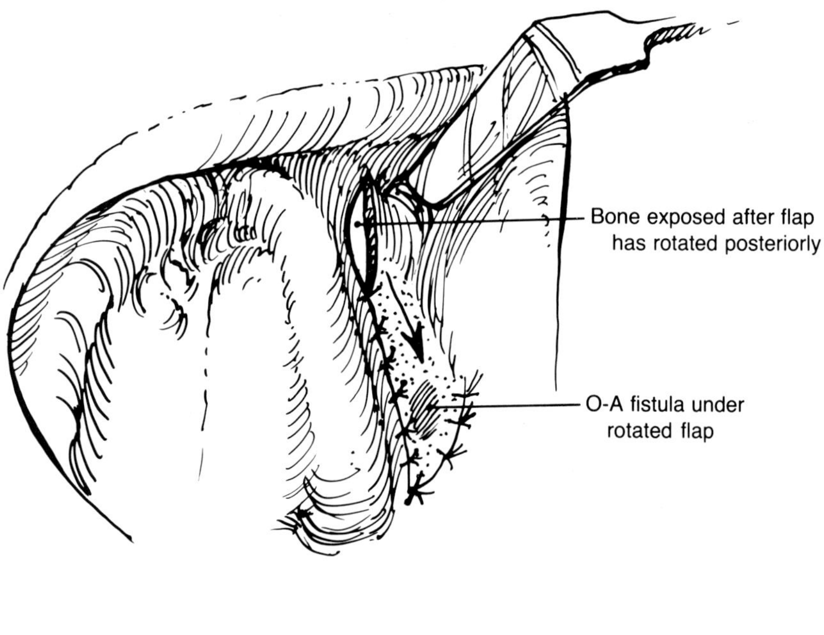

Figure 12–32. *Moczair buccal sliding flap, moved distally to cover a posteriorly positioned oroantral fistula. Its advantage is that it does not decrease the buccal vestibule.*

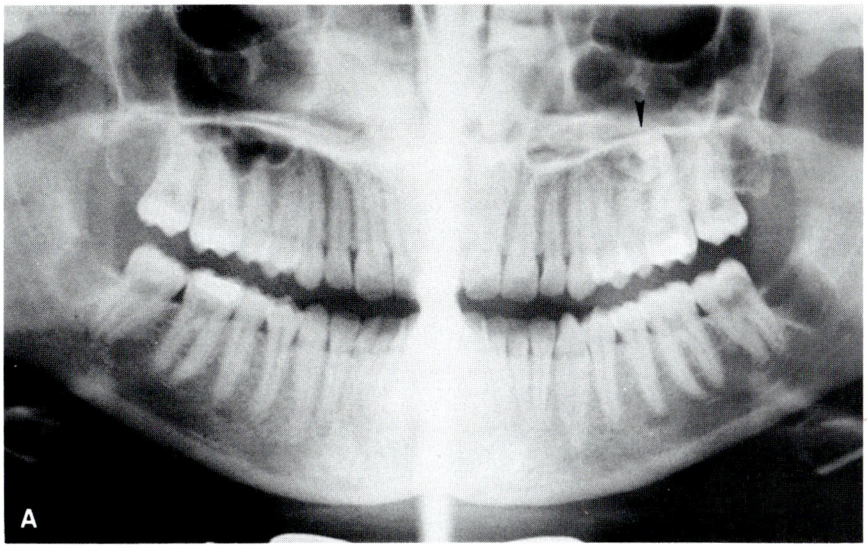

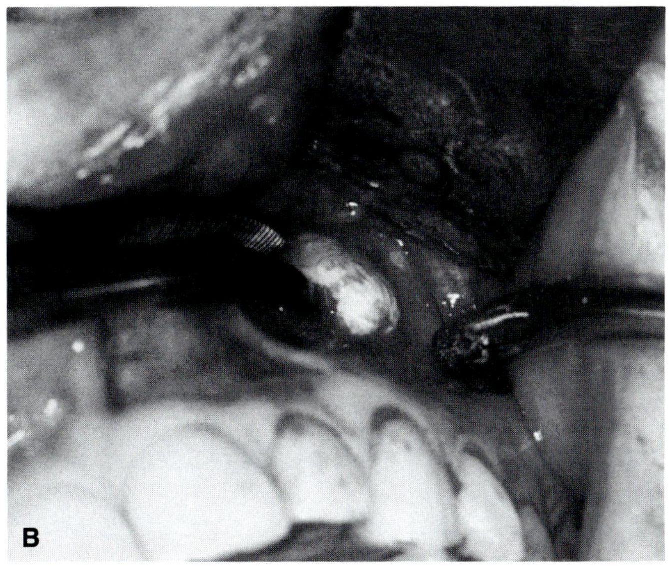

Figure 12–33. *(A) This radiograph shows a third molar that has been displaced into the antrum and lies over the first molar roots. (B) A Caldwell-Luc operation is used to remove the third molar from the antrum.*

Standard precautions after sinus surgery should be followed, and an antibiotic and nasal decongestant should be given to the patient.

If a large piece of root, infected root, or tooth is displaced into the antrum, it should be removed. Third molar surgery is the most common cause of displacement of a tooth into the antrum. Irrigation and suction should be attempted through the existing perforation to retrieve the root or tooth. This procedure is seldom successful. A Caldwell-Luc operation is the procedure of choice to remove a large piece of root or tooth from the sinus (Fig. 12–33). Enlargement of the alveolar antral opening for retrieval of a root or tooth predisposes the patient to the formation of an oroantral fistula and should be avoided.

Management of Chronic Oroantral Openings

Patients who present with a chronic oroantral fistula not only require closure of the fistula but also require management of the inflammatory sinus disease that co-exists with the fistula.[67–71] Various surgical techniques for closure of chronic oroantral fistulas have proved successful. The size of the defect is not a determining factor in selecting a technique.[61, 71] Elimination of chronic sinus disease with the Caldwell-Luc operation and creation of a nasal antral window, in addition to closure of the defect without tension, is much more important than the size of the defect. Patient compliance regarding standard precautions after sinus surgery and medication administration is imperative after surgery. Awang[68] has categorized the techniques for closure of oroantral fistula into:

1. Local flaps
2. Distant flaps
3. Grafts

Local Flaps

The Rehrmann and Moczair buccal flaps are local flaps that were described previously. Various palatal flaps have been described for closure of oroantral fistulas. The palatal tissue is thick and has a rich blood supply when the greater palatine artery is included in the flap. A great deal of bleeding is associated with the palatal flap technique, so an electrocautery should be available when using the procedure. The palatal tissue is less elastic than the buccal tissue.

The palatal rotational or pedicle flap is a popular technique (Fig. 12–34). Care must be taken not to cut the palatine artery when using this technique. Choukas has modified the technique by leaving a band of tissue between the pedicle flap and the fistula on the palatal side.[68] The pedicle flap is then tunneled under the bridge of tissue before closing the fistula. This reduces tension on the flap and helps protect and stabilize it.

Ito and Hara[72] modified the pedicle palatal flap by developing a submucosal connective tissue pedicle flap that has a rich blood supply and is extremely elastic (Fig. 12–35). The bone surface at the donor site does not remain exposed because the epithelial layer is returned to its original position. Healing at the donor site occurs more rapidly than the usual 2 to 3 months for the pedicle palatal flap. Bony palatal necrosis that rarely occurs with the standard palatal flap is prevented (Fig. 12–36). The dissection, however, is technically difficult and injury to the blood supply is possible.

The island flap is another modification of the ped-

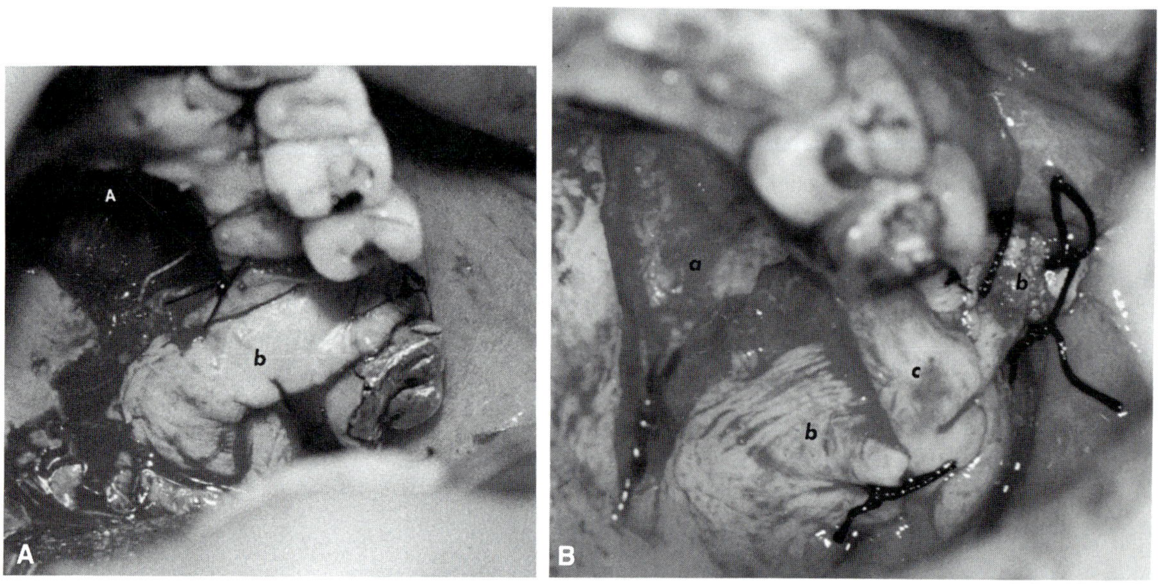

Figure 12–34. *(**A**) This photo shows a donor site (a) and palatal pedicle flap (b) rotated to close an oroantral fistula. (**B**) This photo shows a donor site (a), palatal pedicle flap (b) rotated to close an oroantral fistula, and Choukas' band of tissue (c) that the pedicle flap is tunneled under for stabilization.*

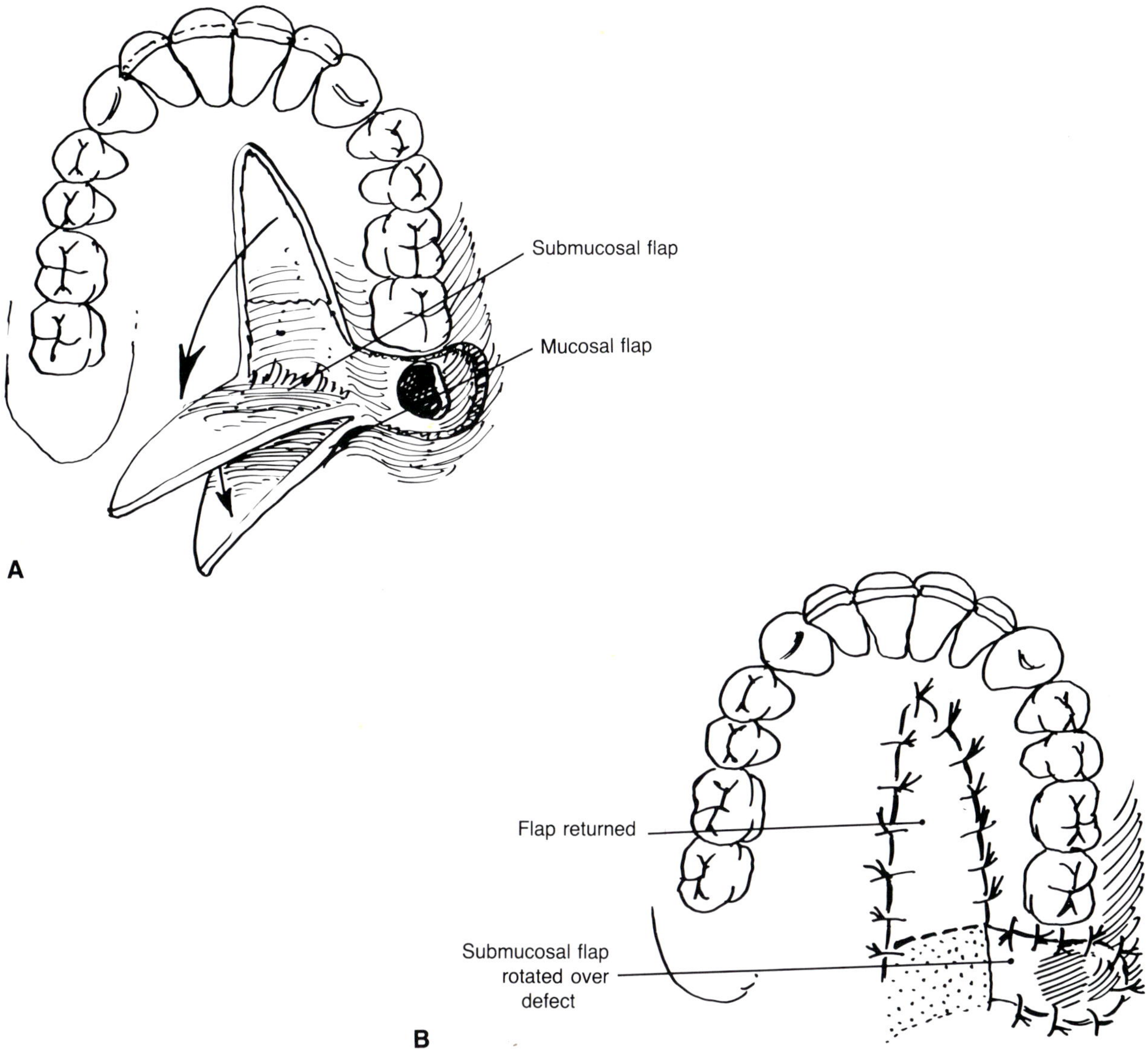

Figure 12–35. *Ito and Hara modified pedicle palatal flap. (**A**) Closure of oroantral fistula with a submucosal connective tissue flap dissected from the primary flap. (**B**) Primary flap sutured back to its original position and the submucosal flap sutured over the oroantral fistula.*

icle palatal flap. The primary indication for its use is a fistula in the second molar area where a palatal pedicle flap cannot reach. In this technique a pedicle palatal flap is elevated. The greater palatine artery is located at the greater palatine foramen and dissected from the palatal flap from a proximal to distal direction. The distal end of the palatal flap with the attached artery is cut off, creating an island flap (Fig. 12–37). The island flap is then tunneled under the bridge of palatal tissue and sutured to the prepared fistula tract site. The palatal bridge of tissue protects the artery. The proximal flap is repositioned back into its original donor site to help promote healing. To provide 8 to 10 cm^2 of tissue coverage, 75% of the pal-

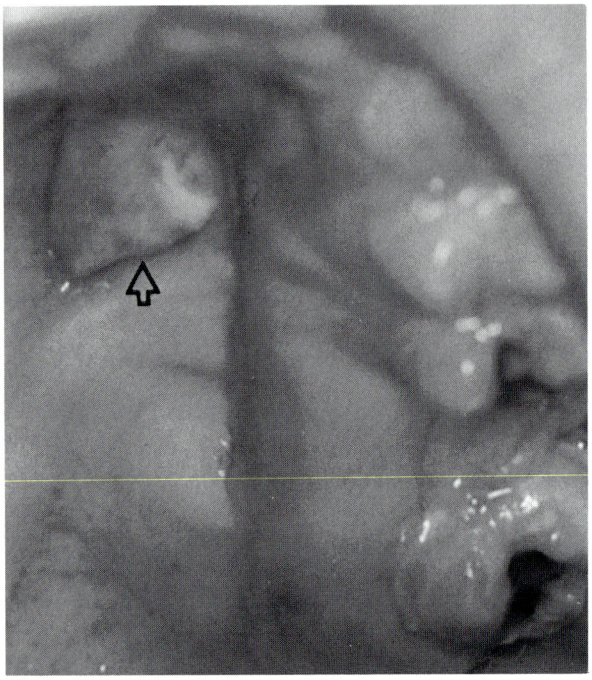

Figure 12–36. *Two months after closure of an oroantral fistula, a rare bony sequestrum was removed from the donor site of a pedicle palatal graft.*

ate may be pedicled and rotated 180° in position.[73] Additional length (up to 1 cm) may be gained by freeing the greater palatine vessels at the foramen. James[74] claims that the island flap provides excellent bulk and blood supply. It also provides good mobility and avoids tethering. Possible complications include excess trauma to the artery, or kinking, with necrosis of the island.

Distant Flaps

Distant flap procedures are used for the closure of large oroantral fistulas. Extremity and forehead flaps are rarely used today because of the poor aesthetic result. The nasolabial tunnel skin flap may be used to close large or resistant oroantral fistulas.[75] The flap is created in the skin of the cheek at the nasolabial fold closest to the oroantral fistula (Fig. 12–38). The flap is superiorly based and is passed through a tunnel created by the blunt dissection of the deeper tissues into the mouth. Because of the lush blood supply of the flap, its repositioning should not be delayed. The flap is sutured to the defect, and the nasolabial defect is sutured primarily. The pedicle flap is left in place for 2 to 3 weeks and then detached. It is close to the defect, and an excellent anesthetic result can be achieved. Hair growth is a frequent finding.

Tongue flaps have also been advocated for the closure of large oroantral fistulas. They may be either anteriorly based dorsal tongue flaps or anteriorly based lateral tongue flaps.[76,77] Tongue mobility may disrupt the flap and should be stabilized by suturing the tongue to the anterior maxillary teeth or by using intramaxillary fixation.[78] The base of the flap should be 2.5 to 3 cm in width and can be extended 5 to 6 cm. The flap should be 5 to 7 mm thick and include mucosa and closely adhering subjacent muscle elements. Posteriorly based dorsal or lateral tongue flaps are indicated when less flap movement is imperative and tongue immobilization is undesirable (Fig. 12–39).[78,79]

Grafts

Grafting procedures include the use of bone and alloplastic materials. The indications for cancellous bone grafting procedures are the presence of a bony defect 5 mm or greater in size, failure of conservative methods, and the need for recontouring of the alveolar ridge before construction of a prosthesis.[80] Most defects can be closed with soft tissue procedures, and the main indication for bone grafting is reconstruction of the alveolar ridge in conjunction with closure of an oroantral fistula.

Gold foil has been advocated for the closure of oroantral fistulas.[67,81–83] The apparent advantage of the technique is that prosthetic construction can be performed before, during, or immediately after surgery. Buccal and palatal flaps are reflected to expose the bone surrounding the oroantral fistula. The gold foil is placed over the defect. The flaps are sutured but need not totally cover the gold. The gold may be left in position but usually becomes exposed over time and may be easily removed when this occurs. Soft tissue granulates under the foil closing the fistula. The disadvantage of gold foil is the expense. Soft polymethylmethacrylate has been recommended as a substitute for gold.[84]

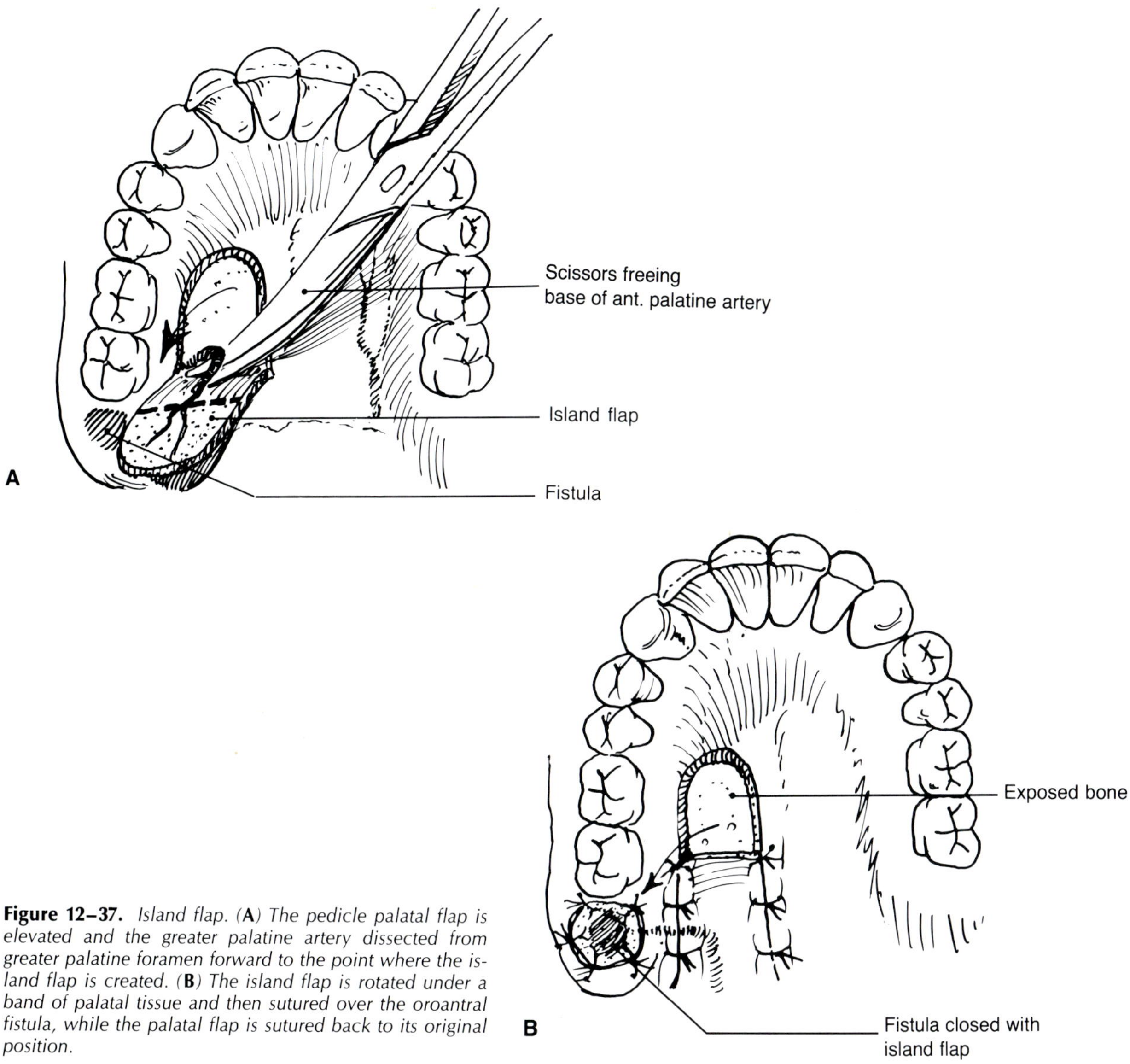

Figure 12–37. *Island flap. (**A**) The pedicle palatal flap is elevated and the greater palatine artery dissected from greater palatine foramen forward to the point where the island flap is created. (**B**) The island flap is rotated under a band of palatal tissue and then sutured over the oroantral fistula, while the palatal flap is sutured back to its original position.*

Management of Odontogenic Cysts of the Maxillary Sinus

The maxillary sinus offers the least path of resistance for the growth of cysts or tumors. Cysts of the maxillary sinus may reach a large size before they become clinically evident. Panoramic radiography is useful to initially identify cysts of the maxilla. Waters' projection and CT scanning provide a more precise view of odontogenic cysts of the antrum.

Odontogenic cysts are often associated with impacted teeth, and the maxillary third molars are most commonly associated with cyst that extend into the antrum. The third molars may be well displaced into the antrum (Fig. 12–40). Apical periodontal cysts or residual cysts may expand into the antrum. Radiographically, these cysts may have a radiopague outline above the lesion (Fig. 12–41). Clinically, when an odontogenic cyst reaches a large size, it may erode the maxillary bone, obstruct the maxillary ostium,

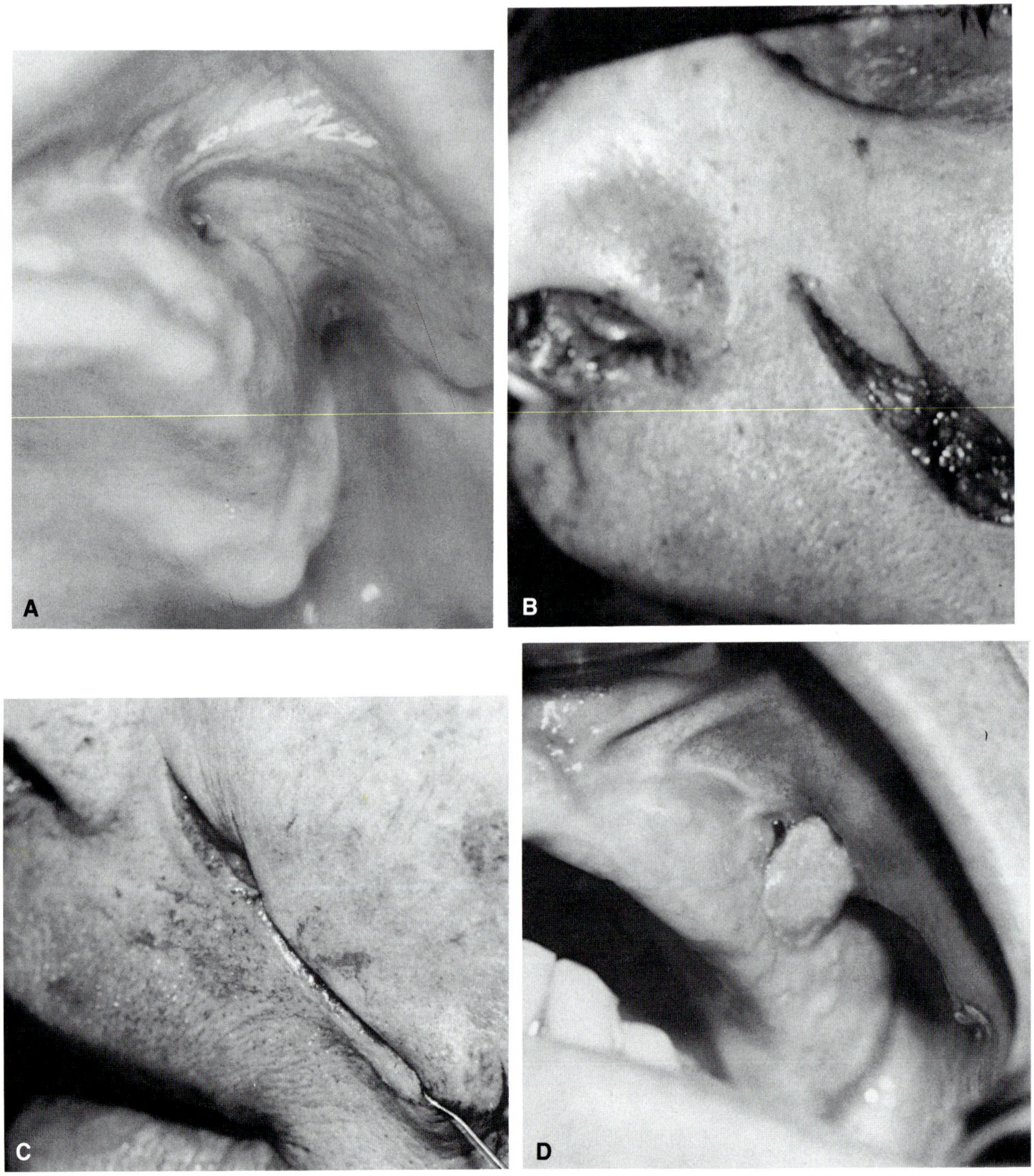

Figure 12–38. *(**A**) An oroantral fistula that has resisted two previous closures. (**B**) The development of a nasolabial fold–skin flap for closure of an oroantral fistula. (**C**) The nasolabial flap is tunneled through the cheek for closure of the fistula. The donor site is closed primarily. (**D**) The successful closure of the fistula with the skin flap at 3 weeks. (**E**) The nasolabial skin flap is taken down, and the base of the flap is revised.*

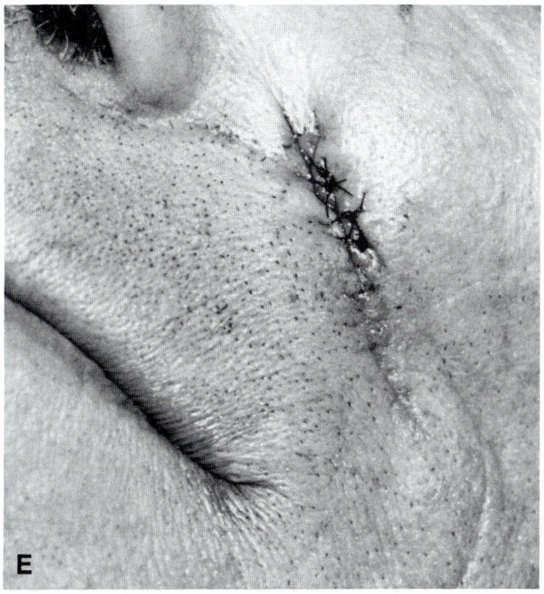

Figure 12–38 *(continued)*

and occlude the nasal passage. When maxillary bone erosion occurs, the patient may complain of fluid drainage into the oral cavity from small perforations in the cyst lining.

The best approach to enucleation of odontogenic cysts from the maxillary sinus is the Caldwell-Luc operation. There is less chance of producing an oroantral fistula by this approach. If a tooth is associated with the cyst, it can also be removed with the Caldwell-Luc operation. The opening into the sinus is made through the lateral wall near the site of origin of the cyst. The cyst is most often tenaciously attached at its site of origin, and this allows direct access for removal. If the cyst is small and the maxillary ostium appears patent, a nasal antral window is not necessary. If the ostium has been obstructed by the cyst and the sinus membrane appears damaged, a nasal antral window should be created. Close follow-up care with radiographic examinations is necessary to detect recurrence or the development of chronic sinusitis. Patients with odontogenic keratocysts have a higher rate of recurrence for the first 5 years after enucleation.[85] Odontogenic keratocysts associated with basal cell nevus syndrome have a high rate of recurrence. These patients require extremely close follow-up.

In cases in which a lesion of the maxillary sinus is excessively large or locally aggressive, such as an odontogenic keratocyst, myxoma, or ameloblastoma, a LeFort I osteotomy may be performed to achieve excellent access to the lesion after down fracturing of the maxilla (Fig. 12–42).[86] The lesion can be removed after the osteotomy and the maxilla repositioned and stabilized with bone plating.

COMPLICATIONS ASSOCIATED WITH SINUSITIS

Infections of the sinuses may spread to the orbits or cranial cavity. Sinus infections may spread by direct extension, by bony dehiscences, through fracture sites in the walls of the sinuses, or through an ophthalmic venous system that is devoid of valves. The superior

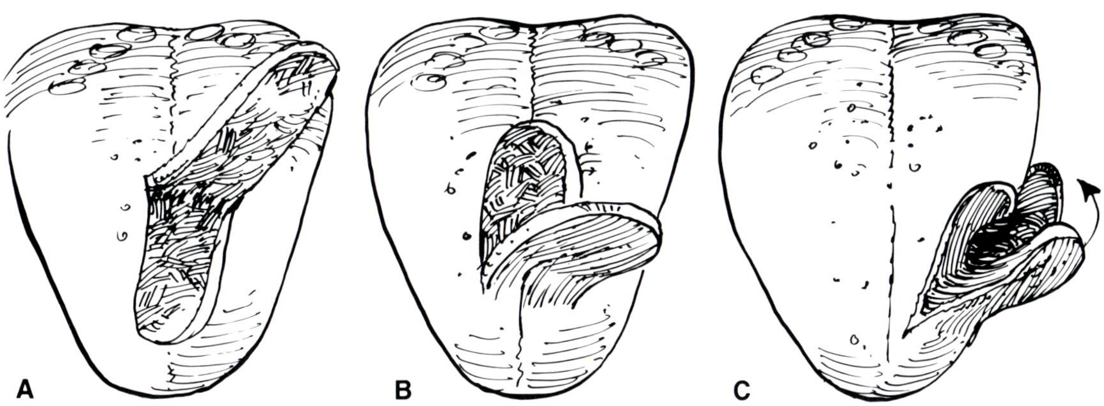

Figure 12–39. *Tongue flaps for palatal and antral fistulas. (**A**) Posteriorly based dorsal flap. (**B**) Anteriorly based dorsal flap. (**C**) Anteriorly based lateral flap.*

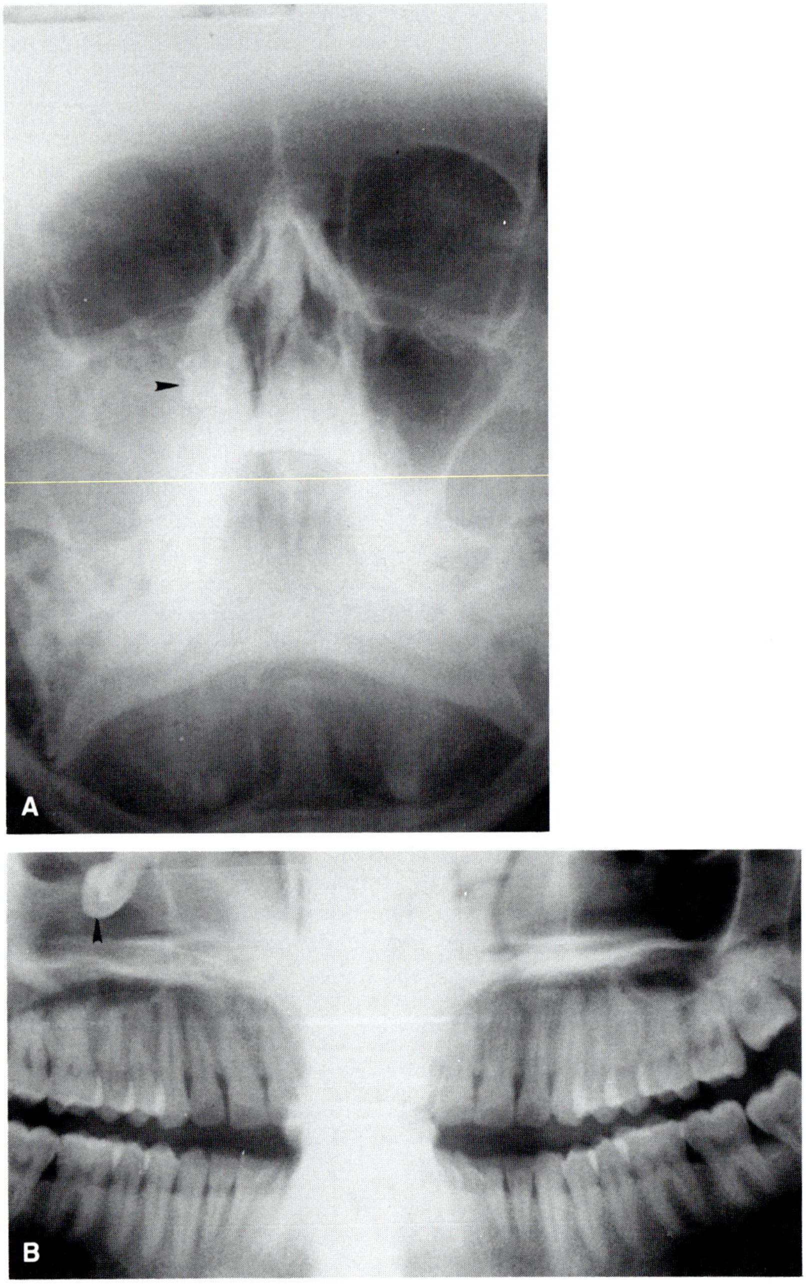

Figure 12–40. *(**A**) This Waters' view shows a maxillary right third molar displaced into the antrum near the medial wall. The antrum is also cloudy because it is filled with a large dentigerous cyst. (**B**) A panoramic view of the same patient shows the maxillary third molar missing from its normal position and displaced into the antrum.*

ophthalmic vein is in communication with the angular vein of the face. It picks up tributaries from the orbit, passes through the superior orbital fissure, and ends in the cavernous sinus. The inferior ophthalmic vein begins as a network in the orbital floor. As it passes posteriorly through the orbit, it divides into two branches. One branch passes through the inferior orbital fissure and joins the pterygoid plexus. The other passes

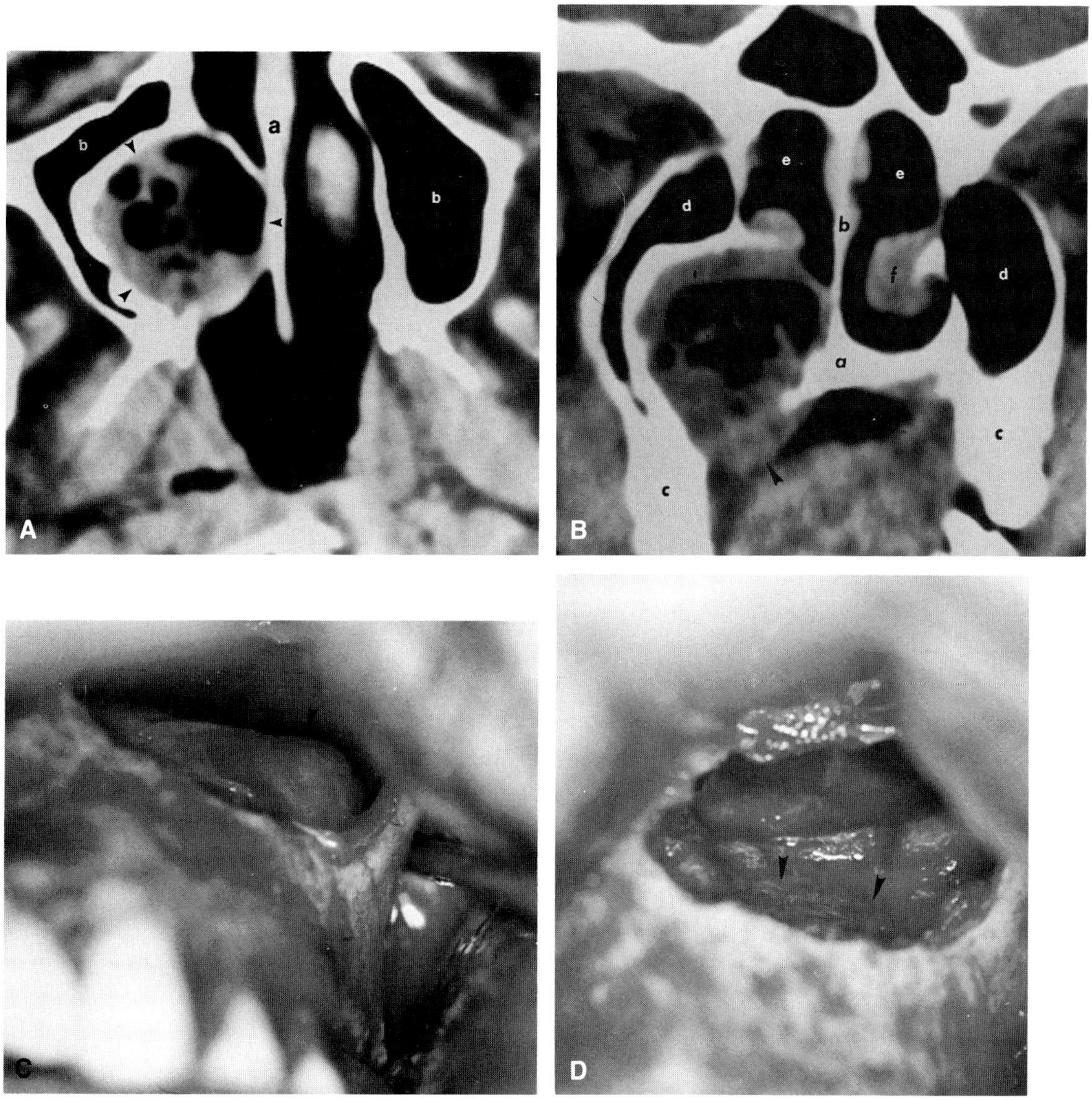

Figure 12–41. *(***A***) An axial CT scan shows the nasal septum* (a)*, maxillary sinuses* (b)*, cystic structure (*small arrows*) surrounded by bone in the antrum (*medium arrows*) and extending to the nasal septum. (***B***) A coronal CT scan also shows the same large cyst with bony outline plus erosion of the palate (*small arrow*), resulting in swelling of the palate and drainage.* a *indicates palate;* b*, nasal septum;* c*, alveolus;* d*, maxillary sinuses;* e*, nasal cavity;* f*, turbinate. (***C***) The antrum was entered through the Caldwell-Luc operation. A large, firm mound (*small arrows*) was found within the antrum, covered by normal sinus membrane and bone overlying the enlarging cyst. (***D***) The sinus lining was incised and the underlying bone was opened. A large cyst was found and enucleated. The CT scans were instrumental in the management of this case. The diagnosis was a residual apical periodontal cyst.*

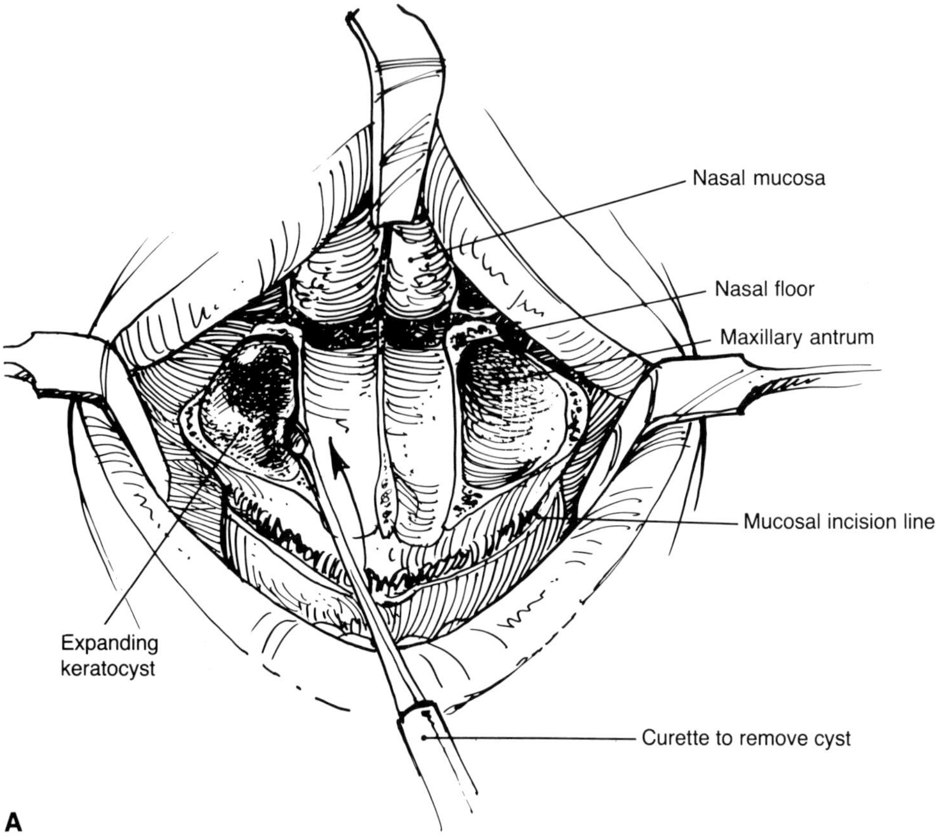

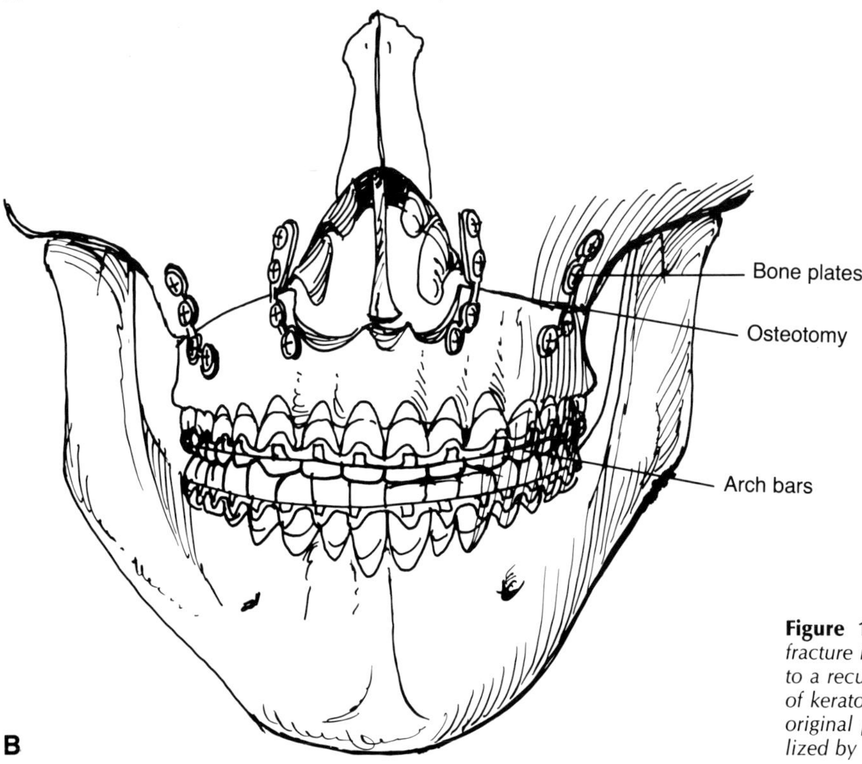

Figure 12–42. *(**A**) LeFort I osteotomy down fracture is performed to achieve excellent access to a recurrent keratocyst. (**B**) Following removal of keratocyst, the maxilla is repositioned into its original position and occlusion. It is then stabilized by bone plating.*

through the superior orbital fissure to join the cavernous sinus. There is also a communication between the ophthalmic veins and the ethmoid veins.[88]

Orbital Complications

There are five types of orbital complications that occur secondary to sinusitis[89]:

1. Inflammatory edema (periorbital edema or preseptal edema): This is edema of the eyelid that is not tender. There is no limitation of the extraocular movements and no impairment of visual acuity. There may be slight proptosis of the globe as a result of edema of the orbital contents.
2. Orbital cellulitis: There is diffuse edema of the orbital contents and acute infiltration of the adipose tissue with inflammatory cells and bacteria; however, there is no discrete abscess formation. There may be some impairment of visual acuity.
3. Subperiosteal abscess: This refers to a collection of pus between the periorbita and the bony wall of the orbit. The orbital contents and globe are displaced by the expanding periosteum.
4. Orbital abscess: A discrete collection of pus forms within the orbital tissue and may be secondary to a progressive and localized orbital cellulitis. There is exophthalmos, chemosis, and visual impairment.
5. Cavernous sinus thrombosis: There is extension of phlebitis posteriorly into the cavernous sinus with symptoms progressing to the opposite eye. Prostration occurs and meningitis occurs frequently.

Acute sinusitis is the most common cause of orbital or periorbital cellulitis. The reported incidence ranges from 60% to 84%.[90–92] In a study by Fearson et al., 80% of the patients had symptoms of upper respiratory tract infection 2 weeks before developing sinusitis with orbital complications.[93]

The majority of orbital complications occur in children under the age of 6 years.[93, 94] Signs in children include fever, an elevated white count, and positive blood cultures. In older children and adults, blood cultures are not as useful. Although younger children may have more frequent orbital involvement, the orbital complications of older children and adults are more severe when they do occur.

The ethmoid sinuses are the most common origin of orbital complications. The maxillary sinuses are next, followed by frontal sinuses. The sphenoid sinuses are rarely involved. The involvement of the frontal sinuses may herald a more ominous course.

Hospitalization and medical therapy, including intravenous antibiotics with systemic and topical decongestants, are imperative in the management of sinusitis with orbital complications. In most instances, the infection resolves without sequelae, especially in children. Surgery is indicated if the condition worsens or visual acuity decreases. According to Schramm et al. surgical drainage of the orbit and involved sinus or sinuses is indicated for patients who have demonstrated abscesses of the orbit, visual acuity worse than 20/60 from normal, or progression of infection for more than 24 hours or lack of resolution with antibiotic therapy after 48 to 72 hours.[95] Delay in surgical drainage may result in permanent blindness or spread of the infection to the brain.

CT scanning is useful in evaluating the soft tissue changes in the orbit. It can indicate orbital abscess formation; however, this should not be used as a criteria for surgery because, as Goodwin et al.[96] have shown, patients have recovered following intravenous antibiotic therapy despite identification of orbital abscess on CT scans.

Intracranial Complications of Sinusitis

Intracranial complications of sinusitis are of major significance. Infections can spread to the cavernous sinus from the veins of the orbit. Cavernous sinus thrombosis is characterized by the spread of septic thrombophlebitis to the contralateral sinus. Paralysis of cranial nerves III, IV, and VI may occur, producing proptosis. Meningitis, blindness, and death may occur. The orbit and paranasal sinus veins also communicate with the emissary veins that enter the skull diploë and leptomeninges.[97] The spread of infection through these veins may give rise to epidural infection, subdural infection, and brain abscess.

Frontal sinusitis may lead to intracranial complications by direct passage through the posterior wall of the sinus as a result of dehiscence, congenital defects, previous fractures, or erosion from osteomyelitis of the frontal bone. Most commonly the extension of infection is through the posterior wall, leading to epidural, subdural, or brain abscess (Fig. 12-43). Erosion and extension of infection through the anterior wall

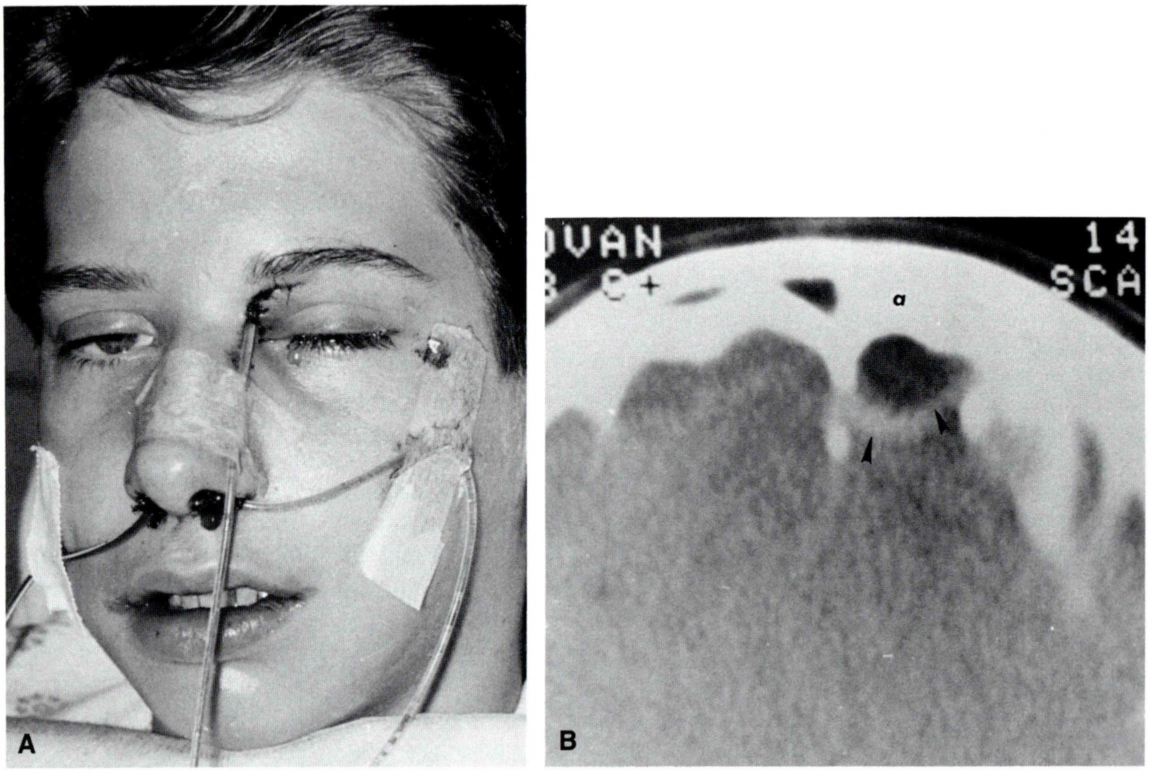

Figure 12–43. *(**A**) This patient underwent a left frontal sinus trephination and bilateral Caldwell-Luc operations with nasal antral windows for pansinusitis and frontal lobe brain abscess secondary to the acute pansinusitis. He developed tonic/clonic seizures from the brain abscess. (**B**) The CT scan demonstrates the frontal lobe brain abscess (arrows) and obliteration of the (a) left frontal sinus secondary to acute sinusitis.*

cause puffiness of the soft tissue of the forehead and is called Pott's puffy tumor.

Intravenous antibiotic therapy and frontal sinus trephination is indicated for intracranial extension of infection. Definitive neurosurgical drainage may be necessary. Osteomyelitis of the frontal bone requires wide resection with a bicoronal flap.

BIBLIOGRAPHY

1. Schaefer JP. The Nose, Paranasal Sinuses, Nasolacrimal Passageways, and Olfactory Organs in Man. Philadelphia: Blakiston's Son & Co., 1920.
2. Alberti PW. Applied surgical anatomy of the maxillary sinus. Otolaryngol Clin North Am 1976; 9:12.
3. Peter van Nostrand AW, Goodman WS. Pathologic aspects of the maxillary sinus. Otolaryngol Clin North Am 1976; 9:21.
4. Mosher HP. Symposium of the ethmoid: The surgical anatomy of the ethmoidal labyrinth. Trans Am Acad Ophthalmol 1929; 34:376.
5. Ritter FN. The Paranasal Sinuses, ed 2. St. Louis: CV Mosby, 1978:34.
6. Bilaniuk LT, Zimmerman RA. Computed tomography in evaluation of the paranasal sinuses. Radiol Clin North Am 1982; 20:501.
7. Caldwell EW. Skiagraphy of the accessory sinuses of the nose. Am J Roentgen 1918; 5:569.
8. Yanagisawa E, Smith HW, Thaler S. Radiographic anatomy of the paranasal sinuses. Arch Otolaryngol 1968; 87:100.
9. Matsubara K. Application of CT in diagnosing carcinoma of the maxillary sinus. I. Clinical evaluation of CT and frontal tomography in diagnosing carcinoma of the maxillary sinuses. Nagoya J Med Sci 1982; 44:57.
10. Sataloff RR, Grossmon CB, Gonzales C, Naheedy MH. Computed tomography of the face and paranasal sinuses. I. Normal anatomy. Head Neck Surg 1984; 7:110.
11. Osborn AG, Anderson RE. Direct sagittal computed tomographic scans of the face and paranasal sinuses. Radiology 1978; 129:81.

12. Hesselink JR, New PF, Davis KR, et al. Computed tomography of the paranasal sinuses and face. II. Pathologic anatomy. 1978; 2:586.
13. Schalz CJ, Becker TS. Normal CT anatomy of the paranasal sinuses. Radiol Clin North Am 1984; 22:107.
14. Alberti PW. Inflammatory disease of the maxillary sinus. Otolaryngol Clin North Am 1976; 9:153.
15. Blitzer A, Lawson W, Fridman WH. Surgery of the Paranasal Sinuses. 1. Philadelphia, Saunders 1985:33.
16. Gardner DG. Pseudocysts and retention cysts of the maxillary sinus. Oral Surg Oral Med Oral Pathol 1984; 58:564.
17. Halstead GL. Mucosal cysts of the maxillary sinus: Report of 75 cases. J Am Dent Assoc 1973; 87:1435.
18. Gardner DG, Gullane PJ. Mucoceles of the maxillary sinus. Oral Surg Oral Med Oral Pathol 1986; 62:538.
19. Som PM, Shugar JM. Antral mucoceles: A new look. J Comput Assist Tomogr 1980; 4(4): 484.
20. Gray WC, Blanchard CL. Sinusitis and its complications. American Family Physicians-Practical Therapeutics 1987; 35:232.
21. Dingle JH, Badger GF, Jordan WS. Patterns of illness. In: Illness in the Home. Cleveland: Press of Western Reserve University, 1964:347.
22. Deutschman CS, Wilton P, Sinow J, Dibbel D, Konstantinides F, Cerra FB. Paranasal sinusitis associated with nasotracheal intubation: A frequent unrecognized and treatable source of sepsis. Crit Care Med 1986; 14:111.
23. Grindlinger GA, Niehoff J, Hughes L, et al. Acute paranasal sinusitis related to nasotracheal intubation of head-injured patients. Crit Care Med 1987; 15:214.
24. Deutschman CS, Wilton PB, Sinow J, et al. Paranasal sinusitis: A common complication of nasotracheal intubation in neurosurgical patients. Neurosurgery 1985; 17:296.
25. Eliasson R, Mossberg B, Cammer P, Afzelius BA. The immotile-cilia syndrome: A congenital abnormality as an etiologic factor in chronic airway infections and male sterility. N Engl J Med 1977; 297:1.
26. Arden GB, Fox B. Increased incidence of abnormal nasal cilia in patients with retinitis pigmentosa. Nature 1979; 279:534.
27. Shurin PA. Etiology and antimicrobial therapy of paranasal sinusitis in children. Ann Otol Rhinol Laryngol 1981; 90(84): 72.
28. McGill T, Simpson G, Healy GB. Fulminant Aspergillosis of the nose and paranasal sinuses: A new clinical entity. Laryngoscope 1980; 90:748.
29. Van Cauwenberge P, Verschraegen G, Van Renterghem L. Bacteriological findings in sinusitis. Scand J Infect Dis [Suppl] 1978; 9:72.
30. Jousimies-Somer HR, Savolainen S, Ylikoski JS. Bacteriological findings of acute maxillary sinusitis in young adults. J Clin Microbiol 1988; 26:1919.
31. Evans FO, Sydnor JB, Moore WEC, et al. Sinusitis of the maxillary antrum. N Engl J Med 1975; 293:735.
32. Gwaltney JM, Syndor A, Sande MA. Etiology and antimicrobial treatment of acute sinusitis. Ann Otol Rhinol Laryngol [Suppl] 1981; 90(84): 68.
33. Nelson JD. Changing trends in the microbiology and management of acute otitis media and sinusitis. Pediatr Infect Dis 1986; 5:749.
34. Wald ER, Milmoe GJ, Bowen DA, et al. Acute maxillary sinusitis in children. N Engl J Med 1981; 304:749.
35. Savolainen S, Ylikoski J, Jousimies-Somer HR. The bacterial flora of the nasal cavity in healthy young men. Rhinology 1989; 24:249.
36. Frederick J, Braude AI. Anaerobic infections of the paranasal sinuses. N Engl J Med 1974; 290:135.
37. Brooke I. Bacteriology of chronic maxillary sinusitis in adults. Ann Otol Rhinol Laryngol 1989; 98:426.
38. Carenfelt C. Pathogenesis of sinus empyema. Ann Otol Rhinol Laryngol 1979; 88:16.
39. Shahin J, Gullane PJ, Doyal VS. Orbital complications of acute sinusitis. J Otolaryngol 1987; 16:23.
40. Lew D, Southwick FS, Montgomery WW, et al. Sphenoid sinusitis. N Engl J Med 1983; 309:1149.
41. Hamory BH, Sande MA, Sydnor A, Seale DL, Gwaltney JM. Etiology and antimicrobial therapy of acute maxillary sinusitis. J Infect Dis 1979; 139:197.
42. Melen I, Lindahl L, Andreasson L, Rundcrantz H. Chronic maxillary sinusitis. Acta Otolaryngol 1986; 101:320.
43. Jaffe BF. Chronic sinusitis in children. Clin Pediatr 1974; 13:944.
44. Chapnik JS, Bach MC. Bacterial and fungal infections of the maxillary sinus. Otolaryngol Clin North Am 1976; 9:43.
45. Bjorkwall T. Bacteriologic examination in maxillary sinusitis. Acta Otolaryngol [Suppl] 1950; 83:1.
46. Brook I. Aerobic and anaerobic bacterial flora of normal maxillary sinuses. Laryngoscope 1981; 91:372.
47. Stanton MB. Actinomycosis of the maxillary sinus. J Laryngol Otol 1966; 80:168.
48. Gonty A, Page L. Aspergillosis of the maxillary sinus: Review of the literature and report of a case. Oral Surg Oral Med Oral Pathol 1977; 43:350.
49. Veress B, Malic O, Tayeb A, et al. Further observations of the primary paranasal aspergillus granuloma in the Sudan: A morphological study of 46 cases. Am J Trop Med Hyg 1973; 22:765.
50. Wright R. Two cases of granuloma invading the orbit, due to an Aspergillus. Br J Ophthalmol 1927; 11:545.
51. Miloshev B, Mahgoub E, Abdel O, Hassan A. Primary aspergilloma of paranasal sinuses in the Sudan: A review of seventeen cases. Br J Surg 1969; 56:132.
52. McGill T, Simpson G, Healy G. Fulminent aspergillosis of the nose and paranasal sinuses: A new clinical entity. Laryngoscope 1980; 90:748.
53. Parfrey N. Improved diagnosis and prognosis of mucomycosis—A clinicopathologic study of 33 cases. Medicine 1986; 65:113.
54. Morgan M, Wilson W, Neel B, Roberts G. Fungal sinusitis in healthy and immunocompromised individuals. Am J Clin Pathol 1984; 82:597.

55. Messerklinger W. Endoscopy of the Nose. Baltimore: Urban and Schwertzenber, 1978.
56. Naumann H. Pathologische Anatomie der chronischen Rhinitis und Sinusitis. In: Proceedings of the VIII International Congress of Otorhinolaryngology. Amsterdam: Excerpta Medica, 1965:80.
57. Schaefer S, Manning S, Closes L. Endoscopic paranasal sinus surgery. Laryngoscope 1989; 99:1.
58. Friedman W, Katsantoris G. The role of standard techniques in modern sinus surgery. Otolaryngol Clin North Am 1989; 22(4): 759.
59. Murray J, Jackson MS. Complications after treatment of chronic maxillary sinus disease with Caldwell-Luc procedure. Laryngoscope 1983; 93:282.
60. Martensson G. Operative method in fistulas of the maxillary sinus. Acta Otolaryngol 1957; 48:253.
61. Von Wowern N. Correlation between the development of an oroantral fistula and size of the corresponding bony defect. J Otolaryngol [Suppl] 1973; 31:98.
62. Schuchardt K. Treatment of oro-antral perforation and fistulae. Int J Oral Surg 1955; 5:157.
63. Von Wowern N. Closure of oroantral fistula with buccal flap: Rehrmann versus Moczair. Int J Oral Surg 1982; 11:156.
64. Peterson L. Prevention and management of surgical complications. In: Peterson, Ellis, Hupp, Tucker (eds). Contemporary Oral and Maxillofacial Surgery. St. Louis: CV Mosby, 1988:265.
65. Rehrmann A. Eine methode zur schliessung von kieferhohlen perforationen. Dstch Zahnaerzth Wochenschr 1936; 48:1136.
66. Moczair L. Nuovo methodo operatiopela chisura della fistole del seno mascella se di origina dentale. Stomatol (Roma) 1930; 28:1087.
67. Skolnik E, O'Neill J, Baim H. Closure of oroantral fistula. Laryngoscope 1979; 89:844.
68. Awang M. Closure of oroantral fistula. Int J Oral Maxillofac Surg 1988; 17:110.
69. Mainous E, Hammer D. Surgical closure of oroantral fistula using gold foil technique. J Oral Surg 1974; 32:528.
70. Choukas N. Modified palatal flap technique for closure of oroantral fistula. J Oral Surg 1974; 32:112.
71. Anderson M. Surgical closure of oroantral fistula: Report of a series. J Oral Surg 1969; 27:862.
72. Ito T, Hara H. A new technique for closure of oroantral fistula. J Oral Surg 1980; 38:509.
73. Gullane P, Arena S. Palatal island flap for reconstruction of oral defects. Arch Otolaryngol 1977; 103:598.
74. James R. Surgical closure of large oroantral fistulas using a palatal island flap. J Oral Surg 1980; 38:591.
75. Georgiade N, Maldick R, Thorne F. The nasolabial tunnel flap. Plast Reconstr Surg 1969; 43:463.
76. Guerrero-Santos J, Altamirano J. The use of lingual flaps in repair of fistulas of the hard palate. Plast Reconstr Surg 1966; 38:123.
77. Vaughan E, Brown A. The versatility of the lateral tongue flap in the reconstruction of defects of the oral cavity. Br J Oral Surg 1983; 21:1.
78. Steinhauser E. Experience with dorsal flaps for closure of defects of the hard palate. J Oral Maxillofac Surg 1982; 40:787.
79. Carlesso J, Mondolfi P, Flicki E. Hemi-tongue flaps. Plast Reconstr Surg 1986; 66:574.
80. Whitney J, Hammer W, Elliott M, Tucker D. The use of cancellous bone for closure of oroantral and oronasal defects. J Oral Surg 1980; 38:679.
81. Goldman E, Stratigos G, Arthur A. Treatment of oroantral fistula by gold foil closure: Report of a case. J Oral Surg 1969; 27:875.
82. Meyerhoff W, Christiansen T, Rontal E, Boerger W. Gold foil closure of oroantral fistulas. Laryngoscope 1973; 83:940.
83. Shapiro D, Moss M. Gold plate closure of oroantral fistula. J Prosthet Dent 1972; 27:203.
84. Al-Sibahi A, Shanoon A. The use of soft polymethylmethacrylate in the closure of ora-antral fistula. J Oral Maxillofac Surg 1982; 40:165.
85. Cioffi G, Terezhalmy G, Del Balso A. Odontogenic keratocysts of the maxillary sinus. Oral Surg Oral Med Oral Pathol 1987; 64:648.
86. Keller E. Resection of a myxoma of the maxilla via LeFort I osteotomy. J Oral Maxillofac Surg 1988; 46:609.
87. Norje C, Ferman A, Joubert J. Pathological conditions involving the maxillary sinus: Their appearance on panoramic dental radiographs. Br J Oral Surg 1979–80; 17:27.
88. Gamble R. Acute inflammation of the orbit in children. Arch Ophthalmol 1933; 10:483.
89. Chandler J, Langenbrunner D, Stevens E. The pathogenesis of orbital complications in acute sinusitis. Laryngoscope 1970; 80:1414.
90. Williamson-Noble F. Disease of the orbit and its contents secondary to pathological conditions of the nose and paranasal sinuses. Ann R Coll Surg Engl 1954; 15:46.
91. Goodwin WJ. Orbital complications of ethmoiditis. Otholaryngol Clin North Am 1985; 18:139.
92. Schramm V, Meyers E, Kennerdell J. Orbital complications of acute sinusitis: Evaluation, management and outcome. ORL J Otorhinolaryngol Relat Spec 1978; 86:221.
93. Fearson B, Edmonds B, Bird R. Orbital facial complications of sinusitis in children. Laryngoscope 1979; 89:947.
94. Hawkins D, Clark R. Orbital involvement in acute sinusitis. Clin Pediatr 1977; 16:464.
95. Schramm V, Curtin H, Kennerdell J. Evaluation of orbital cellulitis and results of treatment. Laryngoscope 1982; 92:732.
96. Goodwin WJ, Weinshall M, Chandler J. The role of high resolution computerized tomography and standardized ultrasound in the evaluation of orbital cellulitis. Laryngoscope 1982; 92:728.
97. Zimmerman R, Bilaniuk L. CT of orbital infections and its cerebral complications. AJR 1980; 134:45.

V

PRINCIPLES OF MANAGEMENT OF MAXILLOFACIAL TRAUMA

13

Initial Assessment and Management of the Trauma Patient

Michael Powers

The initial assessment and management of the injured patient must be completed in an accurate and systematic manner to establish quickly the extent of injury to vital life-support systems. Nearly 25% to 33% of deaths caused by injury can be prevented when an organized and systematic approach is used.[9]

Significant data exists to suggest that death from trauma has a trimodal distribution.[11] The first peak on a linear distribution of deaths is within seconds or minutes of injury. Invariably these deaths are due to lacerations of the brain, brain stem, upper spinal cord, heart, aorta, or other large vessels. Few of these patients can be saved, although in areas with rapid transport, some of these deaths have been avoided. The second death peak occurs within the first few hours after injury. This period following injury has been called the "golden hours" because these patients may be saved with rapid assessment and management of their injuries. Death is usually due to subdural and epidural hematomas, hemopneumothorax, cardiac tamponade, a ruptured spleen, lacerations of the liver, a fractured femur, or multiple injuries associated with significant blood loss. These patients, whose numbers are significant, benefit most from regionalized trauma care. The third death peak occurs days or weeks after the injury and is almost always due to sepsis and multiple organ failure.

Patients are assessed and treatment priorities are established based on their injuries and the stability of their vital signs. In any emergency involving a critical injury, logical and sequential treatment priorities must be established on the basis of overall patient assessment. Injuries can be divided into three general categories: severe, urgent, and nonurgent.[11] Severe injuries are immediately life-threatening and interfere with vital physiologic functions such as airway inadequacy, breathing, hemorrhage, and circulatory system damage or shock. These injuries constitute approximately 5% of all injuries, but represent over 50% of all trauma deaths. Urgent injuries make up approximately 10% to 15% of all injuries and immediately offer no threat to life. These patients may have injuries to the abdomen, orofacial structures, chest, or extremities that will require surgical intervention or repair, but their vital signs are stable. Nonurgent injuries account for approximately 80% of all injuries and are not immediately life-threatening. This group of patients will eventually require surgical or medical management, although the exact nature of the injury may not become apparent until after significant evaluation and observation. Laboratory studies, additional physical findings, radiographic examinations, and observations for several days or weeks may be required.[12] The goal of initial emergency care is to recognize life-threatening injuries and to provide lifesaving and support measures until definitive care can be initiated.

ASSESSMENT OF THE SEVERITY OF THE INJURY

The primary goal of triage is to prioritize victims according to the severity of injury and urgency and the availability of the required care. With regional trauma centers in modern trauma systems, the goal of triage is to rapidly and accurately identify patients with life-threatening injuries and to treat those patients appropriately, while at the same time avoiding unnecessary transport of less severely injured patients (Fig. 13–1).[10]

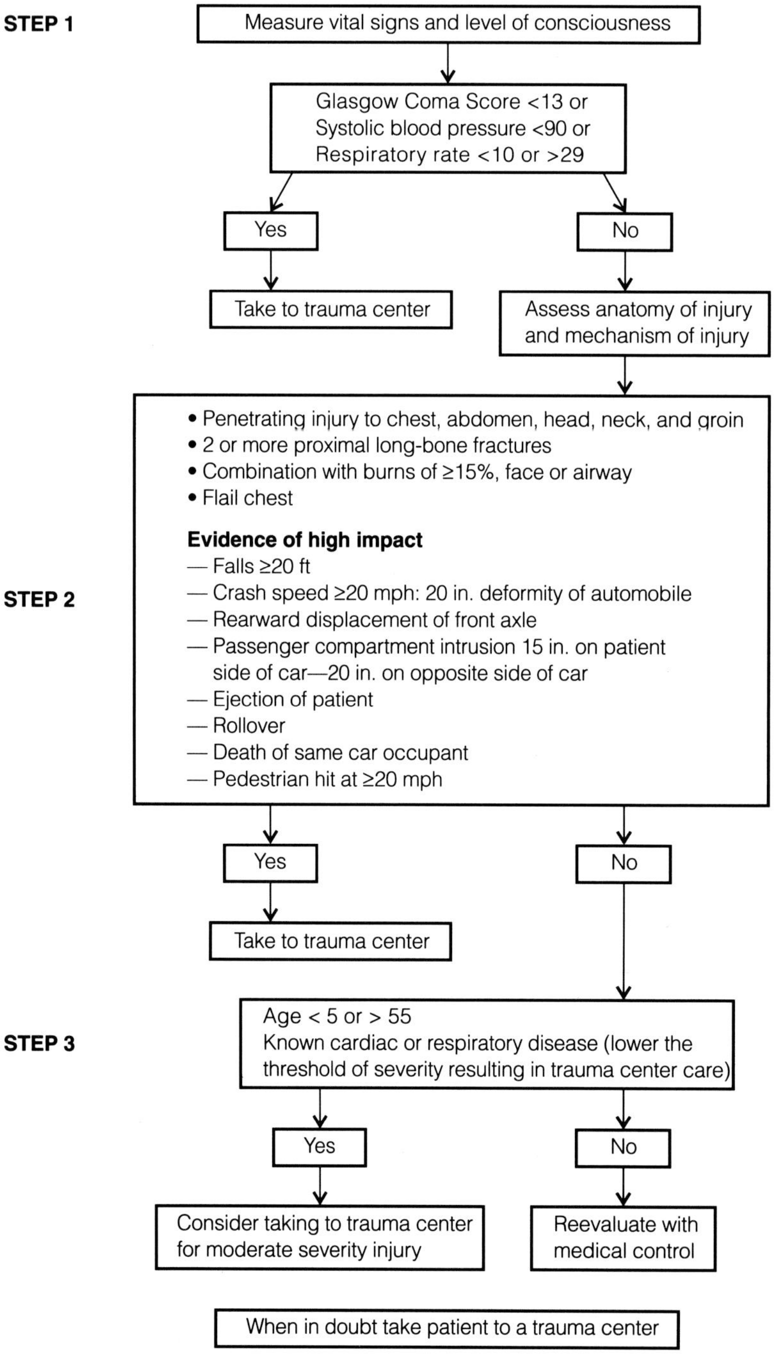

Figure 13–1. *Triage evaluation summary for trauma patients as proposed by the American College of Surgeons Committee on Trauma. (Modified from the Committee on Trauma of the American College of Surgeons. Bull Am Coll Surg 71:10, 1986)*

Trauma Score

The trauma score (Table 13–1) was developed by Champion et al.[1] to quickly assess the extent of injury to vital systems and the severity of the injury to provide proper triage and treatment of the patient.

The trauma score provides a means of characterizing the physiologic status of injured patients' cardiovascular, respiratory, and neurologic systems. The Glasgow Coma Scale (GCS)[4] is incorporated to evaluate the neurologic status and assess the degree of craniocerebral injury. The GCS evaluates the eye-opening response, best verbal response, and best motor response, with a score given for each response. Scores range from 3 to 15 with a higher number representing an increased degree of consciousness.

Similar scales are used to quickly evaluate the cardiovascular system (capillary refill rate and systolic blood pressure) and the respiratory system (rate and effort). The total points are added to give a trauma score of 1 to 15; in this instance also, the higher the score, the better the estimated prognosis. Thus, an injured patient who exhibits eye opening to painful stimulus (score 2), a verbal response that is incomprehensible (score 2), and withdrawal from a painful stimulus (score 4) would have a GCS of 8 points and would contribute 3 points to the trauma score.

Trauma scores of around 8 have approximately a 50% probability of survival.[5] In 1986, the Major Trauma Outcome Study consisted of analysis of 33,308 trauma patients submitted by 89 hospitals across the United States and Canada with survival probabilities associated with admission trauma scores determined for 25,327 patients (Table 13–2).[5] Patients likely to benefit from prompt diagnosis and definitive care at level I trauma centers are those with a trauma score of 12 or less.[1]

CRAMS Scale

The CRAMS system was developed by Gornican in 1982[7] and modified by Clemmer et al. in 1985[6] as another means for nonphysician personnel (emergency medical technicians and paramedics) to quickly assess the injured patient in triage and properly direct the patient to an appropriate facility for treatment. CRAMS is an acronym for *c*irculation, *r*espirations, *a*bdomen, *m*otor, and *s*peech (Table 13–3). Scores are made for clinical findings in each category; the total CRAMS score ranges from 0 to 10.

Clemmer et al.[6] reported that 94.5% of patients studied had CRAMS field scores of 7 or greater. Patients with field scores of 6 or less had a mortality rate of 62%, and the authors felt that the mortality rate could be greatly reduced if these patients were quickly transported to a level I trauma center. Using a CRAMS score of 8 or less as a criterion for transporting patients to a level I trauma center would result in approximately 18% of trauma patients being transported and would encompass all the patients with potentially lethal injuries.[2]

Injury Severity Score

The Injury Severity Score (ISS) was developed to deal with multiple traumatic injuries and compare death rates from blunt trauma using data that rated the severity of injury in each of the three most severely injured organ systems. Each injury is evaluated and categorized according to the organ system (respiratory, central nervous system [CNS], cardiovascular, abdominal, extremities, and skin) injured and graded according to the severity of the injury (*1* is minor; *2*, moderate; *3*, severe, nonlife-threatening; *4*, life-threatening, survival probable; *5*, survival not probable; *6*, fatal cardiovascular, CNS, or burn injuries). The three highest scores are then squared and added to give the ISS. The lowest total possible is 3 ($1^2 + 1^2 + 1^2$) and the highest ISS score possible is 108 ($6^2 + 6^2 + 6^2$). Mortality rates have been found to increase with increased severity of injury and age (Table 13–4).

In addition to the field scales that measure abnormal physiologic signs for assessment of injury for triage decisions, mechanism-of-injury factors and anatomic factors are also important considerations. Mechanism-of-injury factors can provide insight to possible significant injury that has not yet resulted in significant changes in vital signs. Those mechanisms-of-injury factors that have a high correlation with life-threatening injuries include evidence of collisions involving high-energy dissipation or rapid deceleration, a fall of 20 ft. or more, evidence that the patient was in a dangerous environment when injured (i.e., a burning building or icy water), or an automobile accident that involves more than 20 minutes to remove the patient, significant damage to the passenger compartment, rearward displacement of the front anxle, ejection of the patient,

Table 13–1. The Trauma Score*

		Rate	Codes	Score
RESPIRATORY RATE				
Number of respirations in 15 seconds; multiply by four		10–24	4	
		25–35	3	
		≥ 36	2	
		1–9	1	
		0	0	A____
RESPIRATORY EFFORT				
		Normal	1	
Retractive Use of accessory muscles or intercostal retraction		Retractive/none	0	B____
SYSTOLIC BLOOD PRESSURE				
Systolic cuff pressure Either arm, auscultate or palpate		≥ 90	4	
		70–89	3	
		50–69	2	
		0–49	1	
No carotid pulse		0	0	C____
CAPILLARY REFILL				
Normal Forehead or lip mucosa color refill in 2 seconds		Normal	2	
Delayed More than 2 seconds capillary refill		Delayed	1	
None No capillary refill		None	0	D____
GLASGOW COMA SCALE (GCS)		*Total GCS points*	*Score*	
Eye-opening				
Spontaneous	____4	14–15	5	
To voice	____3	11–13	4	
To pain	____2	8–10	3	
None		5–7	2	
		3–5	1	E____
Verbal response				
Oriented	____5			
Confused	____4			
Inappropriate words	____3			
Incomprehensible sounds	____2			
None				
Motor response				
Obeys commands	____6			
Localises pain	____5			
Withdraws (pain)	____4			
Flexion (pain)	____3			
Extension (pain)	____2			
None	____1			
TOTAL GCS POINTS (1 + 2 + 3) ________			Trauma score________ (Total points A + B + C + D + E)	

* *The Trauma Score incorporates the Glasgow Coma Scale for evaluation of neurologic status with physiologic parameters of respiratory rate and effort, systolic blood pressure level and capillary refill time to estimate the severity of injury. (Champion HR, Sacco WJ, Carnazzo AJ, et al. Crit Care Med 1981; 9(9): 672–676*

Table 13–2. *Probability of Survival (P_s) for Trauma Score Values**

Trauma Score on Admission	*No. of Patients*	*P_s (%)*
1	529	2.3
2	131	6.1
3	81	6.2
4	84	14.3
5	116	21.6
6	186	31.7
7	350	38.3
8	312	52.2
9	277	61.7
10	357	66.7
11	509	75.2
12	790	80.4
13	1139	90.7
14	1878	95.0
15	3782	97.6
16	14806	99.1

** The probability of survival was evaluated from data obtained in the Major Trauma Outcome Study (1986) on 25,327 patients. The trauma score attempts to assess quickly the extent of injury by characterizing the physiologic status of the patient's cardiovascular, neurologic, and respiratory systems. Trauma scores have been found to directly correlate with probability of survival. (Champion HR, Sacco WJ. Trauma scoring. In: Mattox KC, Moore EE, Feliciano DV, eds.* Trauma. *Norwalk, CT: Appleton and Lange, 1988)*

Table 13–3. *The CRAMS Scale*

CIRCULATION	
Normal capillary refill and BP > 100	2
Delayed capillary refill or 85 < BP < 100	1
No capillary refill or BP < 85	0
RESPIRATION	
Normal	2
Abnormal (labored or shallow)	1
Absent	0
ABDOMEN	
Abdomen and thorax nontender	2
Abdomen or thorax tender	1
Abdomen rigid or flail chest	0
MOTOR	
Normal	2
Responds only to pain (other than decerebrate)	1
No response (or decerebrate)	0
SPEECH	
Normal	2
Confused	1
No intelligible words	0

Score ≤ 8 = Major trauma
Score ≥ 9 = Minor trauma

(Clemmer TP, Orne JF, Thomas F, Brooks KA. J Trauma *1985; 25(3): 188–191)*

Table 13–4. *Mortality Rates for Various Injury Severity Scores (ISSs) by Age Groups*

Age (yr)	*n*	*15*	*25*	*35*	*45*	*55*
0–49	1540	3%	8%	32%	61%	89%
50–69	316	5%	21%	56%	68%	100%
70+	109	16%	45%	82%	100%	100%

(Wilson RF. Accidental and Surgical Trauma. In Shoemaker, WC, Ayres S, Grenvich A, Holbrock PR, Thompson WC, eds. Textbook of critical care, *ed. 2. Philadelphia: WB Saunders Co, 1989)*

rollover, or death of other passengers.[2,13] Anatomic factors that correlate with mortality include a penetrating trauma to the head, neck, torso, groin, or thigh; flail chest; major burns; amputations; two or more proximal long bone fractures; or paralysis. Concurrent disease or factors such as age of less than 5 years or greater than 55 years and known cardiac or respiratory disease may sharply worsen a patient's prognosis even in the presence of only moderately severe injury.[2,13]

The American College of Surgeons Committee on Trauma Subcommittee on Advanced Trauma Life Support has developed a schematic, orderly assessment of the injured patients. The Advanced Trauma Life Support (ATLS) system consists of a rapid primary evaluation, resuscitation of vital functions, a more detailed secondary assessment, and finally the initiation of definitive care (Fig. 13–2).[8]

PRIMARY SURVEY: ABCs

During the primary survey, life-threatening conditions are identified and reversed quickly. This period calls for quick and efficient evaluation of the patient's injuries and lifesaving intervention done almost si-

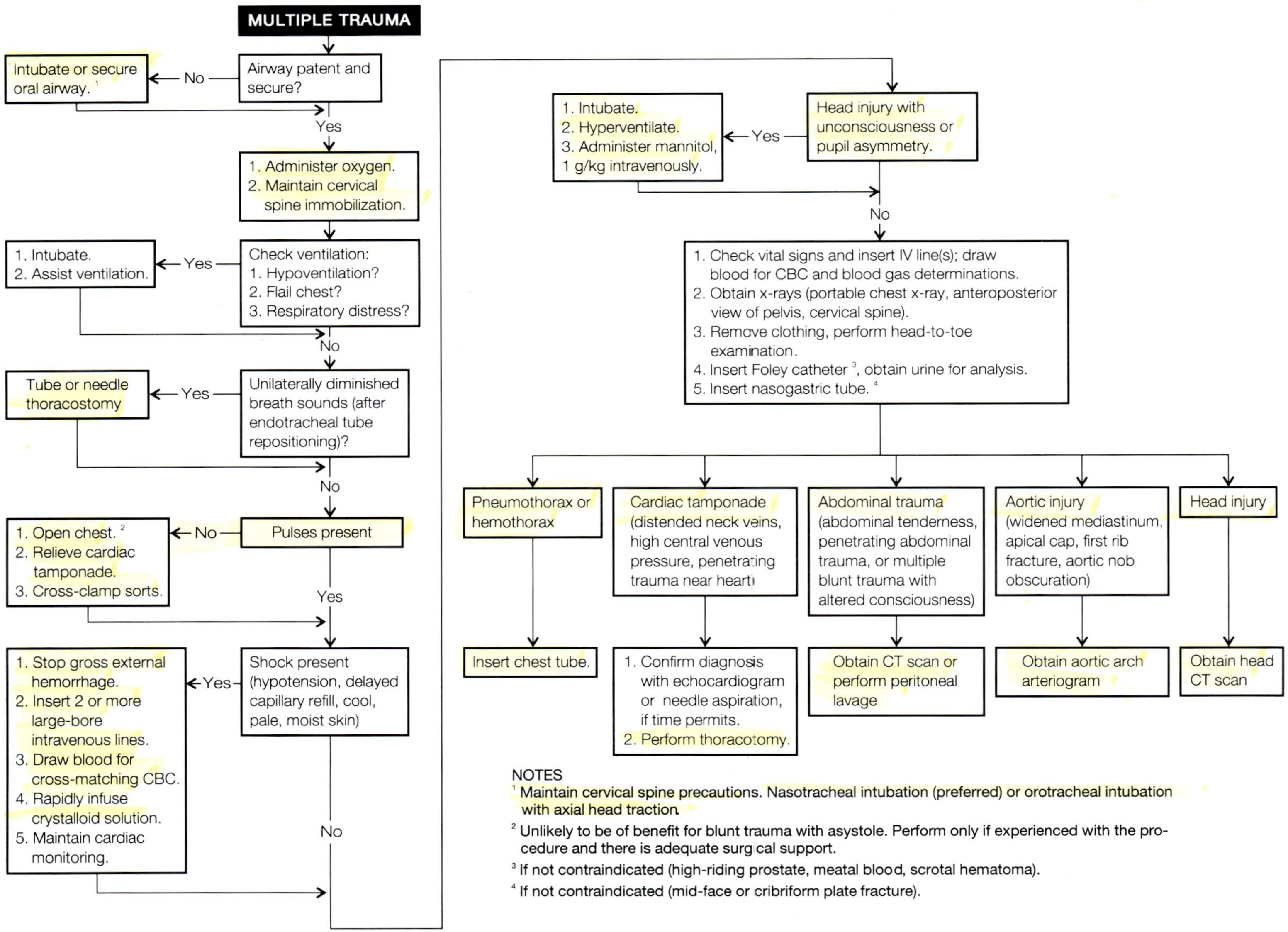

NOTES

[1] Maintain cervical spine precautions. Nasotracheal intubation (preferred) or orotracheal intubation with axial head traction.

[2] Unlikely to be of benefit for blunt trauma with asystole. Perform only if experienced with the procedure and there is adequate surgical support.

[3] If not contraindicated (high-riding prostate, meatal blood, scrotal hematoma).

[4] If not contraindicated (mid-face or cribriform plate fracture).

Figure 13–2. *Flow diagram for initial systematic evaluation and stabilization of the multiply-injured patient. (Trunkey DD. In: Ho M, Saunders CE, eds.* Current emergency diagnosis and treatment, *ed. 3. Norwalk, CT: Lange Publishing Co., 1990)* multaneously. The primary survey progresses in a logical manner based on the ABCs:

A: Airway maintenance with cervical spine control
B: Breathing and adequate ventilation
C: Circulation with control of hemorrhage
D: A brief neurologic examination to establish degree of consciousness.
E: Exposure of the patient by complete undressing to avoid missing injuries camouflaged by clothing

Airway Maintenance with Cervical Spine Control

The highest priority in the initial assessment of the trauma patient is the establishment and maintenance of a patent airway. In the trauma patient, upper airway obstruction may be due to bleeding from oral or facial structures, aspiration of foreign materials, or regurgitation of stomach contents. Commonly, the upper airway is obstructed by the position of the tongue, especially in the unconscious patient (Fig. 13–3). Initially, a chin-lift or jaw-thrust procedure may position the tongue and open the airway. The chin-thrust procedure is performed by placing the thumb over the incisal edges of the mandibular anterior teeth and wrapping the fingers tightly around the symphysis of the mandible. The chin is then lifted gently anteriorly and the mouth opened if possible. The other hand can be used to assist with access to the oral cavity, using the fingers in a sweeping motion to remove such things as debris, vomitus, blood, and dentures that may be responsible for the obstruction. A tonsilar suction tip is helpful to remove accumulations from the pharynx. Patients with facial injuries who may have basilar skull fractures or fractures of the cribriform

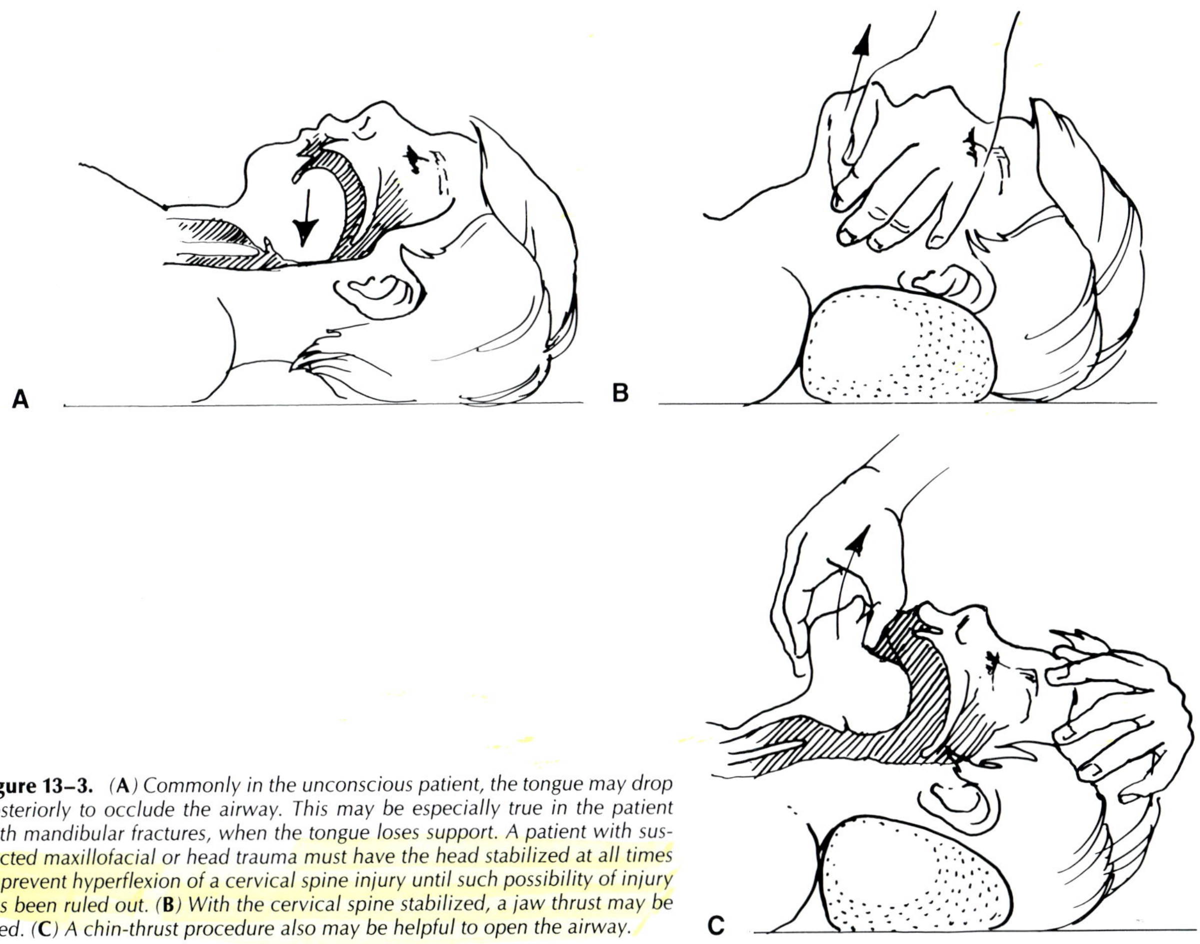

Figure 13–3. *(**A**) Commonly in the unconscious patient, the tongue may drop posteriorly to occlude the airway. This may be especially true in the patient with mandibular fractures, when the tongue loses support. A patient with suspected maxillofacial or head trauma must have the head stabilized at all times to prevent hyperflexion of a cervical spine injury until such possibility of injury has been ruled out. (**B**) With the cervical spine stabilized, a jaw thrust may be used. (**C**) A chin-thrust procedure also may be helpful to open the airway.*

plate may, with the routine use of a soft suction catheter or nasogastric tube, be compromised as these tubes may inadvertently be passed into the contents of the cranial vault during attempts at pharyngeal suction. If the chin-lift procedure is not successful, a jaw-thrust procedure should be tried. The jaw-thrust procedure requires the placement of both hands along the ascending ramus of the mandible at the mandibular angle. The fingers are placed behind the inferior border of the angle, and the thumbs are placed over the teeth or chin. The mandible is then gently pulled forward with the fingers at the angle and rotated inferiorly with pressure from the thumbs. The elbows may be placed on the surface alongside the patient to assist with stability. The jaw-thrust procedure is the safest method of jaw manipulation of a patient with suspected cervical injury. The jaw-thrust procedure does require two hands and assistance must be available to clear the debris and other obstructions. After the jaw is opened, it may be possible to place a bite lock or large suction device to wedge the teeth open. An oral or nasal airway should be placed to elevate the base of the tongue and maintain the patient airway.

With any patient sustaining injuries above the clavicle, one should assume there may be cervical spine injury and should avoid hyperextension or hyperflexion of the patient's neck during attempts to establish an airway. Excessive movement of the cervical spine can turn a fracture without neurologic damage into a fracture that causes paralysis. Maintenance of the cervical spine in the neutral position is best achieved with the use of a backboard, bindings, and sandbags. The use of soft or semirigid collars allows, at best, only 50% stabilization of movement.[29] Cervical spine injury should be assumed present and should be protected against until the patient can be stabilized and cervical injury ruled out during the secondary survey.

Breathing

With establishment of an adequate airway, the pulmonary status must next be evaluated. If the patient is breathing spontaneously—confirmed by feeling and listening for air movement at the nostrils and mouth—supplemental oxygen may be delivered by face mask. Exchange of air does not guarantee adequate ventilation. The chest wall of a patient with a pneumothorax, flail chest, or a hemothorax may move but not ventilate effectively. Also, shallow breaths with minimal tidal volumes do not ventilate the lungs effectively. Very slow or rapid rates of respiration usually suggest poor ventilation. The patient's status should be constantly reevaluated, and if signs of adequate ventilation deteriorate, an airway (preferably an endotracheal tube) should be placed and assisted ventilation begun. If the patient is not breathing after establishment of an airway, artificial ventilation should then be provided with a bag-valve device connected to a mask or to an endotracheal tube or with a time-cycled positive-pressure ventilator to an endotracheal tube. The patient who requires assisted positive-pressure ventilation from an ambu bag or ventilator must be carefully monitored if the chest status has not been completely evaluated. Changes in intrathoracic pressure may convert a simple pneumothorax into a tension pneumothorax. The chest should be exposed and inspected for obvious injury and open wounds. There should be equal expansion of the chest wall without intercostal and supraclavicular muscle retractions during respiration. The rate of breathing should be evaluated for tachypnea or abnormal breathing patterns. The signs of chest injury or impending hypoxia are frequently subtle and include an increased rate of breathing and a change in breathing pattern—frequently toward more shallow respirations.[8] The chest wall should also be inspected for bruising, flail chest, and bleeding, and the neck should be evaluated for evidence of tracheal deviation, subcutaneous emphysema, and extended jugular veins. The chest should be palpated for the presence of rib or sternal fractures, subcutaneous emphysema, and wounds. Asculation of the chest may reveal a lack of breath sounds in an area suggestive of inadequate ventilation. Distant heart sounds and distended neck veins may be suggestive of cardiac tamponade. Arterial oxygen tension (PaO_2) should be maintained between 70 and 100 mm Hg. Aside from airway obstruction, the causes of inadequate ventilation in the trauma victim result from altered chest wall mechanics. Open pneumothorax, flail chest, tension pneumothorax, and massive hemothorax are immediate life-threatening conditions and should be quickly identified and treated.

Open Pneumothorax

An open pneumothorax is due to a defect in the chest wall, allowing the air to be moved in and out of the pleural cavity with each respiration (Fig. 13–4). Be-

Figure 13–4. *(**A**) A pneumothorax develops from damage to the chest wall or laceration of the lung pleura with resulting loss of negative intrapleural pressure. A pneumothorax may be graded as small (15% or less of the pleural cavity), moderate (15% to 60%), or large (greater than 60%). (**B**) An open or communicating chest wound occurs with an open wound in the chest wall. Air can often be heard moving in and out of the wound during respirations and may be referred to as a "sucking chest wound." An open pneumothorax may be converted to a simple pneumothorax with the use of an occlusive dressing over the chest wall wound. Care must be taken not to create a "trap door" effect and developing tension pneumothorax.*

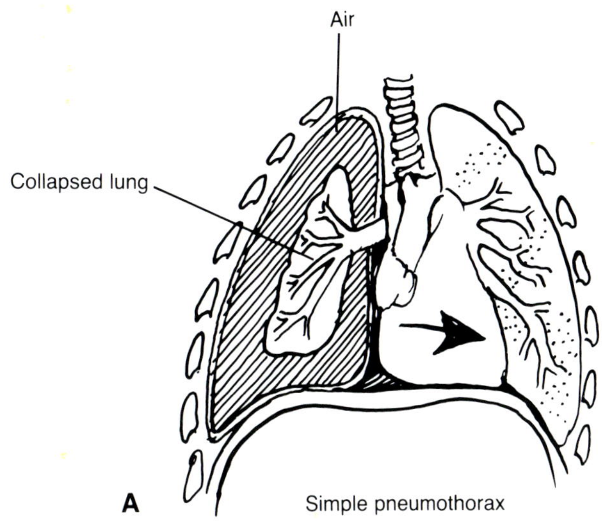

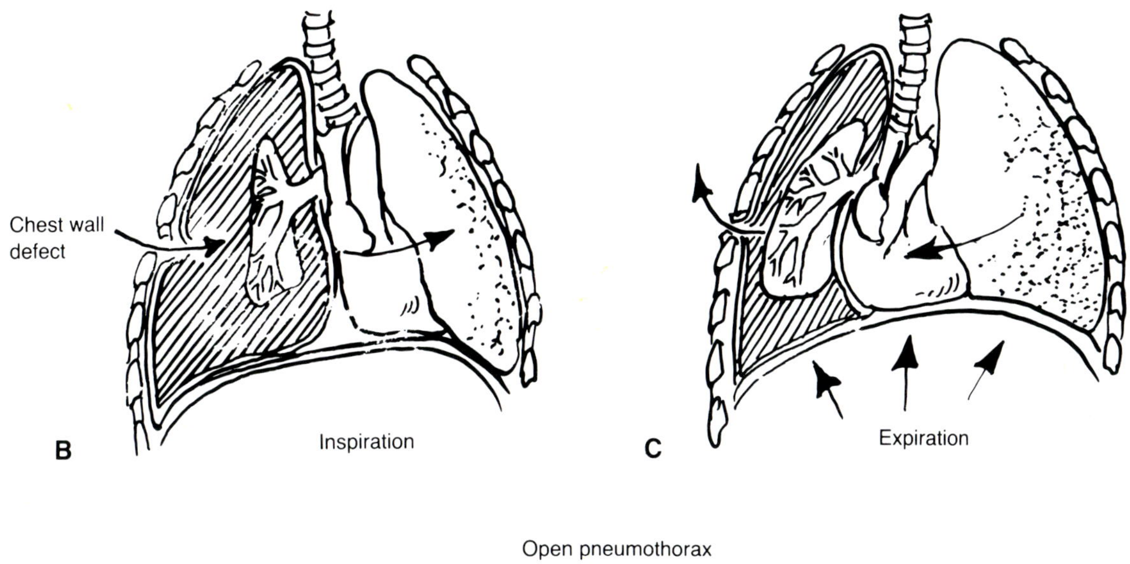

cause of the loss of chest wall integrity, equilibrium develops between intrathoracic pressure and atmospheric pressure. The involved lung collapses on inspiration and slightly expands on expiration, causing air to be sucked in and out of the wound. The sound of the air movement has led to the application of the term *sucking chest wound* to this injury. If the opening in the chest wall is approximately two thirds of the diameter of the trachea, air will pass through the route of least resistance—the chest wall defect. With collapse of the involved lung and loss of negative-pleural pressure, the expired air from the normal lung passes to the involved lung instead of out the trachea, and it returns to the normal lung on inspiration. This eventually results in a large functional dead space in the normal lung and, combined with loss of the involved lung, may develop into a severe ventilation-perfusion problem.

An open pneumothorax should be treated with coverage of the defect with sterile occlusive dressing that is secured on three sides of the dressing to the chest. The unsecured side of the dressing acts as a one-way valve, allowing air to escape the pleural cavity on expiration. Secure taping of all edges of the dressing results in accumulation of air within the thoracic cavity and subsequent tension pneumothorax.

Occlusive dressings such as Vaseline gauze may be used as a temporary measure during initial examination or over large defects. A chest tube must be placed in a distant site on the affected chest wall to avoid development of a tension pneumothorax, and the wound must eventually be closed in the operating room. If the lung does not expand after closure of the defect or if signs of poor ventilation persist, the patient should be placed on a ventilator with positive-end expiratory pressure (PEEP) to expand the lung. The patient should be carefully monitored and have a chest tube in place to avoid development of a tension pneumothorax caused by a tear in one of the bronchi or in the lung parenchyma. Signs of tension pneumothorax with patients on ventilators are increased airway resistance and diminished total volume.

A closed pneumothorax may develop from blunt trauma to the chest and lung laceration, possibly from a fractured rib. Air from the lung to the pleural space equalizes the pressures, and the lung collapses. A ventilation-perfusion deficit occurs because the blood circulated to the affected lung is not oxygenated. With a pneumothorax, percussion of the chest shows hyperresonance. Breath sounds are usually distant or absent. Confirmation and evaluation of management of the pneumothorax is done through upright chest radiographs. An open pneumothorax that has a dressing placed over the chest wound becomes a closed pneumothorax.

Pneumothoraces that are traumatically induced are usually treated with tube thoracostomy, regardless of size, to correct any respiratory compromise. A small pneumothorax may be treated by hospitalization and careful observation if the patient is otherwise healthy, symptom free, and does not need general anesthesia or positive-pressure ventilation and if the size of the pneumothorax is not increasing as measured on serial 24-hour chest radiographs.[43] This is rarely the case with the trauma victim, and a chest tube should be immediately placed in the multiply-injured patient with a pneumothorax.

A moderate-sized chest tube (32 to 40 French in adults or 26 to 30 French in children) is generally placed either anteriorly in the second intercostal space midclavicular line or in the fourth or fifth intercostal space midaxillary line. The midaxillary line is generally preferred for cosmetic reasons, and it can effectively remove both fluid and air if the tube is positioned properly and superiorly toward the apex of the lung (Fig. 13–5).

A skin incision of approximately 3 cm in length is made one intercostal space below the intended placement of the tube. If the tube is to be placed through the fourth intercostal space, an incision is made through the skin along the fifth intercostal space. A gloved finger is then used to make a transverse tunnel through the subcutaneous tissue to the inferior margin of the fourth rib. The intercostal muscles are separated with a large Kelly clamp, and the chest tube is inserted superiorly and posteriorly into the pleural cavity. The tube should be secured to the skin with sutures and an occlusive dressing such as Vaseline gauze should be used to cover the chest defect about the tube. The tube is then connected to underwater sealed drainage to remove the air or fluid. The intrathoracic position of the tube, the last drainage hole on the tube, and the position and amount of air or fluid remaining in the pleural cavity should be checked with an upright posteroanterior and lateral chest radiograph as soon as possible. Serial daily auscultations and chest radiographs should be done to monitor management or removal of air or fluid from the pleural cavity. If the tube becomes blocked and significant fluid or air remains, a new chest tube should be put in place rather than an attempt made to remove the blockage.

Tension Pneumothorax

A tension pneumothorax develops when the injury acts as a "one-way valve" through the chest wall or from the lung into the pleural cavity without equilibration with the outside atmosphere (Fig. 13–6). A dangerous progressive increase of intrapleural pressure develops as air enters the pleural cavity on inspiration but cannot escape on expiration, causing complete collapse of the affected lung. As the pressure increases, the trachea and mediastinum are displaced to the opposite pleural cavity and impinge on the normal lung. The positive-intrapleural pressure compresses the vena cava, leading to decreased cardiac output. The compression of the normal lung causes shunting of blood to nonventilated areas and severe ventilatory disturbances. These changes develop into a rapid onset of hypoxia, acidosis, and shock.[43]

The most common causes of tension pneumothorax are mechanical ventilation with PEEP; spontaneous pneumothorax in which emphysematous bullae have failed to seal; and blunt chest trauma in which the

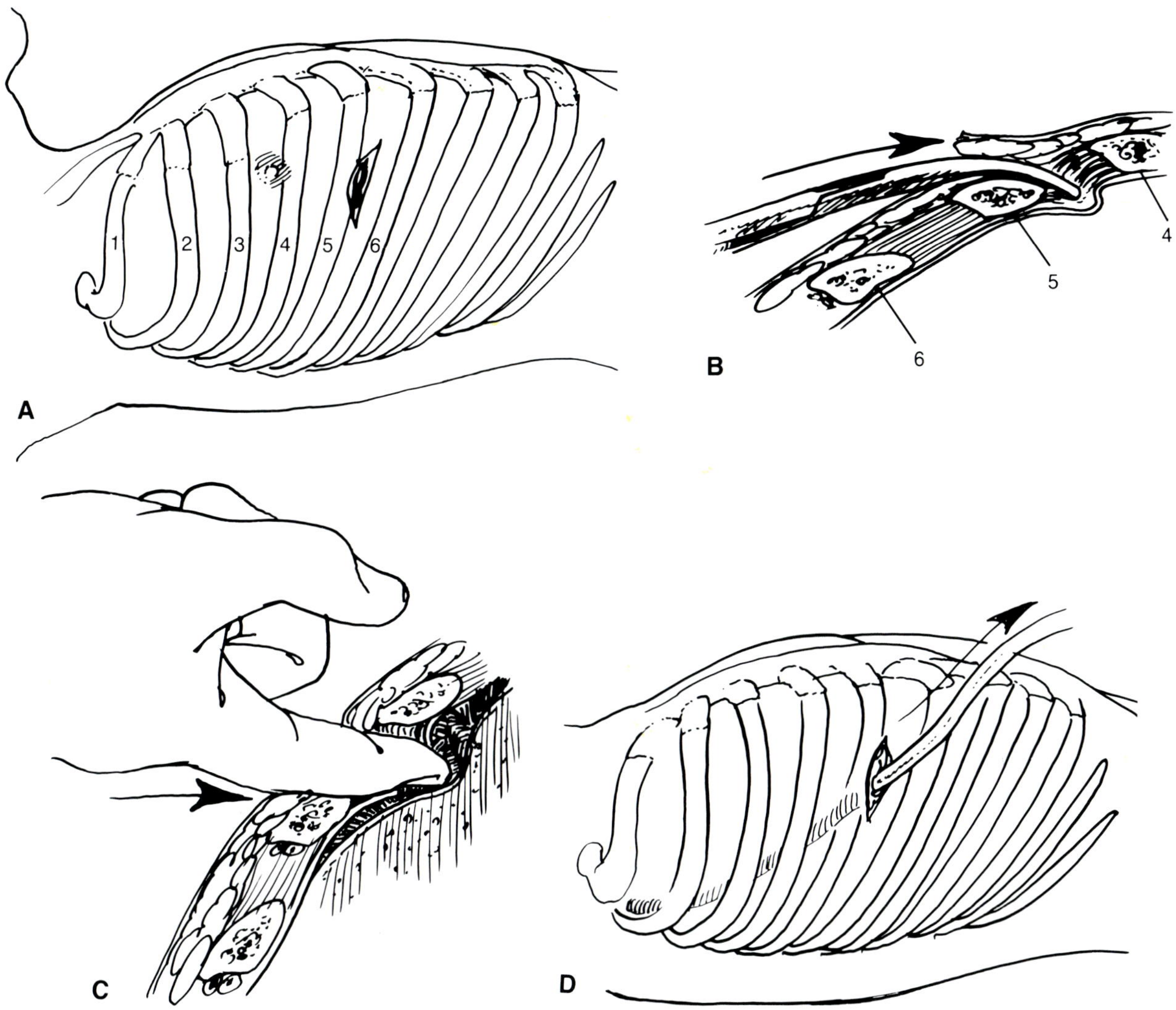

Figure 13–5. *Chest tube placement. The patient should be supine with the arm positioned superiorly to assist with access to the midaxillary line. (**A**) An incision is made through the skin and subcutaneous tissue along the inferior aspect of the fifth rib. (**B**) A large Kelley clamp is used, with the tips placed inferiorly, to bluntly dissect over the fifth rib into the intercostal space between the fourth and fifth rib. (**C**) A gloved finger should be used to enter the pleural space to avoid possible laceration of structures within the pleural space, such as the lung or possible abdominal contents in the case of a ruptured diaphragm. (**D**) The chest tube is then passed along the finger, superiorly and posteriorly within the pleural cavity. The tube should be secured to the chest with sutures, covered with an occlusive dressing, and used for suction under water seal, following verification of tube position by chest radiographs.*

parenchymal lung injury has failed to seal. Occasionally, traumatic defects in the chest wall may lead to tension pneumothorax.[8] The presence of pneumothorax should be considered in patients who rapidly become acutely ill, develop severe respiratory distress, and exhibit decreased breath sounds, hyperresonance on one side of the chest, distended neck veins, and deviation of the trachea away from the involved side (Fig. 13–7A, B). If untreated, a tension pneumothorax is rapidly fatal. If a developing tension pneumothorax is suspected, the positive-intrapleural pressure should be released as quickly as possible. The pressure can be released by inserting a large-bore needle (14 to 16 gauge) anteriorly in the affected hemithorax through the second or third intercostal space in the midclavicular line. This quickly converts the tension pneumothorax to a pneumothorax that can be treated with placement of a chest tube.

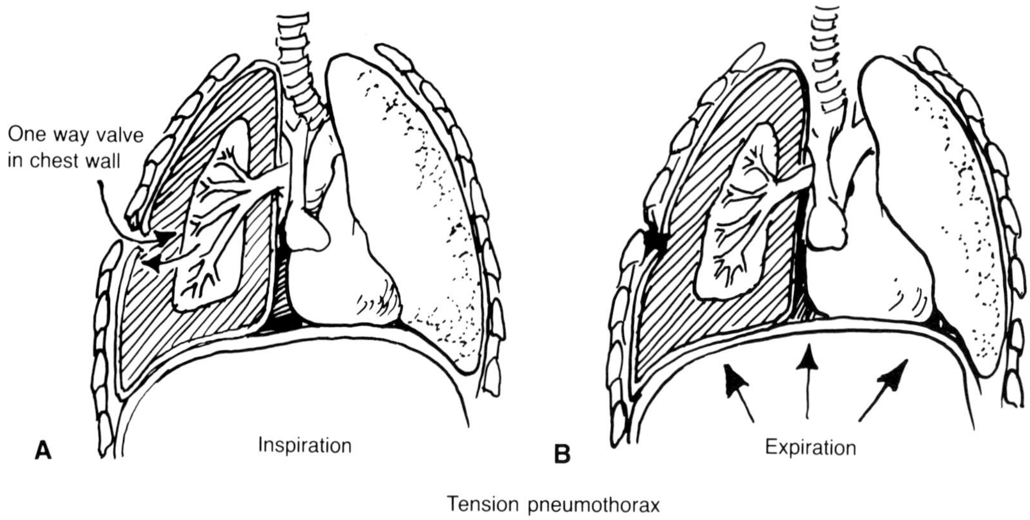

Figure 13–6. *(**A**) A tension pneumothorax develops as air enters the pleural cavity on inspiration but cannot be removed during expiration (**B**), and a progressive increase in intrapleural air pressure develops. The injury in the chest wall or trachea acts like a one-way valve, and the increasing intrapleural pressure results in a shift of the trachea and mediastinal structures away from the injury. The pressure on the vena cava does not allow for adequate return of blood to the heart, and compression of the opposite lung (added to the injured lung) causes severe ventilatory disturbance. (From Uvkich DJ, Markovchick VJ. Pulmonary and chest wall injuries. In Rosen R, ed.* Emergency medicine: Concepts and clinical practice. *St. Louis, CV Mosby Co., 1988)*

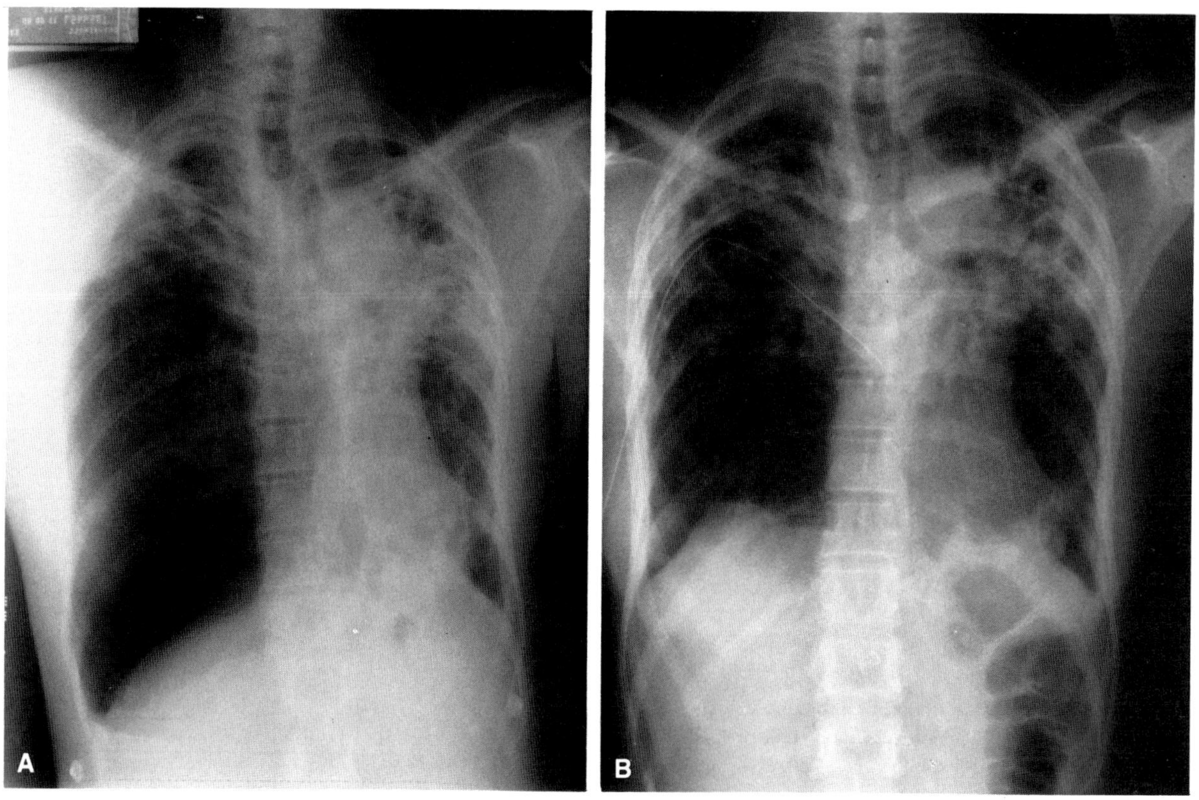

Figure 13–7. *(**A**) A developing tension pneumothorax in a 30-year-old man with a penetrating injury to the right chest wall. Note the shift of the trachea, bronchus, heart, and major vessels to the left lung fields with the expanding tension pneumothorax. (**B**) Placement of a chest tube into the right plural space converts a tension pneumothorax into a simple pneumothorax. The trachea, heart, major vessels, and bronchus are beginning to move back into normal anatomic position from the shift to the left (noted on the previous radiograph).*

Hemothorax

Hemothorax is the collection of blood in the pleural cavity. It is commonly the result of penetrating injuries that disrupt the vasculature but can result from blunt trauma that tears the vasculature. Initial loss of blood collected in the pleural cavity may come from lung injuries, but because of low pulmonary arterial pressure, the blood loss is usually slowed. Massive hemothorax usually results from injuries to the aortic arch or pulmonary hilum; it may also result from injuries to the internal mammary arteries or intercostal arteries, which are branches of the aorta. A hemothorax may dangerously reduce the vital capacity of the lung and contribute to hypovolemic shock. A hemothorax usually is associated with pneumothorax, and the subsequent blood loss causes hypotension, a decreased cardiac output, and metabolic acidosis, which, when combined with the ventilatory compromise, results in hypoxia and respiratory acidosis.

A hemothorax should be suspected following penetrating or blunt chest trauma if the patient is in shock with reduced breath sounds and with the chest dull to percussion on one side. The neck veins may be flat because of severe hypovolemia or distended as a result of the mechanical effects of a chest full of blood.[8] With the loss of a small amount of blood (less than 400 mL) the diagnosis is difficult because there may be little or no change in the patient's appearance, vital signs, or physical findings. Fluid collections greater than 250 mL can usually be seen on a good upright chest radiograph with a blunting of the costophrenic angle. The supine radiograph is less accurate and as much as 1000 mL of blood may not be detectable.[43] Treatment of a hemothorax consists of restoration of the circulating blood volume with transfusion of fluids, volume expanders, blood, or blood products through large-bore intravenous lines, controlling of the airway and support of the ventilation as required, and drainage of the accumulated blood from the pleural cavity. A large chest tube (36 to 40 French) should be inserted in the fifth or sixth intercostal space in the midaxillary line and the tube directed posteriorly and superiorly to avoid damage to a possibly elevated diaphragm. The chest tube should be connected to an underwater seal and steady suction (20 to 30 cm of H_2O). If the chest tube becomes clotted and fails to drain, another chest tube should be put in place rather than an attempt made to irrigate the first tube. With massive bleeding, autotransfusion of the drained blood is possible until bank blood is available.[44] A persistent hemorrhage requires surgical exploration. Thoracotomy for intrathoracic bleeding is indicated if the patient's vital signs remain unstable, if more than 1500 to 2000 mL of blood is lost from the chest in the first 12 to 24 hours, if the drainage of blood from the chest tubes exceeds 300 mL/hour for 3 to 4 hours or longer, or if the chest stays more than half full of blood on radiographs.[45] In a few instances, emergency thoracotomy in the emergency room may be necessary for control of blood loss. However, mortality from this procedure is very high.[8]

Flail Chest

A flail chest results when there are multiple rib fractures, usually at multiple sites along the rib (Fig. 13–8). The resulting unstable segment of chest wall moves paradoxically during respirations—moving inward with inspiration and outward with expiration. A flail chest may affect respiratory ability to the point that hypoxemia occurs. The pain associated with the respiratory effort may also compromise the ventilatory compliance of the patient. The fractured ribs may have punctured the lung, causing a tension pneumothorax or hemothorax. A problem with flail chest and hypoxemia is the underlying pulmonary contusion from the injury. The contused lung may be asymptomatic in the initial presentation but develop complications later with gas exchange. Immediately after the injury, little abnormal breathing may be apparent. Later, as fluid moves into the lung, contusion and lung compliance falls, and more pressure is needed to inflate the lungs. The pulmonary contusion underlying major chest wall injuries may be the primary cause of hypoxia and morbidity in patients with flail chest. Mortality in patients sustaining severe blunt chest trauma remains relatively high at 12% to 50%.[46]

A flail chest is usually apparent on visual examination of the unconscious patient. Flail chest may not be initially apparent in the conscious patient because of splinting of the chest wall. The patient moves air poorly as a result of paradoxical breathing, and movement of the thorax is asymmetrical and uncoordinated. The region of the fracture(s) may be tender to palpation.

Recommended management of flail chest is in three stages.[22] The first step is to initially stabilize the loose segment with an external splint such as a sandbag,

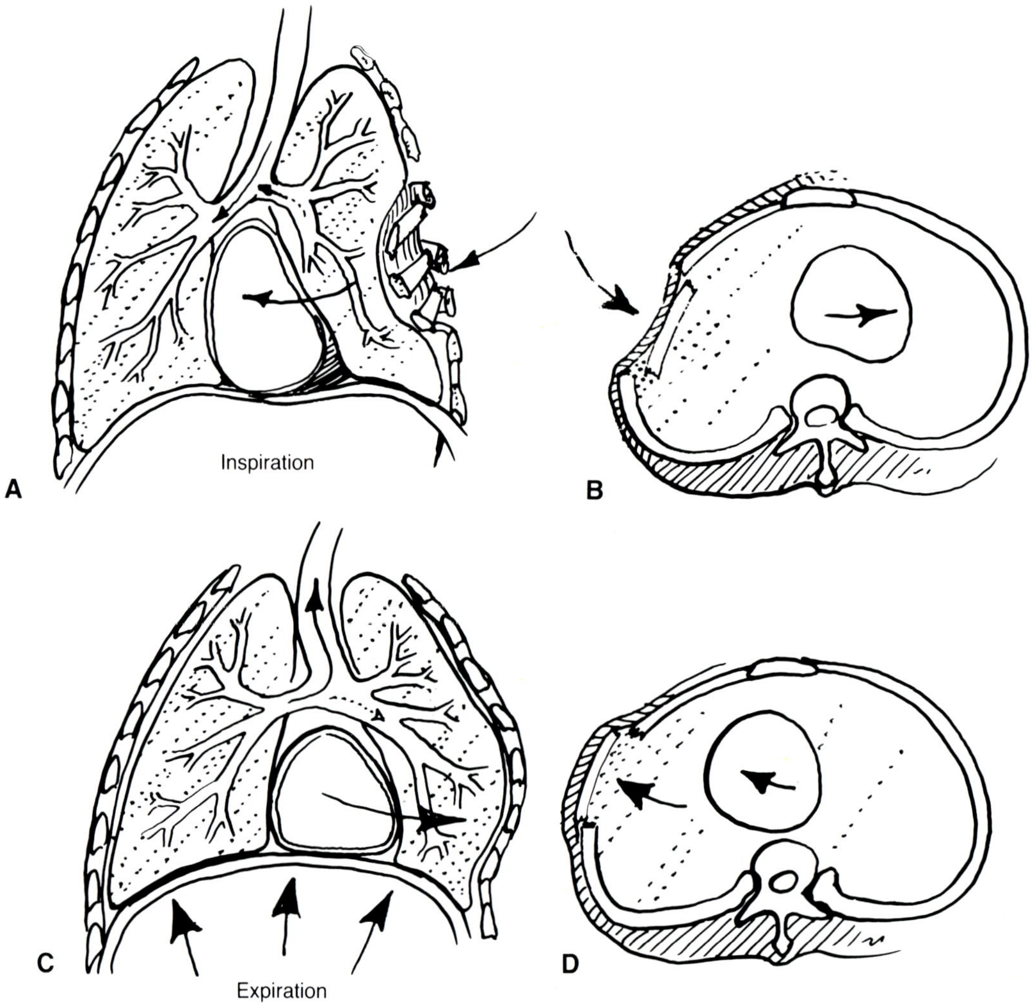

Figure 13–8. *A flail chest occurs when three or more adjacent ribs are fractured at at least two locations, resulting in a freely moving segment of chest wall during respirations. The chest wall moves paradoxically during inspiration and expiration due to the flail segment. (***A***) On inspiration, the flail segment sinks inward as the chest wall expands, impairing the ability to produce negative intrapleural pressure. (***B***) The heart and other contents of the mediastinum shift toward the noninjured side. (***C***) During expiration, the flail segment is pushed outward (***D***) and the chest wall cannot efficiently force air from the lungs. Air may shift uselessly from lung to lung. (From Vukich DJ, Markovchick VJ. Pulmonary and chest wall injuries. In Rosen P, ed.* Emergency medicine: Concepts and clinical practice. *St. Louis, CV Mosby Co., 1988)*

rolled sheet, or intravenous bag taped over the location of the paradoxical movement to both stabilize that segment and to reduce the pain associated with movement of the broken segment. Although this tends to reduce the vital capacity of the lung, it increases the efficiency of ventilation. This form of treatment can produce atelectasis if used for a prolonged period but is adequate for the first 30 minutes until more definitive treatment can be obtained.

The next step for prolonged relief are intercostal nerve blocks to block the pain from the fractured ribs and allow the patient to breathe deeply and cough. The final step involves the use of a volume-cycled respirator with endotracheal intubation to provide PEEP and intermittent mandatory ventilation (IMV). This use of "internal splinting" with ventilatory support effectively manages the inadequate depth of ventilation, improves oxygen absorption in the segments of pulmonary contusion, and decreases atelectasis. If proper management with ventilatory assistance is initiated early, the respiratory support may be required for only 2 to 4 days. If management is delayed until the patient demonstrates respiratory difficulty, prolonged therapy for up to 14 days may be necessary.

Oxygenation

After establishment of a patent airway and sustained breathing, the patient should be given supplemental oxygen to assist with reversing decreased tissue oxygenation during the immediate posttraumatic period. The patient has diminished oxygen-carrying capacity as a result of injuries to the pulmonary or cardiovascular system. Respiratory compromise may be due to head injury and disruption of cerebellar reflex systems, to airway distress from maxillofacial or neck injuries, and to pulmonary injuries such as pulmonary contusion, flail chest, and tension or open pneumothorax that mechanically do not provide for proper delivery of oxygen to the cardiovascular system. Oxygen can be delivered through nasal cannula, face mask, and an endotracheal tube. A person breathing 100% oxygen can move five times as much oxygen into the alveoli with each breath as he can when breathing normal air. Oxygen therapy can increase available oxygen to as much as 400% above normal.[66]

Oxygen administered through a nasal cannula at 2 to 8 L per minute can increase the inspired oxygen concentration (FIO_2). A higher FIO_2 can be delivered by a Venturi mask system or the use of a properly applied bag and mask system. With the bag and mask system, the greatest difficulty is in maintaining an adequate mask-face seal. The seal over the face with the mask is held with the thumb and index finger over the mask and the other fingers curled beneath the inferior border of the mandible. The FIO_2 can be increased in a bag-mask system with a rebreathing mask and an oxygen accumulator to deliver high concentrations of oxygen. Ventilation with the bag-mask system is difficult in patients with possible maxillofacial, cervical spine, and thoracic injuries, and the patient should be intubated if oxygen resuscitation is required.

Endotracheal intubation helps to protect the airway and facilitates adequate lung inflation with high FIO_2 in the injured patient. Oxygen administered through the endotracheal tube should increase the FIO_2 100% in the injured patient (especially if the patient is comatose) until arterial blood gas measurements confirm hemoglobin saturation (PAO_2 > 60 to 70 mm Hg) when FIO_2 can be lowered to between 40% and 60%.[65] Pulmonary oxygen toxicity may result if 100% oxygen is administered continuously for 24 hours; therefore 100% oxygen delivery is acceptable only until PAO_2 levels can be ascertained. Some concern exists about suppression of the respiratory drive with oxygen therapy, but the hypoxic drive can be reestablished following stabilization of the injured patient.

The most important mechanism of delivery of oxygen to the tissues is the hemoglobin within the erythrocytes in the cardiovascular system. With the traumatized patient, hemorrhage may decrease the available hemoglobin to the point of hypooxygenation of vital organ tissues and cell death. A normal hemoglobin of 15 gm/100 mL provides transport of 20% volume of oxygen, whereas a hemoglobin of 7 gm/100 mL carries only a 10% volume of oxygen, which is the critical reserve level of oxygen consumption for most tissues, especially the myocardium and brain.[66] The treatment of shock in the multisystem-injured patient is directed toward restoring cellular and organ perfusion with adequately oxygenated blood, rather than merely restoring the patient's blood pressure and pulse rate.[8]

Circulation

Following establishment of an adequate airway and breathing in the injured patient, the cardiovascular system of the patient must be assessed and control of baseline circulation to the tissues must be quickly restored. The most common cause of shock in the traumatized patient is hypovolemia caused by hemorrhage, either externally or internally into body cavities. Assessment of the degree of shock is important because inadequate tissue perfusion can cause irreversible damage to vital organs, such as the brain or kidneys, in a very short time period. During the primary assessment, a minimum of two large-bore (14- to 16-gauge) intravenous catheters should be placed peripherally if fluid resuscitation is required. At the time of placement of the intravenous catheter, blood should be drawn from the catheter to allow for type, cross-matching, baseline hematologic, and chemical studies. If there is a question of adequate ventilation, arterial blood should be obtained for blood gas analysis.

Tissue perfusion and oxygenation are dependent on cardiac output and are best initially evaluated by physical examination of skin perfusion, pulse rate, urinary output characteristics, and mental status of the patient. Blood pressure levels are commonly used to measure cardiac output and define hypovolemia, but in the emergency situation, time does not permit blood pressure level measurement and the physical signs of hypovolemia are more sensitive to developing shock. The response of the blood pressure level to intravascular loss is nonlinear because compensatory mechanisms of increased cardiac rate and contractility along with venous and arteriolar vasoconstriction maintain the blood pressure in the young healthy adult during the first 15% to 20% of intravascular blood loss. After blood loss of 20%, the blood pressure level may drop significantly. In the elderly patient with less efficient compensating mechanisms, the decline in blood pressure level may begin to develop after a 10% to 15% blood loss. The patient may arrest at 40% intravascular blood loss.[49] Measurement of the blood pressure level may be insensitive to the early signs of shock, and the patient's blood pressure level may quickly drop following initial assessment, as the compensating mechanisms no longer can provide for the intravascular volume loss. Also, the usual baseline blood pressure level of the patient is usually unknown. A patient who has a systolic pressure of 120 mm Hg and who is normally hypertensive may have significant loss, whereas a healthy young athlete may have a normal systolic pressure of 90 mm Hg.

Skin perfusion is the most reliable indicator of poor tissue perfusion during the initial evaluation of the patient. The early physiologic compensation for volume loss is vasoconstriction of the vessels to the skin and muscles. The cutaneous capillary beds are one of the first areas to shut down in response to hypovolemia because of stimulus from the sympathetic nervous system and the adrenal gland through epinephrine and norepinephrine release. The release of the catecholamines cause sweating, and during palpation, the skin may feel cool and damp. The lower extremities are usually first affected, and the first indication of intravascular loss may be paleness and coolness of the skin over the feet and kneecaps. A check of the capillary filling time by a "blanch test" will give an estimate of the amount of blood flowing to the capillary beds. In this test, pressure is placed on the fingernail, toenail, or hypothenar eminence of the hand (to evacuate blood from the capillary beds), followed by a quick release of the pressure. The time required for the blood to return to the capillary beds is noted by restoration of normal tissue color. A time period of less than 2 seconds is usually found in the normovolemic patient and indicates that the capillary beds are receiving adequate circulation.[22]

The rate and character of the pulse is a good measure of the cardiac rate. The pulse rate is a more sensitive measure of hypovolemia than the blood pressure level, but it may be affected by other factors commonly associated with the trauma situation such as the patient's pain, excitement, and emotional response, resulting in tachycardia without underlying hypovolemia. However, in adults with tachycardia above 120 beats per minute, hypovolemia should be expected and investigated further. Older patients generally are unable to exceed rates of 140 beats per minute in the hypovolemic state, whereas younger patients may present rates of 160 to 180 beats per minute with severe intravascular loss. In patients who have pacemakers, are taking heart-blocking medications such as propranolol or digoxin, or have conduction abnormalities within the heart, hypovolemic status may not be represented by increased pulse rates.

The location of the pulse may give some indication of the cardiac output. Generally, if the radial pulse is palpable, the patient's systolic blood pressure is greater than 80 mm Hg. If the femoral pulse is palpable, the patient's systolic blood pressure is 70 mm Hg or higher, and if the carotid pulse is noted, the systolic blood pressure is greater than 60 mm Hg. Pulse rhythm and regularity may also provide clues to increasing hypovolemia and cardiac hypoxia. Cardiac dysrhythmias such as premature ventricular contractions (PVCs) or arterial fibrillations produce an irregular rate and rhythm, signaling loss of compensating mechanisms maintaining myocardial oxygenation.

Decreased intravascular volume is immediately reflected in decreased urinary output because the compensatory mechanisms of the body decrease blood flow to the kidneys in favor of blood flow to the heart and brain. Any patient with significant trauma should always have an indwelling urinary bladder (Foley) catheter inserted to monitor urine volume every 15 minutes.[49] A minimally adequate urine output is 0.5 mL/1 kg/hour (35 cc/hour for a typical 150 lb person), and fluid therapy should be initiated to at least maintain this level of urinary output. If the patient's injuries include pelvic fractures or blunt trauma to the groin, a urinary catheter should not be placed until a urethrogram can be obtained to evaluate urethral injury. If the likelihood of urethral injury is small (for instance, in cases of gunshot wounds to the chest), the urinary catheter may be placed with minimal concern. Classic signs of urethral injury are physical findings of blood at the meatus, a scrotal hematoma, or a high-riding boggy prostate discovered during a rectal examination.

Alterations in the mental status of the trauma patient caused solely by hypovolemia is a very uncommon finding except in the most progressive, preterminal stages of intravascular fluid loss. Compensatory mechanisms maintain blood flow to the brain, and hypoperfusion to the brain does not develop until the blood pressure falls below 60 mm Hg (systolic). The mental changes usually seen are agitation, confusion, uncooperativeness, anxiety, and irrationality. These alterations in mental status can also be seen in patients with head trauma, spinal injury, drug or alcohol indulgence, hypoxia, or hypoglycemia. In the emergency situation, these other causes of mental status changes should also be investigated when hypovolemia is suspected in agitated patients who have suffered or possibly could have suffered substantial blood loss.[49]

Hypovolemia caused by hemorrhage may commonly cause flat neck veins. Distended neck veins, on the other hand, suggest either tension pneumothorax or cardiac dysfunction. As discussed earlier, with tension pneumothorax, an examination of the chest may reveal absent breath sounds and a hyperresonant chest. Cardiac dysfunction results from cardiac tamponade, myocardial contusion or infarction, or air embolus. Cardiac tamponade presents a clinical picture that is very similar to tension pneumothorax—distended neck veins, decreased cardiac output, and hypotension. Blunt or penetrating trauma may cause blood to accumulate in the pericardial sac. The blood in the pericardial sac results in adequate cardiac filling during diastole, diminished cardiac output, and circulatory failure. Cardiac tamponade usually is associated with penetrating wounds to the chest that have injured the tissues of the heart. The classic Beck's triad of decreased systolic blood pressure levels, distended neck veins, and muffled heart sounds may be observed. The expected distended neck veins caused by increased central venous pressure may be absent because of hypovolemia. The neck veins, if distended, may become distended even more during inspiration (Kussmaul's sign), and the pulsus paradoxus (lowering of the systolic pressure more than 10 mm Hg on normal inspiration) may be accentuated or absent. Tension pneumothorax may mimic cardiac tamponade or, because of the nature of the penetrating injury, may develop at the same time as cardiac tamponade, thus presenting a confusing clinical presentation.

Cardiac tamponade is initially managed by prompt pericardial aspiration through the subxyphoid route (Fig. 13–9). Because radiographs and physical examination are not helpful, a positive pericardial aspiration along with a history of chest trauma is frequently the only method a correct diagnosis can be made. Because of the self-sealing qualities of the myocardium, aspiration of pericardial blood alone may temporarily relieve symptoms. All trauma patients with a positive pericardial aspiration require open thoracotomy and inspection of the heart. Pericardial aspiration may not be diagnostic or therapeutic if the blood in the pericardial sac has clotted. This is found in 10% of patients with cardiac tamponade—usually in injuries from blunt trauma.[49] If aspiration does not lead to diagnosis or improvement of the patient's condition, only an emergency thoracotomy can solve this problem.

Pericardial aspiration through the subxyphoid route involves insertion of a needle, preferably covered by a plastic catheter (e.g., an angiocatheter), at 90° slightly to the left of the xyphoid process. The needle is inserted until it clears the sternal border and then is directed at 45° toward the right scapula to attempt to enter the pericardium and myocardium or at 45° toward the left scapula to directly enter the pericardium. Suction is placed on the needle hub to identify with blood return when the needle has entered the pericardial sac. If the needle is properly placed, as little as 50 cc of blood should result in marked improvement in the patient's condition.

Control of Bleeding

Hemorrhage is defined as an acute loss of circulating blood. Normally, the blood volume is approximately 7% of the adult ideal body weight. A 70-kg male has approximately 5 L of circulating blood volume. The

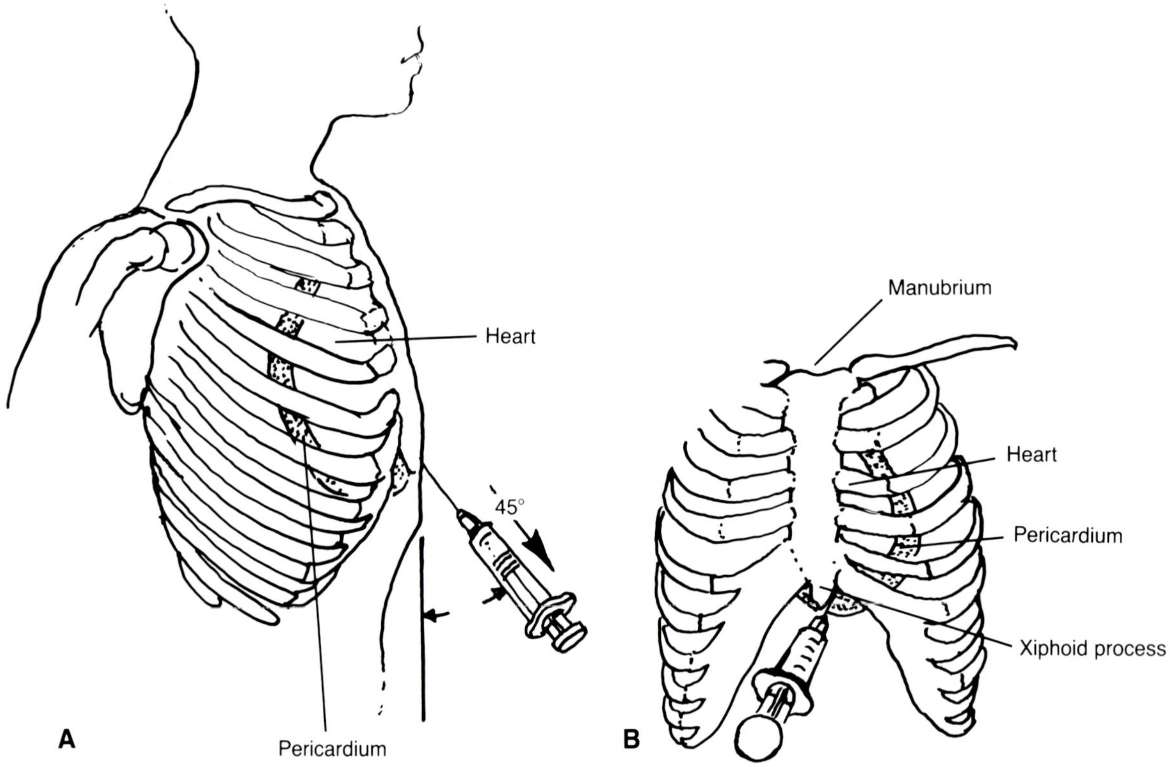

Figure 13–9. *Pericardiocentesis can be transiently lifesaving when significant cardiac tamponade develops. The patient is supine and a 16- or 18-gauge needle on a 60-cc syringe is introduced just to the left side of the xiphoid process. The needle should be introduced at a 45° angle to the chest wall, 45° off the midline and directed toward the posterior aspect of the left shoulder. A popping sensation may be felt as the pericardium is entered. The blood within the pericardial sac may be slightly clotted and relief of a depressed systolic blood pressure level should be immediate, caused by an increased stroke volume. The procedure may be required several times until definitive treatment can be initiated.*

blood volume usually does not increase significantly in obese patients, and in children, the blood volume is usually between 8% and 9% of body weight (80 to 90 mL/kg).[8] Bleeding may be external or internal into body cavities. Most external hemorrhage can be controlled with direct pressure to the wound. If an extremity is involved, it should be elevated. Firm pressure should be continuous, and if the dressings become soaked, they should not be removed but covered with other dressings. Removal of a dressing may disrupt any initial clot formation and promote further bleeding. Firm pressure on the major artery in the axilla, antecubital space, wrist, groin, popliteal space, or at the ankle may assist with control of arterial hemorrhage distal to the site. Pressure points should only be used if direct wound pressure is not effective alone. Pressure bandages include the use of air-pillow splints, blood pressure cuffs, pneumatic antishock garments (PASGs), and medical (military) antishock trousers (MASTs). Scalp or skin wounds may best be managed with immediate closure with large monofilament sutures (without cosmetic closure considerations) and direct pressure until the hemorrhage is controlled.

The PASGs and MASTs may be used as a temporary measure for splinting and hemorrhage control in pelvic fractures, tamponading soft tissue hemorrhages, stabilizing multiple leg fractures, and maintaining perfusion of the upper torso when volume replacement is not adequate in extreme hypovolemic states.[8] The garment may be applied for periods of 3 to 4 hours at 40 to 100 torr to maintain blood pressure above 90 torr systolic.[48] The PASG was originally believed to raise systolic blood pressures by forcing blood from the lower extremities to the central circulation. The major action is a tamponade effect that increases peripheral vascular resistance of the lower body and use of PASGs or MASTs must be considered a temporary measure.[8] The garments have been shown to tamponade bleeding of the extremities and stabilize subdiaphragmatic fractures, but they have shown little overall effect on venous return in hypovolemic or normovolemic subjects in animal studies.[61] Absolute contraindictions to the use of the PASG or MAST include pulmonary edema, pericardial tamponade, tension pneumothorax, hemopneumothorax, pregnancy, open abdominal injury, myocardial dysfunction, and head injuries because of increased myocardial afterload.[49] Because the garments are used to increase peripheral vascular resistance, sudden hypovolemic shock may develop if the garments are not removed properly or before the initial hypovolemic state is adequately managed with fluid resuscitation. Removal of the garment must be done gradually, and the patient's blood pressure should be monitored carefully. Deflation is stopped if the systolic blood pressure drops 5 mm Hg and is not begun again until intravenous fluid therapy restores the blood pressure.[8] The abdominal compartment is slowly deflated first, and then each extremity is deflated. Use of PASGs and MASTs is controversial. In studies reported by Bickell et al.[58] and Mackersie et al.,[59] use of PASGs demonstrated no statistically significant beneficial effect on trauma score, blood pressure index, and mortality. Both of these studies were done on patients in urban settings with rapid EMS transport. The garments may have provided an increased chance of surviving transport to a trauma hospital in the rural setting, but this is unproven.[60]

Currently, use of the PASG is recommended in trauma situations in which the patient is having difficulty maintaining a systolic blood pressure above 70 mm Hg and transport time to the trauma center is greater than 10 minutes. If the hemorrhage appears to be arterial, as with a gunshot wound to the abdomen or a ruptured aortic aneurysm, the garment should be inflated to 90 to 100 torr. If, on the other hand, the injury is confined primarily to the pelvis and the injury is most likely to be venous, inflation to 40 torr may be more effective.[48]

Because of the rich blood supply to the face and neck, significant hemorrhage may be assoiciaged with large scalp wounds, nasal or midface fractures, and penetrating neck wounds. In a short period of time, the scalp may lose a large amount of blood, which oozes from the galea and loose connective tissue layers. The wound can be approximated rapidly with 2-0 nonresorbable sutures without regard to cosmetic closure. Direct pressure should then be placed over the wound to control the hemorrhage and minimize hematoma formation. After the patient has been stabilized, the sutures may be removed and a more cosmetic closure with resorbable sutures may be used to close the galeal layer and to achieve good approximation and orientation of the hair-bearing dermal and skin layers.

Nasal or midface fractures may hemorrhage from tears of the ethmoidal arteries that arise from the internal carotid system or from branches of the maxillary artery system (Fig. 13–10). Most hemorrhages from facial injuries can be controlled with direct pressure or packing. Internal maxillary artery bleeding from posterior maxillary wall fractures associated with LeFort I or II level fractures[52] usually can be controlled by pressure with gauze packing for extended periods (Fig. 13–11). Liquid thrombin or epinephrine may be added to the gauze packing, and the head may be elevated to assist with hemostasis. If direct control of the vessel is necessary, good visualization of the damaged vessel is required. Blind clamping may cause further bleeding from vessels and soft tissues, as well as possible nerve damage. Ligation of the external carotid artery may be required only in extreme cases and usually is ineffective when used alone and without direct control of hemorrhage because of the collateral circulation of the face.[56]

The potential internal sites of hemorrhage are the thoracic cavity, abdomen, retroperitoneum, and extremities (Figs. 13–12 and 13–13). A complete physical examination with radiographic and/or CT examination is useful to identify hemorrhages into these areas. When there is no evidence of external or intrathoracic bleeding, continued severe hypovolemia is usually the result of bleeding into the abdomen or at fracture sites. Blood loss with fractures should be considered to be at least 1000 to 2000 mL for pelvic fractures, 500 to 1000 mL for femur fractures, 250 to 500 mL for tibia or humerus fractures, and 125 to 250 mL for fractures of smaller bones. A hematoma the size of an apple usually contains at least 500 mL of blood. Control of hemorrhage into internal spaces is not done in the primary survey unless the hemorrhage may have damaging effects on the cardiovascular or

Text Continued on Page 290

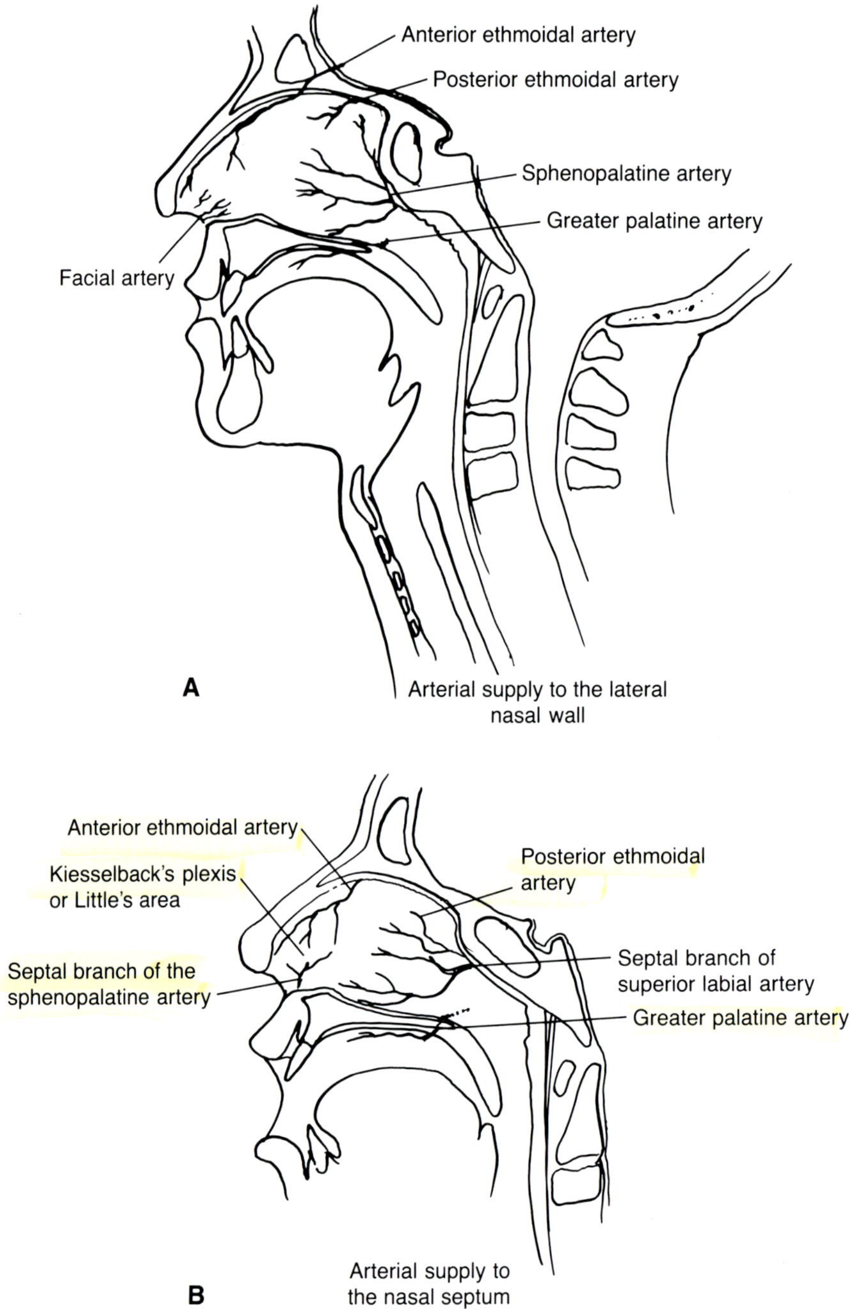

Figure 13–10. *(**A** and **B**). The lateral wall of the nasal cavity and the nasal septum receive a rich blood supply from both the internal and external carotid artery system. The superior aspect of these structures receives a blood supply through the internal carotid system from the anterior and posterior ethmoid arteries. The middle and inferior aspects are supplied by vessels from the external carotid artery: the facial artery and the nasopalatine, greater palatine, and sphenopalatine arteries from the maxillary artery. The region commonly referred to as Kiesselbach's plexis, or Little's area, in the anterior inferior portion of the nasal septum receives an abundant blood supply from all the vessels and is a region where most epistaxis originates.*

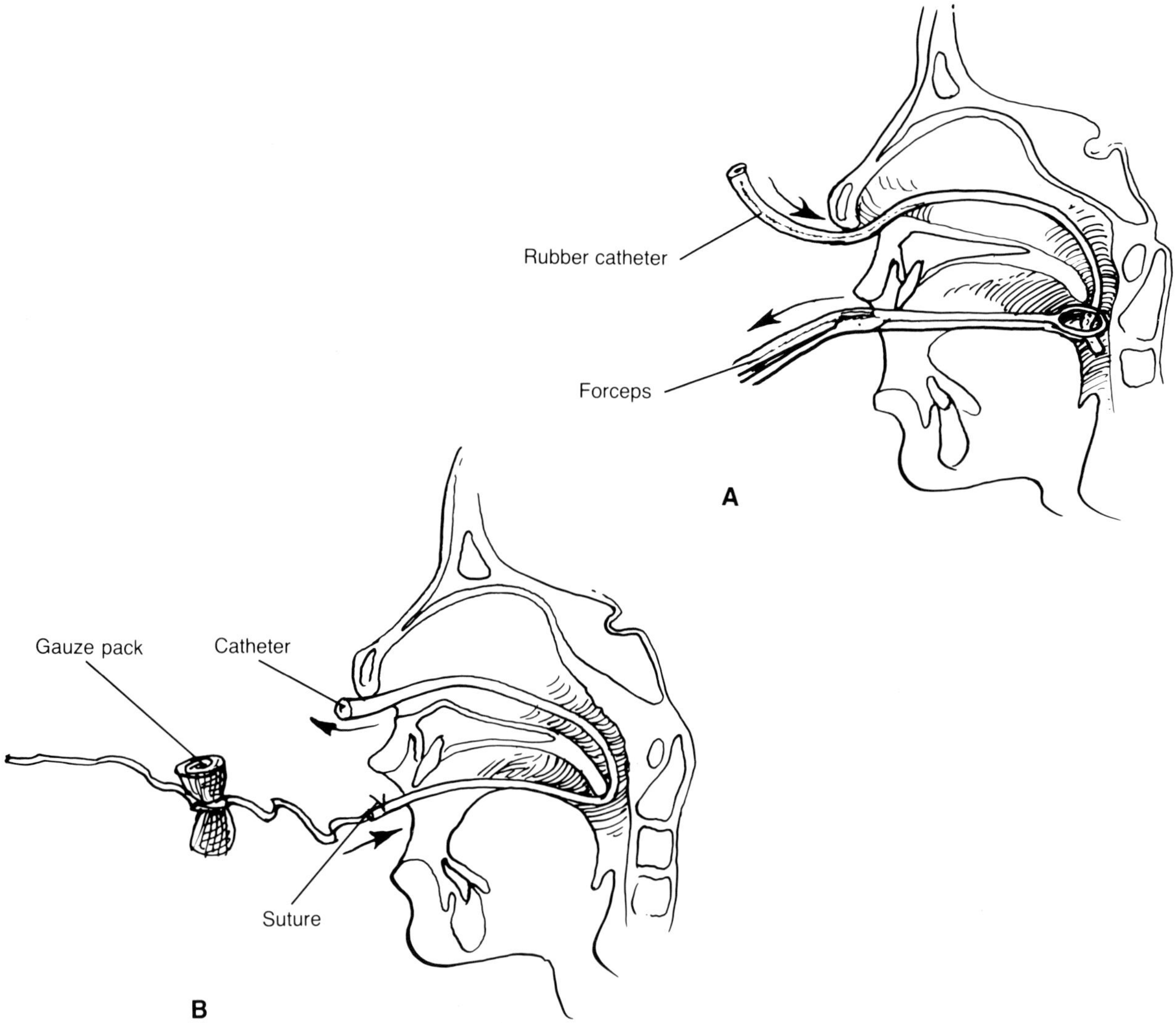

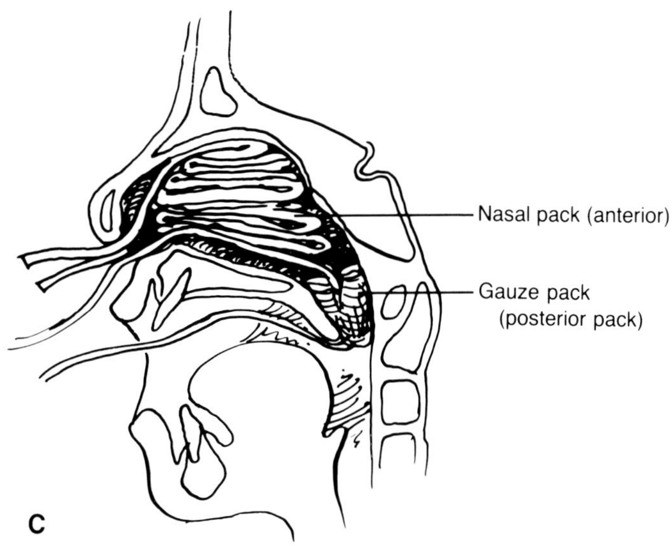

Figure 13–11. *A combined technique used for anterior and posterior packing of the nasal cavity involves the following. (**A**) A small red rubber catheter is introduced through the nostrils and carefully passed the catheter, posteriorly along the floor of the nose until visualized in the oropharynx. Care must be taken with LeFort II level, nasoethmoid, or other fractures involving the cibriform plate that the catheter does not pass through the fracture site into the cranial vault. Once the catheter is visualized, a forceps may be used to grasp the catheter and the catheter pulled into the oral cavity. (**B**) The catheter is then sutured to a tape that is secured to a wad of gauze packing material. The catheter is drawn from the nasal cavity through the nostril to pull the gauze pack into position in the nasopharynx against the posterior aspect of the nasal cavity. (**C**) Once the posterior pack is in place, the anterior pack (consisting of ½-inch ribbon gauze) is packed in an orderly fashion along the nasal floor, building superiorly, which allows for easy removal and efficient packing of the nasal cavity. (From Leigh JM. Primary care. In Rowe NC, Williams JC, eds.* Maxillofacial Injuries. *Edinburgh: Churchill-Livingstone, 1985)*

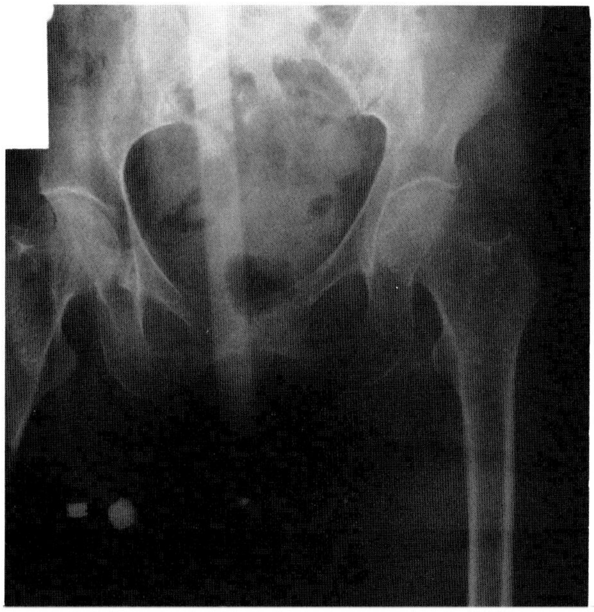

Figure 13–12. *Excessive hemorrhage may be associated with pelvic fractures, and up to 4 L of blood may be lost from the vascular space into the retroperitoneal space. Blood loss should be considered at least 1 to 2 L in a patient with a pelvic fracture.*

pulmonary system. A slow internal hemorrhage may be controlled by secondary fixation of fractures, by the defense mechanisms of vascular occlusion, refraction, and clot formation, or by open exploratory surgery.

Hypovolemic Shock in the Multisystem-Injured Patient

The most common cause of shock seen in the multisystem-injured patient is hypovolemia caused by hemorrhage. Virtually all multisystemic injuries are accompanied by a degree of hypovolemic shock that presents as a graded physiologic response to hemorrhage; this response can be classified based on the percentage of acute blood loss (Table 13–5).[8]

Class I Hemorrhage: Blood Loss of Up to 15%

The clinical symptoms of blood loss of up to 750 mL in the 70-kg adult male are minimal, with a mild tachycardia noted as the compensatory mechanisms of the body retain normal blood pressure levels, pulse pressure, respiratory rate, and tissue perfusion.

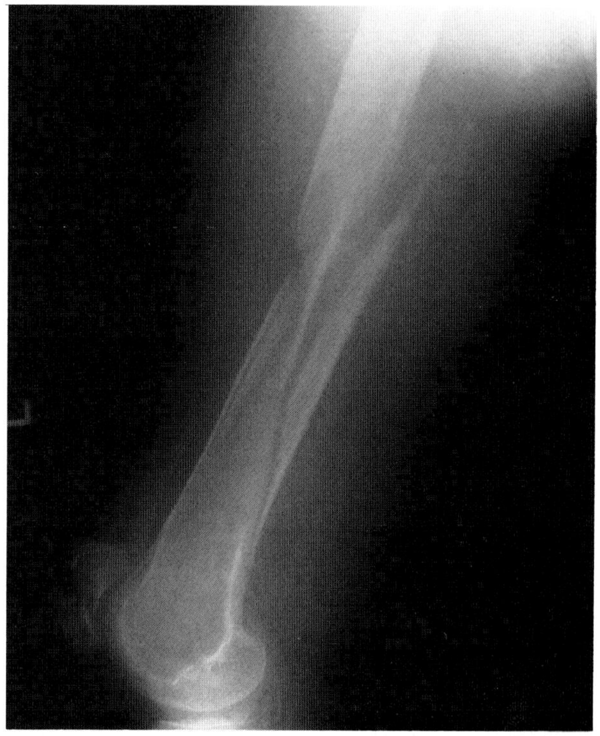

Figure 13–13. *The femur is surrounded by large muscle groups with a rich vascular supply. Femoral fractures may result in the loss of 1 L or more of blood into the soft tissues of the thigh and possible hypovolemic shock.*

Class II Hemorrhage: Blood Loss of 15% to 30%

Blood loss of 15% to 30% represents a 800 to 1500 mL loss in the 70-kg adult male. Clinical symptoms commonly expected with this level of blood loss are tachycardia, tachypnea, and a decrease in the difference between systolic and diastolic blood pressure or pulse pressure levels. The decrease in pulse pressure level is due to the elevation of catecholamines and increased peripheral vascular resistance in response to the decreased intravascular components. The increase in diastolic pressure suggests hypovolemia, because there is no noticeable increase in the systolic pressure in the early stages of blood loss. The peripheral vasoconstriction may show an elongated capillary refill time, and the skin may feel cold and moist.

Class III Hemorrhage: Blood Loss of 30% to 40%

In the 70-kg adult male, a 30% to 40% blood volume loss represents a 1500 mL to 2000 mL loss, which is

Table 13–5. *Estimated Fluid and Blood Requirements* (Based on Patient's Initial Presentation)*

	Class I	*Class II*	*Class III*	*Class IV*
Blood loss (mL)	Up to 750	750–1500	1500–2000	2000 or more
Blood loss (% BV)	Up to 15%	15%–30%	30%–40%	40% or more
Pulse rate	<100	>100	>120	140 or higher
Blood pressure	Normal	Normal	Decreased	Decreased
Pulse pressure (mm Hg)	Normal or increased	Decreased	Decreased	Decreased
Capillary blanch test	Normal	Positive	Positive	Positive
Respiratory rate	14–20	20–30	30–40	>35
Urine output (mL/hr)	30 or more	20–30	5–15	Negligible
CNS-mental status	Slightly anxious	Mildly anxious	Anxious and confused	Confused-lethargic
Fluid replacement (3:1 rule)	Crystalloid	Crystalloid	Crystalloid + blood	Crystalloid + blood

* *For a 70-kg male (Collicott PE. Life support course for physicians. Chicago: The American College of Surgeons Committee on Trauma, Subcommittee on Advanced Trauma, 1984)*

fairly detrimental to the survival of vital organ tissues. Patients present with the classic signs of inadequate tissue perfusion, including marked tachycardia (120 to 140 beats per minute), tachypnea, marked vasoconstriction, a decreased systolic pressure level, diaphoresis, anxiety, restlessness, and decreased urinary output.

Class IV Hemorrhage: Blood Loss of Greater than 40%

Blood losses approaching half of the intravascular volume produce an immediately life-threatening situation. Symptoms include marked tachycardia, a significant decrease in the systolic blood pressure level to less than 60 mm Hg, marked vasoconstriction with a very narrow pulse pressure level, marked diaphoresis, obtunded mental state, and no urinary output.

In managing the trauma patient in shock, the speed with which resuscitation is initiated and the time required to reverse shock are the factors crucial to the patient's outcome.[67] Two large-bore, 16-gauge (or larger) short angiocatheters are a minimum for beginning fluid therapy. Initial attempts should be made to percutaneously place the catheters in the basilic or cephalic veins in the antecubital fossa of both arms. Percutaneous placement of femoral vein catheters may also be used if there are no abdominal injuries or pelvic or femur fractures. When the patient is in an extreme hypovolemic state, placement of percutaneous catheters may be difficult and venous cutdown procedures to expose the saphenous vein at the ankle, the cephalic vein in the upper arm, or the antecubital vein at the elbow provide venous access for fluid resuscitation. With cutdown procedures, the intravenous tubing should be directly inserted and secured within the vein to provide a large bolus of fluid. Subclavian and internal jugular access routes are used primarily for placement of monitoring lines, such as Swan-Ganz catheters or central venous pressure (CVP) lines, and should rarely be used as primary resuscitation lines. The standard CVP line does not provide any significant advantage over peripherally placed intravenous lines in the delivery of fluid to the patient in hypovolemic shock. Flow is directly dependent on the internal diameter and inversely dependent on the length of the catheter. Therefore a catheter of the same length and diameter, whether inserted peripherally or centrally, gives the identical flow rate, with the longer central catheter delivering a lower possible maximum flow rate as compared to a shorter peripherally placed catheter. A centrally placed line through the subclavian or internal jugular vein routes usually takes longer to place than peripheral lines, may require disruption of other resuscitation measures such as chest compressions during placement, and may further complicate resuscitation of the trauma victim by causing or aggravating a developing pneumothorax or hemothorax or other potential complications associated with the placement of central lines.

Peripheral intravenous lines are the access of choice in the primary management of the trauma patient; central lines are reserved for monitoring, after the patient has been stabilized.

Circulatory support and proper oxygenation of tissues requires adequate systolic and diastolic blood pressure levels, pulse pressure levels, pulse rate characteristics, and capillary refill times. The clinical observations of these parameters are difficult to quantitate, as is measuring improvements of stabilization of the circulatory system.

Adequate urine production is a predictable sign of renal function, except in cases in which urine production may be enhanced by use of diuretics. For this reason, urinary output is a prime monitor of resuscitation and patient response. A Foley catheter should be placed in the bladder as soon as possible to measure urinary flow. There are three contraindications for insertion of a Foley catheter, and the catheter should not be placed until all have been ruled out (Fig. 13–14). These contraindications for insertion of a Foley catheter in the traumatized patient are the presence of blood at the urethral meatus, of hemorrhage into the scrotum, and of a high-riding prostate.[71-73] Attempts to pass a catheter up an injured urethra can convert an incomplete laceration into a complete laceration and can introduce infection into the perineal and retropubic hematoma.[71] A rectal examination should be performed in all traumatized patients with suspected pelvic trauma before placement of a Foley catheter. With posterior urethral disruption, the prostate may be forced superiorly by hematoma and, if the prostate cannot be palpated, a urethral injury should be suspected.[70]

The initial intravenous resuscitation fluid used in most hospitals is a balanced electrolyte solution such as lactated Ringer's solution. During prolonged shock, isotonic fluid is lost from the intravascular and interstitial spaces to the extracellular space. Initially, the patient should be given 2 L of intravenous fluid rapidly over 10 to 15 minutes and then observed. If this maneuver does not raise the systolic blood pressure to at least 80 to 100 mm Hg, the patient requires additional fluid, blood, and control of blood loss.

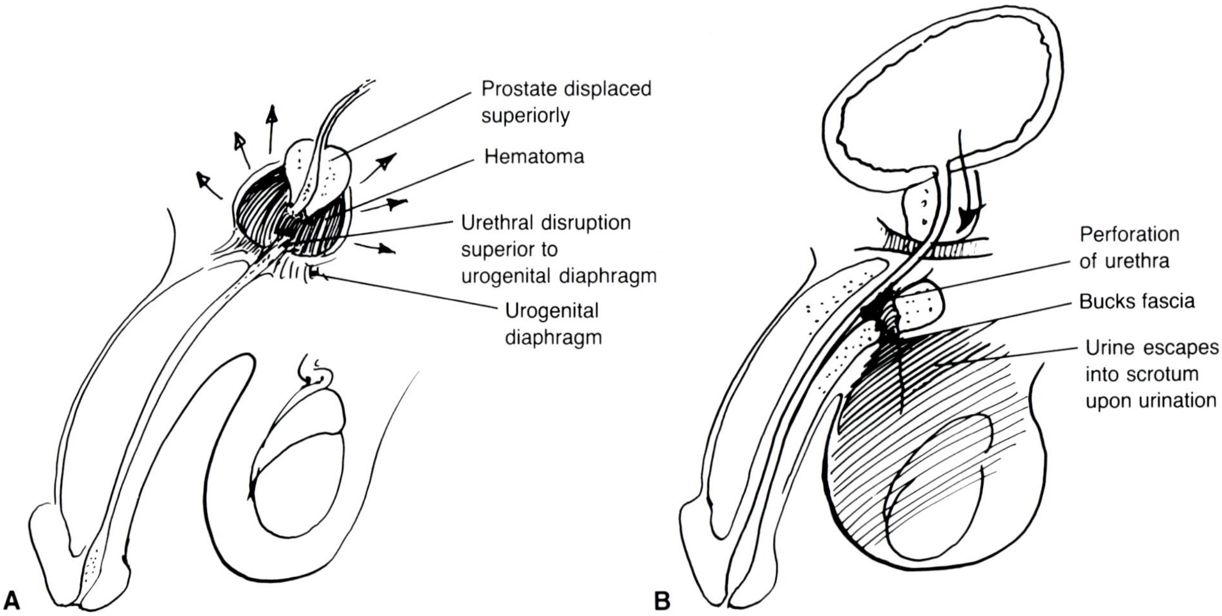

Figure 13–14. *(**A**) The contraindications for placement of a Foley catheter in the trauma patient are the presence of blood at the urethral meatus, hemorrhage into the scrotum, and a high-riding prostate. Blood at the urethral meatus may be a significant enough disruption of the urethra to prohibit passage of a catheter safely. (**B**) A hematoma developing within the scrotum or urine collection within the scrotum typically results from anterior urethral disruption from perineal blunt trauma with perforation of Buck's fascia. With posterior urethral disruption, the prostate may be forced superiorly by the developing hematoma.*

There is much controversy about the use of colloids (albumin, plasma protein fraction) and artificial plasma expanders (dextran, hemastarch) to treat hypovolemia; the cost of these materials does not appear to be justified by clinical data.[74] However, there is increasing support for their use, particularly if blood replacement is delayed or inadequate or in patients with severe head injuries that require fluid restriction therapy to control rising intracranial pressure levels.

Most patients respond to initial fluid administration, but this improvement may be transient—especially in patients who have lost more than 20% of their blood volume.[8] With excess hemorrhage, red blood cells must be replaced into the intravascular circulation to maintain an optimum oxygen-carrying capacity. The safest type of blood to administer is blood that has been fully cross-matched. Cross-matching of blood usually requires 30 minutes or more and is usually not possible immediately in the trauma situation. With whole blood loss and requirements for early blood replacement, O-negative blood may be given in patients with excessive hemorrhage.[12] The O-blood group is the most common and contains no cellular antigens. Theoretically, O-negative blood can be given to persons with any blood group with a minimal risk of antigen-antibody hemolytic reaction. No more than 4 U of O-type blood should be given.[75] Fresh frozen plasma (FFP) is frequently used as a volume expander and provides all of the clotting factors except platelets. It also provides opsonins and some complement, which may be deficient in patients with severe trauma or shock. Because of the cost and the risk of transmission of viral hepatitis and acquired immunodeficiency syndrome (AIDS), it should only be used for specific indications, including thrombotic thrombocytopenic purpura (TTP), antithrombin deficiency, specific immunodeficiencies, and nonplatelet coagulopathies. During massive transfusions, a unit of FFP is often given after every 4 U of blood, especially if packed red blood cells are administered in an attempt to prevent coagulation abnormalities.

If the patient initially responds to therapy, blood may not be required immediately, but the patient requires blood as hypovolemic shock continues to develop. A blood sample should be sent to the blood bank and a type-specific or "saline cross-matched" blood usually can be provided within 10 minutes. The patient who is resuscitated initially with O-negative unmatched blood may also be switched to type-specific blood if additional units are required. Such blood is compatible within the AB-positive and Rh blood groups but may contain minor antigenic incompatibility. Once properly cross-matched blood is available, it should be used for transfusion to limit the risk of major hemolytic reactions.[76] Ideally, the amount of blood given should be closely equal to the amount lost by the patient, which is difficult to assess with the trauma patient. In critically ill or injured patients, the ideal hemoglobin (Hgb) is probably 12.5 g/dL (hematocrit [Hct] of 38% or higher). Although an Hct of 30% to 35% has been recommended in the past, higher Hgb levels improve oxygen-carrying capacity, and the increased viscosity seems to cause relatively little reduction in cardiac output until the Hct exceeds 45% to 50%.

If the patient does not respond to initial fluid resuscitation and blood transfusions, either surgical intervention is required to control continued hemorrhage or the initial diagnosis of hypovolemia is incorrect. Measurement of the central venous pressure with a catheter or evaluation of the neck veins may assist with assessment of hypovolemic shock. Those patients with exsanguinating hemorrhage should have a low central venous pressure, and those with other causes should have a normal or elevated central venous pressure.[8] The ultimate hemodynamic criterion in the treatment of hypovolemic shock is the patient's response. Adequate resuscitation is indicated when adequate circulation and urine output is restored.

The patient is usually placed in a head-down or Trendelenburg's position in the treatment of hypovolemic shock to empty the large capacitance or venous side of the peripheral circulation back to the heart. Frequently, the patient with multisystem trauma has injuries to the abdomen or chest that may cause the Trendelenburg's position to interfere with respiratory capacity. The same effect can be obtained easily by elevating both legs while maintaining the trunk in a supine position.[68]

Neurologic Examination (Disability)

On completion of the assessment of the cardiovascular system and control of external hemorrhage, a brief neurologic evaluation is performed to establish the patient's level of consciousness and pupillary size and reaction. This brief neurologic examination quickly identifies any severe central nervous system problems that require immediate intervention or additional diagnostic evaluation. A lack of consciousness with altered pupil negativity to light requires an emergent computed tomography (CT) scan of the head and initiation of immediate patient management with steroids, mannitol, or fluid restrictions.

The Committee on Trauma of the American College of Surgeons[8] recommends the use of mnemonic AVPU System. In this system, each letter describes a level of consciousness in relation to the patient's response to external stimuli.

A: *A*lert
V: Responds to *v*ocal stimuli
P: Responds to *p*ainful stimuli
U: *U*nresponsive

A more detailed quantitative neurologic examination is part of the secondary survey work-up of the trauma patient. The primary survey establishes a baseline; if the patient's neurologic condition varies from the primary to the secondary survey, then a change in intracranial status may be present. A decrease in the level of consciousness may indicate decreased cerebral oxygenation or perfusion.

The reactivity of the pupils to light provides a quick assessment of cerebral function. The pupils should react equally. Changes represent cerebral or optic nerve damage or changes in intracranial pressure. Further changes in pupil reactivity or levels of consciousness may be due to alterations in ventilation or oxygenation status. The most common cases of coma or depressed levels of consciousness are hypoxia, hypercarbia, and hypoperfusion of the brain.[22] Depressed levels of consciousness with narrow pinpoint pupils may be the combination seen with opiate overdose. In overdose with meperidine hydrochloride (Demerol) the pupils may appear normal or dilated. Treatment requires the narcotic antagonist naloxone hydrochloride (Narcan), 0.4 mg initially. Care should be taken to avoid a quick, violent withdrawal phase in the opiate abuser, which is accompanied by profound distress, nausea, agitation, and muscle cramps. Both hypoglycemia and hyperglycemia can cause depressed levels of consciousness. If a quick blood glucose level cannot be obtained—and depending on other injuries—the patient can be given an immediate bolus of 25 g of glucose to manage the more critical hypoglycemia. A benefit of the glucose load is the hyperosmolar status that may, for a short time, reduce cerebral edema.[22]

Exposure of the Patient

The patient should be completely disrobed so that all of the body can be visualized, palpated, and examined for injuries or bleeding sites. The clothing must be completely removed even if the patient is secured to a spinal board. The easiest method is to cut the clothing down the midline of the torso, arms, and legs to facilitate the examination and assessment. Frequent, careful reevaluation of the injured patient's vital signs is important to monitor the patient's ability to maintain adequate airway, breathing, and circulation (Fig. 13–15).

SECONDARY ASSESSMENT

The secondary assessment does not begin until the primary assessment has been completed and management of life-threatening conditions has begun. During the secondary assessment, the patient's vital signs and condition should be constantly monitored to evaluate the therapeutic interventions initiated during the primary assessment and to further assess the patient for any other life-threatening problems not evident during the primary survey. Changes in the patient's vital signs, respiratory and circulatory status, and neurologic functions are expected in the first 12 hours.[8] The secondary assessment includes a subjective and objective evaluation of the injured patient.

A subjective assessment should include a brief interview of the patient, if possible. A brief health history, including medications, allergies, previous surgery, a history of the injury, and the location, duration, time frame, and intensity of the chief complaint can be useful. Obviously, the comatose patient cannot provide useful subjective information, but family members, bystanders, or other victims may provide some information. The objective assessment should involve inspection, palpation, percussion, and auscultation of the patient from head to toe. Each segment of the body (head and skull, maxillofacial, neck, chest, abdomen, extremities, and neurologic condition) are evaluated to provide a baseline of the patient's present condition. Special procedures such as peritoneal lavage, radiographic studies, and further blood studies may be done at this time.

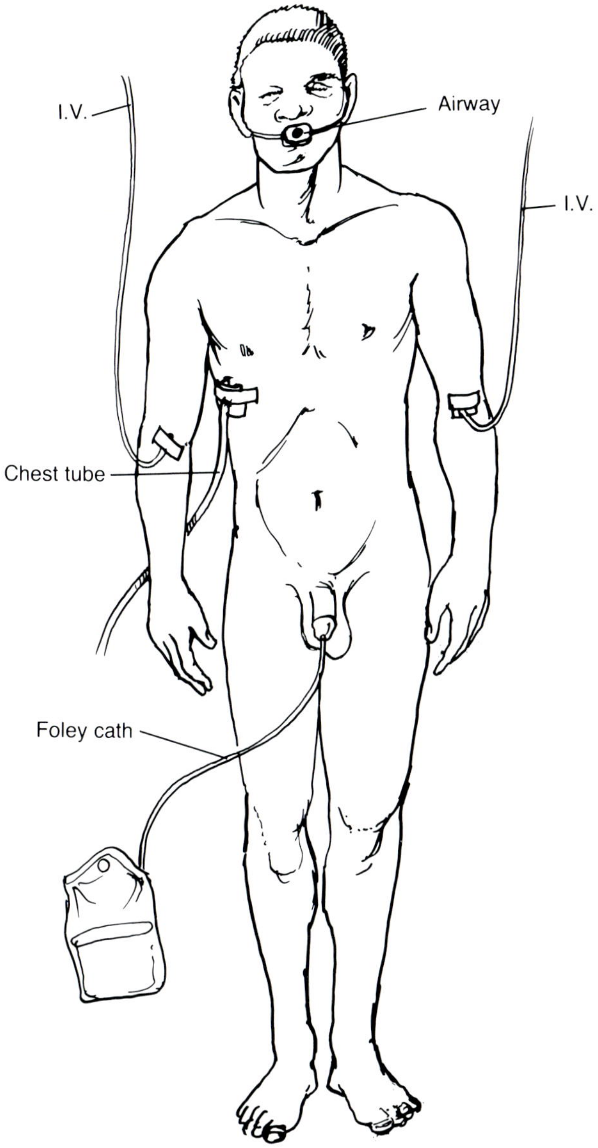

Figure 13–15. *The primary assessment of the multiply-injured patient requires evaluation and maintenance of an adequate airway with cervical protection, adequate breathing (including placement of chest tubes to correct alterations in normal lung and chest wall physiologic conditions), and adequate circulation and hemodynamics, with placement of two large-bore intravenous lines peripherally and insertion of a Foley catheter after ruling out possible urethral damage. The patient should be totally exposed so that the entire body can be examined for possible injury.*

Head and Skull

Primary injuries to the head and skull may involve lacerations, abrasions, avulsions, and contusions of the scalp, fractures of the cranium and cerebral contusions, lacerations, and shearing injuries with intracranial bleeding to the brain. The brain may also suffer secondary insults from intracranial bleeding, hypoxia, and ischemia. Hypoxia is due to impaired delivery of oxygen to the brain, whereas ischemia can result from arterial hypotension, elevated intracranial pressure (ICP), or pressure on intracranial vessels from expanding hematomas resulting in herniation of the brain from the cranial vault (Fig. 13–16). The secondary insults of hypoxia and various forms of ischemia are usually preventable. About one half of patients with head injuries have some degree of reversible injury caused by increased ICP that can be controlled with aggressive management. Failure to prevent increased ICP is the most frequent cause of death in hospitalized patients with severe head injury. Hypertension with concomitant bradycardia may indicate increasing intracranial pressure (Cushing's triad). Hypotension with tachycardia usually indicates blood

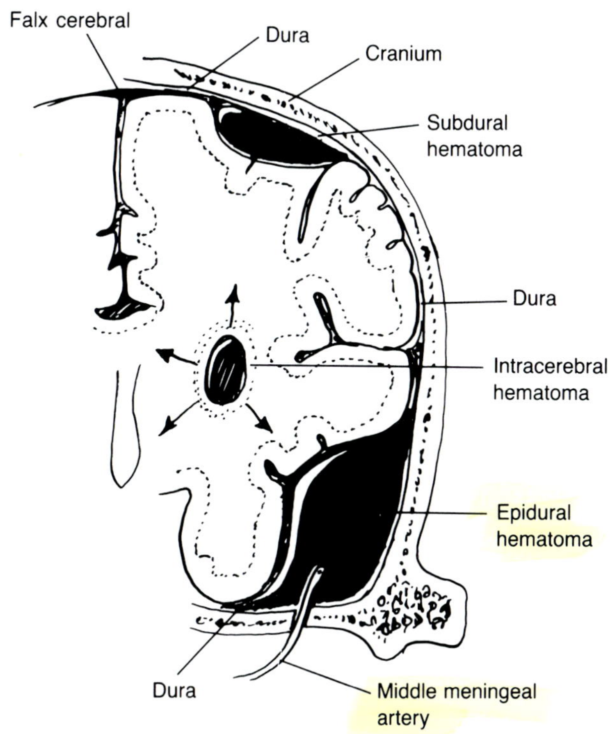

Figure 13–16. *Mass lesions commonly associated with head trauma include epidural hemorrhage, subdural hemorrhage, and intracerebral hemorrhage. A subdural hematoma is usually caused by venous bleeding with progressive loss of neurologic function. The epidural hematoma is usually associated with skull fractures near the temporoparietal region, with tearing of the middle meningeal artery.*

loss. Shock is rarely associated with primary neurologic injury, and systemic sources of blood loss should be investigated. Classic findings of Cushing's triad usually are present less than 25% of the time, even when the ICP was found to be greater than 30 mm/Hg and a value of greater than 15 mm/Hg is considered abnormal.

Accurate continuing neurologic assessment and examination for mass lesions with CT scans are rapid noninvasive techniques that cause no life-threatening risk for the head-injured patient and that establish a baseline examination for future studies. When intracranial injury is suspected, CT scans can quickly and easily diagnose localized intracranial hemorrhage, contusion, foreign bodies, and skull fractures. In addition, CT scans can demonstrate secondary effects of trauma such as edema, ischemia, infarction, brain shift, and hydrocephalus. In the acutely traumatized patient, CT scans can diagnose intracerebral and extracerebral blood collections with nearly 100% accuracy. A significant lesion mass can cause cerebral ischemia by elevating ICP or compressing vasculatory structures. A CT scan should be done immediately following stabilization of the injured patient rather than waiting for signs of an expanding intracranial hematoma. The possibility of a lesion mass has been reported to be about 40% in adults and 25% in children under 18 years of age. Indications for CT scan include seizure activity, unconsciousness lasting for more than a few minutes, abnormal mental status, abnormal neurologic evaluation, and evidence of a skull fracture found on physical examination. Brief loss of consciousness alone or mild amnesia in an awake, alert patient is rarely an indication and does not require a CT scan if observation of positive changes in mental status can be provided. Negative changes in mental status during the 24-hour observation period require a follow-up CT scan (Figs. 13–17 and 13–18).

Extreme care should always be taken in moving a head trauma patient to the CT machine because of the high incidence of associated cervical spine fractures in patients with head and facial trauma.[27] If spine trauma is suspected, the cervical spine should be immobilized before movement of the patient, and the CT examination should be extended to study the cervical spine as well. In addition, any suspected facial inju-

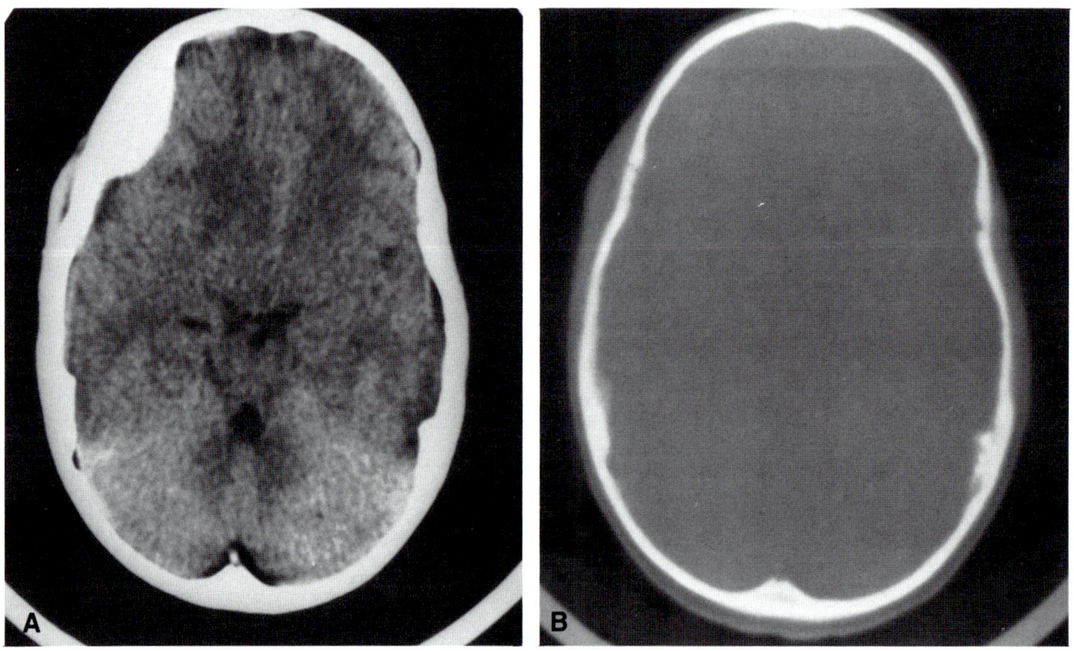

Figure 13–17. *(**A**) This CT scan reveals a typical epidural hematoma, with a lenticular shape from a tear of the middle meningeal artery, and a collection of blood between the inner table of the skull and the dura. Note the considerable shift from the midline of the brain as a result of increasing intracranial pressure (soft tissue window). (**B**) The bone window CT scan reveals the linear supratentorium skull fracture near the course of the middle meningeal artery, which caused the epidural hematoma.*

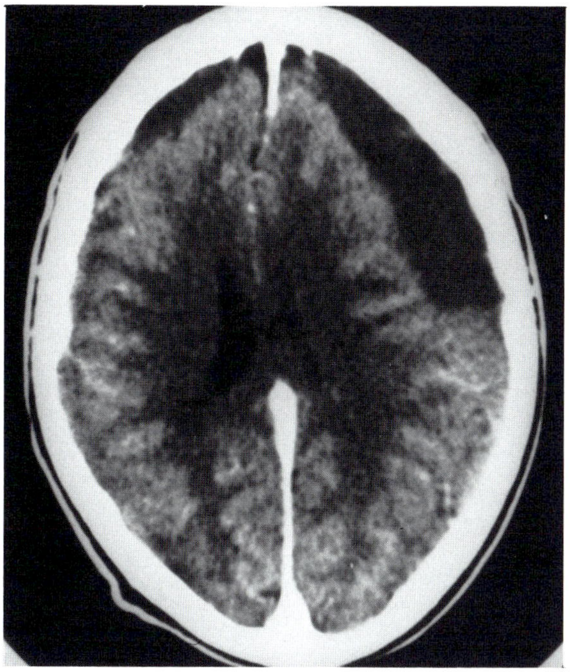

Figure 13–18. *This CT scan reveals a developing subdural hematoma with significant midline shift and ipsilateral ventricular collapse. Expansion of the hematoma with cerebral edema and increasing intracranial pressure accounts for progressive deterioration of neurologic status.*

ries should be examined by extending the CT examination inferiorly—as low as the inferior border of the mandible. Unfortunately, in many cases evaluation and treatment of facial injuries must be delayed for a significant time, and the patient is needlessly transported back for further radiologic studies because of failure to extend the CT examination.

As ICP increases above normal, a fairly standard progression of neurologic abnormalities insues, involving (in order): the cerebral cortex, producing an altered state of consciousness; the midbrain, producing dilation and then fixation of the pupils, initially on the side of the lesion, with varying degrees of bilateral hemiparesis; the pons, resulting in loss of the corneal reflex and abnormal "doll's eyes" findings (Fig. 13–19); and the medulla, producing, in sequence, apnea, hypotension, and death.

The physical examination of the head should include examination of the scalp for lacerations and foreign bodies. The rich vascular supply of the scalp, especially in children, may result in significant blood loss. Lacerations may overlie an injury to the cranium, or intracranial hemorrhage may be present. An untreated scalp wound with cranial injury may eventually act as a port for bacteria to enter the injured area, causing meningitis or brain abscess. The head should be examined for signs of basilar skull fracture: bilateral periorbital ecchymosis (raccoon's eyes), hematoma over the mastoid process behind the ears (Battle's sign), hemotympanum, cerebrospinal fluid (CSF) rhinorrhea or otorrhea, and subscleral hemorrhage. Whenever a basilar skull fracture is suspected, a nasogastric tube should not be used because the tube may inadvertently pass into the cranial vault.

The neurologic examination should be brief and should evaluate the level of consciousness, motor and cranial nerve function (suggestive of developing mass lesions), brain stem findings, and trends in the neurologic status. Alcohol and drug intoxication are frequently associated with injured patients in the trauma situation and may complicate the neurologic examination. A decreased level of consciousness should not be attributed to alcohol or other drugs until intracranial pathologic conditions have been ruled out.

Thomas and Jennett[4] developed a clinical scale, commonly known as the Glasgow Coma Scale, which assesses the depth and duration of impaired consciousness and coma (Table 13–6). The Glasgow Coma Scale (GCS) provides a simple grading of consciousness and functional capacity of the cerebral cortex. The GCS can be used both in the field and as a reassessment tool to assess brain function, brain damage, and patient progress, based on three behavioral responses: eye opening, best verbal response, and best motor response. Two regions of the brain, if injured, can produce unconsciousness: the cerebral cortices bilaterally and the brain stem reticular activating system above the level of the midpons near the opening. Increased ICP and decreased cerebral blood flow, regardless of the cause, can also depress the level of consciousness.[8]

Examination of the motor function is part of the GCS and gives information about any asymmetry of function. The conscious patient should be asked to move the extremities in response to commands. Inability to do so may represent damage to the limb or spinal cord. In the unconscious patient, deep tendon reflex and plantar response testing can assess both sensory input and motor output. Of special concern is abnormal posturing and nonpurposeful movement to stimulus. Abnormal flexor activity (decorticate) in-

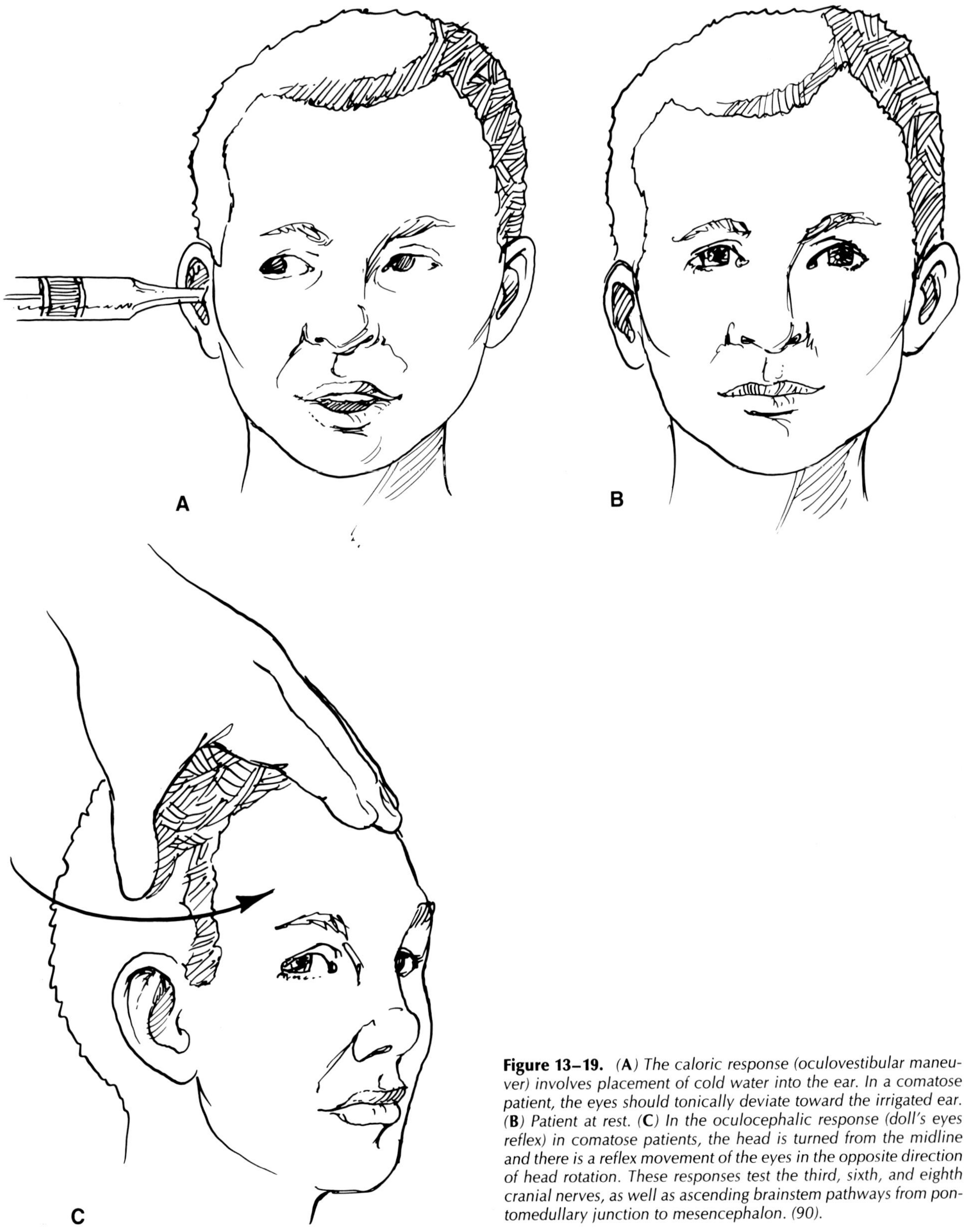

Figure 13–19. *(**A**) The caloric response (oculovestibular maneuver) involves placement of cold water into the ear. In a comatose patient, the eyes should tonically deviate toward the irrigated ear. (**B**) Patient at rest. (**C**) In the oculocephalic response (doll's eyes reflex) in comatose patients, the head is turned from the midline and there is a reflex movement of the eyes in the opposite direction of head rotation. These responses test the third, sixth, and eighth cranial nerves, as well as ascending brainstem pathways from pontomedullary junction to mesencephalon. (90).*

Table 13–6. *The Glasgow Coma Scale*

	Response	Score
EYES		
Open	Spontaneously	4
	To verbal command	3
	To pain	2
	No response	1
BEST MOTOR RESPONSE		
To verbal command	Obeys	6
To painful stimulus (pressure to nailbeds)	Localizes pain	5
	Flexion-withdrawal	4
	Flexion-abnormal (decorticate rigidity)	3
	Extension (decerebrate rigidity)	2
	No response	1
BEST VERBAL RESPONSE		
(Arouse patient with painful stimulus if necessary)	Oriented and converses	5
	Disoriented and converses	4
	Inappropriate words	3
	Incomprehensible sounds	2
	No response	1
	Total	3–15

(Teasdale G, Jennett B. Lancet 1974; 2:81–83)

volves flexion of the forearms on the chest with flexion of the wrists and fingers; in abnormal extensor posturing, the arms, hands, and fingers are extended, with the hands abducted. In both cases, the lower extremities are extended and no attempt is made to localize the point of stimulation. Although bilateral extensor plantar responses are nonspecific, a unilateral Babinski's sign points to corticospinal tract damage. Pupillary function, eye movements, and eye opening can provide information about the level of consciousness, as well as about brain stem function. The size, shape, and reactivity of the pupil to light provides information about the second and third nerve function and midbrain activity. A sluggishly reactive or a dilated, nonreactive (blown) pupil on one side indicates compression of the third cranial nerve by brain herniation in the unconscious patient. The pupillary light reflex can be used to evaluate cranial nerve function and possible elevated ICP with brain herniation.

In normal activity, when light is shone in one eye, both pupils will constrict equally. The optic, or second cranial, nerve carries both visual and pupillary fibers. The optic nerves connect shortly after they leave the retinae to form the optic chasm. At the optic chasm, the nasal fibers cross to join the temporal fibers from the other eye and the visual fibers to the visual occipital cortex. The pupillary fibers are relayed bilaterally to the Edinger-Westphal nucleus of the oculomotor, or third cranial, nerve. The third cranial nerve supplies the sphincter muscle of the iris, allowing it to contract. There is also automatic innervation of the eyes. The iris is supplied by both sympathetic and parasympathetic fibers. Stimulation of the sympathetic fibers causes the pupil to dilate and elevation of the upper eyelid.

Thus, looking into the eyes can give significant information about the trauma patient. If a light is shone into the right eye and the left eye does not respond, there may be disruption of the right optic nerve or left oculomotor nerve. Next the light should be shone in the left eye; if the left eye does not respond, disruption of the third cranial nerve should be suspected. Pupillary dilation of one eye may be due to developing brain herniation on the ipsilateral side, with bilateral pupillary dilation suggestive of significant midbrain injury or loss of parasympathetic function. Conversely, pinpoint pupils after head trauma may indicate drug overdose or loss of sympathetic tone as seen in Horner's syndrome.

The function of the brain stem may also be assessed by evaluating the corneal reflex, which involves sensory input from the trigeminal (fifth) nerve. The oculocephalic maneuver, or "doll's eyes" test, requires an intact vestibular or acoustic (VIII) nerve to permit head rotation to evaluate reflexive movement of the eyes. Obviously this maneuver is not to be used with patients with suspected cervical spine injury. The oculovestibular response test evaluates the same third, fourth, sixth, and eighth cranial nerves, as well as brain stem activity. In this test the external auditory canal is irrigated with cold water; there should be full eye movement toward the ear canal lavaged with cold water. If not, there may be disruption along any of the neural tracts or of tympanic membrane.

Lumbar puncture should not be performed in patients with acute head injuries. The change in pressure associated with removal of cerebrospinal fluid from the lumbar region may precipitate cerebral herniation in the patient with elevated ICP.

Cerebrospinal fluid (CSF) emerging from the nose or ear is commonly associated with a basilar skull fracture. Clear or red-tinged fluid that drains from the nose or ear should be considered to be CSF. There is no reliable method available in the emergency department for distinguishing cerebrospinal fluid from nasal mucosa. The use of glucose indicator sticks is associated with a high incidence of false positive results. A useful aid may be a "ring sign." A drop of blood from the nose or ear is placed on a piece of filter paper. The blood components of the fluid remain in the center and rings of clear fluid may develop about it.[8]

A CT scan should be performed to determine if there is a fracture site. The head of the bed should be elevated to 90°. If indicated, the fracture should be reduced and the leakage should cease after 7 days. If not, neurosurgical procedures may be indicated to repair the dural tear.

A rectal examination is an essential part of the examination of the patient with a head injury. Rectal sphincter tone is present if the injury is intracranial only; if there is no rectal tone, coexisting spinal cord injury is present. Coexisting head and spinal injury should be expected until proven otherwise.

LaHay, Gade, and Becker have developed a categorization of patients with brain injury and the emergency room management to initiate accordingly.

The grade I (GCS-15) patient has a mild head injury with no depression in the level of consciousness and no abnormal neurologic signs on examination. Most grade I patients should be admitted to the hospital for 12 to 24 hours of observation, although a completely asymptomatic patient may be permitted to return home in the company of a responsible adult after several hours of observation. Skull radiographs are indicated when significant scalp injury is present or there are signs of basilar skull fracture. Depressed or open fractures or CSF rhinorrhea or otorrhea require special management.

Grade II (GCS 13 to 10) patients have moderate head injury, are lethargic, and may have abnormal neurologic signs. A CT scan must be obtained, including the cervical spine through C7. If no intracranial mass is noted on the CT scans, the patient is admitted to the intensive care unit. Most grade II patients do not require ICP monitoring. However, ICP monitoring should be considered for patients with mass lesions for which nonsurgical treatment is indicated and for patients requiring general anesthesia for other operative procedures. They should also receive prophylactic diphenylhydantoin (Dilantin) at a loading dose of 18 mg/kg intraveneously over 30 minutes while blood pressure levels and electrocardiogram (ECG) results are monitored to control possible seizure activity. Ongoing seizures may be controlled with diazepam.

Grade III (GCS <9) patients have a severe head injury and are unable to obey any commands because of a disordered level of consciousness. In grade III patients, intubation and controlled ventilation improve outcome and should be promptly carried out. Following establishment of an airway, 100% oxygen is administered, pending proof that lower concentrations will provide adequate oxygenation, and moderate hyperventilation to a P_{CO_2} of 25 to 30 torr is employed to reduce the ICP. Correction of systemic hypotension by vigorous volume expansion must be initiated, avoiding hypotonic fluids. The circulatory system must be adequately maintained for oxygenation of tissues, but excess fluids augment cerebral edema and elevated ICP. Hyperosmolar diuretics such as mannitol are widely used for severe brain injury. A urinary catheter should be placed to monitor urine output. As quickly as possible, a CT scan should be obtained, seizure prevention initiated, and neurosurgical consultation for possible surgical intervention obtained.

Chest

Throughout the secondary assessment of the multiply-injured patient, the primary evaluation of airway, breathing, and circulation must be monitored for development of difficulties or overlooked problems. The immediate life-threatening chest injuries—tension pneumothorax, open pneumothorax, hemothorax, flail chest, and cardiac tamponade—may develop after primary assessment and must be treated accordingly. Chest injuries are directly responsible for over 25% of the 50,000 to 60,000 fatalities that result annually from automobile accidents, and they contribute significantly to at least 25% more of these fatalities.

The secondary assessment of chest trauma involves evaluation of an upright view chest radiograph for the presence of air in the mediastinum or under the diaphragm, widening of the mediastinum with shift toward the midline, thoracic injuries and fractures of lung expansion, and the presence of fluid (Fig. 13–20). An ECG, arterial blood gas analysis, hematocrit, and urinalysis should be obtained. Six potentially lethal injuries to consider in the secondary assessment are pulmonary contusion, aortic disruption, tracheobronchial disruption, esophageal disruption, traumatic diaphragmatic hernia, and myocardial contusion.[8]

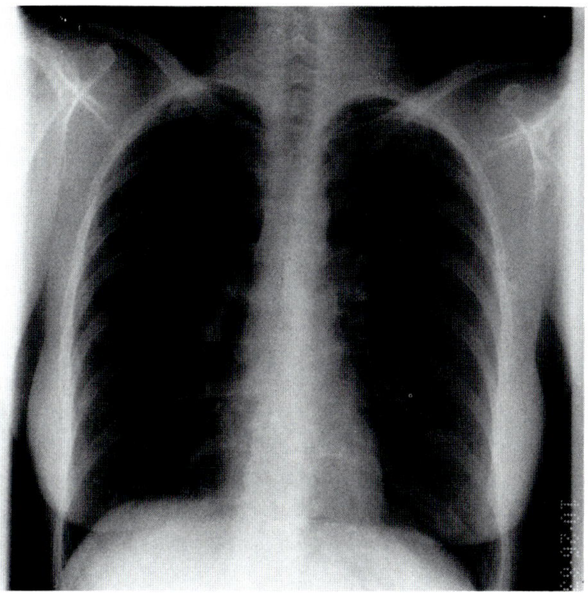

Figure 13–20. *Normal chest radiograph. Note the silhouette of the breast margin. The chest radiograph should be evaluated in a systematic manner, with evaluation of the soft tissues, ribs, sternum and spine, and neck structures and position of the trachea along the midline, abdominal structures, diaphragm and costraphrenic angles, mediastinum and heart structures, and bronchus and lung fields. Any abnormalities should be identified and, if possible, compared with previous radiographs.*

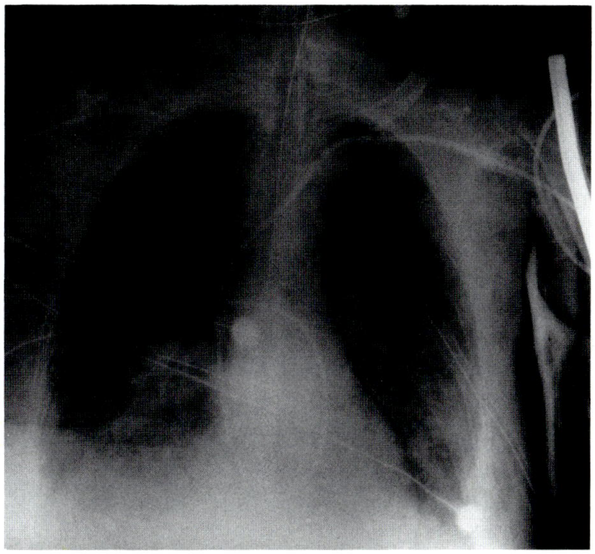

Figure 13–21. *Pulmonary contusion following blunt chest trauma. Unlike the classic form of adult respiratory distress syndrome, pulmonary contusions involve a limited portion of the lung. The pulmonary contusion may cause severe hypoxia as the result of extensive interstitial hemorrhage with alveolar collapse.*

Pulmonary contusions with or without accompanying flail chest are treated in the same manner. Pulmonary contusions are very common in blunt chest trauma because the capillary damage within the lungs results in interstitial and intraalveolar edema and shunting. Pulmonary contusions and adult respiratory distress syndrome (ARDS) are the most common potentially lethal chest injury seen in the United States because the resulting respiratory failure does not occur instantaneously but develops in 24 to 72 hours (Fig. 13–21).

The patient may complain of pain and dyspnea, and blood gas levels tend to deteriorate progressively over the initial 48 to 72 hours as increasing edema develops in the alveoli. Chest radiographs reveal a developing opacification of the involved areas. Treatment involves adequate ventilation of the lungs, including chest physiotherapy, supplemental oxygen, coughing with deep breathing, and nasotracheal suction. If ventilatory assistance is required, spontaneous ventilation with intermediate mechanical ventilation provides much better ventilation-perfusion matching, better hemodynamics, and quicker weaning than assisted ventilation. The use of steroids is controversial.[46] Injury to intrathoracic large arteries or veins may develop with blunt or penetrating trauma, and this is the most common cause of sudden death after an automobile accident or a fall from a great height.[8] Common sites of injury are the aortic root and the descending aorta at the origin of the ductus arteriosus and at the diaphragm. These injuries are fatal within a few minutes—only 15% of patients with thoracic aortic injuries reach the hospital alive. It is not uncommon for the aortic intima and media to be fractured circumferentially, with only the adventitia and surrounding mediastinal tissues preventing fatal hemorrhage. The patient may appear clinically stable, yet failure to recognize this vascular injury leads to eventual death. Adjunctive radiographic signs found on chest radiographs that are suggestive of thoracic vascular injury include a widened mediastinum, fractures of the first and second ribs, obliteration of the aortic knob, deviation of the trachea to the right, presence of a pleural cap, deviation of the esophagus to the left, and downward displacement of the left mainstem bronchus.[8] If an aortic rupture is suspected on clinical or radiographic examination, an aortogram should be performed. While waiting for the aortogram, it is important not to let the patient become hypertensive or cough or gag excessively (e.g., as may occur with the placement of a nasogastric tube).

Maxillofacial Injuries

Maxillofacial injuries may cause airway compromise from blood and secretions, from mandibular fracture that allows the tongue to fall posteriorly against the posterior wall of the pharynx, from midface injury that causes the maxilla to fall down and back into the nasopharynx, and from foreign debris, such as avulsed teeth or dentures. A large tonsilar suction should be used to clear the oral cavity and pharynx. An oral airway assists with tongue position; however, care must always be taken to avoid manipulation of the neck and to provide for access to the oral cavity and dentition for reduction and fixation of any fractures requiring some period of intermaxillary fixation. Neither midface fractures nor cerebrospinal rhinorrhea are contraindications to nasal intubation. Care should be taken to pass the tube along the floor of the nose into the pharynx, and the tube should be visualized before intubation of the trachea.

The physical examination should begin with an evaluation for soft tissue injury. Lacerations should be debrided and examined for disruption of vital structures such as the facial nerve or parotid duct. The eyelids should be elevated to evaluate the eyes for neurologic and possible ocular damage. The face should be symmetric without discolorations or swelling suggestive of bony or soft tissue injury. The bony landmarks should be palpated, beginning with the supraorbital and lateral orbital rims, infraorbital rims, malar eminences, and zygomatic arches, and nasal bones should be palpated. Any steps or irregularities along the bony margin may be suggestive of a fracture. Numbness over the area of distribution of the trigeminal nerve is usually noted with fractures of the facial skeleton.

The oral cavity should be inspected and evaluated for lost teeth, lacerations, and alterations in the occlusion. Any teeth lost at the time of injury must be accounted for because the tooth may have been aspirated or swallowed.

Spinal Cord

There are approximately 10,000 spinal cord injuries per year in the United States, usually caused by motor vehicle accidents. Multiple studies have reported a 10% to 20% association of cervical spine injury in the multiply traumatized patient with maxillofacial injuries, with at least 25% to 30% of these having some nerve damage.

A description of the mechanism of injury may give possible clues to injury of the spine, especially high-velocity accident and whiplash injury. The patient may experience little discomfort from major injury to the chest, abdomen, and extremities as a result of sensory loss from spinal injury. Because of the loss of sympathetic tone with cervical injuries, the patient may present with a systolic blood pressure level of 70 to 80 mm Hg without the tachycardia, cool extremities, poor perfusion, and decreased urinary output noted in the patient in hypovolemic shock. The neurologic shock is due to dilation of the arterial system, loss of muscle tone, and loss of reflexes. It is recommended that secondary physical examination of the cervical spine be deferred until the screening cervical spine radiograph has been reviewed. If results from this study are normal, the protective measures to the axial spine can be removed to allow a thorough examination of the posterior neck. If a helmet is worn by the victim, the helmet should be secured to the long spine board with 3-in cloth tape, and cervical spine radiographs should be taken and cleared for cervical spine injury before attempted removal of the helmet.

Physical examination of the patient with a suspected spinal injury should be done carefully, with the patient in a neutral position and with minimal movement of the spine and head (Fig. 13–22). The presence of an unstable cervical spine injury must be considered in the evaluation and resuscitation of every patient with injuries suffered from blunt injury. The catastrophic physical consequences of irreversible quadriplegia, as well as the huge economic costs required to care for this lifelong disability, make a single missed unstable cervical spine injury an unacceptable disaster. The neck and spine should be carefully examined for deformity, edema, ecchymosis, muscle spasm, or tenderness.

Subcutaneous air may be visualized if massive; if subtle, it may only be detected by palpation. The presence of air in the soft tissues may be the result of tracheal damage. Any externally expanding edema or hematoma of the neck must be observed closely for continued expansion and airway compromise. Carotid pulses should be assessed. Palpation for abnormalities in the contour of the thyroid cartilage and for the midline position of the trachea in the suprasternal notch should be performed.

The neurologic examination of the patient with spinal injury is similar to that of the patient with closed head trauma. The mental status, motor function, sensation over dermatomes, brain stem reflex, and spinal reflexes should all be evaluated and charted. The patient should be carefully examined for rectal tone and bladder control as evidence of autonomic function. Hypoventilation caused by paralysis of the intercostal muscles results from injury to the lower cervical or upper thoracic spinal cord. If the upper or middle cervical spine is injured, the diaphragm will also be paralyzed as a result of involvement of the C3 through C5 spinal cord segments. Abdominal breathing and the use of the respiratory accessory muscles will be evident.[8]

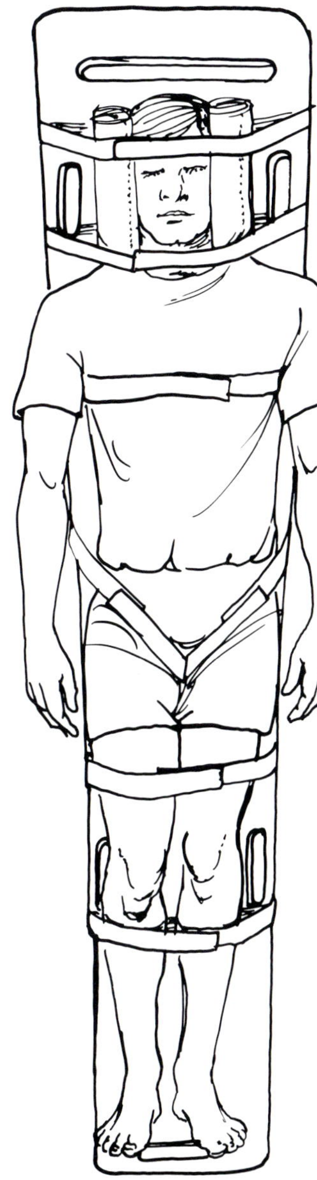

Figure 13–22. *Stabilization of the trauma victim for transportation is best achieved with the use of a long backboard with bindings and sandbags to control the head in a neutral position.*

Cervical Spine Radiographs

Bachulis et al.[27] evaluated 4941 trauma victims between February 1981 and July 1985 and found that 1823 (38%) had radiographs taken of their cervical spines. Injuries to the cervical spine were detected in 94 patients (5%). Ninety of the patients had cervical spine fractures; four had disruption of the cervical longitudinal ligaments without bony injury, and all four were quadriplegic. In the study the overall incidence of cervical spine injury in the trauma patient was 2%. Neurologic deficit did not develop in any patient with a neurologically intact spinal cord at the time of admission. The researchers found that, of the 94 patients, there were 65 alert patients with no neurologic deficits who had unstable cervical spine injuries. Without exception, these patients either complained of neck pain or of pain on palpation of the neck. Other studies have reported that no alert patient without neck pain was found to have any cervical injury.[28] Fischer et al. concluded that a screening radiographic examination of the cervical spine is not indicated in the alert, sober, cooperative patient with no complaints of neck pain and no tenderness to palpation of the neck, even when significant injury is present; however, they do recommend screening for all patients with decreased levels of consciousness and a history of an injury that could have conceivably injured the cervical spine, for all patients with neurologic deficits compatible with a cervical origin, and for all patients with neck pain or tenderness.

In this same study lateral cross-table cervical spine radiographs were obtained in all injured patients and demonstrated cervical spine injury in 70 patients, but not in the other 24, for an unacceptable false-negative rate of 26%. The authors recommended that all patients at risk for cervical spine injury must have a complete initial radiographic examination, including lateral, anteroposterior, odontoid, and right and left oblique views of the cervical spine. CT scanning was found to be the most useful modality to confirm a cervical spine injury in those patients with a suspected injury to the cervical spine not confirmed by plane radiographs. They recommend the use of CT scans of the neck in patients with possible neck injury and associated head injury that requires CT scan of the brain, in patients in whom radiographic visualization of C6 or C7 are difficult, and in cases of suspected cervical injury that are not detected in screening radiographs.

Visualization of all seven cervical vertebrae is important (Fig. 13–23). The shoulders must be distracted inferiorly and it is usually necessary to obtain diagnostic lateral views of C6 and C7. If visualization of C7 and T1 cannot be obtained, the radiographic view may be improved by placing the arms in a swimmer's position with downward traction on one arm and upward traction on the other and with the radiograph beam aimed through the axilla of the upward arm. Radiographs should be examined for fractures and fracture dislocations of the spine by evaluating the anteroposterior diameter of the spinal canal, the contour and alignment of the vertebral bodies, displacement of bony fragments into the spinal canal, linear or comminuted fractures of the laminae, pedicles, or neural fascicles, and soft tissue swelling.[1,8] Three-way cervical views (anteroposterior, oblique cervical, and lateral cervical) plus an open-mouth odontoid view or a CT scan of the neck coupled with adequate cervical spine immobilization during evaluation and resuscitation should allow the cervical spine to be safely viewed.

Cervical spine injuries may result from axial loading, flexion, extension, rotation, lateral bending, and distraction or combinations of these mechanisms of injury.

When examining a lateral cervical spine radiograph, the soft tissue thickness between the pharynx and osseous C3 should be less than 5 mm. An increase in this area suggests fracture. The distance may vary with inspiration or expiration.[8] On the lateral view, the features to be examined are the general contour of the spine, the vertical alignment of the anterior and posterior margins of the vertebral bodies, the midlaminar line, the width of the spinal column, and evidence of compression or fracture of individual vertebrae. On anteroposterior views, the height and alignment of the spinous processes and the interspinous distances are examined. The discovery of any findings suggesting the presence of a cervical spinal injury mandates the use of protective measures. It has been demonstrated that stabilization devices such as the soft cervical collar and Philadelphia collar allow significant movement of the cervical spine. Ligamentous injuries to C5 and C6 from extension of the head on the neck were found to occur with aggressive chin-lift or jaw-thrust procedures, insertion of an esophageal obturator airway, and oral endotracheal intubation. The halo vest has been judged to have the greatest overall immobilizing ability, but the device is difficult to apply and not appropriate for the emergency situation. The recommended stabilization for patients with cervical fractures is a Philadelphia collar in combination with a long spinal board. Sandbags should be used bilaterally to support the neck later-

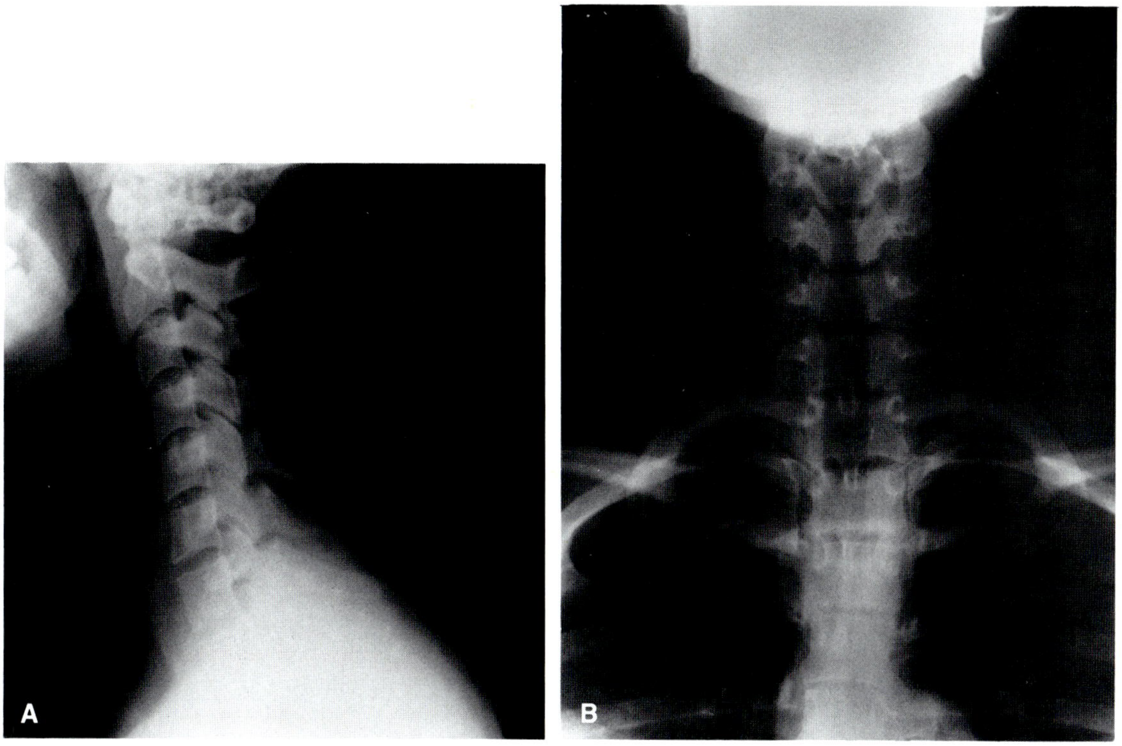

Figure 13–23. *(**A**) On the lateral view of the cervical spine, all seven cervical vertebrae (including the C7 to T1 junction) must be visualized. If the shoulders are in the way, they should be pulled slightly inferiorly by the arms or a swimmer's view should be attempted. The prevertebral soft tissues should be evaluated and a distance of 5 mm or greater down to the C3 or C4 level suggests a hematoma caused by normal fracture. All vertebrae should be evaluated for fracture and the normal lordotic curve should be followed. (**B**) The AP view of the cervical spine should be evaluated for height and alignment of the vertebral bodies, the diameter and contour of the spinal canal, and the intervertebral spaces.*

ally, and the head should be secured with 3-in cloth tape across the forehead and around the board. If protection is needed, a nasal airway should be placed. Nasotracheal intubation or cricothyroidotomy should be performed in that order if required.

Genitourinary Trauma

When injury to the genitourinary tract is suspected, urologic consultation is required to further evaluate and diagnose the extent of injury. The major cause of urethral rupture is blunt trauma. Pelvic fracture is associated with posterior urethral rupture in over 95% of patients. The force of the injury causes a shearing effect between the urethra and the urogenital diaphragm.[72] Anterior urethral ruptures are also commonly associated with blunt trauma. Most of these injuries occur in men.[25]

Blood at the urethral meatus is the single best indicator of urethral trauma.[73] The meatus must be carefully inspected for even the slightest amount of blood before inserting a urethral catheter. Attempts to introduce a Foley catheter up an injured urethra can convert an incomplete laceration into a complete transection with subsequent retropubic or perineal hematoma.[71] A rectal examination should be performed on all patients. With posterior urethral disruption, the prostate may be forced superiorly by hematoma. If the prostate is not palpable, genitourinary injury should be suspected.[70]

Absence of blood at the meatus and palpability of the prostate on rectal examination are sufficient evidence to allow passage of a urethral catheter. If resistance is noted, the catheter should be removed. Retrograde urethrography is the best method to establish continuity or damage to the urethra.[71]

Urine should be obtained and evaluated for the presence of blood. A urinalysis of 10 or more red blood cells on a high-power field (RBC/HPF) is suggestive of urinary system injury. Hematuria is the best indicator of renal injury, and the degree of hematuria may not correlate with the degree of injury.

The initial imaging study in patients with hematuria following trauma should be excretory urography or intravenous pyleogram (IVP). Injection of 150 ml of intravenous contrast medium during initial fluid therapy permits prompt radiographic visualization of the kidneys, renal pelvis, collecting system, ureters, and bladder without extravasation of contrast medium (Fig. 13–24). Should the IVP be abnormal or indeterminate and the patient stable, a CT scan may be helpful in the evaluation of renal injuries.[73]

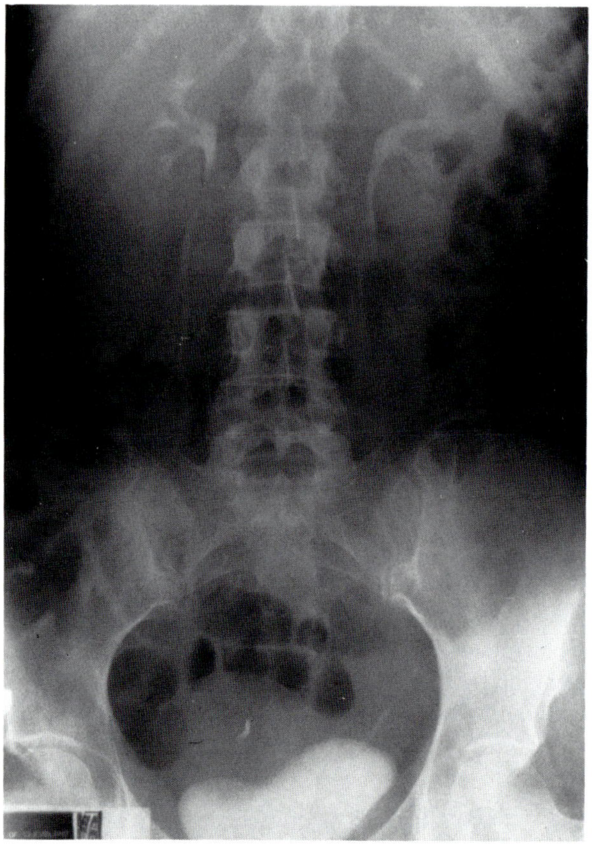

Figure 13–24. *An intravenous pyelogram (IVP) is obtained to evaluate the presence of functioning kidneys and the integrity of the ureters and bladder. This normal IVP demonstrates the bilateral renal cavity, ureters, and the bladder. No extravasation of dye is noted.*

A retrospective study of Oakwood et al.[26] reviewed the contribution of the intravenous urogram (IVU) in the management of patients with hematuria associated with blunt abdominal trauma. Most of the injuries were sustained in automobile accidents (59%), falls (25%), and sports accidents (13%). Of the 79 patients, 30 exhibited hematuria that was visible to the naked eye and 49 had microscopic hematuria. Of the 30 patients with visible hematuria, 8 had "acute abdomens" and underwent emergency laparotomy. The remaining 22 were treated conservatively. Intravenous urography was done on all of these patients, and abnormalities were revealed in 12 of them. Intravenous urography was performed in 35 of 49 patients with microscopic hematuria. Only one patient was found to have an abnormality and had persistent microscopic hematuria for 7 days; in the remaining 48, the hematuria was resolved within 1 week. The authors of this study recommended that, when hematuria is present following renal trauma, the decision to perform an IVU should be made for patients with acute abdomen during trauma (either before laparotomy or in those hemodynamically unstable patients with an expanding loin mass); for patients with visible hematuria; and for patients with prolonged microscopic hematuria that persists beyond 7 days.

Abdominal Trauma

With abdominal trauma, the physical examination is usually the most informative portion of the diagnostic evaluation. Penetrating wounds must be identified, and most surgeons believe that the safest management of penetrating wounds is a laparotomy.[8] The abdominal girth should be measured at the umbilicus soon after admission to establish a baseline against which to evaluate possible bleeding intraabdominally. Abdominal rigidity and tenderness are important signs of peritoneal irritation by blood or intestinal contents, and they may be the main indications for laparotomy for patients injured by blunt trauma. Rectal and pelvic examinations are essential if there is a question of pelvic or perineal injury.

Flat and upright radiographic films of the abdomen and posteroanterior and lateral chest radiographic

Table 13–7. *Parameters for Evaluation of Peritoneal Lavage Fluid*

Positive	20mL gross blood on free aspiration (10 mL in children)
	≥100,000 RBC/mm^3
	≥500 WBC/mm^3 (if obtained ≥3 h after the injury)
	≥175 U amylase/100 mL
	Bacteria (Gram's stain)
	Bil (by inspection or chemical determination of bilirubin content)
	Food particles (microscopic analysis of strained or spun specimen)
Intermediate	Pink fluid on free aspiration
	50,000–100,000 RBC/mm^3 in blunt trauma
	100–500 WBC/mm^3
	75–175 U amylase/100 mL
Negative	Clear aspirate
	≤50,000 RBC/mm^3
	≤100 WBC/mm^3
	≤75 U amylase/100 mL

(Hill AC, Schecter WP, Trunkey DD. Abdominal trauma and indications for laparotomy. In: Mattox KC, Moore EE, Feliciano DV, eds. Trauma. *Norwalk, CT: Appleton and Lange, 1988)*

films or CT scans should be obtained. An IVP should be done if there is a question of renal or urinary tract injury. A nasogastric tube should be passed, if possible, into the stomach to remove gastric contents.

Diagnostic peritoneal lavage is indicated in patients with a history of blunt abdominal trauma and increased pain response, patients with unexplained hypovolemia following multiple trauma, patients who are candidates for laparotomy but who have questionable findings, and patients who have experienced severe trauma and who may require an extended period under general anesthesia.[8] Absolute contraindications to peritoneal lavage are a history of multiple abdominal operations and obvious indications for exploratory laparotomy—free air and penetrating trauma (Table 13–7). A peritoneal lavage is usually performed with a sterile intravenous catheter inserted percutaneously through a small midline incision about 1 to $1\frac{1}{2}$ inches below the umbilicus. The catheter is advanced into the pelvis after the bladder has been emptied. If no blood, bile, or intestinal fluid is aspirated, the abdominal cavity is irrigated with 1 L of saline. The fluid is then drained from the abdomen through the IV tubing. One criteria for laparotomy has been the ability to read newsprint through the fluid return. It is generally felt that the presence of 100,000/mm^3 red blood cells or 500/mm^3 white blood cells after blunt trauma is sufficient to make a laparotomy mandatory.

Extremities and Fractures

Pelvic fractures, fractures of the femur, and multiple fractures of other long bones may cause hypovolemic shock and life-threatening blood loss, the primary site of which may be difficult to determine. Typical closed fractures of the pelvis may lose from 1 to 5 L of blood; femur fractures may lose 1 to 4 L; and arm fractures may lose 0.5 to 1 L from the vasculature.[16] Certain extremity injuries are considered life-threatening because of associated complications—massive, open fractures with ragged, dirty wounds; bilateral femoral shaft fractures (open or closed); vascular injuries, with or without fractures, proximal to the knee or elbow; crush injuries of the abdomen and pelvis; major pelvic fractures; and traumatic amputations of the arm or leg.[8]

The physical examination should consist of inspection and palpation of the chest, abdomen, pelvis, and all four extremities. Areas of tenderness, discoloration, swelling, and deformity should be inspected and proper radiographs obtained. All peripheral pulses should be examined for evidence of vascular injury. Pulse rates should be equal and any abnormality of distal pulse rates suggests a vascular injury and must be explained. Doppler examination of the extremity is useful, but angiograms are the best test for definitely evaluating a suspected vascular injury when the diagnosis is in doubt.[8]

Direct pressure should be used to control hemorrhage, and fractures should be splinted as quickly as possible. Splints should generally include joints above and below the site of injury. Prompt orthopedic consultation should be obtained.

Fat embolism syndrome is usually associated with major long-bone fractures, especially of the femur, in which the patient does well for 24 to 48 hours and then develops progressive respiratory and CNS deterioration. Concomitant laboratory value changes include hypoxemia, thrombocytopenia, fat in the urine, and a slight drop in hemoglobin. Fat enters the venous sinusoids at the fracture site and becomes lodged in the lung alveolae. Fat embolism syndrome was reported to occur in 30% to 50% of major long-bone and pelvic fractures. However, with current coordinated management of multiply injured patients, both the incidence of the fat embolism[17] and adult respiratory distress syndrome (ARDS) are decreased by expeditious femoral shaft and pelvic fracture treatment. The primary treatment is ventilatory assistance. Steroid and aspirin therapy have been shown to be helpful, possibly because of a reduction of platelet aggregation.

With a better understanding of fluid and electrolyte therapy, early aggressive management of hemorrhagic shock and prompt surgical treatment are now possible. However, in the interest of acute resuscitation, orthopedic injuries are often overlooked initially and are treated at a later date. When these injuries involve the spine, pelvis, or femur, they necessitate the immobilization of the patient for the purposes of traction. In immobilized patients with unstable fractures, there is an increased morbidity caused by respiratory failure or sepsis with related multiple organ failure.[15] If the severely injured patient with orthopedic fractures survives the acute phase of treatment, it is generally followed by a prolonged course in the intensive care unit, leading to morbidity secondary to decreased musculoskeletal function (muscle wasting, stiff joints, limb length loss) caused by delays in fracture stabilization and subsequent patient mobilization.[14]

Studies have shown that early fracture stabilization can significantly lower mortality, decrease musculoskeletal morbidity, and decrease cardiopulmonary and metabolic consequences commonly associated with polytrauma-patient care.[16]

Long-bone fractures are a common cause of fat embolism and ARDS. Many cases of fat embolism can be prevented by operative fixation of long-bone fractures in patients with multiple injuries within the first few days of injury.[17] Primary rigid fixation allows the patient to get out of bed and assume the upright position, thus improving pulmonary and musculoskeletal function. Early mobilization, along with the use of mechanical ventilation with PEEP, lowers the incidence of ARDS and remote organ failure.[14]

BIBLIOGRAPHY

1. Champion HR, Sacco WJ, Carnazzo AJ, Copes W, and Fouty WJ. Trauma score. Crit Care Med 1981; 9(9): 672–676.
2. Saletta JD, Geis WP. Initial assessment of trauma. In: Moylan JA, ed. Trauma surgery. Philadelphia: JB Lippincott Co, 1988.
3. Burke JF, Boyd RJ, McCabe CJ eds. Trauma management: Early Management of visceral, nervous system and mucoskeletal injuries. Chicago: Year Book Medical Publishers, Inc., 1988.
4. Teasdale G, Jennett B. Assessment of coma and impaired consciousness: A practical scale. Lancet 1974; 2:81–83.
5. Champion HR, Sacco WJ. Trauma scoring. In Mattox KL, Moore EE, Feliciano DV, eds. Trauma. Norwalk, CT: Appleton & Lange, 1988.
6. Clemmer TP, Orme JF, Thomas F, Brooks KA. Prospective evaluation of the CRAMS scale for triaging major trauma. J Trauma 1985; 25(3): 188–191.
7. Gornican SP. CRAMS scale: Field triage of trauma victims. Ann Emerg Med 1982; 11:132–135.
8. Collicott PE. Advanced trauma life support course for physicians. Chicago: American College of Surgeons (ACS), Committee on Trauma, Subcommittee on Advanced Life Support, 1984.
9. Cales RH, Trunkey DD. Preventable trauma deaths: A review of trauma care systems development. JAMA 1985; 254:1059.
10. West JG, Eastman AB. Field triage. In Mattox KC, Moore EE, Feliciano DV, eds. Trauma. Norwalk, CT: Appleton & Lange, 1988.
11. Committee on Trauma of the American College of Surgeons. Hospital and prehospital resources for optimal care of the injured patient. Bull Am Coll Surg 1983; 68:11.
12. Shires GT. Principles of trauma care, ed 3. New York: McGraw-Hill, 1985.
13. Committee on Trauma of the American College of Surgeons. Field categorization of trauma patients. Bull Am Coll Surg 1986; 71:10.
14. Johnson KD, Cadambi A, Seibert GB. Incidence of adult respiratory distress syndrome in patients with multiple musculoskeletal injuries: Effect of early operative stabilization of fractures. J Trauma 1985; 25(5): 375–384.
15. Baker CC, Oppenheimer C, Stephens B, Lewis FR,

Trunkey DD. Epidemology of trauma deaths. Am J Surg 1980; 140(1): 144–150.
16. LaDuca JN, Bone LL, Seibel RW, Border JR. Primary open reduction and internal fixation of open fractures. J Trauma 1980; 20(7): 580–586.
17. Riska EB, VonBonsdorff H, Hakkinen S, Jaroma H, Kiviluoto O, Paavilainen T. Prevention of fat embolism by early internal fixation of fractures in patients with multiple injuries. Injury 1976; 8:110–115.
18. Gertler JP, Cameron DE, Shea K, Baker CC. The esophageal Obturator airway: Obturator or obtundator? J Trauma 1985; 25(5): 424–426.
19. Kastendieck JG. Airway management. In Rosen P, ed. Emergency medicine: Concepts and clinical practice. St. Louis: CV Mosby Co, 1988.
20. Committee on Trauma of the American College of Surgeons. Early care of the injured patient. Philadelphia: WB Saunders Co, 1973.
21. Baxt WG, ed. Trauma: The first hour. Norwalk, CT: Appleton-Century-Crofts, 1985.
22. McSwain NE, Kerstein MD, eds. Evaluation and management of trauma. Norwalk, CT: Appleton-Century-Crofts, 1987.
23. Birzle H, Bergleiter R, Kuner EH. Radiology of trauma. Philadelphia: WB Saunders Co, 1978.
24. Dolan KD, Jacoby CG, Smoker WRK. Radiology of facial injury. Philadelphia: Field and Wood, Inc, 1988.
25. Condon RE, Nyhus CM, eds. Manual of surgical therapeutics, ed 5, Boston: Little Brown and Co, 1981.
26. Oakwood CDH, Britton JM, Charlton CAC. Renal trauma and the intravenous urogram. J R Soc Med 1987; 80(1): 21–22.
27. Bachulis BC, Long WB, Hynes GD, Johnson MC. Clinical Indications for cervical spine radiographs in the traumatized patient. Am J Surg 1987; 153(5): 473–477.
28. Fischer RP. Cervical radiographic evaluation of alert patients following blunt trauma. Ann Emerg Med 1984; 13: 905–7.
29. Cline JR, Scheidel E, Bigsby EF. A comparison of methods of cervical immobilization used in patient extraction and transport. J Trauma 1900; 25(7): 649–653.
30. Danzl DF. Advanced airway support. In Tintinalli JE, Krome RC, Ruiz E, eds. Emergency Medicine: A comprehensive study guide. New York: McGraw-Hill, Inc, 1988.
31. Michael TAD, Lambert EH, Mehran A. Mouth-to-lung airway for cardiac resuscitation. Lancet 1968; 2:1329.
32. Auerbach PS, Geer EC. Inadequate oxygenation and ventilation using the esophageal gastric tube airway in the prehospital setting. JAMA 1900; 250(22): 3067–3071.
33. Phillips TF, Goldstein AS. Airway management. In Mattox KL, Moore EE, Feliciano DV, eds. Trauma. Norwalk, CT: Appleton & Lange, 1988.
34. Gatrell CB. Unrecognized esophageal intubation with both esophageal obturator airway and endotracheal tube. Ann Emerg Med 1984; 13(8): 624–626.
35. Niemann JT, Rosborough JP, Myers R, Scarberry EN. The pharyngeo-tracheal lumen airway: Preliminary investigation of a new adjunct. Ann Emerg Med 1984; 13(8): 591–596.
36. Iserson KV. Blind nasotracheal intubation. Ann Emerg Med 1981; 10(9): 468–471.
37. Magill IW. Technique in endotracheal anesthesia. Br Med J 1930; 2:817–819.
38. Gallagher TJ. High-frequency ventilation. Med Clin North Am. 1983; 67(3): 633–643.
39. McGill J, Clinton JE, Ruiz E. Cricothyroidotomy in the emergency department. Ann Emerg Med 1982; 11(7): 361–364.
40. Jackson C. High tracheotomy and other errors: the chief causes of chronic laryngeal stenosis. Surg Gynecol Obstet 1921; 32:392.
41. Brantigan CO, Gron JB Cricothyroidotomy: Elective use in respiratory problems requiring tracheotomy. J Thorac Cardiovasc Surg 1976; 71:72.
42. Brantigan CO, Gron JB. Subglottic stenosis after cricothyroidotomy. Surgery 1982; 91:217–221.
43. Vukick DJ, Markouchick VJ. Pulmonary and chest wall injuries. In Rosen P, ed. Emergency medicine: Concepts and clinical practice, ed 2. St. Louis: CV Mosby Co, 1988.
44. Symbas PN. Autotransfusion from hemothorax: Experimental and clinical studies. J Trauma 1972; 12(2): 689–695.
45. Wilson RF, Steiger Z. Thoracic trauma. In Tintinalli JE, Krome RC, Ruiz E, eds. Emergency medicine: A comprehensive study guide, ed 2. New York: McGraw-Hill, Inc, 1988.
46. Shuck JM, Snow NJ. Injury to the chest wall. In Mattox KC, Moore EE, Feliciano DV, eds. Trauma. Norwalk, CT: Appleton & Lange, 1988.
47. Lewis FR. Initial assessment and resuscitation. Emerg Med Clin North Am 1984; 2:733–748.
48. Trunkey DD, Lewis FR. Abdominal trauma. In: A current therapy of trauma, 1984–1985, Philadelphia: BC Decker, 1984.
49. Jacobs LM Jr, Jacobs BB. Management of the multisystem injured patient. In: Tintinalli JE, Krome RC, Ruiz E, eds. Emergency medicine: A comprehensive study guide, ed 2. New York: McGraw-Hill, Inc, 1988.
50. Luce EA. Maxillofacial trauma. Curr Probl Surg 1984; 2(21): 1–68.
51. Bivins BA, Proctor CD, Bell RM. Arguments against mandatory exploration of penetrating wounds of the neck. In Dailey RH, Callahan M., eds. Controversies in trauma management. New York: Churchill Livingstone, 1985.
52. LeFort R. Experimental study of fractures of the upper jaw. P Tessier, translator. Plast Reconstr Surg 1972; 50:497.
53. Woodburne RT. Essentials of human anatomy, ed 7. New York: Oxford University Press, 1983.
54. Saunders WH. Epistaxis. In: Paparella MM, Shumrick

DA, eds. Otolaryngology. Philadelphia: WB Saunders Co., 1988.

55. Alling CC, Osbon DB. Maxillofacial Trauma. Philadelphia: Lea & Febiger, 1988.
56. DeWeese DD, Saunders WH, Shuller DE, Schleuning AJ. Otolaryngology: Head and neck surgery. St. Louis: CV Mosby, 1988.
57. Burke RH. A simplified nasal packing. J Oral Maxillofac Surg 1985; 43(7): 555.
58. Bickwell WH, Pepe EH, Wyatt CH, et al. Effect of antishock trousers on the trauma score: A prospective analysis in the urban setting. Ann Emerg Med 1985; 14:218–222.
59. Mackersie RC, Christensen JM, Lewis FR. The prehospital use of counterpressure: Does MAST make a difference? J Trauma 1984; 24:882–887.
60. Wayne MA, McDonald SC. Clinical Evaluation of the antishock trouser: Retrospective analysis of five years of experience. Ann Emerg Med 1983; 12(6): 342–347.
61. Holcroft JW, Link DP, Lantz BMT, Green JF. Venous return and the pneumatic antishock garment in hypovolemic baboons. Ann Emerg Med 1984; 24(11): 928–937.
62. Johnson RM, Owen JR, Hart DC, Callahan RA. Cervical orthoses: A guide to their selection and use. Clin Orthop 1981; 154:34–45.
63. Podolsky S, Baraff LJ, Simon RR, Hoffman JR, Carmon B, Ablon W. Efficacy of cervical spine immobilization methods. J Trauma 1983; 23(16): 461–465.
64. Aprahamian C, Thompson BM, Finder WA, Darin JC. Experimental cervical spine injury model: Evaluation of airway management and splinting techniques. Ann Emerg Med 1984; 13(8): 584–587.
65. Pope PE, Hudson LD. Acute respiratory failure. In Callaham ML, ed. Current therapy in emergency medicine. Toronto: BC Dĕcker Inc, 1987.
66. Guyton AC. Textbook of medical physiology, ed 5. Philadelphia: WB Saunders, 1976.
67. Sohmer PR, Dawson RB. Transfusion therapy in trauma: A review of the principles and techniques used in the MIEMSS program. Am Surg 1979; 45: 109–125.
68. Guntheroth WG, Abel FL, Mullins GC. The effect of trendelenburg's position on blood pressure and carotid flow. Surg Gynecol Obstet 1964; 119:345.
69. Dawson RB. Colloid versus crystalliod. In Cowley RA, Conn A, Dunham CM, eds. Trauma care: Surgical management. Philadelphia: JB Lippincott Co, 1987.
70. Devine PC, Devine CJ Jr. Posterior urethral injuries associated with pelvic fractures. Urology 1982; 20:467.
71. McAninch JW. Traumatic injuries to the urethra. J Trauma 1981; 21:291.
72. Pokorny M, Pontes JE, Pierce JM Jr. Urologic injuries associated with pelvic trauma. J Urol 1979; 21:455.
73. McAninch JW. Assessment and diagnosis of urinary and genital injuries. In McAninch JW, ed. Trauma management: urogenital trauma. New York: Thieme-Stratton, 1985.
74. Collicott PE. Initial assessment of the trauma patient. In: Mattox KL, Moore EE, Feliciano DV, eds. Trauma. Norwalk, CT: Appleton & Lange, 1988.
75. Barnes A. Status of the use of universal donor blood transfusions. Clin Lab Sci 1973; 4:147.
76. Garvin AS, Fisher RP. Resuscitation of trauma patients with type specific uncross-matched blood. J Trauma 1984; 24:237.

14

Airway Management

Jon P. Bradrick

Airway management assumes the highest priority in a trauma scenario. Facial injury occurs in 70% of all motor vehicle accidents and in only 11% of athletic and 8% of home injuries.[1] The World Health Organization reports that 15% of all motor vehicle deaths are due to respiratory obstruction.[2] Of patients requiring intubation in emergency departments, 28% are trauma victims.[3]

SPECIFIC CIRCUMSTANCES OF AIRWAY COMPROMISE

Cervical Injuries

Any patient with evidence of trauma above the clavicles, of head injury resulting in unconsciousness, or of injury caused by high-speed vehicles is assumed to have a cervical spine injury until proven otherwise.[4] Traditional maneuvers of opening the airway have recently been questioned as to their aggravation of existing cervical spine injury. Whereas the "head-tilt maneuver" is obviously contraindicated, lesser maneuvers such as chin-lift and jaw-thrust procedures, which supposedly minimally affect the cervical spine, have been reexamined. In his study on fresh cadavers with surgically created C5 and C6 instability, Aprahamian et al. found the only maneuvers that did not effect stability of the model were insertion of a nasopharyngeal airway or a blind nasoendotracheal intubation. Application of a soft cervical collar or a two piece semirigid collar failed to immobilize the neck during chin-lift, jaw thrust, or endotracheal intubation procedures using direct laryngoscopy. He concluded that collars may serve only as a warning sign to physicians that a neck injury may be present.[5] The American College of Surgeons has developed a decision algorithm for airway management in the patient who is suspected of having cervical injury (Fig. 14–1).[4]

In-line cervical traction as an aid to intubation requires that an assistant be present on the patient's right, facing the head. The assistant's hands are placed on the patient's shoulders, applying pressure toward the top of the head.[6] Alternatively a person standing behind the patient may apply superior traction by grasping the temporomastoid area.

Flail Mandible

Maxillofacial trauma by itself is not life-threatening unless it results in airway embarrassment or profuse bleeding. It is important to recognize a few fracture situations that are likely to cause airway obstruction. A combination of fractures involving the symphysis and bilateral body, rami, or condyles violates the arch integrity of the mandible, causing loss of support to the tongue, hyoid, and associated musculature. Unopposed posterior traction by these muscles causes posterior displacement, thereby occluding the airway. This set of circumstances is termed the *flail mandible*. Bilateral body fractures of the atrophic mandible produce identical results, which Seshul referred to as the "Andy Gump fracture."[7] Emergency treatment, as-

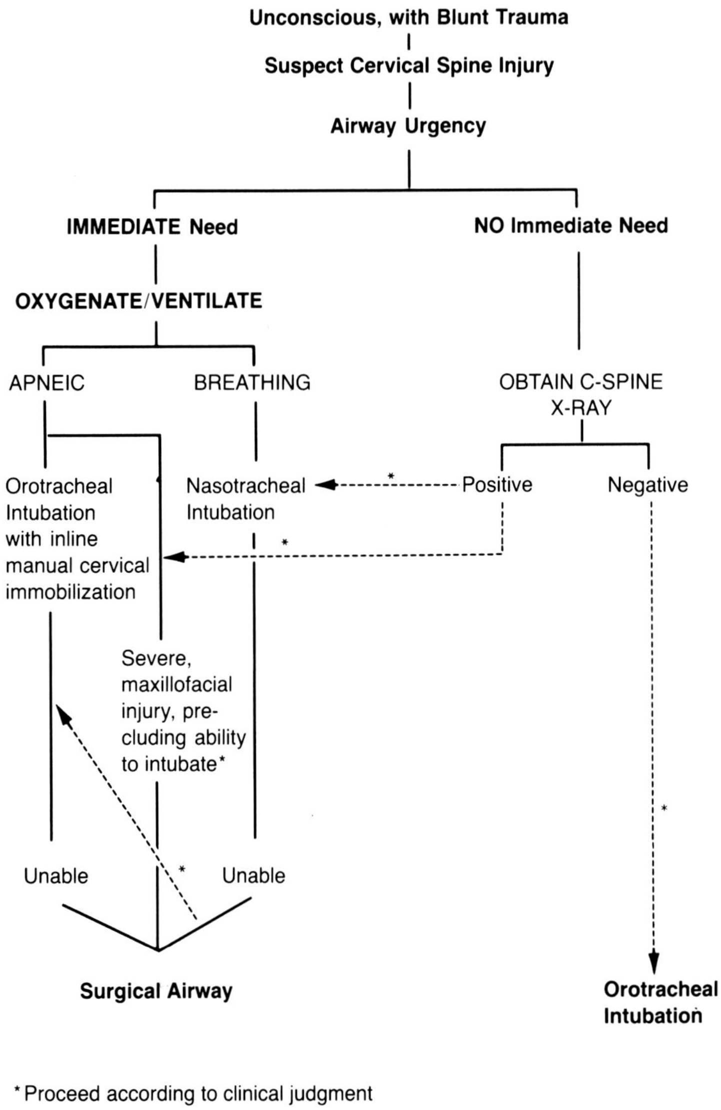

Figure 14-1. *Indications for intubation and surgical airway. (Reprinted with permission from* Advanced Trauma Life Support Course Student Manual, *American College of Surgeons, Committee on Trauma.)*

suming cervical injury is not present, consists of opening the airway by forward traction on the tongue, mandible, floor of the mouth complex, and by maintenance of the airway by temporary stabilization of the fracture with an arch bar, interdental fixation, or Kirschner's (K-wire) insertion. If tongue traction sutures are used, they should always be placed in the midline sagittal plane to avoid damage to the lingual vasculature or the hypoglossal nerve.[1] Severe airway compromise in these situations demands immediate endotracheal intubation or surgical airway maneuvers.

Gagged LeFort Fractures

The factors that cause airway obstruction in patients who present with midface (LeFort) fractures are due to the displacement force of the injury and the muscular distraction from the pterygoid muscle group. Richly vascular nasal and sinus mucosa contribute to hemorrhagic airway compromise. In a series of 117 LeFort fracture patients, Thompson showed that 26.5% required emergency treatment for airway obstruction. Of this group, 43.6% exhibited LeFort III types of fractures, either alone or in combination with other lower level LeFort fractures. In this series the presence of a LeFort III injury almost doubled the likelihood that a patient would present with airway compromise. This reflects the fact that patients with high-level LeFort fractures are more likely to also have other respiratory complicating injuries.[8]

Foreign Bodies

In a trauma patient the most likely items to obstruct the airway are broken teeth, avulsed bone fragments, and broken dental prostheses. Initial examination of a trauma patient should involve manual sweeping of the airway (with a gloved hand), followed by suctioning with a large tonsillar (Yankauer) suction. If stridor, dysphasia, dyspnea, and suprasternal and intercostal retractions are present, a laryngotracheal obstruction is likely. These patients, as is the case with all trauma patients, should be administered 100% oxygen. Positioning of the patient in Trendelenburg's position further decreases distal migration of any foreign body. Careful direct laryngoscopy usually reveals any supraglottic obstructions and renders them easily retrievable. One should resist the temptation for immediate intubation because this could impact the obstruction further in the airway. If the patient is deteriorating, surgical airway maneuvers are indicated as lifesaving. If the patient's other injuries allow transportation to the operating room, bronchoscopy is indicated. Radiographic localization has a role only after an airway emergency no longer exists. In rare instances esophageal foreign bodies can compress the trachea causing extrinsic compression of the trachea.[9] Ventilation with 70% helium and 30% oxygen has been reported to be a temporary method to maintain oxygenation in tracheal obstruction cases. Helium is less dense than nitrogen and can pass through a narrowed airway easier, resulting in increased oxygen delivery.[10]

Laryngeal Fractures

Laryngeal trauma occurs infrequently largely because of protection from the mandible and face.[1] Preventable complications from a laryngeal fracture such as airway obstruction and voice abnormalities should invoke a high degree of suspicion for these injuries during examinations of all head and neck trauma victims. The oral and maxillofacial surgeon needs to be well versed in initial evaluation because facial fractures are the most frequent concomitant injuries.[11] Thompson et al. showed that 37% of laryngeal injuries are delayed in diagnosis and many have symptoms that are subtle or late in onset.[12] In a review of the mechanism of injury, Meislin et al. found that the majority of laryngeal injuries are caused by blunt trauma in automobile accidents, yet the overall frequency rate was only 1%. Drivers of recreational vehicles may suffer laryngeal injury by striking unsuspected impediments producing the so-called clothesline injury.[1] Gunshot or knife wounds produce the majority of penetrating laryngeal injuries. Signs of laryngeal injury include hemoptysis, odynophagia, dysphagia, hoarseness, stridor, suprasternal and intercostal retractions with inspiratory effort, suprasternal air emphysema, superficial neck injuries, and loss of normal landmarks on palpation. If the patient is conscious, they usually attempt to sit up because a supine position worsens their already compromised airway.[11,13]

Diagnoses of laryngeal injuries rely on a high-level of clinical suspicion. Observation of the hypopharynx and glottic opening is critical in making the diagnosis. Indirect laryngoscopy with a dental mirror and forward traction of the tongue can be performed in the stable and cooperative patient. Alternatively, fiberoptic laryngoscopy, either orally or nasally, may provide a better view and a less-hurried inspection. Topical anesthetic agents greatly facilitate these examinations. Direct laryngoscopy may be necessary in the unstable patient but caution should be exercised because laryngeal injury may prevent elevation of the epiglottis. In addition, manipulation with direct instruments may worsen the obstruction by further displacement or edema. Radiographic examination has a role only in the stable patient or in one who has a secure airway. Xerograms of the neck provide improved definition of cartilaginous structures over plain radiographs. Computed tomography (CT) scans have been used to evaluate the injured larynx, but the patient must be very stable to tolerate supine positions in the scanner gantry.[14] Further workup in the stable patient includes a chest radiograph to evaluate the presence of subcutaneous air, pneumomediastinum, pneumothorax, and other tracheobronchial injuries. Finally, a contrast study of the esophagus may reveal trauma-induced occult pathologic conditions.

Most laryngeal injuries from blunt trauma are mild and can be managed conservatively with bedrest, observation, humidified oxygen, and inhaled respiratory dilators and steroids—although patients with these injuries should be hospitalized because signs of worsening obstruction can occur as long as 48 hours after the accident. In contrast, patients that present with emergency airway obstruction caused by laryngeal trauma need aggressive, lifesaving treatment. If a surgical airway is required, tracheotomy is the preferred procedure in the patient with laryngeal trauma. Techniques such as needle transtracheal or cricothyroid membrane puncture with percutaneous ventilation may provide temporary oxygenation. Oral intubation may be difficult or impossible because of distorted anatomic features, and a blind tissue passage may result from intubation attempts.[11] The administration of paralysis agents to facilitate intubation may acutely collapse an airway held open by muscle splinting. Otolaryngology consultation is mandatory because, if surgical repair of the damaged larynx is indicated, better function is obtained if treatment is provided within 24 hours of the injury.[15]

EVALUATION OF THE OBSTRUCTED AIRWAY

The acute nature of airway obstruction demands immediate response. Failure to recognize or adequately treat an obstructed airway has only one, swift outcome: death or extreme disability. Rapid clinical accessment to determine airway patency and ventilation adequacy is of paramount importance.

Plain radiographic films may demonstrate decreased tracheal space (steeple sign), tongue edema, epiglottic edema, tracheal shift, subcutaneous emphysema, and some foreign bodies. The indications for these studies are extremely limited and should be restricted to persistent or congenital stridor where anatomic variants are sought.[16]

CT scans can demonstrate the amount of edema located centrally in the pharyngeal and laryngeal areas to facilitate the assessment of airway patency.[17] These studies are usually of secondary gain in stable patients being studied for other reasons or in follow-up studies on the resolution of edema surrounding already indwelling endotracheal tubes.

Arterial blood gas analyses provide little practical information on acute airway obstruction. The time for obtaining blood gas analyses is after the airway is secured when they can help evaluate the adequacy of ventilation.

INITIAL MANAGEMENT OF THE COMPROMISED AIRWAY

The American College of Surgeons Committee on Trauma outlines basic management objectives for airway obstruction as the following: Maintain an intact airway; protect the airway in jeopardy; and provide an airway when none is available.[4] The patient suffering from facial fractures has, by default, injury to the upper airway as well. Management of the trauma victim's airway, which has been complicated by concurrent facial fractures, increases the urgency, complexity, and difficulty of the situation. The British learned in World War I that simply keeping a patient with facial injuries out of the supine position could be lifesaving.[1] Compromise of the airway of a supine patient with facial injuries or an unconscious patient is often caused by posterior tongue displacement occluding the pharynx. In addition, posterior displacement of the epiglottis compounds airway occlusion at the level of the larynx.[4] Boiden demonstrated epiglottic airway obstruction in the anesthetized, unconscious patient using the fiberoptic laryngoscope. He concluded that anterior traction on the hyoid bone would clear the airway. Three simple maneuvers to aid in relieving the obstructed airway have evolved since Heiberg first described forward displacement of the mandible in 1874.[18]

1. Chin lift: Only one hand is required to grasp the chin, pull the mandible forward, depress the lower lip, and open the mouth.
2. Jaw thrust: Both hands are required to grasp the mandibular angles, push the mandible forward, and open the mouth.
3. Head-tilt: Both hands hyperextend the neck, thereby aligning the pharyngeal and laryngeal axis to clear the airway.

These maneuvers may be applied by themselves, in combination, or as a prelude to the use of adjunctive airway devices. It is important to emphasize that the practitioner must always suspect that the patient may have a cervical spine injury. The chin-lift maneuver is advocated as the method of choice with unknown cervical spine status, whereas the head-tilt procedure is obviously contraindicated.[19] However, as noted earlier, the safety of the chin-lift procedure can be questioned.[5]

ENDOTRACHEAL INTUBATIONS

Endotracheal intubation is the most frequently employed airway control maneuver. Indications are: obtaining airway patency, tracheobronchial toilet, aspiration prevention, ventilation control, and administration of resuscitation medication. The ideal setting for intubation is in an operating room. With proper preoxygenation, a 70-kg adult can tolerate 5 to 8 minutes of apnea without becoming hypoxic, allowing more than enough time for routine intubation.[20] In contrast, the trauma victim never is preoxygenated when first seen and is probably hypoxic, thereby providing considerably less time for intubation. Routine intubation techniques in uncomplicated patients are familiar to most health care practitioners. The goal of this section is to describe alternatives and variations of routine intubations to provide a portfolio of contingency plans.

Oral Intubation

In cases of hypoplastic mandibles or pharyngeal edema the use of the Jackson anterior commissure laryngoscope has some advantages. It is commonly used by otolaryngologists for laryngoscopy and biopsy. It is a hollow, fiberoptic-lighted tube with two connected handles, one perpendicular to the tube, the other parallel (Fig. 14–2). Exposure of the glottis is from an angle, approached from the right lip commissure. A swollen tongue can not "fold over" into the field of view and obscure it as with standard laryngoscopic blades. The Jackson laryngoscope presents a constricted field of view and requires special rigid suction catheters and a fiberoptic light source. Once the glottic opening is visualized the endotracheal tube may be passed directly in alone or in combination with a

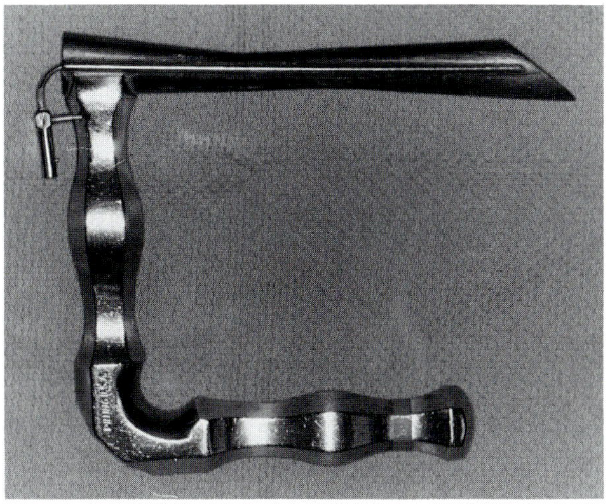

Figure 14-2. *Jackson anterior commissure laryngoscope.*

lighted internal stylet.[21,22] Alternatively a nasogastric tube may be passed, with the laryngoscope removed over the nasogastric tube and the endotracheal tube passed over the nasogastric tube as a guide. Oxygen may be delivered through the nasogastric tube during this time to decrease hypoxia.[22,23]

"Tactile" oral intubation is a blind technique performed in *comatose* patients in which the clinician's left hand advances over the midline of the patient's tongue and palpates the epiglottis. An oral endotracheal tube with a stylette bent into the shape of a J, with an additional small "hook" bent at the end is passed between the middle and index fingers to the epiglottis. The hooked end of the tube lifts the epiglottis anteriorly, while the tube is sandwiched between the fingers and epiglottis. The tube is then guided through the glottic opening, and the stylette is immediately removed to prevent anterior tracheal wall abrasion (Fig. 14–3). Advantages of the technique are that no head or neck movement is necessary (good in potential cervical-spine injuries); that secretions in the pharnyx cannot interfere; that it works well in obese or short-necked patients; that it can be used in field situations where space or positioning of the patient is compromised; and that it provides a good backup procedure in the event of a malfunctioning laryngoscope.[24]

Direct laryngoscopy and oral intubation can be performed with the patient in the sitting position if

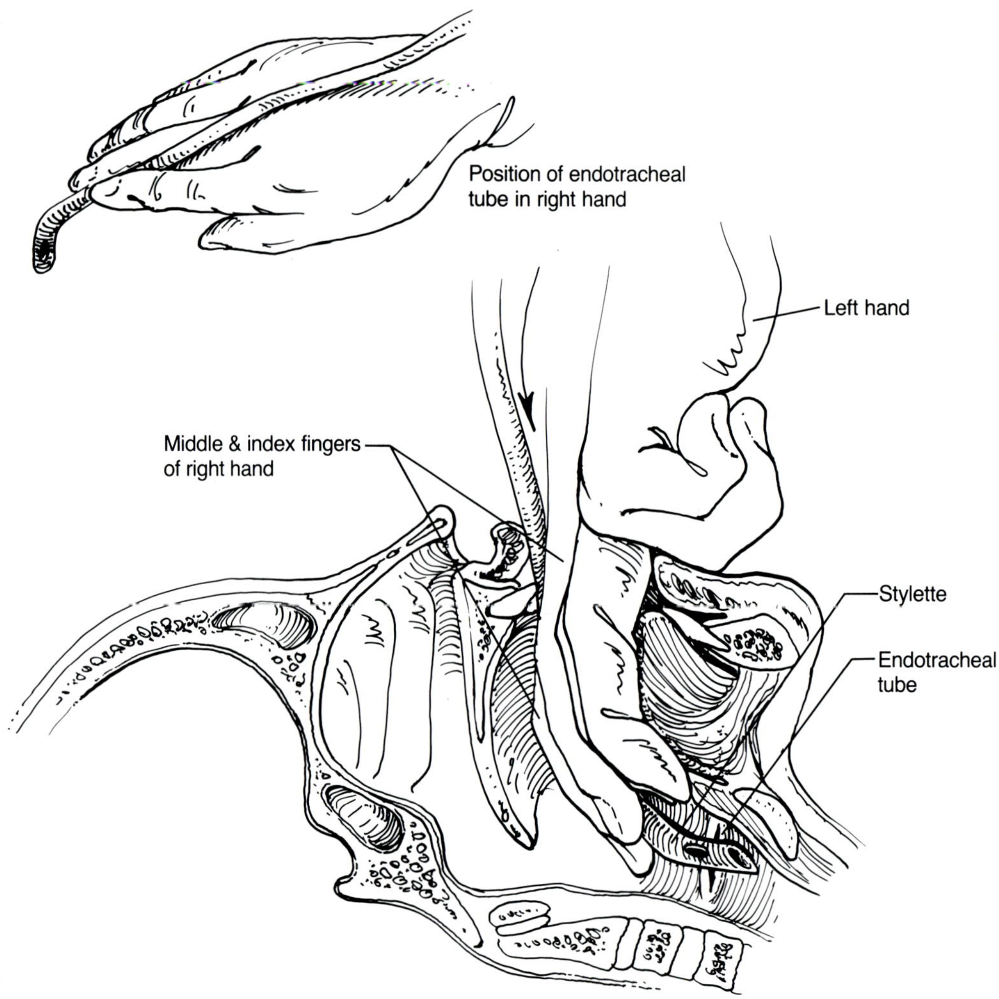

Figure 14-3. *Blind tactile oral intubation. A stylette deforms the end of the endotracheal tube to aid in lifting the epiglottis. The left hand lifts the tongue and epiglottis, while the right hand guides the tube in place.*

the practitioner stands behind the patient on a bedrail or step stool and bends over the patient's head. Positioning of the patient's head on folded sheets to assure the "sniffing" position (8 to 10 cm off the bed) applies here, as in supine intubations.[10]

Nasal Intubations

The oral and maxillofacial surgeon is familiar with nasal endotracheal intubation. Contraindications are coagulopathies, basilar skull fracture, upper airway foreign body in an unknown position, obstructed nasal passages, and patients who have had pharyngeal flap surgery. Blind awake nasoendotracheal intubation sometimes seems to depend on an element of luck. However, with proper technique and attention to details a success rate of 90% with less than a 1% complication rate has been reported.[6] Proper application of topical vasoconstrictors and anesthetics eases nasal passage and provides a bloodless field. If topical cocaine is used, a 4% solution applied with cotton sticks or pledgets placed near the anterior ethmoid neurovascular bundle and the sphenopalatine ganglion for *10 to 15 minutes* is necessary. The maximum dose for adults is 200 to 300 mg, or 5 to 7.5 cc of 4% solution.[25] Elevation of intracranial pressure is common during intubation in head injury patients, especially with any awake technique. To attenuate the hemodynamic response to intubation, small doses of narcotic, 1 μg/kg fentanyl, and lidocaine, 1.5 to 2 mg/kg, can be administered intravenously (IV). This regimen acts quickly; the narcotic can be reversed if necessary; and the lidocaine is quickly redistributed.[20] If epitaxis is encountered during nasal transit and rapid intubation is not possible, inflate the cuff with water or air and withdraw the tube until the tube is in the posterior portion of the nose. In effect, a posterior nasal pack is created that protects the airway from hemorrhage. The patient can still be ventilated through the nasal tube by digitally occluding the nose and mouth.[6] Blind awake nasal intubations depend on the ability to follow the sounds of respirations as a guide to proximity of the glottic opening. For a patient with shallow respirations, special devices are available that fit the end of the endotracheal tube and that amplify respiratory noise.[26]

Fiberoptic Laryngoscopes

Taylor first reported the use of a fiberoptic bronchoscope as an aid to difficult intubations in 1972.[27] Since then, improvements in optics and instrumentation have enabled the successful intubation of airways previously resigned to tracheotomies. The technique of fiberoptic laryngoscopy and intubation require training and practice to perform well. They are not routinely efficacious in situations of extreme urgency, such as those involving an unstable patient on whom multiple traditional intubation attempts have failed. Acute trauma scenarios have few instances where fiberoptic intubation techniques can be used to primarily secure the airway. Various authors have described helpful adjunctive procedures to aid in difficult fiberoptic laryngoscopic intubations.[28-32]

Translaryngeal Guided Intubation

In 1960 Butler first described *retrograde tracheal intubation* after he orally intubated a patient with a guide passed cephalad through a tracheotomy wound.[33] A more descriptive term, *translaryngeal guided intubation*, was suggested by King in 1987. The technique has applications in the trauma airway because head and neck movement is not required. Following sterile preparation and local anesthetic infiltration, cricothyroid membrane puncture is accomplished with a needle or a catheter-needle combination. Puncture is initially directed 30° to 40° caudad, then cephalad once aspirated air signals laryngeal entrance. The spraying of 2 cc of 4% topical lidocaine through this puncture topically anesthetizes the laryngeal mucosa and vocal cords. Caution should be exercised because the patient will cough during this maneuver. A long, plastic catheter or a small angiographic guide wire with a J tip may then be passed through the needle, cephaladly into the oral pharynx or nose. Either guide must be at least 60 to 70 cm long. This allows for insertion into an endotracheal tube while retaining control of the guide. A well-lubricated endotracheal tube may be passed over the guide into the trachea (Fig. 14–4). Passing these guides through the Murphy hole of the endotracheal tube allows an extra 1 cm of tube to be within the trachea before the end of the guide is reached. Alternative techniques are to pass a large suture through a guide catheter and secure it to the Murphy hole on the tube and use it to pull the tube into the trachea. This suture can then be cut at the skin level of the cricothyroid membrane puncture or left in place during extubation, which allows for reintubation immediately if airway difficulty is encountered. Problems with this technique are the following: superficial infections of soft tissue over the cricothyroid membrane; dislodgement of the endotracheal tube once the tip reaches the cricothyroid membrane (only 1 to 1.3 cm from the vocal cords in adults); and taut introducers impacting a tube on the narrow anterior commissure of the vocal cords.[34,35] Gold reviewed 17,500 translaryngeal anesthetic punctures and found that serious complications were limited to two broken needles, two laryngospasms, and four soft tissue infections.[36]

PERCUTANEOUS TRANSTRACHEAL VENTILATION

Percuntaneous transtracheal ventilation (PTV) by small gauge needles distal to the vocal cords was first described in the 1950s. This technique, which involves positive-pressure ventilation, should not be confused with "high-frequency jet ventilation," which uses very small amounts of air at a high frequency (a

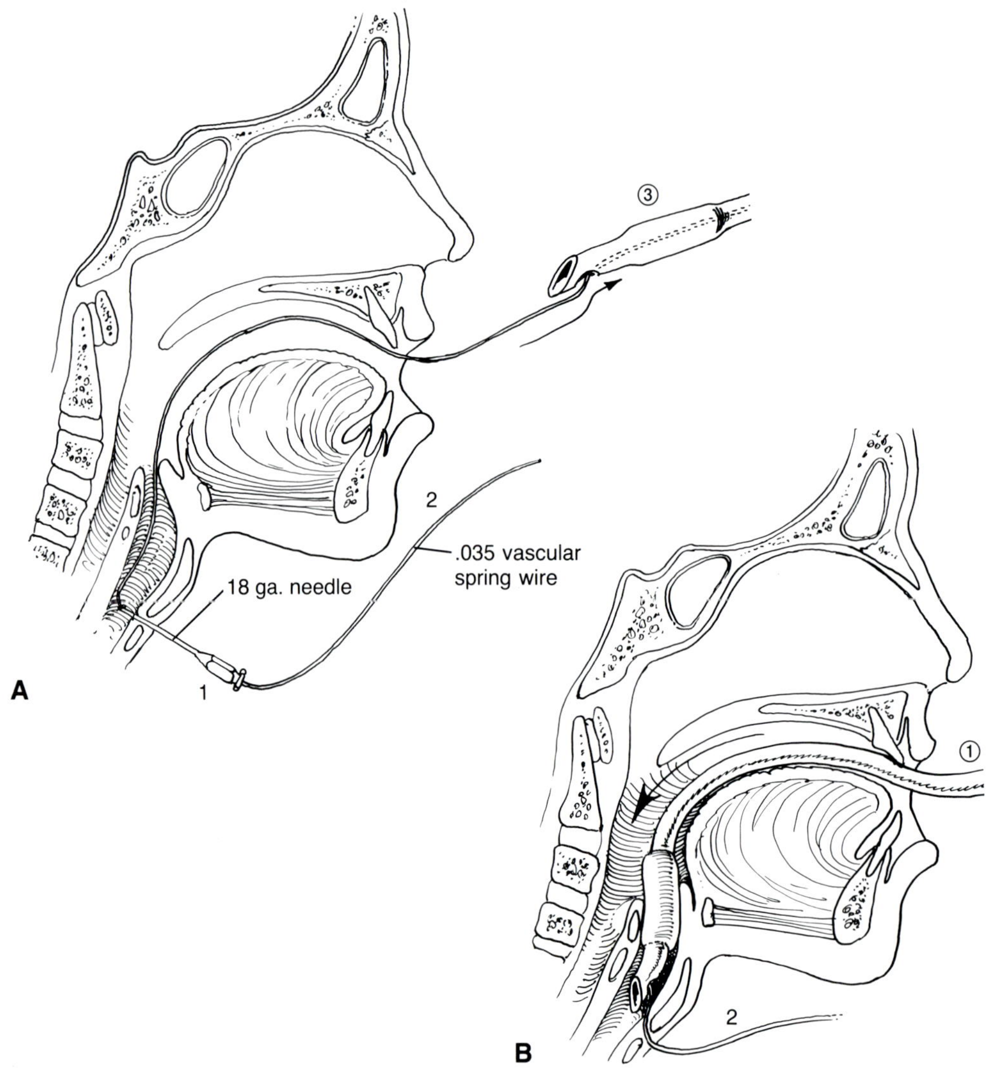

Figure 14-4. *(A) Translaryngeal guided intubation; retrograde passage of guide wire through cricothyroid membrane. (B) Translaryngeal guided intubation; passage of endotracheal tube.*

minumum of 150 breaths per minute).[37,38] Indications are the same as for cricothyroidotomy. The technique is useful in trauma victims with airway compromise and potential cervical spine injuries who cannot be normally intubated. It should be considered a temporary maneuver, providing stabilization for the patient until radiographs of the neck or intubation can be obtained. PTV may also be used to salvage the airway of a patient undergoing emergency tracheotomy that is failing. The puncture technique is identical to that described in translaryngeal guided intubation. Sterile preparation and local anesthesia may be used if time permits. A 14-gauge catheter that is inserted through the cricothyroid membrane *to the hub* and digitally held in place is the *minimum* size adequate for oxygenation (Fig. 14–5). The catheter should be connected to a soure of 100% oxygen at 40 to 50 psi (15 L per minute) or, if in the operating room, to the fresh gas line of an anesthesia machine bypassing the CO_2 absorber. Use of the oxygen flush control provides adequate flow. The connection line should have an in-line Y connector or a side hole cut in the tubing

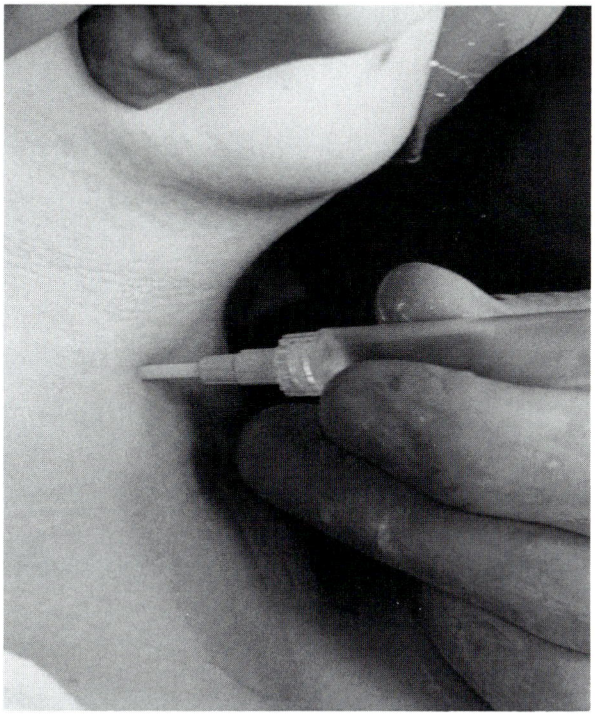

Figure 14-5. *Percutaneous puncture of cricothyroid membrane with 14-gauge catheter. Connection to oxygen line can be made with a 3-cc plastic syringe with the end cut off.*

to allow finger control of ventilation (Fig. 14–6). A three-way stopcock or a plastic syringe with the plunger end cut off can be used to connect the oxygen line to the catheter.[39,40]

A review by Jordan showed that ambu-bag ventilation does not provide adequate ventilation when using PTV.[37] Inflation (using the high-pressure oxygen source) should be for 1 second, alternating with 4 second deflations.[4] Auscultation for breath sounds during inflation is not an adequate measure of ventilation. The chest should be observed for expansion, and audible exhalation noises should be apparent in the pharynx. Topical lidocaine instilled through the catheter may be necessary to eliminate the cough reflex. Complications may originate from bent catheters, incoordination of respiratory effort in an awake patient, distal secretions, and exhalation obstruction. Complete airway obstruction is a contraindication to PTV because barotrauma such as pneumothorax or pneumomediastinium may occur without an exhalation portal. PTV should be discontinued immediately after the first inhalation if the chest fails to deflate. Animal studies have shown that to maintain a P_{CO_2} of 40 to 50 mm Hg, secondary puncture with at least a 10-gauge catheter is necessary for adequate exhalation in the presence of complete obstruction.[41]

Subcutaneous emphysema may develop if the catheter is not completely within the airway of a patient with laryngeal injuries. PTV does not protect the airway against aspiration, unless high-frequency jet ventilation greater than 60 breaths per minute is used as a pressure barricade.[37,42]

The previously described techniques can be useful adjuncts in the management of emergency airway obstruction. However, they will fail if not planned for. A frantic last minute attempt to locate the necessary equipment or unfamiliarity with its use will doom the patient. Nothing can substitute for adequate training, practicing the techniques (in an animal laboratory), and isolation of the proper equipment with nonemergency "dry-run" testing.

SURGICAL AIRWAYS

In emergency situations in which an airway cannot be established by the previous techniques, a surgical airway must be created. It is important for the surgeon to realize that, in many situations, time spent attempting to perform conservative techniques may ultimately condemn the patient to a hastily performed "last ditch" surgical attempt. Surgical airways are not the first management technique to try; however, as soon as the surgeon begins to suspect that a surgical airway is necessary, it should be performed.

Cricothyroidotomy

Brantigan and Graw initiated a resurgence of interest and confidence in cricothyroidotomy.[43] Currently in emergency rooms, 50% of patients undergoing cricothyroidotomy require it because of multiple trauma. Of those patients, 18% have isolated head and neck injuries.[44] Cricothyroidotomy's acceptance as an emergency airway technique—and in some centers as long-term airway management—is secondary to its ability to be rapidly performed, the relative lack of proximity of significant structures, and the low-complication rate. It takes a surgeon 3 to 20 minutes to

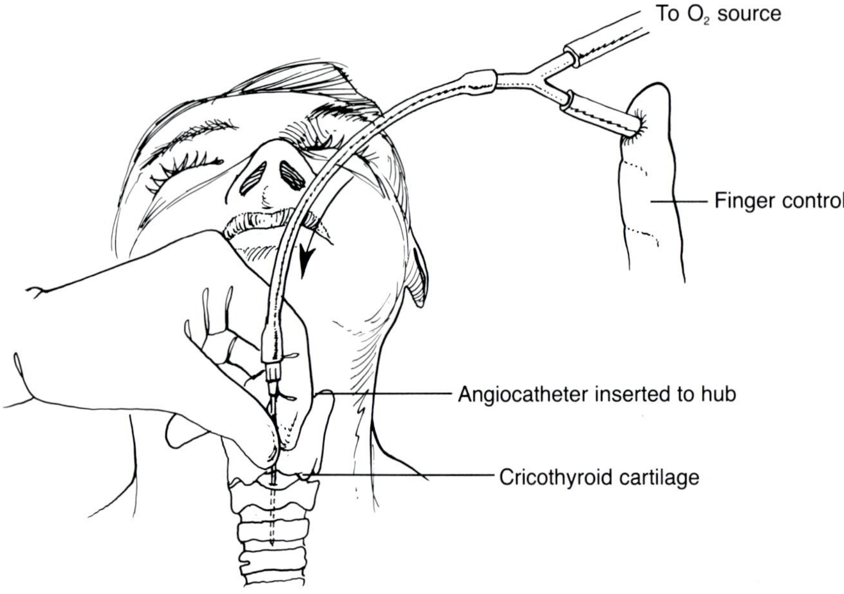

Figure 14-6. *Percutaneous transtracheal ventilation. The catheter must be held firmly in place at all times. The oxygen delivery tube must have a side port to manually control gas flow.*

perform a dissection tracheotomy, whereas a cricothyroidotomy is significantly faster.[45]

Indications for emergency cricothyroidotomy include situations where intubation is contraindicated or cannot be accomplished in maxillofacial trauma and patients with clenched teeth, cervical spine injuries, and gross oral pharyngeal obstruction from edema, mass lesions, or foreign bodies.[46–48] In addition, a cricothyroidotomy is easier to perform than a tracheotomy in extremely obese patients.[49]

Absolute contraindications include any patient who can undergo normal intubation without risk or children less than 12 years of age.[4] Relative contraindications are injuries, infections, or tumors of the larynx.[49] The list of contraindications is longer with regard to elective cricothyroidotomy; however, none outweigh hypoxic death as the alternative in emergency situations.

The anatomic guides and technique of an emergency cricothyroidotomy are as follows (Fig. 14–7). Hyperextension of the neck is unnecessary. If time permits, sterile preparation and local anesthetic infiltration can be used. A 4% topical lidocaine (2 cc) injection through the cricothyroid membrane abates the cough reflex. Palpation of the hyoid bone, thyroid prominence, and cricoid cartilage is essential for orientation. The larynx is stabilized with the operator's left hand, while the left index finger palpates the cricothyroid space, which lies 1 to 1.5 finger widths (2 to 3 cm) inferior to the thyroid prominence.[50,51] A vertical midline incision 2 to 3 cm in length is initiated from below the thyroid prominence and carried inferiorly. The vertical incision avoids the paramedian, anterior jugular veins, and sternohyoid strap muscles. To reach the cricothyroid membrane, the knife must pass through skin, subcutaneous tissue, superficial cervical fascia, superficial layer of deep cervical fascia, midline anastomosis of middle cervical fascia, and pretracheal fascia.[52] A No. 11 blade is then used to make a 1.5 cm *horizontal* stab incision through the inferior aspect of the cricothyroid membrane and tracheal mucosa. This incision avoids the anastomosis of the right and left cricothyroid arteries (branches of superior thyroid artery) that pierce the membrane superiorly.[6, 44, 49] In a cadaver study, Little et al. showed that only 9% of his subjects had this classic pattern of bilateral cricothyroid arteries—32% had a vertical artery in the midline as a branch of the cricothyroid artery; 47% had a variety of veins vertically over the membrane; 62% had one or more vertical vascular structures.[53] These vascular structures likely account for the fivefold increase in the incidence of hemorrhage from emergency versus elective cricothyroidotomies.[48,49]

The average skin to lumen distance in adults is 10 mm.[54] The cricothyroid membrane incision should be made in a 30° to 40° angulation caudad to avoid dam-

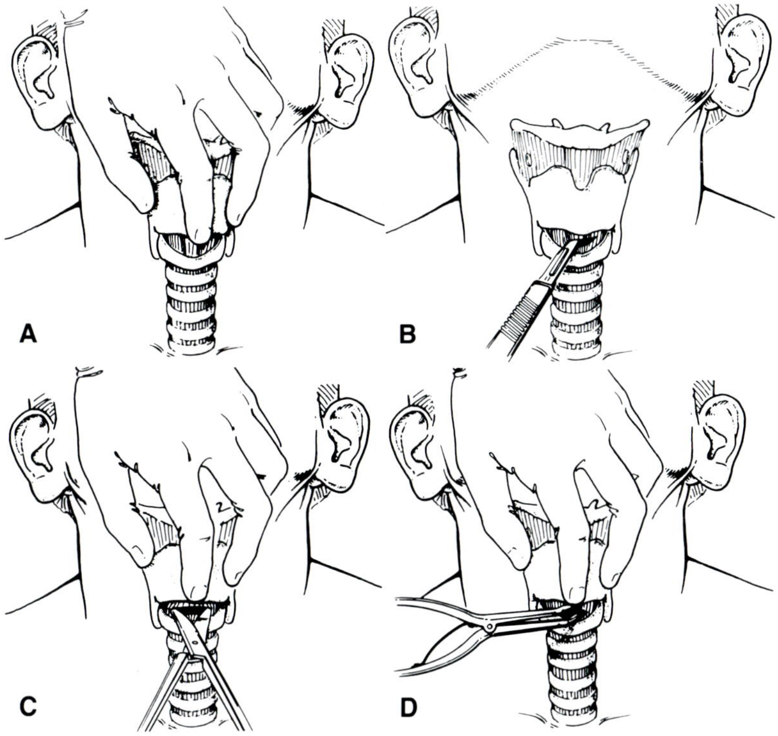

Figure 14-7. *Surgical cricothyroidotomy. (**A**) Palpation of landmarks. (**B**) Horizontal incision through cricothyroid membrane. (**C**) Horizontal dilation. (**D**) Vertical dilation in preparation for tube placement. (Feinberg SE, Peterson LJ. Use of cricothyroidotomy in oral and maxillofacial surgery. J Oral Maxillofac Surg 1987; 45:876.*

age to the vocal cords, which lie an average of 1.5 to 2 cm cephalad.[51] The wider posterior aspect of the cricoid ring protects against esophageal perforation. Dilation of this incision is in two planes—horizontal spreading with Mayo scissors, followed by vertical spreading with a Trosseau dilator. If these instruments are not available, dilation may be rapidly accomplished by inserting the scalpel handle into the wound and rotating it 90°. A well-lubricated tracheotomy tube no greater than 8 mm in outer diameter or a cuffed endotracheal tube no greater than 6 mm in outer diameter can then be inserted.[49] The tube size is limited by the size of the cricothyroid space, which is 9 mm vertically by 30 mm horizontally in the adult.[55] Insertion of a larger tube invites laryngeal fracture.

A simple cricothyroid puncture device has been described by Fisher; it consists of the sharp end of an IV drip set connected to the 15-mm adaptor from a 5.5- to 6.5-mm endotracheal tube. This device provides a 2-mm ventilation lumen, and the finger rest on the IV component prevents excessive penetration (Fig. 14–8).[56]

An excellent review of cricothyroidotomy complications was given by Feinberg and Peterson. They reviewed 11 studies, encompassing 1558 patients, revealing a total complication rate of 10.8%—1.5% with subglottic stenosis, 1.7% with hemorrhage, 5.5% with temporary voice changes, and 2.4% with miscellaneous complications.[49] However, McGill et al. reported on 38 emergency cricothyroidotomy procedures with a complication rate of 32%—three times more than the preceding review. In this study the most frequent complication of emergency cricothyroidotomy was incorrect placement of the incision through the thyrohyoid membrane, thereby creating a supraglottic tube placement. Of these emergency cricothyroidotomy procedures, 87% occurred after failure of conservative maneuvers; 13% were immediate.[48]

The issue of the necessity of changing an emergency cricothyroidotomy to an elective tracheotomy is still unresolved in the literature. Otolaryngologists recommend conversion as soon as possible.[51] Because of their experience with elective cricothyroidotomy both bedside and in the operating room, other surgical specialties believe they are well tolerated for weeks

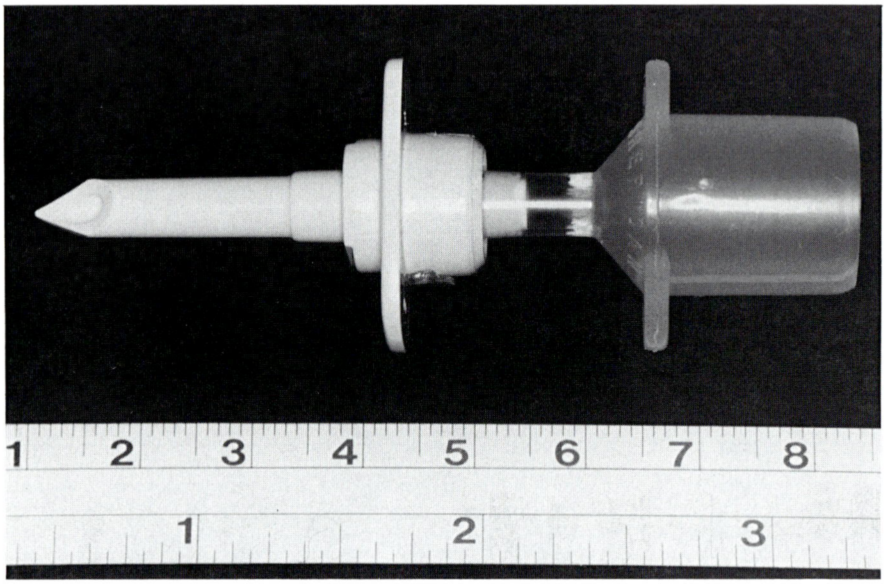

Figure 14-8. *Simple cricothyroid puncture device.*

without significant subglottic stenosis.[43] Some authors advocate circumventing the issue by elective conversion before 72-hours after cricothyroidotomy.[50]

Tracheotomy

Facial injuries are seldom an indication for emergency tracheotomy unless the patient has associated maxillofacial, cervical spine, or laryngeal injuries. Blunt laryngeal trauma with disruption of landmark anatomic features and obstruction is one of the true indications for emergency tracheotomy.[57] In a study by Zacharides et al., only 2.4% of patients presenting with maxillofacial injuries required tracheotomy, with 45.5% of these for respiratory distress.[58] In most situations the airway can be stabilized by intubation, percutaneous needle ventilation, or cricothyroidotomy. A literature review by Skaggs et al. revealed that the complication rate of emergency tracheotomy (29.2%) was two to five times higher than elective tracheostomy. If possible, emergency tracheotomies should be performed in an operating room environment. If performed elsewhere, inadequate lighting, equipment, and assistance combined with a struggling patient will increase complications.[59]

There is no absolute contraindication to emergency tracheotomy; however, the procedure may be difficult in patients with cervical obesity, neck swelling, a short neck, cervical arthritis, kyphoscoliosis, previous neck surgery, or history of cervical radiation therapy.[60] As with cricothyroidotomy, avoidance of hypoxic death takes priority over any of the above considerations.

The technique of emergency tracheotomy and its associated anatomic guides are described. If the condition of the cervical spine permits, a rolled towel is placed under the scapulas to hyperextend the neck. Sterile skin preparation and local anesthesia with vasoconstrictor are helpful if time allows. To avoid bilateral neurovascular structures, a vertical midline incision is indicated, starting at the inferior edge of the cricoid cartilage and extending inferiorly 3 to 4 cm (Fig. 14–9, A).[61] Many surgeons advocate a horizontal skin incision as being more cosmetic. Meade states that the final scar depends not so much on the orientation of the incision but more on the length of cannulation time.[62] When faced with performing an

Figure 14-9. *Surgical tracheotomy. (**A**) Landmarks and vertical skin incision. (**B**) Superficial dissection. (**C**) Exposure of the thyroid isthmus and its associated suspensory ligament to the cricoid cartilage. (**D**) Division and ligation of the thyroid isthmus. (**E**) Tracheal opening with stay sutures.* ►

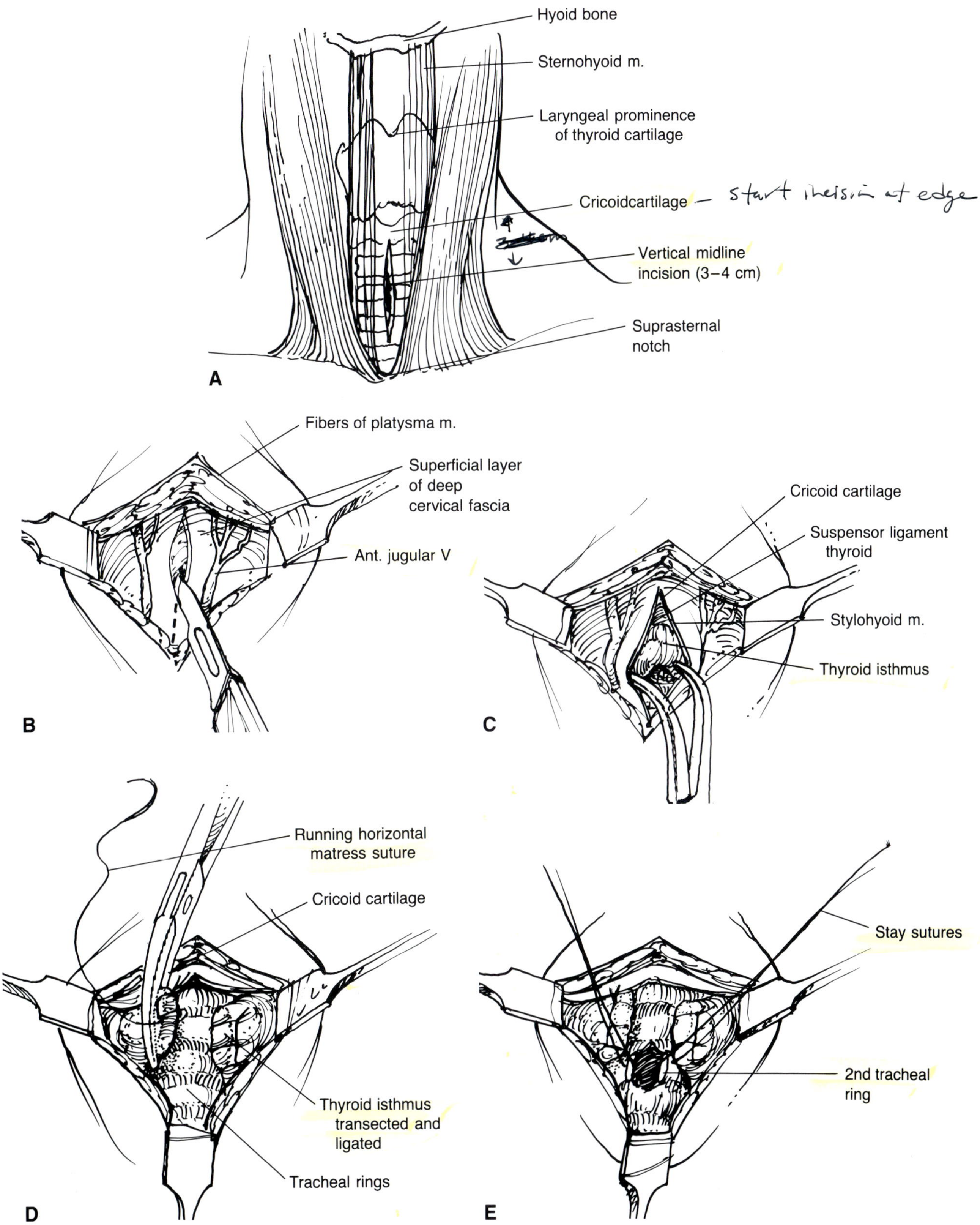
Hyoid bone
Sternohyoid m.
Laryngeal prominence of thyroid cartilage
Cricoidcartilage
Vertical midline incision (3–4 cm)
Suprasternal notch
A
Fibers of platysma m.
Superficial layer of deep cervical fascia
Ant. jugular V
B
Cricoid cartilage
Suspensor ligament thyroid
Stylohyoid m.
Thyroid isthmus
C
Running horizontal matress suture
Cricoid cartilage
Thyroid isthmus transected and ligated
Tracheal rings
D
Stay sutures
2nd tracheal ring
E

emergency tracheotomy, cosmetic appearance of the resulting scar deserves no consideration. McKelvie feels the horizontal incision may provide improved access to a trachea that is severely deviated from the midline.[63] If a horizontal incision is not directly over the tracheal opening because of an error in incision location or retraction of the trachea inferiorly after neck hyperextension is released, the cannula can be displaced anteriorly or posteriorly within the trachea by skin-wound–margin pressure. Finally a vertical incision allows for movement of the cannula with the trachea during swallowing.[61]

Dissection is continued through the subcutaneous tissue and the superficial cervical fascia. This fascia divides 3 to 4 cm superior to the manubrium to form the suprasternal Burns' space. The anterior jugular veins and their transverse connections (arcus venosus) will be either in this fascia layer or immediately below it.[52] If those veins are seen crossing the surgical field, they should be clamped and divided. Definitive ligature should be deferred until the airway is secured in urgent situations (Fig. 14–9, B).

Next, the sternohyoid and underlying sternothyroid strap muscles with their investing middle cervical fascia should be split apart in the midline and retracted laterally. Frequent palpation of the trachea will ensure a midline surgical course. Exposure of the thyroid isthmus and its suspensory ligament to the cricoid cartilage is important because division of this ligament opens a surgical plane to the trachea (Fig. 14–9,C). If the procedure is being performed with local anesthetic alone, it will be necessary to put 1 to 2 cc under the ligament as this area cannot be otherwise anesthetized.[64] If the patient is awake and the airway is not secured by other means, the local anesthetic infiltration should be confined to the midline, avoiding lateral diffusion to the recurrent laryngeal nerves.[13] The resulting partial vocal cord paralysis could further endanger an already compromised airway. In the majority of cases the thyroid isthmus crosses the trachea anteriorly from the second to the third tracheal rings.[61, 64] The isthmus should be undermined caudad through the previously cut suspensory ligament, clamped, and divided in the midline. A running 2-0-resorbable suture is preferred for ligature of the thyroid isthmus because complicating hemorrhage is possible from the vascular thyroid tissue (Fig. 14–9, D). Again, definitive ligature may be delayed until the airway is secured. Avoid dissection lateral to the trachea as recurrent laryngeal nerve damage could result.

It is important to palpate the cricoid cartilage (which a vertical incision facilitates) as the tracheal rings must be counted for orientation. Before opening the trachea, needle aspiration of air confirms the proper structure. If time permits, placement of a tracheal hook stabilizes the surgical field. The trachea should be opened somewhere between the confines of the second and third rings (Fig. 14–9,E). Opening below the third ring increases the risk of tracheal-innominate artery fistula, whereas opening above the second ring predisposes the patient to stenosis.[57,59,65]

The design of the incision through the trachea is controversial. A vertical midline tracheal incision is advocated for emergency procedures because it is quick and allows larger tube insertion. However, a tracheal window facilitates emergency recannulation should the need arise. Natvig et al. showed in rabbits that the design of tracheal incisions plays only a minor role in stenosis. Window or vertical incision access openings resulted in less stenosis than any flap technique.[66] Regardless of how the trachea is opened, two large nonresorbable sutures should be placed on either side of the surgically created tracheal stoma to function as stay sutures. Should emergency recannulation become necessary in the immediate postoperative period, these sutures act as a guide to the tracheal fenestration, while providing retraction of wound margins.[65]

The trachea should be cannulated with a high-volume, low-pressure cuffed tracheotomy tube, but if one is not immediately available, a modified endotracheal tube can be temporarily used. The modifications include splitting the tube vertically along its long axis and reinserting the 15-mm ventilating connector. Strings to secure the tube can be attached to the split sides of the tube (Fig. 14–10). This modification works especially well in morbid obese patients in whom increased tracheocutaneous thickness renders standard tracheotomy tubes impractical.[67] Once the airway is secure and the patient can be adequately ventilated, total hemostasis of the wound should be obtained. Only the peripheral skin margin should be loosely approximated.

After surgery, the patient should be administered humidified oxygen either by ventilator or tracheotomy collar. Immediate chest radiographs are mandatory. The tracheotomy should be suctioned ag-

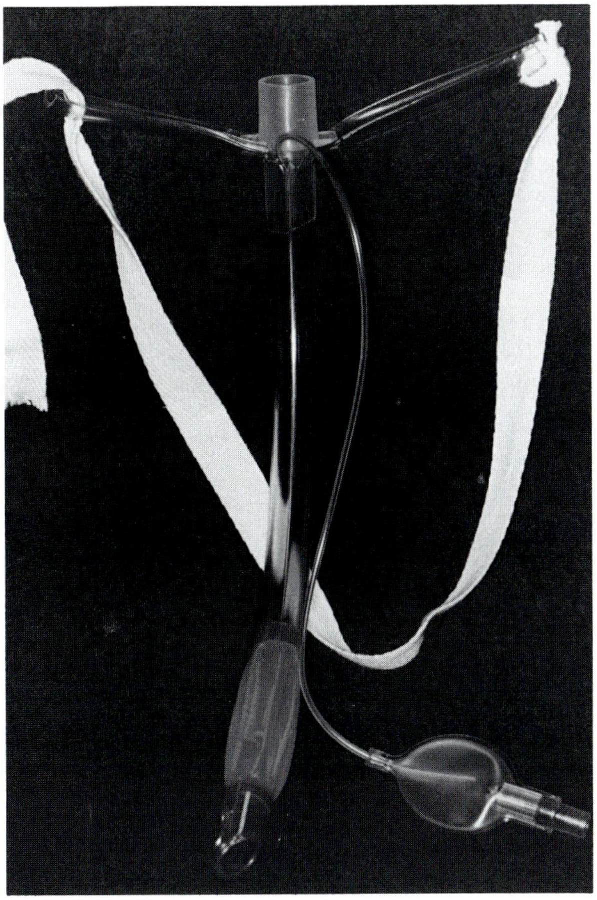

Figure 14-10. *Endotracheal tube modification to allow function as tracheotomy tube.*

gressively, using saline irrigation for thick secretions, immediately after surgery every 15 minutes for 4 hours, tapering to once per hour as needed. The inner cannula should be removed and cleaned along with a sterile dressing change three times per day.[68] Stay sutures may be removed and string ties changed 7 days after surgery. The temptation to suture the tracheotomy tube to the skin should be avoided because this is associated with an increased incidence of necrotizing tracheotomy infections.[69]

Chew et al. reviewed seven series of tracheotomy complication reports encompassing a total of 1928 cases resulting in a 15.8% complication rate and a 1.6% morality rate. Death was frequently secondary to hemorrhage and tube displacement. The most frequent complications were delayed hemorrhage, 3.7%; infection, 3.3%; tube obstruction, 2.7%; displaced tubes, 1.5%; and pneumothorax, 0.9%.[65] The most common sites of immediate hemorrhage are from the anterior jugular veins with their midline anastomosis, inferior thyroid vein, thyroid isthmus, communication branch of superior thyroid artery along the upper edge of the isthmus, thyroid ima artery (rare), and the occasional innominate artery visible above the manubrium.[61] Jugular venous distension resulting from respiratory obstruction can be a cause of increased hemorrhage during tracheotomy. Delayed hemorrhage usually occurs between 1 to 2 weeks after surgery.[70] The differential diagnosis of bleeding after tracheotomy includes tracheitis, local wound bleeding, upper airway surgery bleeding, and vascular erosion. The most feared late hemorrhage is a tracheal-innominate fistula. Yang et al. reviewed 36 cases and found it to have less than a 1% incidence but a 75% mortality. All originated from a low tracheotomy below the third ring. Emergency treatment includes overinflation of the tracheotomy cuff or insertion of a finger through the stoma to compress the innominate artery against the sternum, followed by immediate surgery. Alternatively, an oral endotracheal tube may be placed, which allows for improved access for digital compression through the stoma.[71] Of the 32% of patients who died after tracheal-innominate hemorrhage, 3% died in the operating room, and of those that rebled after emergency surgery, there was a 100% fatality rate.[72] Jones et al. state that "all patients having greater than 10 cc of blood from a tracheotomy 48 hours or more after a tracheotomy, a tracheal-innominate fistula is assumed until proven otherwise."[73]

Displaced tracheotomy tubes cause 25% mortality. Blind reinsertion usually fails. A careful but rapid reexploration of the wound is indicated to locate the tracheal orifice.[65] Subcutaneous emphysema occurs with increased lateral dissection during the tracheotomy or when the deeper layers of the wound are approximated. Pneumothorax or pneumomediastinum occurs with inferior dissection or placement of the tube in a false passage accompanied by ventilation attempts. In patients with respiratory obstruction or with chronic obstructive pulmonary disease (COPD), the dome of the pleura may be higher in the neck, increasing the risk of pleural cavity violation.[61,74]

If difficulty is expected in changing a tracheotomy tube, remove the old tube over a well-lubricated nasogastric tube and slide the replacement tube into place using the nasogastric tube as a guide.[75]

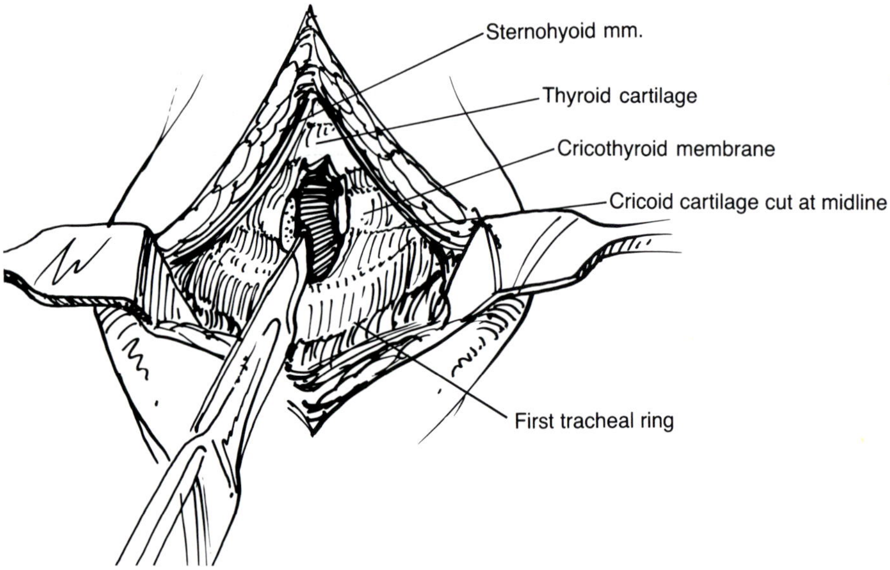

Figure 14-11. *Division of pediatric cricoid cartilage. In extreme emergencies, surgical division of this readily palpable landmark is indicated for rapid airway procurement.*

PEDIATRIC AIRWAY

Differences in anatomic and physiologic features of the pediatric airway, as compared with the adult, obligate management alterations in both elective and emergency situations. Compared with the adult, the most prominent airway structures palpable in children are the hyoid bone and cricoid cartilage. The cricothyroid membrane is not readily palpable in 7- to 8-year-old patients. The cricoid is the narrowest part of the pediatric airway as compared to the glottic opening in the adult airway.[76]

Intubation of the pediatric patient is challenging because of the small size, altered anatomic features, and decreased time available to perform intubation. Estimation of the size of uncuffed tubes (necessary in patients who are less than 12 years of age) can be by age or by comparison with the diameter of the child's small finger or nostril orifice.[77] Laryngoscopy and intubation of the awake and struggling patient when general anesthesia is contraindicated or unavailable can be facilitated by topical lidocaine or cocaine in maximum dosages of 3 mg/kg, each.[11] Intravenous sedation also may be used.[78] In trauma scenarios, oral intubation for airway control is preferred. If cervical spine injuries cannot be excluded, then in-line cervical traction with oral intubation is indicated.[4] Nasal intubation in the pediatric population is difficult because of small nasal passages, hemorrhage from adenoid hypertrophy, and lack of rigidity of small endotracheal tubes.[9,76]

Surgical airway techniques must be used in those patients with failing airways who are unable to be intubated. Cricothyroidotomy is contraindicated in patients who are less than 12 years of age because of the difficulty of locating palpable landmarks and the restrictive size of the cricothyroid space. Percutaneous needle ventilation may be safely employed through the cricothyroid membrane with a 14 gauge catheter as a temporizing maneuver until a definitive airway is obtained.[11] Increased awareness of barotrauma with this technique is essential in the pediatric population.

Emergency pediatric tracheotomy is rarely used because of its difficulty and the increased complication rate. Experience with this procedure is mandatory because it should be reserved only for life-threatening emergencies. The procedure seems to be rarely necessary in trauma situations.[57,79] Because only 2% of pediatric tracheotomies are done on an emergency basis, the airway should be temporally stabilized with intubation, a ventilating bronchoscope, or needle cricothyroidotomy. This will allow the tracheotomy to be converted to a semiemergent procedure in the proper operating environment.[57,78,80,81]

The technique of pediatric tracheotomy is well-described by Tucker.[80] Extension of the neck (if the cervical spine allows) should not be severe because excessive hyperextension distorts the trachea cephalad exposing more tracheal rings from the thoracic outlet.[78] Palpation of landmarks and initial vertical incision is the same as in the adult. Blunt dissection with conservative lateral retraction of strap muscles and tissue layers maintains a narrow midline field. This is important as the carotid sheath is extremely close to the trachea in infants and young children and has been mistaken for the trachea.[57] In cases of extreme urgency the cricoid cartilage may be divided in the midline for rapid airway access (Fig. 14–11). Advantages of this technique include an anatomically exact approach, an easily palpable landmark, a noncompressible structure, avoidance of lateral neurovascular structures, and decreased risk of lung injury. The site may be electively lowered later to decrease the chances of stenosis. Dissection may be continued below the thyroid isthmus; however, clamping, division, and ligation of the isthmus may be necessary. Unlike in the adult, the trachea should be opened at the fourth and fifth tracheal rings.[80] Controversy still abounds over the design of the tracheal fenestration.[82,83]

Pediatric tracheotomy carries with it significant mortality and morbidity, with younger patients experiencing the highest mortality and incidence of complications. The most frequent complications are pneumothorax, pneumomediastinum, and subglottic stenosis. Wetmore et al. reviewed 420 cases coupled with a literature review and concluded that a mortality rate of 3.2% to 8.5% can be directly attributable to the tracheotomy procedure itself.[84]

REFERENCES

1. Meislin HW, Iserson KV, Kaback KR, et al. Airway trauma. Emerg Med Clin North Am 1983; 1(2): 295.
2. WHO. Human factors in road accidents. Report on a symposium in Rome, Italy, convened by the Regional Office for Europe of the WHO, Copenhagen, 1967.
3. Danzil DF, Thomas DM. Nasoendotracheal intubation in the emergency department. Crit Care Med 1980; 8:677.
4. American College of Surgeons. Advanced trauma life support course: Student manual. 00000: The American College of Surgeons, Committee on Trauma, Chicago, Illinois, 1988, p. 39.
5. Aprahamian C, Thompson BM, Finger WA, et al. Experimental cervical spine injury model: Evaluation of airway management and splinting techniques. Ann Emerg Med 1984; 13:584.
6. Dauphinee K. Nasotracheal intubation. Emerg Med Clin North Am 1988; 6:715.
7. Seshul MB, Sinn DP, Gerlock J. The Andy Gump fracture of the mandible: A cause of respiratory obstruction or distress. J Trauma 1978; 18:611.
8. Thompson JN, Gibson B, Kohut RI. Airway obstruction in LeFort fractures. Laryngoscope 1987; 97:275.
9. Badgwell JM, McLeod ME, Friedberg J. Airway obstruction in infants and children. Can J Anaesth 1987; 34:90.
10. Fontanarosa PB, Goldman GE, Polsky SS. Sitting oral-tracheal intubation. Ann Emerg Med 1988; 17:336.
11. Hartmann PK, Mintz G, Verne D, et al. Diagnosis and primary management of laryngeal trauma. Oral Surg Oral Med Oral Pathol 1985; 60:252.
12. Thompson JN, Strausbaugh PL, Koufman JA, et al. Penetrating injuries of the larynx. South Med J 1984; 77:41.
13. Flood LM, Astley B. Anaesthetic management of acute laryngeal trauma. Br J Anaesth 1982; 54:1339.
14. Mancuso AA, Hanafee WN. Computed tomography of the injured larynx. Radiology 1979; 133:139.
15. Leopold DA. Laryngeal trauma: A historical comparison of treatment methods. Arch Otolaryngol 1983; 109:106.
16. Mellis CM. Lateral neck x-rays: Useful or dangerous in acute infective upper airways obstruction. Aust Fam Physician 1987; 16:1490.
17. Frame JW, Wake MJC. Evaluation of maxillofacial injuries by use of computerized tomography. J Oral Maxillofac Surg 1982; 40:482.
18. Boiden MP. Airway patency in the unconscious patient. Br J Anaesth 1985; 57:306.
19. Hochbaum SR. Emergency airway management. In: Kobernick MS, Burney RE, eds. Emerg Med Clin North Am 1986; 4(3): 411.
20. Dauphinee K. Orotracheal intubation. Emerg Med Clin North Am 1988; 6:699.
21. MacIntosh R, Richard H. Illuminated introducer for endotracheal tubes. Anaesthesia 1957; 12:223.
22. Handler SD, Keon TP. Difficult laryngoscopy/intubation: The child with mandibular hypoplasia. Ann Otol Rhinol Laryngol 1983; 92:401.
23. Wolf C, LeJeune FE, Douglas JR. A technique for intubation of the difficult airway. Otolaryngol Head Neck Surg 1987; 96:278.
24. Stewart RD. Tactile orotracheal intubation. Ann Emerg Med 1984; 13:175.
25. Verlander JM, Johns ME. The clinical use of cocaine. In: Johns ME, Rice DH, eds. Otolaryngol Clin North Am 1981; 14(3): 521.
26. Jantzen JAH. Letter to editor. Anesth Analg 1985; 64:646.
27. Taylor PA, Towey RM. The broncho-fiberscope as an aid to endotracheal intubation. Br J Anaesth 1972; 44:611.
28. Childers WF. New method for fiberoptic endotracheal intubation of anesthetized patients. Anesthesiology 1981; 55:581.
29. Ford RWJ. Adaptation of the fiberoptic laryngoscope for tracheal intubation with small diameter tubes. Can Anaesth Soc J 1981; 28(5): 479.
30. Wai WI, Siu KF, Lau WF, et al. Emergency endotracheal intubation under fiberoptic endoscopic guid-

ance for malignant laryngeal obstruction. Otolaryngol Head Neck Surg 1988; 98:10.
31. Stella JP, Lageler WV, Epker BN. Fiberoptic endotracheal intubation in oral and maxillofacial surgery. J Oral Maxillofac Surg 1986; 44:923.
32. Anderton JM. Letter to editor. Br J Anaesth 1978; 50:1267.
33. Butler FS, Cirillo AA. Retrograde tracheal intubation. Anesth Analg 1960; 39:333.
34. King HK, Wang LF, Kahn AK, et al. Translaryngeal guided intubation for difficult intubation. Crit Care Med 1987; 15:869.
35. Orringer MB. Endotracheal intubation and tracheostomy indications, techniques, and complications. In: Bartlett RH, ed. Surg Clin North Am 1980; 60(6): 1447.
36. Gold MI, Bucchel DR. Translaryngeal anesthesia: A review. Anesthesiology 1959; 20:181.
37. Jorden RC. Percutaneous transtracheal ventilation. In: Campbell WH, ed. Emerg Med Clin North Am 1988; 6(4): 745.
38. O'Rourke PP, Crone RK. High-frequency ventilation: a new approach to respiratory support. JAMA 1983; 250:2845.
39. Roven AN, Clapham MCC. Cricothyroidotomy. Ear Nose Throat J 1983; 62:489.
40. Suderi PE, McLeskey CH, Comer PB. Emergency percutaneous transtracheal ventilation during anesthesia using readily available equipment. Anesth Analg 1982; 61:867.
41. Rone CA, Pavlin EG, Cummings CW, et al. Studies in transtracheal ventilation catheters. Laryngoscope 1982; 92:1259.
42. Weymuller EA, Pavlin EG, Paugh D, et al. Management of difficult airway problems with percutaneous transtracheal ventilation. Ann Otol Rhinol Laryngol 1987; 96:34.
43. Brantigan CO, Grow JB. Cricothyroidotomy: Elective use in respiratory problems requiring tracheostomy. J Thorac Cardiovasc Surg 1976; 71:72.
44. King HK, Wand LF, Khan AK. Translaryngeal guided intubation for difficult intubation. Crit Care Med 1987; 15:869.
45. Toye FJ, Weinstein JD. Clinical experience with percutaneous tracheostomy and cricothyroidotomy in 100 patients. J Trauma 1986; 26:1034.
46. Morain WD. Cricothyroidotomy in head and neck surgery. Plast Reconstr Surg 1979; 65:424.
47. Kress TD, Balasubramaniam S. Cricothyroidotomy. Ann Emerg Med 1982; 11:197.
48. McGill J, Clinton JE, Ruiz E. Cricothyrotomy in the emergency department. Ann Emerg Med 1982; 11:361.
49. Feinberg SE, Peterson LJ. Use of cricothyroidotomy in oral and maxillofacial surgery. J Oral Maxillofac Surg 1987; 45:873.
50. Walls RM. Cricothyroidotomy. In: Campbell WH, ed. Emerg Med Clin North Am 1988; 6:725.
51. Esses BA, Jafek BW. Cricothyroidotomy: A decade of experience in Denver. Ann Otol Rhinol Laryngol 1987; 96:519.
52. Gray H, Goss CM. Gray's anatomy, ed 100. Philadelphia: Lea & Febiger, 1962: 426, 430.
53. Little CM, Parker MG, Tarnopolsky R, et al. The incidence of vasculature at risk during cricothyroidotomy. Ann Emerg Med 1986; 15:805.
54. McDowell DE. Cricothyroidotomy for airway access. South Med J 1982; 75:282.
55. Caparosa RJ, Zavatasky AR. Practical aspects of the cricothyroid space. Laryngoscope 1957; 67:577.
56. Fisher JA. A "last ditch" airway. Can Anaesth Soc J 1979; 26:225.
57. Piotrowski JJ, Moore EE. Emergency department tracheostomy. Emerg Med Clin North Am 1988; 6(4): 737.
58. Zachariades N, Rapidis Ad, Papademetriou J, et al. The significance of tracheostomy in the management of fractures of the facial skeleton. J Maxillo Fac Surg 1983; 11:180.
59. Skaggs JA, Cogbill CL. Tracheostomy: Management, mortality, and complications. Am Surg 1969; 35:393.
60. Shugar MA. Fiberoptic tracheotomy guide. Otolaryngol Head Neck Surg 1982; 91:335.
61. Kirchner JA. Tracheostomy and its problems. Surg Clin North Am 1980; 60(5): 1093.
62. Meade JW. Tracheostomy: Its complications and their management. N Engl J Med 1961; 265:519.
63. McKelvie P. How to do an emergency tracheostomy. Br J Hosp Med 1981; 25:640.
64. Kirchner JA. Avoiding problems in tracheotomy. Laryngoscope 1986; 96:55.
65. Chew JY, Cantrell RW. Tracheostomy complications and their management. Arch Otolaryngol 1972; 96:538.
66. Natvig K, Olving JH. Tracheal changes in relation to different tracheostomy techniques. J Laryngol Otol 1981; 95:61.
67. Ghorayeb BY. Tracheotomy in the morbidly obese patient. Arch Otolaryngol Head Neck Surg 1987; 113:556.
68. Price HC, Postma DS. Tracheostomy. Ear Nose Throat J 1983; 62:474.
69. Snow N, Richardson D, Flint LM. Management of necrotizing tracheostomy infections. J Thorac Cardiovasc Surg 1981; 82:341.
70. Potondi A. Pathomechanisms of haemorrhages following tracheostomy. J Laryngol Otol 1969; 83:475.
71. Cooper JD. Trachea-innominate artery fistula: Successful management of three consecutive patients. Ann Thorac Surg 1977; 24:439.
72. Yang FY, Criado E, Schwartz JA, et al. Trachea-innominate artery fistula: Retrospective comparison of treatment methods. South Med J 1988; 81:701.
73. Jones JW, Reynolds M, Hewitt RL, et al. Trachea-innominate artery erosion: Succesful management of a devasting complication. Ann Surg 1976; 184:194.
74. Oliver P, Richardson JR, Clubb RW, et al. Tracheotomy in children. N Engl J Med 1962; 267:631.

75. Gilsdorf JR. Facilitated endotracheal and tracheostomy tube replacement. Surg Gynecol Obstet 1984; 159: 589.
76. Barkin RM. Pediatric airway management. Emerg Med Clin North Am 1988; 6(4): 687.
77. Jorden RC. Airway management. Emerg Med Clin North Am 1988; 6:671.
78. Goldthorn J, Badgwell JM. Upper airway obstruction in infants and children. Int Anesthesiol Clin 1986; 24(1): 133.
79. Line WS, Hawkins DB, Kahlstrom EJ, et al. Tracheotomy in infants and children: The changing perspective. Laryngoscope 1986; 96:510.
80. Tucker JA. Obstruction of the major pediatric airway. In: Yarington CT, ed. Otolaryngol Clin North Am 1979; 12(2): 329.
81. Mayer TA. Emergency tracheostomy: A technique in search of an indication. Ann Emerg Med 1987; 16:606.
82. Fry TL, Jones RO, Fisher ND, et al. Comparisons of tracheostomy incisions in a pediatric model. Ann Otol Rhinol Laryngol 1985; 94:450.
83. Gilmore BB, Mickelson SA. Pediatric tracheotomy. Otolaryngol Clin North Am 1987; 19(1): 141.
84. Wetmore RF, Handler SD, Potsic WP. Pediatric tracheostomy: Experience during the past decade. Ann Otol Rhinol Laryngol 1982; 91:628.

15

Soft Tissue Injuries of the Face

Jonathan S. Jacobs
John A. Dean

The face is the window through which we perceive the world around us and the world sees us. The face serves a crucial role in human interaction, and injuries to it can result in devastating emotional sequelae. This exposed area is commonly injured by a variety of different methods (e.g., flash, chemical, and scald burns, and abrasions) while the rest of the body is protected. The face is a common target for assault and is commonly injured in motor vehicle accidents (Fig. 15–1).

Successful treatment of facial injuries depends on excellent initial management. The acutely damaged face is free of scarring, infection, and secondary skeletal changes that will preclude optimal results when these injuries are treated secondarily. Facial injury, more than any other area of the body, requires accurate acute care. The many delicate structures of the face must be repaired initially to minimize tissue loss, functional loss, scarring, and contracture. Although scar revision may sometimes be necessary even after excellent initial therapy, the results of the scar revision will be predictably better if the acute care was properly performed.

PRINCIPLES OF MANAGEMENT

The injured patient is initially evaluated for more crucial injuries than those to the face. Life-threatening injuries must obviously be addressed first. Even after life-threatening problems have been attended to and treatment of facial injuries in under way, life-threatening problems may arise again; thus, constant monitoring and rechecking of the injured patient is mandatory. Post-repair sequelae, such as edema, must be kept in mind when considering adequacy of the airway. Hemorrhage from facial wounds is seldom enough to cause hypotension.[1] Significant blood loss in major facial injuries, however, must be closely monitored in patients with marginal circulatory reserve. Early, accurate management of facial soft tissue injuries is needed for optimal results, but it must be performed while the patient as a whole is being treated in the safest possible way. The exceptions to treating facial injuries secondarily are patients with upper airway obstruction, posterior nasal hemorrhage, massive facial contamination, and cerebrospinal fluid leak from the nose or ear.

Just as the patient as a whole must be managed on a priority basis, so must injuries to the face. Areas that require early management include globe and eyelid injuries, nasolacrimal system injuries, and injuries of the parotid and its duct. Early wound closure and coverage of underlying tissues minimizes bacterial contamination and subsequent infection. There is a general treatment protocol applicable to facial injuries. Examination of all facial structures is performed first. Debridement of devitalized tissue is carried out next; then layered closure of the wound.

There are several treatment pitfalls. Documentation with carefully kept records and pre- and postoper-

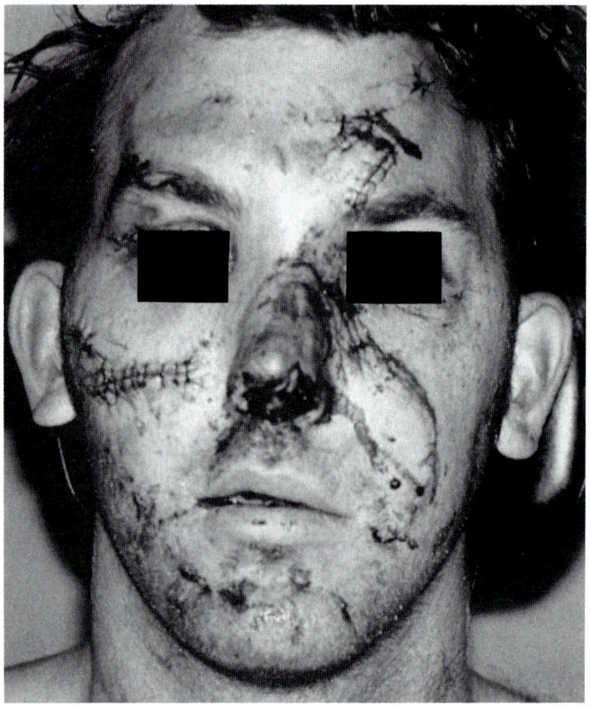

Figure 15–1. *Patient with multiple lacerations, abrasions, and underlying facial bone fracture. (Courtesy of Dr. A. Thomas Indresano, Cleveland Metropolitan General Hospital, Cleveland, Ohio)*

ative photographs is essential. Facial soft tissue is well vascularized and redundancies are limited, especially in young patients. Excessive debridement should thus be avoided. Cartilage and bone that are stripped from their attachments should not be discarded, because they may be subcutaneously "banked" for use in secondary reconstruction.[2] Intricate flaps for primary wound closure should be avoided. Residual foreign bodies left in wounds lead to infection and tattooing. Misaligned wound edges, rough tissue handling, and delayed suture removal leads to tissue necrosis and increased scarring.

ANATOMICAL EVALUATION

A systematic examination of the injured area is needed to plan the treatment approach and to avoid missing occult injuries. This examination must precede the initiation of treatment in all facially injured patients. Thorough knowledge of facial anatomy is imperative.[3]

Early testing of vision and extraocular motion prior to progressive visual obstruction by periorbital edema is mandatory. The eye must be examined in order to rule out injury to the globe, corneal abrasions, hyphema, or traumatic changes in visual acuity. All patients with significant head trauma should have their vision documented in the emergency room and undergo ophthalmoscopic examination. When indicated, fluorescein testing and slit-light examination are needed to document corneal abrasions or foreign bodies. All eyes that have been exposed to chemical irritants must be copiously irrigated. Patients with eyelid injuries are vulnerable to developing acute dry eye and should be protected with saline irrigation. Extraocular motion must be examined to determine whether entrapment exists or whether there has been damage to extraocular muscles or cranial nerves. The superficial position of the inferior oblique muscle lends itself to injury. The patient will not notice diplopia unless tested while looking superiorly and medially when this muscle has been unilaterally injured. The patient should be examined for diplopia in all visual fields. Limitation of upward gaze may indicate entrapment of the inferior oblique–inferior rectus apparatus, attenuated orbital septal strands attached to periosteum, or orbital contents herniation through a fractured orbital floor. Disconjugate gaze is a common finding in intoxicated patients, which corrects spontaneously. Isolated injury to the abducent nerve, manifested by lateral rectus palsy, may indicate a closed head injury.

The nasolacrimal system may be injured when there have been lacerations of the medial canthus region or as a consequence of nasoorbital fracture (Fig. 15–2), a common result of motor vehicle accidents in which the midface strikes the steering wheel or dashboard.[4] When offending bone fragments pierce the medial canthus, telecanthus, with almond-shaped palpebral fissures, may result.[5] The examiner should suspect lacrimal system damage in all patients with medial canthal displacement. Bone fragments may also compress the lacrimal apparatus without actually lacerating it. Unrecognized trauma to the canalicular system will eventually result in epiphora and recurrent dacryocystitis. In some cases a pyocele of the sac will develop.[6] All lacerations involving the medial third of the eyelids must be carefully examined for canicular injury. Under magnification, the structures are probed and identified. Air can be insufflated through a cannula in the upper canaliculus, and the lower canaliculus can

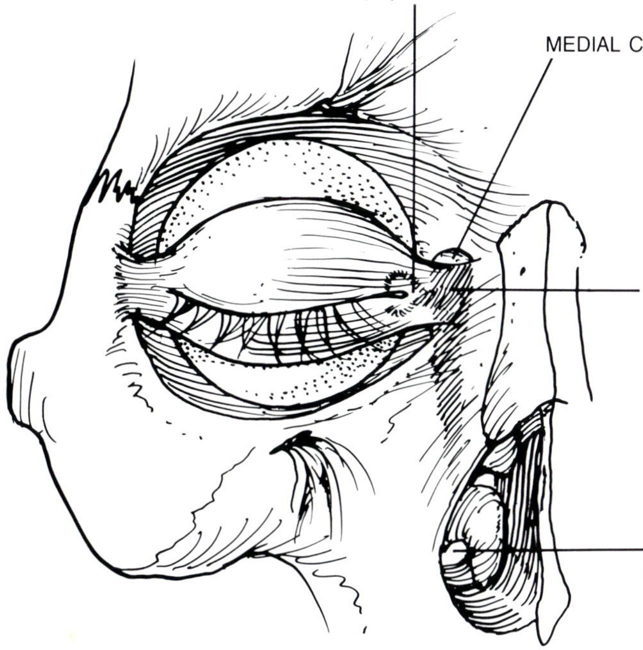

Figure 15–2. *Nasolacrimal system anatomy.*

be sought by flooding the area with irrigating solution and looking for air bubbles. Early recognition and treatment of these injuries, when possible, may obviate the need for later treatment with more extensive surgery such as dacryocystorhinostomy.

The bone structures must be examined for evidence of fracture. This examination includes radiologic evaluation when there is doubt as to the integrity of the facial bone structure. Initial examination is visual and includes assessment of facial symmetry and evidence of distortions. Palpation allows for analysis of bone movement, underlying tenderness, and bone "step-offs." Assessment of occlusion may indicate the presence of an otherwise occult fracture. Testing for evidence of infraorbital nerve palsies will indicate fracture impingement into the foramen of these nerves.

The nose must be carefully examined for evidence of fracture. Tenderness and displacement are cardinal signs. Radiographs of the nasal bones are not as reliable as the clinical examination.[7] All patients with nasal trauma must undergo inspection of the internal nasal anatomy using a nasal speculum. Septal perforation or saddle nose deformity may be the result of cartilage resorption secondary to untreated nasal septum hematoma.

The function of the muscles supplied by the branches of the facial nerve must be examined prior to the initiation of any therapy. Facial nerve dysfunction needs to be documented prior to any invasive treatment to heighten awareness during wound examination and to obviate later claims that facial nerve palsy resulted from therapy rather than initial trauma. Examination must be performed prior to the administration of local anesthetics, because these agents may cause temporary paralysis of facial musculature. The frontal (or temporal) branch of the facial nerve is tested by having the patient wrinkle his or her forehead and raise the eyebrows. The zygomatic branch is tested by the patient closing the eyelids tightly. The buccal branch is tested by the patient smiling or sneering, and the marginal mandibular branch is tested by smiling or pursing of the lips. The cervical branch is examined by having the patient contract the platysma.

The most common cause of facial nerve palsy, incurred as a result of external trauma, occurs with temporal fractures associated with motor vehicle accidents. One fourth of patients with temporal fractures develop facial paralysis. A careful history is needed in these patients. Patients who have a sudden and complete loss of facial nerve function must be presumed to have suffered transection of the nerve. The most common location of transection in these patients is at the level of the geniculate ganglion. Computed tomography may reveal markedly disrupted temporal bone fragments. These patients deserve early exploration. More commonly, patients with temporal bone fractures have a history of delayed or partial facial nerve dysfunction. Fair to complete recovery of facial motor function in this situation is expected without operative therapy.[8] Patients with temporal fractures often have an altered level of consciousness, and thus facial nerve function may not be easily assessed. Painful stimuli may evoke facial grimacing, which the clinician may observe for facial motor function.

Treatment of significant facial lacerations requires strict attention to the position of the branches of the facial nerve (Fig. 15–3). Areas of particular concern include deep lacerations over the temporal area where the frontal branch may be easily damaged. Lacerations of the parotid gland and its duct, due to their immediate proximity to the facial nerve, should also heighten awareness.

Examination for injury to the parotid gland and its duct must be performed in all lacerations involving the cheek. Stenson's duct occupies the region represented by the middle third of a line drawn from the tragus to the midpoint of the upper lip (Fig. 15–4). Documentation of glandular injury can only be confirmed at wound exploration. To test for ductal injury, the oral papilla of the duct can be cannulated with a fine tube and injected with 0.5 mL of methylene blue while observing the wound[9] (Fig. 15–5).

Sensory nerve territories should be examined not only when concerned about facial fractures but also when lacerations may have injured these important structures. Key sensory areas to be examined include areas supplied by the infra- and supraorbital nerves, the infra- and supratrochlear nerves, the mental nerve, and the great auricular nerve. Sensory deficits should be documented prior to anesthetizing the wounds.

When examining soft tissue lacerations the depths of the wounds must be carefully checked. Palpation for underlying fractures is important, as is looking for

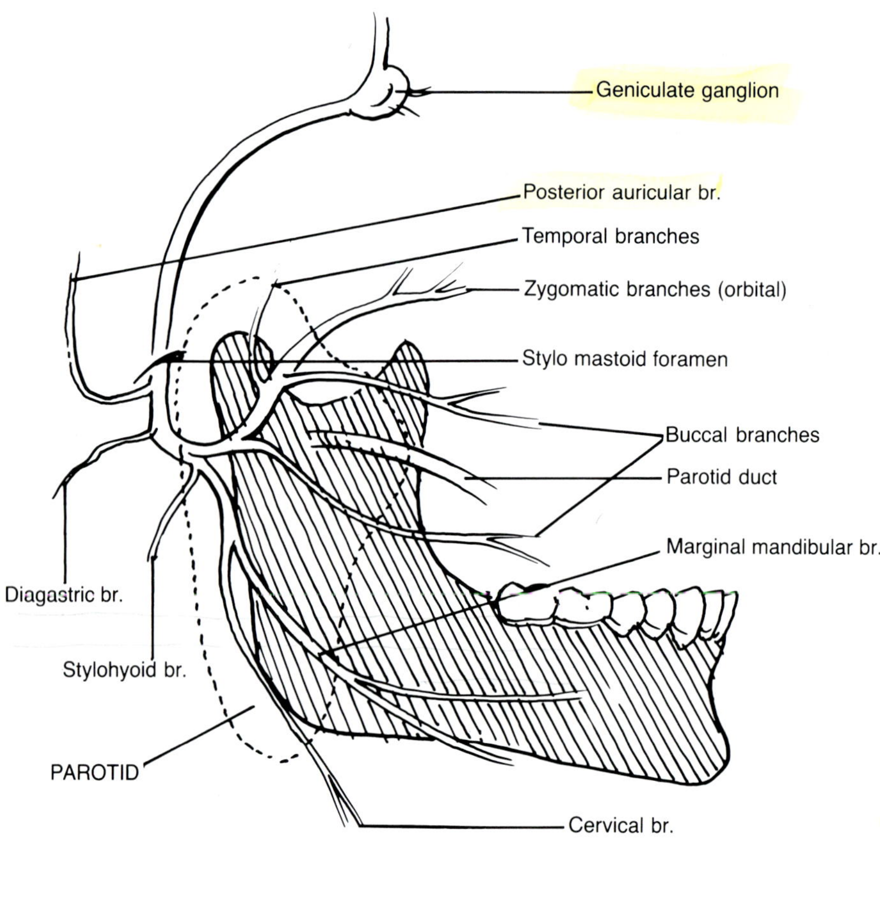

Figure 15–3. *Anatomy of facial nerve.*

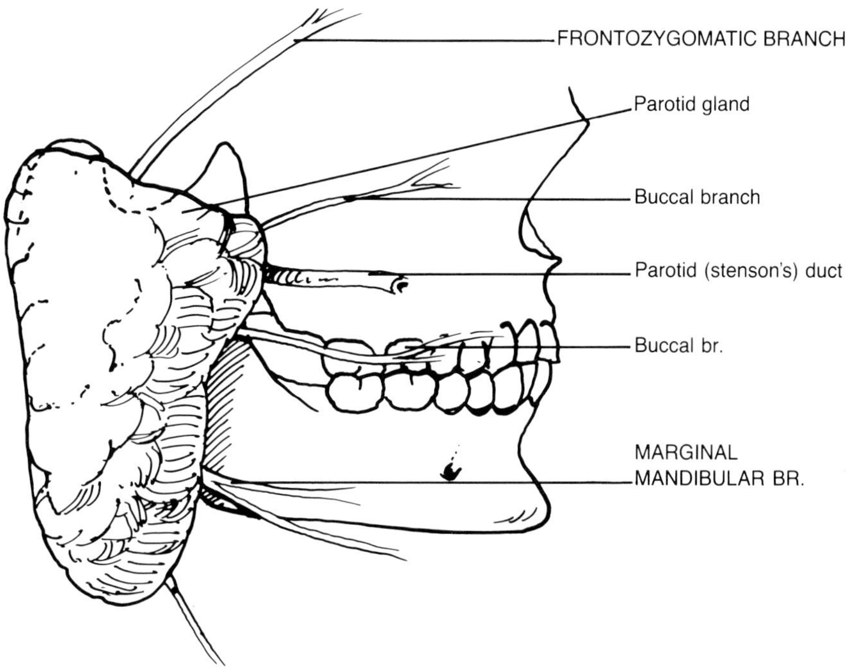

Figure 15–4. *Anatomy of parotid (Stenson's) duct and gland and their relation to the facial nerve.*

cartilaginous and muscular disruption. Retained particulate matter must be sought and removed. The degree of tissue devitalization must be ascertained. There is little damage to adjacent structures in clean, sharp lacerations, but the zone of injury may be significant in lacerations resulting from blunt trauma.

SEQUENCE OF REPAIR

After systematic evaluation of the patient and the facial injuries, operative repair of wounds should follow a logical sequence.

Complex facial injuries may be best treated under

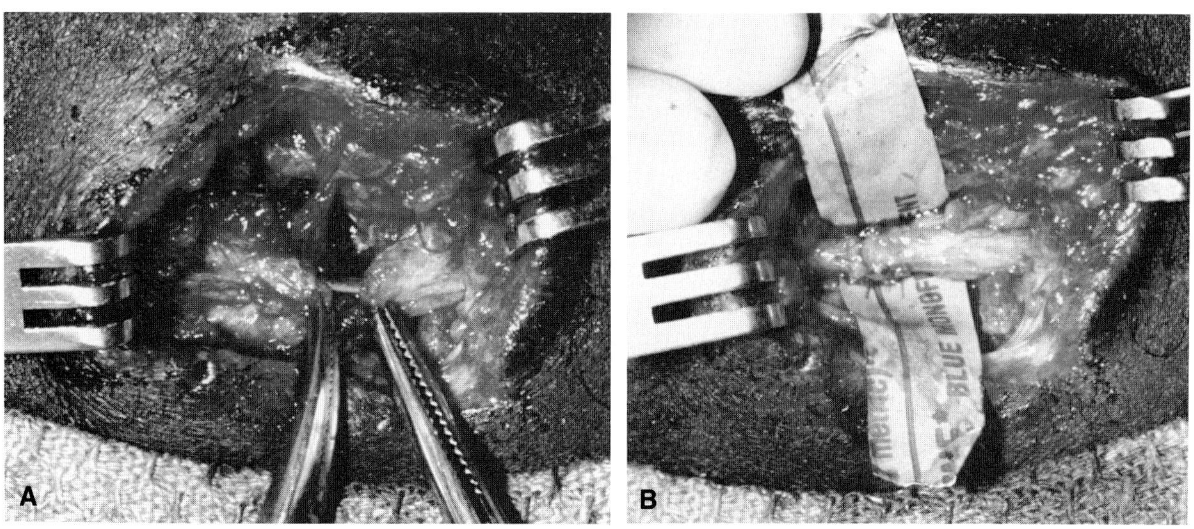

Figure 15–5. *(**A**) Laceration shows Stenson's duct severed and cannulated with polyethylene tubing. (**B**) Duct is sutured over tubing.*

general anesthesia, especially if the airway is in jeopardy, the injuries are extensive, or the patient will not cooperate with local anesthesia. Most injuries of lesser severity may be managed with local anesthetics. One percent lidocaine with epinephrine is used for most wounds. Although epinephrine acts to lessen local bleeding, its use must be carefully monitored in those patients with hypertension. Epinephrine-containing solutions should not be used in the base of precarious flaps of tissue, but the hemostatic properties of these solutions may be used with general anesthesia. One-half percent lidocaine may be needed if a very large field must be infiltrated. Four percent cocaine on cotton pledgets is excellent for shrinking the nasal mucosa and lessening the bleeding in the nose. Initial infiltration of the nerve supplying the traumatized area may lessen the amount of anesthetic required and diminish the amount of pain incurred with subsequent injections. Infraorbital and supraorbital nerve blocks work especially well. Sensation should be checked before cleansing of the wounds.

The face is scrubbed to remove dirt and blood. Prior anesthetization allows for more vigorous cleansing of the wounds. Deeper injuries are copiously irrigated. Although saline or hydrogen peroxide are all that are needed to remove most contaminants, other agents may sometimes be necessary. Tar, asphalt, grease, or gunshot powder staining may require the use of specific solvents. These solvents must be removed immediately after they are applied so as to avoid chemical injury to the facial tissue. Scrubbing with a wire brush may be necessary to remove some types of particulate matter. With this method care must be taken to avoid conversion of a partial-thickness abrasion injury to a full-thickness injury. A number-11 scalpel can also be used to pick out embedded debris. Retained foreign material may result in increased scarring, infection, and tattooing. After removing the debris, the face is washed with bactericidal skin preparation, such as Betadine. If the mouth, nose, or ear is injured, these cavities should also be cleansed.

After the entire face has been thoroughly cleansed and covered with a sterilizing preparation it is isolated with sterile towels and devitalized tissue is debrided. Care must be taken to avoid both over- and under-debridement. In burst-type lacerations resulting from blunt trauma, there is commonly a zone of injury at the edges of the wound. If this area is not debrided initially, the patient may return for follow-up with sutures joining necrotic tissue edges and unfavorable scarring. To avoid this problem, the edges of these wounds must be sharply removed, using a number-15 scalpel, orienting the incision vertically with the skin. Almost all facial wounds require some degree of debridement unless caused by a very sharp instrument. Beveled wound edges must be squared (Fig. 15–6) to avoid rolled up scars. Subdermal undermining will allow for later placement of everting sutures and may decrease the tension on the wound edge (Fig. 15–7). The face is remarkably well vascularized, so that excessive debridement is not indicated. Areas supplied by what may seem to be very small soft tissue bridges often survive, and thus should be preserved, especially if debridement of the area would result in a significant soft tissue deficit.

When multiple adjacent lacerations occur, the surgeon may consider debridement of the central wound to create a single large laceration, if closure can then be comfortably achieved. This limits the number of scars at the expense of possible tissue distortion.

Absolute hemostasis is necessary prior to wound closure. Large vessels should be individually ligated with 5-0 Vicryl or Dexon sutures. Bipolar electrocautery or the use of fine-tipped, nontoothed forceps and a Bovie electrosurgical unit results in pinpoint cauterization. When these tools are not available, a battery-powered, disposable ophthalmic cautery pen can be used.

If indicated, facial fractures should be reduced and stabilized acutely at the time of soft tissue repair. If treatment is left until later, the initial soft tissue re-

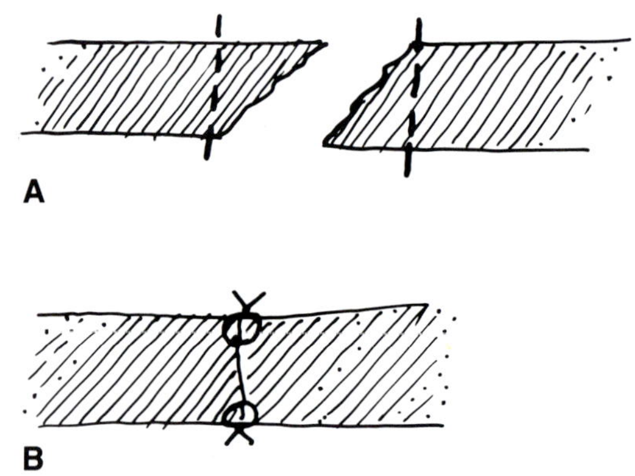

Figure 15–6. *Correction of wound beveling. (**A**) Debridement of beveled wound edges to perpendicular. (**B**) After closure.*

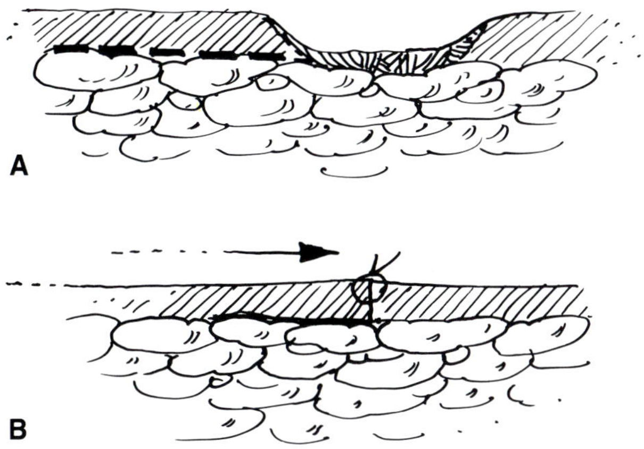

Figure 15–7. *(**A**) Subdermal undermining of wound edges. (**B**) After closure.*

pair often needs to be reopened, which may lead to increased scarring. In the event of soft tissue avulsion, it is imperative that fractures be reduced prior to attempting wound closure.

Specialized structures that were found to be damaged in the initial systematic evaluation should be repaired next. These repairs are discussed later in this chapter. The remaining wounds are then closed in layers. Cartilage, muscle, subcutaneous tissue, and finally skin are individually reapproximated to allow obliteration of dead space and independent motion of these anatomically distinct structures. Drains may be necessary in some situations in which fluid collections are anticipated. Appropriate bandaging is then applied.

SUTURE TECHNIQUE

There are several basic rules that need to be followed to help ensure the best scar result possible. Wound edge debridement is necessary in order to achieve perfect skin edge approximation. The edges that are traumatically crushed apart are sharply resected to clean, viable skin margins to avoid reapproximating devitalized tissue. Lacerations that traverse the skin plane at an angle should be recut so that the wound is oriented vertically. Failure to create vertical skin edges will result in a "rolled up" scar. After creating sharp, vertical skin margins, the dermis should be slightly back-cut to allow skin advancement over underlying soft tissue and to allow placement of correctly oriented sutures. When planning skin closure, the relaxed skin lines must be considered (Fig. 15–8): incisions closed along these lines will result in less conspicuous scars, while closure perpendicular to these lines will leave very prominent scars. It is sometimes possible to orient closures along skin lines or reorient lacerations using Z-plasty techniques in order to improve results.

Delicate handling of tissue is required throughout the course of debridement and wound closure. Fine-toothed forceps or skin hooks must be used to grasp tissue in order to minimize tissue devitalization. The minimum amount of sutures necessary to achieve accurate closure should be used. The size of suture material should be only the minimum necessary to approximate tissue. In general most facial lacerations are closed with 5-0 or 6-0 Vicryl in deep layers (if needed), and 6-0 or 7-0 monofilament nylon is used for skin closure. Fine, sharp cutting needles, such as PC-3 or P-3, allow sutures to be placed with minimal trauma. Sutures are removed from facial lacerations which are free of tension as early as 4 days post repair, in order to lessen the chance of "cross-hatch" marks.

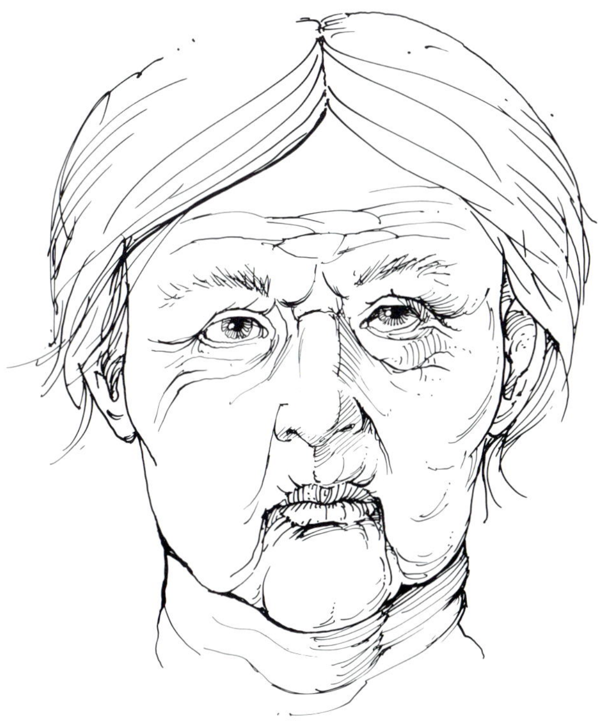

Figure 15–8. *Relaxed skin lines of the face are the best places to hide incisions and scars.*

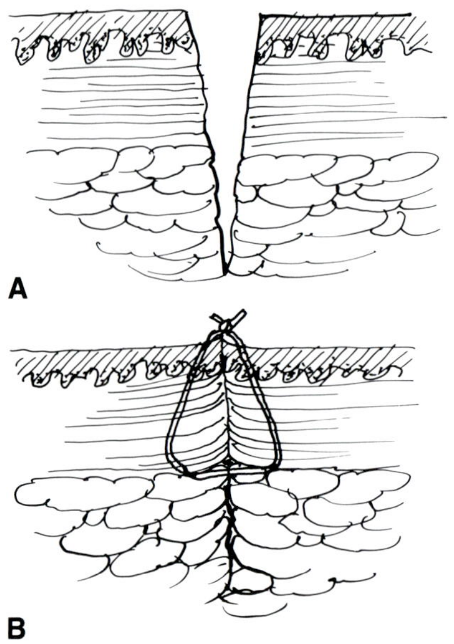

Figure 15–9. *Wound edges are everted with properly placed simple sutures. (**A**) Typical full-thickness wound. (**B**) To achieve epidermal eversion, suture is made wider at the base than superficially.*

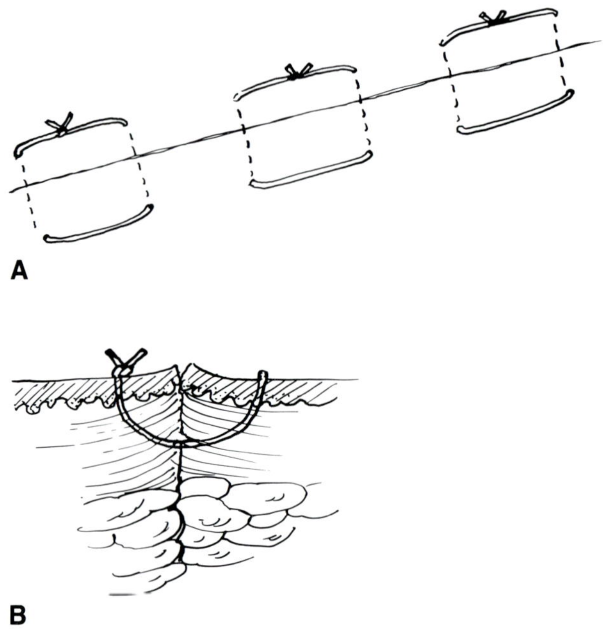

Figure 15–10. *(**A**) Horizontal mattress sutures. (**B**) Sectional view.*

Skin edges must be approximated in eversion so that tensile forces will eventually result in a flat scar; a flat closure will result in depressed scars. There are several suture techniques that may be used to achieve eversion and each are useful in different situations (Figs. 15–9, 15–10, 15–11).

TYPES OF INJURIES

Soft tissue injuries of the face can be categorized into several types. Treatment depends on the understanding of the mechanism of injury and the usual clinical course associated with each type of trauma.

Facial ecchymosis (Fig. 15–12) usually results from blunt trauma, which causes disruption of a soft tissue blood vessel. Hematoma can also occur in avulsion flaps, but these hematomas are easily evacuated at wound debridement. Hematomas not associated with facial lacerations are usually best treated with head elevation and cool saline compresses over the affected area. Unusual cases require needle aspiration. Careful examination for occult injuries, masked by the facial hematoma, must be performed.

Abrasions (Fig. 15–13) are a common type of facial injury in motor vehicle accidents that result in sliding

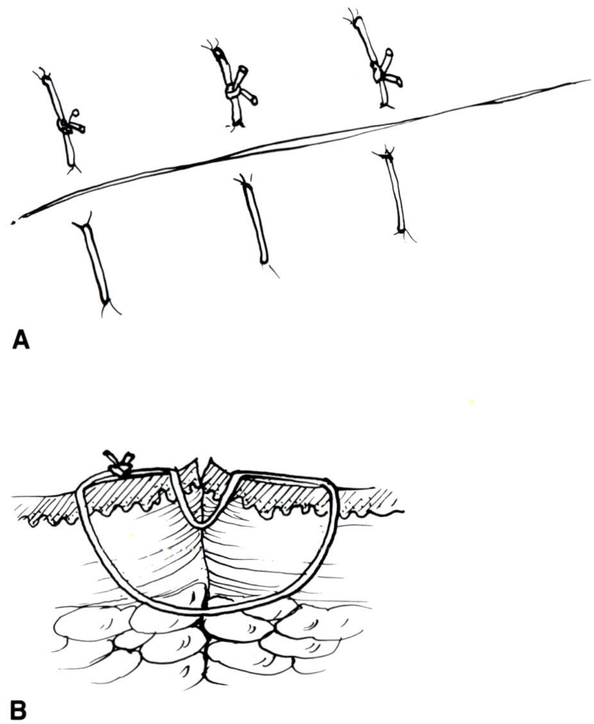

Figure 15–11. *(**A**) Vertical mattress sutures. (**B**) Sectional view.*

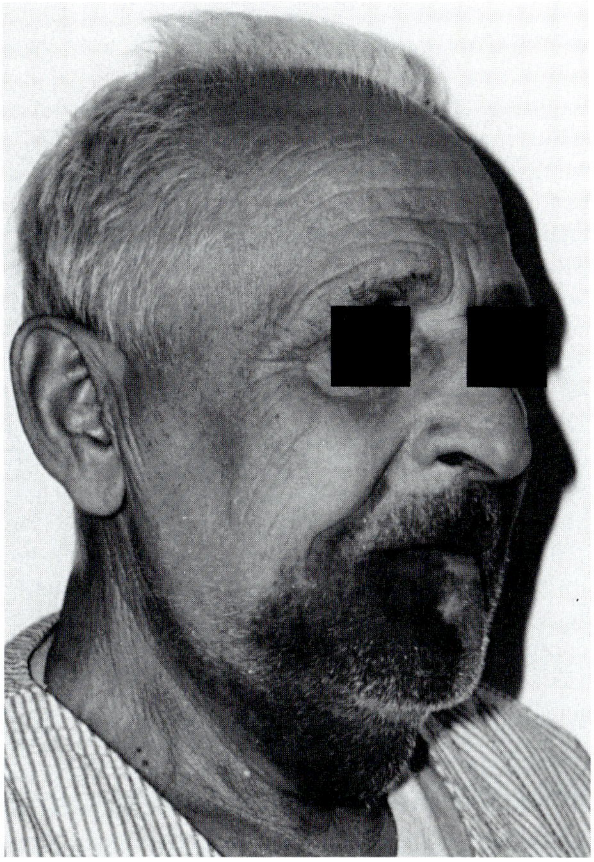

Figure 15–12. *Patient with extensive ecchymosis. (Courtesy of Dr. A. Thomas Indresano, Cleveland Metropolitan General Hospital, Cleveland, Ohio)*

forces transferred to the face. These injuries result in variable degrees of skin loss. Commonly, abrasions result in partial-thickness loss only. These abrasions may be treated with topical antibiotics, as a second-degree burn would be treated, after careful cleansing of the wound. Excellent healing is expected in this situation. Deeper abrasions may result in full-thickness skin loss. When deep gouges permeate more superficial abrasions, the deep gouges may be debrided and closed with interrupted 6-0 chromic sutures, and the abrasion will then be converted into a more favorable superficial type. When larger patches of full-thickness loss occur, initial therapy should be limited to cleansing and serial dressing placement, because often there are more intact dermal elements remaining than initially apparent clinically. Wounds may use a variety of dressing materials, xenografts, or homografts. Early

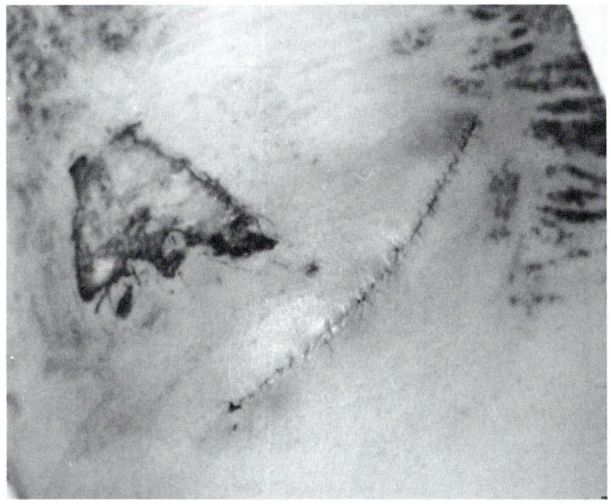

Figure 15–13. *Patient with trapezoidal abrasion at angle of mandible. (Courtesy of A. Thomas Indresano, Cleveland Metropolitan General Hospital, Cleveland, Ohio)*

skin grafting in this situation results in epithelial inclusion cysts, and because most of these abrasions do not occupy specific anatomical units, the grafting is very conspicuous. If skin grafting is eventually required, it should be done prior to the onset of contracting scar tissue and should be placed as an anatomical unit using a single piece of nonexpanded skin.

Traumatic tattooing occurs when foreign material is introduced into the dermal and subdermal layers. If this foreign material is not removed, permanent tattooing will result. Common offending agents include gravel, asphalt, and gunshot powder. Abrasion wounds are commonly contaminated with potentially tattooing material. Wounds must be meticulously cleaned to remove the foreign substance. A number-11 scalpel blade may be useful to pick out gravel or similar particles. A surgical scrub brush helps remove particles from abrasions. Sometimes petroleum-based solvents are necessary, but these substances should contact normal tissue as little as possible. Occasionally, heavily contaminated tissue is best treated with sharp debridement of the entire tissue. When brushing out particulate matter from an abrasion care must be taken to avoid conversion of the wound into a full-thickness injury.

Puncture wounds must be evaluated carefully. Knowledge of the offending weapon helps in diagnosis of the extent of the injuries. Retention of foreign bodies after this type of injury is common. If a puncture wound must be explored because of an expanding hematoma, an underlying neural deficit, or the suspicion of foreign body retention, then extensions of the wound should be made in the direction of relaxed skin creases (see Fig. 15–8). Puncture wounds secondary to bites should not be closed tightly and should be drained carefully.

Simple lacerations (Fig. 15–14) of the face occur from a variety of causes. Cuts that result from sharp instruments can be treated with minimal debridement and closure. Lacerations from blunt trauma have a much larger margin of devitalized tissue at the wound edges. Much more aggressive debridement is necessary, with evaluation for underlying fractures and other injuries. Lip lacerations commonly result from blunt trauma that forces the cutting of the lip with the patient's own teeth. This type of injury again requires appropriate debridement and assessment of the patient for dental injury.

Avulsion flaps (Fig. 15–15) occur when segments of soft tissue are elevated from their underlying beds and remain attached by soft tissue bridges. Many scalp injuries are of this type. Due to the excellent blood supply of the face, most avulsion flaps survive even if supplied by minimal amounts of intact soft tissue. Wound edges still need careful sharp debridement. Traction on the intact soft tissue bridges is avoided. Failure to drain blood or fluid from beneath a wound may result in loss of tenuous flaps.

Burns (Fig. 15–16) are divided into partial and full-thickness types. Partial-thickness injuries involving the epidermis only, without blistering, are termed first degree and heal completely in a few days without treatment. Deeper (second-degree) partial-thickness burns involving the superficial dermis are treated with gentle cleansing and application of triple antibiotic ointment two to three times daily. Second- and third-degree burns to the ear may require treatment with Sulfamylon which has excellent eschar penetration abilities. This helps protect against the devastating sequelae or ear chronditis. Superficial partial-thickness burns, defined as those that heal within 2 weeks of injury, have a hypertrophic scarring rate of 20%. Deeper partial-thickness burns (taking over 2 weeks to heal) have hypertrophic scarring in nearly 80% of cases. Deep partial-thickness burns may heal with contracture, especially in areas of unopposed soft tissue laxity such as the lateral commissures, the lower eyelids, and the neck. Specialized splinting in these areas may minimize the contraction process. Compression garments are custom measured and used to treat hypertrophic scarring. Split-thickness, nonexpanded, single piece skin grafts placed as facial aesthetic units (Fig. 15–17) are used in very deep partial-thickness burns and full-thickness injuries. Very limited full-thickness burns may be amenable to local excision and primary closure. Despite advances in therapeutic techniques, severe facial burns remain as one of the most disfiguring types of facial injury.

Timing of wound closure is important. The vast

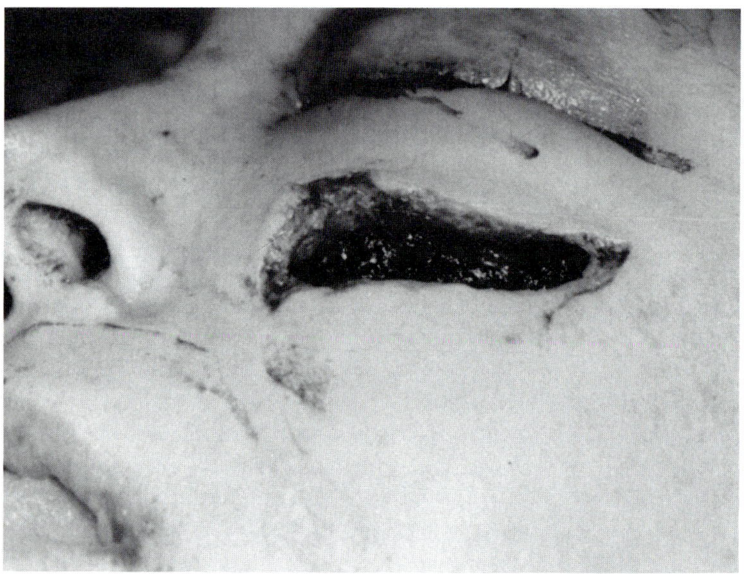

Figure 15–14. *Simple laceration of cheek. (Courtesy of Dr. A. Thomas Indresano, Cleveland Metropolitan General Hospital, Cleveland, Ohio)*

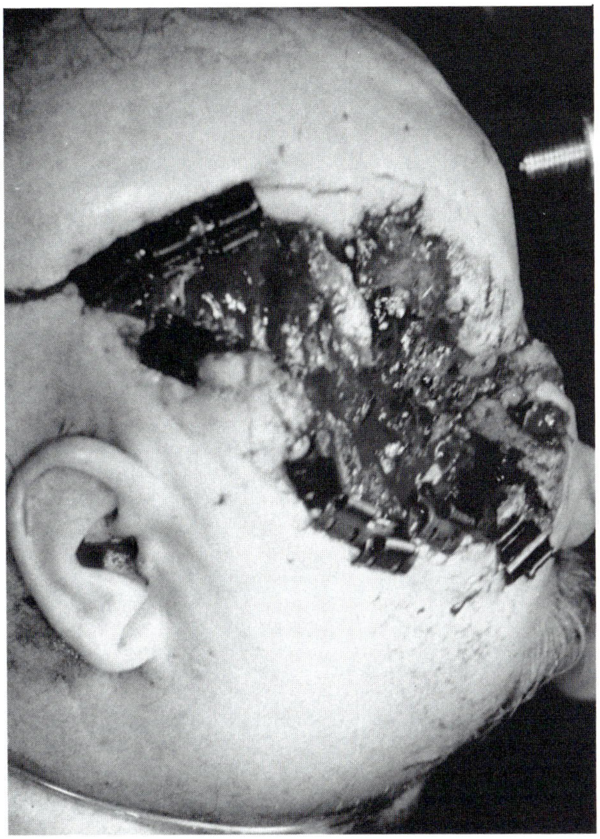

Figure 15–15. *Large avulsion of soft tissue. (Courtesy of Dr. A. Thomas Indresano, Cleveland Metropolitan General Hospital, Cleveland, Ohio)*

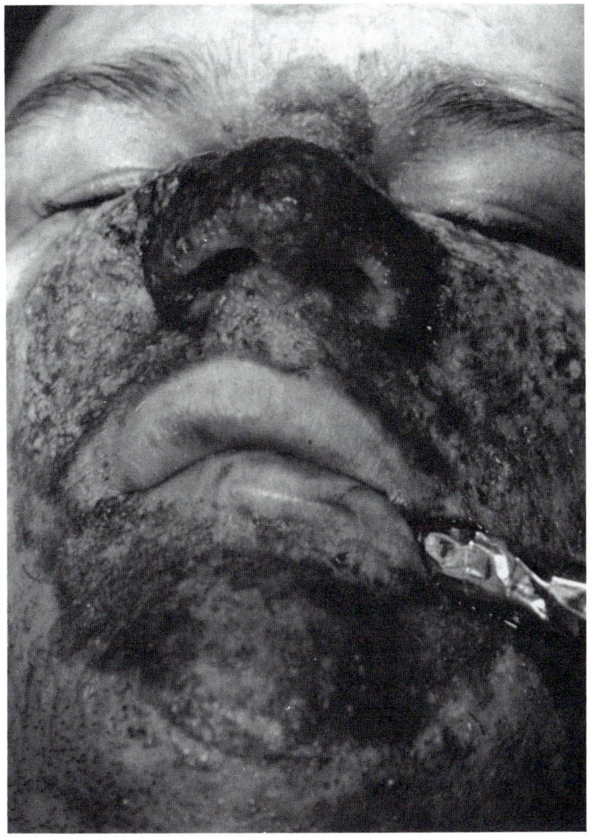

Figure 15–16. *Facial burn. (Courtesy of Dr. J. Bradrick, Cleveland Metropolitan General Hospital, Cleveland, Ohio)*

majority of facial wounds are closed primarily. Because of the rich vascular supply to this region, facial wounds may be closed 24 hours after injury without an excessive infection rate. Rarely, wounds are closed secondarily, such as when there is massive wound contamination. Wounds should be closed as soon as they have been cleansed with local wound care. When patient instability precludes initial treatment, closure should be performed when the status of the patient permits. The use of homograft skin as a biological dressing to cover contaminated soft tissue is useful to help minimize contact of the tissue with the environment, to maintain moisture in the wound, and to test the degree of contamination in the wound. In situations where skin grafting is needed, homograft can be changed as often as needed and, once it has become adherent, skin grafts will reliably "take" in the soft tissue bed.[10]

REGIONAL CONSIDERATIONS

Scalp

Lacerations and avulsions of the scalp are very common injuries. These injuries are often overlooked in patients with other injuries, because they are often hidden in matted hair. The scalp has an extremely rich vascular supply, which may result in a large initial blood loss, but this rich vascularity does allow for survival of large scalp flaps on small soft tissue pedicles. When repairing scalp lacerations, the cranium should be palpated to rule out associated fractures. Subgaleal hematomas should be evacuated and all foreign material debrided away. After minimal debridement, full-thickness closure must be performed; otherwise, hemorrhage from retracted galeal edges

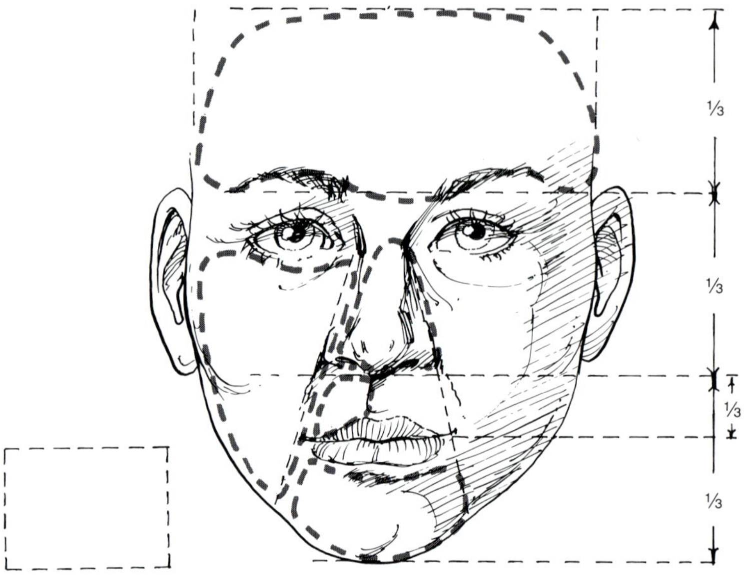

Figure 15–17. *Facial aesthetic units.*

may occur. A running, locked "baseball" suture may be required using 3-0 or 4-0 nylon to aid in hemostasis.

Forehead

In treating forehead injuries (Fig. 15–18) basic soft tissue repair techniques are employed. The specific innervation by the supratrochlear and supraorbital nerves lends this area to nerve blocking. Care must be taken to reapproximate injured frontalis and orbicularis oculi muscle to minimize functional deformity and lessen the chance for depressed scar formation. Horizontal forehead creases, when present, should be carefully realigned. All severe injuries to the upper face should be evaluated for evidence of concomitant paranasal fractures.

Eyebrow

The eyebrows are commonly lacerated in motor vehicle accidents in which the supraorbital rim strikes a stationary object. This hair-bearing area requires special attention to enhance the scar result. Eyebrow hair should not be shaved because it grows back haphazardly. The area is very difficult to perfectly reconstruct, if lost, and conspicuous if missing; thus, all efforts must be made to conserve even marginally viable brow tissue. When debriding the edges of the brow laceration, the wound edges should be cut at an angle parallel to the brow hair follicles (Fig. 15–19). This prevents damage to the hair follicles which would leave an area of alopecia adjacent to the brow scar. When reapproximating the brow, care must be taken to align the wound edges correctly so as to avoid a step-off in the line of the brow. This is made easier by making sure all dried blood and other distracting material is off the field and by making frequent comparisons to the brow over the opposite eye.

Eyelid

Through-and-through margin injuries of the eyelid must be repaired meticulously in order to avoid eyelid notching. If debridement of this highly vascular area absolutely must be performed, it should be done in such a way that the cut tarsus plate will be vertically oriented during repair. The inverted pentagon shape used in excision of lid neoplasms demonstrates the ideal remaining wound design if devitalized tissue must be removed (Fig. 15–20). Wedging of the lid must be avoided. The conjunctiva and tarsus can be

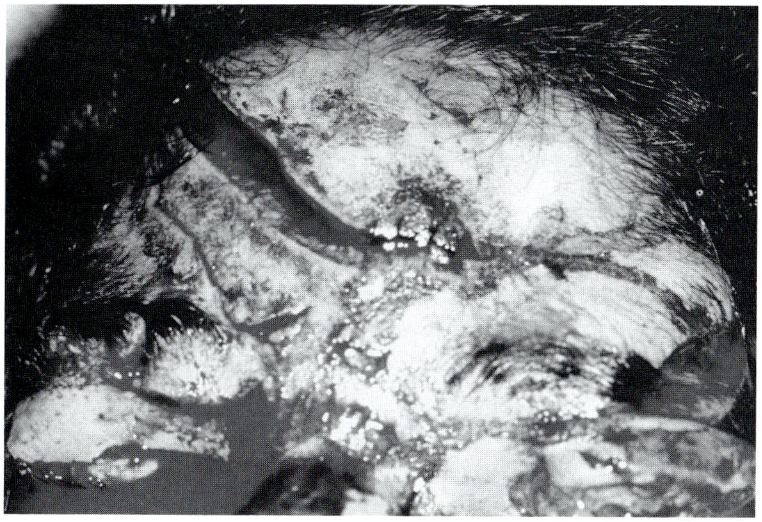

Figure 15–18. *Laceration of forehead. (Courtesy of Dr. Richard Haug, Cleveland Metropolitan General Hospital, Cleveland, Ohio)*

closed together with 6-0 chromic sutures with the knots tied toward the soft tissue. The ciliary margin and gray line must be approximated accurately (Fig. 15–21). The orbicularis oculi muscle is then closed with 5-0 chromic sutures and the skin is reapproximated.

Nasolacrimal Apparatus

After identification of nasolacrimal lacerations early repair is advocated. In cases of bone–nasolacrimal canal impingement it is reasonable to wait 3 to 6 months after initial reduction and fixation of fractures before treating persistent epiphora. The traditional method of repair is suturing over a metal or stiff silk stent with fine absorbable suture material. Alternatively, fine silicone tubing wedged onto metal probes (Crawford tubes) can be introduced into the injured canaliculus, with the end of the tubing allowed to curl up into the lacrimal sac. The stent should be left in place for at least 6 months. Early removal is indicated if there is punctal irritation or cheese wiring of the puncta. The patient should be informed that the longer the stent remains in place, the better the chance of maintaining successful repair.

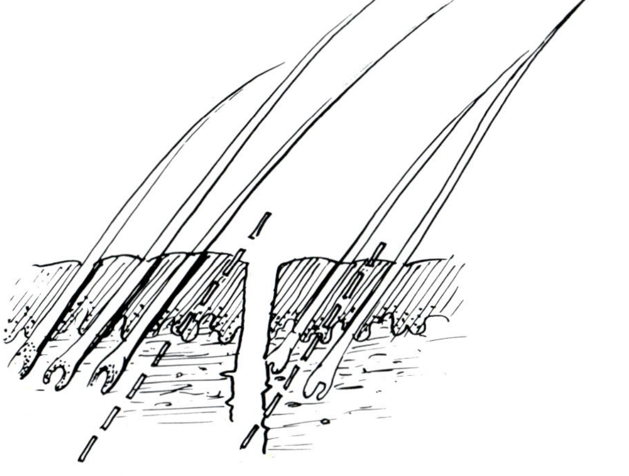

Figure 15–19. *Correct debriding of brow wounds.*

Patients with unsuccessful early repair or unrecognized injury may incur epiphora, recurrent dacryocystitis, or pyocele of the sac. Drainage of the lacrimal apparatus is achieved, in this situation, by dacryocystorhinostomy (DCR). This technique entails opening the bony widow between the lacrimal sac and the nose and anastomosing the nasal mucosa to that of the lacrimal sac. In those patients with total canalicular occlusion, conjunctivodacryocystorhinostomy (CDCR) may be necessary. In this procedure a bypass tube is placed between the lacrimal lake and the nose in addition to performing a DCR.[6]

Telecanthus as a result of medial canthal laceration is best treated immediately, since later reconstruction is more difficult and the results are not as good. The repair consists of open reduction and internal fixation of the medial canthal ligament to the opposite side, if stable. Underlying comminuted fractures often require fixation with transnasal wiring, traditional external lead splinting, or more recently, plate fixation.[5]

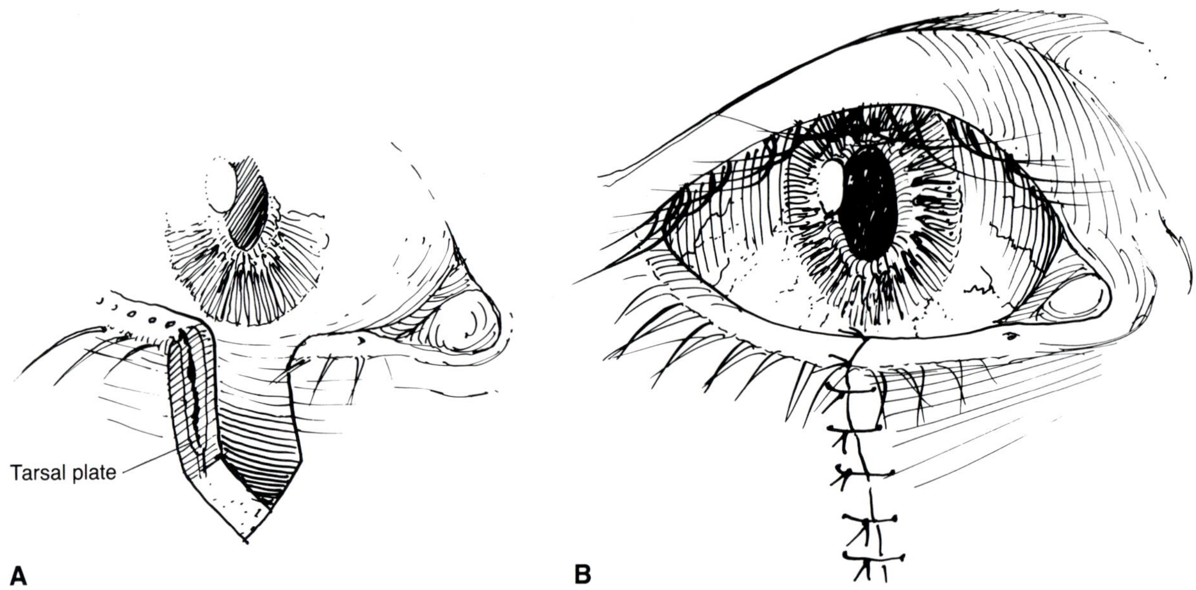

Figure 15–20. *(**A**) Pentagon resection of lower lid allows straight closure of tarsal plate. (**B**) Closure is made with no suture material through conjunctiva.*

Nose

Injuries to the nose generally fall within three categories: lacerations, hematoma, and fractures.

Lacerations (Fig. 15–22) may accompany fractures, usually oriented transversely over the root of the nose and pose no special problems. When lacerations traverse the mucosa and cartilages, then there are special considerations. This area is highly vascular and hemostasis may be difficult, especially in an apprehensive patient in the emergency room. The use of local anesthesia containing epinephrine is extremely useful, as is 4% cocaine nasal packing. It is important to be comfortable with the cartilaginous anatomy of the nose so that lacerated and avulsed portions of nasal cartilage may be returned to their anatomical position and secured with 5-0 chromic suture. Chromic suture is also useful for the nasal mucosal closure. Nasal packing should be placed to keep mucosal flaps in place, splint the nose, and help prevent hematoma accumulation.

Hematomas involving the nasal septum are not common, but when left untreated may result in infection, scarring, and severe nasal deformities such as the "saddle" nose. Saddle nose occurs because the septal cartilage is separated from its blood supply in the mucoperichondrium by the dissecting hematoma. All patients who sustain nasal trauma should undergo nasal speculum examination. Once a hematoma has been diagnosed, it should be evacuated and nasal packing placed to help prevent reaccumulation.

Nasal fractures due to direct blows are very common. When seen acutely, nasal deviation may be visibly obvious, but as swelling increases it becomes less apparent. Palpation over the area reveals nasal bone displacement and tenderness. Nasal obstruction may also be present. These findings are much more sensitive and important than those found on radiographs. Nasal fractures seen quite early may be reduced using local anesthetic, cocaine packs, and sedation in the emergency room. Once edema becomes significant, closed reduction will likely require general anesthesia. Once closed reduction is achieved, internal splinting with nasal packing and an external splint are used to retain reduction.

In less severe injuries in which the bone fragments are in general proximity to each other early malunion will occur in 10 days to 2 weeks. In more severe injuries in which bone fragments are widely displaced the time period before malunion may be extended to 2 weeks or longer.

The main growth center of the nose is in the sep-

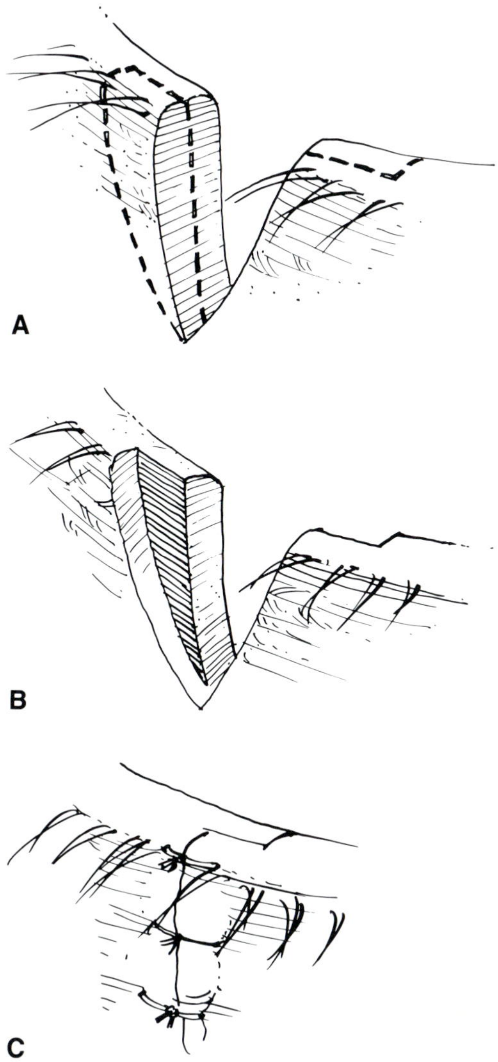

Figure 15–21. *Surgical repair of the eyelid. (**A**) Excision of outer lamina on one side and inner lamina on the other. (**B**) After excision. (**C**) Closure. Inner sutures are buried to avoid suture material coming through conjunctiva.*

tovomerine angle and is responsible for the development of the normal cartilaginous nasal septum. Nasal fractures due to birth trauma should therefore be reduced, if diagnosed. The nose cannot be packed bilaterally because of the newborn's obligate nasal breathing.[11] Parents must be warned of the potential for growth disturbance secondary to fracture in growing children.

Chronically twisted noses that result from nasal trauma are a difficult surgical problem. Severe cases may have a fracture dislocation of the nasal septum combined with a fracture of the nasal bone or frontal porcess of the maxilla. Scarring, malunion, and compensatory growth and curvature of the septal cartilage worsen the external appearance of the nose with time, especially after childhood injuries. Each of these areas must be approached during the surgical correction. The framework of the nose must be released from scar tissue initially. A submucous resection of the septum, preserving a dorsal and caudal strut, is used to relieve nasal obstruction and release the curved cartilage torsional forces on the nasal dorsum and tip. Next, the cartilaginous nasal dorsal hump is reduced and the bony hump removed. The tip may need refinement with resection and sometimes contouring of the lower lateral cartilages. Finally, osteotomies and fractures are performed to reduce the bony pyramid of the nose. Mucosal incisions are then closed, and internal and external splinting is applied.[12]

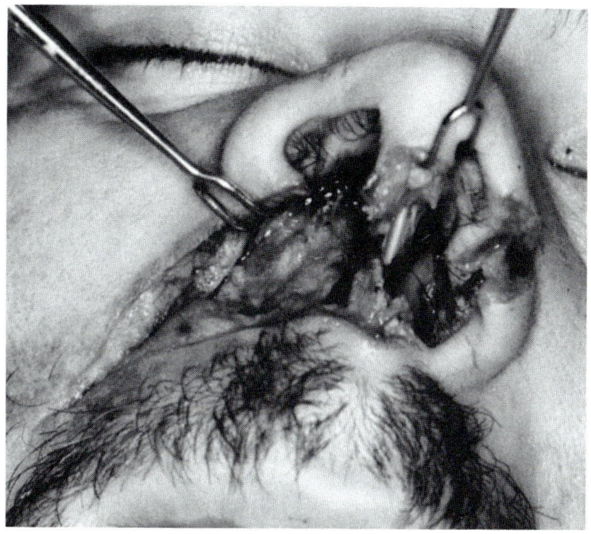

Figure 15–22. *Laceration through base of nose. (Courtesy of J. Prather)*

Lip

Injuries of the lips (burst-type injuries and lacerations) are common secondary to blunt trauma due to force applied to the lip that causes cutting by the

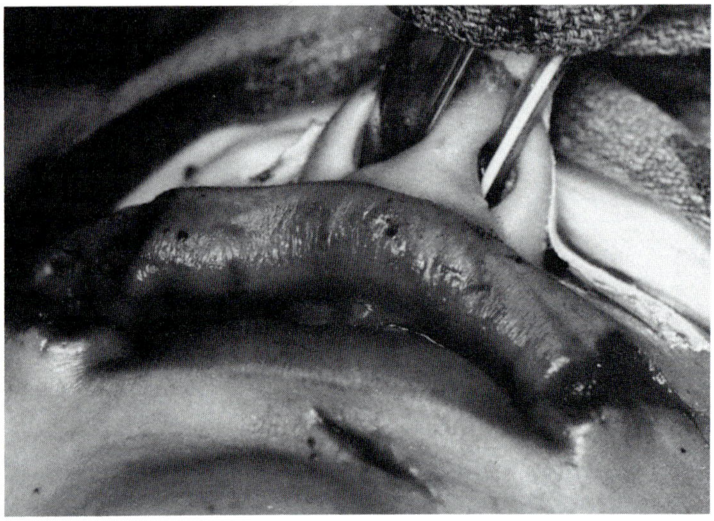

Figure 15–23. *Multiple lacerations of the upper lip.*

teeth. There may be associated damage to teeth, gingiva, or alveolus.

Lacerations (Fig. 15–23) can generally be aggressively debrided to remove devitalized tissue, straighten wound edges, and help remove contaminated tissue. Up to one third of the lower lip can be removed, if necessary, with acceptable cosmetic results. The upper lip is anchored at the columella, alar bases, and oral commissars, which makes it prone to distortion with even minimal tissue loss. If significant lip loss occurs, this defect can be reconstructed at a second stage with tissue borrowed from the opposite lip. In this situation, the mucosa can be closed to the skin while awaiting secondary reconstruction, if primary closure cannot be achieved.[13] Avulsion flaps survive well even when only a small soft tissue bridge exists, especially when the labial artery lies within the pedicle.

After debridement, closure should be performed in layers. The key suture is that which reapproximates the vermilion border. After this line is accurately realigned, the wet-dry line should be aligned next. After these important landmarks are secured, the remaining lip laceration is closed. Lacerated muscle should be accurately opposed with fine absorbable sutures, mucosal edges should be reapproximated with fine chromic sutures, and the skin should be closed with 6-0 nylon.

Due to the high bacterial concentration in the mouth, lip lacerations should be thoroughly cleansed, and antibiotic prophylaxis should be considered. A liquid diet and use of antiseptic mouthwash after repair are encouraged.

Facial Nerve

Several questions arise in the management of traumatically acquired facial palsy. These include indications for exploration, timing of exploration, and operative approach. The expected results of treatment should be known as well as the therapeutic options if these results are not obtained.

If there is any indication that the facial nerve has been transected, it should be explored within 30 days, since results of repair after this time are much less encouraging. Nerve transections that are the result of lacerations are approached by careful identification of the cut ends of the nerve at initial exploration. In a relatively clean wound, primary repair should be carried out under an operating microscope. The cut ends of the nerve are transected to an undamaged area. End-to-end coaptation is performed with epineural sutures of 9-0 or 10-0 nylon. If a gap exists between the ends that precludes a tension-free anastomosis, interposition nerve grafts should be used. The greater auricular nerve is useful for gaps of up to 10 cm in length, and the sural nerve is used for larger gaps.[8,9] Repair of nerve transections anterior to a vertical line drawn from the lateral canthus are unnecessary, because the widely arborizing nerve branches in this region will allow for spontaneous reinnervation

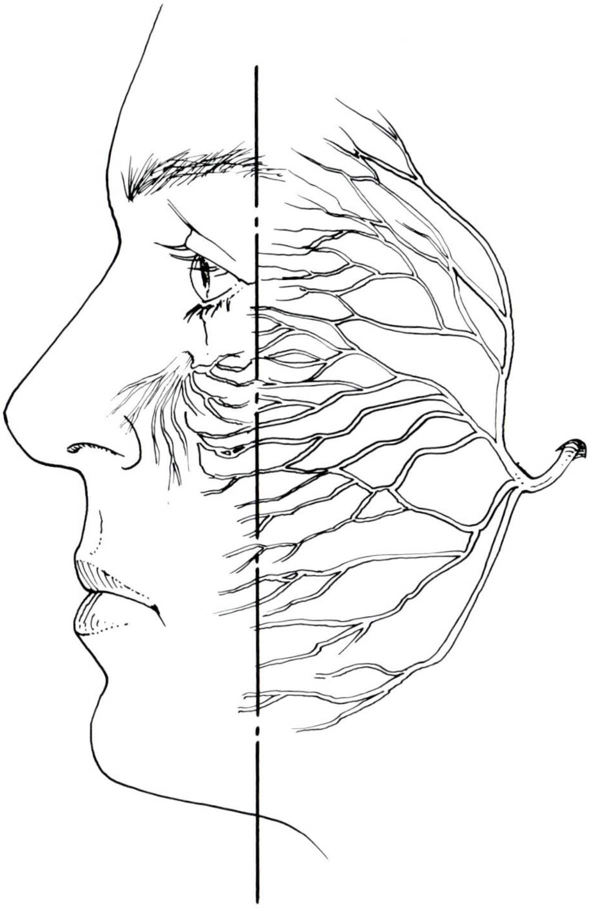

Figure 15–24. *Zone of arborization of facial nerve.*

(Fig. 15–24). Early facial nerve repair results in a 75% favorable result with return of nerve function in 6 to 18 months.[9]

In patients with nerve transection in a severely contaminated wound, the nerve ends should be tagged with fine nonabsorbable suture, which will aid in their identification at secondary repair. The nerve should be repaired within the 30-day period known to offer the most favorable results.

Therapeutic options available to those who do not improve with the above techniques include re-exploration of the nerve coaptation, hypoglossal-to-facial-nerve cross-over for very proximal lesions, and replacement of damaged nerve segments with interposition grafts. For those patients in whom the remaining facial nerve has fibrosed and electrical studies indicate a poor prognosis, facial reanimation by means of muscle transposition reanimation surgery is available.[14] Finally, static support of the eyelids and oral commissure using fascial grafts may be used in otherwise untreatable patients. Facial nerve repair should only be undertaken by those who have the expertise to treat patients with less than optimal initial results.

Parotid Gland and Stenson's Duct

After documentation of injury to the parotid duct and gland, meticulous repair must be performed in order to avoid the disastrous sequelae of salivary fistulae, sialoceles, and salivary cysts. Ductal injuries must be adequately exposed without damaging surrounding facial nerves or the facial artery. After limited debridement of the cut ends of the duct, repair should be performed using very fine interrupted sutures over an indwelling Silastic catheter used as a stent (see Fig. 15–5). Obstruction due to postoperative edema is avoided and parotid drainage is ensured with the use of a stent. The Silastic catheter is sutured to the oral mucosa and removed in 10 to 14 days.[9] The necessity of an indwelling "dowel" to stent the duct was popularized by Bornstein and Simon in the first successful series of parotid duct repairs.[15] When the distal duct cannot be used, a secure ligation of the proximal duct will avoid problems with salivary wound contamination but will result in atrophy of the parotid gland.[2,16] Diversion of the proximal duct into a more posterior portion of the oral cavity has also been described, but this carries a higher complication rate.[17]

With glandular injury, the capsule overlying the parotid gland should be carefully reapproximated. With both ductal and glandular injury, the wounds should be closed in layers and a drain should be used.

In patients who develop complications following injury to the parotid gland and its duct, several treatment modalities are available. These problems are best studied using sialography. If a small salivary fistula develops after a known limited injury to the gland, spontaneous closure can be expected.[1] The use of antisialagogues to decrease salivary flow may be useful. Radiation has been used to temporarily decrease salivary flow, but the risk of cancer induction with this technique discourages its use in an otherwise normal gland. In a more extensively injured gland, without ductal injury, a superficial parotidectomy may be required. Ductal fistulae can be treated by posterior diversion or ligation of the proximal duct, as already described.[9]

Ear

Care of this unique organ initially requires that every effort be made to preserve tissue. Reconstructive efforts to match color and architecture may be difficult and, thus, even a badly traumatized ear should be carefully cleansed, minimally debrided, and given the benefit of time prior to more radical debridement. If chondritis arises, more radical debridement is indicated in order to prevent progression of infection and further loss of tissue.

Lacerations of the ear (Fig. 15–25) are treated with cleansing, minimal wound edge debridement, and reapproximation in layers. There must be a tension-free closure or dehiscence is risked. Relaxing incisions may be necessary. Reapproximation of cut cartilaginous edges to their anatomical position helps to preserve contour. Questionably viable avulsed skin flaps should be used, if necessary, though they may only survive as full-thickness skin grafts. In order to prevent chondritis, exposed cartilage must be covered. If exposed cartilage cannot be covered with remaining tissue, the effected portion of the ear should be resurfaced with pre- or postauricular skin flaps on an acute basis (Fig. 15–26). At a later stage the posterior ear may be released and covered with a skin graft.

When there is a segmental loss of less than 3 cm, several methods have been devised to allow primary closure with contour preservation, though the ear will be a smaller size. These techniques include conversion into a wedge-type deformity, use of Burrow's triangles, and creation of a star-type defect and closure (Fig. 15–27).

Ears with a larger amount of tissue loss may benefit from composite grafting from the contralateral ear. This not only partially retains the size of the traumatized ear but also reduces the size of the contralateral ear, which may help achieve symmetry. These grafts generally should be no larger than a centimeter and a half in length, and the donor area must be meticulously repaired so as not to create a second deformed ear. Alternatively, the injured ear can be buried in pre- or postauricular skin and cartilaginous support can be added at a second stage.

When total or near total ear avulsion has occurred, primary reattachment is indicated in selected circumstances. If a significant skin bridge is intact and there is bleeding at the distal aspect of the ear, success can be expected. If the ear is avulsed with a large scalp injury in continuity, larger vessels are available for microvascular replantation. At the present level of

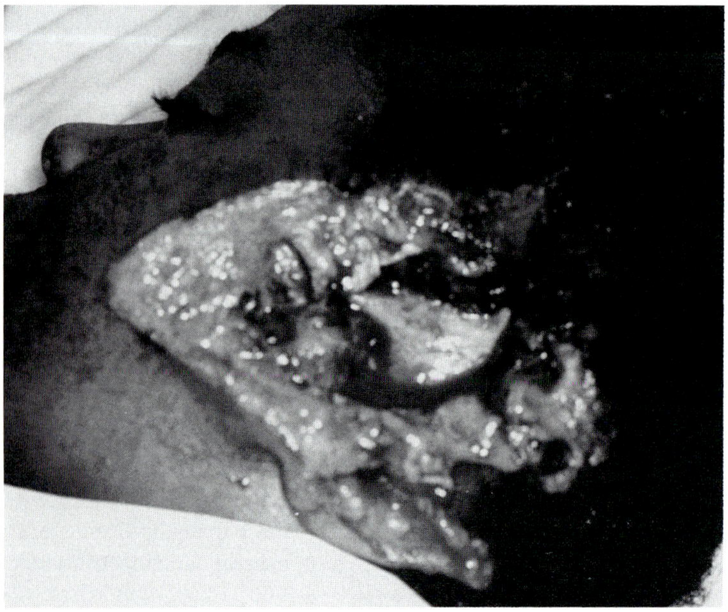

Figure 15–25. *Large avulsive flap includes the ear.*

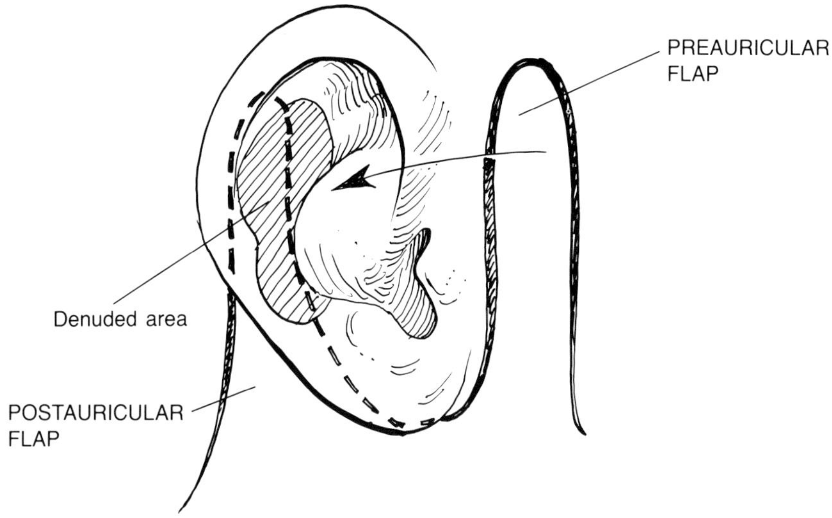

Figure 15–26. *Design of post- and preauricular skin flaps.*

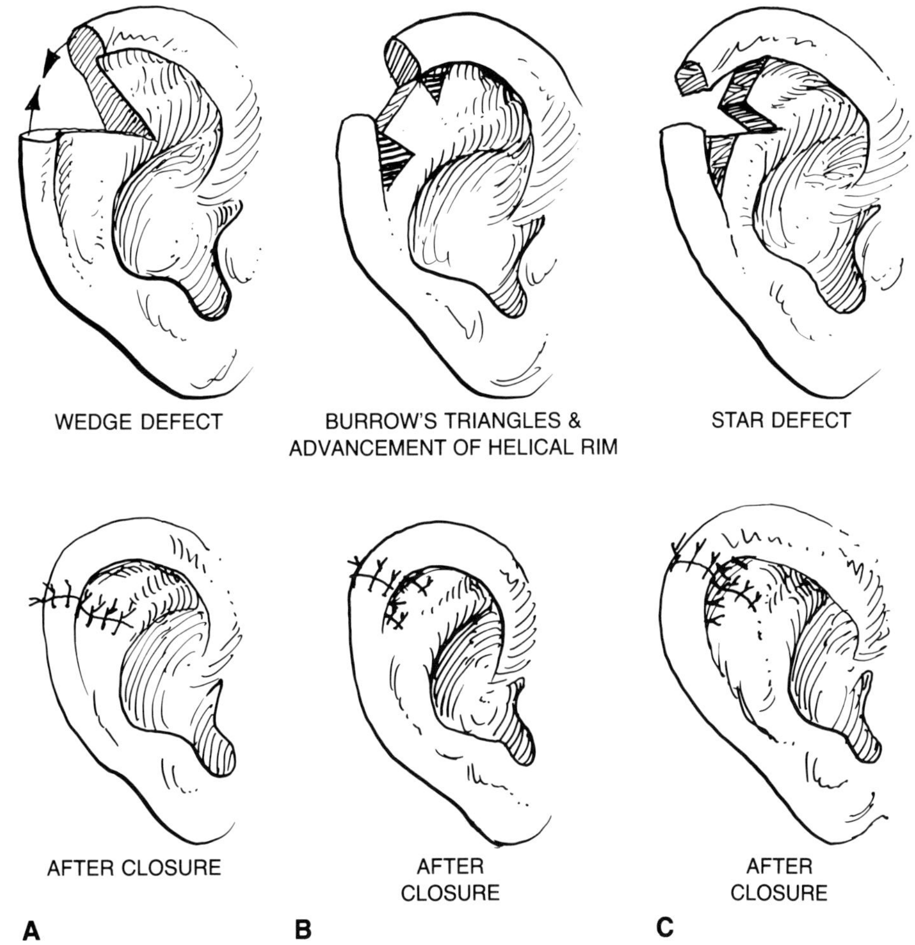

Figure 15–27. *(**A**) Conversion of defect to a wedge. (**B**) The use of Burrow's triangles. (**C**) Conversion of defect to a star.*

microvascular expertise, reimplantation of a severed ear alone is not as reliable as other methods.[18]

The use of the "Pocket Principle" to treat the avulsed ear also may be of use.[19,20] The ear is dermabraded to allow maximal capillary contact. It is reattached at its base and covered with postauricular or scalp flap skin. Bolster placement ensures maximum skin flap contact. After the blood supply to the ear has been reestablished at its base, the covering flap is returned to its original bed and the ear is allowed to reepithelialize. This is normally performed 2 weeks after burial in the ear pocket, since more prolonged burial may require skin graft coverage of the ear when it is exposed.

Hematomas of the ear result in separations of ear cartilage from its cutaneous blood supply. Hematomas must be properly evacuated when found; otherwise, the "cauliflower" ear deformity will result. Reaccumulation is avoided with careful short-term drainage and gentle pressure bandaging. All patients with significantly injured ears, especially in contaminated settings, should be treated with appropriate antibiotic therapy to help prevent the devastating problem of chondritis.

POSTOPERATIVE CARE

Expert care of the injured face after repair helps ensure optimum results. Pressure dressings are indicated when flaps are used that are prone to hematoma or seroma collection. When drains have been placed for fluid evacuation, they should be removed promptly after they have served their purpose so as to minimize potential wound contamination through the drain tract and to prevent organization of the tract around the drain, which causes increased scarring in this area.

Suture lines are kept clean with twice-daily cleaning with hydrogen peroxide and a coating of Bacitracin ointment to help seal the wound and minimize crust formation. This wound care regimen removes blood collection, which may serve as a culture medium for bacteria, and makes suture removal vastly easier.

Appropriate antibiotic coverage is needed when there is wound contamination from external soilage or from contact with the oral or nasal cavity or the ear canal. When there is cartilaginous exposure, especially when blood supply is minimal, the risk of chondritis is high. Antibiotic prophylaxis is indicated. Although infection rates ranging from 6%[21] to 29%[22] have been reported after debridement and closure of animal bites, far worse rates have been appreciated with human bites.[13] Due to the high complication rate of primary closure for human bites, these wounds are best treated with local wound care, antibiotics, and secondary operative closure.

Suture removal should be performed once the tensile strength of the wound is adequate to maintain approximation and preferably prior to the epithelialization of suture tracts, which causes permanent scarring. The use of fine monofilament nylon minimizes tissue reaction and allows for prolonged suture retention in wounds under tension. If doubt exists whether the wound is strong enough to allow suture removal, every other suture may be removed as a preliminary test of the adequacy of wound healing. Generally the minimal cross-hatch scarring that results after prolonged suture retention is preferable to the depressed widened scar that results after wound dehiscence.

SCAR PROGNOSIS

The normal sequence of tissue healing must be understood in order to help in the management of facial injuries. The first 3 to 4 days encompass the substrate phase. Inflammation occurs with dilation of blood vessels and the accumulation of lymphocytes, polymorphonuclear leukocytes, and macrophages. The exudation of fibrin that occurs appears to function as a temporary tissue glue. This initial phase allows for enough wound strength for removal of sutures in wounds not subject to tension. The second phase of wound healing, the proliferation phase, occurs over the next 10 to 14 days. Fibroblasts proliferate and lay down collagen. At the end of this phase a second plateau of wound strength is reached, after which only slight further strength is gained during the third, or remodeling, stage of wound healing (Fig. 15–28).[23] This phase lasts from 6 months to 2 years. In open wounds, two other phases exist: epithelialization and contraction. During the proliferation phase, wounds take on a characteristic red and raised appearance, which is often disconcerting to the patient. Scar revision should be delayed until the remodeling phase has been completed and the final residual scar can be evaluated.

Before proceeding with scar revision the objectives the surgeon hopes to achieve must be understood and

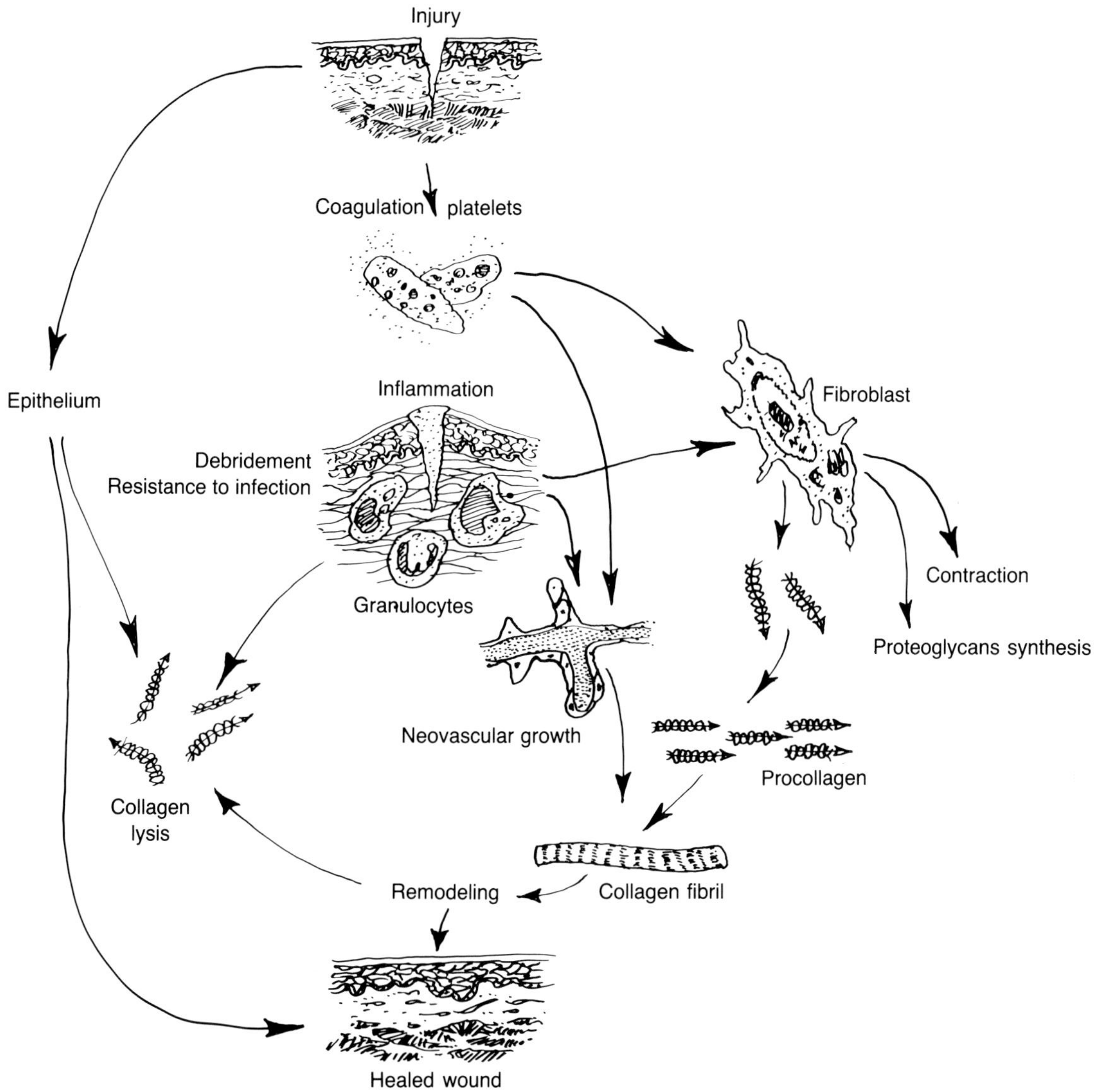

Figure 15–28. *Stages of wound healing.*

conveyed to the patient. As mentioned above, if the objective of revision is to correct a raised scar, then one should wait until the phase of wound remodeling has been completed. Similarly, areas of depigmentation may return to normal with time. If scar revision is necessary to correct a misaligned brow, forehead crease, or vermilion border, little is to be gained from waiting beyond the initial few months of tissue reaction. These landmarks will obviously not realign spontaneously.

After linear scar contraction, long straight wounds shorten and may become prominent, especially if their axis is not oriented parallel to lines of facial expression. This may result in cosmetic deformity, especially when the wound is adjacent to a movable structure such as the lower eyelid or oral commission. Wound contracture is also responsible for the deformity seen with "trap door" flaps. These semicircular or horseshoe-shaped flaps contract along their edges causing lymphatic blockage and edema of the flap. These edematous flaps are difficult to treat but may respond to lengthening of the scars with certain techniques to be described.

One simple form of scar revision is excision of the

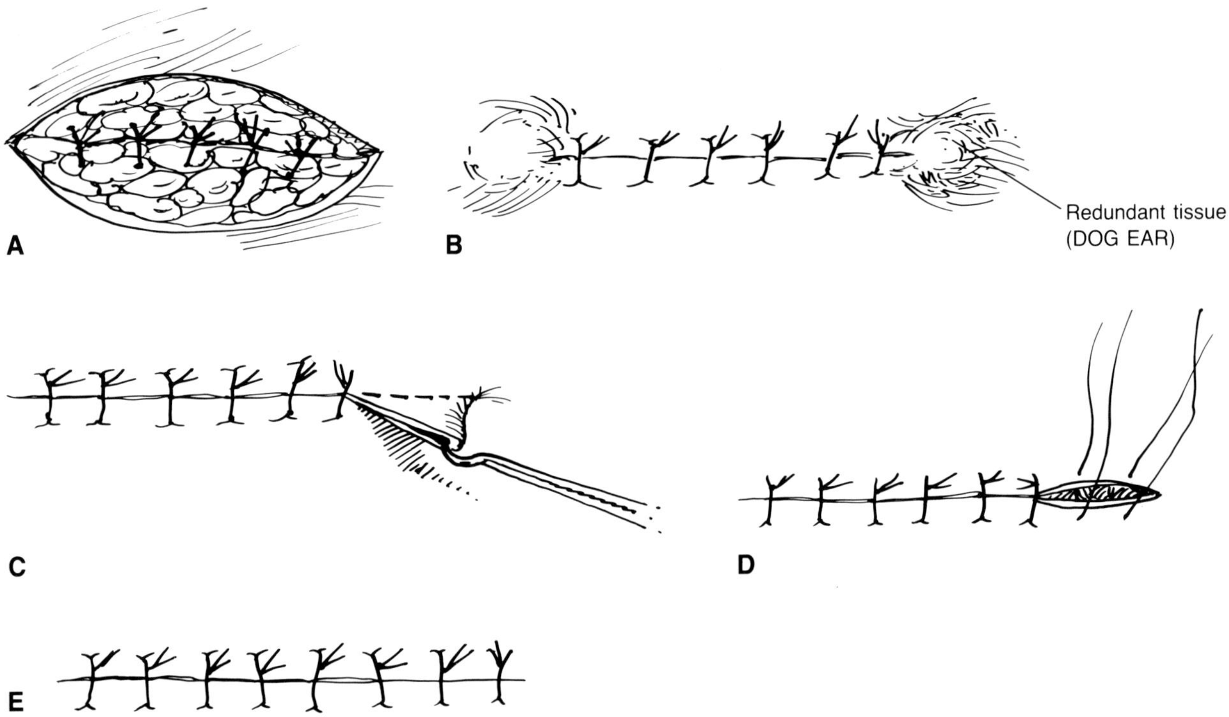

Figure 15–29. *One simple method of scar removal eliminates redundant tissue at incision ends. (**A**) Deep sutures. (**B**) Redundant tissue. (**C**) Use of skin hook to delineate problem. (**D**) Defect after excision of redundant tissue. (**E**) Correction requires lengthening of wound.*

scar and reclosure. This is appropriate therapy only if the factors that caused the initial unfavorable scarring are controlled after the revision. For example, if initial wound healing was impaired by poor initial debridement, poor closure, wound dehiscence, or wound infection and the lines of the scar lie in appropriate skin direction and can be closed after excision without tension, good results can be expected with scar excision. After elliptical excision of a depressed scar, deep sutures must be approximated beneath the wound prior to closure. The ellipse must be fashioned in such a way as to avoid redundant raised tissue at each end of the ellipse (Fig. 15–29).

The technique of Z-plasty is useful to lengthen a contracted scar and to reorient the lines in the scar toward the correct lines of tension. This method may be useful occasionally during primary repair of wounds that are at high risk of developing a disfiguring contracture. Triangular flaps are created at 60° angles to the line of the wound and then are transposed, thus borrowing lateral tissue laxity in order to achieve increased wound length. Simultaneously the prominent portion of the scar is reoriented by 90° (Fig. 15–30). In longer wounds, in which large triangular flaps would be inappropriate and radical changes in overall wound orientation are undesirable, multiple Z-plasties can be used to increase scar length and break up the visual impact of a long, linear scar.

Another technique that is useful to break up the visually obvious straight line scar is the W-plasty technique (Fig. 15–31). This technique does add length to the scar by breaking up the linear contraction forces involved in wound shortening.

Various treatments of depressed scars, such as acne scars, have been advocated. These include injection with subdermal collagen or autologous fat. The advantages of this technique include the fact that treatments are fast and easily performed in the office under local anesthetic. Disadvantages include possible allergic reactions to collagen, the high cost of collagen, and results that have not proven to be long-standing with either substance. Patients should be given a test

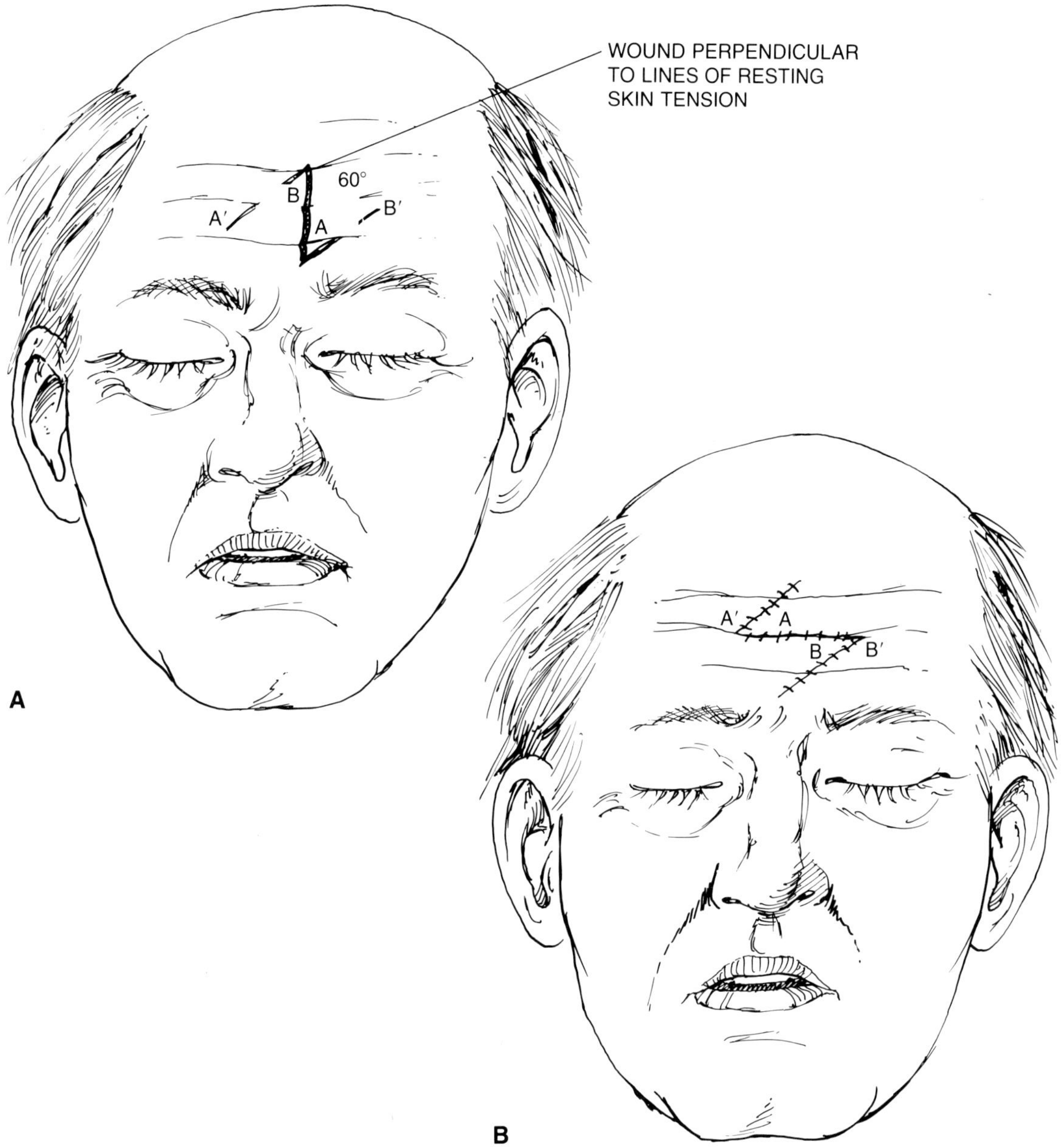

Figure 15–30. *Z-plasty technique. (**A**) Proposed Z-plasty. (**B**) After transposition of flaps and changing axis of wound 90°.*

dose of collagen prior to injection. Prior to filling the depression with autologous fat or collagen, the bevel of the needle used to cut binding scar between dermis and deeper structures.

Some posttraumatic facial scars, acne scars, and wrinkling can be successfully treated with dermabrasion with or without chemical peeling. These techniques are best suited for lesions involving a relatively wide expanse of facial skin, such as those seen after severe facial abrasions which result in uneven ridgelike scars. The outer layers of skin and scar are surgically planed away, allowing the remaining dermis

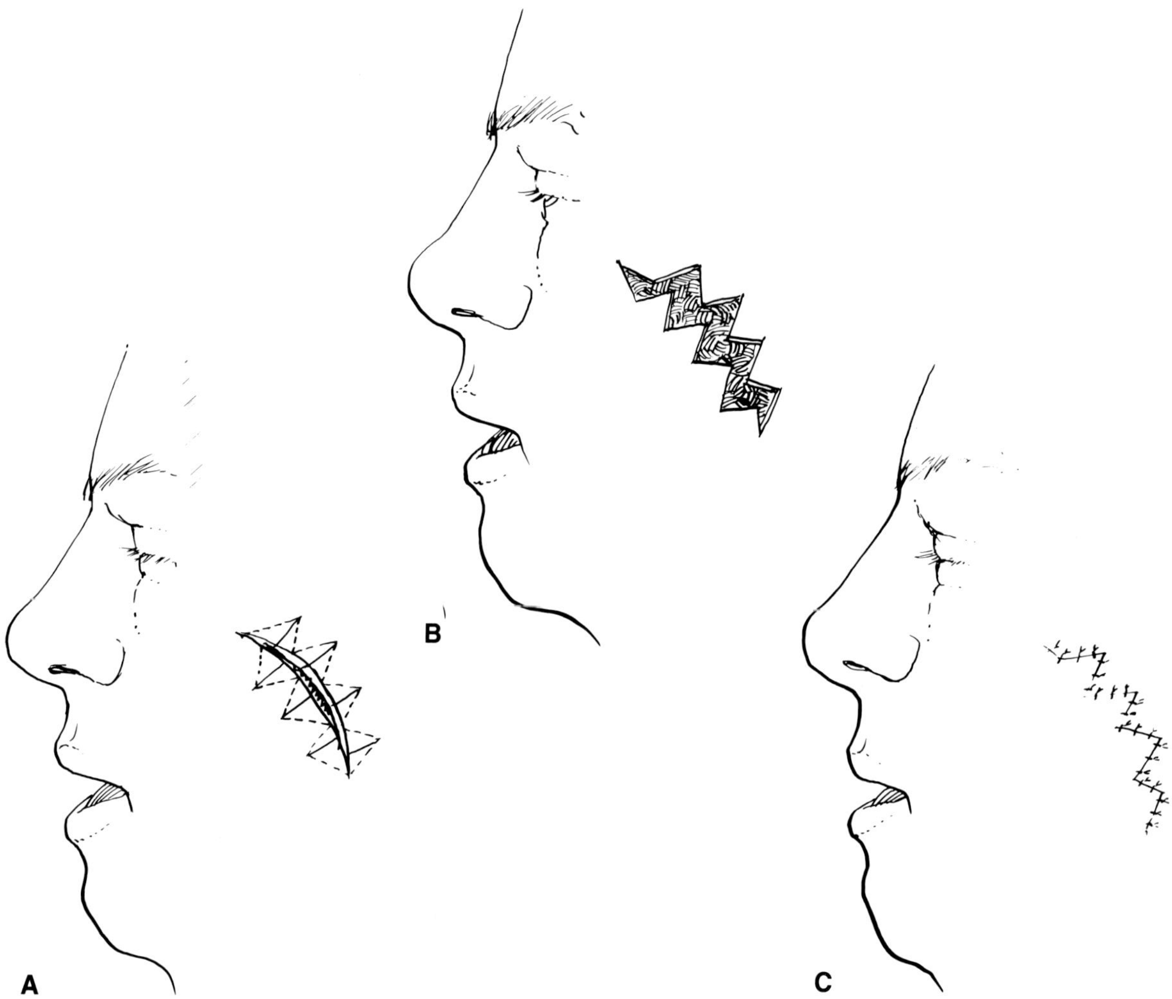

Figure 15–31. *W-plasty technique. (**A**) Planned W-plasty excision. (**B**) After excision and raising of skin edges. (**C**) Initial closure.*

and epidermis to reepithelialize in a more uniform fashion. Phenol use has the disadvantage of causing permanent depigmentation of the skin.[24,25] It should not be used in dark-skinned individuals or those who enjoy sun tanning. After skin planing with phenol is completed the resultant defect is treated like a partial-thickness burn. Reepithelialization occurs in approximately 2 weeks.

When pigmentation has occurred after soft tissue facial trauma the use of tattooing may improve the cosmetic defect. Depigmentation may also occur as the result of burns, chemical irritants, abrasions, or severe lacerations. There are many shades of tattoo dye now available to match most facial complexions. Multiple applications may be necessary in order to cover all depigmented areas.

SUMMARY

The face is the area of the body most commonly displayed and is thus quite conspicuous when disfigured. Knowledge of the modes of trauma and the anatomy of the region injured allows for accurate diagnosis and initiation of treatment. Optimum results—minimal facial scarring and maximal facial function—depend on expert initial treatment and follow-up wound care.

REFERENCES

1. Schultz RC, Oldham RJ. An overview of facial injuries. Surg Clin North Am 1977;57:987.
2. Curtin JW. Basic plastic surgical techniques in repair of facial lacerations. Surg Clin North Am 1973;53:33.
3. Smith TE Jr. Surgical anatomy of the face. Otolaryngol Clin North Am 1982;15:3.
4. Converse JM, Smith B. Symposium: Midfacial fractures. Nasoorbital fractures. Trans Am Acad Ophthalmol Otol 1963;67:622.
5. Bertz JE. Maxillofacial injuries. Clin Symp 1981;33:1.
6. Della Rocca RC, Arthurs B, Silverstone P. Nasolacrimal disorders and their treatment. Clin Plas Surg 1989;15:195.
7. Bailey BJ. Management of maxillofacial trauma. Res and Staff Phys 1982; 57.
8. May M. Trauma to the facial nerve. Otol Clin North Am 1983;16:661.
9. Barton NV, Miller SH, Graham WP III. Managing lacerations of the parotid gland, duct and facial nerve. Am Fam Physician 1976;13:130.
10. Teh BT. Why do skin grafts fail? Plast Reconstr Surg 1979;63:323.
11. Maniglia AJ, Kline SN. Maxillofacial trauma in the pediatric age group. Otolaryngol Clin North Am 1983; 16:609.
12. McCarthy JG, Wood-Smith D. Rhinoplasty. In: McCarthy JG, ed. Plastic Surgery. Philadelphia: WB Saunders, 1990, p 1862.
13. Lawson W. Management of soft tissue injuries of the face. Otolaryngol Clin North Am 1982;15:35.
14. Terzis J. Microreconstruction of Nerve Injuries. Philadelphia: WB Saunders, 1987.
15. Bornstein LA, Simon BE. Successful primary repair of severed parotid duct. Plast Reconstr Surg 1949;6:217.
16. Schultz RC. Soft tissue injuries of the face. In: Smith JW, Aston SJ, eds. Grabb and Smith's Plastic Surgery. Boston: Little, Brown & Co, 1991.
17. Wilkie TF. The problem of drooling in cerebral palsy: a surgical approach. Can J Surg 1967; 10:60.
18. Lacher AB, Blitzer A. The traumatized auricle. Otolaryngol Clin North Am 1982;15:225.
19. Mladick RA, Horton CE, Adamson JE, Cohen BI. The pocket principle; a new technique for the reattachment of a severed ear part. Plast Reconstr Surg 1971;49:219.
20. Mladick RA, Carraway JH. Ear reattachment by the modified pocket principle. Plast Reconstr Surg 1973; 51:583.
21. Schultz RC, McMaster WC. The treatment of dog bite injuries, especially those of the face. Plast Reconstr Surg 1972;49:494.
22. Thomson HG, Svitek V. Small animal bites. The role of primary closure. J Trauma 1973;13:20.
23. Berlinger NT. Wound healing. Otol Clin North Am 1982; 15:29.
24. Hugo NE. Videotape discussion on dermabrasion procedures. In: Gouliam D, Courtise EH, eds. Symposium on Surgery of the Aging Face. St. Louis: CV Mosby, 1978.
25. Horton CE, Sadove MD. Refinements in combined chemical peel and simultaneous abrasion of the face. Ann Plast Surg 1987;19:504.

16

Rigid Internal Fixation of Facial Fractures

Leon A. Assael

The main goal in the treatment of fractures of the facial skeleton is to predictably restore preinjury form and function. This goal must be accomplished by means that will produce the least disability, smallest risk, and shortest recovery period for the patient. In seeking to improve this treatment equation for fracture patients, techniques were sought that would address some of the problems related to traditional methods.

A facial fracture treated by traditional methods is reduced and fixed. Immobilization is normally accomplished by intermaxillary fixation. During the 6 to 8 weeks of immobilization normally employed, the patient must consume a liquid diet, and speech and respiration are made more difficult.

Restoration of preinjury form and function in fractures treated by traditional methods is mitigated by *fracture disease*, described by Danis in 1949.[1] This phenomena produces atrophy and fibrosis of the immobilized muscles. The mineralized portion of the immobilized bones is decreased.[2] Cicatrization and resorption of bone across the fracture sites may result in a loss of position of the bone in space, with resulting deformity or malocclusion. In traditional treatment of midfacial fractures, this has sometimes resulted in loss of vertical dimension and a class III open-bite tendency. Zygoma fractures may be directed inferomedially by this action. This may result in late flattening of the malar eminence. Movement of the body of the zygoma may also increase orbital volume, thereby resulting in late enophthalmos.

Fracture disease and its associated cicatrization in mandible fractures may also result in malunion. This malunion may result in changes in the occlusion that require secondary theraputic intervention. Rotation of the proximal segment in angle fractures can result in eventual union but loss of mandibular angle contour. The retromolar pad and maxillary tuberosity may be in contact, although there is no malocclusion. When symphyseal fractures are associated with condylar fractures, flaring of the ramus of the mandible can result, although no malocclusion is noted (Fig. 16-1).[3]

Condylar fractures of the mandible that are treated by closed reduction and immobilization may result in a functionally shortened mandibular ramus. This causes deviation to the side of injury during function. Although a malocclusion in maximum intercuspation may not be present, there is often a poor contralateral-lateral excursion with loss of cuspid guidance. Compensatory canting of the occlusal plane upward on the side of injury may result.[4]

To counteract the clinical effects of these events, intermaxillary fixation is usually used to maintain the occlusion. As a result, the teeth may move through bone, creating new periodontal and occlusal problems. Although the appearance of the resulting occlusion may be adequate, the loss of skeletal position can produce other functional or aesthetic problems.

For most patients undergoing traditional fracture treatment, fracture disease remains subclinical. Com-

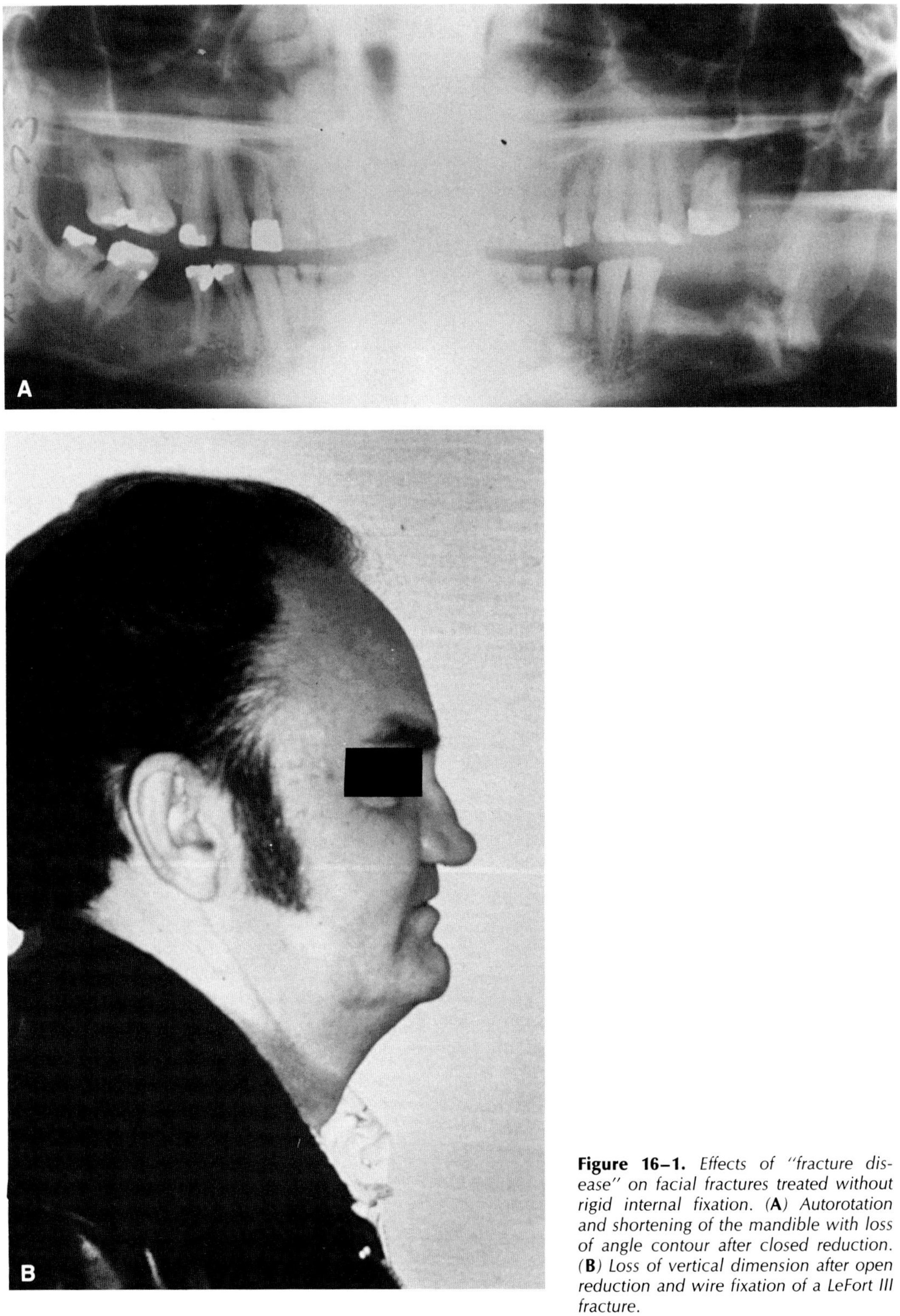

Figure 16–1. *Effects of "fracture disease" on facial fractures treated without rigid internal fixation.* (**A**) *Autorotation and shortening of the mandible with loss of angle contour after closed reduction.* (**B**) *Loss of vertical dimension after open reduction and wire fixation of a LeFort III fracture.*

promises in the position of teeth and bone may not produce a visible deformity or clinically evident functional derangement. Hence, conservative nonsurgical management remains the standard treatment option for many facial fractures.

Through the evaluation of treatment failures, however, means were sought to identify those cases that would likely have functional and aesthetic defects. Research into the biophysics of the facial bones, mechanical aspects of fixation, bone healing physiologic characteristics, and biomaterials has produced methods that identify those cases at risk and provide the means to avoid these problems effectively.[5] This scientific and clinical effort has been very productive in offering improved treatment in the science of rigid internal fixation.

With the development of modern techniques to ensure safe operative procedures, pioneers of modern orthopedic surgery—including Lambotte in 1907 and Danis in 1949—began to advocate surgical fracture management with the goal of early functional mobilization.[1,6] The healing of fractures with rigid fixation was first observed in 1914 by Hicks. In postwar Europe, surgeons interested in the development of methods to improve the surgical management of fractures organized the Association for the Study of Internal Fixation (ASIF) in Switzerland in 1956. The use of rigid internal fixation of long bones became an important part of orthopedic surgery with the publication of Muller, Allgower, and Willenegger's *Technique of Internal Fixation of Fractures* in 1965.[7] The methods developed by the ASIF were refined with important modifications for maxillofacial use by Luhr in 1968 and by Spiessl in 1971.[8,9]

Rigid internal fixation is a method of fracture treatment that relies on fixation modalities that provide absolute stability of the fracture segments during the healing period. It is implicit in the technique that the patient is placed immediately into function. Hence, the fixation device must continuously resist functional forces. The proper use of rigid internal fixation also implies immediate restoration of very precise preinjury anatomic form. When restoration includes dental occlusion, these tolerances are the most extreme of any employed in the human skeleton.

To understand the use of rigid fixation in facial fracture management, a knowledge of the biomechanics of the facial skeleton, factors influencing fracture stability, the biologic features of fracture healing, and the physical characteristics of fixation devices is necessary.

BIOMECHANICS OF THE FACIAL SKELETON

The facial skeleton is arranged in a fashion that efficiently resists function forces. Forces are transmitted through the facial skeleton by means that efficiently distribute the loads applied.

The mandible receives its greatest function forces on the occlusal surfaces of the teeth during mastication. When such a load is placed, vectors are produced that distribute the force. This causes a distractory force along the alveolar ridge and external oblique ridge, termed the *tension zone*. If a fracture exists in this area, it tends to separate when an occlusal load is placed on it. Force applied to the occlusal surface is transmitted along the middle of the body of the mandible and through the lingula to the condyle. The *neutral zone* closely follows the course of the inferior alveolar nerve. The portion of a fracture passing through the neutral zone does not have a displacement force on it when an occlusal load is placed on it. When the same occlusal load is placed, a compressive force is applied to the inferior border of the mandible and the mentum. In this *compression zone*, a fulcrum occurs when force is applied to the occlusal surface, allowing for a point around which a fracture will rotate (Fig. 16–2).[10]

Transmission of occlusal forces in the midface create

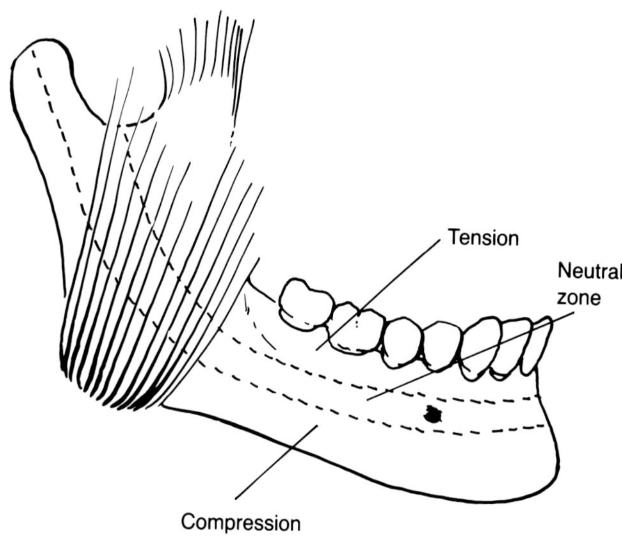

Figure 16–2. *Force zones of mandible. The forces produced by the muscles of mastication create natural zones of tension (superior border) and compression (inferior border) in the mandible.*

similar compression, neutral, and tension zones. The natural buttresses for transmission of these forces are the piriform rim, the zygomatic buttress, and the pterygoid plates. On the upper midface, the zygomaticofrontal region, infraorbital rim, and nasomaxillary complex further transmit occlusal forces and muscular forces. Vertical forces placed on the maxilla during masticatory function generally create compression zones along these buttresses. However, the zygomaticofrontal region is a tension zone, because of the inferior medial pull of the powerful masseter muscle.[11,12]

FRACTURE STABILITY

In determining the ability of a fracture to remain stable, an analysis of the usual functional forces applied to the fracture is necessary. Stability is the key in determining the need for surgical management with rigid internal fixation. Fracture segment displacement is not a measure of fracture stability. A widely displaced fracture may require no internal fixation once reduced. Conversely, a minimally displaced fracture may be completely unstable without internal fixation.

An examination of the forces applied to the facial skeleton reveals the direction and force (vectors) that are applied during function. During masticatory function, the tension zone of the mandible is along the anterior ramus and alveolar process to the canine region. Hence, the portion of a mandible fracture that is transmitted across this area will be distracted. A simple example is an angle fracture with inferior distraction of the distal segment and superior rotation of the proximal segment. Separation of this fracture will be at the superior border with an associated open bite. The inferior border, a compression zone, will act as a fulcrum around which the displacement of the fracture will rotate. If the fracture passes anteriorly from the external oblique ridge, this is a favorable development because the fulcrum of rotation at the inferior border (compression zone) tends to reduce the fracture.

Fracture stability is also influenced by many other anatomic and biologic factors. Fracture interdigitation may provide the means to prevent fracture displacement. Favorable fractures produce functional forces across fracture sites that tend to reduce the fracture. In these cases the fracture site acts as a buttress across which a force is directed. This produces a beneficial interfragmentary compression in the fracture. Comminution adversely affects buttressing. Hence, the comminuted fracture loses stability.

Biologic factors influence fracture stability. Partial immobilization of a fracture occurs because of the subperiosteal deposition of the clot that subsequently organizes. Early resorption of bone in a fracture site adversely influences stability. Muscle splinting and spasm about a fracture site can affect displacement and produce excessive forces that prevent reduction.

BIOLOGIC FEATURES OF FRACTURE HEALING

Evolution and natural selection of vertebrates has produced a mechanism of fracture healing that reduces interfragmentary mobility caused by the necessary continual functional movement of the organism. In this mode of secondary fracture healing, the fracture is first stabilized by pain, hemorrhage, edema, and muscle splinting. Clot organization and contracture in the fracture site produces initial stabilization of the segments. Fibrous immobilization and callus formation follows to further immobilize the fracture and draw the fracture segments closer together. At this point, woven bone appears in the fracture site and later organizes to efficiently resist functional forces. Preinjury form is not always restored because of shortening of the affected bone. Only in the late stage of healing is function restored.

This mechanism of fracture healing may be disturbed by continued interfragmentary mobility. This produces further hemorrhage and prevents the migration of fibroblasts and osteoblasts. In such situations, a nonunion and pseudoarthrosis may result.

Fractures that are treated with rigid internal fixation with interfragmentary compression heal in a distinctly different manner, termed *primary bone healing*.[13] With the bone placed immediately into function, cutting cones of osteoclasts appear early to pass from one fragment and through the fracture site to another. These cutting cones are followed by osteoblasts that pass woven bone directly across the fracture site. No callus is formed and no fibrous immobilization occurs. Early remodeling of the fracture site completes the restoration of form and function.

Biomechanics and Design of Plates and Screws

Rigid internal fixation is currently applied by means of metal plates and screws fixed to the bone. In combination with the buttressing forces of fracture interdigitation, the use of these devices is designed to create forces that exceed functional forces at all times. The devices are produced from metals that demonstrate appropriate strain characteristics, durability, malleability, and biocompatability. Metals in current use include stainless steel, titanium, and chromium cobalt alloy.

Most bone plates may be adapted both along their flat surface and torsionally. Some bone plates may be three-dimensionally adapted. Bone plates currently in common use in oral and maxillofacial surgery range widely in size and shape and are designed for specific applications. Minifragment systems have been designed for use in the midface with screw diameters ranging between 0.8 and 2 mm. For the mandible, thicker bone plates with screw diameters up to 2.7 mm have been designed.

Screw design for internal bone fixation has a number of parameters. The screw threads act as an inclined plane to drive the screw through bone. The contact between the threads and the bone provides a resistance to forces applied to the long axis of the screw. This axial force can be quantified by examining the pull-out strength of the screw in bone. The difference between the core diameter of the screw and the greatest diameter of the shaft influences the bone contact and pull-out strength. The axial force provided by a screw (dependent on the area of bone contact) also increases with the square of the radius. Hence, small changes in screw diameter may produce great changes in pull-out strength. An example is a 2.7-mm screw that produces twice the axial force as does a 2-mm screw. The screw head design also varies in different systems. The production of torque for placement, maximizing screw-plate contact, and allowing for low profile, all influence screw-head design (Fig. 16–3).[14]

Screws are designed to be either self-tapping or pretapped. When a screw is inserted, debris from the cutting edge is created. This debris increases friction and heat and may cause displacement of the bone at the margin of the screw. To mitigate against these undesirable occurances, modifications of bone-screw application have been made. In self-tapping screws, a

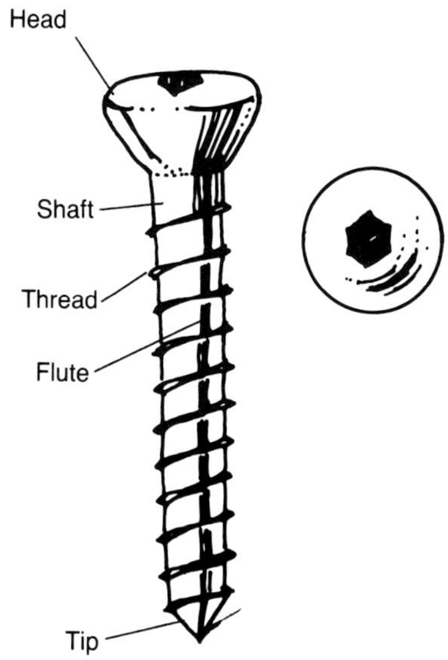

Figure 16–3. *Screw design. The functional characteristics of a screw are dependent on the length, core diameter, thread diameter, and tip, thread, and head design. A flute is present in a self-tapping screw.*

vertical flute along the long axis of the screw fills with bone debris during placement. Pretapped screws have no flute. Instead, a sharp cutting instrument called a *tap* is used to make a screw preparation in the bone and to remove bone debris under copious irrigation. The screw is then passively placed in the prepared hole. There continues to be debate over the optimal screw design for given clinical situations. Research by Phillips indicates that self-tapping screws are superior in thin bones, whereas in bones thicker than 3mm, pretapping provides superior axial force in the screw.[15] Variable evidence exists as to whether axial force is better maintained when a pretapped screw is used and whether greater heat is generated by tapping or using a self-tapping screw. Whatever the results of further research, both types currently are successfully used in a wide variety of clinical situations.[16]

Rigid bone plates are constructed in a manner that permits compressive forces to be applied across the fracture site. In 1969 Perren reported on the dynamic compression hole for bone plates.[17] This hole has an inclined arc of a larger diameter than the screw shaft but a smaller diameter than the screw head. When a screw is placed in the hole eccentrically, it engages the screw head and inclined arc as the screw is being driven home. A lateral moment of force is created that

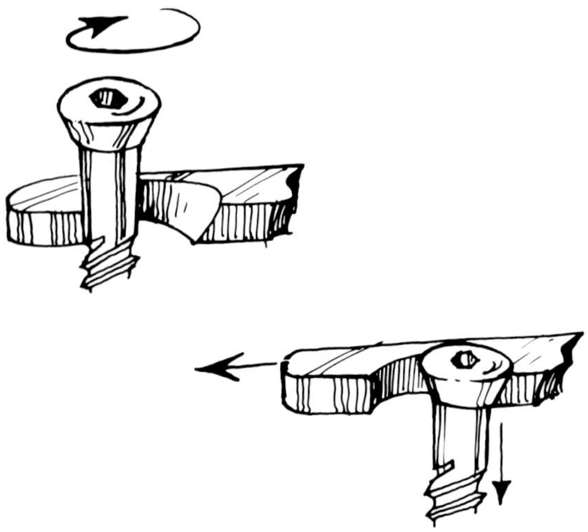

Figure 16–4. *Dynamic compression hole. As the screw is driven home, the screw head engages in an inclined plane within the screw hole. This creates both vertical and lateral moments of force. The vertical moment of force clamps the plate to the bone. The lateral moment of force can be applied to the fracture site to produce compression of the fracture ends.*

compresses the fracture margins together (Fig. 16–4). The main biomechanical advantage of compression is that the frictional forces produced in the fracture site allow for load sharing in function. Hence, a less strong, less bulky plate may be used. With less exposure to functional loads by the plate itself, there is less chance of plate failure. The biomechanics of compression are such that, during healing, compression decreases. Thus, the implant may be exposed to increasing loads in the weeks following surgery. Eventually the healing bone takes up the functional loads.[18]

The necessary size and strength of a plate and screw system used for stable fixation is dependent on the initial and eventual ability of the bone to carry functional loads. This may help to explain why a miniplate on the external oblique ridge with four 2-mm screws may permit uneventful healing of a simple mandibular angle fracture, whereas a comminuted fracture in the same location might require a reconstruction plate with eight 2.7-mm screws (Fig. 16–5).[19]

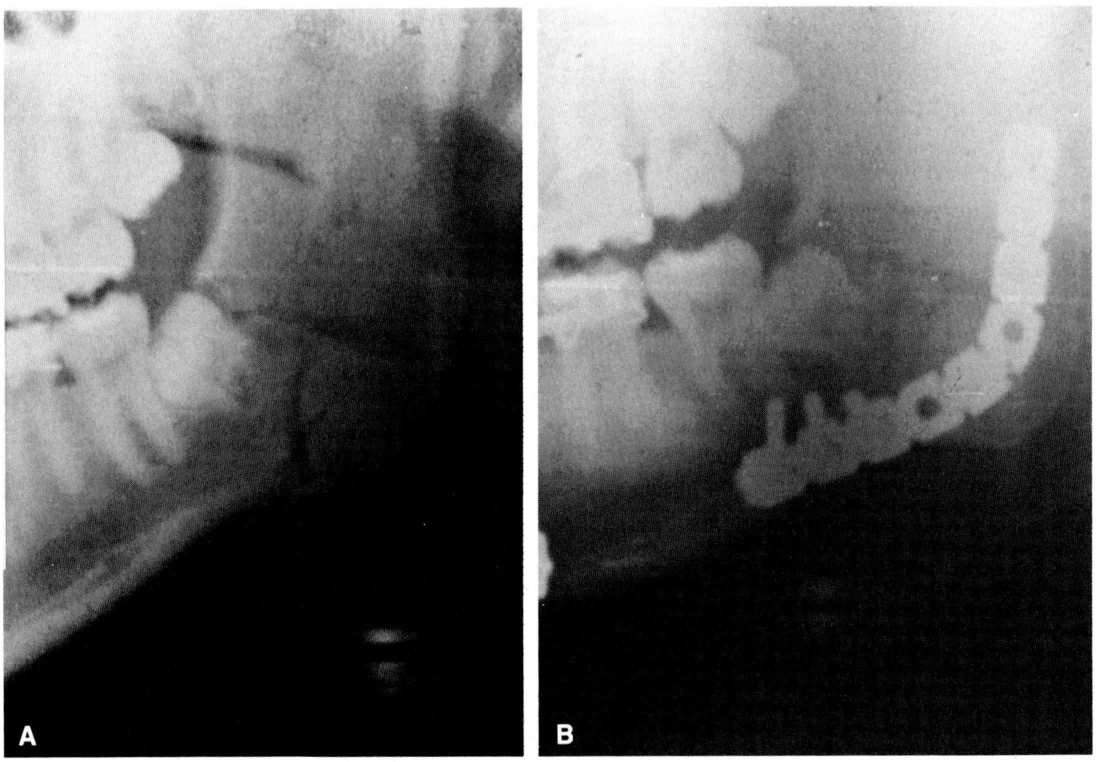

Figure 16–5, A *and* B. *The amount of fixation needed depends on the ability of fracture compression to carry a portion of the functional load. A comminuted angle fracture requries a large reconstruction plate because compression is not possible.*

When adapted for use in mandibular fractures, the compression bone plate was found to have certain limitations. Although compression directly beneath the bone plate on the inferior border was excellent, there was distraction of the fracture in the alveolar process. The presence of teeth uniquely restricted the placement of plates in the alveolar process. In 1973 Schmoker and Spiessl determined that dynamic compression could be obtained in the alveolar process by redirecting the dynamic compression holes of a plate placed at the inferior border. The eccentric dynamic compression plate has become the preferred means of obtaining uniform interfragmentary compression of mandible fractures.[20]

BASIC OPERATIVE TECHNIQUE

The operative procedure for applying rigid internal fixation of a facial fracture requires a logical sequence of steps. This operative technique is unforgiving of omitted steps or inadequately performed components. The procedure may be thought of as a chain in which only one broken link makes the entire chain useless.

Intermaxillary Fixation

The rigid internal fixation of any facial fracture that includes fractures of the mandible or maxilla must begin with the placement of intermaxillary fixation. This portion of the operative procedure must produce the preinjury occlusion with the condyles in their normal position. The occlusion, fixed before the open reduction of facial fractures, determines the ability to obtain precise anatomic reduction with restoration of full masticatory function.

Placement of intermaxillary fixation is best performed with full arch bars and the assistance of skeletal wires, if necessary. Large forces will be placed on the dental arch during the reduction and fixation, and it is important that these forces do not exceed those of the intermaxillary fixation because this may produce a postoperative occlusal derangement. To prevent this, acrylic reinforcement of at least four intermaxillary wires may be used. In addition, periodic examination of the intermaxillary fixation during the operative procedure and avoidance of excessive force prevents many problems.

The use of study models of the teeth and the construction of splints is recommended for partially edentulous patients, patients with panfacial fractures, and those with fractures in the dental arch. Maximum interdigitation of the teeth in centric occlusion with multiple tooth contacts through an occlusal wafer satisfactorily reproduces the preinjury occlusion.

When the facial fracture crosses the dental arch (e.g., in a mandible symphysis fracture) or a split palate, the arch bar may be reinforced with acrylic to prevent reopening of the fracture diastema. Such acrylic reinforcement is best done following the anatomic reduction of the fracture but before the placement of rigid internal fixation.[11] As previously described, the dental alveolus is in a tension zone. By acting as a fixation device to prevent tensile forces from producing fracture distraction, this acrylic reinforcement functions as a "tension band."[21]

Surgical Approach

The exposure of facial fracture sites is designed to reveal sufficient fracture morphologic features and permit careful reduction and fixation of the fracture. This must be accomplished with maximum attention to principles of wound management and facial aesthetics. With these principles in mind, mandibular fractures and LeFort I fractures are often approached through the transoral vestibular approach. This technique has the advantages of eliminating the risks of facial nerve damage and facial scars.[22] No increased incidence of infection has been noted with this approach. The transoral approach has considerable limitations in the mandible, however. Exposure of sufficient fracture morphologic features to make appropriate fixation decisions may not be possible. It is also often more difficult to reduce the fracture and apply fixation through the transoral approach (Fig. 16–6).

Transfacial exposure of fractures need not be greater because of the use of rigid internal fixation (Fig. 16–7). The incision may be shorter than the fixation device. Periosteum should be elevated in a conservative fashion, exposing only the fracture site and the facial aspect of the bone in the area in which the hardware is to be placed. Supraperiosteal placement of hardware may be indicated in areas of compromised blood supply, such as in comminution or mandibular atrophy. Subperiosteal dissection should be carried out after

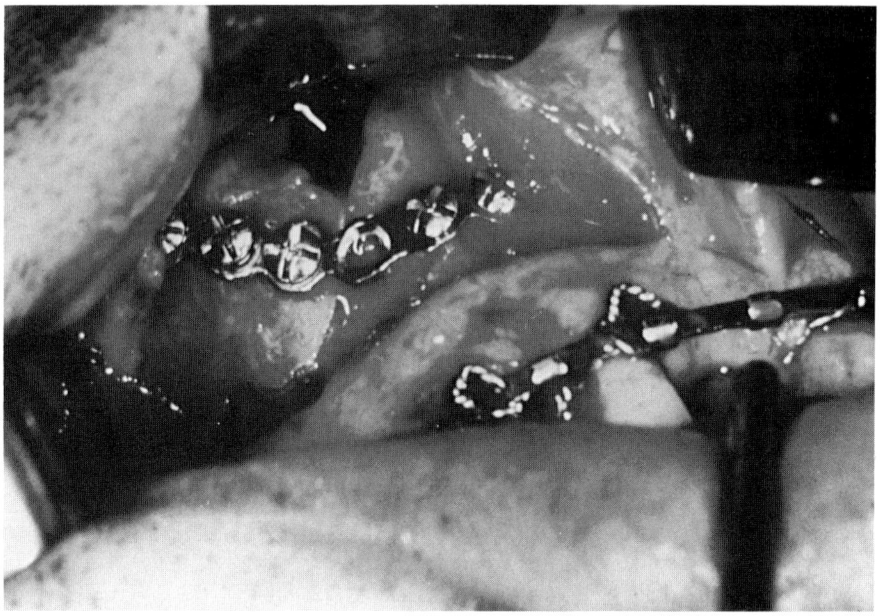

Figure 16–6. *Transoral approach may be used to treat fractures of the mandibular symphysis, mandibular angle, and midface.*

careful examination of radiographs to prevent unnecessary loss of blood supply to fracture segments. By stripping only the edges or the facial aspect of a comminuted segment, some periosteal blood supply may be preserved. If the imaging or fracture exposure is insufficient, incorrect fixation decisions may be made that could result in treatment failure. Failure to completely understand the fracture morphologic features before the selection of a rigid internal fixation modality is a primary reason for treatment failure.[3]

Fracture Reduction and Preload

Reduction of facial fractures is made more complex by the use of rigid internal fixation. The reduced fracture segments must be temporarily immobilized to permit the passive placement of permanent fixation. Temporary transosseous wires have been employed for this purpose. Alternatively, this temporary reduction may be accomplished manually with bone-holding clamps. Pairs of clamps have also been manufactured with a rigid adjustable connector to produce temporary fixation. The ASIF-reduction forceps is also a useful instrument in mandibular fractures.[23]

Preload of the fracture site is often helpful in that it increases interfragmentary friction and makes primary bone healing more likely. A towel clip or reduction forceps applied across the fracture site may be used to produce interfragmentary compression. This compression may then be increased when the fixation is placed (Fig. 16–8).

Not all fracture treatment benefits from the use of preload. Preload may cause overreduction of another site. It should not be employed in areas of comminution. Thin bones may produce iatrogenic fractures if preloaded.

Following reduction and temporary immobilization, it is helpful to recheck the dental occlusion.

Plate Selection

Each of the systems designed for use in facial fractures has a variety of sizes and shapes of plates to accommodate the needs of many different clinical situations. The smallest bone plate that will provide three-dimensionally stable fixation under functional loads during the healing period is selected. Two screws on either side of the fracture site is the least fixation that will achieve this goal; the placement of a third screw on each side increases the fixation stability.

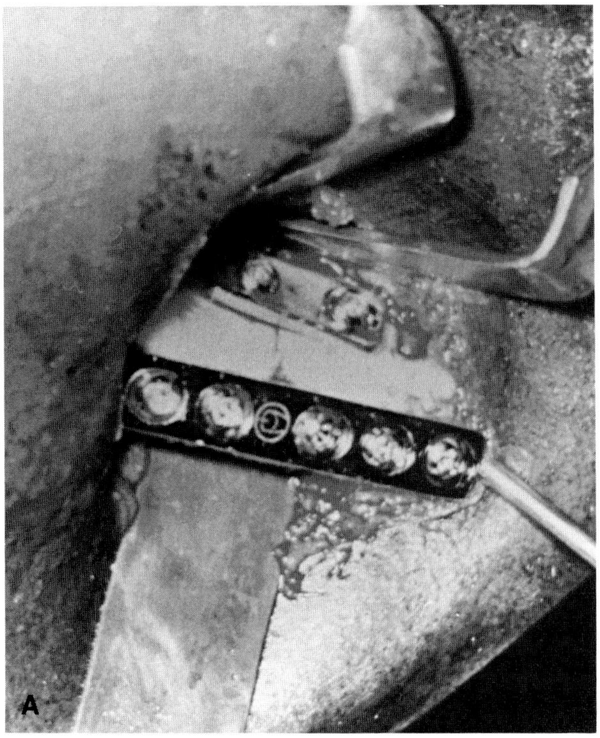

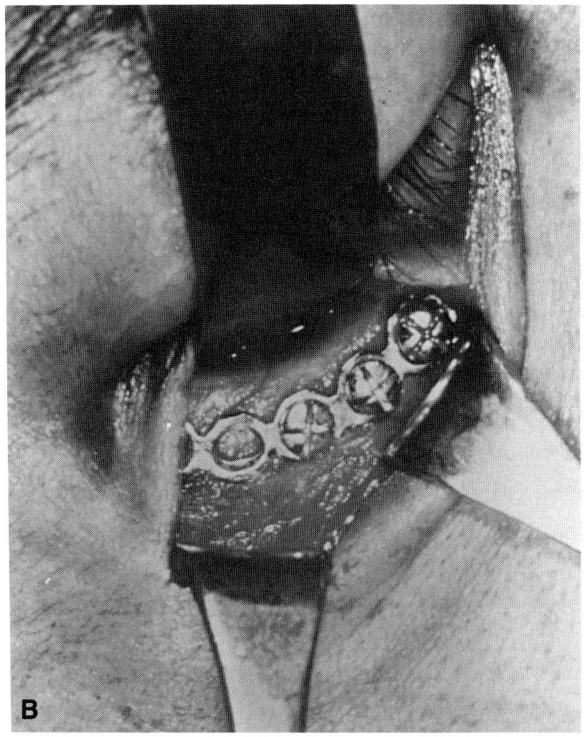

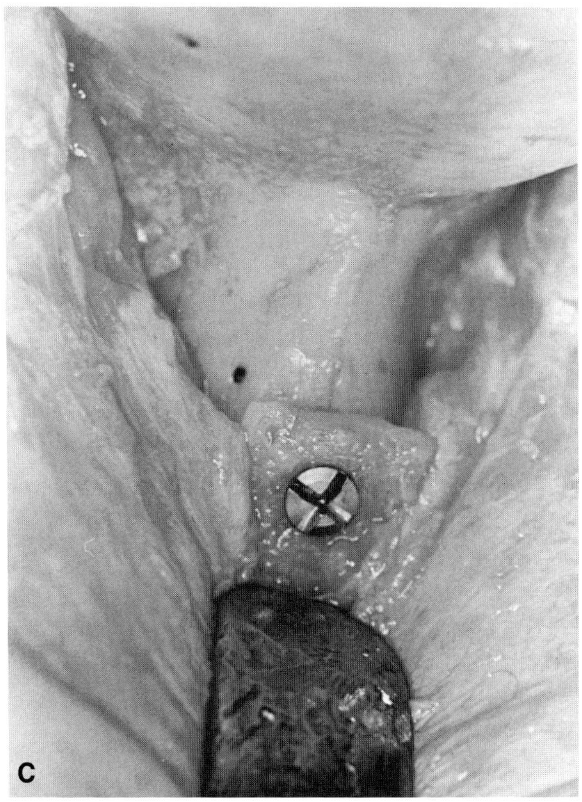

Figure 16–7. *Transfacial approach to fractures. (**A**) The transcervical approach is used for mandibular fractures. (**B**) The subciliary incision reveals fractures of the orbital rim. (**C**) The coronal incision is useful for the nasofrontal region, supraorbit, zygomatic body, and zygomatic arch.*

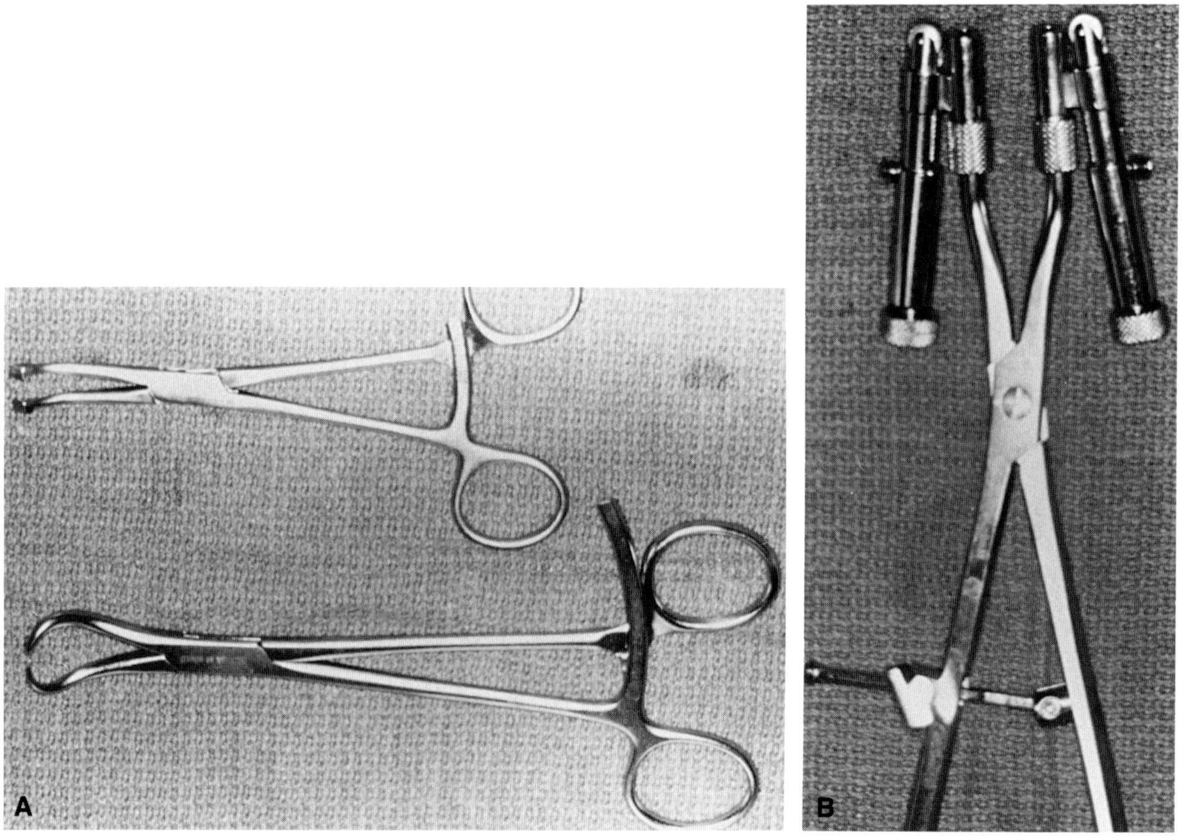

Figure 16–8. *Fracture preload. Preload may be applied to simple fractures with a towel clip, (**A**) clamp, or (**B**) reduction forceps.*

The size of the plate necessary is dependent on many aspects of the clinical situation. A smaller plate can be used when there is a large amount of interfragmentary friction in the fracture site. A smaller plate is more often adequate in a tension zone than in a compression zone because the lever arm of force applied is shorter. Larger plates are necessary where the lever arm of force is longer (e.g., the mandibular angle, compared with the mandibular body). A larger plate is needed where there is comminution or a gap because the buttressing affect of contact and compression of the fracture site is lost (Fig. 16–9).

Plates designed for use in the mandible are generally stronger than those used in the midface. This design is necessary to resist the large forces applied to fixation in the compression zone on the inferior border of the mandible. By using a tension band technique, Champy has employed much smaller plates at the superior border of angle fractures and as pairs in the neutral zone of the symphysis and body.[24] Monocortical screws and softer plates are used. This technique has the advantage of providing easier transoral placement of fixation. Its limitations are in those fractures that have less than adequate interfragmentary friction after reduction. Research by Kroon had indicated that a reversal of forces in the tension zone may occur after a tension band is placed and functional movements are applied.[25] In the mandibular angle this may produce opening of the inferior border with fixation failure in angle fractures treated with tension bands.

In the midface, plate selection may also provide the means to restore facial contour. Curved plates used circumorbitally will permit the restoration of form and provide the matrix for the anatomic placement of bone grafts. The position of the dorsum of the nose is also determined by plate contour (Fig. 16–10).

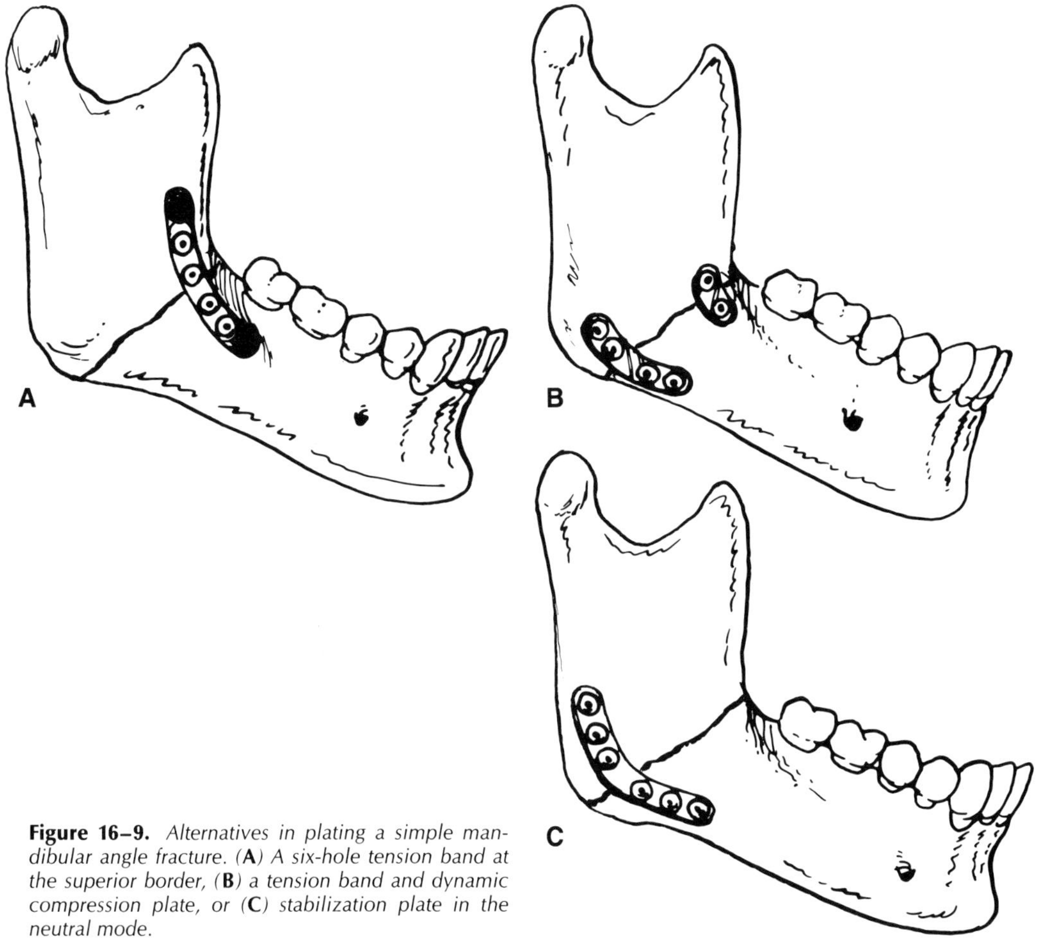

Figure 16–9. *Alternatives in plating a simple mandibular angle fracture. (**A**) A six-hole tension band at the superior border, (**B**) a tension band and dynamic compression plate, or (**C**) stabilization plate in the neutral mode.*

Plate Bending

It is imperative that plates be adapted accurately to precisely accomplish the goal of anatomic reduction. An imprecisely bent plate produces several avenues towards possible clinical failure. If the poorly bent plate is sufficiently stiff, it draws the bone towards it as screws are tightened, disrupting an excellent reduction. If interfragmentary compression is sufficient to prevent this, it will nevertheless set up a force in the screw thread that will result in a loose screw weeks later. If the poorly bent plate is soft, it will adapt to the bone, but the elastic memory of the metal of the plate will produce orthopedic forces that only later will produce movement of the bone and malunion.

A properly adapted plate must rest passively on the bone and have a broad frictional contact with the cortical surface. The use of soft metal templates that are well adapted to the bone surface and carefully removed for examination have assisted surgeons in the precise bending of plates. Many systems have instruments designed specifically for bending plates. Separate attention should be given to each component of bending in sequence; side-shape alteration (if available), flat surface, and torsion. The properly adapted plate must sit passively on the cortical surface with broad bone contact underneath each of the screw holes (Fig 16–11). An exception to this is in thicker bones, such as the mandibular body, in which compression is used. In such cases compression is only active directly under the facial surface of the plate. This may result in distraction of the fracture at the lingual surface. As little as 1 mm of overbending in the fracture site can provide a force active enough to cause compression on the lingual surface.[21]

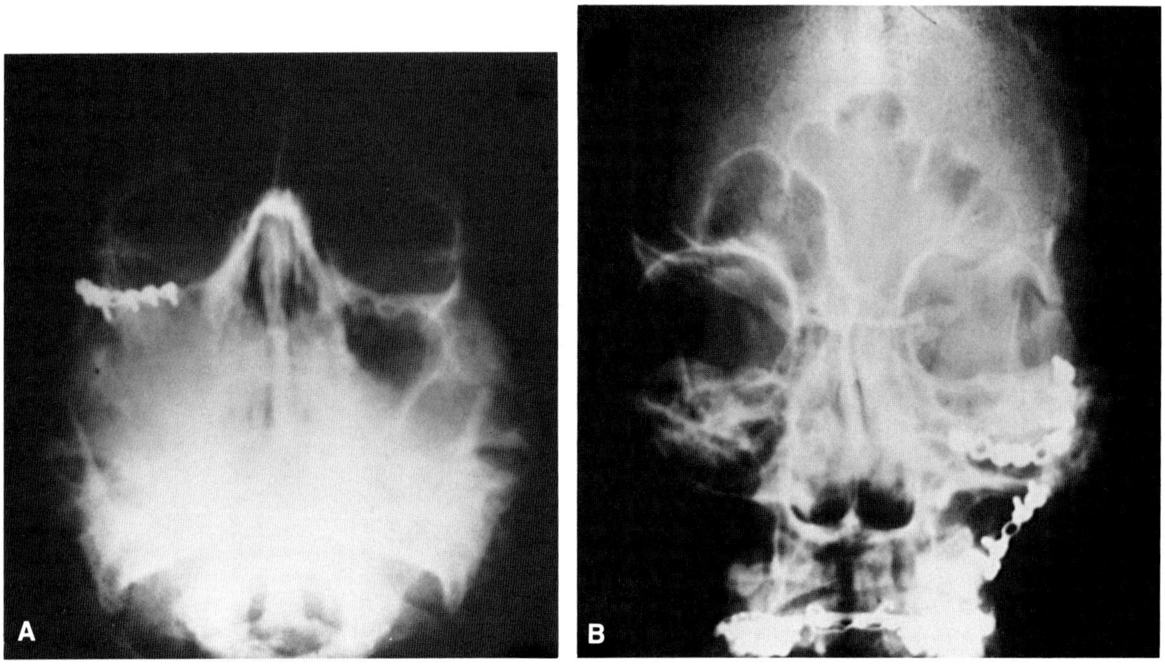

Figure 16–10. *Plate selection in midface fractures. A variety of shapes conforming to the anatomic features of the midface are available in most systems. These may be contoured to permit reconstitution of the (**A**) orbital rim, supraorbital rim, (**B**) malar eminence, maxilla, and nose.*

Screw Placement

Screws are most efficient when their axial force is directed at right angles to the plate and the underlying bone. Clinical situations may dictate that this direction be altered to provide bicortical screw placement without interference. Bicortical screw placement is recommended where possible because this improves both the pull-out strength and lateral stability of the screw. Most systems permit adequate engagement of the screw head in the plate hole through a range of about 30°. A drill hole with a diameter smaller than the screw must be made in the bone to prepare the way for the screw. This is best accomplished with a drill guide to ensure proper placement and direction. To prevent a horizontal moment of force on the plate, the screw hole should be in the center of the hole in the plate. An exception to this is with the dynamic compression hole. In this case a hole eccentrically placed away from the fracture produces a force that compresses the fracture ends together. Measurement of the hole dictates the appropriate screw length. Tapping is then done, if necessary, and the screw is placed passively, under irrigation.

In screw placement, it is better not to tighten the first screw until the second screw on the other side of the fracture is completely placed. This prevents movement of the plate into an undesirable position. If compression holes are used, it is not desirable to place more than one in a given direction. If two compression holes direct the plate in the same direction on the same side of the fracture, the second hole may produce a force greater than the first. In this situation, lateral forces are distributed between the screws in the static site on the same side of the fracture. Because fracture compression cannot distribute these forces, the result may be the loosening and subsequent failure of the hardware. For similar reasons, holes in the neutral position should be placed following the complete activation of dynamic compression holes.

Lag Screws

Functionally stable rigid internal fixation and interfragmentary compression can be achieved without the use of bone plates in selected cases. Oblique fractures, particularly those of the mandible and zygoma may be managed through the use of lag-screw fixation. A lag screw is one which is placed from the outer

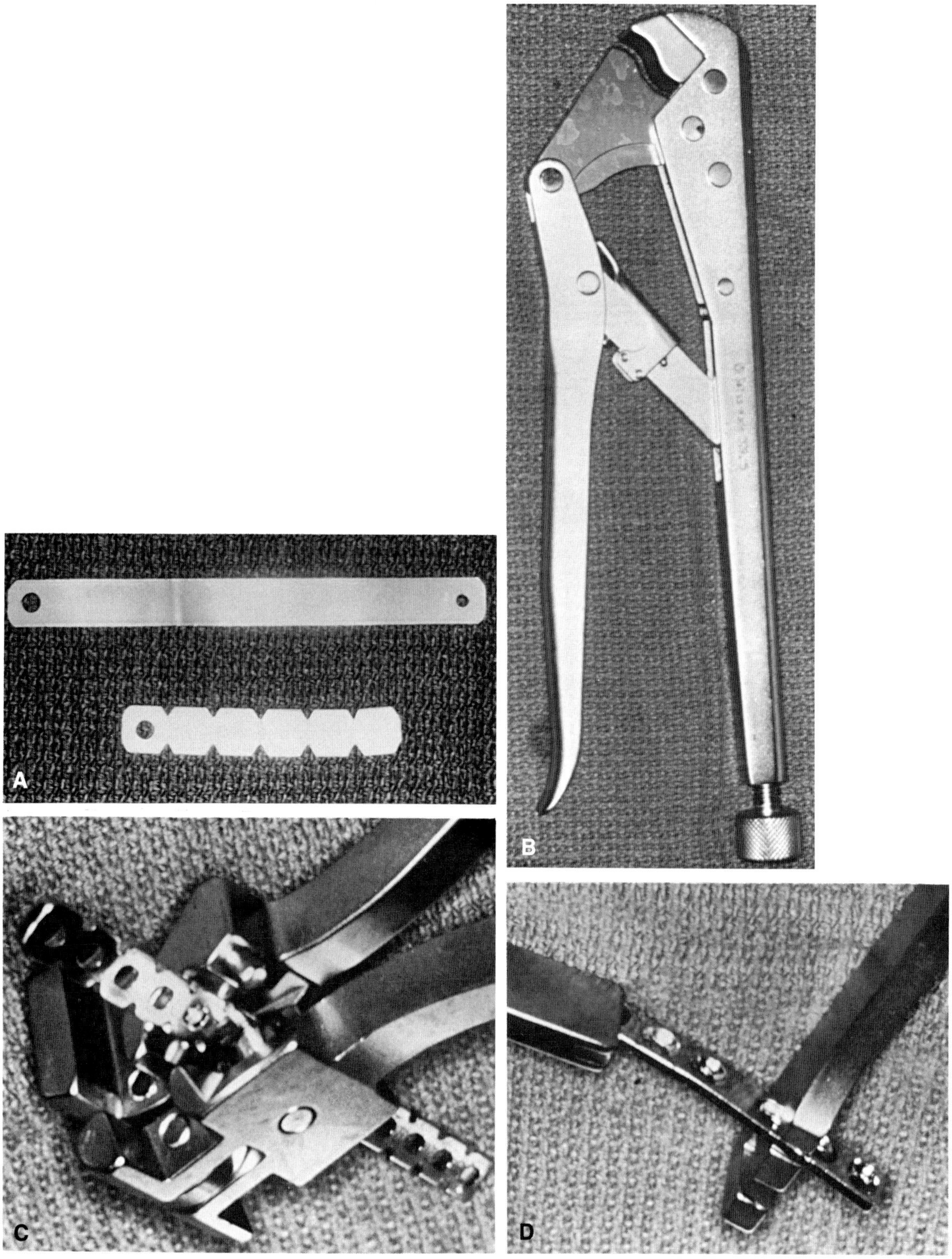

Figure 16–11. *(**A**) Templates are contoured to bone to assist accurate plate bending. (**B**) Bending instruments are designed to precisely bend plates. (**C**) The plate is first bent edgewise and along its flat surface. (**D**) Torsion is applied last.*

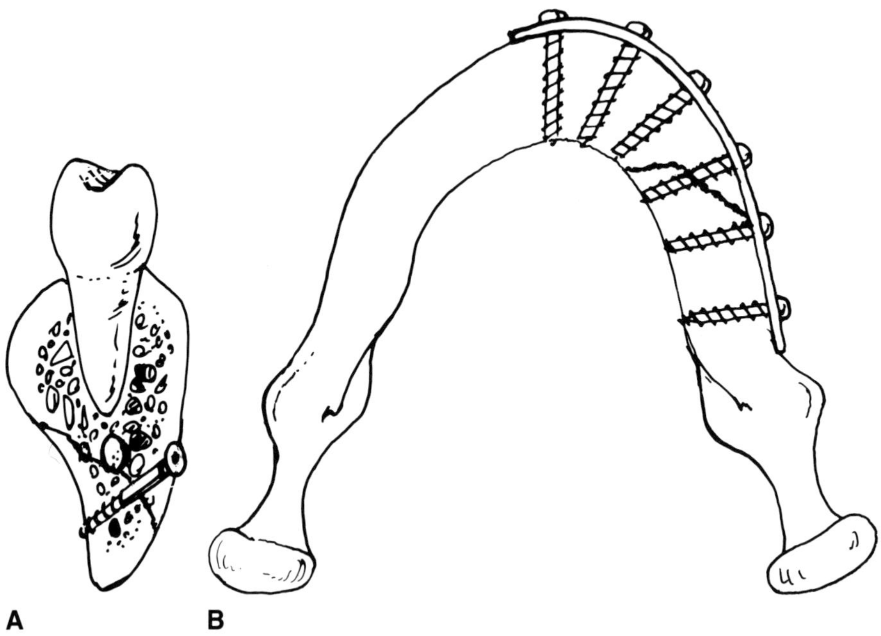

Figure 16–12. *The lag screw principle. (**A**) A lag screw glides through the outer hole and engages the inner hole to provide interfragmentary compression. (**B**) It may be used alone or in combination with plates.*

cortex on one side of the fracture site, then through the fracture site to engage the inner cortex on the other side. The screw threads only engage the bone in the inner cortex opposite the fracture site. The outer cortex is a gliding hole that engages only the screw head. As the screw is tightened, axially directed compression occurs across the fracture site (Fig. 16–12).

Niederdellmann has described successful rigid internal fixation of mandibular fractures with from one to three lag screws.[26, 27] Lag screws are most frequently used in symphysis and body fractures because of their usual fracture morphologic features (Fig. 16–13). To understand the lag screw principle, it is important to note that, if the screw threads engage both outer and inner cortex, the fracture segments may be driven apart or a gap maintained. Lag screws may be combined with the use of plates in complex or comminuted fractures.[28]

A lag screw is placed after the fracture is reduced and preloaded. A hole is drilled in the outer cortex only, at a diameter equalling that of the screw. An inner hole is drilled in the same direction at a smaller diameter. To broaden the area of screw contact in the outer cortex, a countersink is used to make a preparation that will accommodate the screw head. The measured screw then glides through the outer cortex and engages the inner cortex. If more than one lag screw is placed, all screws will need to be tightened further after the last is in position.

Wound Considerations

Care of the wound during and after surgery should be consistent with those principles delineated for contaminated wounds. Be reminded that the presence of hardware provides a surface against which blood and bacteria may rest during the early phases of healing. To reduce the incidence of infection, perioperative antibiotic prophylaxis is generally used. Attention to atraumatic dissection and complete hemostasis is important. Dilutional lavage of the contaminated operative site is helpful. Suction drainage of dead space, particularly in tissues abutting the implant is occasionally indicated. Closure in anatomic layers further reduces dead space.

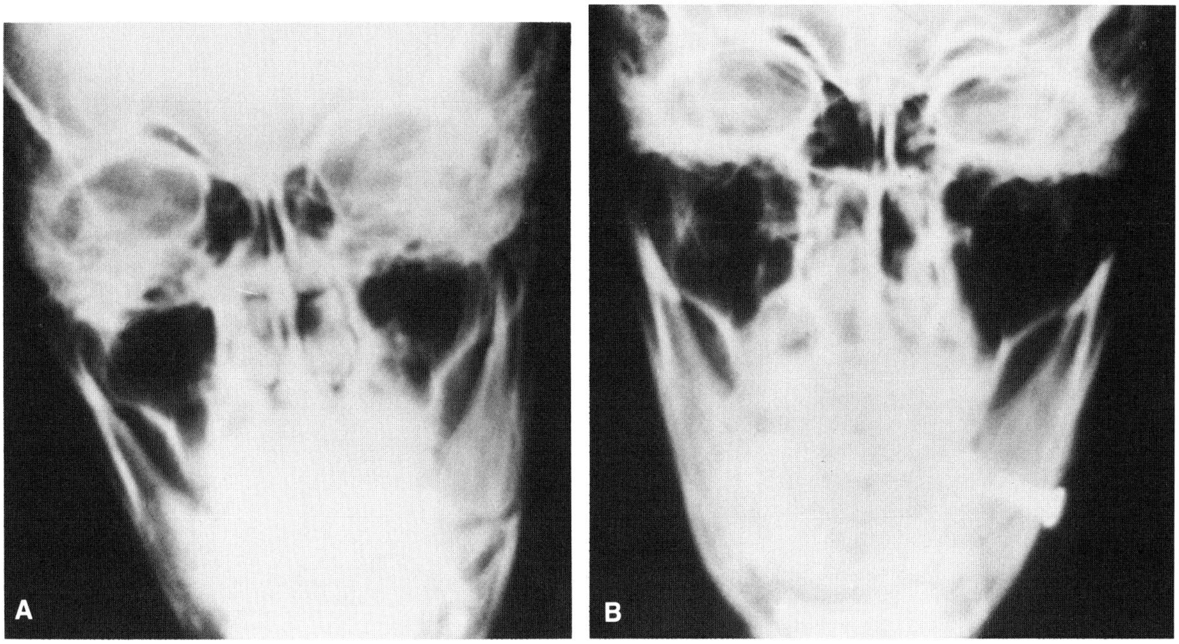

Figure 16–13. *(**A** and **B**) Lag screws are employed commonly as a single mode of fixation for parasymphyseal fractures and angle fractures.*

CLINICAL APPLICATION IN MANDIBLE FRACTURES

Indications for rigid internal fixation of mandibular fractures include anatomic reasons for open reduction and medical and social reasons that indicate a need to avoid intermaxillary fixation. Anatomic reasons include unstable fracture of the mandibular symphysis and angle. Anatomic considerations only rarely dictate open reduction of mandibular body and vertical ramus fractures. Of continued controversy are those indications for open reduction of condylar fractures. Rigid internal fixation maintains anatomic reduction of condylar fractures.

Avoidance of intermaxillary fixation is helpful in fractures associated with temporomandibular joint injury because posttrauma physiotherapy can be employed much earlier without intermaxillary fixation. Neurologic injury and other multiple injuries may also benefit from the avoidance of intermaxillary fixation.

The increased risks of the use of rigid internal fixation appear to be those associated with any surgical procedure in this region. Morbidity of rigid internal fixation of mandible fractures is comparable to other methods of open reduction, except in the incidence of infection—less infections were reported in cases of rigid internal fixation of open reductions of mandible fractures than in other procedures.[29] Rigid internal fixation causes less postoperative infection than does interfragmentary mobility.

Fractures of the mandibular symphysis region have been treated successfully by a number of rigid internal fixation techniques. These include lag screws, paired miniplates with 2-mm screws in the neutral zone, and mandibular bone plates with 2.7-mm screws in the compression zone at the inferior border. Of these methods, the greatest interfragmentary compression occurs with lag screws. The greatest fracture stability is likely with the use of a six-hole mandibular bone plate.

In treating a symphyseal fracture, attention must be given to the lingual aspect of the fracture to ensure proper reduction and screw placement. An open lingual plate in conjunction with a condylar fracture results in flaring of the angle of the mandible and buccal movement of the posterior dentition.

Comminution of symphysis fractures commonly occurs in the area of the digastric muscle attachment

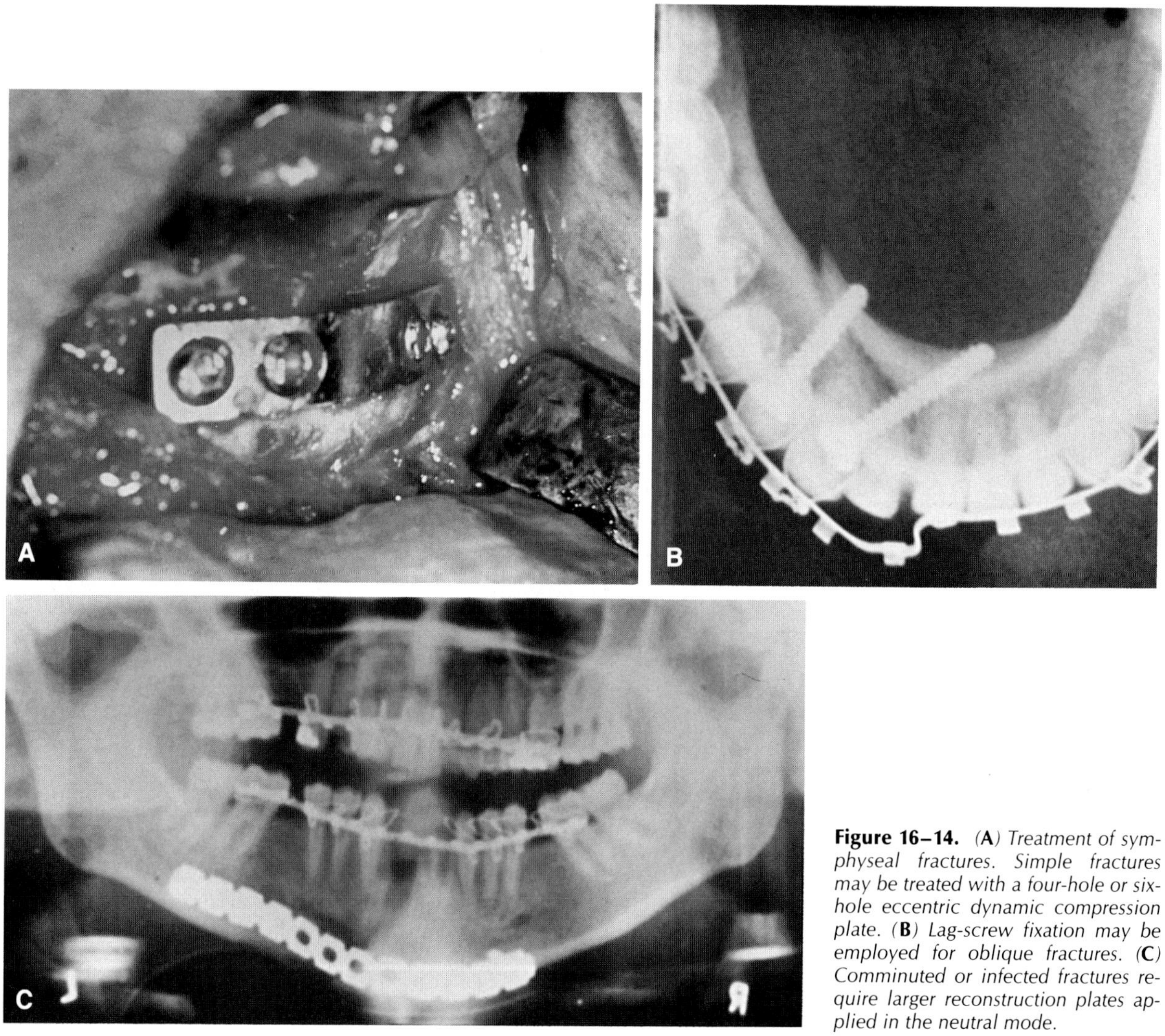

Figure 16–14. *(**A**) Treatment of symphyseal fractures. Simple fractures may be treated with a four-hole or six-hole eccentric dynamic compression plate. (**B**) Lag-screw fixation may be employed for oblique fractures. (**C**) Comminuted or infected fractures require larger reconstruction plates applied in the neutral mode.*

where a triangle of bone often becomes separated. This may be attached to the proximal mandible with a lag screw. The main fracture can then be plated. Fractures of the alveolar process may be fixed to the basal bone by means of a miniplate after the rigid internal fixation of the basal bone (Fig. 16–14).

When indicated, rigid internal fixation of body fractures may be accomplished through the use of lag screws or mandibular bone plates in the compression zone. Monocortical screws with miniplates have also been used in the neutral zone.[30] A detailed understanding of the location of the mandibular nerve is necessary to avoid injury during screw placement. If a mandibular bone plate is used, the screws may be directed inferiorly to pass beneath the nerve. Occasionally, the mandibular nerve appears too low on radiographs to warrant risking its damage with screw placement. In this situation, the plate may be placed high in the neutral zone or a longer plate may be selected.

Fractures of the mandibular angle have been successfully managed with lag screws, miniplates in the tension zone, and mandibular bone plates at the inferior border. Mandibular bone plates are usually placed by a transcervical approach because transoral visualization is difficult. If a mandibular plate is placed transorally, a transbuccal trochar is needed to place the screws (Fig. 16–15).

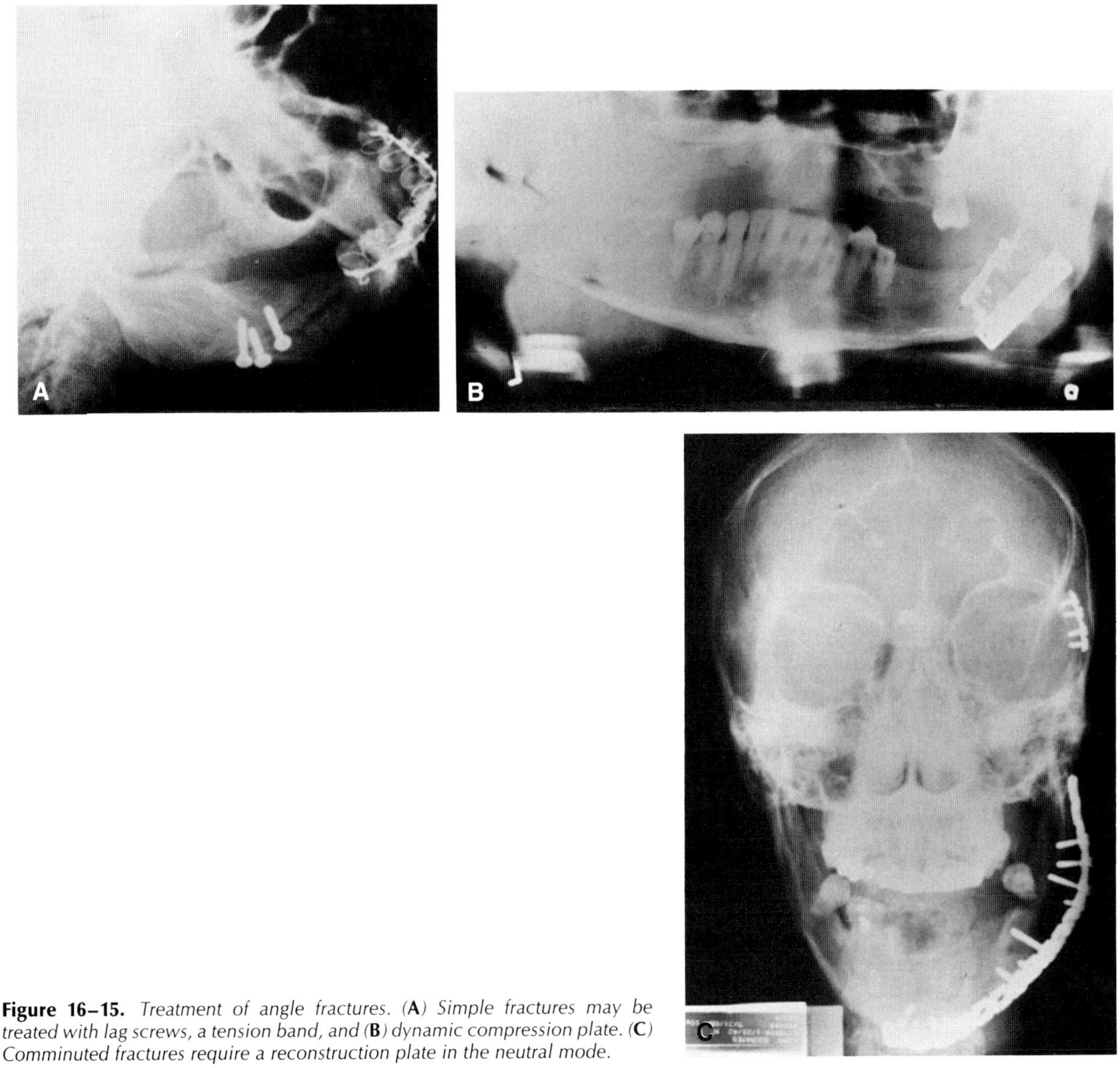

Figure 16–15. *Treatment of angle fractures. (**A**) Simple fractures may be treated with lag screws, a tension band, and (**B**) dynamic compression plate. (**C**) Comminuted fractures require a reconstruction plate in the neutral mode.*

The chief advantage of miniplate fixation in this region is that it is easily done transorally. Miniplate fixation of the mandibular angle is ill-suited to sustaining full masticatory loads in the molar area. For this reason, temporary use of intermaxillary fixation after surgery may be necessary. This technique is often referred to as *semirigid fixation*.

Condylar neck fractures are generally managed with miniplate fixation. Low subcondylar fractures may be approached transorally. The miniplate that is to be applied may be twisted to permit anteroposterior transoral placement of screws in the condylar neck and placement of screws on the lateral ramus with a transbuccal trochar.

CLINICAL APPLICATION IN MIDFACE FRACTURES

The goals of management of midface fractures are both aesthetic and functional. The masticatory system, ocular orbital apparatus, airway, sinuses, and aesthetic contours of the face must all be considered in producing optimal surgical care. Traditional methods of treat-

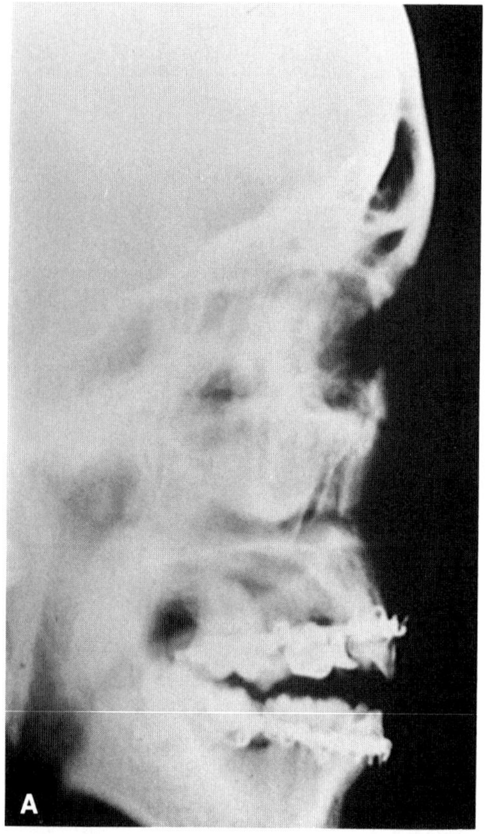

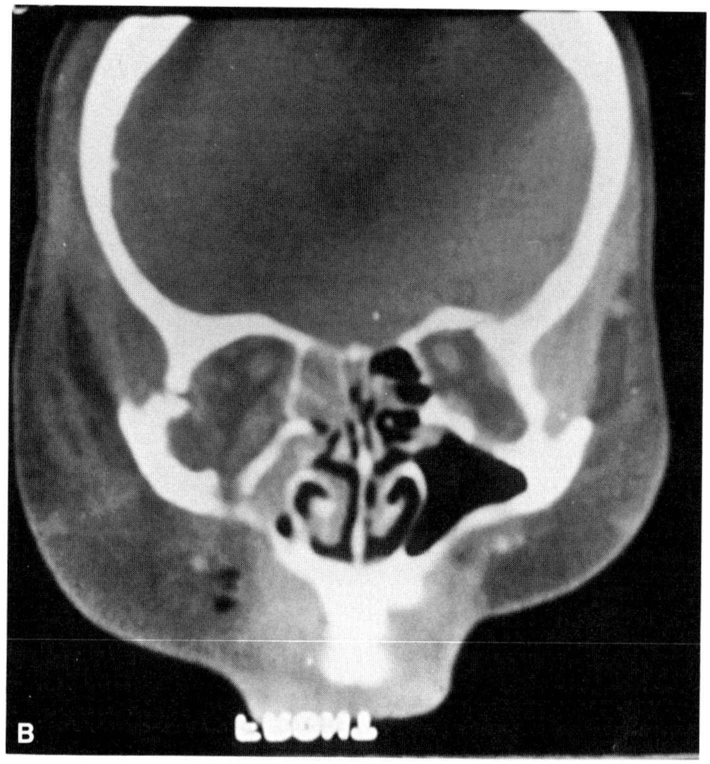

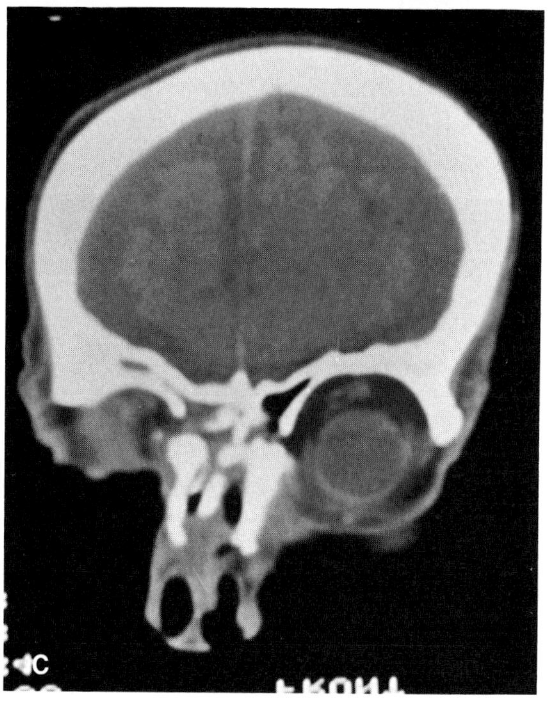

Figure 16–16. (**A**) *A lateral cephalogram reveals changes in the vertical dimension and anterior projection.* (**B**) *Coronal CT scanning assists in the delineation of potential fixation sites at the zygomatic buttress,* (**C**) *orbital rim, and nasofrontal region.*

ment of midface fractures with transosseous and suspension wiring does not offer the means to maintain anatomic restoration of form. Rigid internal fixation provides the force necessary to preserve anatomic reduction obtained at the time of surgery. Although nonunion is not a frequent problem in the management of midface fractures, the loss of substance and cicatrization that occurs to finally permit union has adverse clinical outcomes, which were previously delineated.[11,31]

The LeFort I fracture can be reduced in its anteroposterior and transverse dimensions with the anatomic placement of intermaxillary fixation. Only restoration of the vertical dimension is not addressed by this method. Suspension wiring does not prevent shortening or late posterior movement of the maxilla. Hence, the goal of rigid internal fixation of LeFort I fractures is to restore facial height, permit early primary bone healing, and thereby minimize posterior contracture of the maxilla.

Preoperative clinical examination should reveal whether there is a loss of vertical dimension and whether the maxilla telescopes superiorly. This may be checked by seeing the lip to tooth ratio at rest and checking it again with the patient clenching his or her teeth. If there is no telescoping or loss of vertical dimension, then it is possible that the fracture can be managed without rigid internal fixation. The use of a cephalometric radiograph taken with the patient clenching his or her teeth quantifies the derangements present in the maxillary position.

Preoperative coronal computed tomography (CT) scans of the maxilla should be examined to select the buttresses that are sufficiently cleanly fractured to permit easy anatomic rigid internal fixation (Fig. 16–16). With the condyles serving as two points, a third point that is determined at one reliably anatomic maxillary buttress will precisely position the maxilla. A miniplate of at least four holes should be placed at this point. These three points define a plane identical to the preinjury position of the maxilla (Fig. 16–17).

Debate exists over what degree of further treatment is necessary at the LeFort I level. Plates may certainly be electively placed at other available sutures before intermaxillary fixation is removed. Difficulties in planning therapy arise when, as is often the case, there is a great deal of comminution of the antral walls. Bony parts are always present and waiting to be adapted with a contour restoring plate.[12] Cranial bone grafts with the

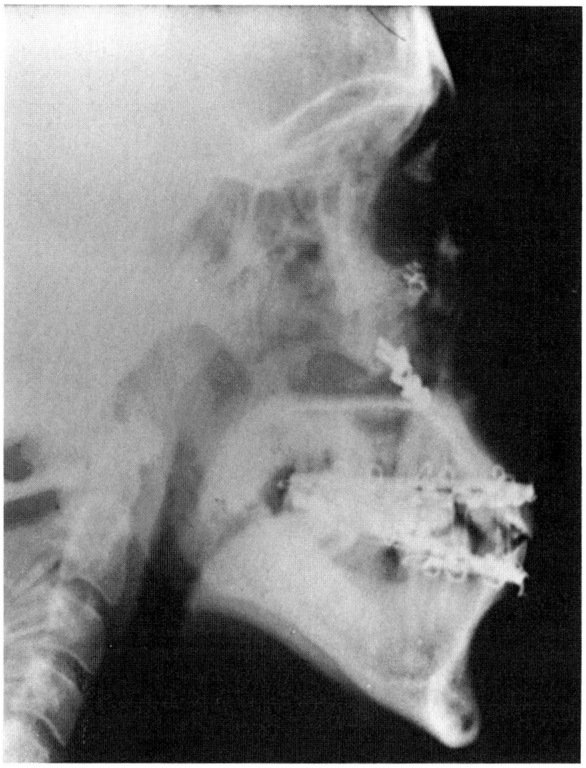

Figure 16–17. *With restoration of a single buttress, the vertical dimension and anterior projection of the face is restored if combined with intact condyles and a normal occlusion.*

application of plates to restore each zygomatic buttress and piriform rim have been used extensively.[32,33]

Zygoma fractures require three-dimensionally stable, rigid fixation to prevent inferior, posterior, and medial movement of the zygoma during function and healing. Before the application of any fixation, exposure of all necessary surgical sites and initial reduction should be carried out. For example, if orbital floor exploration is necessary, exposure of the subciliary site and zygomaticofrontal suture should precede the application of irreversible fixation.

The tension zone of the zygoma is at the zygomaticofrontal suture. A four-holed tension band placed at this site offers sufficient fixation to permit anatomic union even in the presence of comminution elsewhere. Additional plates at the zygomatic buttress or infraorbital rim are necessary only if maxillary or medial orbital fractures are present (Fig. 16–18).

In many zygoma fractures, the frontal component is generated inferior to the attachment of the lateral

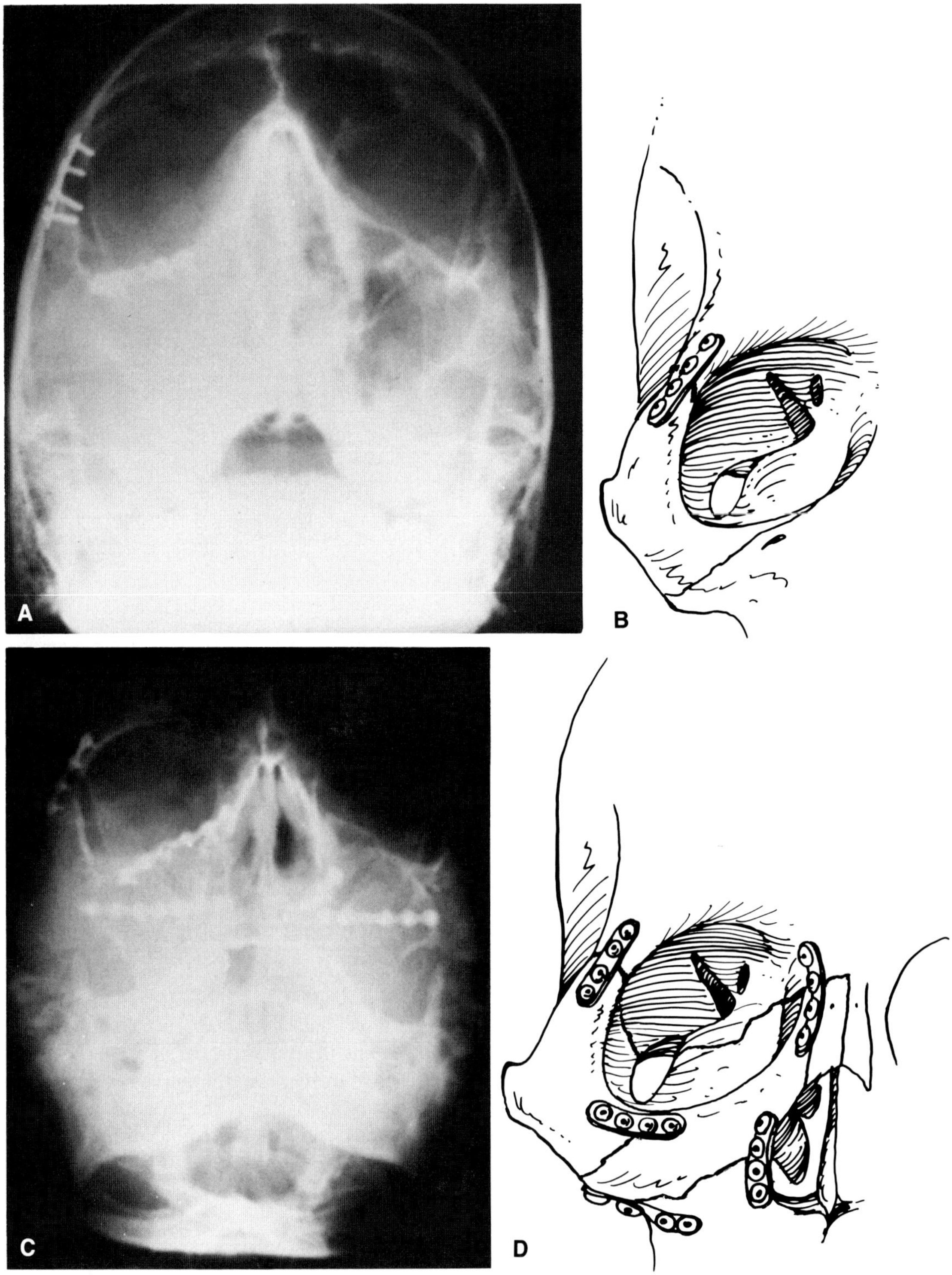

Figure 16–18. *(**A** and **B**) Simple fractures may achieve three-dimensionally stable fixation with a single plate at the zygomaticofrontal suture. (**C** and **D**) Complex fractures of the malar complex and associated bony buttresses require multiple sites of fixation.*

canthal ligament at the orbital tubercle. In these cases a single arc-shaped plate may be used to restore the contour of the zygoma. With a subciliary approach, screws are first placed in the intact bone of the frontal region and the nasomaxillary complex. The reduced zygoma is then attached to the center of the contoured plate. Other alternative sites of fixation include the zygomatic buttress and the piriform rim to zygomatic body.

Inadvertent overrotation of a zygoma fracture reduction may produce a bowing of the zygomatic arch. Where proper positioning of the zygoma is in doubt, the examination of a third site may be necessary to better define the position. The zygomatic buttress or the zygomatic arch (if a bicoronal flap is being used) will serve this purpose. Although an additional site is exposed, no additional fixation is necessary for the sake of the zygoma fracture.

Fractures of the medial orbital rim and nasomaxillary complex are normally reduced after the zygoma is fixed at the zygomaticofrontal site. This permits stabilization with a four-hole miniplate at the now stabilized infraorbital rim. Orbital wall reconstruction should be carried out against the fixed and anatomically reduced zygoma. This offers the greatest stability to bone grafts or alloplasts in the orbit.

Nasofrontal fractures and frontal sinus fractures are also amenable to fixation with contour-restoring plates.[34] Short monocortical screws prevent projection of the screw heads into the frontal sinus or cranium. Bicortical screws may be safely placed if directed into the orbit. An orbital protector should be used when carrying this out.

The integrated management of panfacial fractures with rigid internal fixation can only produce a stable restoration of anatomic form if the sequence of the reduction and fixation is logical. Unlike traditional treatment, the principle of "inside out, bottom up" does not apply.[13,35] It is better to think of the facial skeleton as a jigsaw puzzle in which the edges are treated first, on the top, the bottom, and laterally. A patient with fractures in all major components of the facial skeleton could be successfully managed as follows. After intermaxillary fixation is placed, the mandibular symphysis, body, and angle may be reduced and rigidly fixed. Restoration of the posterior facial height with open reduction of the condyles is necessary in a panfacial fracture. This establishes the position of the maxilla in its anteroposterior and transverse dimensions. Unlike a LeFort I fracture, rigid fixation of the

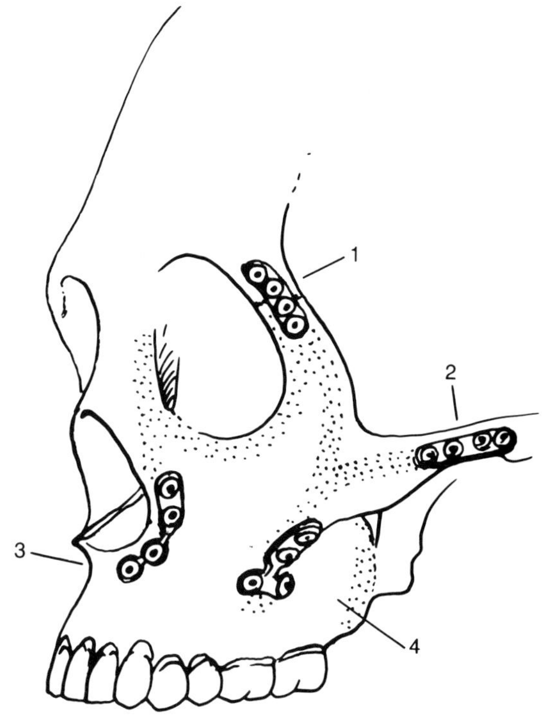

Figure 16–19. *Zygoma and LeFort I fracture order of fixation. After all fractures are grossly reduced and intermaxillary fixation is achieved, plates are placed in the zygomaticofrontal region (**1**), zygomatic arch (**2**), piriform rim (**3**), and zygomatic buttress (**4**).*

maxillary buttresses is not indicated at this time because this would most probably have to be redone later. The anterior vertical dimension of the face must be restored from the top down (Fig. 16–19). Reduction and fixation of the zygoma fractures may then be carried out with the careful restoration of facial height in the zygomatic buttress integrated with this portion of the procedure. With the main aspects of the three dimensions of the face now restored attention can be directed to the center of the face, including the nasal septum, nasomaxillary complex, orbit, and nasofrontal regions (Fig. 16–20).

COMPLICATIONS: ETIOLOGY AND MANAGEMENT

Complications of rigid internal fixation of facial fractures include infection, nonunion, malunion, and malocclusion. Many but not all complications can be traced to failures in techniques or violation of biomechanical principles.

Infection of the operative site in rigid internal fixa-

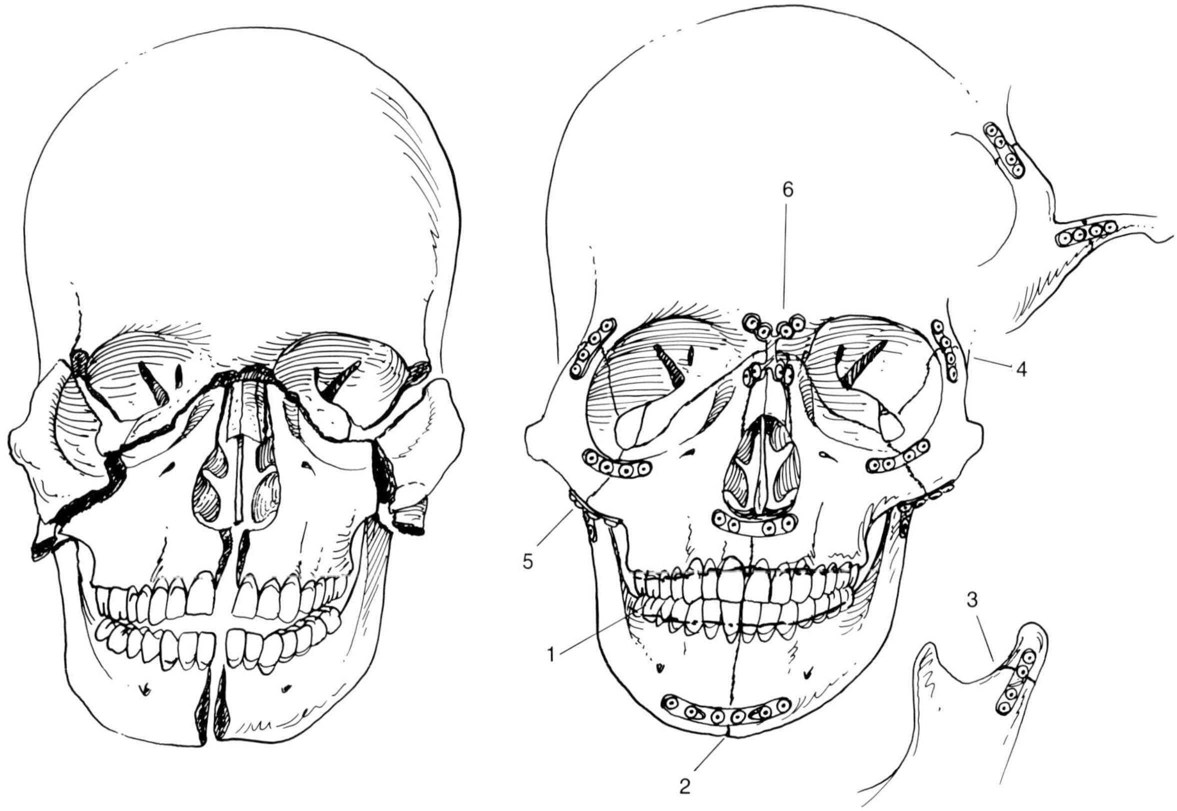

Figure 16–20. *Schematic of panfacial fracture management. After intermaxillary fixation (**1**), open reduction of mandible fractures is accomplished (**2** and **3**). The zygomas are then restored (**4**). Next the maxilla may be fixed to the zygomas (**5**). With the vertical dimension, projection, and width of the face restored, the central midface and nasofrontal regions are treated (**6**).*

tion is usually a result of failure of fixation and interfragmentary mobility. All operative sites in the facial skeleton are colonized by bacteria, and movement about the fracture site causes repeated hemorrhage as young capillaries are torn by movement. Blood provides nutrition to the colonized bacteria resulting in cellulitis.

Restoration of rigid internal fixation and supportive therapy resolves the infection by providing a stable environment for healing. All loose hardware should be removed and replaced with adequate fixation. This may necessitate placing a larger plate with new screws further from the fracture site. Alternatively, external pin fixation may be used. New internal fixation is not normally placed in the presence of acute cellulitis. In some cases of infection, no interfragmentary mobility is evident on clinical examination, and there are no revealing radiographic findings. Exploration of the operative site to perform necessary debridement of necrotic bone and adjustment of hardware is sometimes indicated. If hardware is exposed but not loose it need not be removed.

Nonunion may result from persistent interfragmentary mobility and infection. Rigid internal or external fixation is employed in these cases until the active drainage of pus becomes quiescent. Autogenous bone grafting may be indicated to permit fracture union.

Malocclusion following rigid internal fixation of facial fractures has been noted by Assael to occur in 8% of cases.[29] Unlike nonrigid techniques, orthopedic tractional forces cannot be used to reposition bones once rigidly fixed because the in situ hardware will become loosened. If a malocclusion is noted, clinical examination, imaging, and study models should be used to determine its cause.

Some of the reasons for postoperative malocclusion

include occult fracture, muscle splinting, capsular edema of the temporomandibular joint, dental injury, an improperly bent plate, or orthodontic movement of teeth.[3] Occult fractures include condylar fractures and alveolar fractures.

Muscle splinting and capsular edema often produce an early class III open-bite tendency. Intermaxillary fixation is not recommended for this problem because orthodontic movement of the teeth and a more permanent malocclusion may result. As edema and postoperative pain resolve, so will this malocclusion.

If the malocclusion is thought to be due to incorrectly placed hardware, the replacement of the fixation at the earliest possible time is indicated. This may be avoided only if the discrepancy is small and can be compensated for by conservative means such as orthodontics or restorative dentistry.

Malunion in the midface is an early event, requiring only 4 to 6 weeks. In these cases repositioning of the affected bones may be impossible. In such cases early osteotomy and bone grafting with rigid internal fixation may be indicated.

CLINICAL DECISION MAKING

Rigid internal fixation should not be used for every clinical situation, every patient, or every surgeon. Other means of managing nearly every facial fracture exist. When prescribing therapy, the surgeon must consider what is optimal from a physiologic point of view, as well as from his own ability to effectively employ therapy.

Rigid internal fixation of facial fractures is a demanding and unforgiving technique. It requires the development and maintenance of precise technical skills.

REFERENCES

1. Danis R. Theorie et pratique de l'osteosynthese. Paris: Masson, 1949.
2. Muller M, Allgower M, Willeneger H. Manual of internal fixation. Berlin: Springer-Verlag, 1979.
3. Assael L. Complications of rigid internal fixation of the facial skeleton. Oral Maxillofac Surg Clin North Am 1990; 2:3.
4. Kent J, Neary J, Silvia C, Zide M. Open reduction of fractured mandibular condyles. Oral Maxillofac Surg Clin North Am 1990; 2:1, 69.
5. Rahn B. Biomechanics of fracture treatment. In: Spiessl, ed. Internal fixation of the mandible. Berlin: Springer-Verlag, 1989: 19.
6. Lambotte A. Le Traitment des Fractures. Paris: Masson, 1907.
7. Muller M, Allgower M, Willenegger H. Technique of internal fixation of fractures. Berlin: Springer-Verlag, 1965.
8. Luhr H. Operative behandlungsverfahren bei frakturen des zahnlosen unterkiefers unter besonderer berucksichtigung der kompressions osteosynthese. Chir Plast Recons 1970; 7:84.
9. Spiessl B. Rigid internal fixation of fractures of the lower jaw. In: Chapchal G, ed. Reconstructive surgery and traumatology. Basel: Karger, 1972.
10. Spiessl B. New concepts in maxillofacial bone surgery. Berlin: Springer-Verlag, 1976: 21.
11. Assael L. Considerations in rigid internal fixation of midface trauma. Oral Maxillofac Surg Clin North Am 1990; 2:1, 103.
12. Schilli W. Internal fixation of zygomatic and midface fractures by means of miniplates and lag screws. In: Schilli W, Kruger. Oral and maxillofacial traumatology, vol. 2. Chicago: Quintescence, 1986.
13. Willeneger H, Peren S, Schenk R. Primare und sekundare knochenbrucheilung. Chirurg 1971; 42:252.
14. Rahn B. Paper presented at the Association for the Study of Internal Fixation, Advanced Applications in Maxillofacial Surgery, Phoenix, AZ, February 1990.
15. Phillips J, Rahn B. Comparison and torque measurements of self tapping and pretapped screws. Plast Reconstr Surg. 1989; 83:447.
16. Buchbinder D. Use of rigid internal fixation in the treatment of mandibular fractures. Oral Maxillofac Surg Clin North Am 1990: 41.
17. Perren S, Russenberger M. A dynamic compression plate. Acta Orthop Scand 1969; 125 (Suppl): 29.
18. Perren S. The reaction of cortical bone to compression. Acta Orthop Scand 1969; 125 (Suppl): 17.
19. Prein J. Rigid internal fixation of compound mandibular fractures. In: Spiessl B. New concepts in maxillofacial bone surgery. Berlin: Springer-Verlag, 1976: 35.
20. Schmoker R, Spiessl B. Exczentrisch dynamische kompressionsplatte. Schweiz Mschr Zahnheilk 1973; 83:12.
21. Spiessl B. Internal fixation of the mandible. Berlin: Springer-Verlag, 1989.
22. Schilli W, Harle F. Functionally stable osteosynthesis: A problem of surgical approach. Fortschr Kiefer u Gesichtschir 1976; 21:300.
23. Schmoker R. Experimental studies on the effect of rigidity using an excentric dynamic compression plate (EDCP). In: Spiessl B. New concepts in maxillofacial bone surgery. Berlin: Springer-Verlag, 1976: 41.
24. Champy M, Lodde J, Wilk A. Osteosynthesis mandiublaires selon la technique de Michelet. Rev Stomatol Chir Maxillofac 1976; 77:569.
25. Kroon F. Paper presented at the Association for the Study of Internal Fixation Meeting, Davos, Switzerland, December 1989.

26. Neiderdellmann H. Rigid internal fixation by means of lag screws. In: Schilli W, Kruger. Oral and maxillofacial traumatology. Chicago: Quintescence, 1982: 371.
27. Neiderdellmann H, Shelty V. Solitary lag screw fixation in the treatment of fractures of the mandible: A retrospective study. Plast Reconstr Surg 1977; 80:68.
28. Schwimmer A. Lag screw fixation in maxillofacial trauma. Oral Maxillofac Surg Clin North Am 1990; 195.
29. Assael L, Hammon K. A comparison of rigid internal fixation with wire osteosynthesis of mandibular fractures. J Oral Maxillofac Surg 1987; 45:M5.
30. Champy M, Pape H, Gerlach K, et al. The Strasbourg miniplate osteosynthesis. In: Schilli W, Kruger. Oral and maxillofacial traumatology, vol. 2. Chicago: Quintescence, 1986: 19.
31. Hotte H. Orbital fractures. Springfield: Charles C Thomas, 1970.
32. Gruss J. Naso-ethmoid-orbital fractures: Classification and role of primary bone grafting. Plast Reconstr Surg 1985; 75:303.
33. Gruss J, et al. The role of primary bone grafting in complex craniomaxillofacial traums. Plast Reconstr Surg 1985; 75:17.
34. Manson P. Cranial orbital fractures. Oral Maxillofac Surg Clin North Am 1990: 121.
35. Manson P. Facial injuries. In: McCarthy. Plastic surgery. Philadelphia: WB Saunders, 1990: 867.

17

Management of Alveolar and Dental Fractures

Joseph E. Margarone
Richard Hall

ETIOLOGY AND INCIDENCE

Injuries to the dentoalveolar complex are fairly common and can be caused by a variety of circumstances. The majority of these injuries are produced by vehicle accidents (including automobiles, motorcycles, and bicycles), assaults, falls, and sports-related and work-related injuries (Fig. 17–1).[1] Teeth also can be injured by physicians and dentists, especially in an operating room setting, by an inappropriately directed laryngoscope during intubation for general anesthesia. In addition, iatrogenic trauma also can occur during dentoalveolar surgery. Teeth can be chipped and fractured when struck by instruments during the extraction of teeth.

The frequency and nature of dentoalveolar injuries vary and are largely dependent on the cause and the gender and age of the individual at the time of trauma. Although there is a wide range in the reported incidences, those reporting the highest incidence of alveolar fractures are surveys of fractures in pediatric populations, who constitute only 5% of all facial fractures.[3] This increased incidence may be a reflection of anatomic differences between the adult and pediatric facial skeleton, but most likely it reflects the differences in causes—i.e., assaults and motor vehicle accidents in adults versus sporting or play injuries and falls in children.

Several excellent reviews in the literature report on the cause, pathogenesis, and frequency of injuries to the teeth.[2,4] As with alveolar fractures, the type of dental injury seen and its association with other soft tissue injuries is greatly dependent on the age of the patient and etiologic mechanism. Injuries to the deciduous dentition show a greater occurrence of luxations and exarticulations when compared to injuries to the permanent dentition, in which the most common injury appears to be crown and crown-root fractures.[2] In his review of the causes and pathogenesis of dental injuries, Andreasen reported that, of trauma to the primary dentition, 10% involved crown or crown-root fracture, whereas 75% involved luxations and exarticulations. A similar assessment of injuries to the permanent dentition showed crown or crown-root fracture involvement to represent 39%.[2] It is probable that this difference again is due partly to the anatomic differences between adult and pediatric teeth and supporting structures.

CLASSIFICATION

A number of systems for the classification of dental and dentoalveolar trauma have been developed in an attempt to produce a universally acceptable system that allows for uniformity of description of injuries for

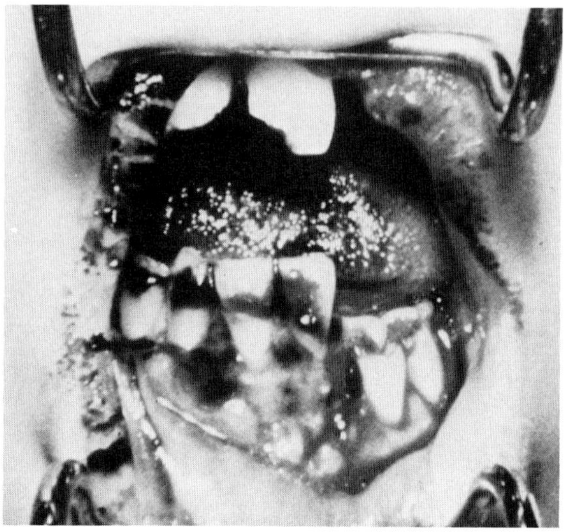

Figure 17–1. *Multiple dentoalveolar trauma secondary to a motor vehicle accident.*

communication purposes and treatment planning.[5-12] These systems vary and are based on classification by anatomic site of the injury, cause, treatment alternatives, or a combination of these. The three most common systems for classifying dentoalveolar injuries currently in use are those developed by Ellis and Davey,[13] Andreasen,[4,14] and Sanders et al.[15]

Ellis and Davey originally developed their classification system to describe injuries to the anterior teeth of the deciduous and permanent dentition, although it can be used to describe injuries anywhere in the dentoalveolar complex.[13] Injuries are divided into eight classes based on the anatomic nature and location of the injury, with no consideration given to the mechanism that produced the injury. Some of the classes contain subdivisions that relate to the magnitude of the injury or various recommended treatment options. The major problem with this system is that it is difficult to remember the specific definition for each of the classes.[15] Information dissemination to other healthcare professionals or lay people is problematic if they are not fully conversant with the system. In addition, the system becomes unwieldy because some injuries can be placed into several classes (e.g., an avulsed tooth can be in class 5 or class 7, division 3), whereas other injury combinations are not categorized (e.g., displacement of a tooth with an accompanying fracture of the crown or the root).

Andreasen developed a comprehensive classification system paralleling the World Health Organization's system for disease classification, using the International Classification of Diseases (ICD) codes.[14] This system was refined to take into account anatomic, therapeutic, and prognostic considerations.[4] In Andreasen's redefined classification, dentoalveolar injuries were divided into four large categories: injuries to the dental tissues and the pulp (Fig. 17–2); injuries to the periodontal tissues (Fig. 17–3); injuries to the supporting bone (Fig. 17–4); and injuries to the gingiva or oral mucosa. The latter is not considered in this chapter. Six types of injuries to the teeth were described (Fig. 17–2A–F). These categories are:

1. Crown infraction, i.e., a craze line or crack in the tooth without loss of tooth substance
2. Crown fracture confined to enamel or enamel and dentin with no root exposure (uncomplicated)
3. Crown fracture producing a pulp exposure (complicated)
4. Fracture involving the enamel, dentin, and cementum without pulp exposure (uncomplicated crown-root fracture)
5. Fracture involving the enamel, dentin, and cementum with pulp exposure (complicated crown-root fracture)
6. Root fracture involving the dentin and cementum and producing a pulp exposure (root fracture)

Injuries to the periodontal tissues were divided into six categories and encompass what are commonly referred to as subluxations and avulsions (Fig. 17–3A–D). These categories are:

1. Concussion, which is defined as an injury to the periodontium, producing sensitivity to percussion without loosening or displacement of the tooth
2. Subluxation, in which the tooth is loosened but not displaced
3. Luxation, dislocation, or partial avulsion, in which the tooth is displaced, with or without an accompanying comminution or fracture of the alveolar socket (Three types of luxation are described by the direction in which the tooth is displaced: intrusive, extrusive, and lateral.)
4. Exarticulation, in which the tooth is completely displaced out of the alveolus

Injuries to the supporting bone were divided into four categories with different ICD code numbers given for fractures located in the maxilla versus the mandible. These are (Fig. 17–4A, B):

1. Comminution of the alveolar housing, often occurring with an intrusive or lateral luxation

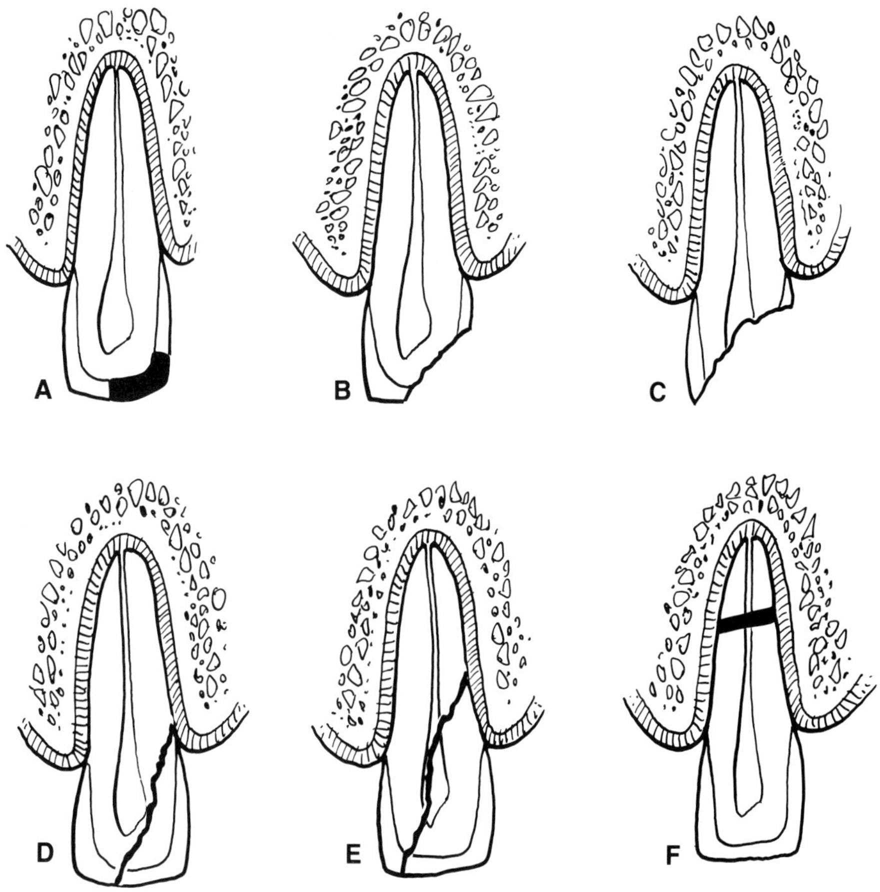

Figure 17–2. *Diagram of injuries to dental tissue and pulp. (**A**) Crown infraction. (**B**) Crown fracture confined to enamel and dentin (uncomplicated crown fracture). (**C**) Crown fracture directly involving pulp (complicated). (**D**) Uncomplicated root fracture. (**E**) Complicated crown root fracture. (**F**) Horizontal root fracture. (After Andreasen JO, ed. Traumatic injuries of the teeth, ed 1. Philadelphia: WB Saunders, 1972).*

2. Fracture of a single wall of an alveolus, i.e., lateral, buccal, or labial (vestibular) and lingual or palatal
3. Fracture of the alveolar process, en bloc, in a patient having teeth, but without the fracture line necessarily extending through a tooth socket
4. Fracture involving the main body of the mandible or maxilla

Finally, injuries to the gingiva or oral mucosa are categorized as:

1. Laceration
2. Contusion
3. Abrasion

One advantage of this system is that the categories are well described and appear to encompass all possible dentoalveolar injuries. Because the system is anatomically based, it also allows for the development of a treatment system within each injury category. In addition, it can be used to classify injuries to both the permanent and deciduous dentition, and by providing ICD codes in its original form, it is useful for medicolegal purposes. The disadvantages of this system are similar to those stated for that developed by Ellis and Davey and, indeed, are even more formidable because there are more levels of injury in the Andreasen system to recall.

To eliminate the disadvantage of memorizing category descriptions in the previous two classification systems, Sanders et al. presented a more simplified scheme based solely on a description of the injury sustained during trauma.[15] They divided traumatic injuries to the teeth and supporting structures into 13 categories depending on: the tooth structures involved; the type of displacement (if any); and the direction of the crown or root fracture. A summary of their classification system is presented in Table 17–1. This system was further simplified by Assael and Ellis who combined several categories into "alveolar process fractures" and eliminated a designation for maxillary and mandibular fractures.[16]

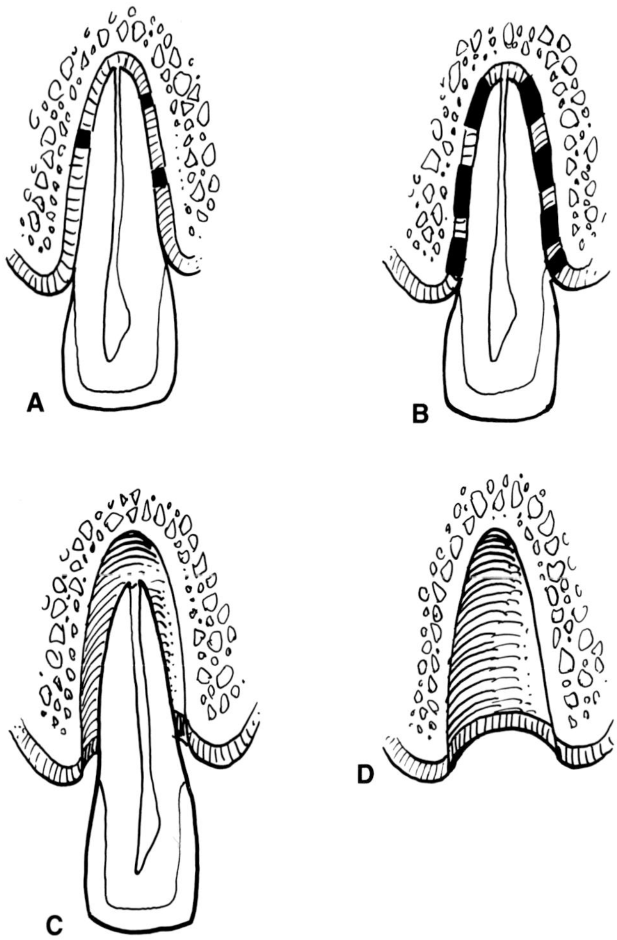

Figure 17–3. *Diagram of injuries to periodontal tissues. (**A**) Periodontal concussion. (**B**) Subluxation. (**C**) Luxation, dislocation, or partial avulsion. (**D**) Exarticulation or avulsion. (After Andreasen JO, ed. Traumatic injuries of the teeth, ed 1. Philadelphia: WB Saunders, 1972.)*

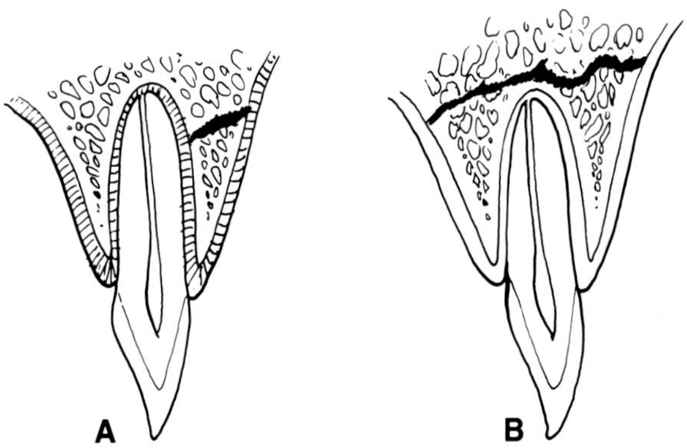

Figure 17–4. *Diagram of injuries to supporting alveolar bone. (**A**) Fracture of single wall of the alveolus. (**B**) Fracture of the alveolar process. (After Andreasen JO, ed. Traumatic injuries of the teeth, ed 1. Philadelphia: WB Saunders, 1972.)*

Table 17–1. *Classification of Dentoalveaolar Injuries**

Crown craze or crack
No loss of tooth structure
Horizontal or vertical
Crown fracture
Only enamel involved
Enamel and dentin involved
Enamel, dentin, and pulp involved
Horizontal, vertical, or oblique
Crown-root fracture
No pulpal involvement
Pulpal involvement
Root fracture
Apical, middle, or cervical third
Horizontal or vertical
Sensitivity or concussion
Mobility, subluxation, or looseness
Tooth displacement
Intrusion
Extrusion
Labial
Lingual
Lateral
Evulsion or exarticulation
Compression fracture of the alveolar socket
Alveolar socket wall fracture
Labial
Lingual
Alveolar process fracture
Maxilla fracture
Mandible fracture

* *Modified from Saunders B, Brady FA, Johnson R. Injuries. In: Saunders B, ed.* Pediatric oral and maxillofacial surgery, *ed 1. St. Louis: CV Mosby, 1979: 330.*

All systems for the categorization of dentoalveolar injuries have intrinsic advantages and disadvantages; the one used depends on which system the individual practitioner feels will allow for a readily understood description of an injury that can be easily communicated to colleagues and lay personnel.

GENERAL EXAMINATION

The history and physical examination performed following injuries to the face or mouth should be comprehensive. An adequate history and physical examination can be lifesaving and may prevent serious, irreversible complications. If the mechanism by which the injury was produced is known, it becomes much easier to predict and confirm the nature of the maxillofacial injury and the probability of the presence of associated trauma. If the traumatic episode was not witnessed, caution is advised because occult injuries may exist. Even if the patient has been examined first at a hospital emergency room, one cannot be complacent and assume that no other injuries exist. Treatment, unless emergent, should be delayed until physical assessment has been completed.

The incidence of associated closed head injury, usually manifesting as a loss of consciousness of less than 1 hour, in conjunction with facial trauma has been reported to occur frequently.[17] Injuries to the cervical spine, scalp and skull, chest, abdomen, and extremities can also occur, and these must be examined. Swelling, bleeding, abrasion, ecchymosis, and tenderness to palpation in areas other than that which is obviously injured must be evaluated. On the basis of the history, visual inspection, and palpation and percussion, other diagnostic aids (such as radiographs) may be necessary to rule out serious associated injuries or impending morbidity. Changes in breathing, such as wheezing and the use of accessory muscles of respiration, could indicate the aspiration of an avulsed tooth, which has not been recovered. The abdomen must be evaluated for evidence of guarding and rebound tenderness. In the case of an unrecovered, swallowed avulsed tooth, one must be cautious and observe the patient over several days for signs of alimentary tract obstruction.

ORAL EXAMINATION

A thorough examination of the oral cavity, including inspection, palpation, percussion, and ancillary diagnostic tests, must be performed. It does not suffice to assess and treat the obvious. During inspection of the oral cavity, one must look for areas of laceration and active bleeding. Immediate measures should be employed to stop serious bleeding. Areas of ecchymosis and hematoma must be evaluated as they may indicate fracture of the underlying osseous structures. One must look for the presence of foreign bodies in the oral cavity, pharynx, or nose. Salivary gland orifices and ducts must be visualized to assess for abrasion, avulsion, or transection. Avulsed or missing teeth could be embedded in the soft tissue of the mouth, be aspirated or swallowed, or be lying in the floor of the mouth under the tongue. Cracked or fractured teeth with or without pulpal involvement must be identified. Displaced teeth and en bloc displacement of tooth and bone may require early temporary reduction (Fig. 17-1). The dental occlusion should be carefully evaluated. Inspection should also include the evaluation of the skeletal position of the maxilla and mandible. Study casts obtained from the patient's general dentist or orthodontist can be of great value in the diagnosis and treatment of maxillofacial trauma.

Palpation of the temporomandibular joint area is essential to rule out injury to the condyle, subcondylar region, or joint structures. Mobile teeth can be indicative of traumatic luxation, root fracture, or en bloc fracture of an alveolar segment with teeth. The palate should be palpated to determine the presence of a palatal fracture. The floor of the mouth should be bimanually palpated to evaluate for the presence of swelling, tenderness, displaced teeth, or other foreign bodies. The submandibular and parotid glands should be compressed to assess the patency of the ducts associated with those salivary glands and the character of the saliva that is expressed from the glands.

Percussion of the teeth should be performed in a gentle manner. The end of the handle of an examining mirror is most often used when performing percussion. One can evaluate the feel, sound, and movement of the tooth, as well as the patient's reaction to the stimulus of percussion. Pain in the absence of other pathologic conditions may indicate that the tooth has been injured. Dullness to percussion in one or several adjacent teeth can be indicative of partially luxated teeth or en bloc fracture of tooth and alveolar bone. Occasionally, percussion of the teeth produces a sound similar to that obtained when a cracked tea cup is struck and, hence, is referred to as the cracked cup sound.[18]

Additional diagnostic modalities to be performed at the time of examination include vitality testing and radiographic studies. Assessing the vitality of traumatized teeth using thermal means (hot and cold) is of questionable value. Pulpal response to heat stimulus is difficult to standardize, but a technique using warmed gutta-percha has been advocated as a reproducible method for assessing pulp vitality.[19]

Electric vitality testing certainly lends itself to ease of standardization over other techniques. One must take into account, however, that electric pulp testing depends on a number of factors including the stage of eruption of the tooth, the presence of a restoration or decay, and the ability to isolate the tooth and keep the area clear of blood and saliva.[20] Importantly, any type of vitality testing immediately after trauma produces responses that are difficult to interpret as most responses are decreased after trauma and may not return to normal for weeks or months. However, electric pulp testing is of significant value in the posttrauma period to assess the potential recovery of the tooth and need for endodontic therapy.

Radiographic imaging of dentoalveolar trauma usually consists of one or more of the routine dental projections: periapical, occlusal, and panoramic. The periapical radiograph is the best image for producing the fine detail necessary to adequately evaluate root structure and surrounding alveolar bone for fractures (Fig. 17–5). At times it is difficult to assess radiographically whether a fracture is present because the

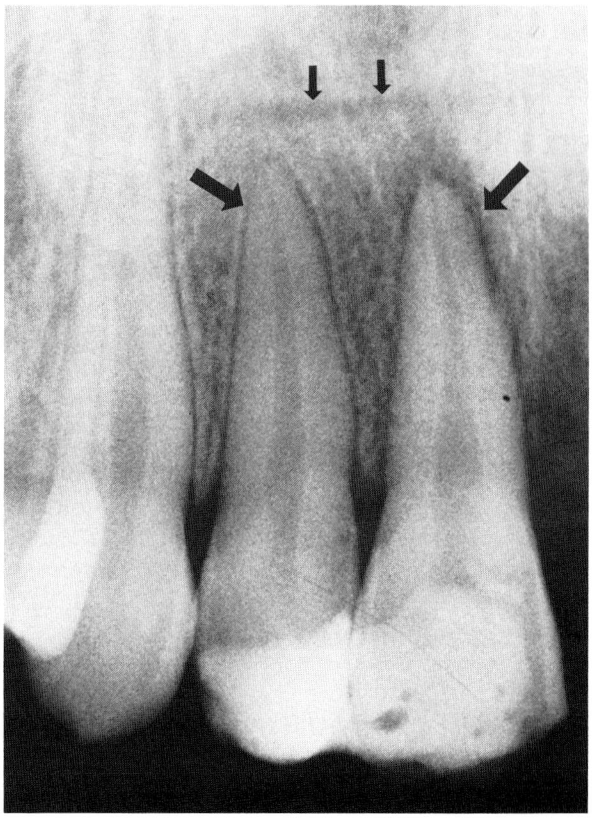

Figure 17–5. *Periapical radiograph of maxillary anterior alveolar fracture demonstrating alveolar fracture* (small black arrows), *widening of periodontal ligament space secondary to luxation* (large arrows), *and acid-etched composite stabilization.*

ability to confirm a fracture on periapical radiographs is highly dependent on radiograph tube-tooth-film geometry. Clinical evaluation, in addition to periapical radiographs, can usually make that determination. Following treatment, the periapical radiograph can confirm the proper repositioning of an avulsed or luxated tooth into the alveolus.

Occlusal radiographs are often made for patient comfort because they place minimal pressure on the traumatized area. In addition, a larger field of view is provided, eliminating the need for multiple periapical radiographs. The detail obtained is almost as sharp as a periapical radiograph, with root and alveolar fractures being readily apparent (Fig. 17–6).

The panoramic radiograph can demonstrate fractures of the mandible and maxilla, in addition to fractures of the alveolar ridges and teeth (Fig. 17–7).[22,23] Fractures of the condyle and subcondylar regions, angle, or body of the mandible that may not clearly be demonstrated clinically can be ruled out with this single screening image. A recent study demonstrated the value of the panoramic radiograph compared with routine head and neck imaging done in a hospital setting.[21] Air-fluid levels in the paranasal sinuses, as well as displaced tooth fragments and other radioopaque foreign bodies, usually can be identified. The projection can be somewhat less diagnostically helpful in assessing the anterior regions of the maxilla and mandible.

Occasionally, access to routine dental radiographs is not available, particularly in the hospital setting,

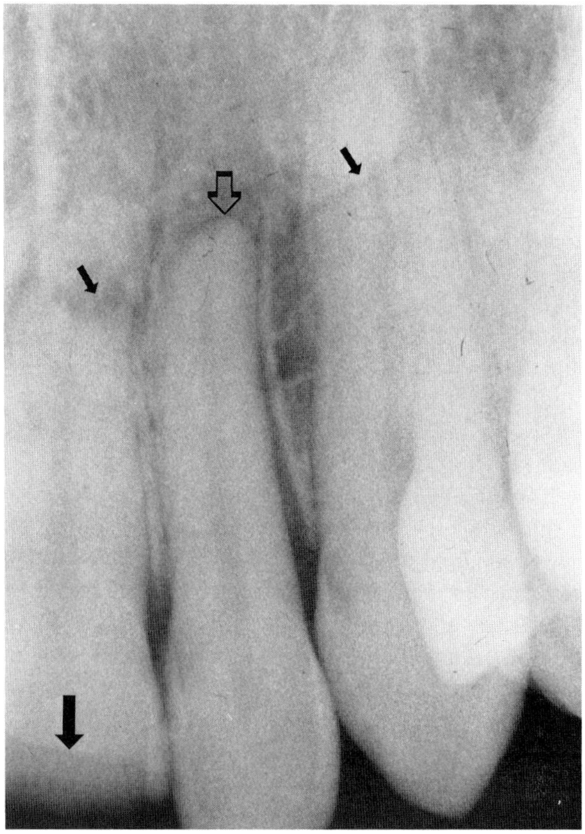

Figure 17–6. *Occlusal radiograph of maxillary anterior dentoalveolar trauma demonstrating horizontal apical root fractures* (small black arrows)*, luxation of lateral incisor* (open arrow)*, and uncomplicated crown fracture* (large black arrow).

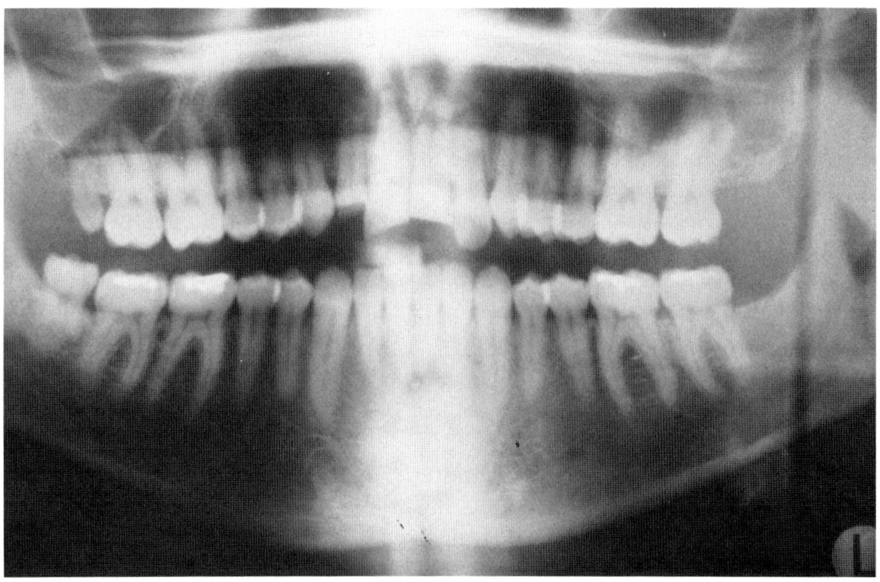

Figure 17–7. *Panoramic radiograph depicting maxillary anterior injuries in the same patient illustrated in Figure 6. Although most injuries are apparent (cuspid root fracture unidentifiable) fine detail is diminished.*

and other radiographic projections are performed in an effort to delineate dentoalveolar trauma. Although not ideal, standard films taken in a facial bone or mandibular series can reveal tooth and alveolar injuries (Fig. 17–8A–C).

Radiographic evaluation may also include lateral and posteroanterior chest and flat plate and upright abdominal films (Fig. 17–9A–C). In a trauma patient who has suffered loss of a tooth that is not accounted for or recovered at the site of the accident, chest films should be made to rule out the possibility of aspiration, even if the patient is asymptomatic. Other foreign bodies such as crowns, bridges, removable prostheses, or orthodontic retainers, brackets, and wires may also be displaced into the pharynx or aspirated. Abdominal radiographic films can determine whether displaced teeth or prosthetic or orthodontic appliances have been ingested. If ingested, follow-up films should be taken in a week to 10 days to ensure that the object has passed through the gastrointestinal tract. Teeth and metal containing crowns and appliances are radioopaque and therefore readily discernible. Objects made of acrylic may be radiolucent and therefore difficult to ascertain on radiographs, even though it has been suggested that all oral prosthetic appliances contain some type of radiodense material.[24]

TREATMENT

Crown Infractions

Crack lines or craze lines in enamel caused by trauma without the loss of any associated tooth structure are referred to as crown infractions or as class I crown fractures.[4,13,25] This type of injury usually occurs as a result of direct trauma to the enamel and manifests as single or multiple craze lines (in horizontal, vertical, or oblique directions) that do not cross the dentinoenamel junction. These injuries can be very difficult to diagnose in direct lighting and are often only seen if indirect lighting or transillumination is used. Although these injuries rarely require immediate treatment, patients may desire aesthetic, bonded restorations if any crack lines are visible. Importantly, although cracks may appear initially to be a minor injury, they are often associated with other dentoalveolar trauma, such as fractures and luxations, and examination should provide for an assessment of these potentially associated injuries. Teeth with craze lines secondary to trauma should be assessed periodically for vitality as a theoretical long-term sequela is pulpal necrosis. If this occurs, appropriate endodontic and restorative treatment is indicated.

Crown Fractures

Crown fractures can be divided into those that are limited to enamel, those that produce dentin exposure, and those that involve enamel, dentin, and pulp. The treatment that is instituted depends on the extent of the injury and whether the traumatized tooth is a permanent or deciduous tooth.

Small fractures confined to enamel may only require smoothing and recontouring with a rotary instrument. Care should be taken to provide an aesthetically pleasing result, with the appearance of the injured tooth compatible with adjacent and contralateral teeth. This can pose some problems in certain areas, such as the mesial-incisal corner of anterior teeth, which anatomically is close to a right angle in configuration. This appearance is very hard to duplicate without removing a great deal of healthy tooth structure. The distal-incisal corner of anterior teeth, on the other hand, usually has an easily reproducible, gently sloping curve. If aesthetics cannot be obtained with grinding, an appropriate restoration is indicated. Deciduous and permanent teeth can be handled in the same manner.

Similar to craze lines, although fractures of the crown limited to the enamel do not seem to lead to pulpal necrosis after injury, the vitality of the tooth should be monitored at regular intervals and endodontic therapy instituted if evidence of pulpal involvement develops in a permanent tooth.[26,27] If it is a deciduous tooth, extraction with space maintenance or pulpotomy with crowning is indicated.

The primary consideration with injuries producing dentinal exposure is to cover the exposed dentin with a calcium hydroxide-containing agent as soon after the injury as possible (Fig. 17–10A–C). This not only decreases symptoms of sensitivity to hot, cold, and pressure, but also allows the pulp to generate secondary dentin.[28,29] Some investigators recommend placement of a temporary restoration of zinc oxide and eugenol to act as a sedative.[30] Rapid treatment intervention is desired because the incidence of posttrauma pulpal

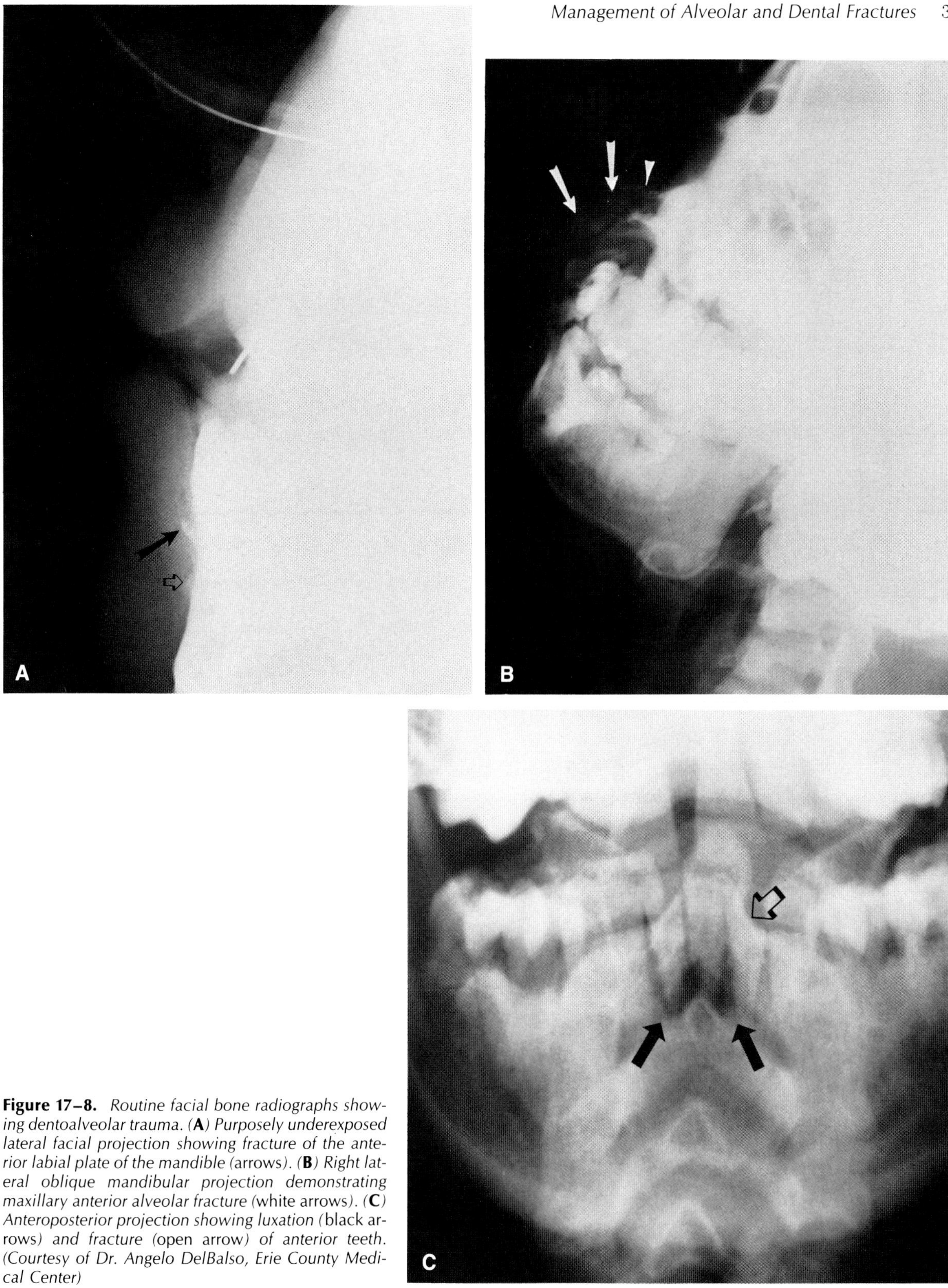

Figure 17–8. *Routine facial bone radiographs showing dentoalveolar trauma. (**A**) Purposely underexposed lateral facial projection showing fracture of the anterior labial plate of the mandible (arrows). (**B**) Right lateral oblique mandibular projection demonstrating maxillary anterior alveolar fracture (white arrows). (**C**) Anteroposterior projection showing luxation (black arrows) and fracture (open arrow) of anterior teeth. (Courtesy of Dr. Angelo DelBalso, Erie County Medical Center)*

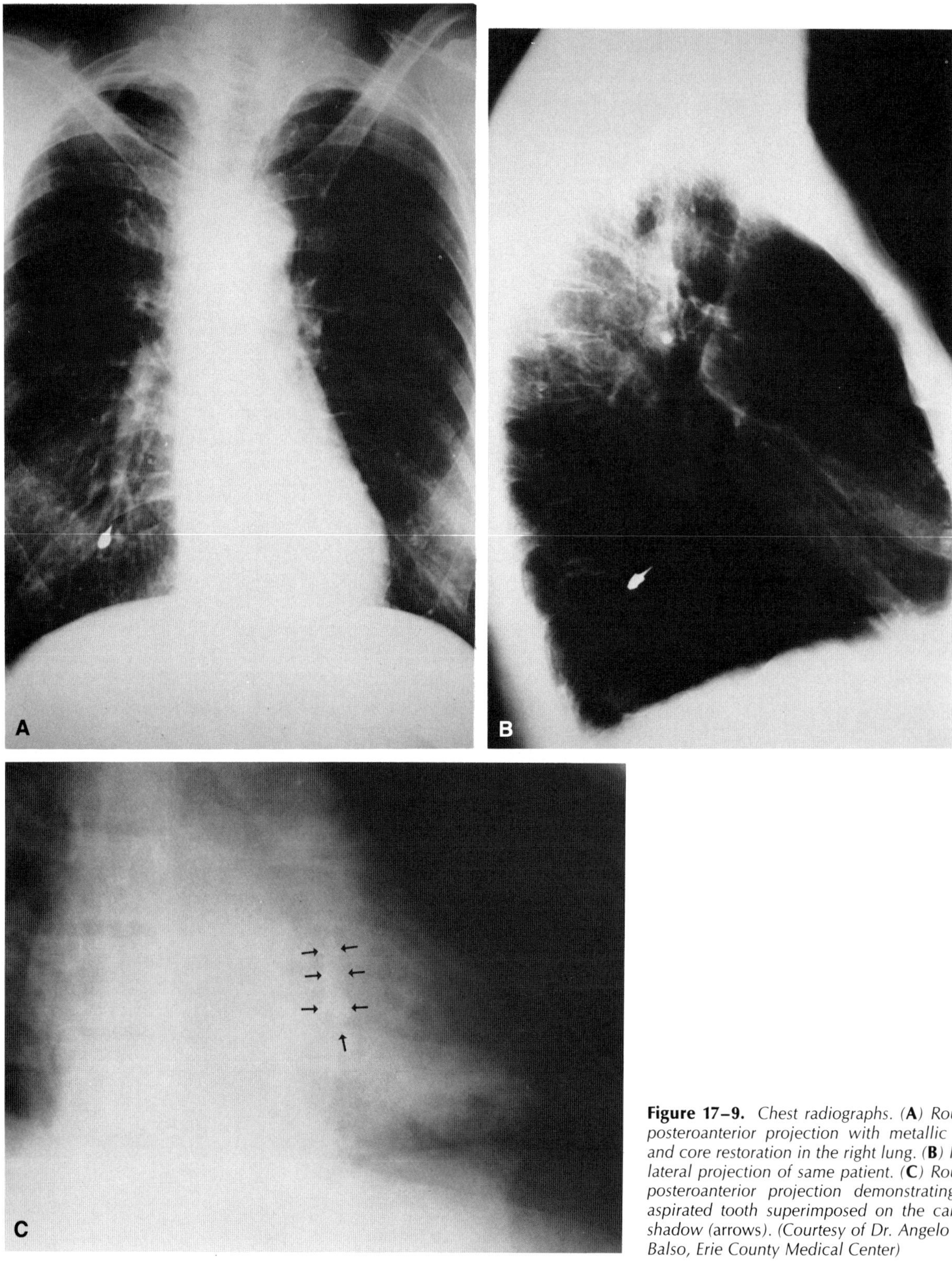

Figure 17–9. *Chest radiographs. (**A**) Routine posteroanterior projection with metallic post and core restoration in the right lung. (**B**) Right lateral projection of same patient. (**C**) Routine posteroanterior projection demonstrating an aspirated tooth superimposed on the cardiac shadow (arrows). (Courtesy of Dr. Angelo Del-Balso, Erie County Medical Center)*

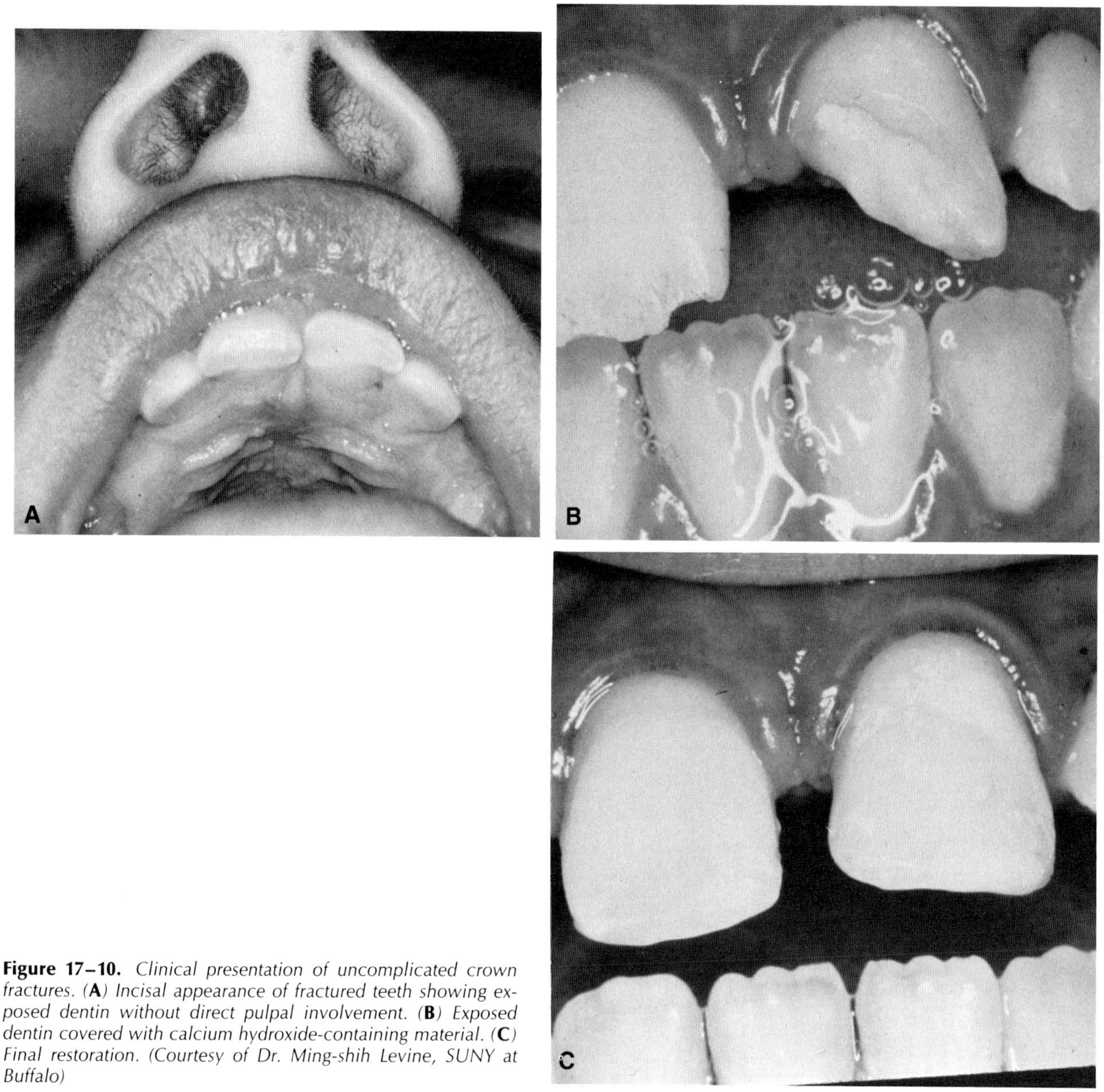

Figure 17–10. *Clinical presentation of uncomplicated crown fractures. (**A**) Incisal appearance of fractured teeth showing exposed dentin without direct pulpal involvement. (**B**) Exposed dentin covered with calcium hydroxide-containing material. (**C**) Final restoration. (Courtesy of Dr. Ming-shih Levine, SUNY at Buffalo)*

necrosis increases if treatment is delayed beyond 24 hours.[26,31]

Following placement of the dentinal coverage, an appropriate temporary restoration can be made. Immediate attempts at a permanent, final restoration is usually contraindicated because a period of at least 8 weeks after the injury is needed for pulp response to return to normal.[26] At this time electric pulp testing can determine whether the pulp has become necrotic and whether endodontic therapy is needed. It has been reported that teeth with this type of injury experience pulpal necrosis in up to 7% of the cases.[31] Unfortunately, it may take up to 7 months for the pulp to recover its normal reaction to electric pulp testing.[32]

Deciduous teeth with dentin exposure can be treated in a similar manner. However, dentin exposure in primary teeth often can be treated by removing any sharp, projecting areas. If the dentin remains sen-

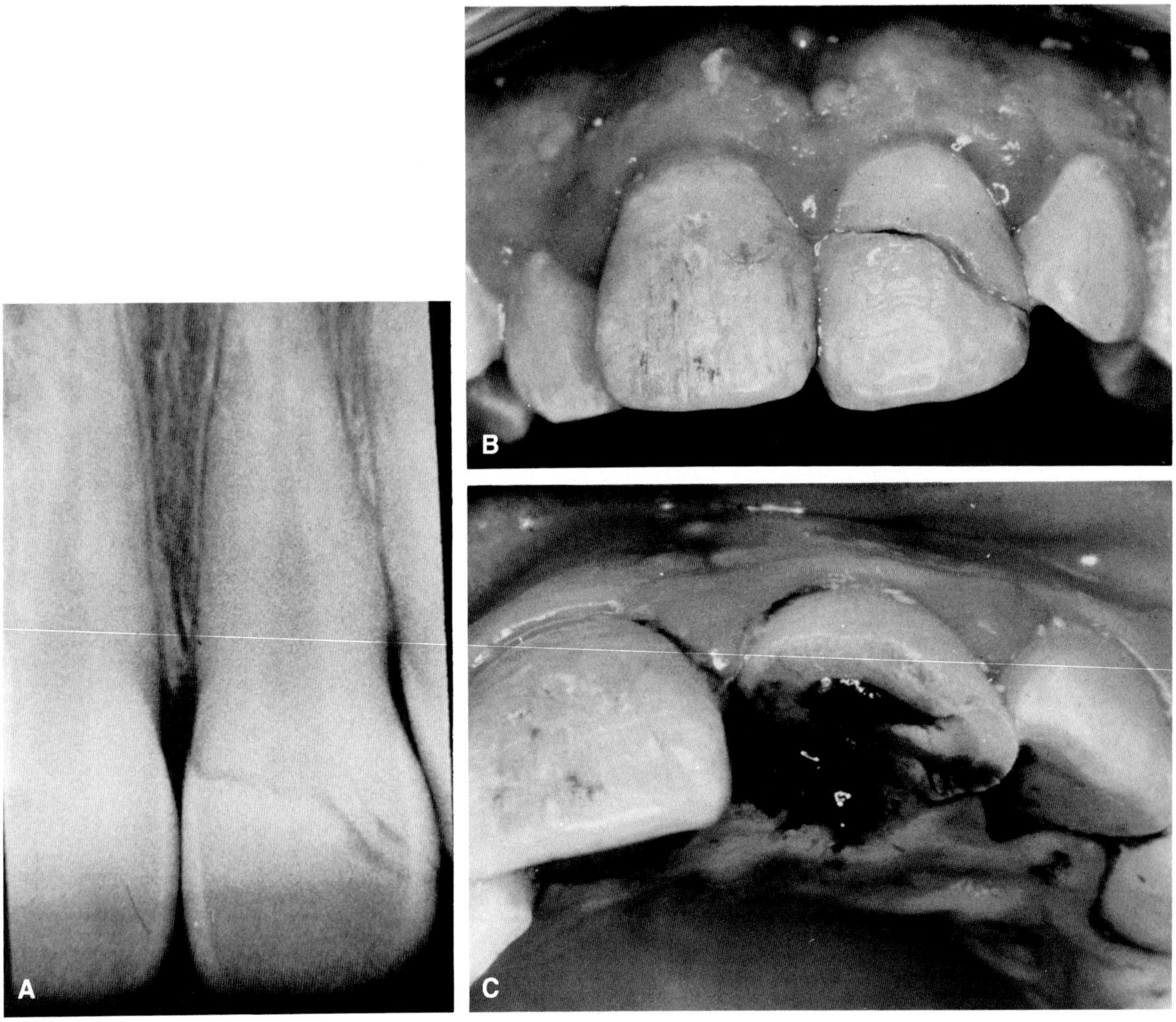

Figure 17–11. *Case series presenting complicated crown fracture. (**A**) Periapical radiograph suggesting direct pulpal involvement. (**B**) Fractured crown in position. (**C**) Fractured crown segment removed revealing pulp exposure. (Courtesy of Dr. Ming-shih Levine, SUNY at Buffalo)*

sitive, it has been suggested that the exposed area be coated with a fluoride-containing varnish.[33]

Crown fractures resulting in pulp exposure (Fig. 17–11A–C) can be handled in one of four ways: pulp capping, pulpotomy, pulpectomy, and extraction. The treatment method chosen depends on a number of factors, including the type of dentition (i.e., deciduous or permanent) determined by the age of the patient; whether the apex of the root is fully developed or still immature, exhibiting a large apical foramen, a reverse taper to the geometry of the canal, and thin root-canal walls; the interval between the time of the injury and the institution of treatment; the size of the pulp exposure; the presence of other dental trauma (e.g., root fracture, luxation, or alveolar fracture); and the presence of any associated dental pathologic conditions (i.e., caries, periodontal disease, or preexisting endodontic involvement).

With permanent teeth, every effort is made to retain the tooth, extraction being the treatment of last resort. In contrast, although deciduous teeth with traumatic pulp exposures can also be treated with pulp capping, pulpotomy, or pulpectomy, the decision is often made to extract the tooth for many reasons. Most important among these are poor patient compliance and cooperation, the small size of the tooth, the presence of large pulp chambers, and the presence of root resorption on the deciduous tooth caused by eruption of the permanent dentition.

Pulp capping is usually reserved for use in the tooth that has a very small exposure, is endodontically healthy, and does not have any other accompanying dentoalveolar injuries. To ensure the greatest chance for success, the tooth should be isolated with a rubber dam, cleaned with an appropriate sterile solution, and covered with a calcium hydroxide-containing material placed onto and around the area of the exposure. This treatment should be instituted within hours of the injury, but small exposures up to 24-hours-old can still be treated with this technique.[34] After placement of the pulp cap, a temporary restoration is fabricated. Following the production of a layer of secondary dentin at the pulpal surface, the appropriate permanent restoration can be achieved unless pulpal necrosis ensues, which can occur in up to 30% of the cases.[33,35]

Pulpotomy, which is the removal of that portion of the pulp tissue located in the coronal portion of the tooth, is used when the size of the pulp exposure is too large to accommodate a pulp-capping procedure or when the injury occurred more than 96 hours earlier.[34] Two types of pulpotomy have been described. The shallow pulpotomy, in which only 2 to 4 mm of pulp tissue in the region of the exposure is removed, can be used in an immature (recently erupted) tooth in which maintenance of sufficient pulpal tissue is desired to allow for dentin deposition to strengthen the tooth. In addition, this procedure allows for continued root apex development and closure.[34] In the conventional pulpotomy, the removal of pulp extends to the level of or below what is the equivalent position of the cementoenamel junction. Following removal of the coronal pulp, the remaining tissue is covered with a calcium hydroxide-containing agent and temporarily restored.

Pulpotomy should be considered only as a temporary, emergency procedure, to be followed by conventional endodontic therapy after the tooth and root apex has fully matured because pulpotomy rendered as the only treatment has a reported success rate of as low as 72%.[36] In addition, obliteration of the pulp canal has been reported as a long-term complication of calcium hydroxide pulpotomy, thereby making future endodontic therapy difficult to impossible. If the tooth becomes symptomatic, the only remaining treatment alternative is extraction.

Pulpectomy, which is the surgical removal of the entire pulp tissue, is usually used in an emergency situation in the treatment of fully formed teeth having mature apices in which pulpotomy or pulp capping is not indicated (e.g., the injury occured over 96 hours earlier). This is then followed by routine endodontic and restorative care at the appropriate time. A pulpectomy can also be performed on newly erupted teeth in which the anatomic configuration of the root canal system makes completion of conventional endodontic treatment difficult. In this instance, calcium hydroxide is placed into the root canal system after the pulpal tissue is removed. The calcium hydroxide then serves as a stimulus for continued apical maturation (apexogenesis or apexification).[37-41]

Root Fractures

Root fractures can occur as an isolated event or in combination with a fracture that extends from the crown onto the root surface (Figs. 17–6 and 17–12). The crown-root fracture often presents one of the more difficult treatment dilemmas. The treatment option chosen depends on the extent of the fracture, that is, how far down the root it extends. If the fracture ends at or above the osseous margin, it is usually possible to remove the fractured crown-root segment, perform a pulpotomy or pulpectomy if needed, and perform a temporary restoration. If the fracture line extends onto the root below the alveolar crest, it is often difficult if not impossible to gain access to the apical limit of the fracture so that a permanent, casted restoration can eventually be made. Certainly, a small amount of gingival and osseous recontouring can be performed. Consideration should be given to orthodontic extrusion of the tooth to gain access to the margin of the fracture, but most often, these teeth are extracted.

Root fractures are most commonly classified on the basis of the anatomic location of the fracture, that is,

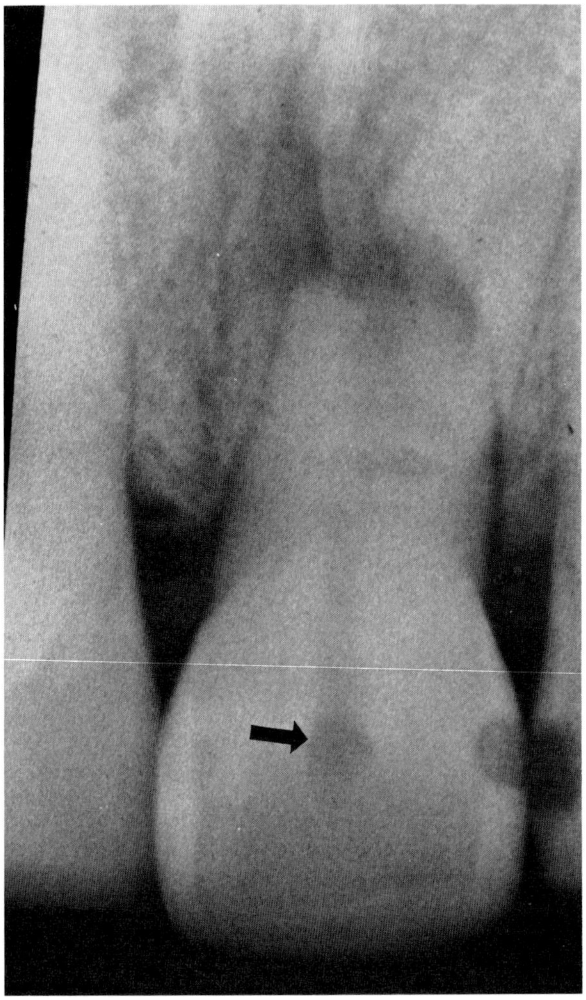

Figure 17–12. *Periapical radiograph demonstrating fracture of the middle third of the root with distal displacement. Note endodontic access evident in crown. (Courtesy of Dr. Ming-shih Levine, SUNY at Buffalo.)*

whether it is located in the coronal, middle, or apical one third of the root. Coronal root fractures most often present with a highly mobile crown and the likelihood that the fracture communicates with the gingival crevice. Theoretically, splinting of the crown to adjacent teeth may lead to healing. Unfortunately, pulp necrosis occurs in about 50% of these injuries, and therefore treatment usually consists of removal of the fractured coronal segment and pulpectomy on the retained root structure followed by prosthetic reconstruction.[42]

Fractures located in the middle and apical one third of the tooth are associated with a pulpal necrosis incidence of only about 20%, and therefore initial therapy should be directed toward repositioning of the tooth and fixation with an appropriate rigid appliance as rapidly as possible after the trauma.[34] Fixation should be maintained for 2 to 4 months to allow for healing to occur by the deposition of calcified dental tissue, fibrous connective tissue, fibrous connective tissue and bone, or granulation tissue between the fragments.[12,16,43] If healing occurs by one of the first three mechanisms, the teeth usually do not exhibit mobility, usually react normally to vitality testing, and require no further treatment other than periodic observation for evidence of pulpal necrosis. If healing occurs by the proliferation of granulation tissue between the fragments, the teeth are usually loose, symptomatic, and may be associated with a fistulous tract. Treatment in this instance is extraction of the affected fragments.

Treatment of root fractures in deciduous teeth usually consists of removing the mobile coronal segment and leaving the apical root segment in position, allowing it to resorb by physiologic processes.

Concussion or Sensitivity

Injuries to teeth caused by forces that are not strong enough to produce serious, visible damage to the tooth and surrounding structures are categorized as a concussion.[15,44] Examination reveals no discernible abnormal movement, and the tooth is not displaced into a nonanatomic position. The crown may show no evidence of infraction or crazing, and the patient may not perceive any differences in occlusion. These teeth are very commonly highly sensitive to percussion from any direction but usually respond normally to vitality testing. Radiographic examination of these injuries yields negative results. Treatment should include elimination of occlusal forces by spot grinding of the opposing tooth or teeth and periodic evaluation and vitality testing during the healing phase. If the pulp becomes necrotic, as demonstrated by radiographic evidence of pulp canal obliteration, or develops periapical pathologic conditions, changes in color of the crown, or a difference in light transmission with transillumination as compared to adjacent teeth, endodontic therapy is indicated.[44]

Subluxation or Mobility

Many times the force that is imparted to a tooth during trauma is sufficient to cause discernible movement of the tooth but not anatomic displacement clinically or radiographically. Clinical evaluation demonstrates abnormal mobility of the tooth to palpation. The force at times is sufficient to cause bleeding from the gingival crevice. Root fracture must be ruled out by radiographic examination. The tooth may or may not be sensitive to percussion and often will produce a dull sound when struck. The tooth may or may not respond normally to vitality testing. Treatment, depending on the extent of the mobility, can be similar to that which is rendered for a dental concussion. The amount of mobility dictates the necessity for stabilization followed by periodic evaluation with observation, radiographs, and vitality testing. If the aforementioned signs of pulpal deterioration are present, endodontic treatment is necessary.

Displacement, Luxation, or Partial Avulsion

Traumatic displacement of teeth can occur in any direction depending on the direction from which the force originated (Figs. 17–5, 17–6, and 17–13). Displacement may be accompanied by fracture of the surrounding alveolar bone. Displacement can present as intrusion, extrusion, labial or buccal, lingual or palatal, or lateral movement.

The cause of intrusion is a traumatic force that is superiorly directed in the maxilla and inferiorly directed in the mandible. Intrusion is much more common in the maxilla as a result of the anatomic configuration of the premaxilla and the character of the bone in the area. The bone of the anterior mandible is denser and less compressible than that of the maxilla, making this area more susceptible to alveolar process fracture. At times the intrusion can be extensive and can appear as if the tooth has been avulsed. Maxillary central incisors, for example, can be displaced straight upward and enter the nasal cavity. Radiographic examination can rule out avulsion and demonstrate the position of the intruded tooth. In general, intruded permanent teeth should be left in place to reerupt. If reeruption does not occur within 2 to 3 months, orthodontic aids may be necessary to facilitate eruption.[30] The treatment approach to intruded deciduous teeth is debatable. Some investigators recommend a conservative approach, allowing the intruded tooth to reerupt, especially if the surgery to retrieve an intruded deciduous tooth will threaten the underlying permanent dentition.[44] Others feel that, because a retained deciduous tooth is likely to damage the underlying permanent teeth, immediate extraction is indicated.[30]

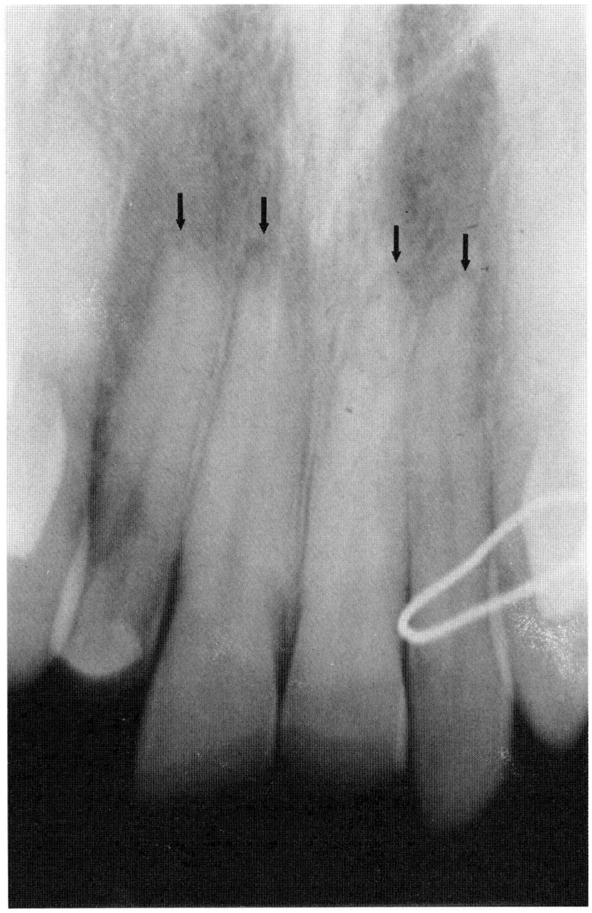

Figure 17–13. *Occlusal radiograph showing evidence of luxation of maxillary anterior teeth with associated crown fractures (*black arrows*). Note temporary stabilization of repositioned exarticulated tooth with a circumdental wire.*

Permanent teeth that have been traumatically extruded or displaced in a direction other than intrusion should be repositioned as soon as possible. At times the displacement is accompanied by fracture or expansion of the surrounding alveolar bone. These teeth respond with a dull sound to percussion, and most often do not respond normally to vitality testing. Radiographs should be taken to rule out root fracture. Digital pressure is usually sufficient to reduce the displacement. One must be careful not to compromise further the blood supply to the area when repositioning displaced teeth by using gentle manipulation of the soft tissue. Suturing of lacerated gingiva, if needed, should place the soft tissue under as little tension as possible. Stabilization of the displaced permanent tooth is accomplished by one of a number of methods, which are discussed later. Periodic clinical and radiograph evaluation should be performed for several months. If evidence of pulpal death becomes apparent, endodontic therapy is indicated.

The treatment for extruded deciduous teeth is extraction. As with intrusion, the treatment approach to deciduous teeth displaced laterally, labially, or palatally (lingually) is debatable, with some investigators advocating a period of observation and others recommending immediate extraction.[30,44]

Avulsion, Exarticulation, or Evulsion

The critical factor in determining the treatment approach to avulsed teeth is the amount of time that the tooth has been out of the alveolus (Fig. 17–14). It has been shown that, although 90% of avulsed teeth replanted within 30 minutes of the injury show no radiographic signs of root resorption on follow-up visits, those that are reimplanted more than 90 minutes after the injury demonstrate resorption in over 90% of the cases.[45] Of equal importance for the long-term survival of the tooth, however, is the care and method by which the avulsed tooth is transported. Ideally, temporary reimplantation should be advised before transportation of the patient. It does not matter if the tooth is not perfectly positioned as long as the tooth is gently handled by the crown and replaced in the alveolus. If temporary replantation cannot be achieved, the tooth should then be stored and transported in the patient's mouth or in a container of milk.[46] Milk is significantly superior to saliva or water as a temporary storage medium for survival of periodontal fibroblasts. The manner in which the avulsed tooth is manipulated by the attending physician is likewise critical for successful replantation. The root surface should not be touched

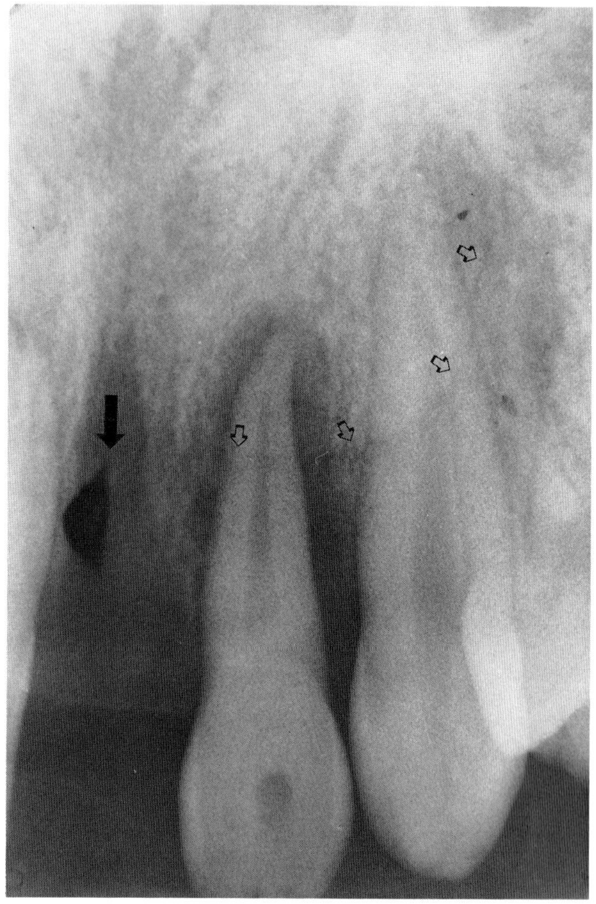

Figure 17–14. *Periapical radiograph showing avulsion of a maxillary anterior tooth* (black arrow). *Note loss of bony support after stabilization and endodontic therapy of the adjacent tooth and apparent alveolar fracture line* (open arrows).

or scraped. No effort should be made to mechanically cleanse the root of the tooth because this damages the remaining periodontal ligament and threatens the success of the reimplantation. Gentle irrigation with saline or gauze soaked with saline may be employed to remove blood clots or foreign objects from the surface of the root.[47] The tooth should be handled only by the crown, thereby avoiding any digital contact with the root surface.

If the apex of the avulsed tooth has not as yet closed, the tooth should be replanted and observed closely, both clinically and radiographically, to determine if revascularization of the pulpal tissues has occurred. If there are any signs of resorption or indication of pulpal necrosis, endodontic therapy should be started immediately in an attempt to arrest the resorptive process. In permanent teeth with closed apices, endodontic treatment should be initiated as early as possible and no later than 2 weeks after replantation. Endodontic therapy before reimplantation is associated with an increased incidence of complications, including resorption and ankylosis, and therefore is contraindicated.[47] Avulsed deciduous teeth should not be reimplanted to prevent damage to the underlying developing permanent tooth.

Care must be exercised when manipulating the alveolus into which the tooth will be reimplanted. One must not cause additional injury to the reimplantation site. The clinician should not curette the alveolus and should not further injure the recipient site with vigorous irrigation and suctioning. The tooth should be placed gently into the socket and properly positioned. The occlusion must be evaluated and occlusal forces against the tooth should be eliminated. Stabilization can be accomplished by one of a number of methods to be discussed. If possible, it is desirable to use two teeth on either side of the reimplanted tooth to secure the stabilization and fixation device. Short-term fixation of 2 to 3 weeks is usually sufficient to obtain support and helps to prevent root ankylosis and subsequent root resorption caused by a prolonged fixation time.[47]

The incidence of infection following reimplantation is low. However, infection and accompanying inflammation can lead to resorption. The use of antibiotics prophylactically can be decided on by the attending doctor based on the presenting circumstances. Tetanus immunization status should be checked and tetanus toxoid administered if necessary.

Fractures of the Alveolar Process

Fractures of the alveolar process usually occur in adult age groups and are usually confined to the anterior areas of the dental arch (Figs. 17–5, 17–6, and 17–14). They are observed in both dentulous and edentulous arches and can involve an isolated tooth, although the fracture usually involves multiple tooth segments.[48] The arch form of the palate is architecturally strong. As a result, alveolar process fractures of the maxilla very often occur in the labial portion of the alveolus while the palatal process acts as a palatal fulcrum for an anterior to posterior traumatic impact. The tooth or teeth crowns will be displaced posteroinferiorly as fracture of the labial plate occurs. Superiorly directed forces can produce intrusion of a tooth in the maxilla, causing fracture and anterior displacement of the labial alveolus. Fracture of both labial and lingual plates occurs more frequently in the mandible because intrusion of a mandibular tooth into the alveolus resulting from an inferiorly directed blow is very uncommon. The alveolar fracture and the tooth or teeth will be displaced either labially or lingually.

Adjacent teeth that move en bloc usually indicates a fracture of the alveolus, with the teeth producing a dull percussive response when struck. Palpation of rough osseous edges and observation of torn gingiva or gingival ecchymosis are all signs of possible underlying bone fracture.

Treatment is usually straightforward. Care must be taken to protect the blood supply of the fractured segment. Irrigation of the area should be carefully performed, and small extruded bone fragments should be removed. The teeth and displaced fractured segment should be gently reduced; stabilization is usually needed. Soft tissues should be approximated and sutured as necessary. The occlusion should be checked and relieved if necessary. Fixation is maintained for a period of 4 weeks.[48] Antibiotic and tetanus prophylaxis is instituted depending on presenting circumstances. Confirmation of tooth and alveolar segment repositioning should be confirmed by radiographic examination.

Fixation Techniques

Many techniques can be used for the stabilization and fixation of dentoalveolar injuries. Some techniques have been used for many years, whereas others are more recent and have become possible as a result of the development of new dental restorative materials.

The goal of stabilization varies slightly depending on the situation. Teeth that have been luxated or avulsed must be stabilized loosely for only a short time—2 weeks or less.[50,51] The goal of fixation is to hold the tooth in place so that the periodontal ligament can heal (i.e., for *soft tissue healing*). It should be loose enough to allow physiologic movement. Rigid stabilization of a loose tooth, especially if left in place for 3 weeks or longer, results in a portion of the root being held tightly against the alveolar process causing ankylosis.[52] Ankylosis leads to root resorption.[53]

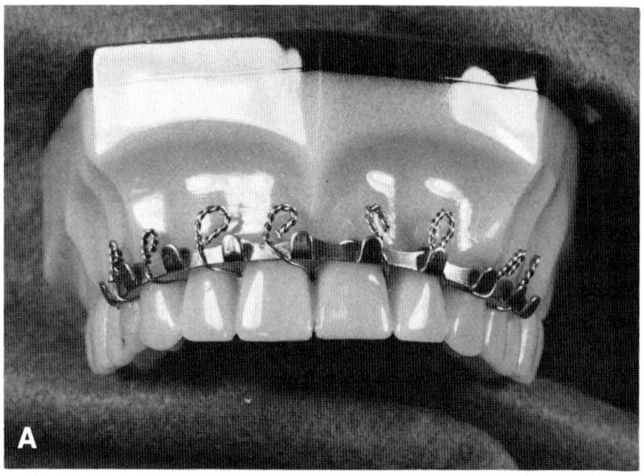

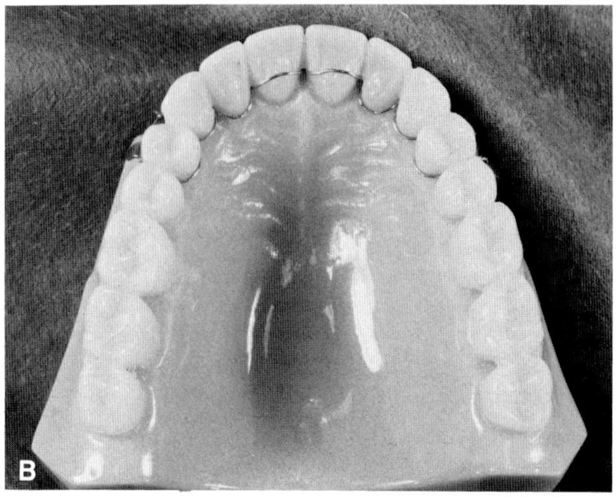

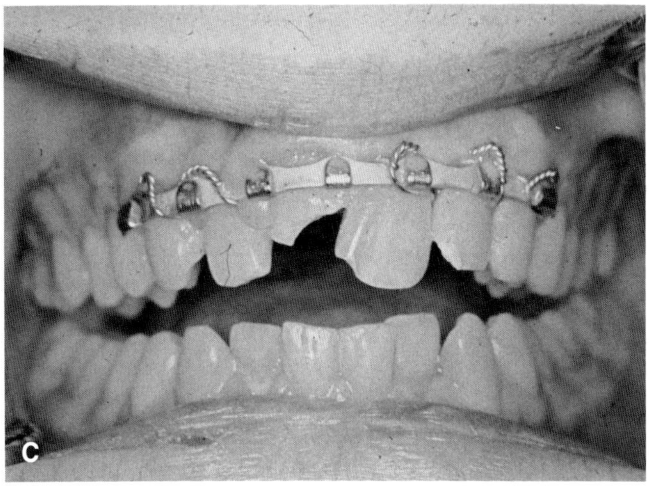

Figure 17–15. *Model demonstrating stabilization and fixation technique using arch bar and circumdental wires. (**A**) Labial view. (**B**) Palatal view demonstrating positioning of wire to prevent mechanical extrusion and to facilitate apical repositioning. (**C**) Clinical use of this technique.*

If an alveolar fracture has occurred, the fixation device must be designed to be more rigid, allowing *bone tissue healing*. The appliance should be left in place for at least 4 weeks.

Root resorption is caused by injury to the root by such factors as: prolonged period of extraarticular time; excess manipulation by the dentist in cleaning the root surface; and wires placed around the tooth being on the root instead of the crown.

Therefore, when planning the method for stabilization, the surgeon must plan for physiologic movement with luxated teeth and no movement with alveolar fractures; for techniques that do not further injure already injured tooth roots; and for the proper time period of stabilization.

The fixation and stabilization methods with the longest history of usage are arch bar and wire fixation. They should be used primarily for alveolar fractures. Figure 17–15A–C demonstrates the application of an Erich arch bar with circumdental wires for fracture stabilization and fixation. Light wire (26 to 28 gauge) is desirable for the circumdental ligatures because it is more easily and more securely adapted to the teeth than heavier gauge wires. Figure 17–15B also demonstrates the positioning of the wire on the palate in a position incisal to the cingulum so that the force of stabilization is directed apically and does not lead to the extrusion of the tooth from the alveolus as the circumdental wire is tightened. This is also done to avoid injury to the tooth root by the wire. Arch bars are indicated *only* for injuries involving bone fractures in which rigid stabilization is required.

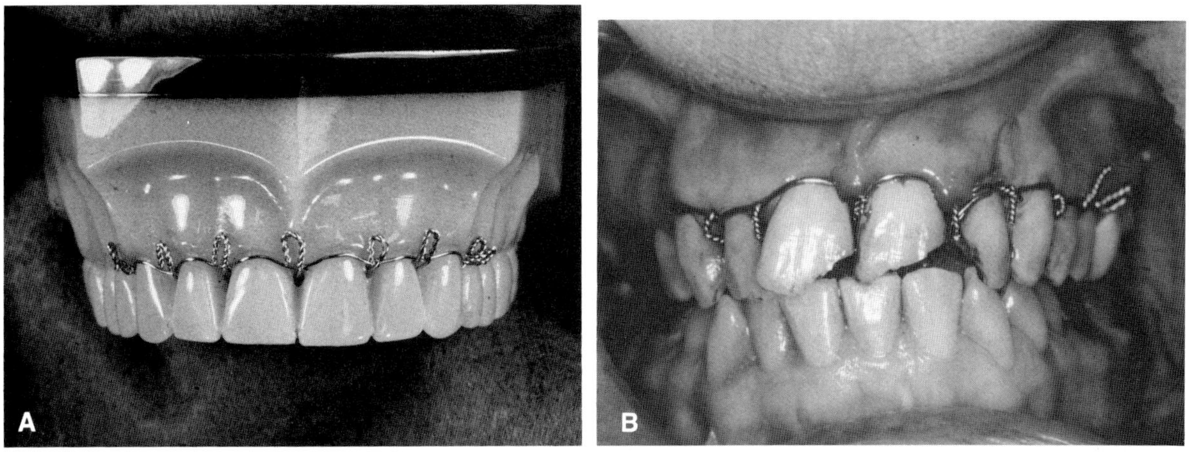

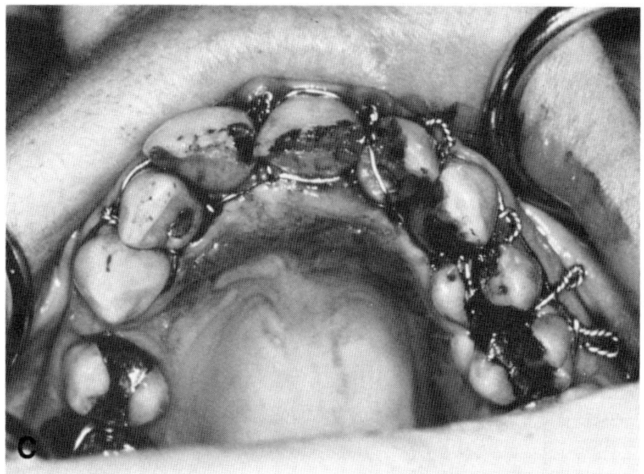

Figure 17–16. *(**A**) Model demonstrating stabilization and fixation technique using the Essig wiring method. (**B** and **C**) When applied to the clinical setting, the surgeon must take care to ensure that the wires do* not *engage the roots of the injured teeth.*

Figure 17–16 shows the use of the Essig method for horizontal wiring.[49] In this technique, a 25-gauge wire is looped to the labial and lingual direction of the fractured segment. Secondary wires are then looped between the teeth, apical to the contact point, with one pass above and the other below the primary wire; these are then tightened in a sequential manner. The labial and lingual wires must be kept off of the tooth roots. Essig wiring is most useful for alveolar fractures but may be used for multiple-luxated teeth if the wires are not tightened too tightly and are removed in 10 to 14 days.

The use of acid-etched composite dental material is an accurate and easy method to use for stabilization and fixation. This technique must be viewed as the standard for management of luxated teeth. It can be used in the treatment of single or multiple displaced teeth, as well as of alveolar process fractures. The advantage of this technique is that it is much less stressful to the injured area because the forces needed to apply the material are far less intense than those needed to apply wires or arch bars. The *preferred* method is to use the composite material to ligate a semirigid wire (braided orthodontic wire) or heavy nylon cord to the injured and adjacent teeth. This method allows for physiologic movement and enhances healing without ankylosis (Fig. 17–17). Figure 17–18A and B shows the use of the acid-etch composite material alone and with a wire embedded to increase its strength. Composite bars like these are indicated for alveolar fractures, but not luxated or avulsed teeth.

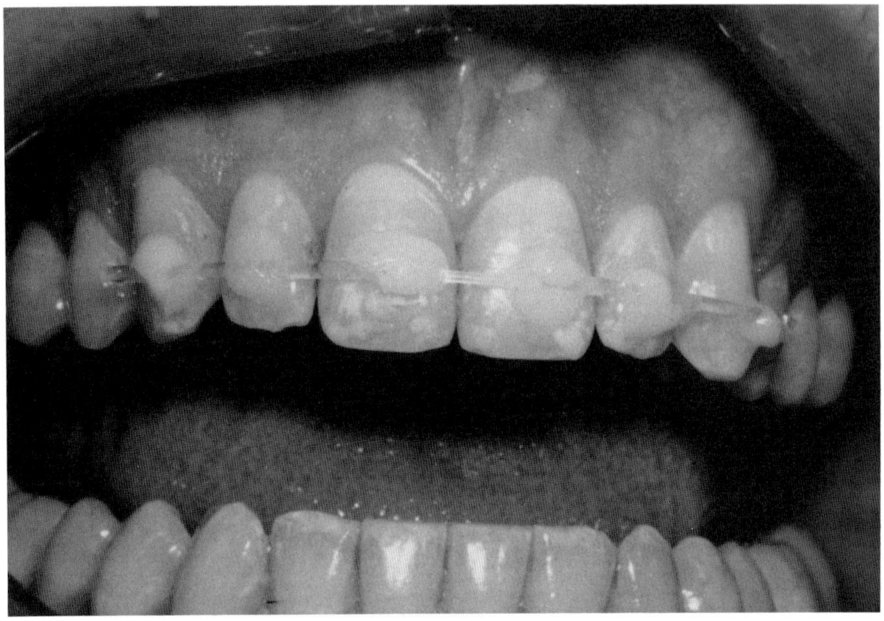

Figure 17–17. *The method of choice for stabilization of an avulsed tooth or teeth is to bind a heavy nylon cord or braided orthodontic wire (flexible wire) to the repositioned tooth and adjacent teeth with acid-etch composites. This technique allows for physiologic movement, thus permitting soft tissue (periodontal ligament) healing but preventing ankylosis. (Courtesy of Dr. Denny McTique)*

COMPLICATIONS

One of the most common complications resulting from dentoalveolar trauma is pulpal necrosis, the incidence of which is dependent on the severity of the injury (Fig. 17–19). Trauma that produces enamel crazing or a fracture confined to the enamel does not seem to be associated with an increased occurrence of pulp necrosis.[27] Exposure of dentin is associated with up to a 7% incidence of pulp necrosis, whereas pulp exposures and root fractures are associated with a 20% to 30% incidence.[32–35] The incidence of pulpal necrosis associated with luxation injuries ranges from a reported low of 15% to as high as 96%, depending on the direction of luxation and the stage of root development of the involved tooth.[44,54,55] Avulsion or exarticu-

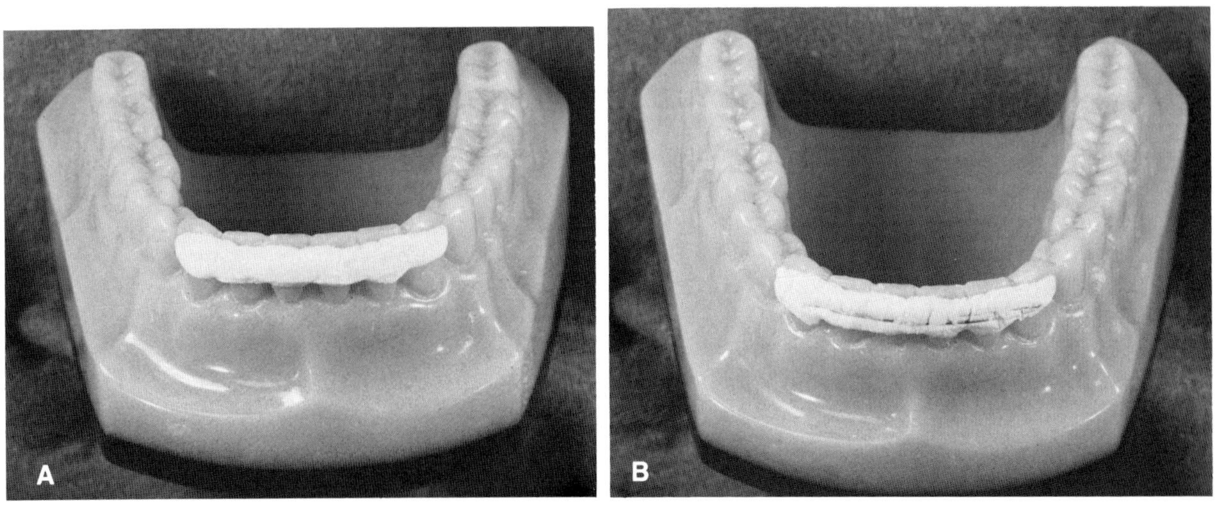

Figure 17–18. *Model demonstrating stabilization and fixation technique using an acid-etched composite resin splint. (**A**) Composite material only. (**B**) Composite material reinforced with wire.*

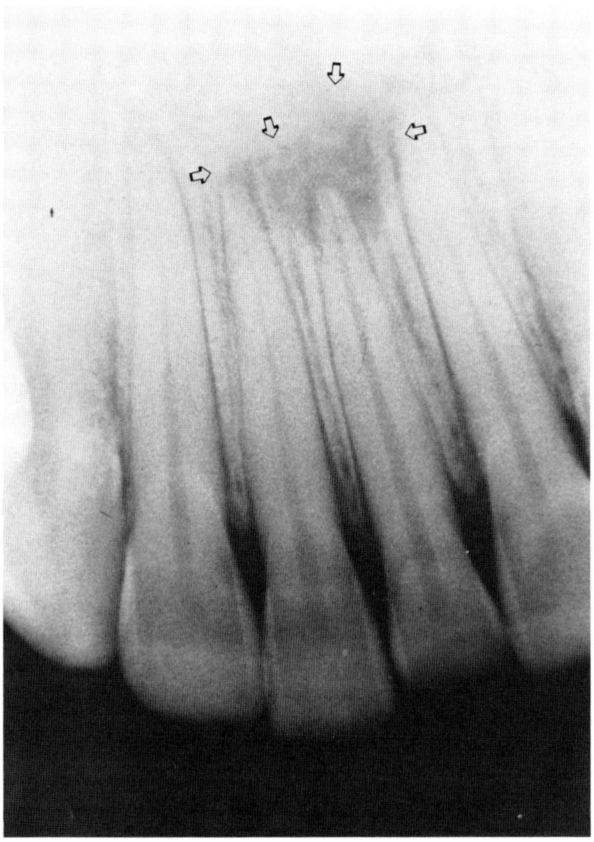

Figure 17–19. *Periapical radiograph demonstrating periapical pathologic features that are secondary to dental trauma and that produced an uncomplicated crown fracture* (arrows).

lation is associated with an incidence of pulpal necrosis of essentially 100% if the tooth is out of the alveolus for greater than 2 hours.[47] If vitality testing suggests that the pulp is necrotic (taking into consideration the previously described difficulties associated with vitality testing in traumatized teeth), the treatment options are endodontic therapy or extraction.

Infection can occur secondary to any facial trauma, but usually it is of low incidence as a result of the excellent blood supply to the head and neck region and the fact that patients are often placed on antibiotics prophylactically subsequent to the trauma. Although the necessity for use of antibiotics in patients with all types of dentoalveolar trauma is debatable, most surgeons administer an appropriate antibiotic to patients following an exarticulation or alveolar process fracture, especially if the injury is not recent or stabilization and fixation is difficult. The infection may be associated with loss of alveolar support, loss of tooth, and subsequent considerations for replacement and space maintenance. Inability to appropriately reposition and stabilize the tooth or dentoalveolar segment can lead to occlusal discrepancies, posttreatment periodontal defects, and similar difficulties, with immediate or subsequent loss of the tooth or teeth and the need for prosthetic replacement.

Although resorption of roots (internal and external) and ankylosis are potential complications from any type of dentoalveolar trauma, they are usually associated with exarticulation, alveolar process fractures, luxations, or root fractures in either the deciduous or permanent dentition (Fig. 17–20A–D). The resorption appears to be caused by an inflammatory process that is produced by damage to the root, the periodontium, or the pulp, either traumatically or iatrogenically. Andreasen has divided the various types of histologically identifiable root resorption into a number of categories.[44] External resorption has been divided into three types:

1. Surface resorption characterized by superficial resorption of the root with replacement by new cementum
2. Inflammatory resorption characterized by resorption of tooth cementum and dentin with an associated inflammatory response in the adjacent periodontium
3. Replacement resorption (ankylosis) characterized by a gradual resorption of the tooth with replacement by bone, thereby inhibiting continued physiologic eruption or reeruption

Internal resorption is similarly divided into two types:

1. Inflammatory resorption characterized by resorption of the dentin with an associated inflammatory response in the pulp
2. Replacement resorption characterized by an irregular enlargement of the pulp chamber with replacement by calcified tissue and obliteration of the canal

Endodontic therapy should be initiated immediately upon radiographic evidence of the development of internal or external root resorption because the resorptive process can be aborted.[43,45] For deciduous teeth, evidence of resorption necessitates extraction and probably space maintenance. An interesting recent development based on animal studies is the suggestion that soaking avulsed teeth in a solution of fibronectin before replantation enhances early replacement of the fibrin clot, increases connective tis-

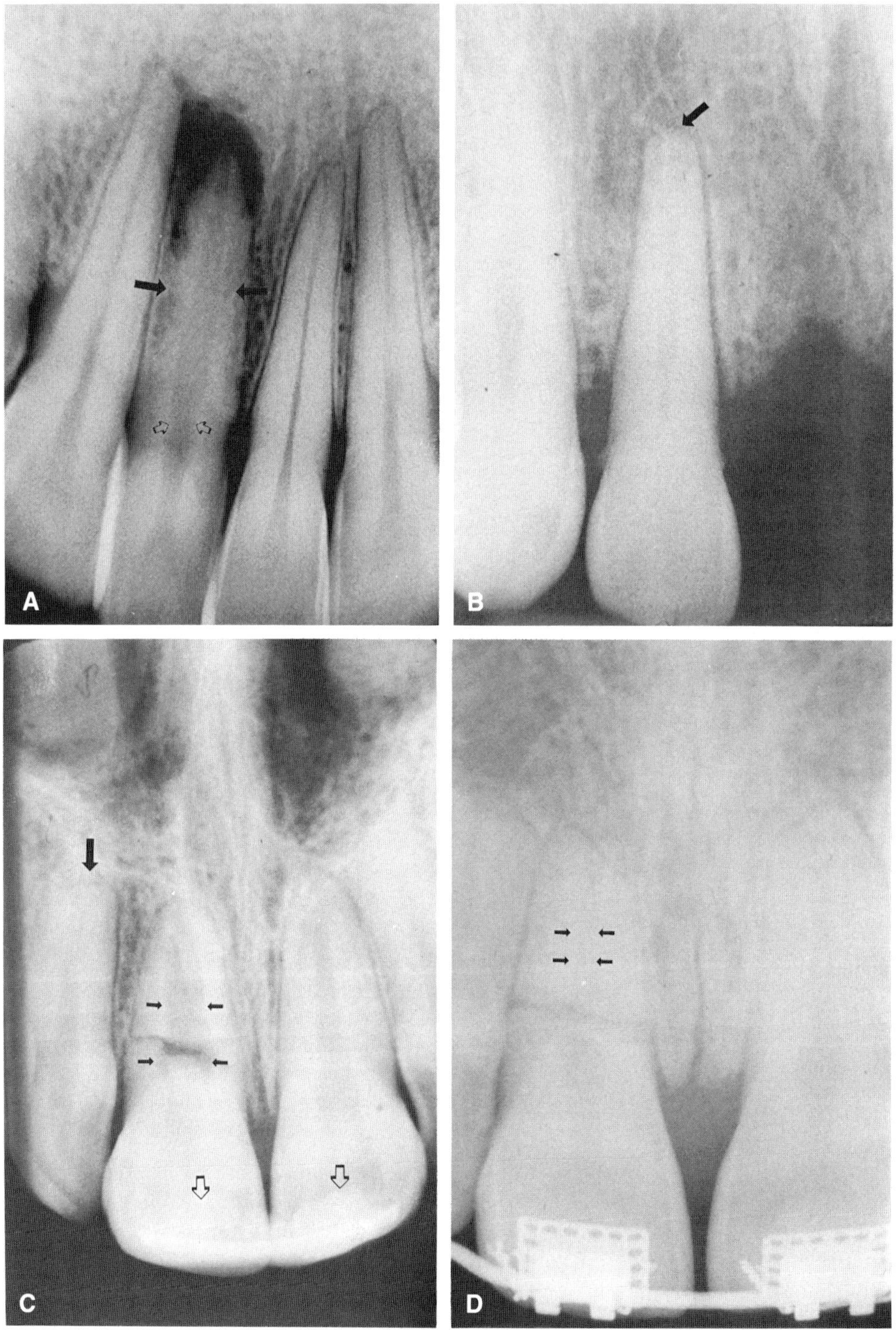

Figure 17–20. *Series of periapical radiographs demonstrating various types of root resorption. (**A**) Demonstration of external replacement resorption (black arrows) and internal inflammatory resorption (open arrows). Also note periapical pathologic features associated with external inflammatory resorption. (**B**) Radiograph demonstrates poorly delineated periapical radiolucency associated with external inflammatory resorption of the root apex (black arrow). (**C**) Radiograph demonstrating central incisor with middle third of horizontal root fracture associated with inflammatory internal resorption (small black arrows). Also note external inflammatory root resorption on adjacent tooth (large black arrow) and acid-etched composite splint reinforced with wire for fixation and stabilization (open arrows). (**D**) Six-month postoperative follow-up radiograph of patient shown in C. Note internal replacement resorption in the tooth with root fracture (arrows). (Courtesy of Dr. Ming-shih Levine, SUNY at Buffalo.)*

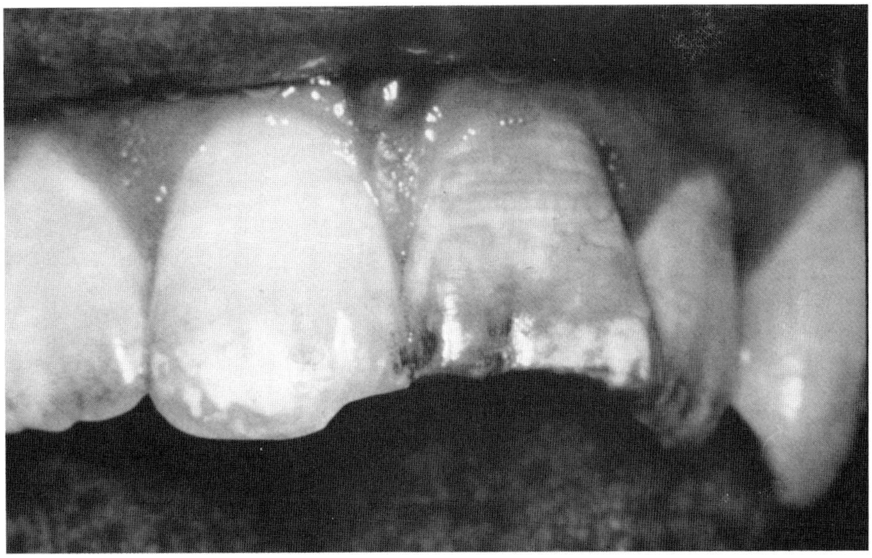

Figure 17–21. *Clinical presentation of a traumatized tooth showing color change secondary to hemoglobin pigment breakdown. (Courtesy of Dr. Ming-shih Levine, SUNY at Buffalo.)*

sue proliferation, reduces the inflammatory response, and most importantly, inhibits the resorption of cementum and subsequent development of dentoalveolar ankylosis.[56]

Luxation and displacement (particularly intrusion) of the deciduous dentition can be associated with injuries to the succedaneous teeth, particularly the development of dilacerated roots.[57] In addition, up to 10% of the permanent teeth demonstrating enamel hypoplasia present with this finding secondary to trauma to the overlying deciduous teeth.[58] Again, treatment for these displaced deciduous teeth is debatable, with some investigators advocating no treatment and others advocating extraction.[30,44]

Color changes in the crowns of teeth can also occur subsequent to trauma, especially as a result of the release of erythrocytes into the pulpal tissue. Initially, the teeth are pink, but as the hemoglobin pigment breaks down and is metabolized, the teeth take on a blue or gray tint (Fig. 17–21).

As described previously in the section on examination, aspiration or swallowing of a tooth can occur with any tooth or tooth segment lost in a traumatic event (Fig. 17–9). Any patient presenting with avulsed dentition and no record of the teeth being accounted for should undergo pulmonary and abdominal radiographic examination, even if the patient is asymptomatic.

REFERENCES

1. Ellis E, Moos KF, El-Attar A. Ten years of mandibular fractures: An analysis of 2,137 cases. Oral Surg Oral Med Oral Pathol 1985; 59:120.
2. Andreasen JO. Etiology and pathogenesis of traumatic dental injuries: A clinical study of 1,298 cases. Scand J Dent Res 1970; 78:329.
3. James D. Maxillofacial injuries in children. In: Rowe NL, Williams JLL, eds. Maxillofacial injuries, ed 1. Edinburgh: Churchill Livingstone, 1985: 538.
4. Andreasen JO. Classification, etiology and epidemiology. In: Andreasen JO, ed. Traumatic injuries of the teeth, ed. 2. Copenhagen: Munksgaard, 1981; 19.
5. Hogeboom FE. Juvenile operative dentistry, ed. 4. St. Louis: CV Mosby 1938: 228.
6. McBride WC. Juvenile dentistry, ed. 3. Philadelphia: Lea & Febiger, 1941: 243.
7. Sweet CA. Fractured anterior permanent teeth. J Am Dent Assoc 1942; 29:97.
8. Adams FR. Traumatized and fractured young teeth. J Am Dent Assoc 1944; 31:241.
9. Cooke C, Rowbotham TC. Treatment of injuries to anterior teeth. Br Dent J 1951; 91:146.
10. Bennett DT. Traumatized anterior teeth. I. Assessing the injury and principles of treatment. Br Dent J 1963; 115:309.
11. Brauer JC. Dentistry for children, ed 5. New York: McGraw-Hill, 1964: 530.
12. Ingle JI, Frank AL, Natkin E, Nutting EE. Diagnosis and treatment of traumatic injuries and their sequelae. In: Ingle JI, Beveridge EE, eds. Endodontics, ed 2. Philadelphia: Lea & Febiger, 1976: 685.

13. Ellis RG, Davey KW. Introduction. In: Ellis RG, Davey KW, eds. The classification and treatment of injuries to the teeth of children: A reference manual for the dental student and the general practitioner, ed 1. Chicago: Year Book Medical Publishers, 1970: 13.
14. Andreasen JO. Classification, etiology, and epidemiology. In: Andreasen JO, ed. Traumatic injuries of the teeth, ed 1. Philadelphia: WB Saunders, 1972: 19.
15. Sanders B, Brady FA, Johnson R. Injuries. In: Sanders B, ed. Pediatric oral and maxillofacial surgery, ed 1. St. Louis: CV Mosby, 1979: 330.
16. Assael LA, Ellis E. Soft tissue and dento-alveolar injuries. In: Peterson LJ, Ellis E, Hupp JR, Tucker MR, eds. Contemporary oral and maxillofacial surgery, ed 1. St. Louis: CV Mosby, 1988: 527.
17. Davidoff G, Jakubowski M, Thomas D, Alpert M. The spectrum of closed-head injuries in facial trauma victims: Incidence and impact. Ann Emerg Med 1988; 17:27.
18. Rowe NL, Killey HC. The clinical examination of fractures of the middle third of the facial skeleton involving the dento-alveolar component. In: Rowe NL, Killey HC, eds. Fractures of the facial skeleton, ed 2. Baltimore: Williams & Wilkins, 1970: 345.
19. Mumford JM. Evaluation of gutta-percha and ethyl chloride in pulp-testing. Br Dent J 1964; 116:338.
20. Fulling HJ, Andreasen JO. Influence of maturation status and tooth type of permanent teeth upon electrometric and thermal pulp testing. Scand J Dent Res 1976; 84:286.
21. Chayra GA, Meador LR, Laskin DM. Comparison of panoramic and standard radiographs for the diagnosis of mandibular fractures. J Oral Maxillofac Surg 1986; 44:677.
22. Hartman LC, Wolfgang L, Hall RE, DelBalso A. The application of panoramic zonography to the diagnosis of maxillofacial fractures. Oral Surg Oral Med Oral Pathol 1989; 67:214.
23. DelBalso A, Hall RE. Trauma of the maxillofacial complex. In: Langland OE, Langlais RP, McDavid WD, DelBalso AM, eds. Panoramic radiology, ed 2. Philadelphia: Lea & Febiger, 1989: 350.
24. Drinnan A. The dangers of using radiolucent dental material. J Am Dent Assoc 1967; 74:446.
25. Hale ML. Traumatic injuries of the teeth and alveolar process. In: Kruger GO, ed. Textbook of oral and maxillofacial surgery, ed 6. St. Louis: CV Mosby, 1984: 357.
26. Andreasen JO. Crown fractures. In: Andreasen JO, ed. Traumatic injuries of the teeth, ed 2. Copenhagen: Munksgaard, 1981: 71.
27. Fialova S, Jurecek B. Urazy zubu u deti a nase zkusenosti s jejich lecenim. Prakt Zubni Lek 1968; 16:171.
28. Zander HA. Reaction of the pulp to calcium hydroxide. J Dent Res 1939; 18:373.
29. Glass RL, Zander HA. Pulp healing. J Dent Res 1949; 28:97.
30. Sowray JH. Localized injuries of the teeth and alveolar process. In: Rowe NL, Williams JL1, eds. Maxillofacial injuries, ed 1. Edinburgh: Churchill Livingstone, 1985: 214.
31. Kroncke A. Uber die Viterhalung der gefahrdeten Pulpa nach Fraktur von Frontzahn-kronen. Deutsch Zahnarztebel 1957; 11:333.
32. Gaare A, Hagen A, Kanstad S. Tannfrakturer hos barn. Diagnostiske og prognostiske problemer og behandling. Norsk Tannloegeforen Tid 1958; 68:364.
33. Cvek DMS. Endodontic treatment of traumatized teeth. In: Andreasen JO, ed. Traumatic injuries of the teeth, ed 2. Copenhagen: Munksgaard, 1981: 321.
34. Antrim DD, Bakland LK, Parker MW. Treatment of endodontic urgent care cases. In: Terezhalmy GT, Antrim DD, eds. The dental clinics of North America, ed 1. Philadelphia: WB Saunders, 1986: 549.
35. Kozlowska I. Pokrycie bezposrednie miazgi preparatem krajowej produkcji. Czas Stomatol 1960; 13:375.
36. Hallet GEM, Porteous JR. Fractured incisors treated by vital pulpotomy: A report on 100 consecutive cases. Br Dent J 1963; 115:279.
37. Martin DM, Crabb HSM. Calcium hydroxide in root canal therapy: A review. Br Dent J 1977; 142:277.
38. Aponte AJ, Hartsook JT, Crowley MC. Indirect pulp capping success verified. J Dent Child 1966; 33:164.
39. Attalla MN, Noujaim AA. Role of calcium hydroxide in the formation of reparative dentin. Can Dent Assoc J 1969; 35:267.
40. Binnie WH, Rowe AHR. A histological study of the periapical tissues of incompletely formed pulpless teeth filled with calcium hydroxide. J Dent Res 1973; 52:1110.
41. Steiner JC, Van Hassel HJ. Experimental root apexification in primates. Oral Surg Oral Med Oral Pathol 1971; 31:409.
42. Andreasen JO, Hjorting Hansen E. Intra-alveolar root fractures: Radiographic and histologic study of 50 cases. J Oral Surg 1967; 25:414.
43. Andreasen, JO. Treatment of fractured and avulsed teeth. J Dent Child 1971; 38:29.
44. Andreasen JO. Luxation injuries. In: Andreasen JO, ed. Traumatic injuries of the teeth, ed 2. Copenhagen: Munksgaard, 1981: 151.
45. Andreasen JO, Hjorting-Hansen E. Replantation of teeth. I. Radiographic and clinical study of 100 human teeth replanted after accidental loss. Acta Odontol Scand 1966; 24:263.
46. Courts FJ, Mueller WA, Tafeling HJ. Milk as an interim storage medium for avulsed teeth. Pediatr Dent 1983; 5:183.
47. Andreasen JO. Exarticulation. In: Andreasen JO, ed. Traumatic injuries of the teeth, ed 2. Copenhagen: Munksgaard, 1981: 203.
48. Andreasen JO. Injuries to the supporting bone. In: Andreasen JO, ed. Traumatic injuries of the teeth, ed 2. Copenhagen: Munksgaard, 1981: 243.
49. Thoma KH. The treatment of traumatic diseases of the jaws. In: Thoma KH, ed. Oral surgery, ed 2. St. Louis: CV Mosby, 1952: 415.
50. Kehoe J. Splinting and replantation after traumatic avulsion. J Am Dent Assoc 1986; 112:224.
51. Hammarstrom L, et al. Tooth avulsion and replantation: A review. Endod Dent Traumatol 1986; 2:1.

52. Andreasen JO. Review of root resorption systems and models: Etiology of root resorption and the homeostatic mechanisms of the periodontal ligament. In: Davidovitch Z, ed. The biological mechanisms of tooth eruption and root resorption. Birmingham, AL: EBSCO Media, 1988: 9.
53. Tronstad L. Root resorption: Etiology, terminology and clinical manifestations. Endod Dent Traumatol 1988; 4:241.
54. Stalkane I, Hedegard B. Traumatized permanent teeth in children aged 7–15 years. II. Swed Dent J 1975; 68:157.
55. Andreasen JO. Luxation of permanent teeth due to trauma: A clinical and radiographic follow-up study of 189 injured teeth. Scand J Dent Res 1970; 78:273.
56. Nasjleti CE, Caffesse RG, Castelli WA, Lopatin DE, Kowalski CJ. Effect of fibronectin on healing of replanted teeth in monkeys: A histologic and autoradiographic study. Oral Surg Oral Med Oral Pathol 1987; 63:291.
57. van Gool AV. Injury to the permanent tooth germ after trauma to the deciduous predecessor. Oral Surg Oral Med Oral Pathol 1973; 35:2.
58. Andreasen JO, Ravn JJ. Enamel changes to permanent teeth after trauma to their primary predecessors. Scand J Dent Res 1973; 81:203.

18

Principles of Management of Fractures of the Mandible

Neil H. Luyk

GOALS OF MANAGEMENT

In the management of any fracture of bone, the goals are to restore function to the affected bone by ensuring union of the fractures and reestablishing prefracture strength of the bone; to restore any contour defect that might arise as a result of the injury; and to prevent infection at the fracture site. Restored function of the mandible, in particular, as part of the masticatory system must include the ability to masticate food properly, to speak normally, and to open the mouth as widely as before the trauma. In order to achieve these goals there must be restoration of the normal occlusion for the patient. Historically, the application of three principles would ensure the achievement of these goals[1]: reduction, fixation, and immobilization.

Reduction can be open or closed. In open reduction, as the name implies, part or all the fracture site is visualized so that the accuracy of the reduction can be seen. Often this is accompanied by the direct application of fixation at the fracture site (Figs. 18–1 and 18–2). A closed reduction takes place when the fracture site is not directly visualized, but the reduction is deemed accurate by palpation of the bony fragments and by restoration of the functioning segments, for example, restoration of the dental occlusion by wiring the teeth together, using splints, or employing external pins (Figs. 18–3 to 18–5).

Fracture union will not take place in the presence of excessive mobility; the fracture site must be stabilized. Fixation must be able to resist the displacing forces acting on the mandible. Fixation can take one of two forms: direct or indirect. When direct fixation is used the fracture site is opened, visualized, and reduced; then stabilization is applied across the fracture site. The rigidity of direct fixation can range from a simple osteal wiring acoss the fracture (i.e., nonrigid fixation), to a mini–bone plate at the area of fracture tension (i.e., semirigid fixation), to a compression bone plate (i.e., rigid fixation). Indirect fixation is the stabilization of the proximal and distal fragments of the bone at a site distant from the fracture line. The most commonly used method for mandibular fractures is the use of intermaxillary fixation. A further example of indirect fixation is the use of external pin fixation.

To achieve fracture union, the fracture site must be stabilized (i.e., immobilized for a sufficient period of time to allow clinical fracture union). The fracture must be able to resist the displacing forces acting on it. When indirect methods of fixation are used in adults, the clinical consolidation occurs by 4 weeks in 80% of patients.[2,3] The immobilization period required is affected by the age of the patient, state of dentulism, cooperation of the patient, the presence of modifying factors such as alcoholism, and the presence of general and local periodontitis.[3,4]

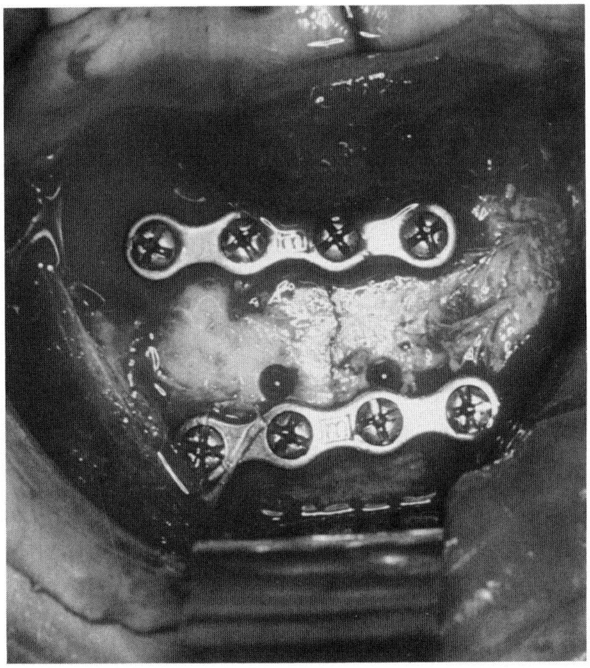

Figure 18–1. *A symphysis fracture treated by open reduction (note holes for reduction forceps) and two miniplates for fixation.*

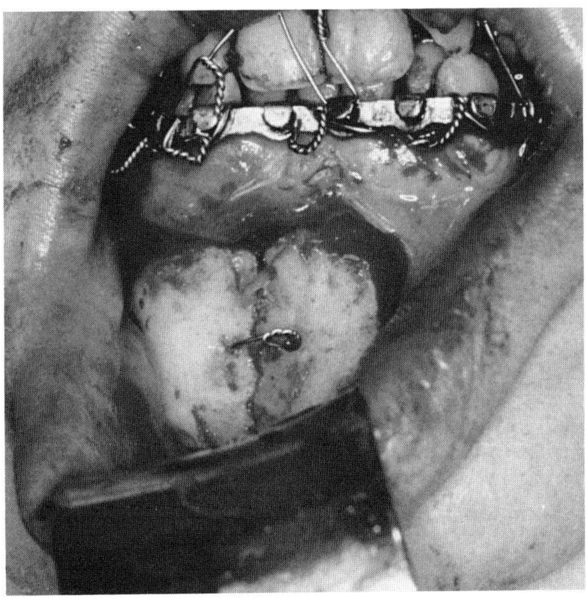

Figure 18–2. *A symphysis fracture treated by open reduction and fixation with a simple wire.*

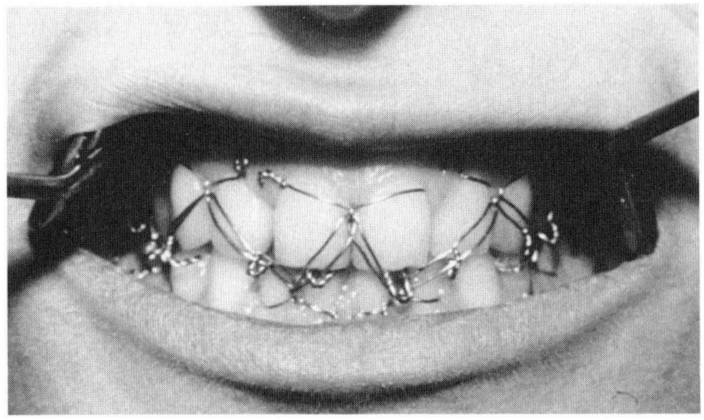

Figure 18–3. *A closed reduction of a mandibular fracture treated with Ivy wires and intermaxillary fixation.*

In the modern era, with so many options at hand, one can be easily caught up in using the current fashionable treatment, but basic principles must not be compromised for convenience. Overall, the simplest, easiest method that is effective should be used to achieve the goals. This rule should always apply.

CLASSIFICATION

Fractures can be displaced or undisplaced at the time of injury. This depends on the force and direction of the blow and the direction line of the fracture, and on the muscular forces acting on the fragments. It is the displacing forces of the muscles of mastication that influence favorability (Figs. 18–6 and 18–7). The principle of favorability is based on the direction of a fracture line as viewed on radiographs in the horizontal or vertical plane. A horizontally favorable fracture line resists the upward displacing forces, such as the pull of the masseter and temporalis muscles on the proximal fragment when viewed in the horizontal plane. A vertically favorable fracture line resists the medial pull of the medial pterygoid on the proximal fragment when viewed in the vertical plane. In the area between the canine teeth of the mandible, the combined action of the suprahyoid and digastric muscles on a bilateral fracture can pull on the distal fragment inferiorly in unfavorable fractures.

Mandibular fracture may be further classified by

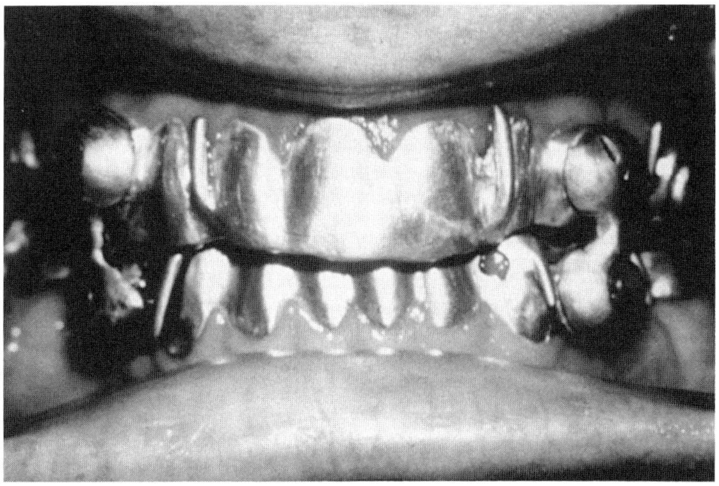

Figure 18–4. *Cast cap splints used to treat a mandibular fracture.*

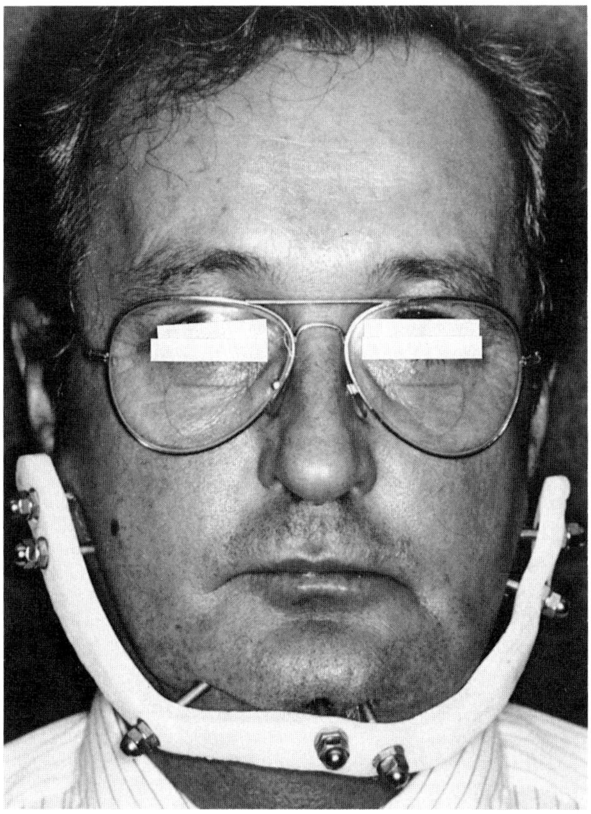

Figure 18–5. *Biphasic pin technique used to treat a fractured mandible.*

the type of fracture (Fig. 18–8) present and by anatomical location.

Types of Fracture

Simple fracture: A simple fracture consists of a single fracture line that does not communicate with the exterior. In mandibular fractures this implies a fracture of the ramus or condyle or a fracture in an edentulous portion with no tears in the periosteum.

Compound fracture: These fractures have a communication with the external environment, usually by the periodontal ligament of a tooth, and involve all fractures of the tooth-bearing portions of the jaws. In addition, if there is a breach of the mucosa leading to an intraoral communication or a laceration of the skin communicating with the fracture site, edentulous portions of the mandible may be involved.

Greenstick fracture: This type of fracture frequently occurs in children and involves incomplete loss of continuity of the bone. Usually one cortex is fractured and the other is bent, leading to distortion without complete section. There is no mobility between the proximal and distal fragments.

Comminuted fractures: These are fractures that exhibit multiple fragmentation of the bone at one fracture site. These are usually the result of greater forces than would normally be encountered in simple fractures.

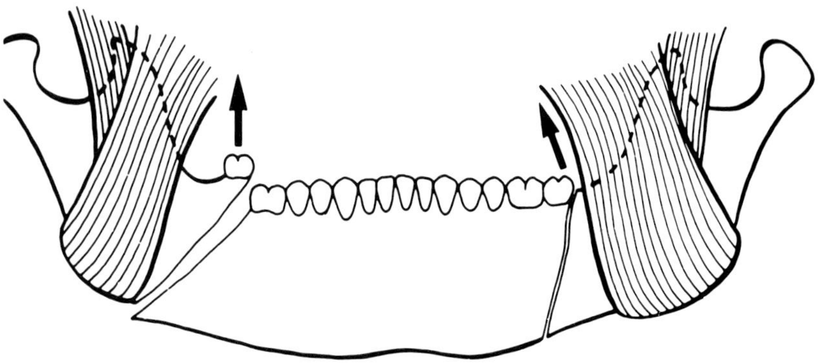

Figure 18–6. *Diagram of horizontally unfavorable* (left) *and favorable* (right) *fracture lines.* Arrows *indicate displacing forces.*

Complex or complicated fracture: This type of injury implies damage to structures adjacent to the bone such as major vessels, nerves, or joint structures. This usually implies damage to the inferior alveolar artery, vein, and nerve in mandibular fractures proximal to the mental foramen and distal to the mandibular foramen. On rare occasions a peripheral branch of the facial nerve may be damaged or the inferior alveolar nerve injured in subcondylar fractures. A recent study has shown that the internal structures of the temporomandibular joint can suffer extensive damage in the presence of fractures elsewhere.[5]

Telescoped or impacted fracture: This type of injury is rarely seen in the mandible, but it implies that one bony fragment is forcibly driven into the other. This type of injury must be disimpacted before clinical movement between the fragments is detectable.

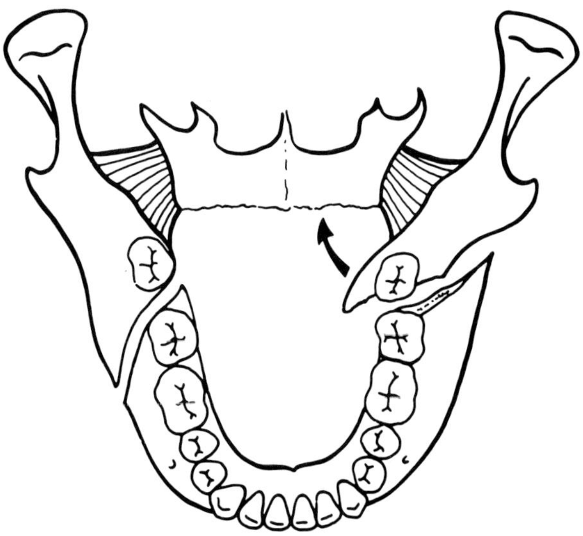

Figure 18–7. *Diagram of vertically favorable* (left) *and unfavorable* (right) *fracture lines.* Arrow *indicating displacing force.*

Indirect fracture: Direct fractures arise immediately adjacent to the point of contact of the trauma, whereas indirect fractures arise at a point distant from the site of the fracturing force. An example of this could be a subcondylar fracture occurring in combination with a symphysis fracture.

Pathologic fracture: A pathologic fracture is said to occur when a fracture results from normal function or minimal trauma in a bone weakened by pathology. The pathology involved may be localized to the fracture site, such as the result of a cyst or metastatic tumor, or as part of a generalized skeletal disorder, such as osteopetrosis.

A further classification of mandible fractures is by site of fracture (Fig. 18–9). Kelly and Harrigan[6] defined the following regions:

Condylar process fracture: A fracture that runs from the mandibular notch to the posterior border of the ramus of the mandible.

Ascending ramus fracture: A fracture in which the fracture line extends horizontally through both the anterior and posterior borders of the ramus or that runs vertically from the mandibular notch to the inferior border of the mandible.

Angle fracture: Any fracture distal to the second molar, extending from any point on the curve formed by the junction of the body and ramus in the retromolar area to any point on the curve formed by the inferior border of the body and posterior border of the ramus of the mandible.

Body fracture: Any fracture that occurs in the region between the mesial portion of the canine and the distal portion of the second molar and extends from the alveolar process through the inferior border.

Symphysis fracture: Any fracture in the region of the incisors that runs from the alveolar process through the

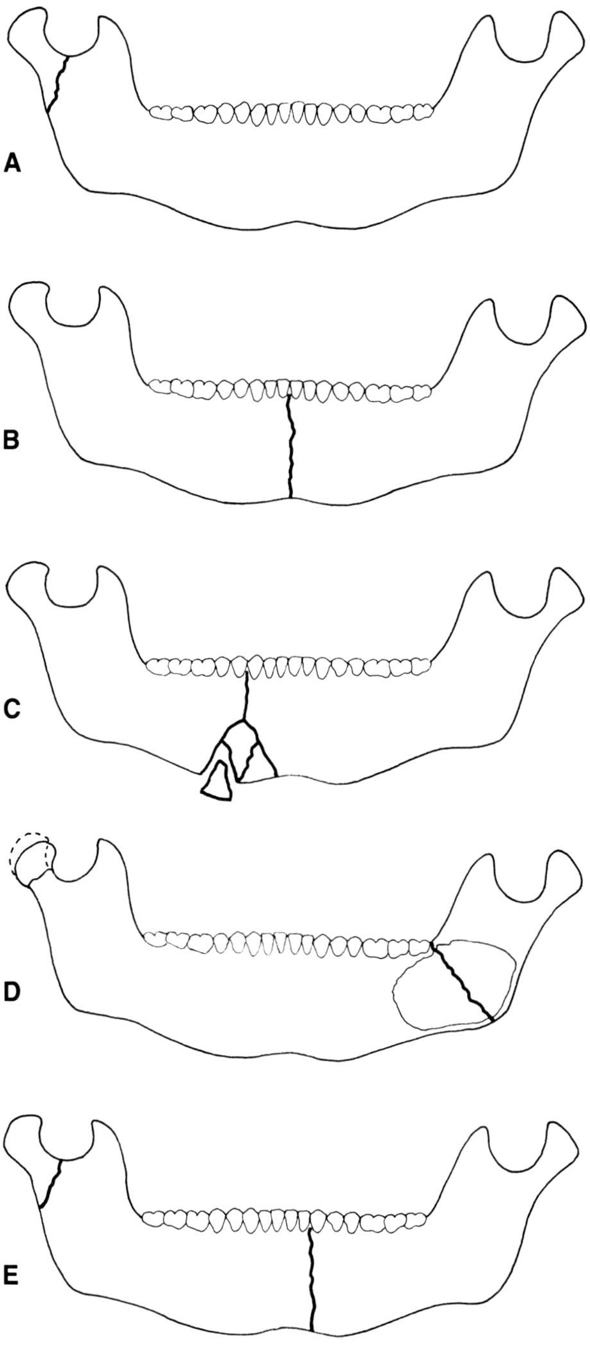

Figure 18–8. *Diagram of types of fractures: (**A**) Simple fracture; (**B**) compound fracture; (**C**) comminuted fracture; (**D**) impacted fracture in the right subcondylar area and a pathologic fracture in the left angle area; (**E**) direct and indirect fractures.*

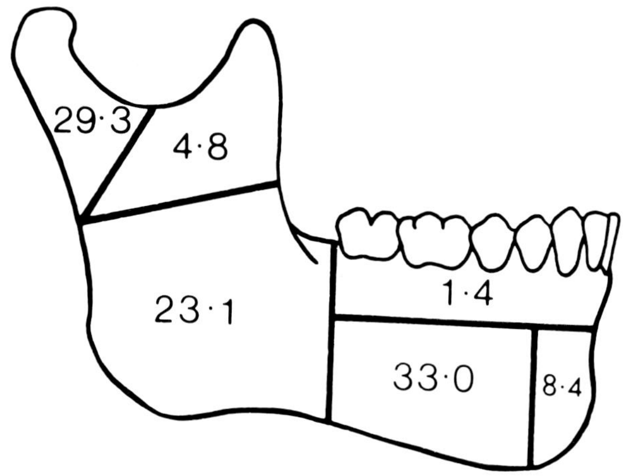

Figure 18–9. *Percentage of mandibular fracture site distribution. (Adapted from Ellis E, Moos KF, El-Attar A. Oral Surg 1985; 59 : 120).*

inferior border of the mandible. Some authors define this area to also include the canine tooth.[7,8]

To this list is frequently added dentoalveolar fractures, which are fractures of the tooth-bearing portion of the jaw not extending to the inferior border.[9,10]

Fractures involving the condylar area can be classified as extracapsular (subcapsular) or intracapsular, depending on the relation of the fracture to the capsular attachment. Extracapsular fractures may have no displacement, deviation, or a fracture dislocation of the condylar head. When displacement of the condylar head occurs it is usually in an anteromedial direction under the influence of the lateral pterygoid muscle. Rarely, the displacement occurs centrally into the glenoid fossa (although usually there is no fracture associated with this displacement)[11] or laterally medial to the zygomatic arch.

Fractures of the mandible have been reported to comprise between 40% and 62% of all facial fractures,[6,10,12] although these figures may not represent the true incidence, because isolated nasal fractures are seldom included in such surveys. Gratten and Hobbs[13] have reported that 39% of patients involved in road traffic accidents sustained facial injuries; this figure included 0.68% of patients with fractured mandibles. Males are reported to be affected more frequently than females in a ratio ranging from 3:1 to 7:1 depending on the survey and especially the country involved.[9,10,12,14] Predictably, such studies reveal the most susceptible age group for both sexes is between

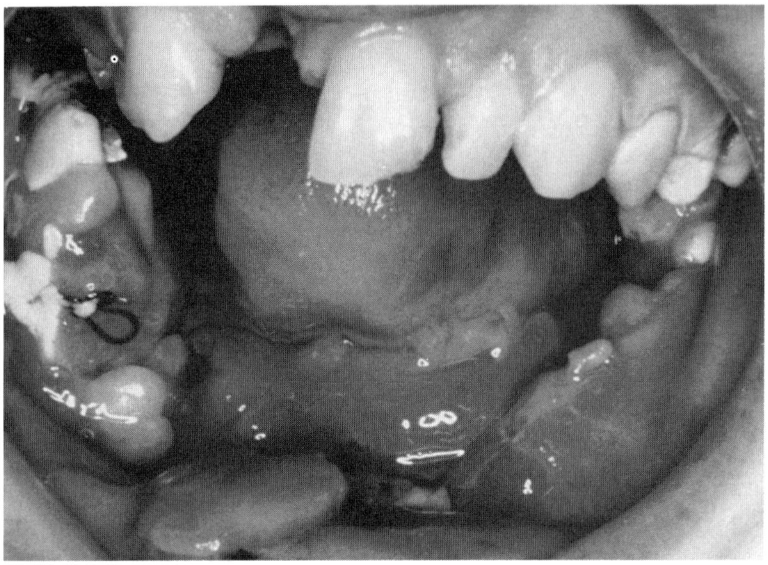

Figure 18–10. *This patient sustained a severely comminuted mandibular fracture with multiple missing teeth.*

ages 21 and 30.[7,9,10,12] There are two principal causes of facial fractures: interpersonal violence and motor vehicle accidents (MVA) (Figs. 18–10 and 18–11); these vary according to the area in which the survey was undertaken and the socioeconomic and ethnic status of the community.[7,9,10,14,15] Other significant causes are falls and sports injuries.

A percentage of patients with mandibular fractures have other facial injuries. Surveys by Ellis et al.,[10] Salem et al.[15] and Haug et al.[16] reported that 20% of patients also sustained fractures in other parts of the facial skeleton, mainly the zygomaticomaxillary complex. Further injury away from the facial region may be present, including multiple-system trauma. In the study by Ellis et al.[10] of 2137 patients with mandibular fractures, 10.5% of subjects sustained other injuries outside the maxillofacial region. Injury patterns are largely dependent on the mechanism of injury, with

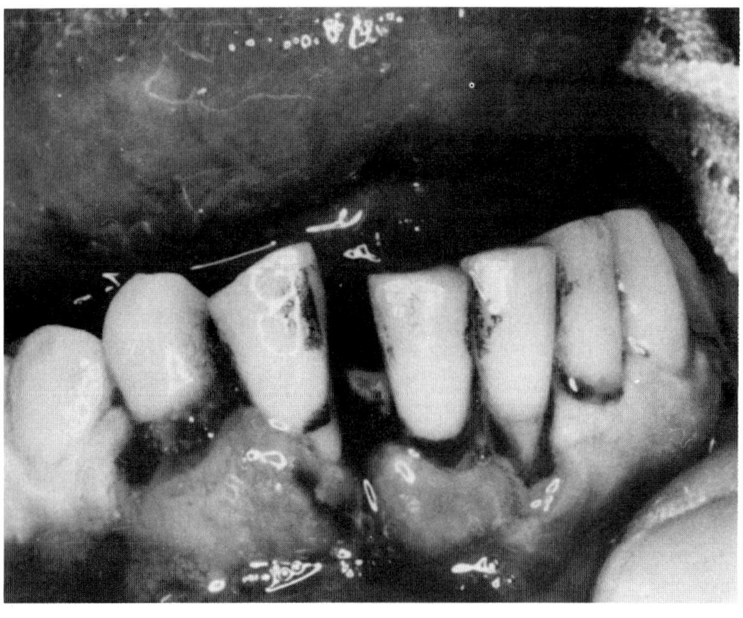

Figure 18–11. *A compound symphyseal fracture sustained from a blow to the jaw. Note the sublingual ecchymosis.*

patients involved in MVA sustaining a greater percentage of other injuries. In one large survey[10] of 3462 mandibular fractures, the distribution of principal fracture sites was reported as 33% involving the body, 29% in the condylar region, 23% the angle, and 8.4% in the symphysis region (see Fig. 18–9). It is not unusual to sustain more than one fracture site in the mandible. Although some studies have reported the majority of patients to have sustained only one fracture,[7,14,15] others[9,10,17] have reported a small majority of patients with multiple fracture sites. The anatomical distribution of the fracture sites is largely dependent on the mechanism of injury, as well documented by Olson et al.,[7] who showed that in MVA 30.9% of fractures occurred in the subcondylar area, 27.7% in the symphyseal region, 17.3% in the angle, 13.9% in the body and the alveolus, and 7.2% in other sites. A different distribution pattern was seen in cases resulting from interpersonal violence: 33.3% of fractures were located in the angle, 23.4% in the subcondylar area, 19.4% in the body, 16% in the symphyseal area, and 4.1% in the alveolar and other sites. The left side is more commonly involved, in particular the left angle, probably because most assailants are right-handed and the left side of the jaw would be the side most likely to be struck.[7] Falls show a greater proportion of subcondylar fractures, as high as 36.3% in one survey.[10] When multiple fractures of the mandible are considered, the most common combinations are angle and opposite body, bilateral body, bilateral angle, condyle, and opposite body[6] (Fig. 18–12).

The site of fracture is also determined by the size, direction, and surface area of the impacting blow. An impact to the chin with a line of force through the symphysis and temporomandibular joints will produce a single subcondylar fracture at 425 lb[18] and a bilateral subcondylar fracture at about 550 lb, whereas symphyseal fractures require force between 550 and 900 lb.[18] An impact to the lateral aspect of the mandibular body using a 1 × 4-inch impact surface will produce a mandibular fracture at 300 to 700 lb.[18,19] When an impact force is delivered to the mandible, the bone bends inwards, producing compressive forces on the impacted (lateral) surface and tensile forces on the lingual (medial) surfaces of the bone opposite the impact site.[19] Fracture results when the tensile strain overcomes the resistance of the bone, beginning on the medial side of the mandible and progressing through the bone toward the impact point.[19]

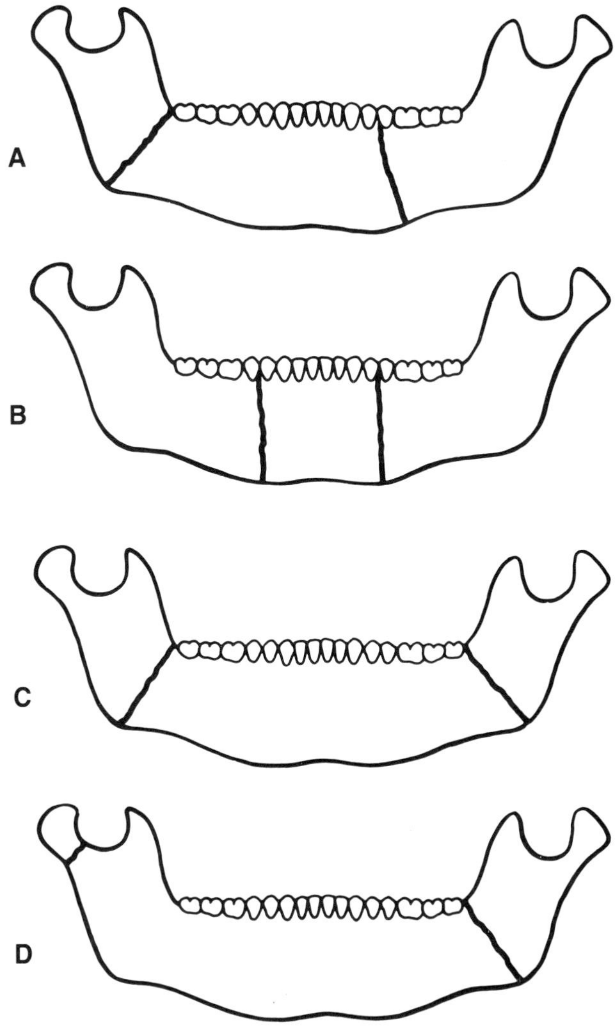

Figure 18–12. *The most common multiple mandibular fracture sites. From top to bottom:* (**A**) *angle and opposite body,* (**B**) *bilateral body,* (**C**) *bilateral angle,* (**D**) *condyle and opposite angle.*

Direct fracture may occur at the site of impact, but additional indirect fractures may result when higher forces are involved. An example would be a blow to the left angle, causing a direct fracture at the left angle region and an indirect fracture in the right body. Occasionally only indirect fracture results, usually in the subcondylar area as, for example, when a blow on the chin results in a fracture of one or other condylar necks. Indirect fractures demonstrate the opposite tensile strain patterns and fracture outcomes from those of the direct fracture; that is, the tensile strain develops on the side opposite to the impact. In the case of greenstick fractures, the fracture occurs on the tension side and bending occurs on the compression side.

Bone Healing

In the 19th century, Wolff postulated that the shape a bone takes conforms to the forces exerted on it. This applies to both the gross shape of the bone and the architecture of the trabeculare within the bone. The bone healing that occurs after a fracture may be considered as an accelerated form of bone remodeling, with the disrupted bone gradually returning to its original size and shape.

Other than bone itself, three tissues are primarily involved in fracture healing: periosteum, endosteum, and fracture hematoma. There are two layers to the periosteum. The outer fibrous layer conveys blood vessels to the cortex and provides limited blood supply to the outer 25% of the cortex. The inner cambium layer, which is usually not more than one cell layer thick, is osteogenic and activated by injury, forming a bridge across and cuff of bone around the periphery of a fracture. This new periosteal bone is termed "callus" as is all new bone formed in a fracture site. The endosteum is similar to the periosteum but is a single-cell layer lining the medullary canal. It is the major source of callus that fills the fracture defect and achieves union. The fracture hematoma forms in and around the fracture site as a result of bleeding from ruptured soft tissues and bone vessels. It is rapidly invaded by blood vessels, fibroblasts, and chondroblasts that quickly organize it into granulation-type tissue.

Based on their histologic and morphologic appearance, three overlapping phases of fracture healing are typically described (Fig. 18–13): the inflammatory stage, the reparative stage, and the remodeling stage. The inflammatory reaction helps to immobilize the fracture. Pain causes the patient to limit mandibular function, and swelling helps to hydrostatically splint the fracture. The inflammatory process is not unique and consists of the typical dilation of vessels, hyperemia in the soft tissues around the fracture, inflammatory cell infiltrate, followed by a nonspecific exudate. Damage to both the adjacent soft tissue and the bone ends undergoes active phagocytosis and lysis by monocytes and osteoclasts later in the inflammatory process.

In the reparative phase, which begins within 1 to 2 days of injury and continues well into the remodeling phase, the key event is osteoblast proliferation. In undisplaced fractures this process is dominated by the endosteum. However, in displaced fractures, the periosteal tissues dominate early but are quickly replaced by the endosteal tissues, which play the major role in fracture healing.[20,21] Within a few days, callus begins to form. Islands of cartilage cells and osteoid begin to form in the granulation tissue. Early bone usually forms in the periosteal area first, forming a collar of callus. Endochondral ossification with osteoid formation by osteoblasts then progresses, and mineralization is sufficiently well developed that callus bridges the fracture site and the callus stiffens, producing what clinicians term "clinical healing"; that is, the manipulation across the fracture site does not produce movement. At this point the remodeling stage is said to begin. During this phase the fracture callus and bone remodel in response to mechanical stimuli to restore normal shape and strength. The mandible takes approximately 20 to 25 weeks to regain preinjury strength.

Primary Bone Healing versus Secondary Bone Union

Secondary (indirect or callus) bone union is the normal process of fracture healing when a mandibular fracture is treated with closed reduction and intermaxillary fixation. In the event of an anatomical reduction and rigid internal fixation with very limited motion between the fracture ends, a primary (direct or osteonal) bony healng is observed (Fig. 18–14). Histologically an intense remodeling of the fragment ends starts in a zone of a few millimeters from the fracture. Groups of osteoclasts locally resorb bone to form tunnels in the compact bone. Vessels and osteoblasts follow the osteoclasts into the tunnel and fill it with new bone. When there is no movement between the fracture ends, the remodeling can proceed across the fracture. The newly formed osteons crossing the fracture plane lead to a step-by-step substitution of the fracture by new bone elements. No intermediate cartilage appears at the union of the fragment, and healing takes place by bone tissue. Compression has been shown by some studies to aid in the achievement of primary bone healing,[22] but others have suggested that axial compression does not augment fracture healing of plated cortical bone.[23]

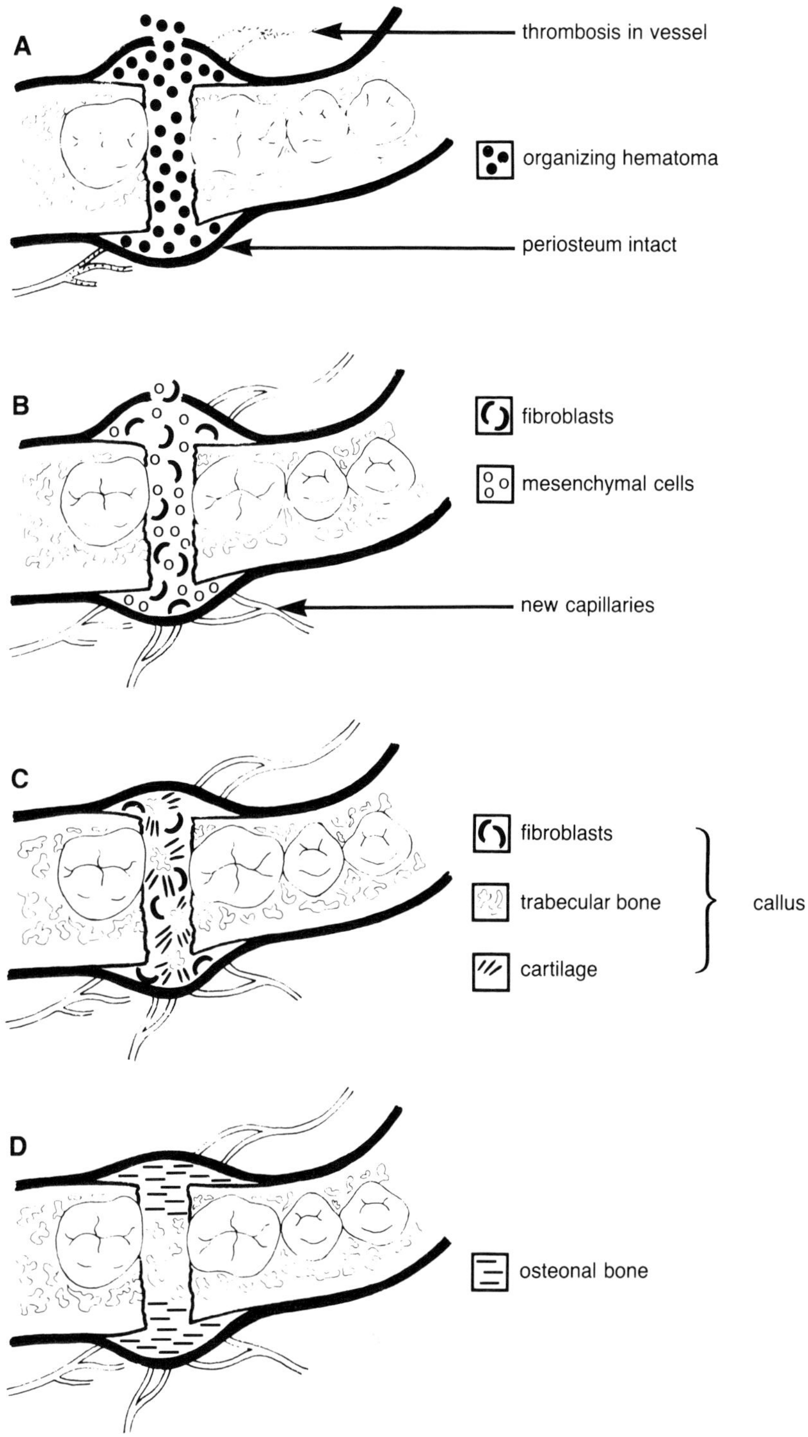

Figure 18–13. *Healing fracture site. (***A***) Inflammatory phase (1–2 days); (***B***) reparative phase (4–12 days); (***C***) reparative phase (7–40 days); (***D***) Remodeling phase (over 50 days).*

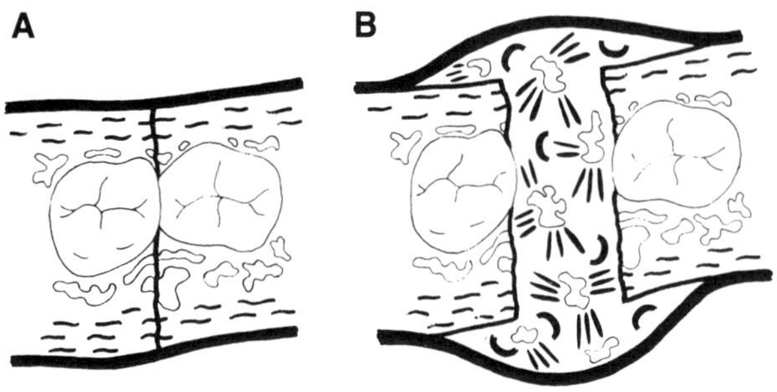

Figure 18–14. *(**A**) Direct bone healing showing direct bridging across the fracture site by osteons. There is no gap present at the fracture site and there must be rigid fixation; (**B**) Indirect bone healing with fibroblasts, trabecular bone, and cartilage making up the callus.*

DIAGNOSIS OF FRACTURED MANDIBLES

Before any local examination of the mandible, consideration must be given to the overall patient. Victims of MVA frequently appear to have gruesome facial mutilation, which may divert the clinician's attention from the fact that these injuries are rarely fatal and that other more critical problems might be present. The advanced trauma life support (ATLS) protocol is to be followed. On the patient's arrival at the emergency department, the first obligation is to make sure that the airway is free. The tongue, which may have a tendency to fall back, must be controlled, and objects obstructing the airway must be removed. If an obstruction cannot be removed, a new airway must be established by endotracheal intubation (remembering possible cervical spine injuries) or cricothyrotomy. After the airway has been secured and respiration is occurring, vital signs must be assessed, including pulse rate and blood pressure. Any significant blood loss is likely to be coming from injuries apart from those of the face. Other critical injuries must be ruled out, including intracranial hemorrhages, cervical and other spinal injuries, chest injuries, abdominal trauma, and fractures of the long bones.

Local examination of the face and jaws should be conducted in a logical sequence. The first objective is to obtain an accurate history from the patient or relative if the patient cannot cooperate. Pertinent to a fractured mandible examination is to note the size, number, and force of any blows to the face. Patients often complain of the following:

Pain or tenderness at the site of a blow with the possibility of a direct fracture, or at a distant site in the case of an indirect fracture.

Difficulty chewing. Pain could be limiting mandibular function or there may be a malocclusion or mobility at a fracture site.

Malocclusion. The patient may be able to tell the clinician of an alteration in the bite from normal, although patients are not always reliable and may claim that the bite feels normal when it is not and vice versa.

Numbness in the distribution of the inferior alveolar nerve. This usually indicates a displaced fracture in the region of the body or angle of the mandible on the affected side. An undisplaced fracture often does not give rise to numbness in the distribution of the inferior alveolar nerve.

Examination should follow the history. The skin of the face and, in particular, the area around the mandible should be inspected for swelling, hematomas, and lacerations. A common site for a laceration is under the chin, and this should alert the clinician to the possibility of an associated subcondylar or symphysis fracture. It is best to begin the examination from behind the seated or supine patient (Fig. 18–15). The fingertips are placed on the inferior border of the mandible, and the mandible is palpated from the symphysis to the angle on each side, noting any areas of swelling, step deformity, or tenderness. Patients with a fracture of the body or angle of the mandible will usually complain of numbness in the distribution of the mental nerve on the affected side due to damage to the inferior alveolar nerve within the mandible. The next part of the examination is undertaken standing in front of the patient. The clinician should palpate the movement of the condyle through the external auditory meatus and observe the movement of the mandible itself (Fig. 18–16). Any significant deviation on opening may be indicative of subcondylar fracture on the side to which the mandible deviates. The fifth finger is placed in each auditory meatus and the patient is asked to open and close the mouth. A fracture in the subcondylar area will produce pain and limitation of movement of the affected condyle. Any limitation of mandibular movement may also be a result of reflex muscle spasm, temporomandibular effusion, or mechanical obstruction to the coronoid process resulting from depression of the zygomatic bone

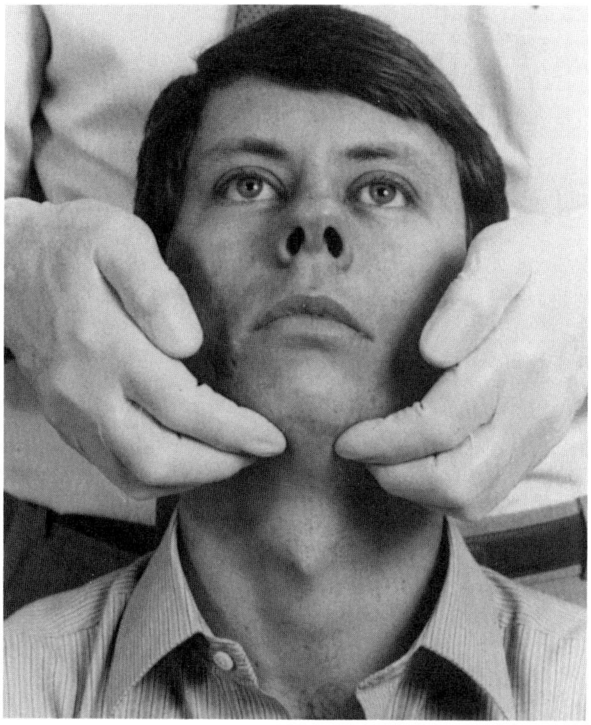

Figure 18–15. *Examination of the suspected fractured mandible from behind the seated patient, with palpation of the inferior border.*

or arch. The external auditory canal is carefully examined for signs of hemorrhage externally and internally with an otoscope. Occasionally a subcondylar fracture will produce a tear in the epithelial lining of the anterior wall of the canal, which produces bleeding from the auditory meatus. It is important to determine that this bleeding is not coming from behind a ruptured tympanic membrane, which may signify a basilar skull fracture.

A detailed intraoral examination should be undertaken with good lighting, following the removal of any artificial dentures (Fig. 18–17). It is important to be systematic, and it is suggested that examination of the soft tissues be undertaken first. The gum tissue should be inspected for tears or lacerations. With the aid of a tongue blade the floor of the mouth is examined; sublingual ecchymosis is almost pathognomonic of a fracture of the mandible. Any areas of bleeding are noted; it is useful to have suction available at this stage. Next the dentition is examined for evidence of broken teeth and for steps or irregularities in the dental arch. The patient is asked to lightly bite the teeth together and say if the bite feels different from normal, following which the occlusion is inspected. Premature occlusal contacts are noted. The three causes of an altered occlusion in the trauma patient are a dis-

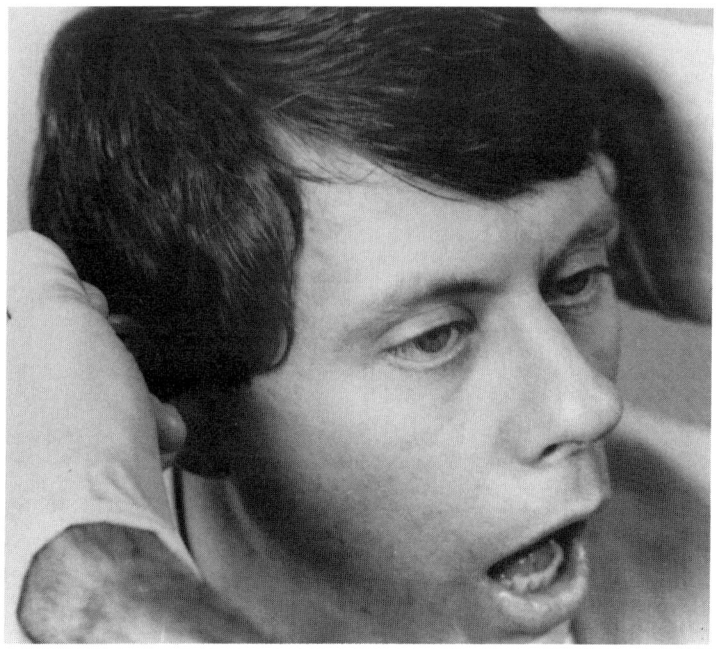

Figure 18–16. *Examination of movement of the condylar head through the external auditory meatus with the fifth digit.*

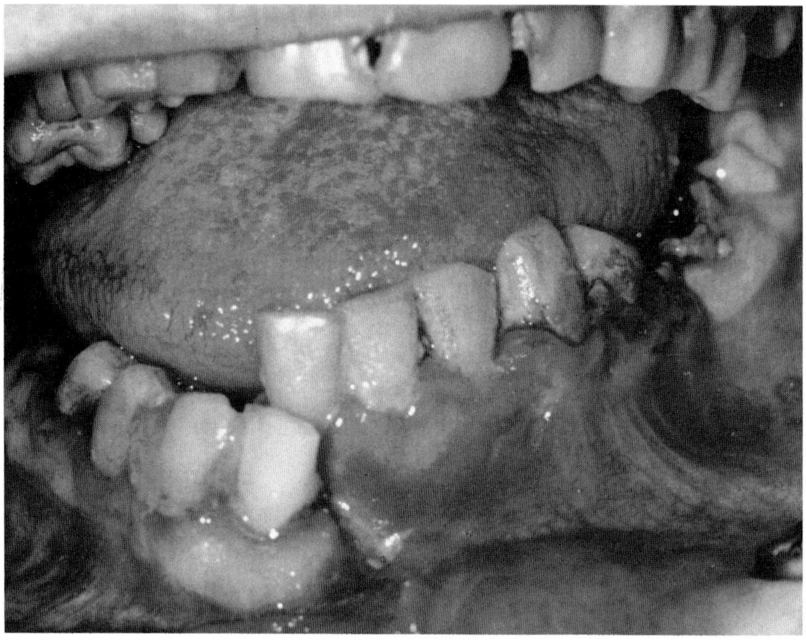

Figure 18–17. *A symphysis fracture between the lower right lateral and central incisor teeth. Note the gingival tear, buccal ecchymosis, malocclusion, and displacement.*

placed fracture, a dental injury such as a displaced tooth, and a temporomandibular joint effusion or dislocation.

If the patient is edentulous and has intact dentures with him, these can be replaced in the mouth and the occlusion inspected. The mandible should then be grasped on each side of any suspected fracture and gently manipulated to assess mobility (Fig. 18–18). If no fracture can be found but clinical suspicion remains high, the mandible may be compressed by applying pressure over both angles (FIg. 18–19). This nearly always gives rise to pain at a fracture site. In the case of subcondylar fractures, firm posterior pressure on the chin will cause pain in the preauricular region.

Radiographs

Radiographic examination of the fractured mandible should include views in three planes of space. The following views are used:

Panoramic radiograph (PR)
Lateral oblique radiographs of the mandible
Posteroanterior (PA) mandibular view
Reverse Townes view
Mandibular occlusal view

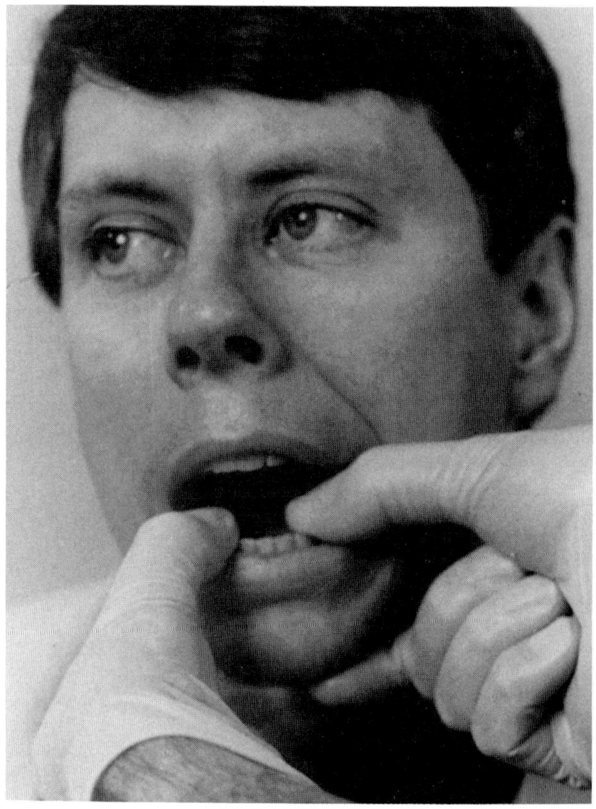

Figure 18–18. *Examination of movement across a suspected fracture site.*

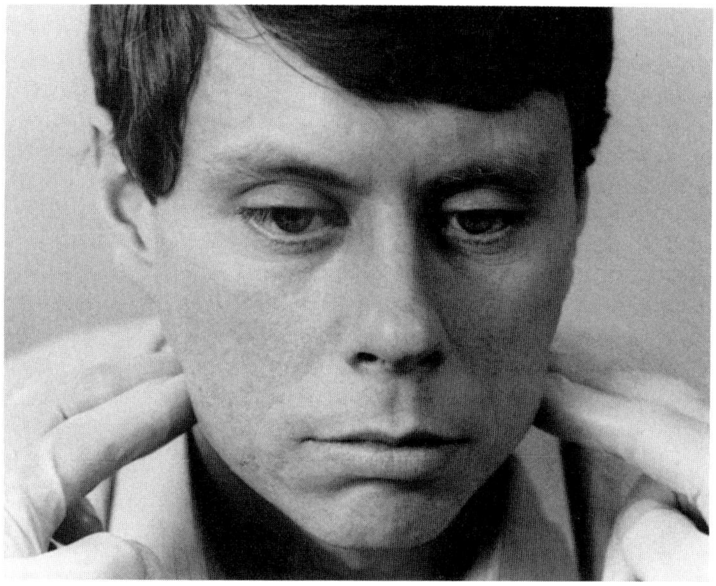

Figure 18–19. *Bilateral compression over the angles of the mandible to elicit pain at a suspected fracture site.*

Periapical radiographs
Temporomandibular joint views including tomography
CT scans

Traditionally the standard views for a suspected mandibular fracture had been the lateral oblique views of the mandible, the PA view of the mandible, and the reverse Townes view. To this list has been added the panoramic radiograph (PR). Recently, Chayra et al.[24] have reviewed the need for a complete series of films. They concluded that the initial screening of patients could be effectively undertaken with a PR alone. Ninety-two percent of fractures were seen on a PR alone, compared with only 66% on a routine radiographic series without a panoramic view. However, in order to accurately visualize displacement it is recommended that the standard mandibular views should consist of a PR, a PA mandibular, and reverse Townes views (Fig. 18–20). The PR usually requires the patient to be able to stand upright and also requires accurate patient positioning for good quality films. In the severely traumatized patient this may be difficult to achieve with some PR machines, although others can accomplish this. Furthermore, mediolateral displacement in the ramus and body and anteroposterior displacement in the symphyseal regions are difficult to visualize and the panoramic technique lacks good resolutional detail compared with plain films. The traditional lateral oblique views of the mandible can be used when PR films are not possible. It requires accurate positioning of the patient and film to obtain useful views particularly in the condylar area. A transcranial temporomandibular view may be helpful in these circumstances. After initial screening further radiographs may be necessary. Following the radiologic principle that radiographs of a fracture are taken at right angles so that any degree of displacement can be visualized, a reverse Townes view is useful in the assessment of condylar and subcondylar fractures, and posteroanterior mandibular views are necessary to assess mediolateral displacement of angle and some body fractures. Accurate assessment of symphyseal fractures can be problematic with the standard views. It is here that a mandibular occlusal view is useful. It also aids in the assessment of the fracture of the lingual plate, particularly in very oblique fractures. Periapical views are necessary for teeth on either side of the fracture line to assess root fractures, periapical and periodontal pathology, and the relationship of the fracture line to the periodontal ligament of each tooth.

Intracapsular fractures of the condylar head are often difficult to visualize accurately on plain films. Axial CT scans with reconstruction in different planes offers an excellent opportunity to study the fracture details. If a CT scanner is not readily available, then tomography of the condylar head area may be useful. However, both these techniques involve high doses of radiation.

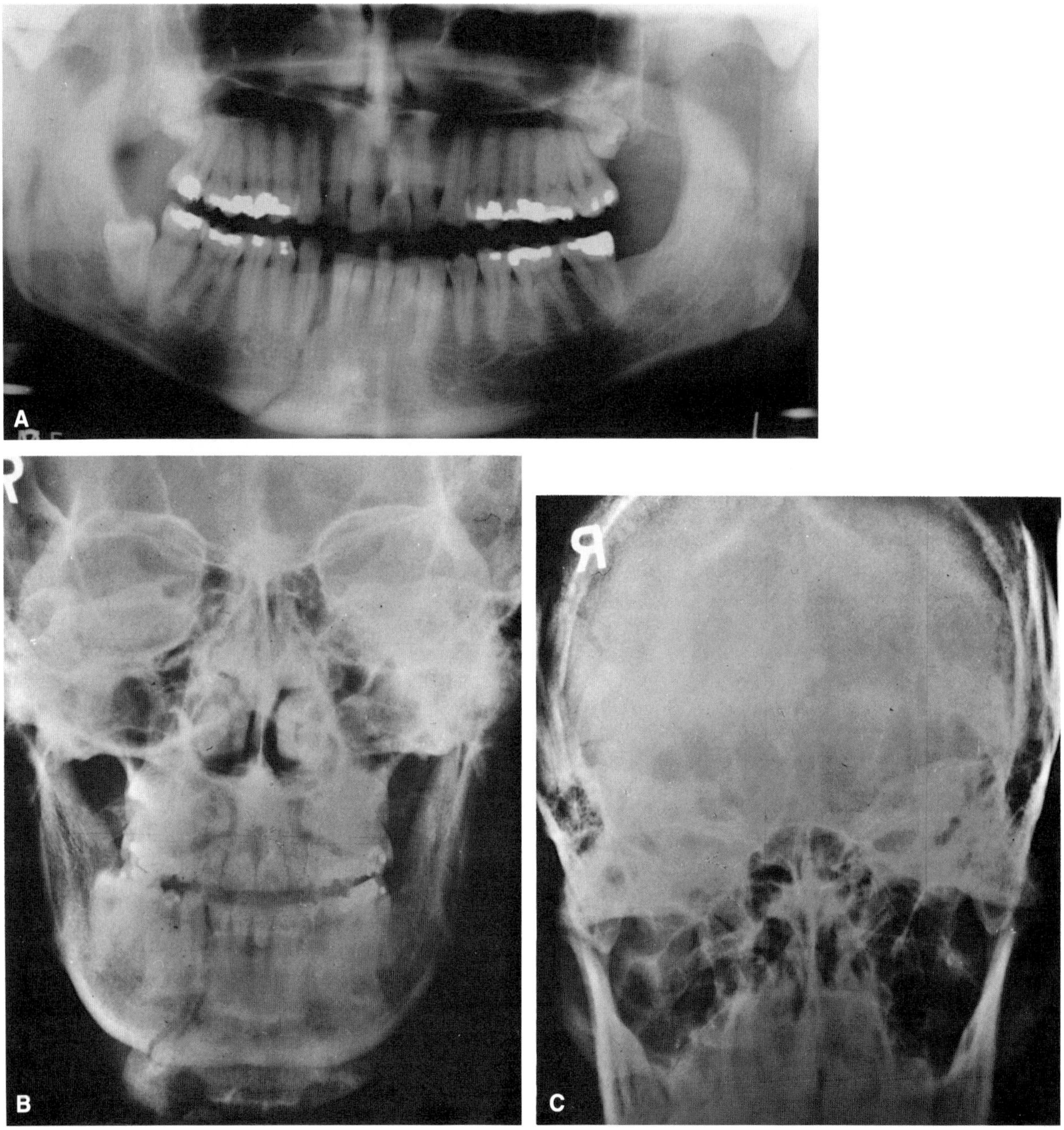

Figure 18–20. *(***A***) A panoramic radiograph of a symphysis fracture between the right lower canine and lateral incisor. (***B***) PA mandibular view of the same patient as in* **A***, minimal displacement of the fracture site. (***C***) Reverse Townes view of the same patient as* **A** *no fracture seen.*

CLOSED REDUCTION

If the principle of using the simplest method to achieve optimal results is to be followed, the use of closed reduction for mandibular fractures should be widely used. According to Bernstein, "It is safe to say that the vast majority of fractures of the mandible may be treated satisfactorily by the method of closed reduction."[25] May et al.[26] go further:

> Many fractures are probably overtreated by open reduction. It is important to realize that the majority of fractures can be successfully managed by conservative means (closed reduction). This concept becomes critical when one considers the economic significance of inflated hospital, operating room material, and personnel costs. Even more important, the need for general anesthesia is obviated. A patient with a mandibular fracture managed by closed technique can be treated as an outpatient or at the most may require two days in the hospital.

Therefore, the indications for closed reduction may simply be stated as all cases in which an open reduction is either not indicated or is contraindicated. Several conditions deserve specific mention:

- Grossly comminuted fractures are, as a general rule, best treated by closed reduction, because using open reduction techniques would jeopardize the blood supply to the small bone fragments and lead to an increased likelihood of infection. This category also includes gunshot wounds, which are particularly prone to infection.
- Fractures in the severely atrophic edentulous mandible represent a difficult clinical situation. On the one hand there is limited osteogenic potential; the majority of the blood supply comes from the periosteum so that an open reduction further disrupts the blood supply. On the other hand, a stable, nonmobile reduction and fixation of these fractures is difficult with closed reduction techniques. Open reduction with limited dissection of the soft tissue and rigid fixation may be the preferred technique.
- Lack of soft tissue overlying the fracture site. When soft tissue flaps have to be transposed to cover a fracture site (particularly if a through-and-through communication exists between the skin and oral cavity) the presence of bone plates, screws, and wires may increase the likelihood of infection.
- Fractures in children involving the developing dentition are difficult to manage by open reduction because of the possibility of damage to the tooth buds or partially erupted teeth.

Closed reduction of fractures of the mandible together with indirect fixation can be achieved by either the application of intermaxillary fixation or by applying a technique to the mandible only.

Intermaxillary Techniques

Dentate Patients

Intermaxillary techniques in dentate patients include application of arch bars (Fig. 18–21 A,B), direct wiring, Ivy loops (Interdental eyelet wiring) (Fig. 18–3),

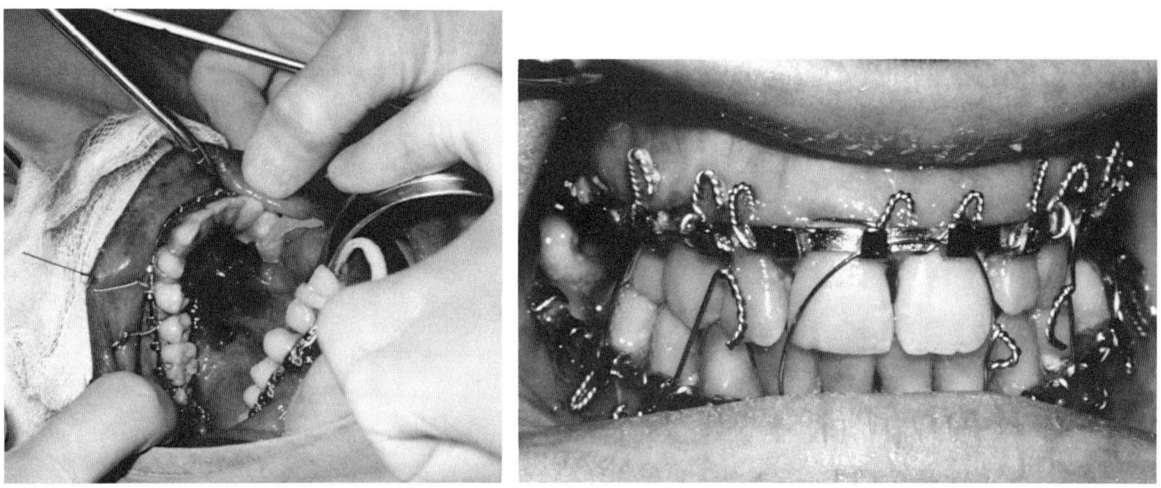

Figure 18–21. *(**A**) Placement of archbars. (**B**) Patient in intermaxillary fixation utilizing archbars.*

continuous wire loop technique (Stout's method, Obwegeser's method), and cast cap splints (Fig. 18–4).

Methods for dentate patients usually include 0.5-mm (25-gauge) soft stainless steel wires around the teeth. In general, the wires should be handled in a similar fashion for all methods, following certain principles:

- Tighten the wires with a continuous tension.
- Direct the force when tightening the wires apically.
- Tighten all wires in a clockwise direction.
- At the end of tightening turn only half a turn at a time.
- Turn the end of the wire into the interproximal embrasure.

These additional rules apply when arch bars are used:

- Adapt the arch bar closely.
- Use a cuspid wrap wire where indicated (Fig. 18–22).
- Avoid placing the wire across the intermaxillary stabilization lugs.
- Use circumferential wires when single teeth stand alone and intraosteal suspension or circummandibular wires in edentulous areas.
- In the area of the fracture, the arch bar may be split or the fracture reduced prior to stabilization of the arch bar on both sides of the fracture.

When intermaxillary fixation is used it may be applied with either elastics or wires. Elastics can be used for fracture reduction and for intermaxillary fixation; however, they apply a constant pressure, which can lead to muscle spasm and pain, particularly in the masseter muscle, and they are difficult to keep clean. Wires, on the other hand, are easier to keep clean and are passive. However, they do loosen over time and need to be tightened or replaced over the period of fixation.

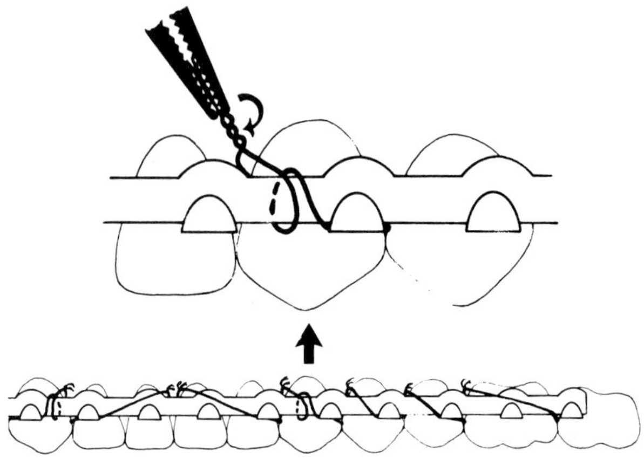

Figure 18–22. *Diagram showing the wiring of a mandibular arch bar.*

Edentulous Patients

Closed reduction in edentulous patients is achieved with Gunning splints or splints made from the patient's own dentures (Fig. 18–23).

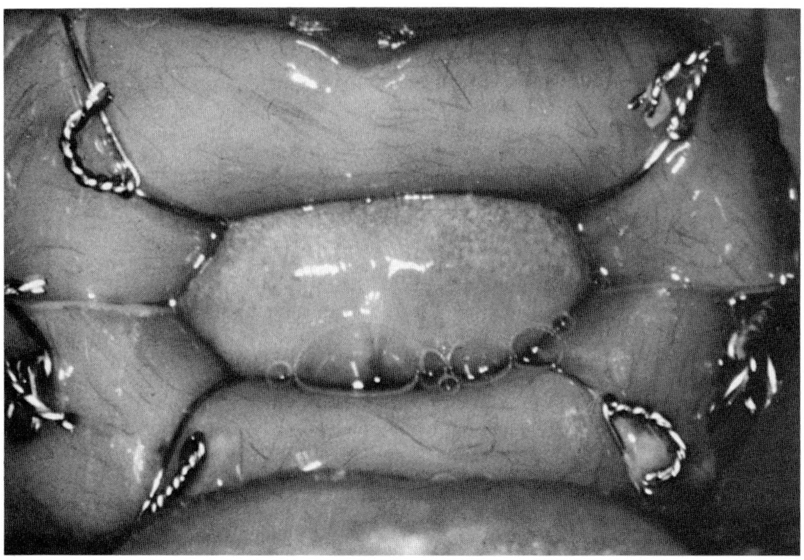

Figure 18–23. *Intermaxillary fixation with Gunning splints.*

Mandibular Arch Only Techniques

Techniques of closed reduction for the mandible only include a mandibular Gunning splint, lingual or labial splint wired to the dentition, acrylic or cast cap splint wired to the mandible, and external pin fixation.

Lingual or Labial Splint

To construct a lingual splint, an impression is taken of the lower arch and a stone model is poured (Fig. 18–24A). If there is displacement of the fracture site an upper impression will also need to be taken. The lower stone model is then sectioned at the fracture site (Fig. 18–24B) and, using the upper model as a guide (Fig. 18–24C), the correct occlusion is reconstructed. Then the sectioned model is waxed together in the correct relationship, and the lingual surface is relieved with a 1-mm thickness of wax (Fig. 18–24D). A hard acrylic splint is then made and holes drilled so that it can be wired to the teeth (Fig. 18–24E,F). Just before placement a thin coating of soft liner is applied. The fracture is reduced and the splint is wired into position.

External Pin Fixation

In external pin fixation (Fig. 18–25A,B) usually two pins on both the proximal and distal fragments are placed, if possible. The biphasic extraoral technique uses a special transbuccal trocar set. This is used for each hole through 7-mm skin incision. A 2.2-mm twist drill is used to drill through both cortical plates at slow speed with constant irrigation. Specially designed self-tapping, coarse-threaded screws are then placed with a socket wrench. A series of locking plates and bars are secured to the four or more pins, and then a self-curing acrylic secondary splint is constructed (see Fig. 18–5). External pin fixation can be used in edentulous fracture sites in which there is bone loss secondary to gunshot injuries, pathologic fractures, or osteomyelitis, or in cases in which a bone grafting procedure has been performed. It can also be used in fractures of the atrophic edentulous mandible or in mandibular fractures associated with midface fractures when a quick and simple method of fixation is required.

MANAGEMENT OF TEETH IN THE LINE OF FRACTURE

In the past, teeth in the line of the fracture were removed.[27–29] Their removal was advocated because fractures of the dentate portion of the jaws are compound via the periodontal ligament and it was believed that this communication fostered infection, osteomyelitis, and nonunion. However, Neal et al.,[30] Kahnberg and Ridell,[31] Schneider and Stern,[32] and Amaratunga[33] have all been able to show that the majority of teeth in the fracture line can be saved if appropriate antibiotic therapy and fixation techniques are used. The impacted mandibular third molar tooth deserves special mention. Most authors have advocated leaving the tooth in situ if the tooth is not in direct communication with the mouth, no pericoronitis exists, and if reduction of the fracture is achievable without removal. Shetty and Freymiller[34] have recently reviewed the indications for removal of teeth in the line of the fracture as follows:

- Teeth grossly loosened, showing evidence of periapical pathology or significant periodontal disease
- Partially erupted third molars with pericoronitis or associated cyst
- Teeth that prevent reduction of fractures
- Teeth with fractured roots
- Teeth with exposed root apices or entire root surface from the apex to the gingival margin
- An excessive delay from the time of fracture to definite treatment

Use of Antibiotics

Zallen and Curry[35] demonstrated that with compound mandibular fractures, an infection rate of 50% can be expected in those patients who do not receive antibiotic therapy. A prospective trial was undertaken in which only dentate compound mandibular fractures were evaluated. Half of the patients in this study received "prophylactic antibiotics," usually penicillin. It was not stated for how long the antibiotic therapy was continued or when it started in relation to the injury. Half the patients who did not receive antibiotics had infections at the fracture site as opposed to only 6% of those who did receive antibiotics. It seemed to make little difference whether the fractures were treated by open or closed reduction. All fractures in

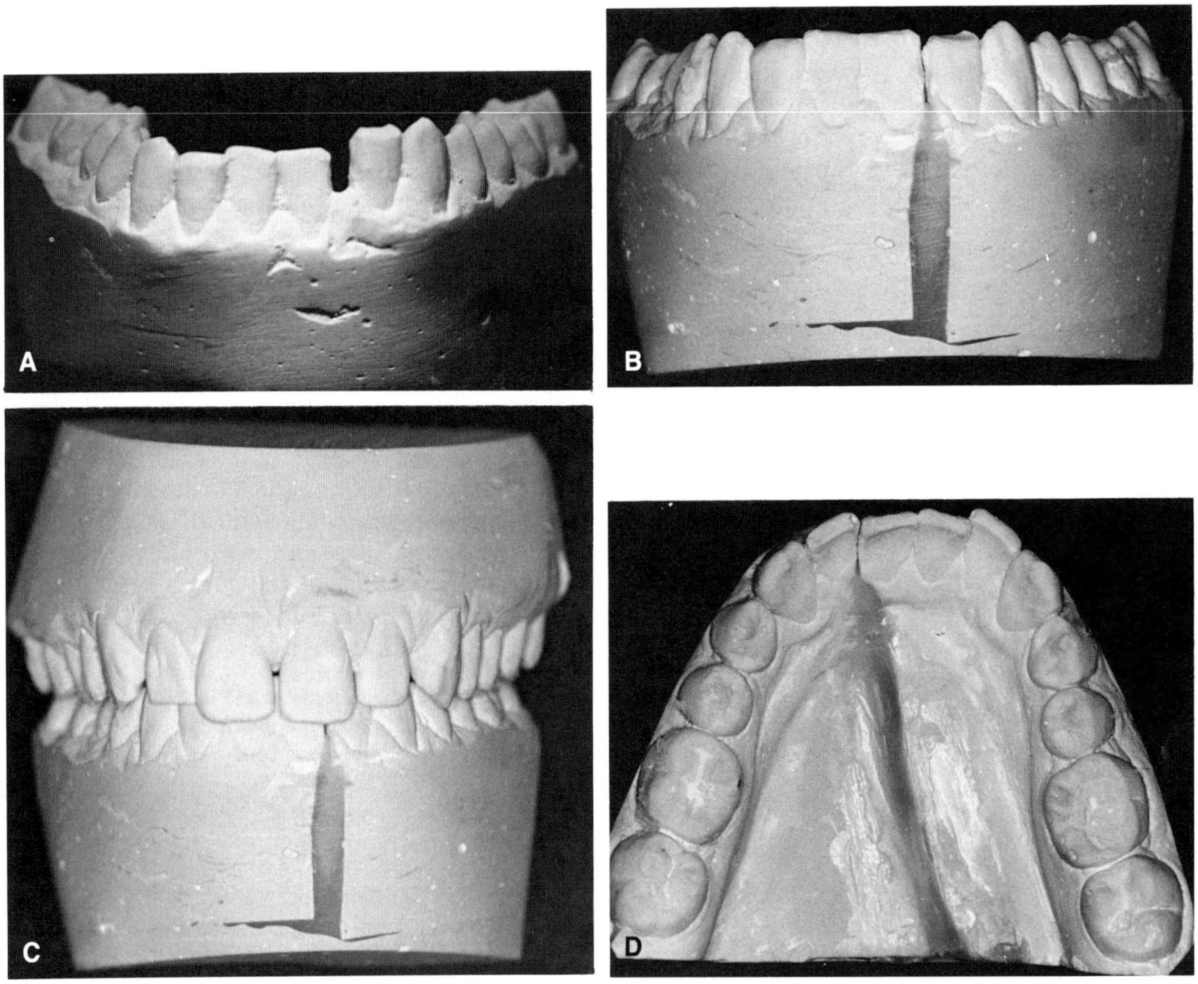

Figure 18–24. *(**A**–**F**) An acrylic lingual splint used in the treatment of a fractured mandible. The different stages of construction. (**A**) Model with separation of teeth at fracture, (**B**) sectioning model, (**C**) lining up occlusion, (**D**) waxing out, (**E**) splint on model, (**F**) completed splint.*

this study were treated within 36 hours. A recent study has confirmed these results in facial fractures and has suggested that short-term prophylaxis as is used in elective surgery may be as effective as the more usual five-day course of antibiotics.[36] This group also found little difference in the incidence of infection whether there was a delay in treatment of mandibular fractures or not.

Penicillin should remain the antibiotic of choice for compound mandibular fractures whether closed reduction or open reduction is contemplated. The antibiotic prophylaxis should begin preoperatively and be continued for not more than 24 hours postreduction.

Length of Fixation

Traditionally the length of intermaxillary fixation (IMF) used for adult mandibular fractures has been 6 weeks. However, this length of IMF is not without penalty. Often patients continue to lose weight during this period, they may not be able to return to work,

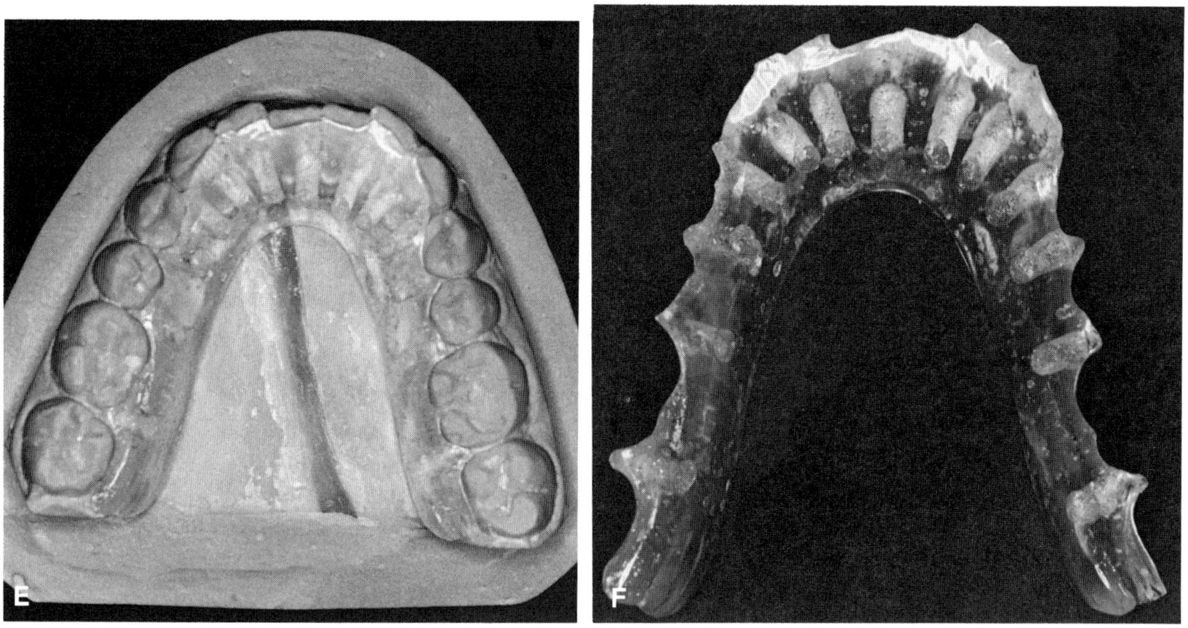

Figure 18–24. *(Continued)*

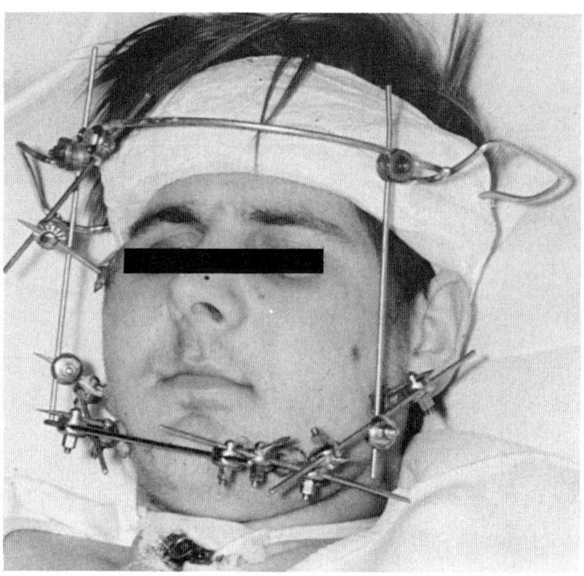

Figure 18–25. *External pin fixation to treat a fractured mandible, combined with a box frame connected to a plaster of Paris head cap.*

and there is some evidence of histologic changes in the temporomandibular joint.[37] Juniper and Awty[2] were able to demonstrate that 80% of mandibular fractures treated by open or closed reduction and IMF were clinically united in 4 weeks. They were also able to demonstrate a clear relation between the age of the patient and the predictability of early fracture union. These results were confirmed by Amaratunga.[3] He found that 75% of mandibular fractures were clinically stable by 4 weeks, that almost all fractures in children healed in 2 weeks, and that a significant number of fractures in older patients took 8 weeks to heal. It appears that each individual case must be judged on its merits, but that most uncomplicated fractures in children are united in 2 to 3 weeks, in adults 3 to 4 weeks, and in older patients in 6 to 8 weeks. Several other factors should be taken into account when deciding on the appropriate regime for a particular patient. The following situations generally require longer periods of IMF: comminuted fractures, fractures in alcoholics, particularly those with nutritional problems, fractures in patients with psychosocial handicaps, fractures treated late, and fractures with teeth in the line of the fracture removed.

OPEN REDUCTION

Indications

The major indications for open reduction of a fractured mandible are summarized in the following paragraphs.

When a closed reduction will not work. This situation arises in several circumstances. When an angle fracture is displaced at the time of injury and is horizontally or vertically unfavorable, it is unlikely that simple IMF will maintain the proximal segment in the correct position. Under the influence of the medial pterygoid or the powerful mandibular elevator muscles (temporalis and masseter) the proximal segment most likely will be displaced. This could lead to delayed healing and possibly permanent disruption of the inferior alveolar nerve. When the fracture is both horizontally and vertically unfavorable, an extraoral approach is recommended; otherwise either intra- or extraoral approaches would be satisfactory. Fractures in the parasymphyseal region also cannot be normally treated satisfactorily by closed reduction because of the pull of the suprahyoid and digastric muscles. Fractures in this region tend to open at the inferior border with the superior aspects of the mandibular segments rotating medially at the point of fixation when closed reduction and IMF are used. With the medial rotation of the horizontal ramus the lingual cusps of all premolars and molars move out of occlusal contact. This results in masticatory inefficiency, and untoward periodontal changes will follow.[38]

Prolonged delay in treatment of the fracture with interpositional soft tissue. Occasionally when there has been an excessive delay in treating a fractured mandible, interpositional tissue between the two bone ends can prevent a satisfactory closed reduction. In this situation an open reduction is necessary to remove the soft tissue between the fragments.

Complex facial fractures. The satisfactory reduction of complex facial fractures requires two stable reference points to which the maxillary complex can be reduced. This includes a stable supraorbital bar of bone and also a stable mandible. This often necessitates open reduction and fixation of the mandibular fractures. Open reduction and fixation of a subcondylar fracture are indicated when there are bilateral subcondylar fractures in the presence of complex middle third fractures, so that a stable vertical platform is provided on which the face can be reconstructed.

Medically compromised patients. Some patients with special medical conditions are best treated without intermaxillary fixation. They may be better treated with an open reduction. This group of patients includes those with decreased pulmonary function. Williams and Cawood[39] have demonstrated significant decrease in pulmonary function associated with intermaxillary fixation. Patients with gastrointestinal disorders who are on a liquid diet, particularly one based on milk products, may have difficulties. Those with severe seizure disorders in which airway difficulties may arise with IMF and patients with psychiatric or neurologic problems may be candidates for open reduction.

Concurrent condylar fracture associated with fractures elsewhere in the mandible. It is often advantageous to be able to mobilize condylar fractures early to prevent possible ankylosis. This is particularly true in cases of intracapsular fractures in which immobilization is more likely to lead to ankylosis. In this situation open reduction and fixation of angle, body, or symphyseal fractures will allow early mobilization of an associated condylar fracture.

There are certain contraindications to the use of open reduction of mandibular fractures. As a general principle, when a simpler means of treating a fracture can be used it should be. This is often more cost-effective for the community at large and often results in fewer complications. However, each individual case must be judged on its merits.

The periosteal blood supply of multiple small fragments of bone can be jeopardized when an open reduction is attempted for comminuted fractures. This can lead to an increased likelihood of infection and delayed healing. Gunshot wounds are best managed by closed reduction whenever possible, because often the bone is comminuted and there is a greater risk of infection in these fractures. Atrophic edentulous mandibles must be treated with care. When an open reduction is necessary the maximal blood supply to the fracture site should be preserved.

Principles of Wire Placement

Intraosteal wiring (wire osteosynthesis) can be placed either by an intra- or extraoral route using one of three basic techniques:

1. A simple straight wire across the fracture site (Fig. 18–26A). This should be placed so that the direction of pull of the wire is perpendicular to the fracture site. This technique can be either through both the buccal and lingual cortical plate or it may be used on the buccal cortical plate only. This is useful in the angle region, where a third molar socket can be quickly and easily used for a simple straight buccal cortex wire.
2. Figure-of-8 wire (Fig. 18–26B). This wiring technique has been shown to have increased strength compared with simple techniques at both the inferior and superior borders in angle fractures.[40]
3. Transosteal circummandibular wiring (Obwegeser's technique) (Fig. 18–26C). This is a useful wiring technique when the fracture runs obliquely compared with the inferior border of the mandible. If the fracture line is too vertical the wire could become displaced into the fracture line.

The wire used should be a prestretched soft stainless steel, and the fracture should be held in a reduced position while the wire is being tightened so that the wire does not reduce the fracture and possibly lead to wire breakage.

Transoral Open Reduction

Open reduction of mandibular fractures prior to the advent of antibiotics was associated with a high incidence of infection. Following the introduction of antibiotics most clinicians used the extraoral approach to the fracture site. This technique, however, is time consuming, results in a visible surgical scar, and can damage adjacent structures, particularly the marginal mandibular branch of the facial nerve. Transoral open reduction (see Fig. 18–2) has been advocated as an alternative.[41–44] The technique is claimed to be quicker to perform, results in no extraoral scar, and does not damage the facial nerve. Less postoperative wound care is required and it is simple to perform the techniques under local anesthesia. Transoral open reduction of mandibular fractures is useful in tooth-bearing portions of the jaw (i.e., in symphyseal, body, and

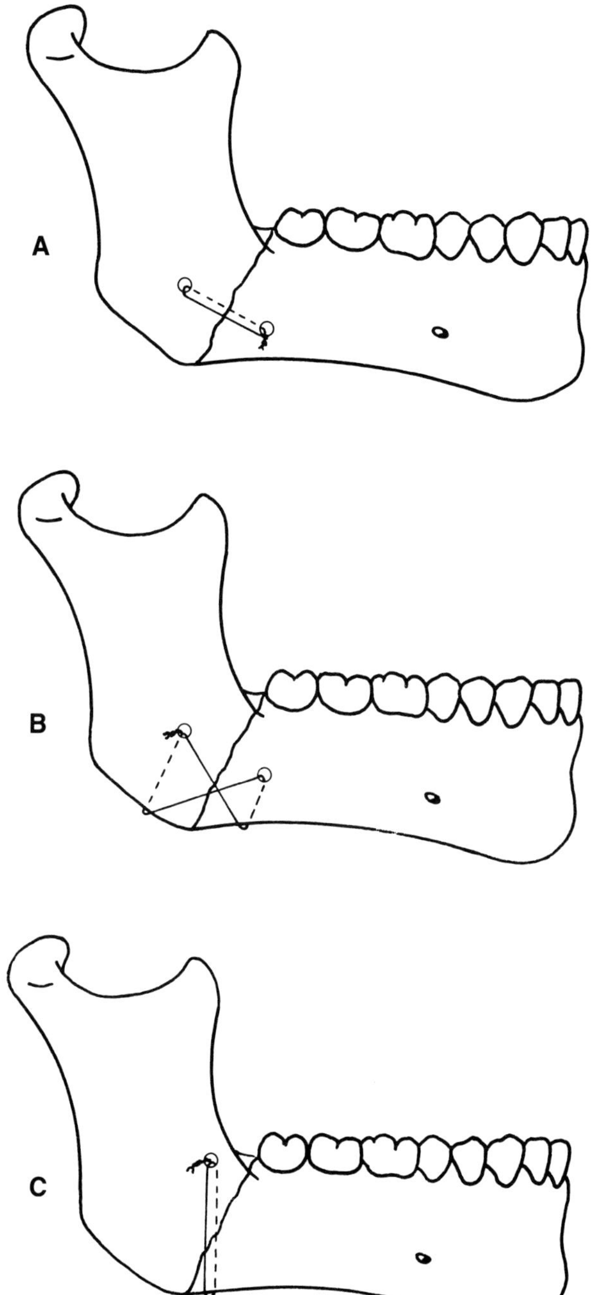

Figure 18–26. (**A**) *Simple wiring technique;* (**B**) *figure-of-8 wire;* (**C**) *transosseous circumandibular wire.*

angle fractures). Complications rates and infection rates appear to be similar between the two techniques when large numbers of cases are studied.[45,46]

Rigid Fixation

Dissatisfaction with the use of IMF as a means of treatment of mandibular fractures has resulted in the development of open reduction and fixation techniques that do not require the teeth to be wired together. Criticism of the disadvantages of prolonged immobilization of the jaws has included patient complaints of panic, insomnia, social inconvenience, phonetic disturbance, loss of effective work time, physical discomfort, weight loss, histologic changes in the condylar head, and difficulty recovering a normal range of jaw movement. This has led some clinicians to seek alternative methods of treatment, including the use of rigid internal fixation.

Rigid fixation is probably best defined as that form of fixation that holds the bone fragments together with absolute stability so that no motion can occur between them; its use results in primary bone healing.[47] On the other hand, less-rigid fixation systems often result in abundant callus formation (secondary healing). Within the maxillofacial area there is much confusion as to what constitutes rigid fixation, and any system of plates and screws has been dubbed as rigid fixation. There is good evidence that rigid fixation with the use of compression results in primary bone healing when applied to the mandible.[48] The principle technique that has been developed was a modification by Spiessl[49] of the Swiss Association for Internal Fixation (ASIF) system. The system involves the use of bicortical screws, an eccentric dynamic compression plate at the inferior border of the mandible, and a tension band at the superior border. The main advantages and purposes of the rigid internal fixation system are primary bone healing, early active pain-free function, avoidance of IMF, safe secured airways without tracheostomies particularly in polytraumatized patients, and shorter absences from work and perhaps shorter periods of hospitalization.[50]

The principal disadvantages of the compression plating systems for mandibular fractures are the use of an external approach, thus giving rise to facial scarring and the potential for damage to the mandibular branch of the facial nerve; and the use of very rigid plates, giving rise to "stress shielding," although this has never been shown to be a problem in mandibular fractures. Also, the position of the teeth and inferior alveolar nerve and the use of bicortical screw fixation necessitate that the compression plates be placed in areas of compression rather than tensile forces and, therefore, additional techniques are required to overcome the tension forces. Another disadvantage is that removal of the plates is advocated.

The second major group of plate fixation techniques is the monocortical miniplate osteosynthesis, which was first described by Michelet et al.[51] and then modified and popularized by Champy et al.[52] The principal advantages of this technique over compression plating systems are the use of the intraoral approach and the positioning of the plates in the juxtaalveolar area where tensile strain occurs when the mandible is loaded. The healing that results from the use of this system in humans has not been demonstrated clearly. At least one group of authors claims that the system gives rise to rigid fixation and that it results in primary bone healing, although no evidence is provided to support this assertion.[53] In view of the small malleable nature of these plates and the fact that the system is monocortical, it would seem more likely that the technique is only semirigid and would result in callus formation and secondary bone repair. This is not to imply that it is an inferior technique, because callus formation generally gives rise to quicker and stronger early bone repair.[47]

MANAGEMENT OF EDENTULOUS FRACTURES

The edentulous mandible in the trauma patient has several factors modifying its behavior that the dentate mandible does not. The loss of the teeth results in resorption of the alveolar bone which weakens the mandible. The loss of bone also means that there is less cross-sectional area of bone in contact in fracture patients and less periosteum and endosteum to supply the osteogenic cells for fracture healing. Because of the aging process the majority of the blood supply to the edentulous mandible is from the periosteum rather than the inferior alveolar artery.[54] A larger percentage of fractures in the edentulous patient are not compound because of the lack of teeth. Minor displacement of the bones can be easily accommodated in the construction of new dentures. The edentulous population also tends to have more health problems. These include conditions such as osteoporosis, diabetes mellitus, and steroid therapy, which may directly affect bone healing. The site distribution of fractures tends to be different in the edentulous patient, with a higher percentage of body fractures (43.5%) and lower percentages of angle (15.2%) and symphyseal (4.3%) fractures[55] (Fig. 18–27). A 20% incidence of nonunion has been reported in the treatment of edentulous fractures, particularly when nonrigid fixation was applied in open reduction cases.[56] Longer periods of immobilization have also shown to be necessary to achieve satisfactory healing.[55,56]

The anatomical site influences treatment. If the location of the fracture is posterior to the denture-bearing area, then either additional fixation (e.g., external pin fixation) or open reduction and fixation may be necessary to control the proximal fragment. Muscle pull on the edentulous jaw is considerably weaker than in a dentate mandible and undisplaced fractures are often closed injuries. Therefore, if the fragments are undisplaced or minimally displaced and not mobile, then conservative therapy may be all that is necessary. More definitive treatment will be necessary if the fragments are displaced or excessively mobile. The bilateral body fracture deserves special mention because the pull of the suprahyoid muscles tend to displace this fracture inferiorly. These usually occur in the pencil-thin atrophic mandible. A variety of treatment modalities have been suggested to treat these difficult fractures including open reduction with rigid internal fixation, closed reduction with and without bone grafts, and external pin fixation. When the edentulous mandible is comminuted again because of the poor blood supply to the bone fragments, those fragments are best managed by closed reduction.

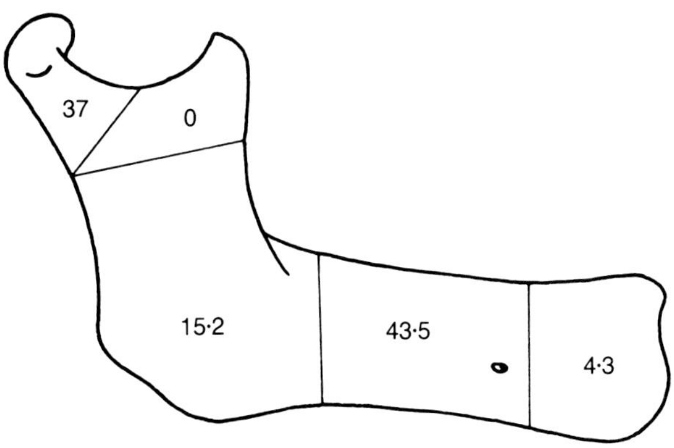

Figure 18–27. *Percentage of fracture sites in edentulous patients.*

External pin fixation by the biphasic technique is often used in edentulous fractures. It obviates the need for IMF, thus allowing early mobilization of the jaw and improving feeding in some patients. It can be used in comminuted fractures without jeopardizing blood supply to the fractures, and it can bridge a bone loss gap before bone grafting.

MANAGEMENT OF FRACTURES IN CHILDREN

Fractures in children are less common than those in adults. Their management is complicated by the presence of deciduous teeth, which may be mobile during the mixed dentition stage and whose shape has little in the way of undercut areas, which means that they do not retain wire as well as adult teeth. The presence of teeth buds reduces the area available for interosteal fixation, and there exists a greater potential for ankylosis and growth disturbances in the younger population. Also, children do not tend to tolerate IMF as well as adult patients. On the other hand, fractures tend to heal quicker in children and slight malocclusion problems can be compensated for by growth of the patient.

Children make up about 5% of all mandibular fractures.[57] These fractures are rare in children under age 5 because of the greater elasticity of the bone and lighter weight of children, which lowers the forces of impact during falls. Condylar fractures appear to be common, affecting about 46% of patients either alone or in combination with other fractures.[57]

Mandibular fractures in children can often be successfully managed by acrylic splint therapy of the mandible only or with eyelet wires and IMF.[57,58] A shortened period of IMF, 2 to 3 weeks, is all that is required. When an open reduction is required, it has been successfullly accomplished by the extraoral route using inferior border wiring in order to avoid the tooth buds.[59,60]

Complications are rare in this group of patients. Malunion, nonunion, and infection tend to have a low incidence.[57] Two serious complications that can occur, however, are ankylosis and growth disturbances. Both these tend to be more common with intracapsular condylar fractures and when the damage is of a crushing nature.[61] The incidence and severity of these complications can be reduced by shorter periods of IMF and close follow-up.

COMPLICATIONS

Delayed Union and Nonunion

Nonunion is distinguished from delayed union by the potential of the bone to heal. Delayed union is a temporary condition in which adequate reduction and immobilization eventually produces bony union. On the other hand, nonunion may persist indefinitely without evidence of bone healing unless surgical treatment is undertaken to repair the fracture. Nonunion is generally characterized by pain and abnormal mobility following treatment. Malocclusion may be present in dentate cases and mobility exists across the fracture line. Radiographs demonstrate no evidence of healing and in later stages show rounding off of the bone ends. Delayed and nonunion occur in about 3% of fractures.[17]

There are several causes and contributory factors. The most common reason is poor reduction and immobilization.[62] This is more likely in edentulous fractures. Infection is often an underlying cause, and any tooth in the line of the fracture must be carefully assessed for root fracture and vitality. A decreased blood supply can lead to delays in healing. Excessive stripping of the periosteum, especially in comminuted and edentulous fractures, can lead to delayed healing. Metabolic deficiencies and alcoholism are also significant contributions to delayed healing. Cannell and Boyd[63] showed a high incidence of delayed union and nonunion in a group of alcoholic patients. These patients were probably also at increased likelihood to sustain a mandibular fracture. Although the exact reasons for delayed healing in this group of patients is not known, they are known to have metabolic and vitamin deficiencies, poor compliance particularly with IMF, poor bony quality, and impaired local blood supply, which could all be contributing factors. These patients should be treated whenever possible with closed reductions, because this treatment has a lower incidence of complications in this group of patients.[63]

Treatment of delayed union and nonunion is aimed at eliminating the underlying cause of the problem. When infection is present it must be managed with debridement of sequestra, drainage, and antibiotic therapy. Loose fixation such as wires and plates must be removed, and adequate fixation with IMF, extraoral pin fixation, or even rigid plate fixation should be applied across the fracture site.[64] If there is a gap between the bone ends, a bone graft may be necessary.

Infection

Infection and osteomyelitis appear to be the most common complication (Fig. 18–28A, B). In some studies, particularly without antibiotics, it may occur in over 50% of cases.[65] Some of the underlying causes have already been discussed. These can be divided into systemic factors, such as alcoholism and no antibiotic coverage, and local factors, such as poor reduction and fixation, fractured teeth in the line of fracture, and comminuted fractures.

Most infections appear to be mixed in nature, with α-hemolytic *Streptococcus* and *Bacteroides* organisms found most commonly.[7] Treatment has already been outlined as for delayed and nonunion of fractures.

Malunion

Malunions can be defined as a bone union of the fracture in which some displacement of the bones still exists (Fig. 18–29). Not all malunions of fractured mandibles are clinically significant. Often malunions in edentulous patients or those involving the ramus and condylar area of the mandible result in no clinically detectable alteration in appearance or function. When, on the other hand, the dentate portion of the jaw is involved a malocclusion can result. The rates of malocclusion in patients treated with IMF tend to be very low. In one prospective trial between rigid internal fixation and standard techniques the rate of malocclusion with the rigid fixation was three times higher. However, as the authors concede, they were initially inexperienced with the technique and others have reported a low incidence of malocclusion.[66,67] Malocclusion can be corrected by further or prolonged IMF in the early stages of healing, and selective tooth grinding, orthodontics, or osteotomies after complete bony union.

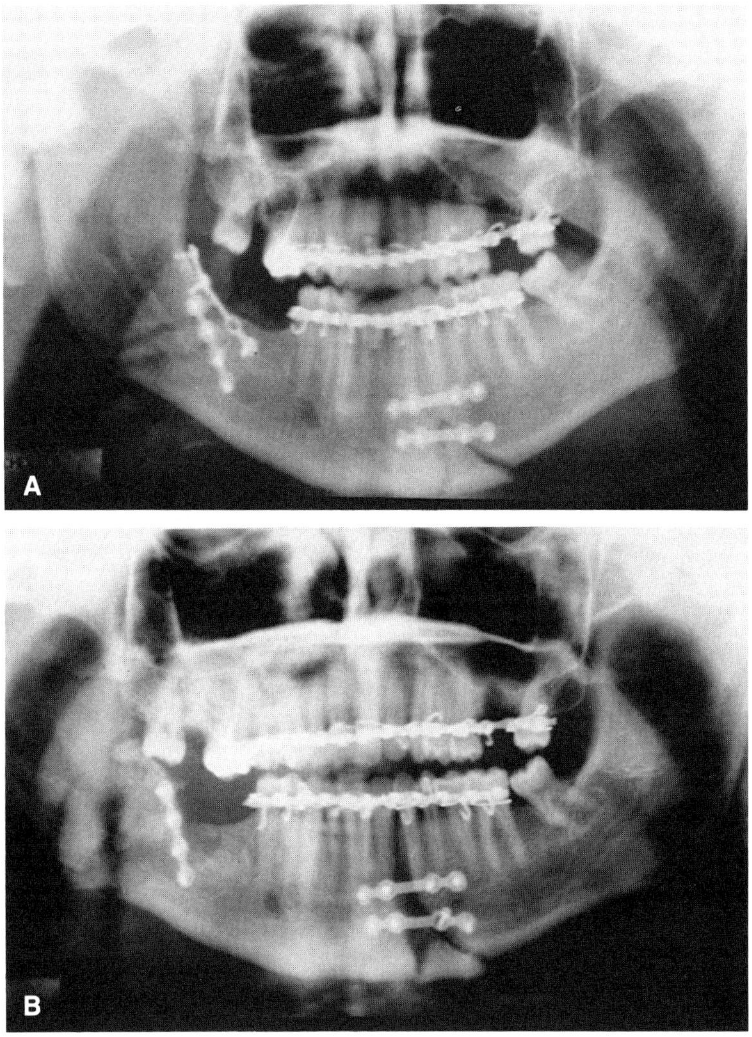

Figure 18–28. *(A, B) Fractured right angle and symphysis with loose fixation and mobility leading to infection and fracture displacement.*

Ankylosis

Ankylosis is a rare complication of mandibular fractures. It is more likely to occur in children and is associated with intracapsular fractures and immobilization of the mandible. The most commonly accepted etiology is of intraarticular hemorrhage, leading to abnormal fibrosis and ultimately ankylosis.[62] In children, if left untreated, it results in disturbed growth and underdevelopment of the affected side. Prevention is easier than cure, and the use of only short periods of IMF in children can help reduce the occurrence of this complication. Management once the condition is established is surgical with a temporomandibular joint arthroplasty, wide resection of the ankylotic portion of bone, coronoidectomy, and reconstruction with a costochondral rib graft, with active early and prolonged mobilization and exercises.[68]

Nerve Injury

Traumatic injury to the inferior alveolar nerve is common in displaced fractures of the body and angle of the mandible. There are few studies documenting recovery of the nerve. Larsen and Nielsen[69] reported a permanent disturbance in mental nerve function in 8% of 229 patients studied. Return of nerve function

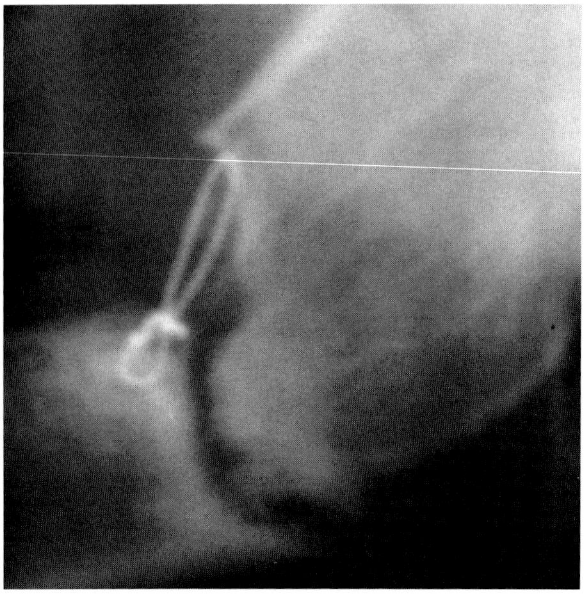

Figure 18–29. *Two-years postreduction and fixation with a displaced nonunion present.*

depends on the degree of initial trauma to the nerve and an accurate reduction and adequate fixation of the mandibular fracture. Rarely other branches of mandibular division of the trigeminal nerve can be affected. These include the masseteric nerve, auriculotemporal nerve (both with condylar fractures), and the buccal and lingual nerves associated with intraoral lacerations with body or angle fractures. Also rare is damage to the marginal mandibular branch of the facial nerve with fractures of the condyle, ramus, and angle of the mandible. It is more common to see this nerve damage caused by a laceration along its course.

Most fractures of the mandible heal with relatively simple management. All clinicians must be wary of overtreatment of simple cases that can lead to an increase in cost of treatment for both the patient and society and also an increase in complication rates.

REFERENCES

1. Thoma KH. Historical review of methods advocated for treatment of jaw fractures with ten commandments for modern fracture treatment. Am J Orthodont Oral Surg (Oral Surg section) 1944; 30:399.
2. Juniper RP, Awty MD. The immobilization period for fractures of the mandibular body. Oral Surg 1973; 36:157.
3. Amaratunga NA de S. The relation of age to the immobilization period required for healing of mandibular fractures. J Oral Maxillofac Surg 1987; 45:111.
4. Adell R, Eriksson B, Nylén O, Ridell A. Delayed healing of fractures of the mandibular body. Int J Oral Maxillofac Surg 1987; 16:15.
5. Goss AN, Bosanquet AG. The arthroscopic appearance of acute temporomandibular joint trauma. J Oral Maxillofac Surg 1990; 48:780.
6. Kelly DE, Harrigan WF. A survey of facial fractures: Bellevue Hospital 1948–1974. J Oral Surg 1975; 33:146.
7. Olson RA, Fonseca RJ, Zeitler DL, Osborn DB. Fractures of the mandible: A review of 580 cases. J Oral Surg 1982; 40:23.
8. James RB, Fredrickson C, Kent JN. Prospective study of mandibular fractures. J Oral Surg 1981; 39:275.
9. Hagan EH, Huelke DR. An analysis of 319 case reports of mandibular fractures. J Oral Surg 1961; 19:93.
10. Ellis E, Moos KF, El-Attar A. Ten years of mandibular fractures: An analysis of 2,137 cases. Oral Surg 1985; 59:120.
11. Copenhaver RH, Dennis MJ, Kloppedal E, Edwards DB, Scheffer RB. Fracture of the glenoid fossa and dislocation of the mandibular condyle into the middle cranial fossa. J Oral Maxillofac Surg 1985; 43:974.
12. Adekeye EO. The pattern of fractures of the facial skeleton in Kaduna, Nigeria. Oral Surg 1980; 49:491.
13. Gratten E, Hobbs JA. In: Rowe NL, Williams J, eds. Maxillofacial Injuries. Edinburgh: Churchill Livingstone, 1985:37.
14. Van Hoof RF, Merkx CA, Stekenlenburg EC. The different pattern of fractures of the facial skeleton in four European countries. Int J Oral Surg 1977; 6:3.
15. Salem JE, Lilly G, Cutcher JL, Steiner M. Analysis of 523 mandibular fractures. Oral Surg 1968; 26:390.
16. Haug RH, Prather J, Indresano AT. An epidemiologic survey of facial fractures and concomitant injuries. J Oral Maxillofac Surg 1990; 48:926.
17. Chuong R, Donoff RB, Guralnick WC. A retrospective analysis of 327 mandibular fractures. J Oral Maxillofac Surg 1983; 41:305.
18. Huelke DF, Compton CP. Facial injuries in automobile crashes. J Oral Maxillofac Surg 1983; 41:241.
19. Huelke DF, Harger JH. Mechanism in the production of mandibular fractures: An experimental study. J Oral Surg 1968; 26:86.
20. Rhinelander FW, Baragry RA. Microangiography in bone healing Part 1. Undisplaced closed fractures. J Bone Joint Surg 1962; 44A:1273.
21. Rhinelander FW, Phillips RS, Steel WM, Beer JC. Microangiography in bone healing. Part II. Displaced closed fractures. J Bone Joint Surg 1968; 50A:643.
22. Perren S: Physical and biological aspects of fracture healing with special reference to internal fixation. Clin Orthop 1979; 138:175.
23. Holmström T, Paavolainen P, Slätis P, Karaharju E.

Effect of compression on fracture healing. Plate fixation studied in rabbits. Acta Orthop Scand 1986; 57:368.
24. Chayra GA, Meador LR, Laskin DM. Comparison of panoramic and standard radiographs for the diagnosis of mandibular fractures. J Oral Maxillofac Surg 1986; 44:677.
25. Bernstein L. Practical points in the management of mandibular fractures. Trans Am Acad Opthalmol Otolaryngol 1970; 74:1068.
26. May M, Tucker HM, Ogura JH. Closed management of mandibular fractures. Arch Otolaryngol 1972; 95:53.
27. Rowe NL, Killey HC. Fractures of the Facial Skeleton, ed 2. London: Williams & Wilkins, 1968.
28. Kruger GO. Textbook of Oral Surgery, ed 3. St Louis: CV Mosby, 1968.
29. Clark HB. Practical Oral Surgery, ed 2. Philadelphia: Lea & Febiger, 1959.
30. Neal DC, Wagner W, Alpert B. Morbidity associated with teeth in the line of mandibular fractures. J Oral Surg 1978; 36:859.
31. Kahnberg K-E, Ridell A. Prognosis of teeth involved in the line of mandibular fractures. Int J Oral Surg 1979; 8:163.
32. Schneider SS, Stern M. Teeth in the line of mandibular fractures. J Oral Surg 1971; 29:107.
33. Amaratunga NA de S. The effect of teeth in the line of mandibular fractures on healing. J Oral Maxillofac Surg 1987; 45:312.
34. Shetty V, Freymiller E. Teeth in the line of fracture: A review. J Oral Maxillofac Surg 1989; 47:1303.
35. Zallen RD, Curry JT. A study of antibiotic usage in compound mandibular fractures. J Oral Surg 1975; 33:431.
36. Chole RA, Yee J. Antibiotic prophylaxis for facial fractures. Arch Otolaryngol Head Neck Surg 1987; 113: 1055.
37. Glineburg RW, Laskin DM, Blankstein DI. The effect of immobilization on the primate temporomandibular joint: A histologic and histochemical study. J Oral Maxillofac Surg 1982; 40:3.
38. Messer EJ, Keller JJ. A rational approach to the mandibular parasymphyseal fracture. J Oral Surg 1976; 34:808.
39. Williams JG, Cawood JI. Effect of intermaxillary fixation on pulmonary function. Int J Oral Maxillofac Surg 1990; 19:76.
40. Fisher JT, Cleaton-Jones PE, Lownie JF. Relative efficiencies of various wiring configurations commonly used in open reductions of fractures of the angle of the mandible. Oral Surg 1990; 70:10.
41. Hooley JR. Reduction of mandibular fractures by intraoral inferior border wiring. J Oral Surg 1969; 27:87.
42. Paul JK, Acevedo A. Intraoral open reduction. J Oral Surg 1968; 26:516.
43. Rontal E, Meyerhoff W, Hohmann A. The transoral reduction of mandibular fractures. Arch Otolaryngol 1973; 97:279.
44. Suzima HJ, Grafft ML, Fulcher CL. Transoral reduction of mandibular fractures. J Oral Surg 1971; 29:247.
45. Dijk LV, Brons R, Bosker H. Treatment of mandibular fractures by means of stable internal wire fixation. Int J Oral Surg 1977; 6:173.
46. Freihofer HPM, Sailer HF. Experience with intraoral trans-osseous wiring mandibular fractures. J Maxillofac Surg 1975; 1:248.
47. Woo SL-Y, Lothringer KS, Akeson WH, et al. Less rigid internal fixation plates historical perspectives and new concepts. J Orthop Res 1984; 1:431.
48. Rahn BA. Direct and indirect bone healing after operative fracture treatment. Otolaryngol Clin North Am 1987; 20:425.
49. Spiessl B. New concepts in Maxillofacial Bone Surgery. New York: Springer-Verlag, 1976.
50. Prein J, Kellmar RM. Rigid internal fixation of fractures. Basis of AO technique. Otolaryngol Clin North Am 1987; 20:441.
51. Michelet FX, Deymes J, Dessus B. Osteosynthesis with miniaturised screwed plates in maxillofacial surgery. J Maxillofac Surg 1973; 1:79.
52. Champy M Lodde JP, Schmitt R et al. Mandibular osteosynthesis by miniature screwed bone plates via a buccal approach. J Maxillofac Surg 1978; 6:14.
53. Johansson B, Knekmanov L, Thomson M. Miniplate osteosynthesis of infected mandibular fractures. J Craniomaxillofac Surg 1988; 16:22.
54. Bradley JC. Age changes in the vascular supply of the mandible. Br Dent J 1972; 132:142.
55. Amaratunga NA de S. A comparative study of the clinical aspects of edentulous and dentulous mandibular fractures. J Oral Maxillofac Surg 1988; 46:3.
56. Bruce RA, Strachan DS. Fractures of the edentulous mandible: The Chalmers J Lyons Academy study. J Oral Surg 1976; 34:973.
57. Amaratunga NA de S. Mandibular fractures in children—A study of clinical aspects, treatment needs and complications. J Oral Maxillofac Surg 1988; 46:637.
58. MacLennan WD, Simpson W. Treatment of fractured mandibular condylar processes in children. Br J Plast Surg 1965; 18:423.
59. Kraulsen AS, Samuel M. Pediatric jaw fractures: Indications for open reduction. Otolaryngol Head Neck Surg 1979; 87:318.
60. Khosla VM, Boren W. Mandibular fractures in children and their management. J Oral Surg 1971; 24:116.
61. Walker DG. The mandibular condyle; fifty cases demonstrating arrest in development. Dent Practit 1957; 7:160.
62. Mathog RH, Rosenberg Z. Complications in the treatment of facial fractures. Otolaryngol Clin North Am 1976; 9:533.
63. Cannell H, Boyd R. The management of maxillofacial injuries in vagrant alcoholics. J Maxillofac Surg 1985; 13:121.
64. Beckers HL. Treatment of initially infected mandibular fractures with bone plates. J Oral Surg 1979; 37:310.

65. Abiose BO. Maxillofacial skeleton injuries in the western states of Nigeria. Br J Oral Maxillofac Surg 1986; 24:31.
66. Dodson TB, Perrott DH, Kaban LB, Gordon NC. Fixation of mandibular fractures: A comparative analysis of rigid internal fixation and standard fixation technique. J Oral Maxillofac Surg 1990; 48:362.
67. Tu HK, Tenhulzen D. Compression osteosynthesis of mandibular fractures: A retrospective study. J Oral Maxillofac Surg 1985; 43:585.
68. Munro JR, Chen YR, Park BY. Simultaneous total correction of temporomandibular ankylosis and facial asymmetry. Plast Reconstr Surg 1986; 77:517.
69. Larsen OD, Nielsen A. Mandibular fractures. 1. An analysis of their etiology and location in 286 patients. Scand J Plast Reconstr Surg 1976; 10:213.

19

Traumatic Injuries of the Condyle

Peter E. Larsen

Injuries to the articular apparatus are common. Fracture of the mandibular condyle accounts for 15% to 30% of all mandibular fractures,[1,2] and more subtle injuries to the surrounding soft tissue are probably even more common but poorly documented.

Of those injuries that are recognized, most are treated with relatively simple methods, and there is little subsequent morbidity in the acute perioperative phase. This has led to the misconception that injuries to this area are less complex and that management of a patient with "just a condyle fracture" is relatively simple. On the contrary, because of the potential long-term morbidity and because the principles for treating fractures in this area are so different from those used in treating fractures elsewhere in the mandible, specific attention must be given to condylar injuries.

As the understanding of temporomandibular joint physiology and pathology has increased, it has become necessary to reevaluate what constitutes a successful outcome of treatment of a given condylar injury. This too has contributed to some of the continued controversy in management of these injuries.

The discussion that follows attempts to outline a reasonable course of management for patients with traumatic injuries of the condyle and articular apparatus.

ANATOMY

Complete anatomy of the joint is covered elsewhere in this text; however, some aspects that are directly related to condylar injury require special emphasis. Because the head of the condyle articulates within the glenoid fossa, injury may involve adjacent structures. Superiorly and through relatively thin bone lies the middle cranial fossa. Posteromedially is the tympanic plate, and posterolaterally lies the wall of the external auditory canal (Fig. 19–1A and B). Although it is encapsulated, the anteromedial aspect of the capsule is relatively weak. This, combined with pull in this direction by the lateral pterygoid muscle (Fig. 19–2), leads to displacement and dislocation of the condylar head in this direction during fracture.[3]

INJURIES OF THE CONDYLE AND ARTICULAR APPARATUS OTHER THAN FRACTURE

The most commonly documented result of trauma to the articular apparatus and mandibular condyle is fracture. Other injuries occur as well, and must be considered in the differential diagnosis (Table 19–1).

Effusion and Hemarthrosis

The temporomandibular joint reacts to trauma in a manner similar to other joints with serous or hemorrhagic effusion.[4] In most cases this leads to a distention of the joint capsule with varying amounts of discomfort. Frequently deviation of the mandible away from the affected side occurs as a result of downward pressure on the condyle from the production of fluid

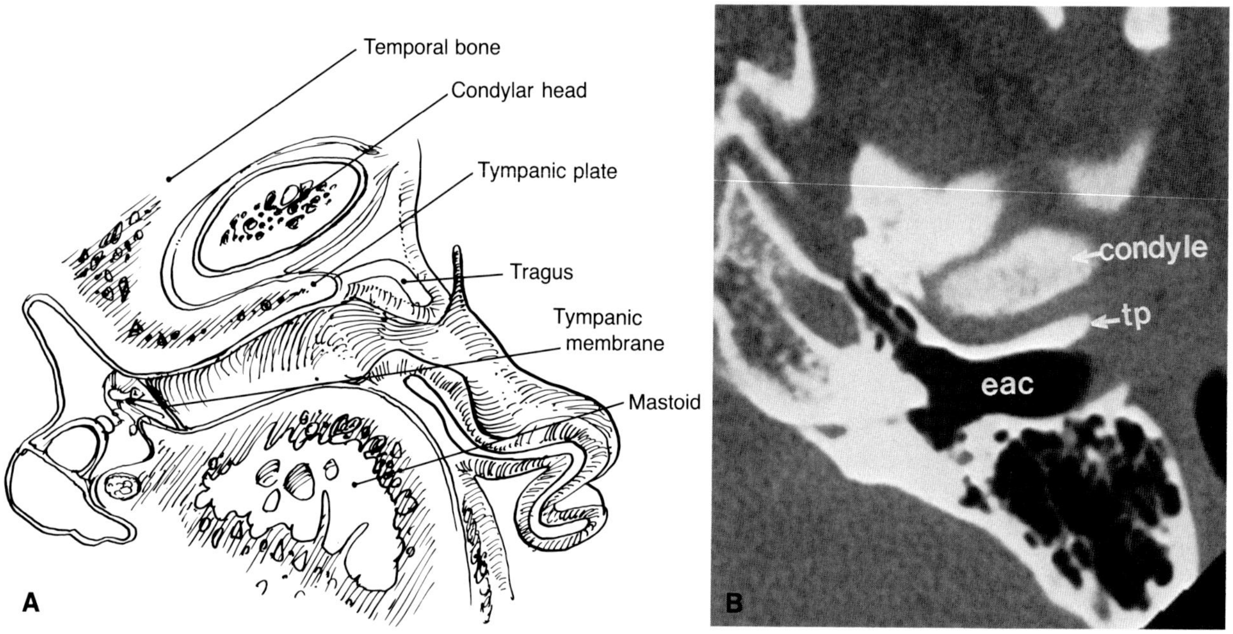

Figure 19–1. *(**A**) Axial section through mandibular condyle and ear. Note the relationship of the tympanic plate to the condylar head and the proximity of the external auditory canal and tympanic membrane to the condylar head. (**B**) Axial computed tomogram through the condylar head. Note the clarity and relationships of the structures outlined in A.*

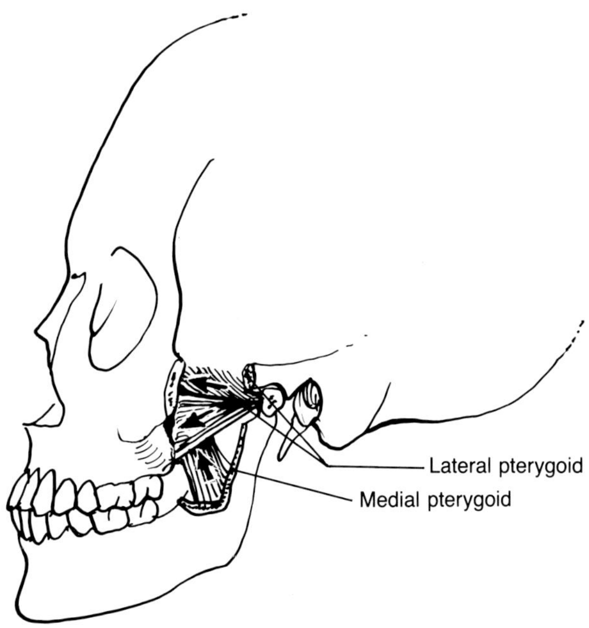

Figure 19–2. *View of the lateral and medial pterygoid muscles with the masseter and a portion of the ramus removed. The direction of pull of the lateral pterygoid muscle (arrow) tends to displace the condyle anteriorly, whereas the medial pterygoid muscle causes superior displacement of the angle of the mandible when a fracture of the condyle leads to loss of vertical support.*

within the joint. This produces facial asymmetry and malocclusion (Fig. 19–3A to C).

The treatment of traumatically induced effusions of the temporomandibular joint is aimed at the restoration of preinjury occlusion with return of function and relief of pain. If the patient presents with the subjective symptoms of a joint effusion but has a stable and reproducible occlusion, the condition may be managed with close daily observation, nonsteroidal anti-inflammatory medications, and a soft diet. Frequently the condition will resolve in a matter of days. If, however, the malocclusion is significant enough that the patient is unable to achieve a stable occlusion without manipulation of the jaw (Fig. 19-3D and E), Ivy loop-wiring or arch bars should be placed and guiding elastics used to produce a stable occlusion. Simple needle aspiration, arthroscopy, or both is a common therapy for hemarthrosis in other joints and may also be considered.[5] Regardless of the therapy chosen, care should be taken to avoid excessive intermaxillary fixation because this may result in a long-term limitation of function. It has been suggested that this limitation in function is due to organization of the blood within the joint space with development of fibrosis and subsequent ankylosis. Many authors have emphasized

Table 19–1. *Injuries of the Articular Apparatus*

Effusion	Hemorrhagic or serous
Soft tissue injury	Disk Capsule Ligaments
Dislocation of the condyle from the fossa	Without fracture With fracture other than condyle With associated condylar fracture
Fracture	Nondisplaced Deviated Displaced Dislocated Comminuted Involving adjacent bony structures
Or combinations of the above	

the importance of this proposed mechanism in the development of ankylosis.[6,7] Aspiration or arthroscopic lavage may alleviate this. It is possible, however, that the development of limited function and ankylosis is more dependent on the inability to maintain a full range of motion during the intermaxillary fixation period rather than on the hemarthrosis. This theory is supported by the failure of experimentally induced hemarthroses to produced ankylosis[8] and by the absence of ankylosis and limited function after iatrogenically induced hemarthroses during joint injections or arthroscopy.[9] Most likely, decreased range of motion after joint effusion is the result of intra-articular fibrosis potentiated by prolonged intermaxillary fixation.

Intracapsular Soft Tissue Injury

Trauma to the temporomandibular joint may result in injury to the articular disk and associated ligaments and muscles. It is well accepted that the development of internal derangement within the temporomandibular joint is often related to a previous episode of trauma.

Dislocation

A dislocation occurs when the head of the condyle moves in such a way that it no longer articulates with the glenoid fossa. When this is associated with a fracture of the condyle, it is termed a *fracture dislocation*. Fracture dislocations are more completely discussed in the section dealing with the management of fractures. The mandibular condyle may also be dislocated as a result of trauma without an associated condylar fracture. Dislocations can occur anteriorly, posteriorly, laterally, and superiorly.

Anterior Dislocation of the Condyle

Anterior dislocation occurs when the condyle moves anterior to the articular eminence. This is by far the most common situation and represents a pathologic forward extension of the normal translational movement of the condylar head. Unlike subluxation, which is also a forward extension of the condyle, dislocation is not self-reducing. Dislocation may be caused by yawning, oral sex, phenothiazine use, and trauma. Traumatically induced anterior dislocation is most commonly bilateral, but it may occur unilaterally (particularly if associated with a concomitant fracture elsewhere in the mandible [Fig. 19–4]). The diagnosis of an anteriorly dislocated mandible is made by the following clinical features (Fig. 19–5A and B): an anterior open bite with the inability to close the mouth; severe pain in the region anterior to the ear; absence of the condyle from the glenoid fossa with a visible and palpable preauricular depression; inability to move the mandible except to open the mouth slightly in a purely rotational manner; difficulty in speaking; and a prognathic appearing lower jaw. Finally, if unilateral dislocation is present, the chin will be deviated to the opposite side.

Patients with anterior dislocation of the mandibular condyles without other mandibular trauma should be approached using the following treatment protocol: 2 cc of local anesthetic solution should be deposited into the joint capsule followed by manual reduction (Fig. 19–6); if this is unsuccessful or the patient is overly apprehensive, diazepam should be carefully titrated intravenously followed by further attempts at manual reduction; if these measures fail, then general anesthesia with the use of a muscle relaxant may be necessary.[10] It is usually possible to reduce an acute dislocation with these maneuvers. In refractory cases or in cases associated with mandibular body and angle fractures in which the dislocated segment is difficult to control by manipulation, surgical intervention may be required. A percutaneous bone hook placed through the sigmoid notch[11] or wires placed through

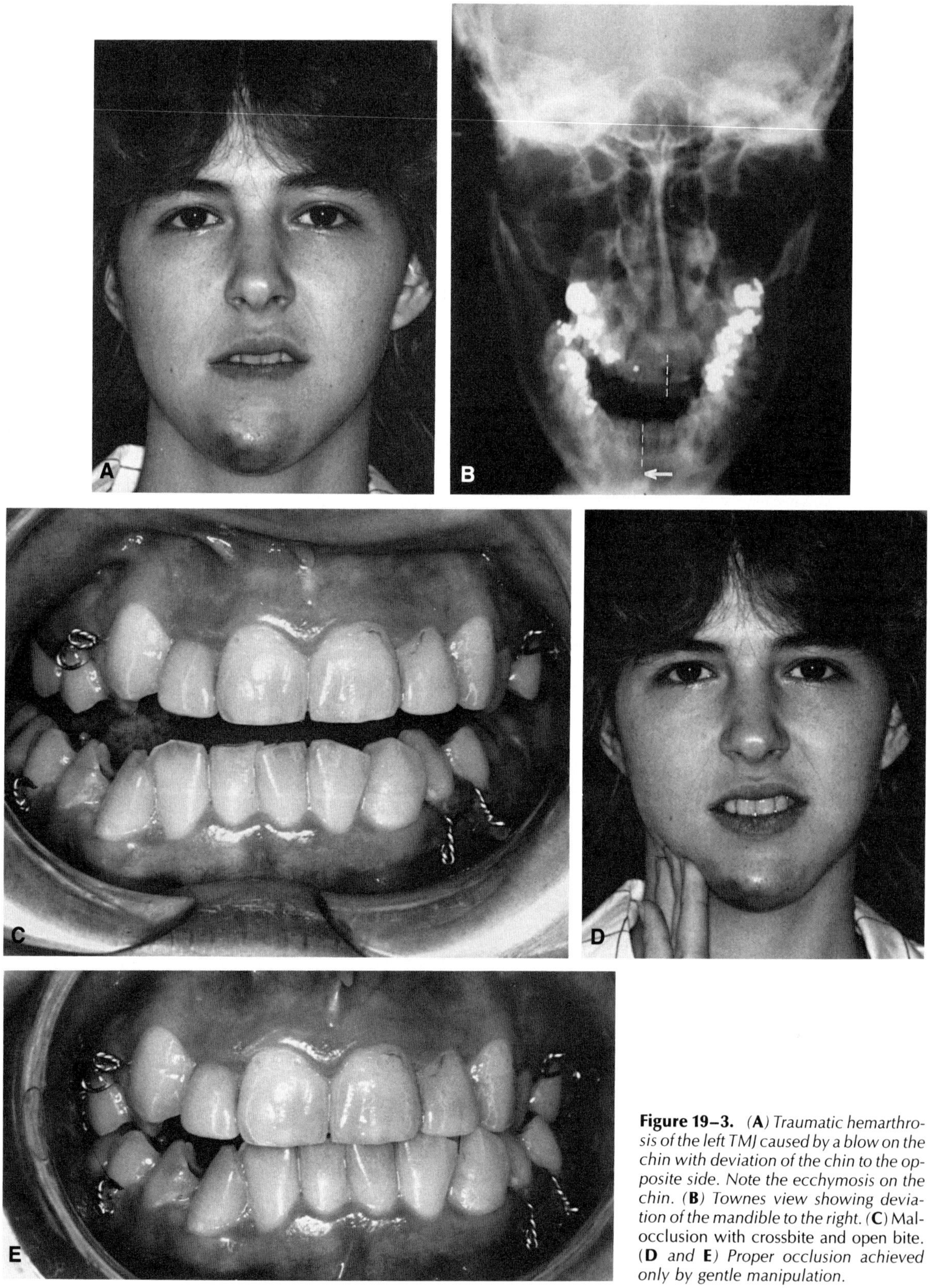

Figure 19–3. *(**A**) Traumatic hemarthrosis of the left TMJ caused by a blow on the chin with deviation of the chin to the opposite side. Note the ecchymosis on the chin. (**B**) Townes view showing deviation of the mandible to the right. (**C**) Malocclusion with crossbite and open bite. (**D** and **E**) Proper occlusion achieved only by gentle manipulation.*

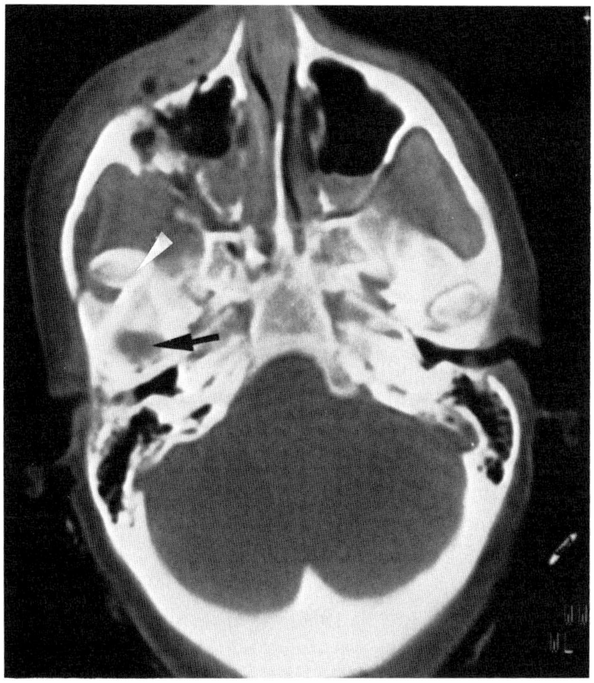

Figure 19–4. *Traumatic unilateral anterior dislocation associated with a body fracture of the mandible. CT shows anterior position of left condyle* (white arrow) *and the empty fossa* (dark arrow).

the angle of the mandible[12] allow for additional downward traction.

Following successful reduction, the patient should be instructed to refrain from opening his or her mouth widely and to support the jaw with a hand under the chin when yawning for a period of 3 weeks to allow for healing of the injured soft tissue in and around the joint. Intermaxillary fixation is not necessary for a first-time acute anterior dislocation of the jaw, unless it persistently dislocates after reduction. In persistent, recurrent dislocation, contributing factors, such as phenothiazine use, should be identified. A soft diet may also be recommended for several days along with a nonsteroidal antiinflammatory analgesic.

Posterior Dislocation

When a blow to the mandible produces primarily a posterior vector of force and does not result in fracture of the condylar neck, the head of the condyle may be forced into a posterior dislocation. This injury is frequently associated with laceration and fracture of the external auditory canal leading to hemorrhage that is visible at the external auditory meatus.[13] In most cases maintenance of the patient's occlusion and treatment of the associated ear injuries are the only management procedures necessary.

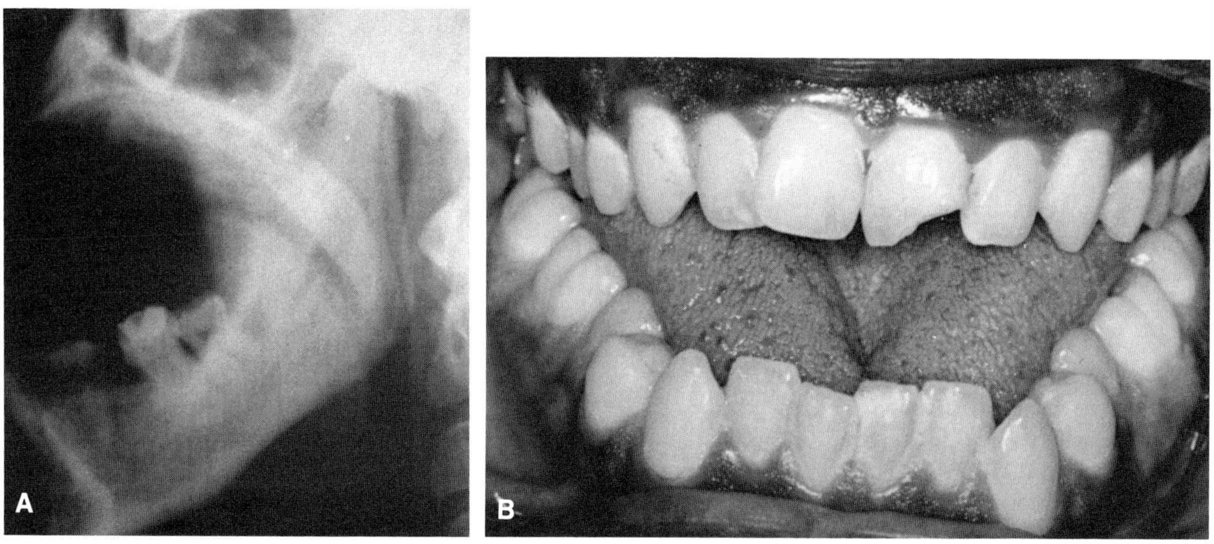

Figure 19–5. *(***A***) Lateral skull radiograph showing bilateral dislocation. (***B***) Anterior dislocation of the condyle with open bite and prognathic mandibular appearance.*

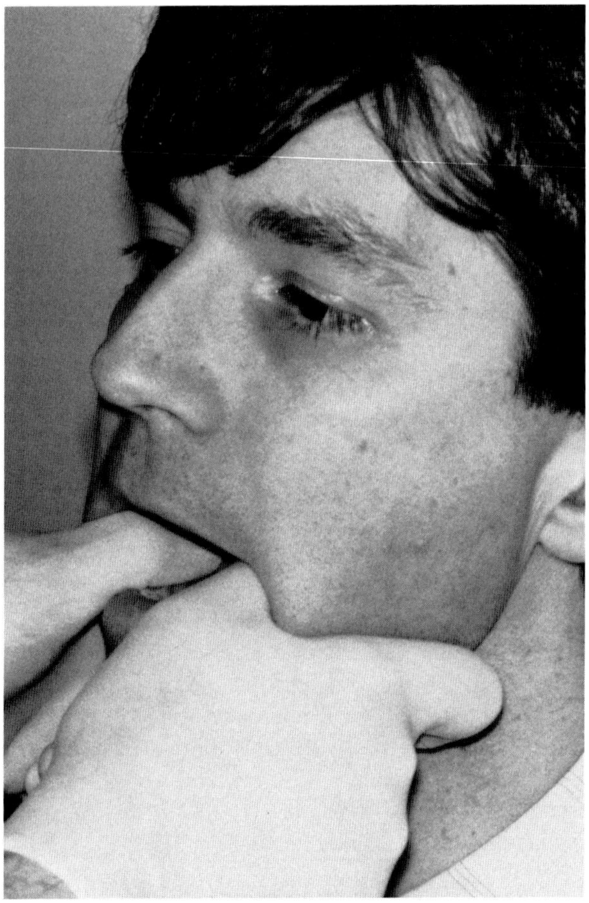

Figure 19–6. *Positioning for manual reduction of anteriorly dislocated mandible. Force is directed downward and posteriorly. Reduction is accomplished one side at a time.*

Lateral Dislocation

Lateral dislocation of the condylar head is always associated with a concomitant fracture either of the condyle or elsewhere within the mandible (Fig. 19–7A and B). The diagnosis of this condition is straightforward. The condylar head is palpable as a hard mass either in the preauricular region or in the lower part of the temporal space. This type of injury is associated with a marked crossbite, which is not attributable solely to the mandibular fracture, but instead is secondary to the displaced condyle. Treatment requires reduction of the dislocation through manipulation of the dislocated segment by grasping it with a thumb on the dentition and with the fingers extraorally along the body of the mandible. If the proximal segment size is inadequate for this maneuver, a percutaneous towel clip through the angle or a small incision with placement of a wire through the angle (as described for anterior dislocation) may be necessary. After reduction of the dislocation, treatment of the associated fracture is accomplished, preferably with rigid internal fixation.

Superior Dislocation

Superior dislocation into the middle cranial fossa without associated fracture of the mandibular condyle has been described. The patient is predisposed to this type of dislocation when the condylar head is small and rounded.[14] This injury is more common when the mouth is open at the moment of impact.[15] This type of injury usually occurs with concomitant midface fractures that are telescoped, causing shortening of the vertical dimension of the face and allowing superior dislocation of the mandibular condyle. Superior dislocation of the mandibular condyle is associated with cerebral contusion and basilar skull fracture with facial nerve paralysis and deafness. These patients present with severe restriction of interincisal opening, pain in the area of the temporomandibular joint, bleeding from the external auditory canal or hemotympanum, and deviation of the jaw to the affected side. A variety of treatment modalities are recommended, including observation, condylotomy, elastic traction, condylectomy, and manual reduction.[16] Neurosurgical consultation is required.

FRACTURE

Classification of Fractures

Many systems of classification have been applied to fractures involving the mandibular condyle.[3,17-22] The recommended classification parallels the comprehensive classification set forth by Lindahl.[22] It requires that radiographs be taken of the suspected injury in two planes at right angles to each other. The following major relations are noted: the level of the fracture; the relation of the condylar fragment to the mandible, termed the *degree of displacement;* and the relation of the condylar head to the fossa, or the *degree of dislocation.* Although it may be difficult to place every

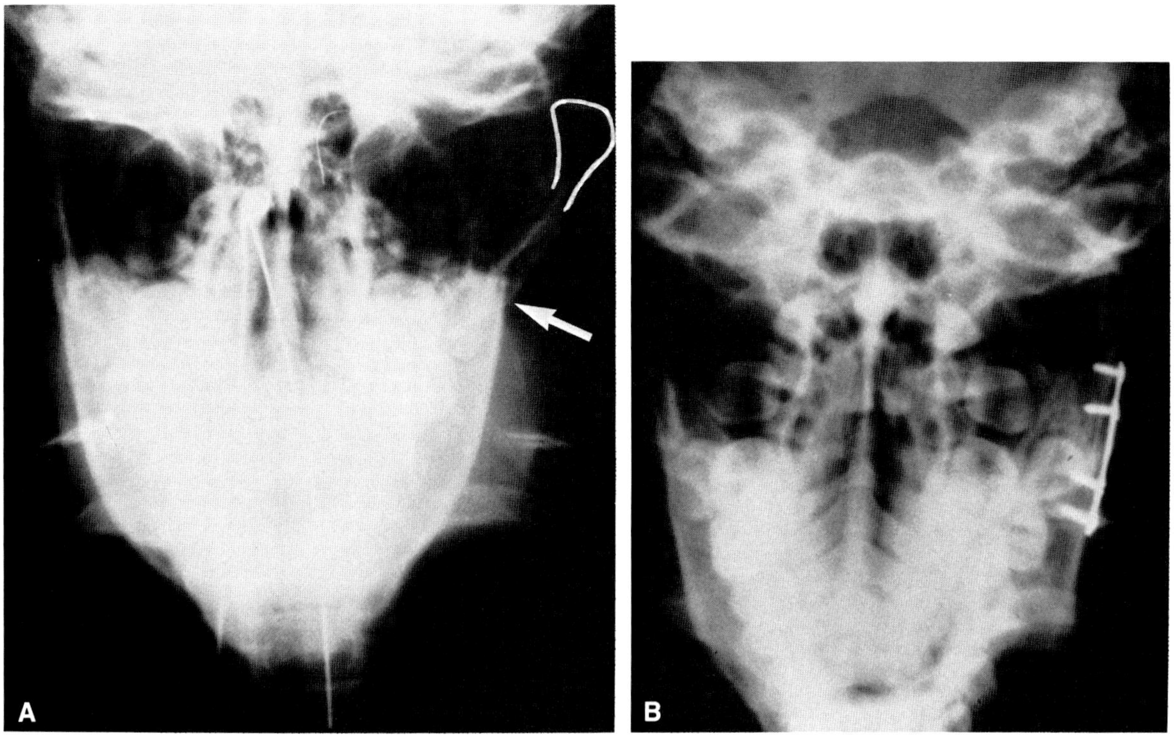

Figure 19–7. *(**A**) Lateral extracapsular dislocation of the left condyle associated with left mandibular angle fracture. (**B**) Reduction of the lateral dislocation with fixation of the fracture.*

fracture into a given classification and there is often no relation between the classification of an injury and its response to a given treatment, this provides a basis of understanding when discussing treatment of fractures.

Level of Fracture

The level of the fracture may be within the condylar head, condylar neck, or subcondylar region (Fig. 19–8). The condylar head is that region defined as the

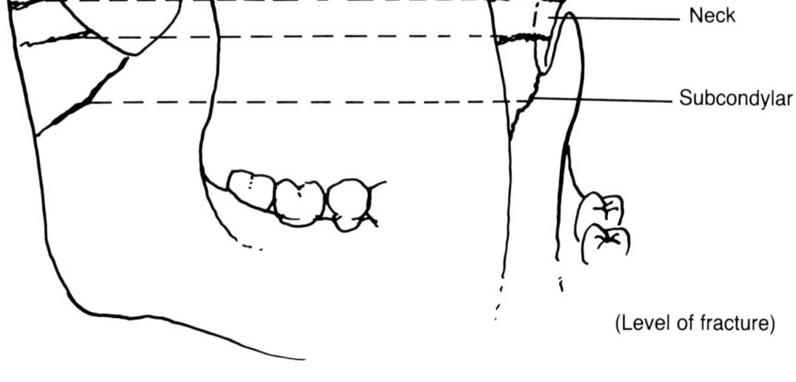

Figure 19–8. *Fracture classification. Condylar fractures can be classified according to the level of fracture; included are the neck, angle, and subcondylar region.*

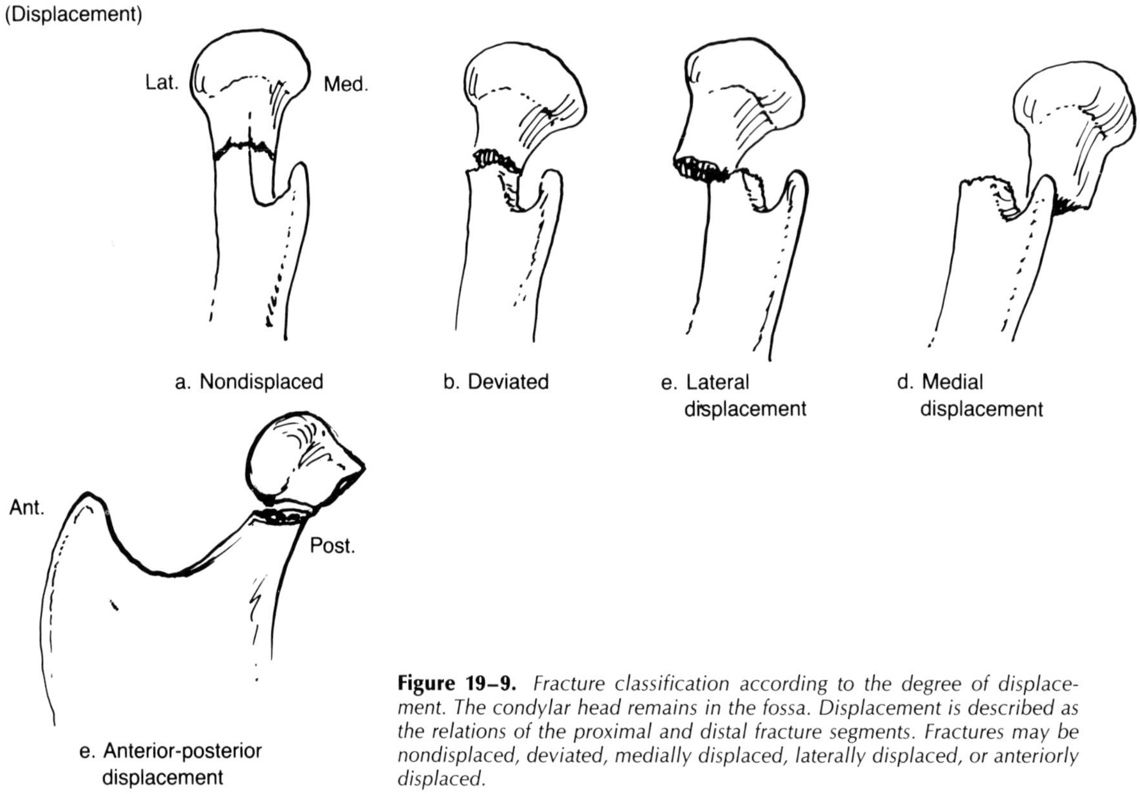

Figure 19–9. *Fracture classification according to the degree of displacement. The condylar head remains in the fossa. Displacement is described as the relations of the proximal and distal fracture segments. Fractures may be nondisplaced, deviated, medially displaced, laterally displaced, or anteriorly displaced.*

area superior to where the head of the condyle begins to taper. Fractures within this area are usually horizontal; rarely they may extend vertically through the articular surface.[4] By definition, these fractures are also intracapsular because the capsule of the temporomandibular joint attaches to the neck of the condyle.

The condylar neck is defined as the radiographic constriction representing (anatomically) the region of the inferior attachment of the joint capsule. A fracture of the condylar neck is extracapsular and lies below the attachment of the external pterygoid to the mandibular condyle.

Those fractures classified as subcondylar occur in the region below the neck, extending down to the most inferior point on the sigmoid notch anteriorly, whereas its posterior limit is situated more inferiorly, corresponding with the point of maximum concavity of the posterior border of the mandible in that region.[21]

Displacement

Fractures may be nondisplaced, deviated, or displaced (Fig. 19–9). A nondisplaced fracture is a linear fracture with the proximal fragment retaining its usual anatomic relation with the distal fragment. In a deviated fracture, a simple angulation of the condylar process exists in relation to the remaining mandibular fragment, without development of a gap or overlap between the two segments. Displacement is defined as movement of the condylar fragment in relation to the mandibular segment with movement at the fracture site. The fragment can be displaced in a lateral, medial, or anteroposterior direction. In displaced fractures the articular surface of the condyle remains within the glenoid fossa and does not herniate through the joint capsule.

Dislocation

If the head of the condyle is outside the fossa and is associated with a fracture of the condylar process, it is termed a *fracture dislocation.* Fracture dislocations may occur in an anterior, posterior, medial, lateral, or superior direction (Fig. 19–10). The most common direction of dislocation is anterior or anteromedial because of the pull of the lateral pterygoid muscle.[18]

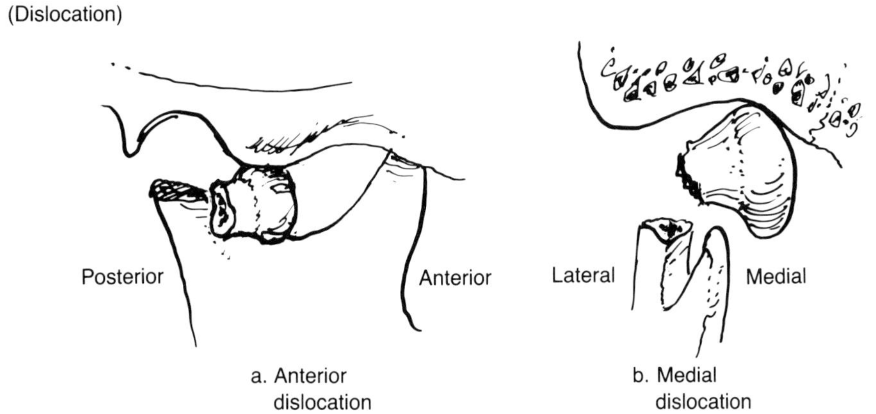

Figure 19–10. *Fracture dislocations are classified according to the direction of dislocation of the condylar head.*

Special Situations

Other types of fractures that do not readily fit the above classification are the following (Fig. 19–11): grossly comminuted fractures or fractures involving adjacent bony structures, such as the glenoid fossa or tympanic plate; open or compound fractures; and fractures in which a combination of several different types of fractures exist. Open fractures of the condyle are usually caused by missiles such as bullets.

Mechanism of Injury

Certain patterns of injury of the condyle occur more frequently. Factors that are considered important in determining the type of fracture and degree of displacement include: the nature, severity, and direction of traumatic force; the occlusion of the teeth and the position of the mandible on impact; and anatomic considerations such as the line of fracture and the influence of muscle pull, ligaments, and other adjacent soft tissue.[1,3,4]

Biomechanical Considerations

Studies of the relation between the nature, severity, and direction of traumatic force on the resultant mandibular injury were made by Huelke.[23-28] Before this, few experimental studies had been done with regard to the mechanism of mandibular fracture. Most literature regarding the mechanism of fracture was based on clinical impressions and opinions.

Early investigators showed that linear fractures in long bones were initiated by bone failure resulting from tensile strain rather than compressive strain.[29] Huelke and Harger applied forces of varying magnitudes and direction to dried mandibles and observed the resultant production of tension and compression.[26] They found that greater than 75% of all experimentally produced fractures of the mandible were in primary areas of tensile strain, which supported a similar observation made earlier in long bones. A notable exception was that comminuted condylar head injury that was produced by a load parallel to the mandibular ramus was primarily the result of compressive force.

In response to loading, the mandible is similar to an arch because it distributes the force of impact throughout its length (Fig. 19–12). However, unlike the arch, the mandible is not a smooth curve of uniform bone, but rather it has discontinuities such as foramina, sharp bends, ridges, and regions of reduced cross-sectional dimension like the subcondylar area. As a result, parts of the mandible develop greater force per unit area, and consequently, tensile strain is concentrated in these locations.

When a force is directed along the parasymphysis-body region of the mandible, compressive strain develops along the buccal aspect, whereas tensile strain develops along the lingual aspect. This produces a fracture that begins in the lingual region and spreads

OTHER FRACTURES:

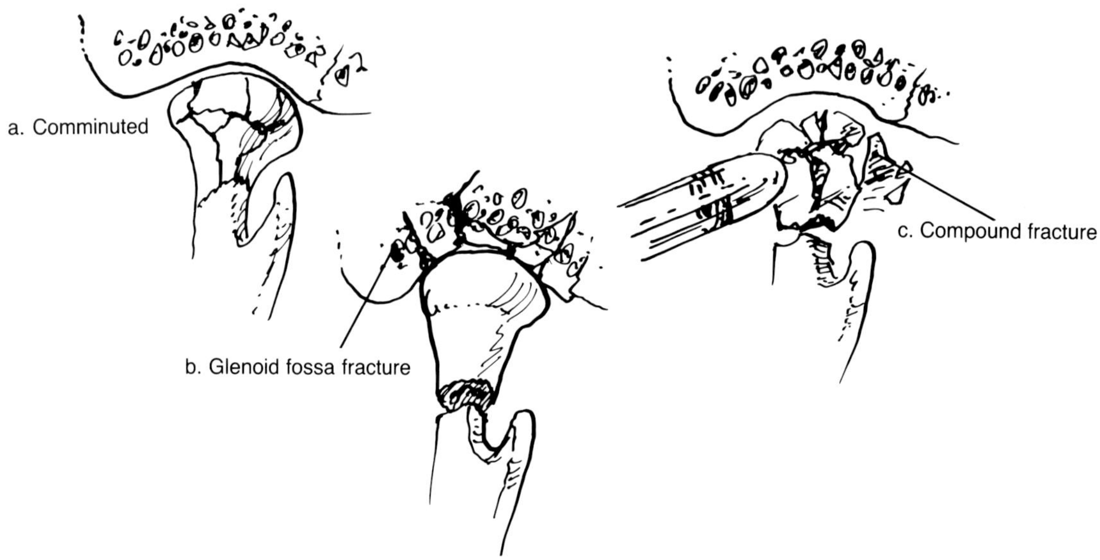

Figure 19–11. *Some fractures do not readily fall into the routine classification. These include grossly comminuted fractures of the condylar head, fractures involving the glenoid fossa, and open fractures.*

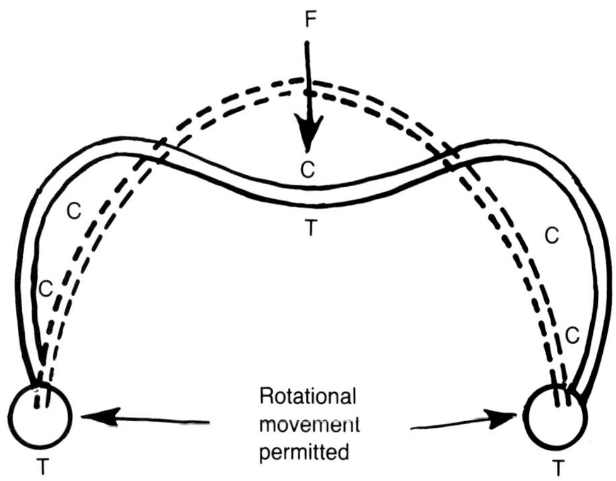

Figure 19–12. *The effect of a load on an arch where the ends are free to rotate. (Reproduced with permission of Huelke DF, Harger JH. Maxillofacial injuries: Their nature and mechanisms of production. J Oral Surg 1969; 27:451)*

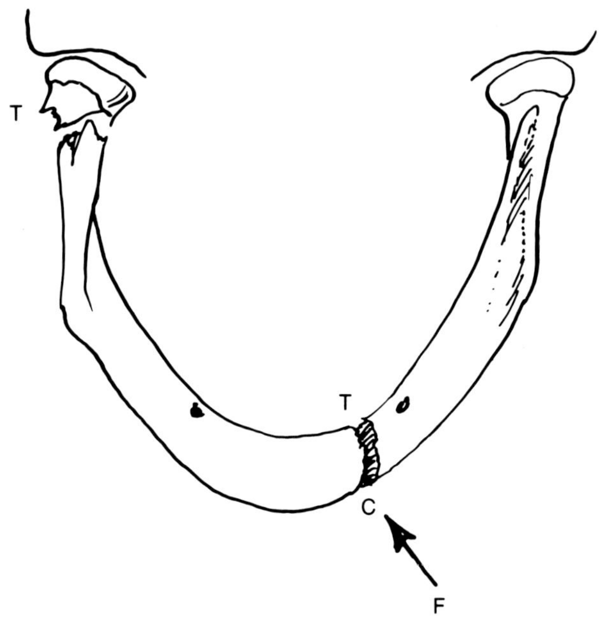

Figure 19–13. *Compression in the parasymphysis region secondary to a blow causes lingual tension and fracture. Forces are distributed along the arch and the contralateral condyle is forced laterally until the ligaments and fossa limit its movement. Tension develops laterally and fracture occurs.*

toward the buccal.[26] The mobile contralateral condyloid process moves in a direction away from the impact point until it is limited by the bony fossa and associated soft tissue. At this point, tension develops along the lateral aspect of the contralateral condylar neck and a fracture occurs (Fig. 19–13). If greater force is applied to the parasymphysis-body region, not only will tension develop along the contralateral condylar neck leading to fracture in this area, but continued medial movement of the smaller ipsilateral mandibular segment will lead to bending and tension forces along the lateral aspect and subsequent fracture of the condylar process on the ipsilateral side (Fig. 19–14). Force applied directly in the symphysis region along an axial plane is distributed along the arch of the mandible. Because the condylar heads are free to rotate within the glenoid fossa to a certain degree, tension develops along the lateral aspect of the condylar neck and mandibular body regions, as well as along the lingual aspect of the symphysis. This leads to bilateral condylar fractures and a symphysis fracture (Fig. 19–15).

Variation from these standard fracture patterns occurs for two general reasons. First, there is a wide range in the possible magnitude and direction of the impact and in the shape of the object delivering the impact. Secondly, the condition of the dentition, position of the mandible, and influence of associated soft tissues could not be controlled for in these studies.

Occlusion and Mandibular Position

Early observers felt that the presence of posterior dentition tended to reduce the incidence of condylar injury.[1,3,4] The implication was that, as the mandible was forced posteriorly and superiorly, the dentition would meet and absorb some of the force, thereby diminishing the force received at the condyle. This was supported by the clinical observation that the posterior dentition was often fractured on the side of the condylar fracture. However, more recent findings do not support this theory and show that all types of fractures occur, irrespective of the occlusion, and that no correlation exists between the degree of dislocation, level of fracture, or type of fracture with the presence of a distal occlusion.[22] Although the presence or absence of a posterior dentition does not correlate with the incidence of fracture, the presence of specific

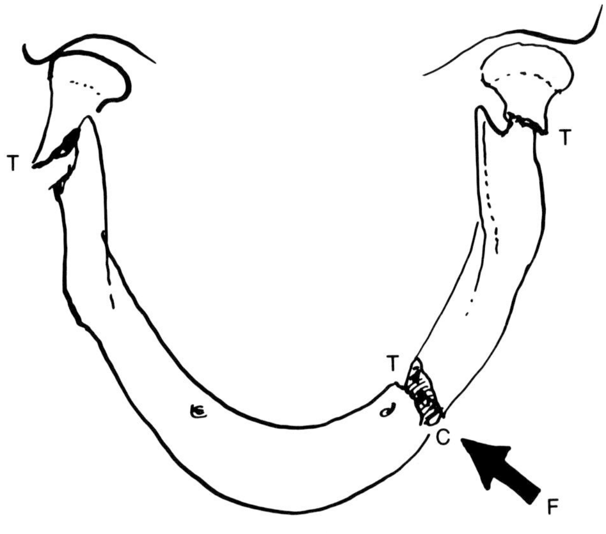

Figure 19–14. *Greater force than that applied in Figure 19–13 will not only fracture at the point of contact and at the contralateral condylar neck, but the smaller mandibular segment will be moved medially to a greater degree, creating tension laterally in the ipsilateral condylar neck, and fracture will occur here as well.*

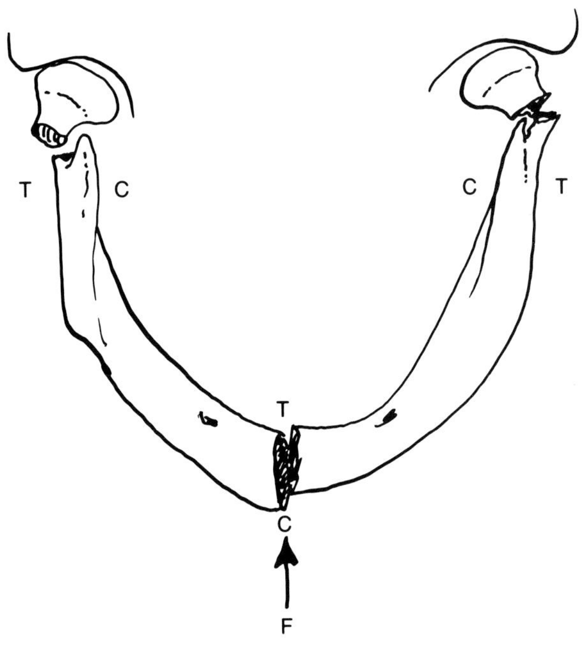

Figure 19–15. *Force directed at the symphysis along an axial plane is distributed along the arch of the mandible. Tension is dissipated along the mandible, and the fracture occurs bilaterally in the area of least stability, the condylar necks. As in other fractures, a symphysis fracture may develop caused by tension from the blow.*

teeth, particularly impacted third molars, has been shown to markedly affect the incidence of condylar fracture. It was shown that, when impacted third molars are present, this area represented a region of inherent weakness and the incidence of condylar fractures decreases, whereas the incidence of mandibular angle fractures increases.[30]

Although unable to show that the occlusion played any role in the type of fracture produced, investigators have found that the relative degree of mandibular opening at the time of impact does play an important role in the type of fracture that occurs.[4,14] More recent studies have shown that, not only is the incidence of fracture higher when the mouth is open, but that, the level of fracture varies with degree of opening. When the mouth is opened, the fractures tend to be located more in the condylar neck or condylar head region, whereas when it is closed, fractures are in the subcondylar area.[30]

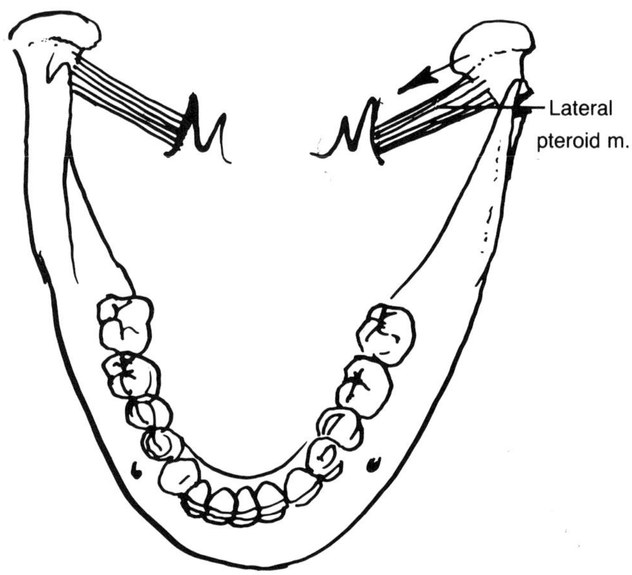

Figure 19–16. *Action of the lateral pterygoid on the proximal segment of fractured condyle tends to pull it anterior and medial.*

Muscle Pull

Once a fracture occurs, the associated soft tissue, particularly the muscles of mastication attached to the various bony segments, determine the degree of displacement or dislocation. The fracture segments tend to override each other as a result of the powerful upward pull of the masseter, medial pterygoid, and temporalis muscles.[3] If the fracture line occurs below the attachment of the lateral pterygoid, which is most common, the medial inferior and anterior pull of this muscle tends to displace the condylar head in that direction.[3] The degree of displacement depends on the line of the fracture. If the fracture is more superior along the medial aspect of the condylar neck than on the lateral aspect, the segment tends to be stabilized against the pull of the lateral pterygoid and is not displaced as much as when the fracture is higher on the lateral aspect.[3] This medial and anterior pull of the condylar fragment is directed toward the weakest area in the temporomandibular joint capsule, explaining why anteromedial displacement and dislocation is by far the most common pattern (Fig. 19–16).

Diagnosis

The definitive diagnosis of condylar fracture must be arrived at through thorough clinical and radiographic evaluation. Although the suspicion of condylar fracture may be high during a clinical examination (Table 19-2), other injuries of the articular apparatus that may mimic fracture must be ruled out with a radiographic examination. Frequently, the severity of the clinical symptoms do not correspond to the severity of the fracture and vice versa.[31] The clinical examination should be performed before the radiographic examination. Information gained from the clinical examination can then be used to determine the most appropriate radiographs to be ordered.

Clinical Examination

The clinical examination should consist of inspection and palpation. It is best to proceed in an orderly fashion and to perform this evaluation as a component part of the entire head and neck examination of the trauma patient. Typically, the patient who has suffered a fracture of the mandibular condyle will present with facial asymmetry (Fig. 19–17). This is due to loss of the vertical height of the ramus on the side with the fracture, resulting in a shift of the mandible to the ipsilateral side. On opening, the mandible frequently shifts even more toward the side of the fracture as a result of decreased translation of the condyle on the injured side. Other less common findings include blood within the external auditory canal and,

Table 19–2. *Clinical Signs of Condylar Injury*

Extraoral	Swelling over joint Blood in external auditory canal Deviation of chin (unilateral conditions) Tenderness to palpation or on mouth opening Inability to palpate condylar movement Limited range of motion
Intraoral	Malocclusion Tooth fracture

in the case of fracture dislocation, development of a prominent preauricular depression. Palpation will frequently confirm tenderness over the lateral pole of the injured condyle with associated crepitation. In the case of fracture dislocations, the condyle may not be palpable. Because of the swelling that accompanies fracture, the most effective means for palpation is to place the little fingers simultaneously into the external auditory canals bilaterally. The pads of the fingers should be directed anteriorly. The patient is then asked to open and close his or her mouth in maximum range of motion. A subjective assessment can then be made between the palpable movement of one side compared to the other. Failure to detect the translation of the condyle—especially when associated with pain on palpation—is highly indicative of a fracture in this area.

The most common intraoral findings are malocclusion, fracture of the dentition, and decreased interincisal opening. In unilateral fractures, there is deviation of the occlusion toward the fractured side, with premature occlusal contact in the posterior region on that side (Fig. 19–18). The midlines no longer coincide, and there is an open bite in the body region on the contralateral side. This is often accompanied by fracture of the posterior dentition on the same side as the condylar fracture (Fig. 19–19). The extent to which the incisal opening is affected depends on the amount of displacement and dislocation of the condyle, as well as on the amount of associated soft tissue trauma. In bilateral fractures, the occlusion may not be deviated. The midlines are often coincident, and premature contact is present bilaterally on the posterior dentition with an anterior open bite. The posterior dentition may be fractured on both sides in these situations.

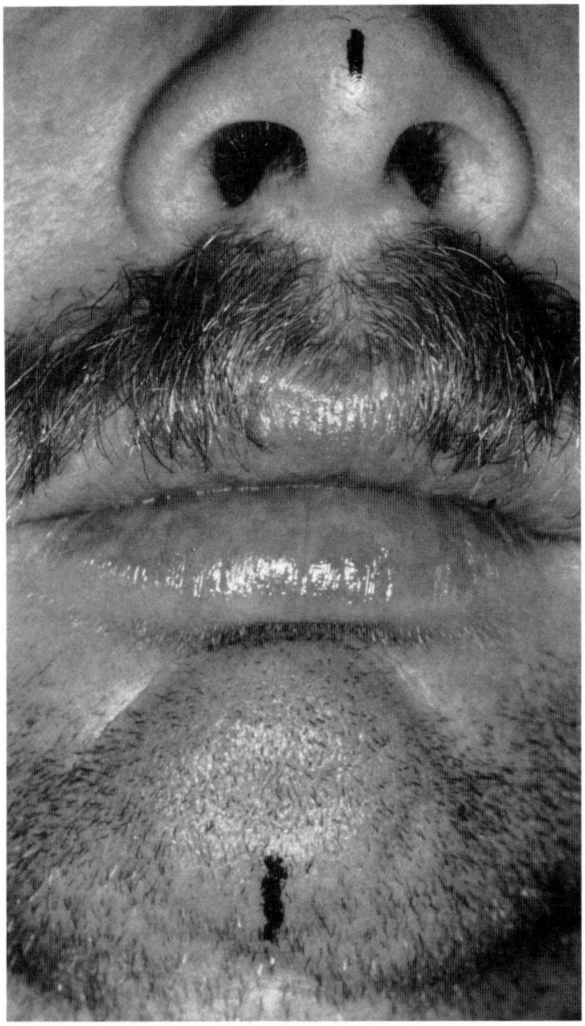

Figure 19–17. *The chin of a patient with a fracture of the right condyle. There is deviation toward the side of injury.*

The patient with a fracture of the condylar process also has a limited range of motion. The limitation is primarily caused by voluntary restriction as a result of pain. In addition, if the patient is asked to protrude the jaw or can open the jaw wider than that obtained by condylar rotation alone, the jaw will deviate to the fractured side. This results because the lateral pterygoid muscle on the fractured side pulls on the fractured segment and does not have any protruding influence on the mandible. The lateral pterygoid muscle on the contralateral side is unopposed and thus causes deviation to the fractured side.

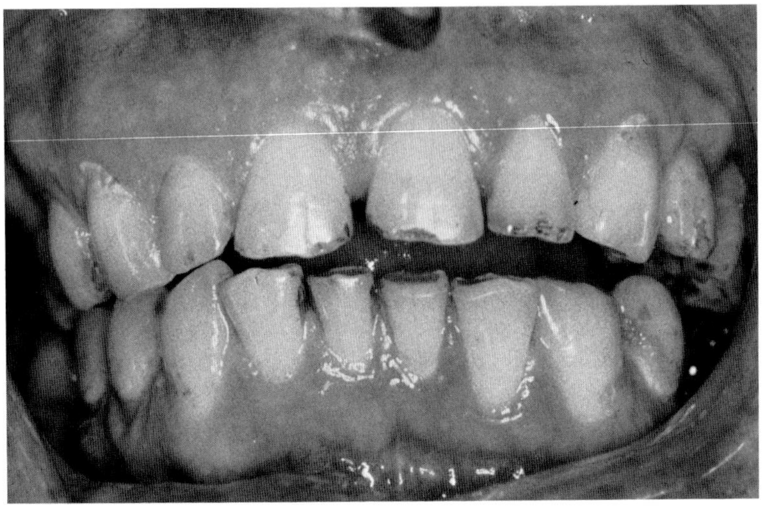

Figure 19–18. *The occlusion of a patient with a fractured right condyle. There is premature occlusal contact of posterior teeth on the ipsilateral side with an open bite on the contralateral side.*

Radiographic Examination

If the patient presents with any of these clinical findings or if the nature of the injury is highly suggestive of potential condylar fracture (e.g., laceration of the chin, presence of other mandibular fractures, or unexplained malocclusion), a thorough radiographic analysis should follow. To adequately screen for the presence of a fracture of the mandibular condyle, at least two views at right angles to each other are necessary. A panoramic radiograph and a modified Townes view (Fig. 19–20) are adequate studies to screen for the presence of condylar fracture. If only one view is used, fractures can easily be missed (Fig. 19–21A and B). In the multiple trauma patient for whom panoramic radiographs are not possible, lateral oblique views may be substituted. The typical findings on panoramic radiograph are the following: a shortened condylar-ramus length; the presence of a radiolucent fracture line or, in the case of overlapped segments, the presence of a radiopaque double density (Fig. 19–22); and evidence of premature contact on the side of the fracture if the radiograph was taken with the patient in occlusion. The modified Townes view shows the degree of medial or lateral displacement of the fracture and allows for the visualization of subtle deviation, such as is seen in greenstick fractures that are not readily evident on panoramic view (Fig. 19–23A and B).

Computed tomography (CT) can be useful in determining the position of the condylar segment, particularly in situations in which a fracture dislocation has occurred (Fig. 19–24A and B). Indications for CT scans are the following:

1. Significant displacement or dislocation, particularly if open reduction is contemplated
2. Limited range of motion with a suspicion of mechanical obstruction caused by the position of the condylar segment
3. Alteration of the surrounding osseous anatomy by other processes, such as previous internal derangement or

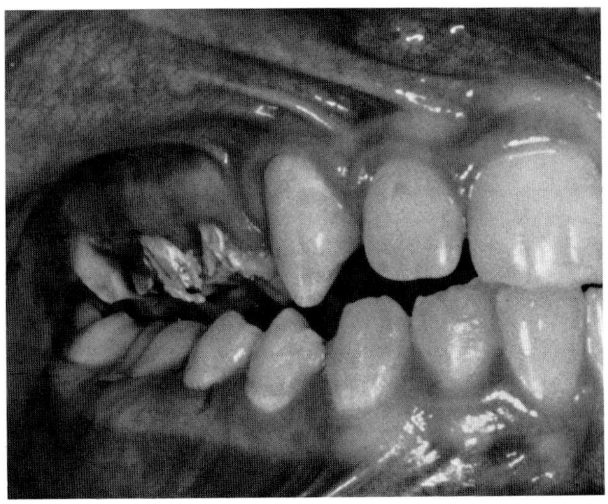

Figure 19–19. *Fractured posterior teeth are occasionally associated with fracture dislocation of the condylar process. This results when mandibular teeth are forced against maxillary teeth during fracture of the condyle.*

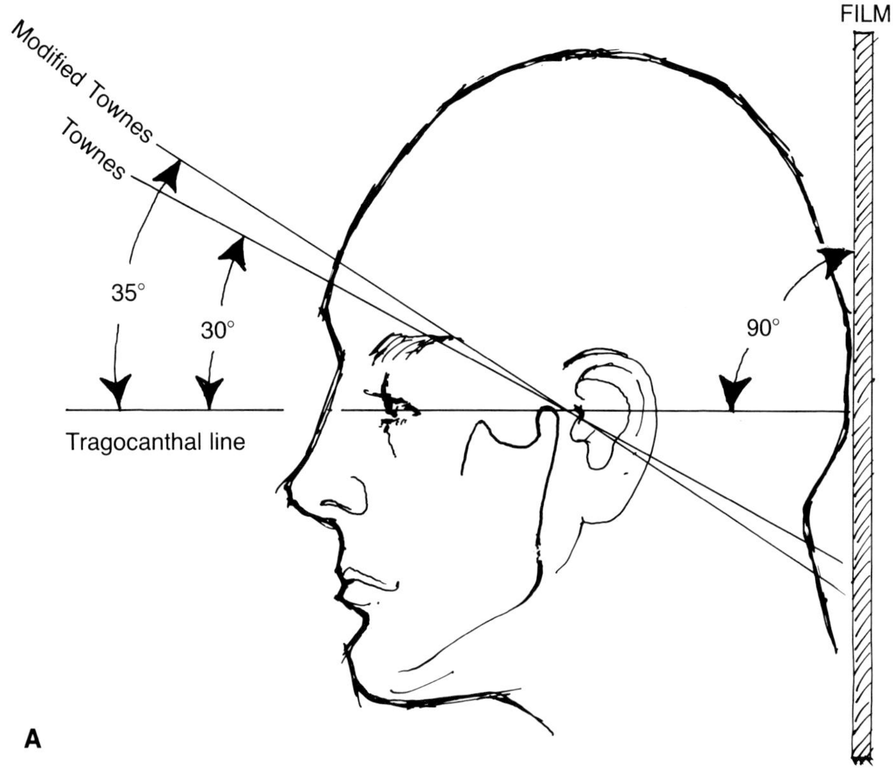

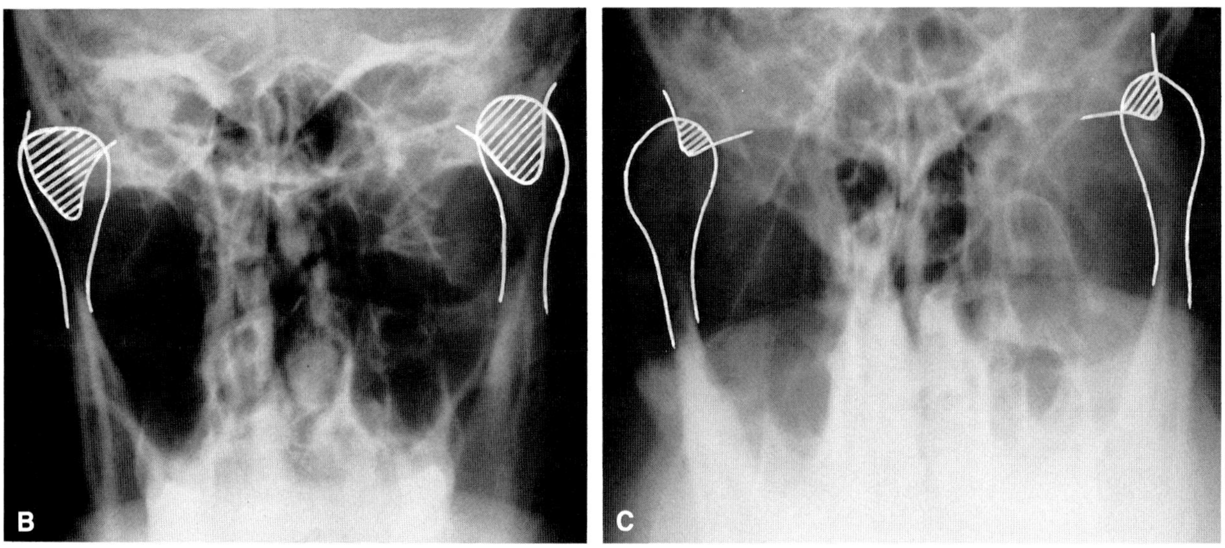

Figure 19–20. *(**A**) The technique for a modified Townes view directs the x-ray beam superiorly an additional 5° to further project the condyles below the mastoid processes. (**B**) A regular Townes view of a patient with no fracture. Much of the condylar head is not clearly visible because of the mastoid process overlying the superior aspect (shaded area). (**C**) A Modified Townes view of the same patient shown in A. Note the improved visualization of the condyle.*

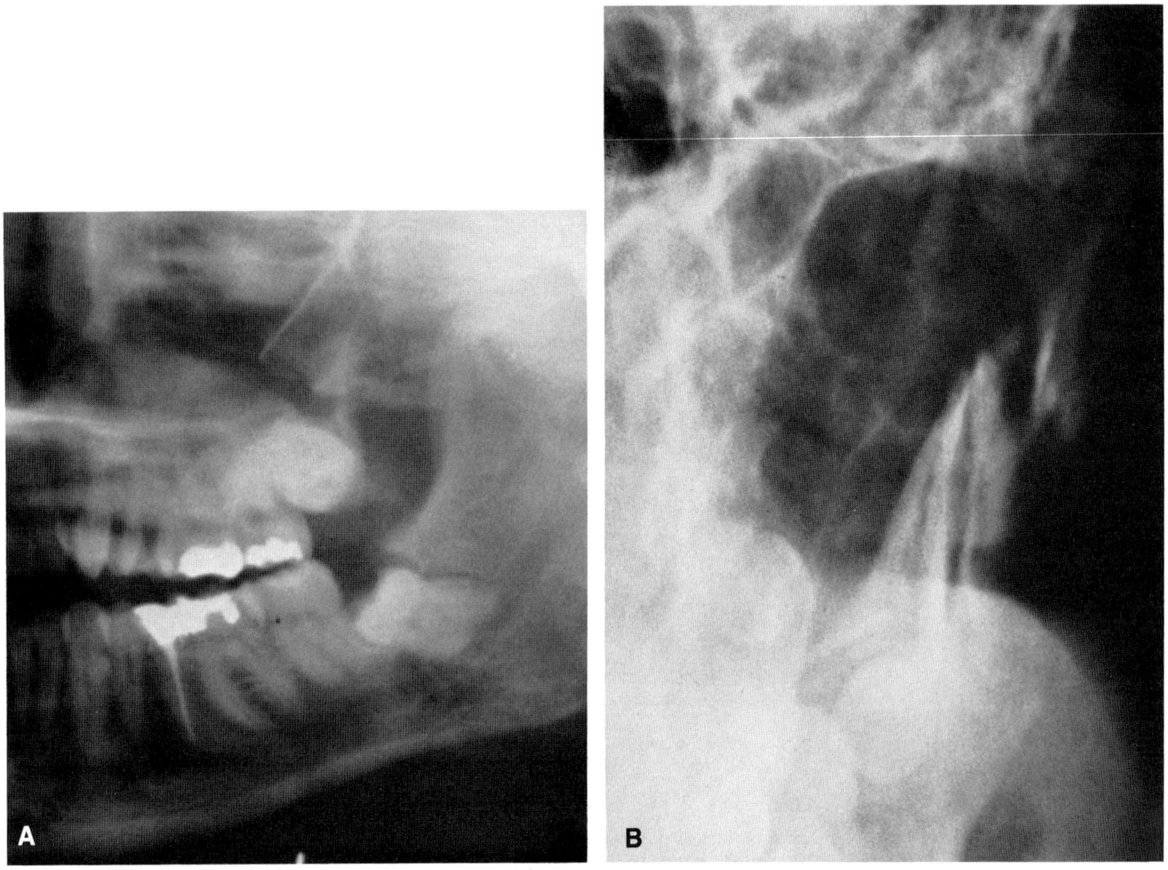

Figure 19–21. *(**A**) Panoramic radiograph fails to show a fractured left condyle. (**B**) Townes view of same patient shows a significantly displaced condyle fracture.*

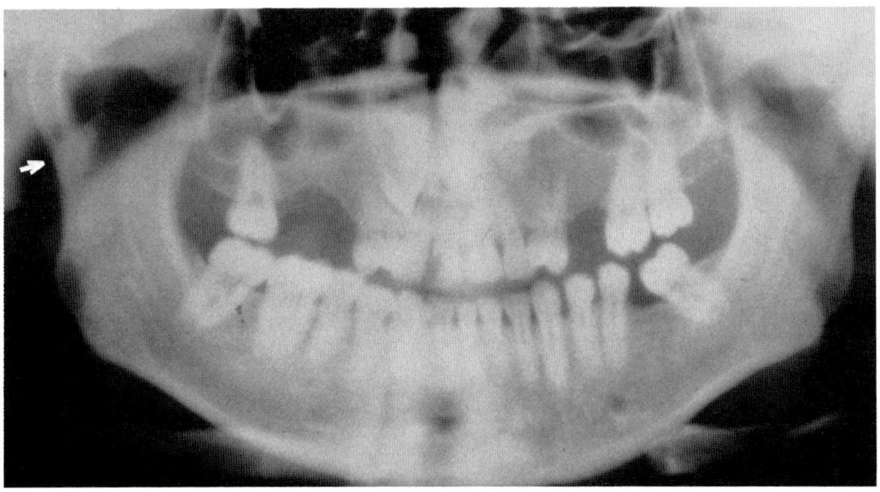

Figure 19–22. *Typical panoramic view of a subcondylar fracture. Note the shortened condylar-ramus height and radiopaque double density associated with overlap of the segments (arrow). Also note the premature occlusion on the right with open bite on the left.*

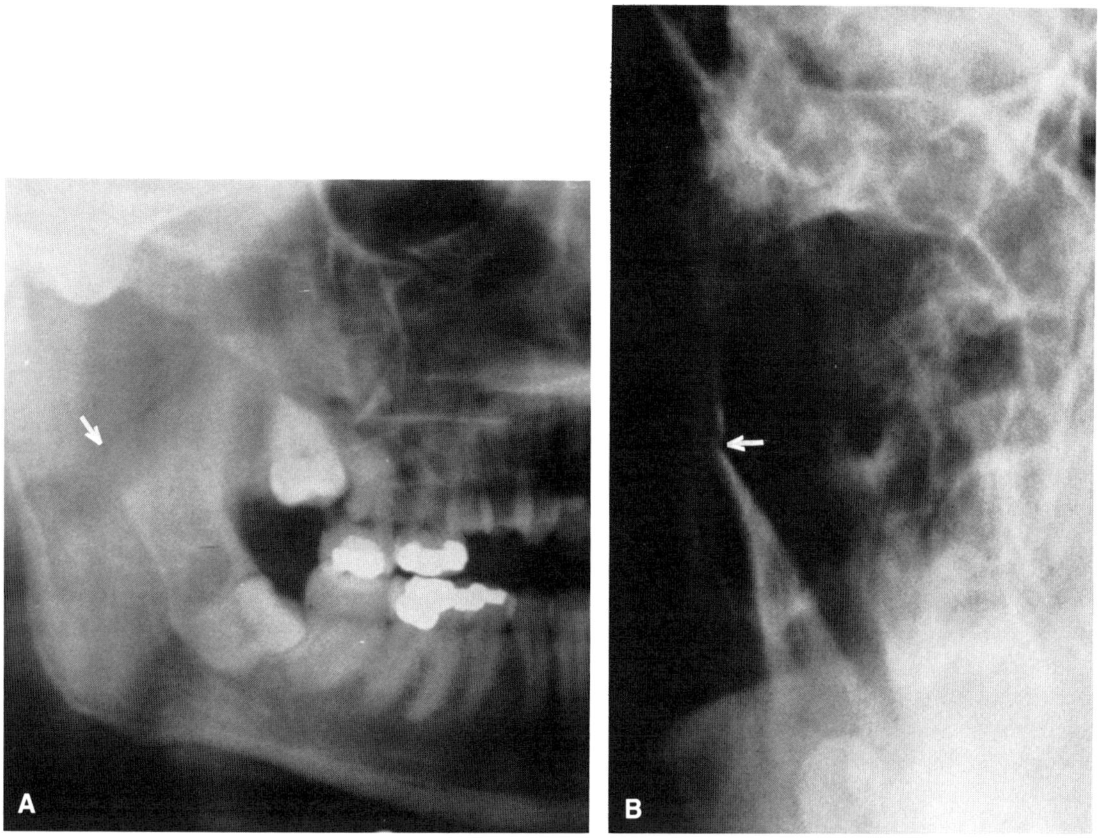

Figure 19–23. *(**A**) Enlarged partial panoramic radiograph with radiolucent line (arrow), indicating a right subcondylar fracture. (**B**) Townes view allows better visualization of the degree of deviation.*

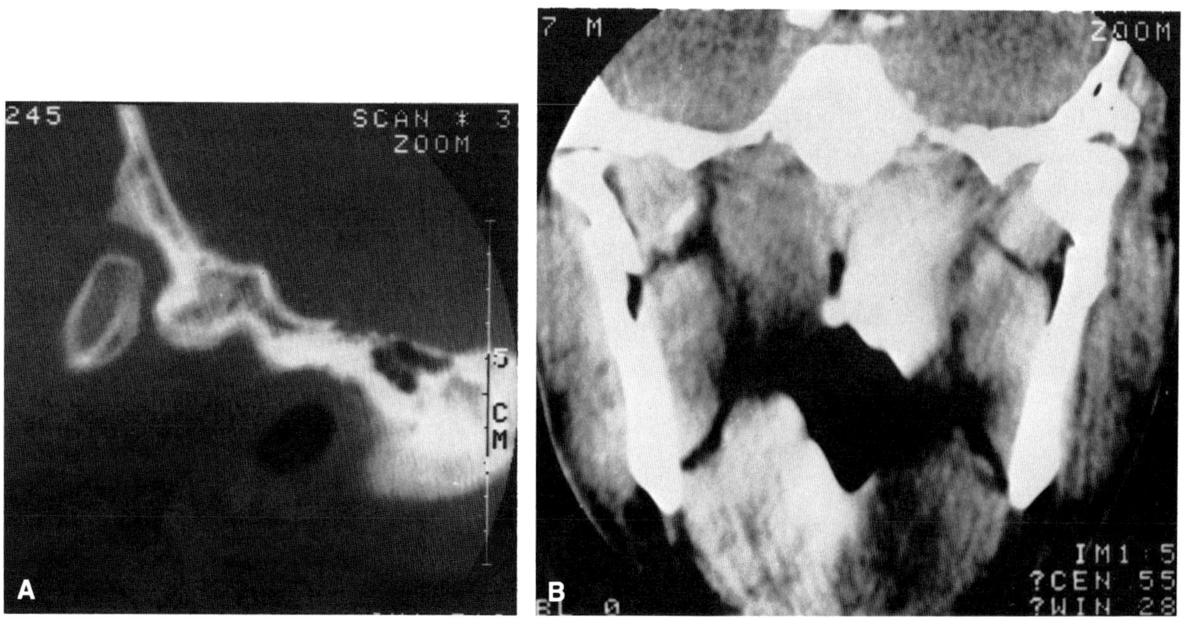

Figure 19–24. *(**A**) Sagitally reconstructed CT of a fracture dislocation of the right condyle. (**B**) Coronally reconstructed CT delineates bilaterally fractured condyles.*

temporomandibular joint surgery, to the degree that a pretreatment baseline is necessary
4. Inability to position the multiple trauma patient for conventional radiographs (CT scans may be the only useful radiograph that can be obtained)

Treatment

General Approach and Goals of Therapy

The decision about what the correct treatment should be is often more difficult to arrive at than performance of the treatment itself. The dilemma concerning the appropriate management of fractures of the mandibular condyle is most exemplary of this. Technically easy procedures such as closed reduction have experienced long-term successful results, whereas more complicated and technically demanding procedures of open reduction have continually and cyclically been employed in an attempt to improve on the results obtained with closed reduction. Although anatomic reduction with rigid internal stabilization of the fracture segments may be desirable, it is essential that the surgeon clearly define the goals of therapy and choose the simplest and most effective surgical method available to reach them.

The goals to be achieved in treatment of fractures of the mandibular condyle are the following (Table 19–3): obtain a stable occlusion; restore interincisal opening and mandibular excursive movements; minimize deviation of the mandible; produce a pain-free articular apparatus at rest and during function; avoid internal derangement of the temporomandibular joint on either the injured side or the contralateral side; and avoid the long-term complication of growth disturbance.

Table 19–3. Goals of Therapy

1. Stable occlusion
2. Restoration of interincisal opening
3. Full range of mandibular excursive movements
4. Minimize deviation
5. No pain
6. Avoid internal derangement of temporomandibular joint
7. Avoid growth disturbance

Maintenance of a stable occlusion is necessary for both functional and aesthetic reasons. Complete range of motion also allows normal mastication and prevents the development of contralateral temporomandibular joint dysfunction. A normal range of motion is most dependent on postoperative retraining of the muscles and elimination of pain. Ideally, the meniscus-condylar relation should remain intact without evidence of internal derangement. Some clinical sign of internal derangement such as joint noise can be tolerated if not associated with pain or decreased range of motion. Growth disturbance can result from ankylosis or from injury to the cartilaginous head of the condyle. A goal of treatment should include early mobilization to prevent ankylosis and close follow-up to identify growth changes early in their development. Attainment of an anatomic bony union is not a primary goal in treatment of condylar fractures, particularly if it must be done at the expense of other more important goals. A malunion or fibrous union that functions normally without pain is preferable to a radiographically exellent reduction that does not eliminate pain or limits motion.

Closed Reduction

INDICATIONS FOR CLOSED REDUCTION. A step-by-step approach can be applied to almost all condylar fractures (Fig. 19–25). Following this, algorithm will allow for the selection of the most appropriate treatment modality, given the clinical situation. The overwhelming majority of published clinical series over the last 40 years strongly promote closed reduction for the management of fractures of the mandibular condyle in both adults and children. A review of these studies (Table 19–4) reveals that, in the treatment of 714 patients with 865 condylar fractures, the total number of complications was 53, which represents a complication rate of approximately 7%.[1,3,19,20,31-34] These uniformly excellent results were obtained in all ages of patients treated. Conclusions drawn by various authors are the following: no correlation exists between the degree of radiographic displacement and the severity of clinical symptoms; no correlation exists between the radiographic alignment of the fracture segments and postoperative function; growth complications and ankylosis are exceedingly rare; open reduction with internal fixation is fraught with complications; and evidence supports the choice of closed

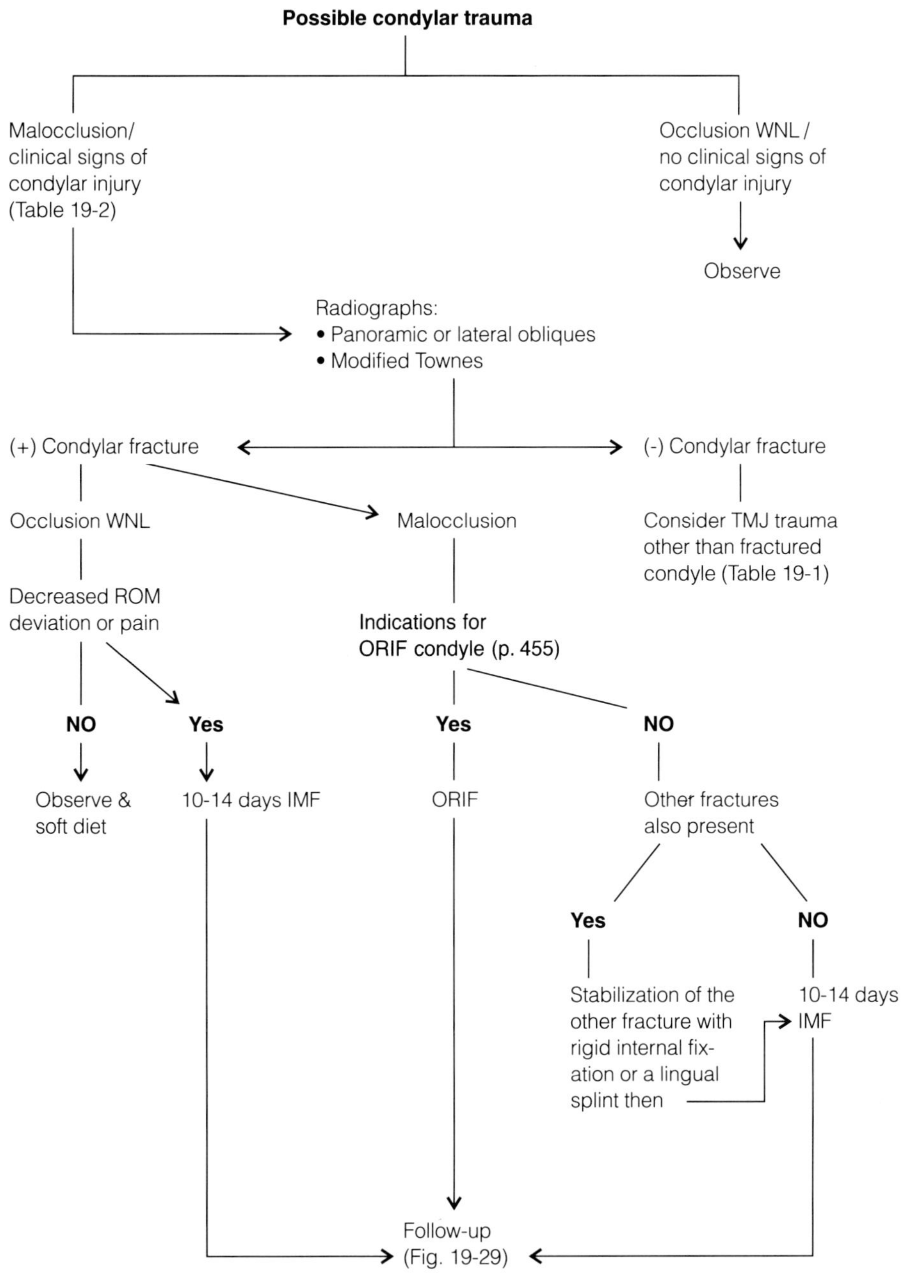

Figure 19–25. *Treatment algorithm for condylar trauma.*

reduction as the primary treatment modality for condylar fractures regardless of the degree of displacement.

Although the majority of the large studies reviewed patients in all age groups, some authors specifically studied children and their response to conservative management of condylar fractures.[35-41] All obtained excellent results with minimal complications when fractures of the condyle in children were treated with closed methods.

Some difficulty with all of these studies exists as a result of limited criteria evaluated. Evaluation was

Table 19–4. Closed Reduction Series

Author	Patients (N)	Fractures (N)	Length of F/U Range	Length of F/U Average	Age Range	Age Average	Complications*
Chalmers-Lyons (1947)[3]	120	156	1–19	5	4–68	28	7
MacLennan (1952)[20]	180	205	1–11	3	<10–35	—	9
Kromer (1953)[1]	154	185	—	—	—	—	14
MacGregor (1957)[32]	26	35	3–13	6	4–56	26	4
Blevins & Gores (1961)[19]	140	185	1–12	—	3–77	28	6
Cook & MacFarlane (1969)[31]	74	74	—	—	—	—	22
Leake, et al. (1971)[33]	20	25	0–17	3.5	2–12	6	0
Lindahl (1977)[30]	67	94	0–4	—	3–>20	—	12
Total	781	959	—	—	—	—	65 (6.8%)

* Complications were defined as decreased range of motion, malocclusion, growth alteration, visible deformity, or pain. They do not include deviation not compromising function, asymptomatic joint noises, or radiographic deformity.

made of long-term interincisal opening and the presence of pain and malocclusion. Some deviation on terminal opening was considered acceptable if the occlusion was stable. No evaluation of temporomandibular joint function other than range of motion and pain was made.

The superiority of closed reduction of condylar fractures is also supported by numerous animal studies. Experimentally induced fracture dislocation in Macaca rhesus monkeys has resulted in "a workable, usable mandibular articulation regardless of whether the condyle was left remaining at right angle to the ramus, pushed medially or anteriorly, or reduced and maintained by transosseous wire. There was little sacrifice of mandibular growth or symmetry."[42,43] Further studies compared three methods of treatment for fracture dislocations in rhesus monkeys.[44] No difference existed between those treated with internal fixation using wire ligature, those treated with maxillomandibular fixation, or those that received no treatment. No incidents of nonunion were reported with any closed technique.

TECHNIQUE FOR CLOSED REDUCTION. Closed reduction of condyle fractures is accomplished through immobilization of the mandible. This is performed most frequently with the use of intermaxillary fixation between arch bars or wires applied to the dentition or with Gunning type splints.

Ideally, the period of intermaxillary fixation should allow for reestablishment of the preinjury occlusion and should not be longer. Increased length of the time of fixation may result in limitation in function or ankylosis of the joint. In practice, a wide variety of opinions exists over the length of time that constitutes an adequate period of fixation. Differences depend on the age of the patient, the type of fracture, and the presence of other fractures. The period of time for intermaxillary fixation has ranged from none to 6 weeks. Most clinicians agree that a shorter period is needed in children, but they are no closer in agreement over what this time should be.

Animal studies have shown excellent occlusion and postoperative function even in fracture dislocations when no intermaxillary fixation is used.[42-44] Some studies in humans also agree with this. However, the inability to occlude the teeth without pain is frequently present in patients and does require some period of fixation. Attempts to predetermine which fractures will need longer intermaxillary fixation than others have been made.[4] The length of time has been based on the presence or absence of teeth, the type of fracture, and the age of the patient. However, Walker has suggested that a relatively short period of intermaxillary fixation is often required for all patients regardless of age, occlusion, and type of fracture.[45,46] Based on these observations, it is best that intermaxillary fixation be discontinued in all patients at approximately 10 to 14 days. If other mandibular fractures are associated with the fractured condyle, it is desirable to treat them with some form of additional stabilization, such as a lingual splint, external pins, or rigid internal fixation. This allows for the early release of intermaxillary fixation without compromising the healing of these other fractures.

Open Reduction

The significance of the rather large number of successfully managed patients using closed reduction is magnified when one considers that no large study on open reduction showed any improvement in the result or any decrease in the rate of complications. Those recommending open reduction have failed to report complication rates for the proposed technique or, when cited, reported complication rates that are greater than those seen historically with closed reduction; they experienced complications that have not been seen with closed techniques; and they allowed inadequate follow-up before assessing the outcome.

A variety of useful techniques for open reduction have been described.[36,47-50] The reason for employing open reduction in each case was to avoid the complications found in closed reduction. No data or follow-up of patients was presented to document this. Tasanen and Lamberg,[51] Zide and Kent,[52] and Raveh[53] followed patients with open reduction for up to 37 months. Complication rates of 85%, 50%, and 10% were seen, respectively, including facial nerve dysfunction and keloid formation. No comparison was made to patients treated with closed reduction during the same time period. Chuong and Piper attempted to compare closed reduction with open reduction, including concomitant disk repair in their study.[54] Eight of nine open reduction patients who were studied for an average of 11 months experienced complications (88%). Six of 12 patients receiving closed reduction were found to have malocclusion at the end of treatment (50%). It is possible that the high incidence of malocclusion in the closed reduction group might be due to prolonged fixation ($3\frac{1}{2}$ weeks), inadequate follow-up (1 to 14 weeks), and lack of supervised postoperative rehabilitation.[46]

There is a lack of any controlled clinical data to indicate the superiority of open reduction techniques as a primary mode of management of condylar fractures in children or adults. Although it is apparent that, in some situations, an unacceptable incidence of complications results when closed reduction is employed, it is inappropriate to assume that an open technique can avoid these complications until this is borne out in controlled clinical trials.

INDICATIONS FOR OPEN REDUCTION. Despite the evidence in favor of closed reduction as the treatment of choice for the majority of fractured condyles in both children and adults, there are indications for the performance of open reduction (see outline).

Indications for Open Reduction of Fractures of the Mandibular Condyle

- **I.** Absolute indications
  - A. Limitation of function secondary to:
    1. Fracture into middle cranial fossa
    2. Foreign body within the joint capsule
    3. Lateral extracapsular dislocation of condylar head
    4. Other fracture dislocations in which a mechanical stop is present on opening, which is confirmed radiographically
  - B. Inability to bring the teeth into occlusion for closed reduction
- **II.** Relative indications
  - A. Bilateral condylar fractures with comminuted midface fractures in which rigid internal fixation of the midface is not possible
  - B. Situations when intermaxillary fixation (IMF) is not feasible as a result of:
    1. Medical restrictions
       - a. Poorly controlled seizure disorder
       - b. Psychiatric disorders
       - c. Severe mental retardation
       - d. Concomitant injuries such as head injury or chest injury (unless tracheostomy is planned)
    2. Displaced fractures where dentures or splints are not feasible because of severe mandibular atrophy
  - C. Bilateral fractures in which it is impossible to determine what the proper occlusion is as a result of loss of posterior teeth or the presence of a preinjury skeletal malocclusion
  - D. In fracture dislocations in adults to restore the position and function of the meniscus (controversial)

In the past the indication for open reduction of a condylar fracture was primarily a radiographic one. Essentially, it was thought that the condyle behaved like other areas of the mandible or other bones in the body and that it would respond better and heal with more satisfactory function if an ideal anatomic reduction were obtained.[49,51,55,56] It has been shown that there is little if any correlation between the degree of displacement or dislocation of the fracture and the ability to obtain satisfactory function with a closed reduction. A more functional approach in assessing the need for open reduction was taken by Zide and Kent.[52,57] According to these investigators, indications for open reduction of condylar fractures should rely on the identification of specific clinical entities that, when treated with closed reduction, would result in a high degree of failure. They also take into account an objective evaluation of function at the time of the planned reduction, the presence and condition of the patient's dentition, the likelihood of successfully performing a closed reduction, and the presence of other modifying factors such as the patient's medical condition or the existence of other facial fractures.

Absolute Indications. Absolute indications for open reduction are present in those situations in which limitation in function is highly probable if a closed reduction is performed or in those situations in which a closed reduction is not possible. Limitation of function may be caused by fracture with dislocation of the proximal segment into the middle cranial fossa, by invasion of the joint by a foreign body (Fig. 19–26A and B), by lateral extracapsular dislocation of the condylar head, or by the presence of any fracture dislocation that produces a mechanical stop, preventing mandibular movement. Inability to perform a closed reduction may result when the fracture is displaced so that it is impossible to manipulate the teeth into an appropriate occlusion (Figure 19–26C).

Possible or Relative Indications. Possible or relative indications for open reduction also exist and should be assessed on the basis of benefit as opposed to risk.

BILATERAL CONDYLAR FRACTURES WITH COMMINUTED MIDFACE FRACTURES. The rationale for open condylar reduction in these situations is that it allows for the establishment of a horizontal and vertical dimension of the midface when this cannot be achieved by other means (Fig. 19–27A and B). If rigid internal fixation of the midface is possible, then open reduction of the condyle may no longer be indicated.

SITUATIONS IN WHICH INTERMAXILLARY FIXATION IS NOT FEASIBLE. Certain medical conditions, such as poorly controlled seizures, psychiatric disorders, or severe mental retardation, make maxillomandibular fixation difficult and possibly dangerous. Also, patients with multiple trauma—particularly head injury or chest injury—are at increased risk for complications if placed in maxillomandibular fixation unless tracheostomy is planned for other reasons. In addition, maxillomandibular fixation is extremely difficult in those patients with displaced condylar fractures in whom dentures are not present and splints are not feasible because of severe mandibular atrophy.

BILATERAL FRACTURES IN WHICH IT IS IMPOSSIBLE TO DETERMINE THE PROPER OCCLUSIONS. Occasionally, a patient with bilateral fractures will have such an ambiguous occlusion that, even with the use of study models and careful clinical examination, it is not possible to determine the appropriate maxillomandibular relation. This may lead to inappropriate placement of the mandible into malocclusion or to placement of a preexisting malocclusion into a normal relation, thereby predisposing the patient to nonunion or long-term functional disability.

FRACTURE DISLOCATION IN AN ADULT PATIENT TO RESTORE POSITION AND FUNCTION OF THE MENISCUS. Previous emphasis on indications for open reduction have centered around the need for bony reduction and fixation without consideration of disk position. The unstated implication of most of the literature is that the position of the dislocated disk is not critical for optimal functional results after condyle fracture.[54] However, this is contradictory, given the present emphasis on the importance of correct condylar disk alignment for management of those patients with internal derangement of the temporomandibular joint. The disk is important in the prevention of posttraumatic ankylosis.[9] An interesting concept has been raised about the possible necessity for disk repositioning, especially in fracture dislocations, to allow for optimal temporomandibular joint function.[54] Some clinicians now believe that "open reduction and internal fixation of condylar fractures in conjunction with disk repair is a biologically sound approach . . ."[54] Based on their experience, it might be recommended that, in fracture dislocations in which open reduction is indicated, an attempt should be made to reposition the disk at the time of the reduction. However, inadequate data

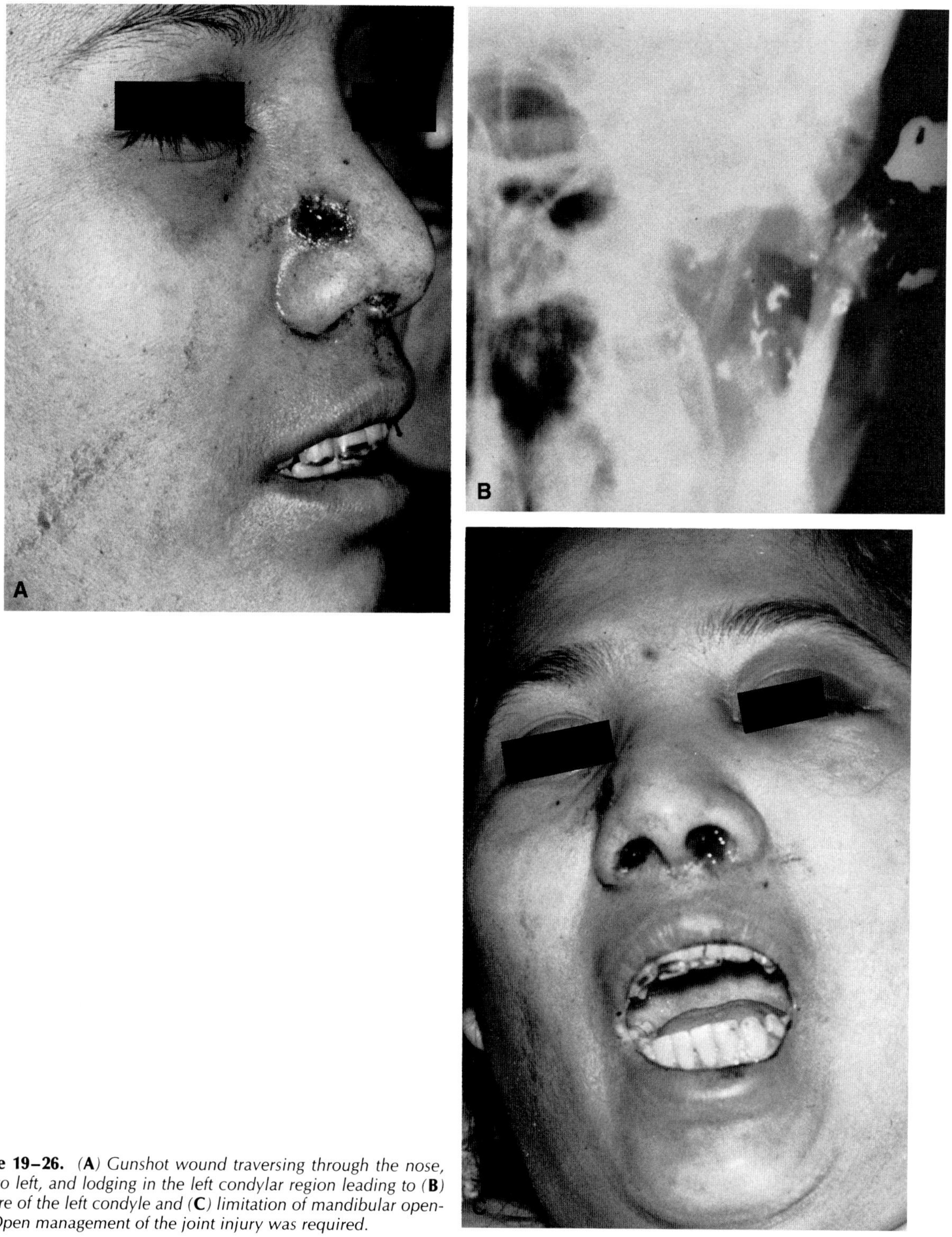

Figure 19–26. *(**A**) Gunshot wound traversing through the nose, right to left, and lodging in the left condylar region leading to (**B**) fracture of the left condyle and (**C**) limitation of mandibular opening. Open management of the joint injury was required.*

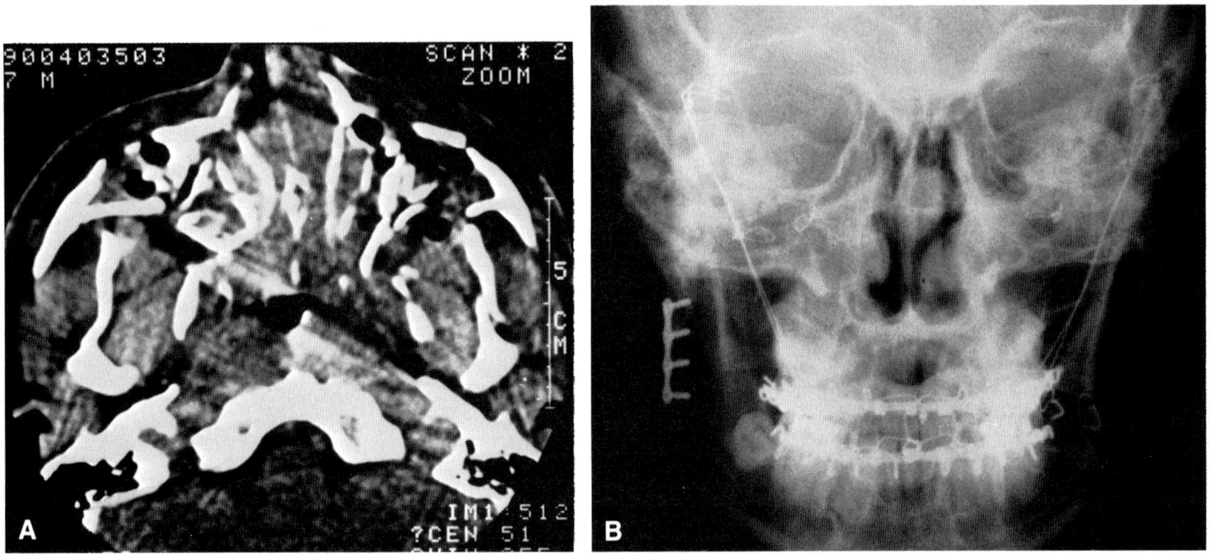

Figure 19–27. *(***A***) CT scan of comminuted midface fractures with bilaterally fractured condyles. (See Fig. 19–24* (B) *for coronal reconstruction of condyle fractures.) Open reduction of the left condyle fracture allowed restoration of a stable vertical dimension to which the remaining fractures are reduced. (***B***) Postoperative PA radiograph.*

exists to suggest that open reduction performed solely for the purpose of disk repositioning is valid.

TECHNIQUE FOR OPEN REDUCTION. Some authors have advocated the performance of open reduction without concomitant fixation of the reduced segments. The potential for complications with this approach are great, because no measures are taken to adequately counteract the instability caused by muscle pull. Maintenance of appropriate reduction may be compromised. Therefore, when open reduction is contemplated, some form of fixation should be attempted to predictably and stably maintain the reduction achieved at surgery. The approach taken should be the one that most effectively gains access to the fracture and the technique of fixation should be the one that most adequately maintains the reduction.

APPROACHES FOR OPEN REDUCTION. A variety of surgical approaches to the fractured condyle have been suggested, including intraoral, submandibular, retromandibular, preauricular, and combinations of the above. The most important factor in determining the approach used is the level at which the fracture has occurred. Modifying factors such as the degree of displacement or dislocation and the planned method of fixation may also have a bearing on the approach selected.

Fractures in the condylar neck and above are best approached through a preauricular or endaural incision.[57] This approach also has the added advantage of allowing for surgical manipulation of the soft tissues within the joint, if desired.

Subcondylar fractures and fractures extending into the upper ramus region are best approached using a retromandibular or Hinds approach.[58] The incision begins approximately 1 cm below the lobe of the ear and 1 cm posterior to the ramus of the mandible. The dissection is carried down to the parotid, which is retracted anteriorly, providing access to the vertical fibers of the masseter muscle overlying the ramus. These fibers are not stripped but instead are separated bluntly along their vertical course, allowing access to the underlying ramus. Access can easily be gained to relatively high subcondylar fractures through this approach, and a variety of fixation techniques are possible without additional percutaneous puncture, as may be needed if a submandibular approach is used. Low subcondylar fractures, especially those without a significant degree of displacement, may be easily approached from an intraoral incision.[59]

In severe anteromedial fracture dislocations in

which the condylar head is not retrievable despite the choice of approach, a vertical ramus osteotomy, followed by removal of the osteotomized segment, has been recommended.[60-62] This allows for access to the proximal condylar head, which is located medially and is also removed. Rigid fixation with plates or screws is carried out between the ramus segment and condylar head (Fig. 19–28). The unit is returned as a free autogenous bone graft, and the osteotomy is plated. This technique is useful for high dislocated fractures and may be accomplished through a retromandibular approach.

Occasionally, a combination of approaches is necessary, particularly in fracture dislocations in which a preauricular approach may be necessary to retrieve the proximal segment, while fixation is performed through another approach.[63]

FIXATION. Once access to the fracture has been achieved, any number of fixation devices may be employed (Fig. 19–28). In a given situation, any one of these techniques may have certain advantages over the other. With the development of sophisticated rigid internal fixation systems and instrumentation for their placement, miniplate fixation of these fractures will be the technique most readily employed in most cases. Miniature bone plates can be applied using any of the previously discussed approaches. These plates have the advantage of being available in a wide variety of shapes and sizes; they are now readily available in most operating rooms; and they provide a more stable form of fixation than do wires or Kirschner's wires. Theoretically, bone plates have another advantage—they can be placed on a relatively small proximal fragment first, allowing for the creation of a handle to more effectively manipulate the proximal segment into an appropriate reduction. Should the incision selected not allow for total access to the fracture, currently available bone-plating systems are equipped with instrumentation for percutaneous placement of screws (see Chap. 23).

Postoperative Management

Regardless of the technique employed for treatment of the condylar fracture, the postoperative management of the patient is important to the long-term successful rehabilitation and return to function. The proper length of maxillomandibular fixation (if used), the duration and frequency of evaluation by the surgeon, the early detection of potential complications, the judicious use of physiotherapy, and proper patient education are all necessary.

In most cases some form of intermaxillary fixation will have been employed. The length of the fixation period (as discussed in the section on closed reduction) usually is about 2 weeks. At the end of this period, a systematic approach for removal of the fixation is desirable. A follow-up regimen similar to that descibed by Walker (Fig. 19–29) can then be instituted.[45,46] This allows for elastic fixation and control of occlusion in those patients who need further stabilization, while encouraging early movement in those patients who have stable occlusions. It is impossible to predict on the basis of the type of fracture which patients will need continued aggressive elastic guidance to maintain their occlusion. Children of less than 12 years of age rarely require more fixation, but patients over the age of 12 years show extreme variability, regardless of fracture type.

If the occlusion is stable and reproducible at the time of intermaxillary fixation release, then aggressive jaw-opening exercises are begun. The patient should be evaluated in 24 hours to confirm the presence of a stable occlusion. The arch bars are left in place and training elastics are used. The purpose of these elastics is to permit function, while maintaining the occlusion. An effective way to accomplish this is to gradually reduce the use of elastics over a period of time. Initially, elastics should be used 24 hours a day. They should be placed lightly during the daytime to assist in guiding the mandible into occlusion, particularly if significant deviation is present, and applied more tightly at night. After 1 week, it may be possible to completely abandon daytime elastic fixation and continue with relatively tight elastic fixation at night. After another 1 to 2 weeks of this therapy, assuming that continued maintenance of a normal occlusion is present, the patient should be allowed to function without any guiding elastic fixation for approximately 1 week. If, at that time, there continues to be a stable occlusion, further evaluation should continue for other problems, such as limited mouth opening or pain, and the arch bars may be removed. If, on the removal of the intermaxillary fixation or at any time during the training period, the occlusion becomes unstable and nonreproducible, an additional period of tight intermaxillary fixation with wires or elastics is indicated for

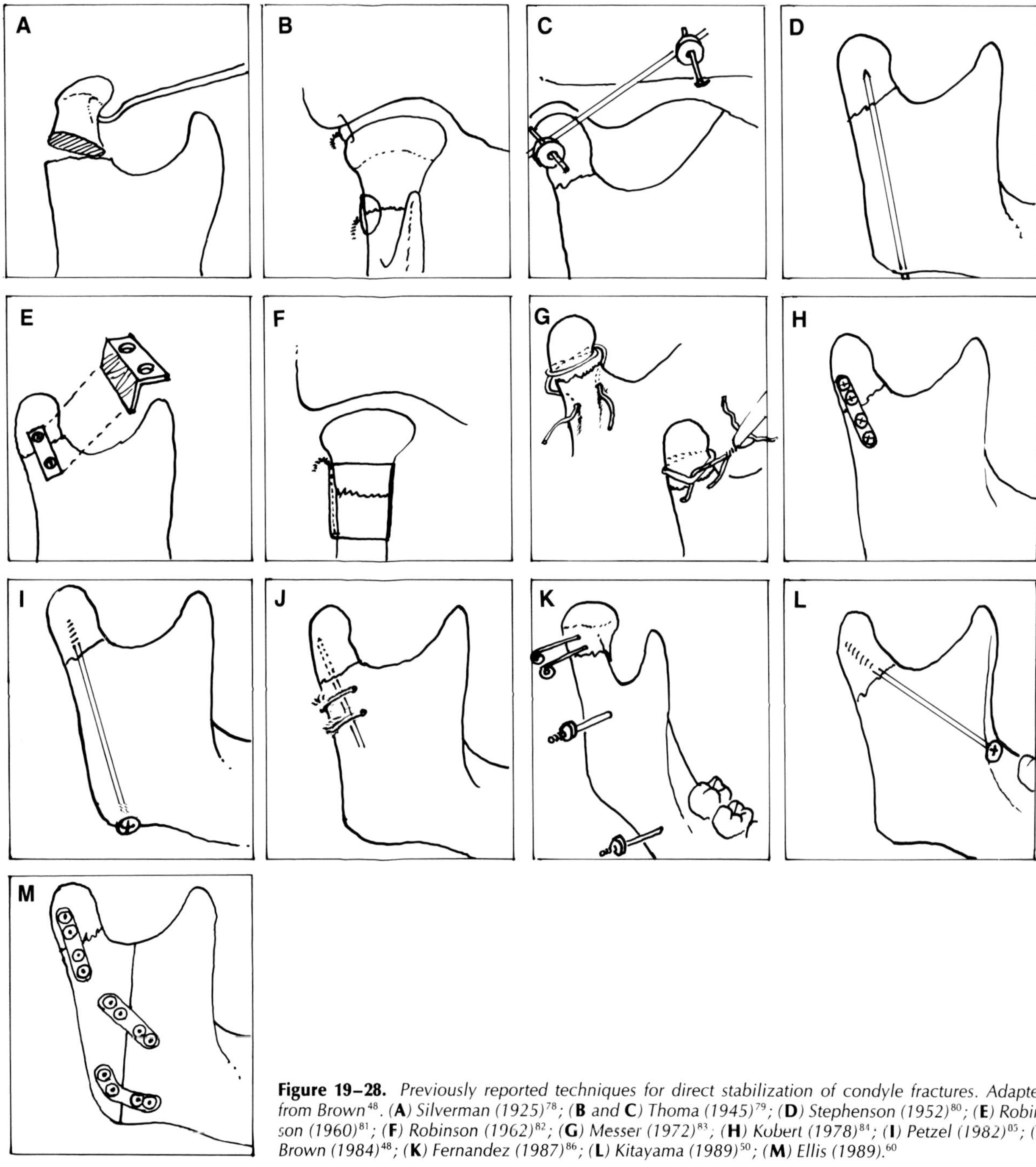

Figure 19–28. *Previously reported techniques for direct stabilization of condyle fractures. Adapted from Brown*[48]. (**A**) *Silverman (1925)*[78]; (**B** and **C**) *Thoma (1945)*[79]; (**D**) *Stephenson (1952)*[80]; (**E**) *Robinson (1960)*[81]; (**F**) *Robinson (1962)*[82]; (**G**) *Messer (1972)*[83]; (**H**) *Kobert (1978)*[84]; (**I**) *Petzel (1982)*[85]; (**J**) *Brown (1984)*[48]; (**K**) *Fernandez (1987)*[86]; (**L**) *Kitayama (1989)*[50]; (**M**) *Ellis (1989)*.[60]

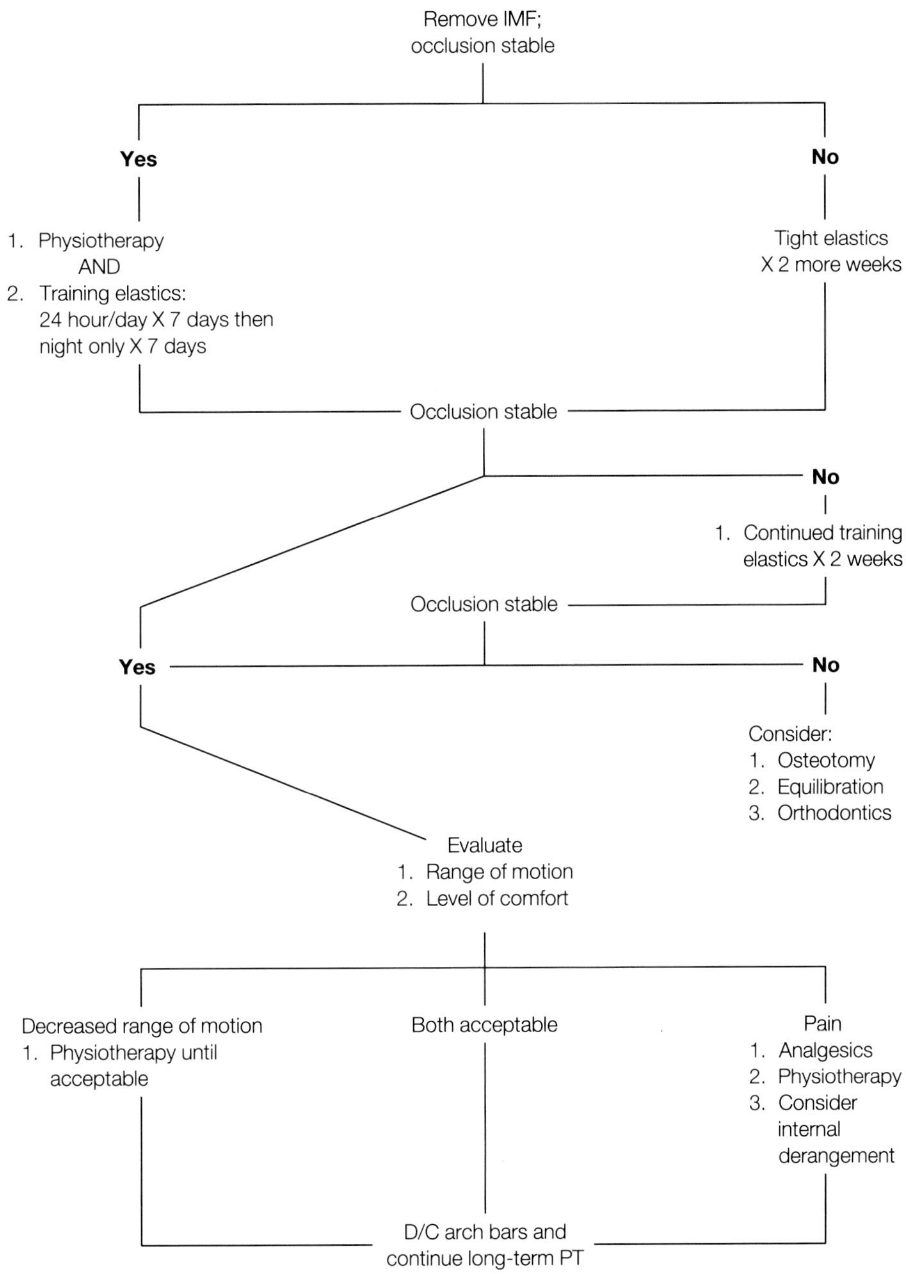

Figure 19–29. *Follow-up of condylar fractures.*

1 or 2 weeks. Clinical experience seems to indicate that a longer period of controlled elastic traction is often needed in adults with displaced or dislocated fractures, particularly if these are bilateral. Even with judicious use of guiding elastic fixation, patient education, and careful continued evaluation, malocclusion persists in some patients. In these cases one must consider equilibration, orthodontics, osteotomies, or a combination of these to correct the malocclusion.

Throughout the postintermaxillary fixation period, aggressive maintenance of range of motion is necessary. In some patients this may be as simple as in-

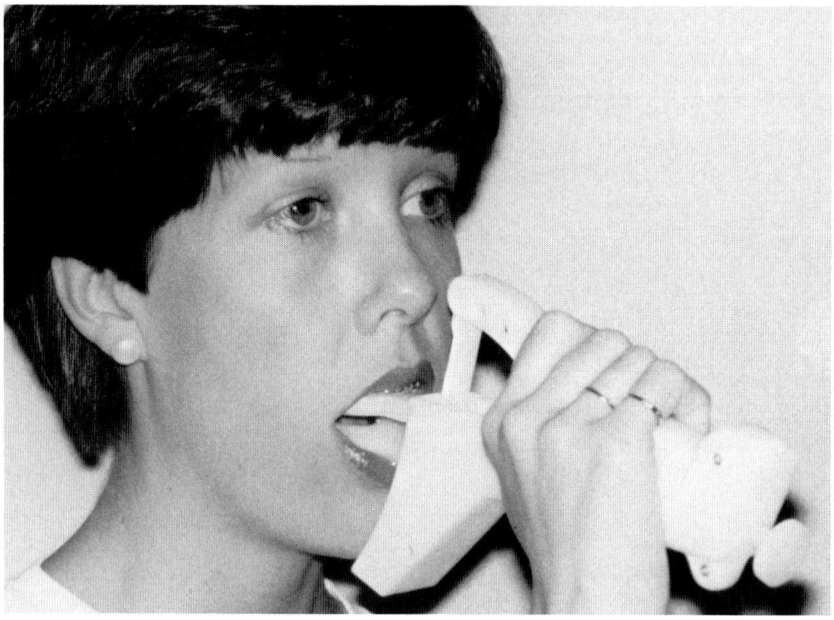

Figure 19–30. *Physiotherapy device for use in regaining or maintaining post-fracture range of motion. (Courtesy of Walter Lorenz Surgical Instrument Company, Jacksonville, FL)*

structing them to open their mouths as wide as possible in a symmetrical manner. Other patients may initially require daily evaluations and forced opening by the surgeon. Manually forcing the teeth apart, use of a rachet mouth props, progressive wedging of tongue blades between the teeth, or other more sophisticated physiotherapy devices (Fig. 19–30) are all effective means of regaining preinjury interincisal opening.

The success or failure of any proposed treatment for the fractured condyle, whether by open or closed reduction, will necessarily hinge on the careful adherence to close postoperative follow-up.

Adverse Sequelae of Condylar Fracture

In considering any treatment, the potential for complications exists. These complications may be divided into those that occur early in the course of injury or treatment and those that occur later (Table 19–5).

Early Complications

When the condylar head is forced posteriorly in the process of fracture, some force is directed against the posterior and superior walls of the glenoid fossa. Fracture of the tympanic plate may occur. In addition, partial obstruction of the external auditory canal may result, causing a conductive hearing loss because of the close proximity of the middle ear (Fig. 19–1). Patients with a history of a condyle fracture should undergo a careful otoscopic examination to evaluate the condition of the anterior wall of the external auditory

Table 19–5. *Complications Associated with Condylar Fracture*

Early	Ruptured tympanic plate or middle ear injury
	Basilar skull fracture
	Cerebral contusion
	CN VII deficit
	CN VIII deficit
	CN V_3 paresthesia
	Traumatic aneurysm
Late	Malocclusion
	Growth alteration
	Chronic pain
	TMJ dysfunction
	Internal derangement
	Degenerative joint disease
	Limited function or ankylosis
	Auriculotemporal syndrome

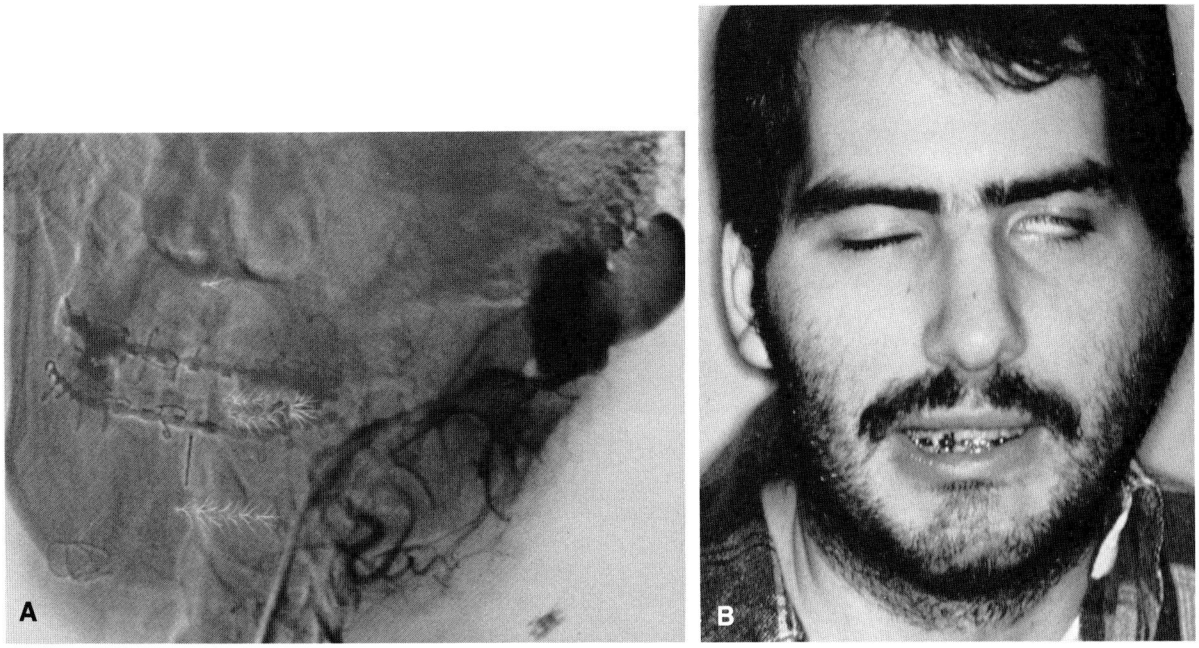

Figure 19–31. *Left condyle fracture with pseudoaneurysm of the superficial temporal artery. (**A**) Digital subtraction arteriography showing pseudoaneurysm. (**B**) Resultant facial nerve paralysis is seen, as well as the large swelling of the left face.*

canal, as well as to observe for signs of potential middle ear injury. Appropriate consultation must be obtained if injuries of this nature are indicated by clinical examination or history.

Basilar skull fracture along the floor of the middle cranial fossa may also occur from a similar mechanism, resulting in cerebral contusion. The fracture may also spread through the petrous portion of the temporal bone, resulting in injury of the seventh and eight cranial nerves and a neurosensory hearing deficit (as opposed to a conduction deficit), facial nerve paralysis, and possibly Battle's sign.

If either of the fracture segments encroach on the infratemporal fossa, trauma to the nerves or vessels in this area may occur. Damage of a large vessel can result in hematoma formation or development of a false aneurysm.[64] This expanding hematoma or false aneurysm may also cause injury to the seventh cranial nerve (Fig. 19–31A and B). The third division of the fifth cranial nerve may also be injured by the displaced condylar segments.[65,66] If aberrant reinnervation occurs from this injury, the late complication of auriculotemporal syndrome may result.[66,67]

Late Complications

MALOCCLUSION. Malocclusion that does not result from growth alterations but from a malunion of the condyle fracture occurs infrequently if an adequate follow-up regimen is followed (Fig. 19–29). If malocclusion does persist, its management is similar to the management of malocclusion from other causes. Judicious use of equilibration, orthodontics, and orthognathic surgery allows for restoration of a functional occlusion. Before reconstructing the occlusion to this new articulation, it is necessary to allow a period of 6 to 12 months for complete healing and for any remodeling of the articular apparatus to occur.

GROWTH ALTERATION. Growth alterations as the result of condylar injury may occur as the result of two mechanisms: Over or under stimulation of normal growth may result from direct injury to the condyle, or a restriction of normal growth may occur secondary to fibrosis or scarring of the surrounding tissue.

It was once thought that fracture of the condyle produced a growth deficit in proportion to the age of

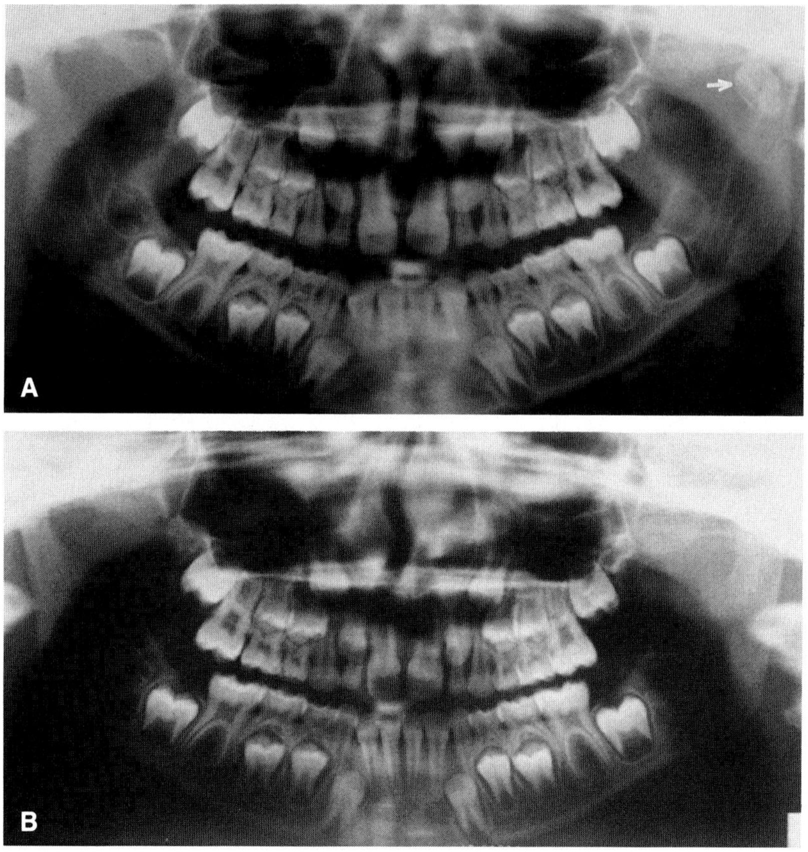

Figure 19–32. *(**A**) Fracture dislocation in a 7-year-old patient (arrow points to the condylar head). (**B**) Radiograph of the same patient taken 6 months later, showing restitution of growth of condyle with remodeling of displaced condylar segment.*

the patient at the time of injury; the younger the child, the greater potential growth problem.[39] However, although it is true that children undergo several periods of rapid growth during their development and that an injury during one of these growth periods may be associated with a higher incidence of growth alteration,[40] other factors are involved that alter this simplistic theory. Frequently, complete regeneration of the condyle occurs in young patients, with no residual deficit following fracture, and better regeneration occurs in actively growing patients, particularly those under the age of 12 years.[68,69] This clinical observation is supported by experimental studies,[60] which found that, following surgically created fracture dislocations in young monkeys, excellent regeneration occurred with no growth disturbance in any of the animals. This ability for restitution of growth in children under the age of 12 years appears to account for the lack of direct correlation between the age of injury and the degree of growth disturbance—a correlation that would be expected if the sole determinant were the amount of growth left at the time of injury.

The concept that the condylar cartilage acts as a growth center has been replaced by the theory that the cartilage acts as a remodeling center.[70] The restitution of growth seen after condylar injury (which at times may actually lead to overgrowth of the affected condyle) is a direct result of this remodeling center within the condylar cartilage reacting to a traumatic episode. It is not unusual for a new condylar apparatus to develop, with resorption of the displaced or dislocated condylar head (Fig. 19–32). This compensatory growth seems to depend on the potential space created by the displacement of the stump of the condylar process.[68] For this reason, it is important to maintain the mandible in its original occlusion—not only for a few weeks during healing, but also for the next several months while bony regeneration and compensatory growth occur. Even when occlusion is maintained and the patient is of the ideal age, there is as high as a 25%

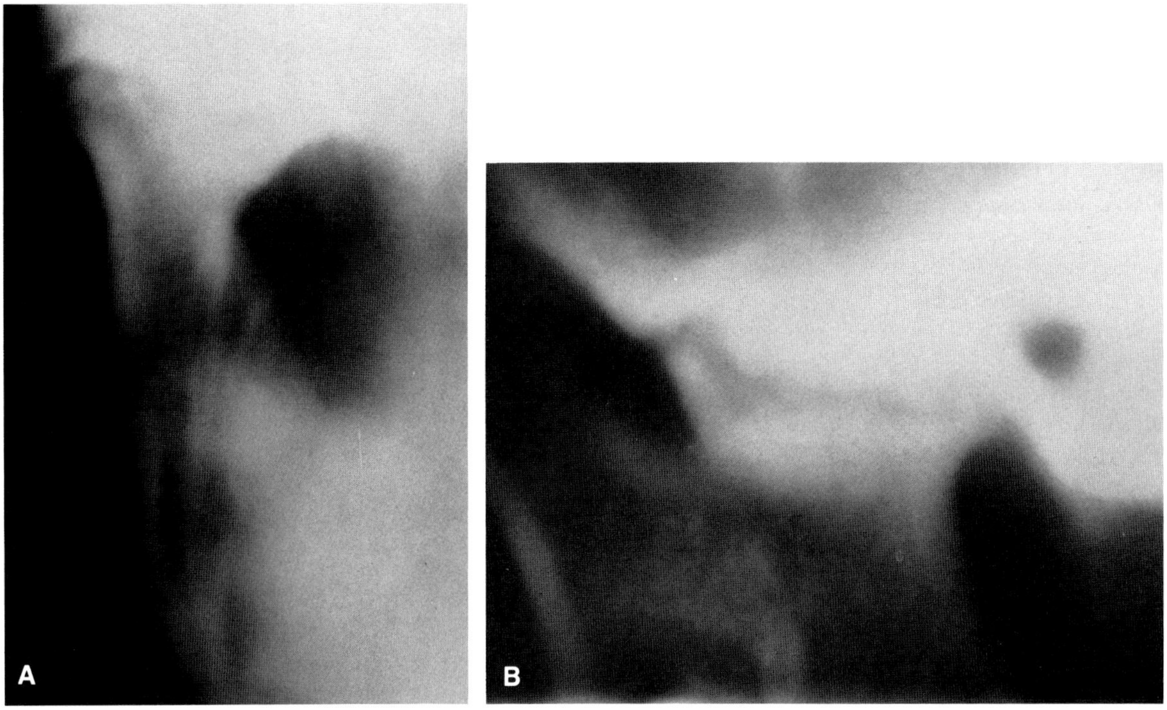

Figure 19–33. *Radiograph of ankylosed temporomandibular joint secondary to condyle fracture. (**A**) Posterio-anterior (PA) view. (**B**) Lateral view.*

occurrence of growth disturbance.[68,69,71] Because of this, adequate patient education and long-term follow-up for several years is necessary in children with fractures of the condyle.

TEMPOROMANDIBULAR JOINT DYSFUNCTION. A wide range of temporomandibular joint problems may result from injuries to the condylar apparatus. Internal derangement and ankylosis are perhaps the two most common.

INTERNAL DERANGEMENT. A correlation exists between previous condylar fracture and the development of internal derangement of the temporomandibular joint. There is a greater incidence of temporomandibular joint pain, deviation on opening, and joint noise in patients with previous condylar fractures.[72] The resultant internal derangement primarily occurs in adults and is of two broad types. The first is internal derangement that occurs on the side of the fracture and is due to soft tissue injury within the joint. Open reduction with direct repair of the injured soft tissues has been advocated by some as a possible means of preventing this problem.[53,54] No long-term data has established that this is effective. The other form of internal derangement occurs contralateral to the condylar injury. This derangement was described by Gerry as the "condylar postfracture syndrome."[18] Patients who develop a unilateral hinge type of joint after fracture can rapidly develop overfunction of the contralateral joint with hypermobility and, ultimately, anterior dislocation of the meniscus.

ANKYLOSIS. Although development of internal derangement seems to occur solely in adult patients, ankylosis is much more common in children (Fig. 19–33A and B).

Factors contributing to the development of ankylosis have been outlined.[21] They include the site and type of fracture, the age of the patient at the time of injury, the duration of intermaxillary fixation, and the extent of damage to the meniscus.

The site and type of fracture may play an important role in whether or not ankylosis occurs. It is widely accepted that intracapsular fractures are more likely to develop ankylosis. The postinjury relation of the condylar stump with the glenoid fossa is also a factor. With fractures of the condylar head, a greater likelihood exists that there will be intimate contact between the proximal portion of the distal segment and the glenoid fossa, predisposing the patient to ankylosis.[9] Failure to produce ankylosis after experimentally induced condylar fractures,[43] coupled with the clinical observation that the incidence of intracapsular fracture is much higher than that of ankylosis, leads one to believe that other factors besides the site of fracture must be operative in the production of ankylosis.

The condyle of a young child is more easily crushed than fractured,[73,74] possibly because the cortical bone of the child is relatively thin and the condylar neck broad.[75] The immediate subarticular layer is also extensively vascularized. An impact leading to a crush injury is more common in a child because of these anatomical differences, and the resulting fragments of highly vascularized osteogenic material that are dispersed throughout the joint space may be the cause of ankylosis.[75] This theory helps to explain the clinical observation that there is a greater predisposition for posttraumatic ankylosis in patients sustaining such injuries before the age of 10 years.[76]

It is widely accepted that the length of the maxillomandibular fixation may play a role in the development of ankylosis. Markey was unable to produce ankylosis after experimentally induced fracture with prolonged maxillomandibular fixation.[77] In studies performed by Beekler and Walker, ankylosis occurred with prolonged fixation, while no ankylosis could be created in a moving jaw.[43] This confirms the observation that the duration of immobilization is contributory to the development of ankylosis, although it is not the primary determinant.

The location and condition of the meniscus may be another determinant in the occurrence of temporomandibular joint ankylosis because one never finds the meniscus in the area of temporomandibular joint ankylosis.[9] Experimentally, ankylosis has been created in a baboon by a combination of bilateral fractures of the condyloid process, meniscectomy, and prolonged immobilization, while the same procedure without meniscectomy did not produce ankylosis.[9]

Thus far, this discussion has been limited to the development of true ankylosis with the formation of a bony or fibrous union within the joint itself. There is also the potential for the development of pseudoankylosis if soft tissue trauma surrounding the joint leads to fibrosis and scarring or (in the case of zygomatic arch and coronoid fractures) a bony union develops between other fractured areas and not within the joint itself.

In summary, it is likely that the following groups of patients will be at high risk for development of ankylosis: patients under the age of 10 years at the time of injury; patients with intracapsular fractures and fracture dislocations with gross telescoping; and patients with compound comminuted fractures, particularly if the coronoid process and zygoma are also involved.[21]

Prevention of temporomandibular joint ankylosis is accomplished by recognition of those patients at risk, brief immobilization periods, and aggressive postoperative physiotherapy and long-term follow-up.

REFERENCES

1. Kromer H. Closed and open reduction of condylar fractures. Dental Record 1953; 73:569.
2. Goldberg MG, Williams AC. The location and occurrence of mandibular fractures. Oral Surg 1969; 28:336.
3. Chalmers J, Lyons Club. Fractures involving the mandibular condyle: A post-treatment survey of 120 cases. J Oral Surg 1974; 9:233.
4. Rowe NL, Killey HC. Fractures of the facial skeleton, ed 2. Edinburgh: Churchill-Livingstone, 1968.
5. Harilainen A, Myllynen P, Anhla H, Seitsalo S. The significance of arthroscopy and examination under anesthesia in the diagnosis of fresh injury haemarthrosis of the knee joint. Injury 1988; 19:21.
6. Fieldhous J. Bilateral temporomandibular joint ankylosis with associated micrognathia: Report of a case. Br J Oral Surg 1974; 11:213.
7. Guralnick WC, Kaban LB. Surgical treatment of mandibular hypomobility. J Oral Surg 1976; 34:343.
8. Hoaglund FT. Experimental hemarthrosis. J Bone Joint Surg 1967; 49(A): 285.
9. Laskin DM. Role of the meniscus in the etiology of posttraumatic temporomandibular joint ankylosis. Int J Oral Surg 1978; 7:340.
10. Luyk NH, Larsen PE. The diagnosis and treatment of the dislocated mandible. Am J Emerg Med 1989; 7:329.
11. Lello J. Treatment of long standing mandibular dislocation. J Oral Maxillofac Surg 1987; 45:893.
12. Hayward JR. Prolonged dislocation of the mandible. Oral Surg 1965; 23:585.
13. Cope MR, Lawlor MG. An unusual mandibular dislocation. Br J Oral Maxillofac Surg 1985; 23:112.
14. Fonseca GD. Experimental study on fractures of

the mandibular condylar process (mandibular condylar process fractures). Int J Oral Surg 1974; 3:89.
15. Ihalainen U, Tasanen A. Central dislocation of the mandibular condyle into the middle cranial fossa: A case report and review of the literature. Int J Oral Surg 1983; 12:39.
16. Musgrove BT. Dislocation of the mandibular condyle into the middle cranial fossa. Br J Oral Maxillofac Surg 1986; 24:25.
17. Gilhuus-Moe O. Fracture of the mandibular condyle in the growth period. Acta Odontol Scand 1971; 29:53.
18. Gerry R. Condylar fractures. Br J Oral Surg 1965; 3:114.
19. Blevins D, Gores RJ. Fractures of the mandibular condyloid process: Result of conservative treatment in 140 patients. J Oral Surg Anesth Hosp Dent 1961; 19:329.
20. MacLennan WD. Consideration of 180 cases of typical fractures of the mandibular condylar process. Br J Plast Surg 1952; 5:122.
21. Bradley P. Injuries of the condylar and coronoid process. In: Rowe NL, Williams JL, eds. Maxillofacial injuries, vol 1. Edinburgh: Churchill-Livingstone, 1985.
22. Lindahl L. Condylar fractures of the mandible. I. Classification and relation to age, occlusion and concomitant injuries of teeth and teeth supporting structures, and fractures of the mandibular body. Int J Oral Surg 1977; 6:12.
23. Huelke, DF. Mechanics in the production of mandibular fractures: A study with the "stresscoat" technique. I. Symphyseal impacts. J Dent Res 1961; 40:1042.
24. Huelke DF, Burdi AR, Eymen C. Mandibular fractures as related to site of trauma and state of dentition. J Dent Res 1961; 40:1262.
25. Huelke DF, Burdi AR, Eymen CE. Association between mandibular fractures and site of trauma, dentition and age. J Oral Surg Anesth Hosp Dent 1962; 20:278.
26. Huelke DF, Harger JH. Maxillofacial injuries: Their nature and mechanisms of production. J Oral Surg 1969; 27:451.
27. Huelke DF, Harger JH. Mechanisms in the production of mandibular fractures: An experimental study. J Oral Surg 1968; 26:86.
28. Huelke DF, Patrick LM. Mechanics in the production of mandibular fractures: Strain-gauge measurements of impacts to the chin. J Dent Res 1964; 43:437.
29. Evans FG, Pedersen HE, Lissner HR. The role of tensile stress in the mechanism of femoral fractures. J Bone Joint Surg 1951; 33:485.
30. Petzel JR, Bulles G. Experimental studies of the fracture behavior of the mandibular condylar process. J Maxillofac Surg 1981; 9:211.
31. Cook RM, MacFarlane WI. Subcondylar fracture of the mandible. Oral Surg Oral Med Oral Pathol 1969; 27:297.
32. MacGregor AB, Fordyce GL. The treatment of fracture of the neck of the mandibular condyle. Br Dent J 1957; 351.
33. Leake D, Doykos J, Habal M, et al. Long-term follow-up of fractures of the mandibular condyle in children. Plast Reconstr Surg 1971; 47:127.
34. Lindahl L. Condylar fractures of the mandible. IV. Function of the masticatory system. Int J Oral Surg 1977; 6:195.
35. MacLennan WD, Simpson W. Treatment of the fractured mandibular condylar process in children. Br J Plast Surg 1965; 18:423.
36. Thomson HG, Farmer AW, Lindsay WK. Condylar neck fractures of the mandible in children. Plast Reconstr Surg 1964; 34:452.
37. Russell D, Nosti JC, Reavis C. Treatment of fractures of the mandibular condyle. J Trauma 1972; 12:704.
38. Hotz RP. Functional jaw orthopedics in the treatment of condylar fractures. Am J Orthod 1978; 73:365.
39. Rowe NL. Fractures of the jaws in children. J Oral Surg 1969; 27:497.
40. Waite DE. Pediatric fractures of the jaw and facial bones. Pediatrics 1973; 51:551.
41. Rakower W, Protzell A, Rosenkrans M. Treatment of displaced condylar fractures in children. J Oral Surg 1961; 19:517.
42. Walker RV. Traumatic mandibular condyle fracture dislocations. Am J Surg 1960; 100:850.
43. Beekler DM, Walker RV. Condyle fractures. J Oral Surg 1969; 27:563.
44. Boyne PJ. Osseous repair and mandibular growth after subcondylar fractures. J Oral Surg 1967; 225:300.
45. Walker RV. The consultant: Condylar fractures. J Oral Surg 1966; 24:367.
46. Walker RV. Open reduction of condylar fractures of the mandible in conjunction with repair of discal injury: Discussion. J Oral Maxillofac Surg 1988; 46:262.
47. Wood GD. Assessment of function following fracture of the mandible. Br Dent J 1980; 149:137.
48. Brown AE, Obeid G. A simplified method for the internal fixation of fractures of the mandibular condyle. Br J Oral Maxillofac Surg 1984; 22:145.
49. Wennogle CF, Delo RI. A pin-in-groove technique for reduction of displaced subcondylar fractures of the mandible. J Oral Maxillofac Surg 1985; 43:659.
50. Kitayama S. A new method of intraoral open reduction using a screw applied through the mandibular crest of condylar fractures. J Craniomaxillofac Surg 1989; 17:16.
51. Tasanen A, Lamberg MA. Transosseous wiring in the treatment of condylar fractures of the mandible. J Oral Maxillofac Surg 1976; 4:200.
52. Zide MF, Kent JN. Indications for open reduction of mandibular condyle fractures. J Oral Maxillofac Surg 1983; 41:89.
53. Raveh J, Vuillemin T, Ladrach K. Open reduction of the dislocated fractured condylar process: Indications and surgical procedures. J Oral Maxillofac Surg 1989; 47:127.
54. Chuong R, Piper MA. Open reduction of condylar fractures of the mandible in conjunction with repair of dis-

cal injury: A preliminary report. J Oral Maxillofac Surg 1988; 46:262.

55. Lund K. Unusual fracture dislocation of the mandibular condyle in a six year old girl. Int J Oral Surg 1972; 1:53.
56. Henny FA. A technique for open reduction of fractures of the mandibular condyle. J Oral Surg 1951; 9:233.
57. Zide MF. Open reduction of mandibular condyle fractures: Indications and technique. Clin Plast Surg 1989; 16:69.
58. Hinds ED, Girotti WJ. Vertical subcondylar osteotomy: A reappraisal. Oral Surg 1967; 24:164.
59. Jeter TS, Vansickels JE, Nishioka GJ. Intraoral open reduction with rigid internal fixation of mandibular subcondylar fractures. J Oral Maxillofac Surg 1988; 46:1113.
60. Ellis E, Reynolds ST, Park HS. A method to rigidly fix high condylar fractures. Oral Surg 1989; 68:369.
61. Boyne PJ. Free grafting of traumatically displaced or resected mandibular condyles. J Oral Maxillofac Surg 1989; 47:228.
62. Mikkonen P, Lindqvist C, Pihakari A, et al. Osteotomy-osteosynthesis in displaced condylar fractures. Int J Oral Maxillofac Surg 1989; 18:267.
63. Takenoshita Y, Oka M, Tashiro H. Surgical treatment of fractures of the mandibular condylar neck. J Craniomaxillofac Surg 1989; 17:119.
64. Kennedy JW, Kent JN. False aneurysm and partial facial paralysis secondary to mandibular fracture. J Oral Surg 1970; 28:854.
65. Schmidseder R, Scheunemann H. Nerve injuries in fractures of the condylar neck. J Maxillofac Surg 1977; 5:186.
66. Laws IM. Two unusual complications of fractured condyles. Br J Oral Surg 1967; 5:51.
67. Martis C, Athanassiades S. Auriculotemporal syndrome (Freye's syndrome) secondary to fracture of the mandibular condyle. Plast Reconstr Surg 1969; 44:603.
68. Proffit WR, Vig KWL, Turvey TA. Early fracture of the mandibular condyles: Frequently an unsuspected cause of growth disturbances. Am J Orthod 1980; 78:1.
69. Gilhuus-Moe O. Fractures of mandibular condyle in the growth period. Oslo: Universitetsforlaget, 1969. Dissertation.
70. Durkin JF, Heeley J, Irving JT. The cartilage of the mandibular condyle. Oral Sci Rev 1973; 2:29.
71. Lund K. Mandibular growth and remodeling processes after condylar fracture. Acta Odontol Scand 1974; 64(Suppl 32): 56.
72. Lindahl L. Condylar fractures of the mandible. IV. Function of the masticatory system. Int J Oral Surg 1977; 6:195.
73. Dufourmental ML. Fractures of the mandible in the region of the joint. Br Dent J 1929; 50:620.
74. Rushton MA. Growth of mandibular condyle in relation to some deformities. Br Dent J 1944; 76:57.
75. Rowe NL. Ankylosis of the temporomandibular joint. J Coll Surg Edinb 1982; 27(2): 67.
76. Topazian RG. Etiology of ankylosis of the temporomandibular joint: Analysis of 44 cases. J Oral Surg 1964; 22:227.
77. Markey RG. Condylar trauma and facial asymmetry: An experimental study. Seattle: University of Washington, 1974. Thesis.
78. Silverman SL. A new operation for displaced fractures at the neck of the mandibular condyle. Dent Cosmos 1925; 67:876.
79. Thoma KH. Fractures and fracture dislocation of the mandibular condyle: A method for open reduction and internal wiring and one for skeletal fixation, with a report of 32 cases. J Oral Surg 1945; 3:3.
80. Stephenson KL, Graham WC. The use of the Kirschner pin in fractures of the condyle. Plast Reconstr Surg 1952; 10:19.
81. Robinson M, Yoon C. New onlay-inlay metal splint for immobilization of mandibular subcondylar fractures: Report of twenty-six cases. Am J Surg 1960; 100:845.
82. Robinson M, Lytle J, Yoon C. Sleeve over interosseous wire to aid in immobilization of jaw fractures. Plast Reconstr Surg 1962; 32:557.
83. Messer EJ. A simplified method for fixation of the fractured mandibular condyle. J Oral Surg 1972; 30:442.
84. Koberg WR, Momma W. Treatment of fractures of the articular process by functional stable osteosynthesis using miniaturized dynamic compression plates. Int J Oral Surg 1978; 7:256.
85. Petzel JR. Instrumentation and technique for screw-pin osteosynthesis of condylar fractures. J Oral Maxillofac Surg 1982; 10:8.
86. Fernandez JA, Mathog RH. Open treatment of condylar fractures with biphase technique. Arch Otolaryngol Head Neck Surg 1987; 113:262.

20

Management of Maxillary Fractures

Richard H. Haug
A. Thomas Indresano

EPIDEMIOLOGY OF MAXILLARY FRACTURES

Epidemiologic surveys of maxillary fractures differ with the geographic region studied, era in time, regional politics, socioeconomic status, population density, and institution reviewed,[1–5] which makes generalizations difficult; yet trends are evident. Maxillary fractures are more frequently associated with motor vehicle accidents and motorcycle accidents than any other cause. The vast majority occur in males. The age group most frequently affected is between 16 and 40 years of age, with the highest density between 21 and 25 years of age. Anatomic location of maxillary fractures according to the LeFort system is not replicated in the literature. Virtually every possible combination of frequency has been reported with no identifiable explanation or reason. Concomitant injury is found more with maxillary fractures than with any other facial fracture.[1,2] The most prevalent associated injuries are lacerations, other facial fractures, orthopedic injury, and neurologic injury. Therefore a high level of concern and management skill is required for the treatment of patients with maxillary fractures.

HISTORY

Although the maxillary fracture commonly bears the name of Rene LeFort, the description and treatment of this fracture existed thousands of years before LeFort was born. The first clinical examination of a maxillary fracture was recorded in 2500 BC in the Smith Papyrus.[6] Many other early records describe treatments for maxillary fractures or the iatrogenic fracture of the maxilla for therapeutic purposes. In 1822 Reiche provided the first detailed treatise of maxillary fractures entitled *De Maxillae Superioris Fractura*.[6] In 1823 Carl Ferdinand van Graefe described the use of a head frame for the treatment of a maxillary fracture.[6] His device was as technically complex as those currently in use. In 1859 Von Langenbeck described a technique for the osteoplastic resection of a maxilla.[7] In 1867 Cheever discussed complete mobilization of the maxilla by chisels.[8] His operation was used for the removal of a nasopharyngeal tumor. In 1893 Lanz also described an iatrogenic maxillary fracture for access to a tumor. It was not until 1901 that Rene LeFort published his landmark works.[9–11]

Rene LeFort was born into a family of physicians in 1869 in Lille, France (Fig. 20-1).[12] LeFort received his doctorate in medicine at the age 21 years with a thesis on cranial anatomy. He began his career as a military surgeon and after 9 years returned to academia and public service. He died in his hometown in 1951. It was because of his landmark anatomic work that the maxillary fracture has become known as the LeFort fracture.

In 1901 LeFort published his three-part experiment, using 32 cadavers that were either intact or decapitated.[9–11] The cadavers or heads were placed in

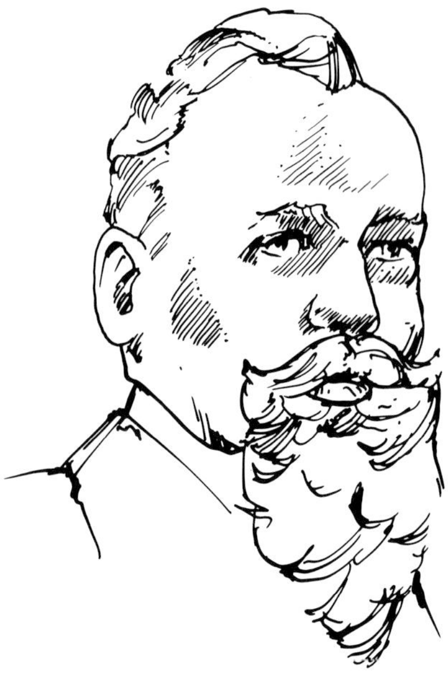

Figure 20-1. *Rene LeFort (1869–1951).*

various positions, some laying on their backs, some with their heads hung over tables, and yet others clamped in vises. They were kicked with the heel of a boot or hit with a wooden stick or steel bar. Decapitated heads were taken and thrown against a marble floor. After each of the episodes of trauma, some requiring multiple blows before the fractured bones could be heard to crepitate, the specimens were inspected. The cranial vault was examined for fracture. The faces were then dissected by hand or boiled in water until the tissues sloughed off. LeFort concluded that buttresses exist in the horizontal and vertical planes to resist forces. He noted that, generally, if the face was fractured, the skull was not. He then disclosed that fractures occurred through weak lines. These lines were those that protect the cranial cavity; those that circumscribe the midface; and those that cut across the face. It is from these three lines that the LeFort classification system was derived. Never since then has a work of this magnitude been performed to verify the anatomic levels of midface fractures.

LEFORT CLASSIFICATION SYSTEM

In his description of maxillary fractures, LeFort considered several factors. He considered the vector of force overcoming the inertia of the face. He investigated the thickness of the bone and buttresses counteracting the mass, velocity, and point of application. Lastly, he noted that the maxilla is unaffected by muscle pull, as are the long bones. These considerations resulted in a classification of three kinds of fracture.

LeFort I Level

Maxillary fractures at the LeFort I level traverse the lateral antral wall, lateral nasal wall, lower third of the septum, and separate at the pterygoid plates. Thus the entire mobilized segment consists of the maxillary alveolar bone, palatine bone, lower one third of the nasal septum, and lower one third of the pterygoid plates. The superior two thirds of the aforementioned bones remain associated with the face (Fig. 20-2).

LeFort II Level

Maxillary fractures at the LeFort II level contain most of the nasal bones, maxillary bones, palatine bones, lower two thirds of the nasal septum, dentoalveolus, and pterygoid plates. Rather than the horizontal separation noted in the LeFort I fracture, this fracture is pyramidal in shape. The fracture extends from below the nasofrontal suture through the nasal bones along the maxilla to the zygomaticomaxillary suture, including the medial inferior one third of the orbit. It then continues along the zygomaticomaxillary suture to and through the pterygoid plates. The septum is also separated superiorly. The segments may not be totally intact below this line of fracture, but instead may be segmentalized or comminuted (Fig. 20-2).

LeFort III Level

The LeFort III level fracture involves the nasal bones, zygomas, maxillae, palatine bones, and pterygoid plates. It is essentially a separation of the face along the base of the skull. The fracture line extends from the nasofrontal suture along the medial wall of the orbit through the superior orbital fissure. It then extends along the inferior orbital fissure and lateral orbital wall to the zygomaticofrontal suture. The zygomaticotemporal suture is also separated. The fracture then ex-

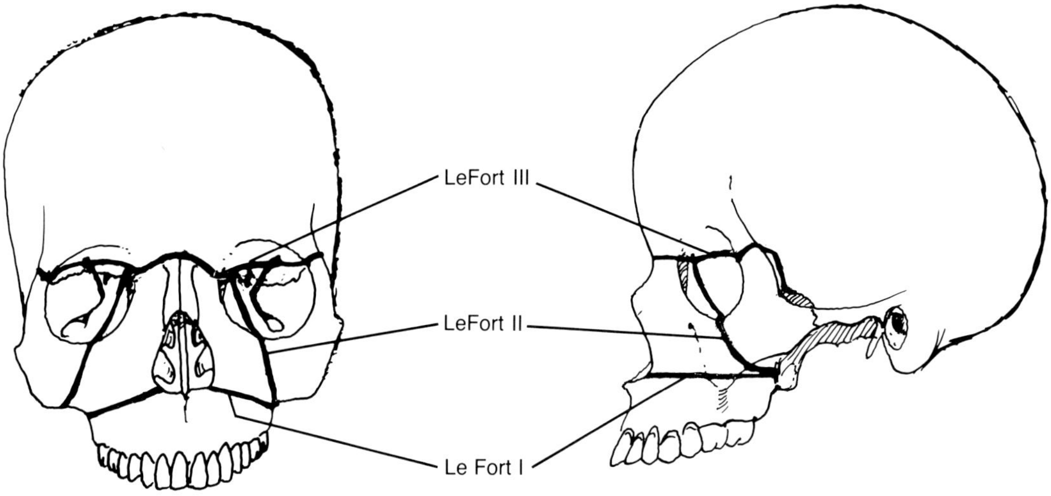

Figure 20-2. *Anterior-posterior and lateral view of skull, showing LeFort classification system of maxillary fractures.*

tends along the sphenoid, separating the pterygoid plates. The septum becomes separated at the cribriform plate of the ethmoid. The LeFort III level fracture is rarely a one-piece fracture. It is usually segmentalized or comminuted (Fig. 20-2).

Combinations

With highly segmentalized and comminuted fractures, patients may sustain combined level fractures. Virtually all right and left combinations of LeFort I, II and III fractures are possible.

ANATOMY OF THE MAXILLA AND CONTIGUOUS STRUCTURES

The clinical examination of LeFort fractures is merely the description of altered anatomy. The treatment of these fractures is the reestablishment of the anatomy. It is therefore necessary that the surgeon be intimately aware of the anatomic features of the maxilla and contiguous structures.

The two maxillae are paired structures connected by a midline suture composing a five-sided pyramid (Fig. 20-3). The anterior surface slopes downward

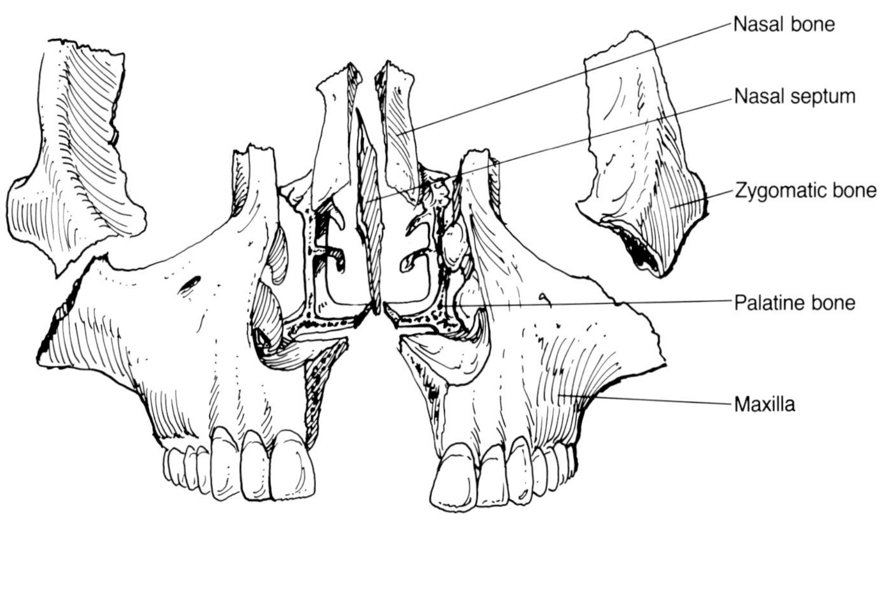

Figure 20-3. *Disarticulated midfacial skeleton demonstrates the anatomy of the maxilla, zygoma, nasal, and volmer bones.*

from its superior contact with the frontal and nasal bones at an angle of approximately 15°. The most prominent point at the anterior surface is the anterior nasal spine. A number of protuberances exist on the maxilla, formed by the alveolar base and origins of the small facial muscles. The lateral surface of the maxillae forms the infratemporal fossae and buccal vestibule and attaches to the zygoma. Most of the superior surface forms the majority of the orbital floor. The medial surface of each maxilla forms the midline suture and lateral nasal walls. The inferior border composes the palatal vault and alveolus, which contain the teeth. The posterior border abuts the sphenoid bone and pterygomaxillary suture.[13] Within the maxilla is the maxillary sinus. This 34.0 × 33.0 × 25.0 mm cavity of air is responsible for the weakness of the maxilla. It is present at birth but does not pneumatize to its mature extent until 14 to 18 years of age. Minor changes continue throughout life.[14] The strong buttresses of the maxilla are the lateral piriform buttress, zygomatic buttress, greater palatine buttress, and floor of the nose.

The palatine bone is L-shaped and abuts the posterior maxilla as a paired structure. These bones assist the maxilla in forming the posterior sinus, posterior lateral nasal wall, and pterygomaxillary suture. When joined to the maxilla, the four bones represent one unit (Fig. 20-3).[13]

The nasal bones are paired structures that abut the frontal bone superiorly, the maxilla laterally, the septum posteriorly and medially, and each other anteriorly and medially. The bones are thicker superiorly, and therefore fractures at the LeFort II level may occur inferior to the nasofrontal suture. The nasal septum is a thin trapezoidal bone lying perpendicular to and joining the maxillae and palatine bones. The superior border is thick and articulates with the ethmoid bone (Fig. 20-3).[13]

The ethmoid bone is cuboidal and extremely pneumatized, allowing easy fracture and comminution. The cribriform plate of the ethmoid composes the roof of the nasal cavity and communicates with the anterior cranial fossae through multiple foramina for the olfactory nerves. Lateral to the crista galli is a slit through which dura mater is exposed. Posterior and superior movements of the midface can easily comminute this bone, disrupting the dura mater and resulting in a cerebrospinal fluid (CSF) leak.[13]

The zygoma abuts the frontal bone at the frontozygomatic suture and the temporal bone at the zygomaticotemporal suture. The maxilla and zygoma form two thirds of the orbital rim and, along with the palatine bone, one third of the walls and floor of the orbit (Fig. 20-3).

The infraorbital nerve traverses the orbital floor and exits through the infraorbital foramen. The maxillary bone, along with the zygoma, forms the inferior orbital fissure. Through this fissure runs the maxillary nerve, infraorbital vessels, and ascending branches of the pterygopalatine ganglion. The frontal process of the maxilla contains the lacrimal apparatus, which is housed between the medial canthal ligaments.

The blood supply to the maxillae and palatine bones is through the periosteum, incisive artery, and greater and lesser palatine arteries. The internal maxillary artery, a source of potentially devastating hemorrhage, lies posterior to the maxillae and palatine bones, anterior to the pterygoid plates of the sphenoid.[15] The blood supply to the nasal septum and lateral nasal walls are the anterior and posterior ethmoidal arteries, the sphenopalatine artery, the greater palatine and superior labial arteries.[13]

Whereas the osteum of the nasolacrimal duct is beneath the inferior concha, the ostea of the antrum and middle ethmoids lie beneath the middle concha. The direct opening or ostea of the nasofrontal duct lies underneath the middle concha.

DIAGNOSIS

History

The initial examination of the patient should begin with the history of the event. Mechanism of injury, point of impact, associated symptoms, and concomitant injury should all be elicited. If the victim was in a motor vehicle accident, the speed, use of restraints, and obstacle impacted should all be identified. If the victim has been assaulted, knowledge of the instrument used, direction of force, and number of impacts is helpful.

Clinical Examination

The clinical examination should begin with the initial observation of the patient. Laceration, abrasion, or ecchymotic areas should be visualized and recorded. Periorbital ecchymosis and edema should be observed.

Epistaxis with "tram lines," indicative of cerebrospinal rhinorrhea, should be identified (Fig. 20-4). Asymmetry of the nose, traumatic telecanthus, a flat nasal bridge, and a dish-shaped face should all be noted.

After control of airway patency, tamponade of hemorrhage, and neurologic stabilization, the "hands-on" maxillofacial examination may begin. The mouth should be opened to look for accumulation of blood, debris, or avulsed anatomic structures that could compromise the airway. Next, the presence of laceration, abrasion, and ecchymosis in the mouth is determined. The posterior prematurities of a *gag bite* should be identified (Fig. 20-5).

The thumb and forefinger of the dominant hand should examine the dentoalveolus for alveolar or segmental fractures. The opposite hand should stabilize the head. The examiner should observe the maxilla for movement as a unit (Fig. 20-6). Next, the opposite hand should be placed at the nasal bridge, while the maxilla is mobilized (Fig. 20-7). Following these steps, the maxilla should be mobilized, while the less dominant hand identifies movement at the frontozygomatic suture (Fig. 20-8). The nose should be examined grossly for contour irregularity. A nasal speculum should be used to identify compound fractures of the septum or septal hematoma. Both hands should be used to examine the orbital rims and, in particular, the zygomaticomaxillary suture.

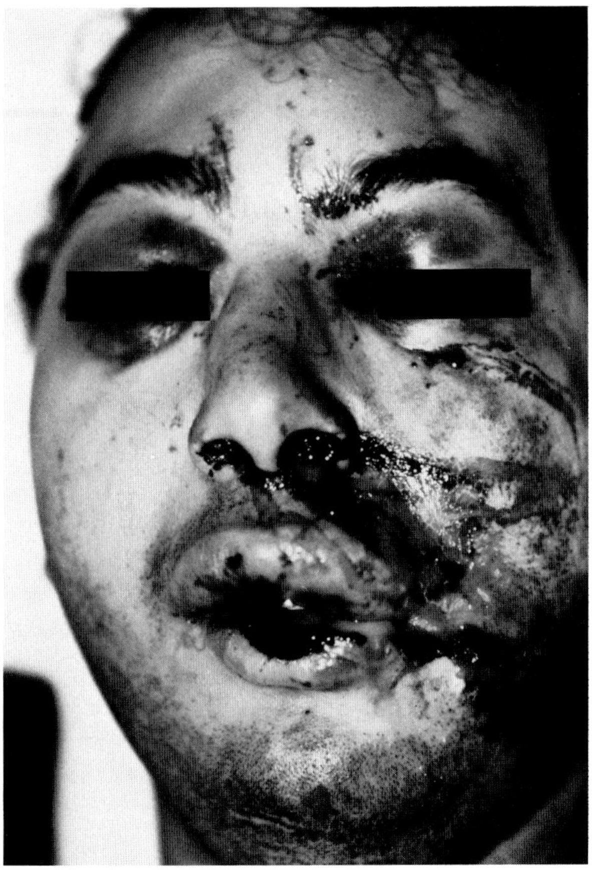

Figure 20-4. *Patient with cerebrospiral fluid leak diagnosed by "tram lines" on the left cheek and traumatic telecanthus with flattened nasal bridge.*

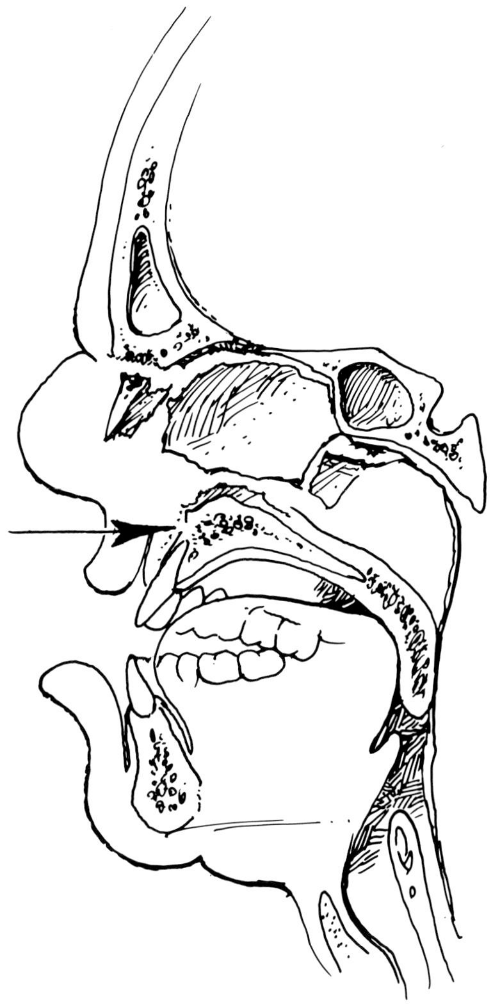

Figure 20-5. *Posterior displacement of a maxillary fracture results in several important sequelae. The soft palate may be displaced, occluding the nasopharynx and leaving the oropharynx as the only airway. The posterior and inferior displacement of the maxilla results in posterior occlusal prematurities, causing an anterior open bite, the so-called gag bite.*

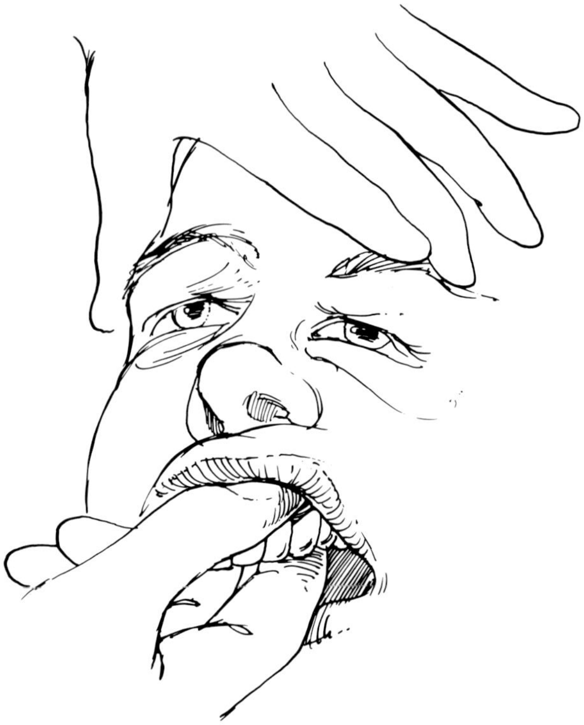

Figure 20-6. *To examine the maxilla for fracture, the head is stabilized and the dentoalveolar process is manipulated to detect gross movements of fractured segments.*

When the "Panda bear" appearance of a flat nasal bridge, periorbital ecchymosis, and round edematous head are noted, additional concern should be registered for a CSF leak or traumatic telecanthus (Fig. 20-4). Often, the "tram line" of dried blood and CSF may be visualized. If the leakage is not blood tinged, CSF may be identified by a colorimetric test using litmus paper, which detects glucose contents higher than that in serum. If 0.1 cc of fluid can be collected, a chloride concentration of less than serum (95 mEq per liter) and a glucose concentration higher than serum (120 mg/100 mL) confirms the presence of CSF.[16]

A ruler or caliper should be used to measure the intercanthal distance. The normal distance for adult females is 28.6 to 33.0 mm and for adult males is 28.9 to 34.5 mm.[17] Increased widths suggest a nasoorbital-ethmoid fracture. Along with these measurements, the Furness test is helpful. In performing this test, a forceps with single teeth is used to grasp the skin overlying the medial canthus. When lifted, lack of creasing or resistance by underlying bone is indicative of an underlying fracture.

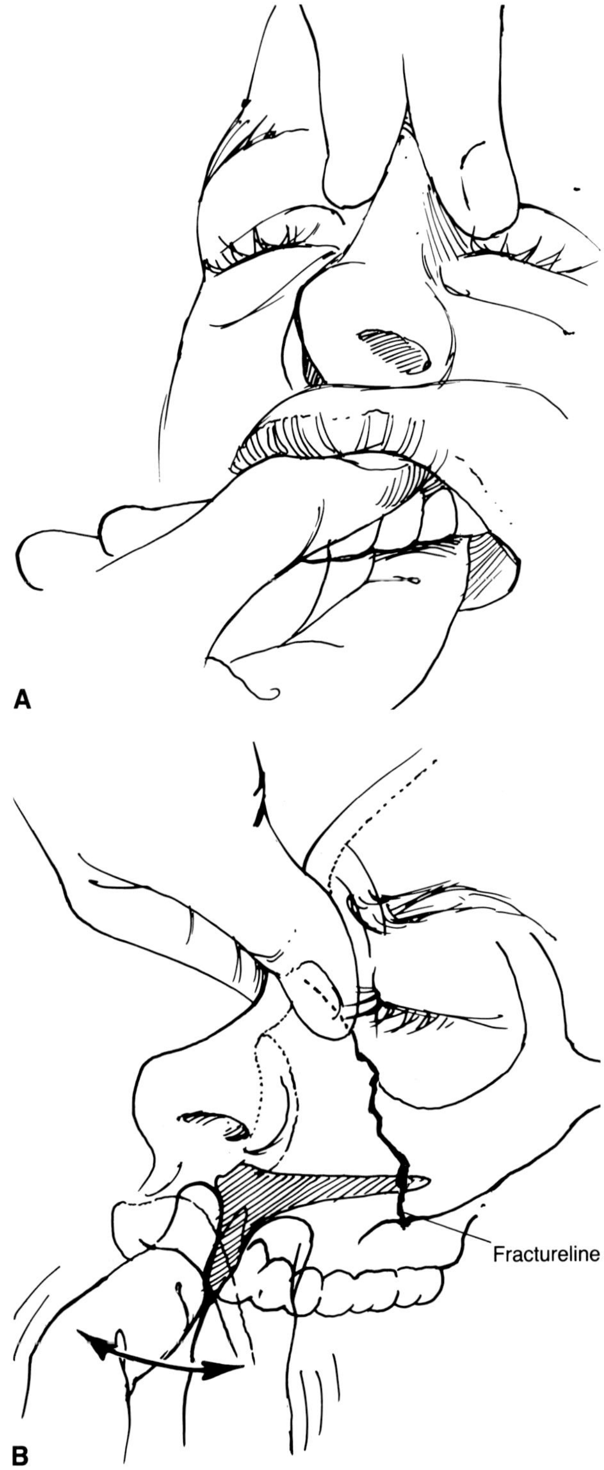

Figure 20-7. *(**A** and **B**) To check for LeFort II or III fractures, one hand is held on the bridge of the nose, while the other manipulates the maxilla. Movement at the nasofrontal suture suggests a LeFort II or III fracture.*

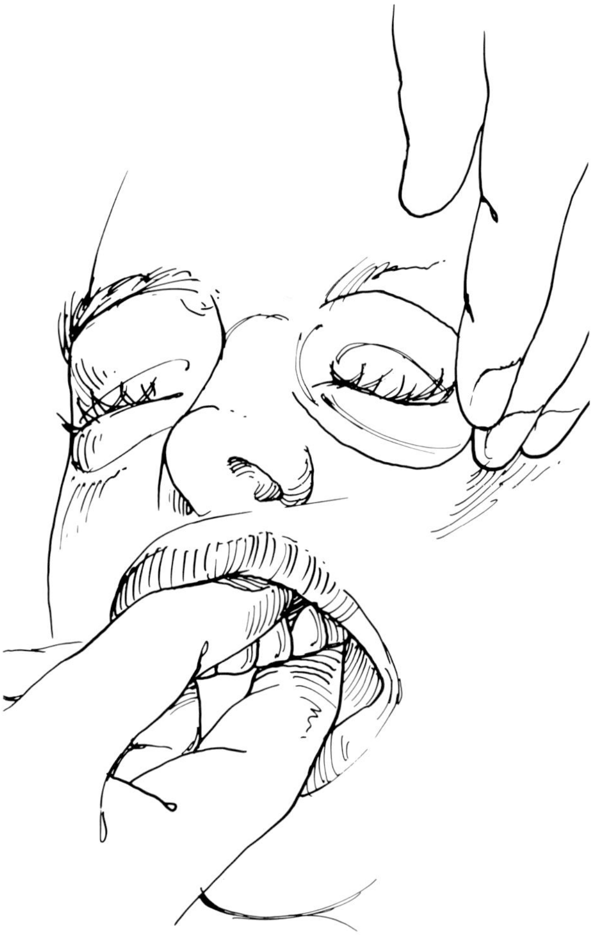

Figure 20-8. *Palpation at the frontozygomatic suture while manipulating the maxilla aids in the diagnosis of a LeFort III fracture.*

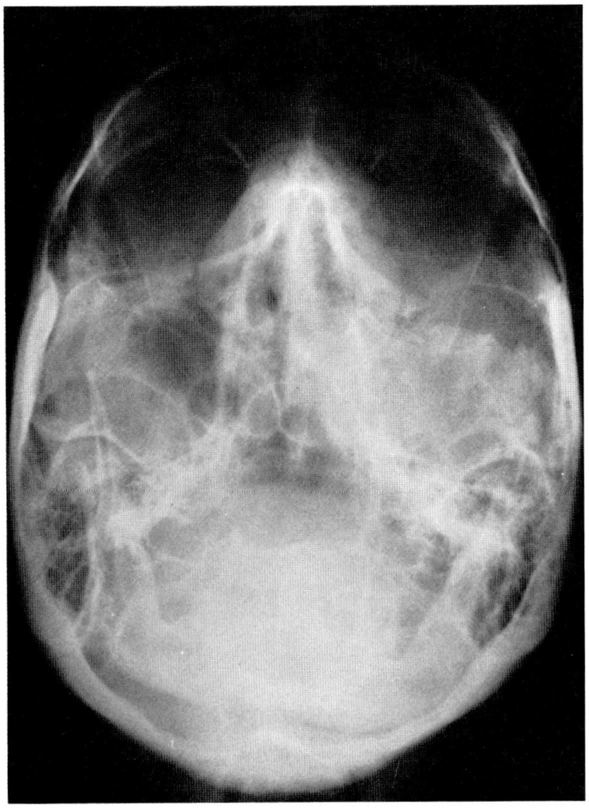

Figure 20-9. *Waters' radiograph is the best single plane radiograph to evaluate maxillary fractures. The frontozygomatic, zygomaticotemporal, and zygomaticomaxillary sutures are visualized, as well as the infraorbital rim and maxillary and frontal sinuses.*

Imaging

Fractures are identified clinically and confirmed radiographically. A Waters' view and lateral facial radiograph (Figs. 20-9 and 20-10) are valuable in identifying maxillary fractures. Their value diminishes, however, when hemorrhage fills the sinuses and soft tissue swelling obliterates identifiable radiographic anatomy. Generally, the time periods when radiographs can be taken with the most value are within 1 hour of fracture or after 5 days. With comminuted fractures and complicated anatomic features, the computed tomography (CT) scan has become the standard (Fig. 20-11). Fractures may be identified, as well as the soft tissue differences of hematoma, edema, muscle, and fat. From a treatment planning standpoint the three-dimensional CT scan has become a valuable tool. The conceptual abilities afforded by this imaging technique are unsurpassed as an aid to surgical treatment planning (Fig. 20-12).

TREATMENT

Prehospital Care

Patients do not die from maxillary fractures, but they may die from concomitant injury or failure to manage the sequelae of maxillary fractures. As with all injuries, initial attention should be directed at establishing patent airways and controlling hemorrhage. The patient's mouth should be suctioned free of debris

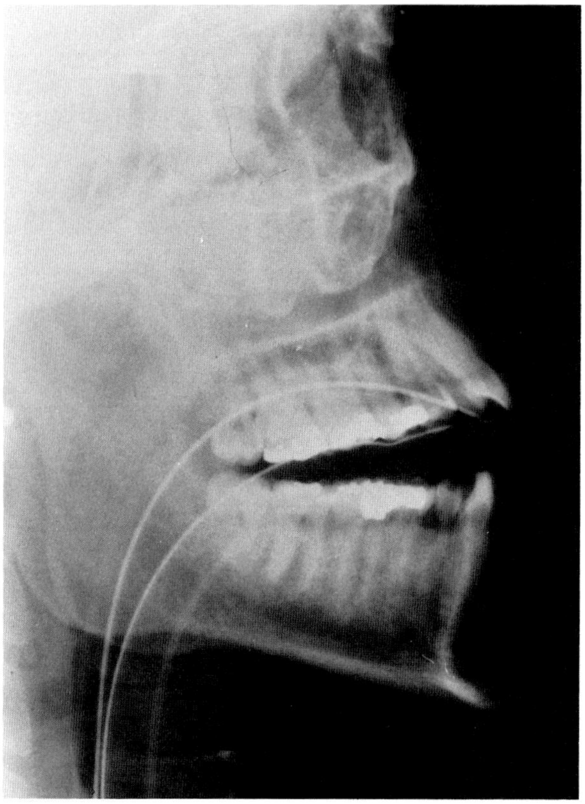

Figure 20-10. *The lateral facial radiograph provides information concerning displacement of the maxilla but provides little information concerning individual fracture lines.*

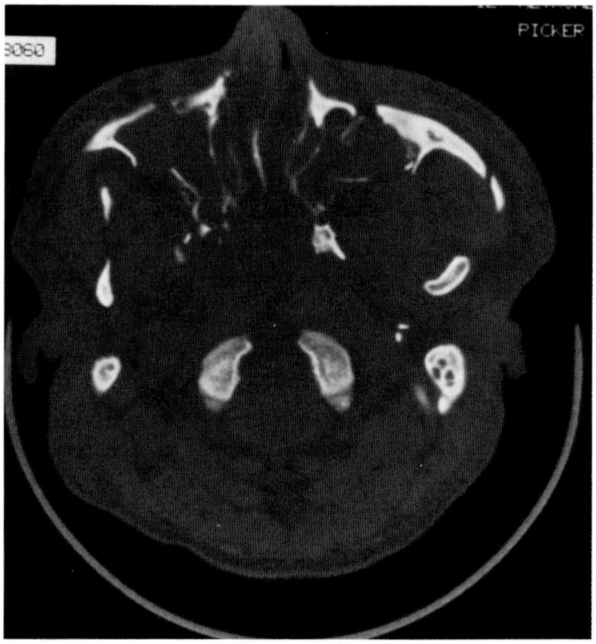

Figure 20-11. *Computed tomography demonstrates clearly the multiple and complex nature of maxillary fractures. The CT scan taken at a soft tissue window demonstrates multiple fracture sites.*

during transport and a patent airway maintained by assistance, endotracheal intubation, or tracheotomy.

The most frequent cause of hemorrhage in LeFort level fractures is due to bleeding from a fractured septum. This may be addressed by the placement of both posterior and anterior nasal packs. Bleeding from sites of laceration or abrasion may be controlled by tamponade. Exsanguinating hemorrhage is rarely encountered with facial fractures, and transfusions for such are generally not required.

Presurgical Care

Upon entrance to the hospital, the history and clinical examination should be performed with imaging used to confirm clinical impressions. After providing a diagnosis, soft tissue injuries may be repaired or dressed with normal saline-soaked gauze for 24 hours. Intra-

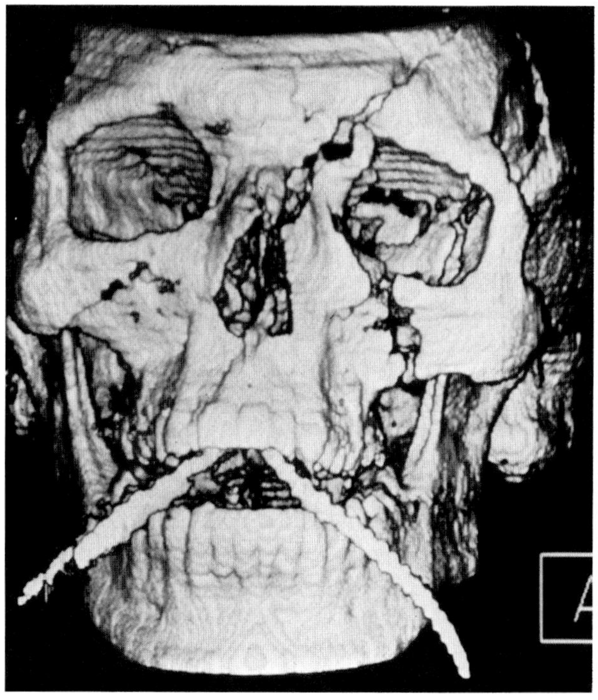

Figure 20-12. *Three-dimensional CT scans provide the most graphic representation of a fracture of the maxilla. The displaced maxilla is readily diagnosed in this example.*

venous antibiotics of a narrow spectrum that are directed at oral and nasal contaminants may be used. Penicillin and clindamycin remain the best choices. The preoperative nutritional, fluid, and electrolyte status should be evaluated and managed. The patient's record of immunizations should be elicited and a tetanus toxoid booster administered if necessary.

If multiple comminuted or segmentalized components of the dentoalveolus exist, dentoalveolar impressions may be obtained. If the mobilized segments induce pain, both local anesthesia and intramuscular analgesia may be administered before definitive care is given. Model surgery and splint or stent fabrication may be undertaken.

Temporary stabilization with Essig wires, Risdon wires, or Barton bandages may provide the patient comfort from painful bone movements. These may also reduce hemorrhage or bone oozing. Definitive treatment should occur within 10 to 14 days for most patients. Children should be treated earlier, and the geriatric patient may be treated later.

Sequence of Treatment

The sequence of treatment of maxillary fractures depends largely on the associated injuries. Nasotracheal intubation is adequate in all cases except those requiring detailed repair of nasal and nasoethmoid injuries. In such cases a tracheotomy should be performed. After securing the airway and administering general anesthesia, arch bars should be placed along with any required splints or stents. If teeth are deemed unsalvageable, they should be removed at this time. Necrotic debris should be removed. If present, the mandible fracture should be addressed. Intraoral lacerations should then be repaired and the maxillary fracture reduced and placed in intermaxillary fixation. Zygomatic injuries, if present, may be addressed next. First, the frontozygomatic suture is exposed, reduced, and fixed. Next, the zygomaticomaxillary suture and floor of the orbit are repaired. The nasal injury and nasoethmoid injury should be addressed after this. The last injuries to be repaired are the lacerations of the skin.

Higher level LeFort fractures are treated as if they are maxillary fractures with associated nasal and zygomatic fractures. The discussion to follow describes methods that can be incorporated into the treatment of all maxillary fractures.

Postoperative Care

Immediate postoperative care should be directed at the evaluation of the surgical treatment and initiation of rehabilitation. A good clinical examination should be performed to evaluate symmetry, occlusion, stability, and adequacy of reduction. Waters', lateral, and submentovertex radiographs should be evaluated for anatomic reduction. Evaluation of nutritional status, fluids, and airways should be performed before discharge.

If intermaxillary fixation is used, it may be released in 4 to 6 weeks for most patients. In older patients, intermaxillary fixation may remain in place longer, whereas in children, the period is shorter. One or two intermaxillary fixation elastics may provide physical therapy, guiding the patient into occlusion and providing resistance to the musculature for a period of 2 weeks after fixation. Evaluation for secondary reconstruction of soft and hard tissue defects may begin in 3 to 6 months.

Surgical Care

Closed Reductions

Closed reductions of maxillary fractures have been performed successfully for more than a century.[18] This method is excellent for patients with a satisfactory complement of dentition (at least three teeth per sextant in occlusion) with no gross neurologic problem and with an isolated LeFort I level fracture. This procedure is accomplished by contouring stainless steel Erich arch bars to fit intimately with the existing dentition. These bars are then ligated to the dentition with 24-gauge surgical stainless steel wire. A smaller diameter wire (26 gauge) may be necessary for the anterior dentition. After removal of any debris and throat pack, the maxillary dentition is placed in maximum intercuspation with the mandibular dentition and ligated with 24-gauge surgical steel wire.

If the maxilla does not mobilize, the use of Rowe disimpaction forceps may be necessary to reduce the fracture (Fig. 20-13). The paired forceps are placed with the flat end in the nose and bowed end on the palate. The surgeon stands over the patient's head and in an inferior anterior movement disimpacts the maxilla. Further assistance may be provided with a Hayton Williams forceps used in conjunction with the

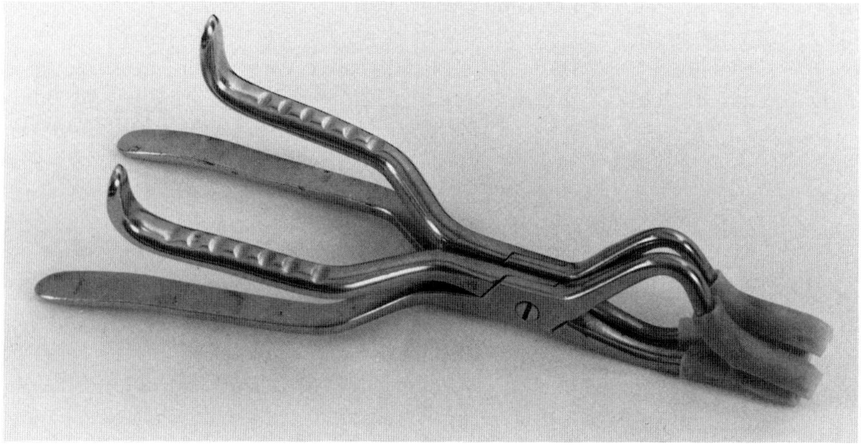

Figure 20-13. *Rowe disimpaction forceps should be used to mobilize and reposition the maxilla anterially in most maxillary fractures.*

Rowe disimpaction forceps. The patient may now be placed in intermaxillary fixation (Fig. 20-14).

Surgical Splints

In cases of multiple segmentation, gross comminution, periodontal disease, or inadequate partial dentition (less than three occluding teeth per sextant), occlusal wafers or palatal splints are useful. After impressions and model surgery, the splint may be fabricated.

If a full-coverage palatal splint is chosen, adequate soft tissue relief should be present so that undue pressure and loss of blood supply does not occur. This type of splint should cover the palate to the vibrating line for strength. It should cover the cingulae and the heights of contour of the teeth, but not the occlusal surface or incisal edge. Interdental ligation holes should be placed in the embrasures (Fig. 20-15).

If an occlusal wafter is to be fabricated, it should cover the occlusal surfaces and heights of contour, but should not encroach on the soft tissues. Holes should be placed between occlusal surfaces in the splint so that it may be ligated separately to the arch bar.

The Gunning type of splint is essentially a denture fabricated to the existing edentulous or partially edentulous jaw with arch bars or suspension brackets.[19] This type of splint can be used to treat any combination of edentulousness that is usually supported with any of the suspension methods outlined in the following discussion.

Methods of Skeletal Fixation

ADAMS WIRING TECHNIQUE. In 1942 the Adams technique of fixation of the facial skeleton was described, and it still has application today.[20] This method of fixation incorporated suspension of the

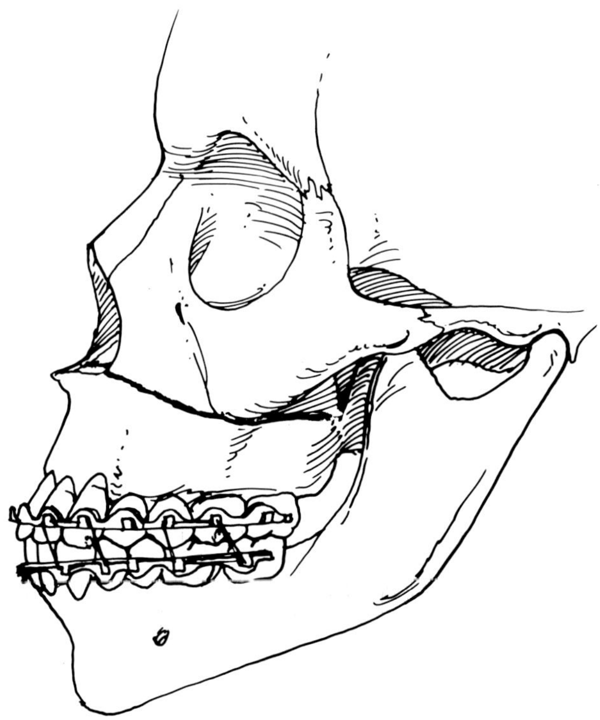

Figure 20-14. *Closed reduction with intermaxillary fixation is usually sufficient for most LeFort I fractures.*

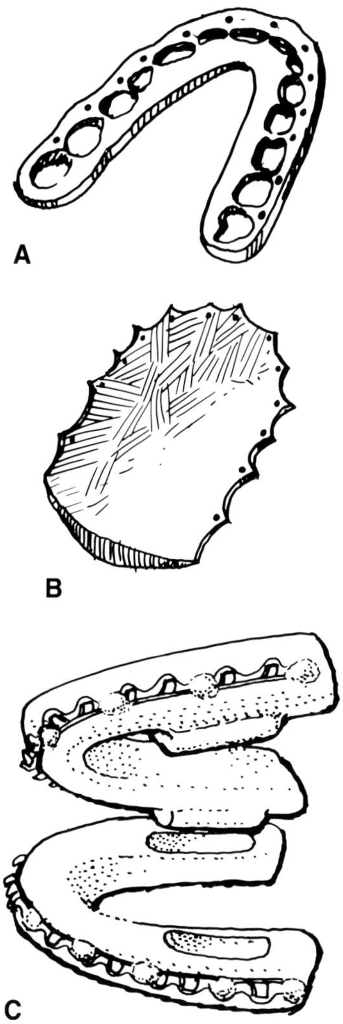

Figure 20-15. *Custom-made acrylic splints are necessary adjuncts to the management of fractures of the jaws, especially when teeth are missing. (**A**) Occlusal wafer. (**B**) Palatal splint. (**C**) Gunning splint.*

midface from the zygomatic process of the frontal bone or maxillary process of the zygoma. With modifications, the technique is as follows. An incision is made through skin, orbicularis oculi, and periosteum to indentify the frontozygomatic suture and fracture site. A drill with a wire-passing burr is then used to create an anteroposterior hole from the superior lateral orbital rim to the temporal fossa. A 22-gauge surgical stainless steel wire is then placed through the hole and adjusted so that equal amounts remain on either side. A zygomatic awl is then used to introduce the wire through the temporal fossae, posterior and medial to the zygoma and into the mouth. The wire is then secured to the arch bar or splint. A wire of a lesser diameter (24 gauge) is then used to secure the superior aspect, serving as a pull-out wire when the fractures are healed. The lesser diameter pull-out wire is used so that it, rather than the skeletal fixation wire, will break upon removal. The wire is then twisted into a braid so that the soft tissues are not incorporated into it. It is secured with a passing awl, passed under the scalp into the hairline for cosmesis, and affixed with a nylon button (Fig. 20-16).

INFRAORBITAL RIM WIRE. Infraorbital rim wires are useful for anteriorly directed suspension.[20,21] A horizontal incision is created in the vestibule inferior to the infraorbital rim. A freer elevator is used to dissect superiorly to the infraorbital rim and over it. The lateral two thirds of the infraorbital rim is identified. This will be at the lowest point of contour, at a distance from the nasolacrimal duct. The tissues are retracted superiorly, and the orbit is protected with a malleable or Seldin retractor. A drill and wire-passing burr are used to create a hole in the thick inferior orbital rim. A 24-gauge stainless steel wire is passed through the hole, repositioned inferiorly, and secured to the arch bar or splint (Fig. 20-17).

PIRIFORM APERTURE WIRE. Piriform aperture wires may not only support a compromised dentition or splint but may help stabilize a LeFort I level fracture if secured properly.[21] The lateral inferior corner of the piriform rim is dissected free and isolated. A hole is placed superior to the fracture in the thick lateral nasal buttress. A 24-gauge surgical stainless steel wire is then placed and positioned inferiorly and is secured to the arch bar or splint (Fig. 20-18).

DIRECT WIRES. Direct wires at the piriform rim and zygomaticomaxillary buttress are used occasionally.[22] The fracture sites are identified, holes are prepared, and 24-gauge wires are passed. After anatomic reduction, the wires are tightened to hold the maxilla in position.

ZYGOMATIC BUTTRESS WIRE. For skeletal fixation in midface fractures not affecting the zygoma, direct zygomatic buttress wires may be placed.[23] The zygomatic buttress is identified and an anteroposterior

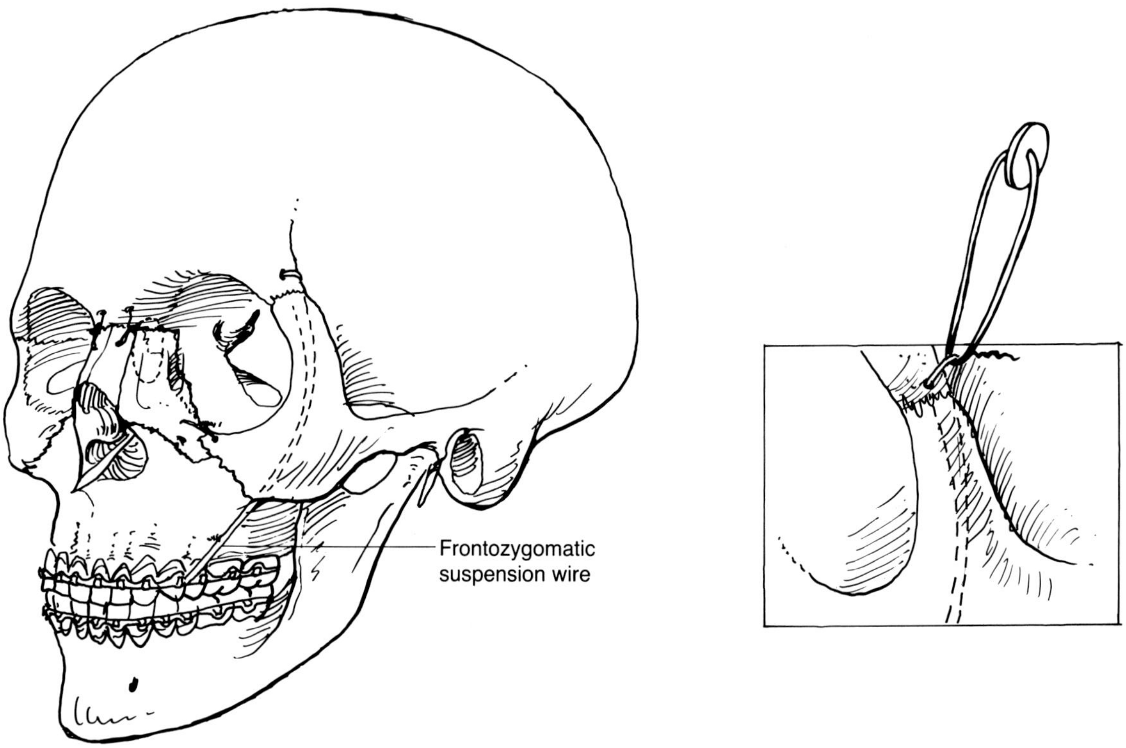

Figure 20-16. *(**A**) Frontozygomatic suspension wires are attached to arch bars to aid in supporting the maxilla. (**B**) A pullout wire attached to the primary wire is attached to a button until needed.*

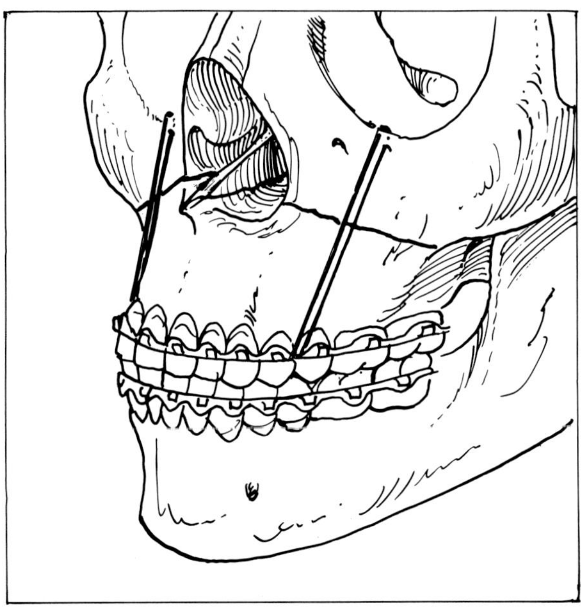

Figure 20-17. *Infraorbital rim wires provide anterior suspension for LeFort I fractures.*

hole is made with a wire-passing burr. A wire is then placed from anterior to posterior and brought inferiorly through the incision so that it can be ligated to the arch bar or splint.

CIRCUMZYGOMATIC WIRE. The lateral orbital rim and zygomatic arch are palpated where they meet at a right angle. The awl is inserted through the skin superior to the anterior aspect of the zygomatic arch and directed medially and anteriorly. After the skin is pierced, the awl passes inferiorly between the skin and the zygomatic arch until the mucosa lateral to the maxillary first molar is pierced. A wire is then placed into the aperture of the awl and secured. The awl is then pulled back superior to the arch and directed medial to the zygomatic arch. The awl is driven inferiorly and anteriorly to exit the same hole created in the mucosa. Care is taken not to pull the awl through the skin on the backstroke, thereby creating a dimple or track debris and bacteria into the wound.[24] Both ends of the wire are then grasped with separate needle

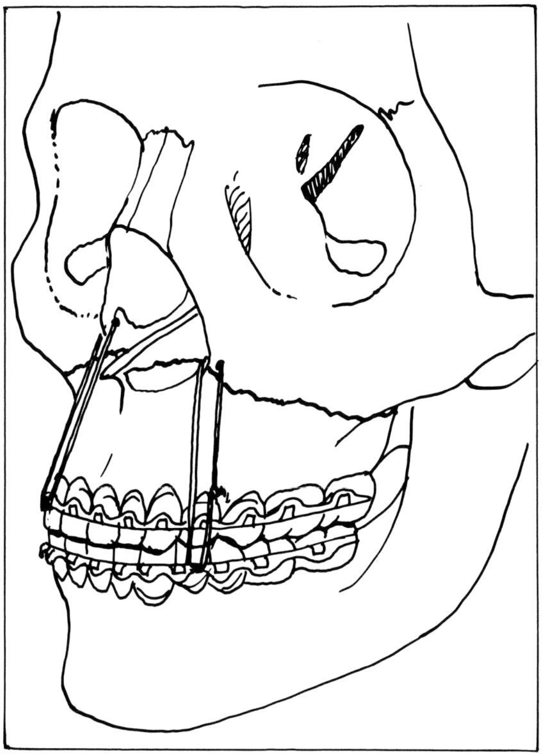

Figure 20-18. *The lateral piriform rim is sufficiently strong to support an anterior suspension wire. It is placed above the fracture line and is tied to the arch bar.*

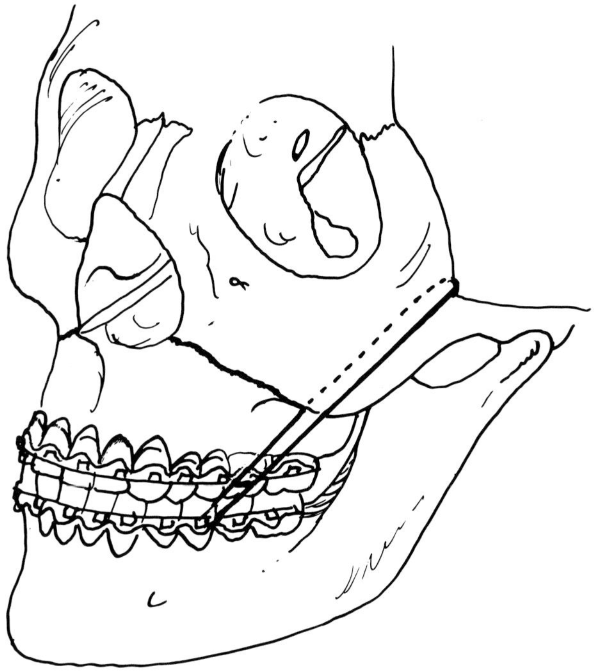

Figure 20-19. *Circumzygomatic suspension wires can be placed without making any incisions. They are useful for LeFort I and II fractures, but not for LeFort III fractures.*

holders and "sawed" so that no soft tissue exists between the wire and the arch. The wire is then secured to the maxillary arch bar (Fig. 20-19). After this procedure is completed, the mandible should be passed through its excursions to ensure that the coronoid was not grasped. Suspension wires of any type are usually unnecessary for treatment of LeFort I fractures if the patient has sufficient dentition to assume a proper anteroposterior reduction.[25] In addition, if mandibular condyles are intact, only one circumzygomatic wire is necessary. If one condyle of the mandible is fractured, the circumzygomatic wire will be effective only on the contralateral side.

CIRCUMPALATAL WIRE. Circumpalatal fixation is useful in securing Gunning splints and dentures and is performed partially "blind."[26] A nasal speculum is first introduced into the aperture through which the wire is to be placed to identify anatomic irregularities. Attention is then directed to the mouth where the same aperture is identified by palpation. A mandibular passing awl is then placed curve down at the most inferior portion of the aperture. The oral mucosa is perforated with the tip of the awl and an attempt is made to pass the instrument along the floor of the nose submucosally. Occasionally, a perforation will occur. The tip of the awl is then felt to slip off the posterior aspect of the maxilla. With the forefinger of the opposite hand, the soft palate is pushed superiorly, and the tip of the awl is palpated. The awl then perforates the soft palate and mucosa. Next, a 22-gauge stainless steel wire is placed in the aperture of the awl and pulled back along the floor of the nose and out the piriform aperture. The two ends of the wire are secured around the splint (Fig. 20-20).

RIGID FIXATION. Recent advances in technology have resulted in the advocacy of bone plating of all facial fractures.[27] In cases of seizures, gross neurologic compromise, or for patient convenience, rigid fixation may be used. Currently, a myriad of plating systems are available to the surgeon, each with a different material design or technique. An outline of rigid fixation of the maxilla follows.

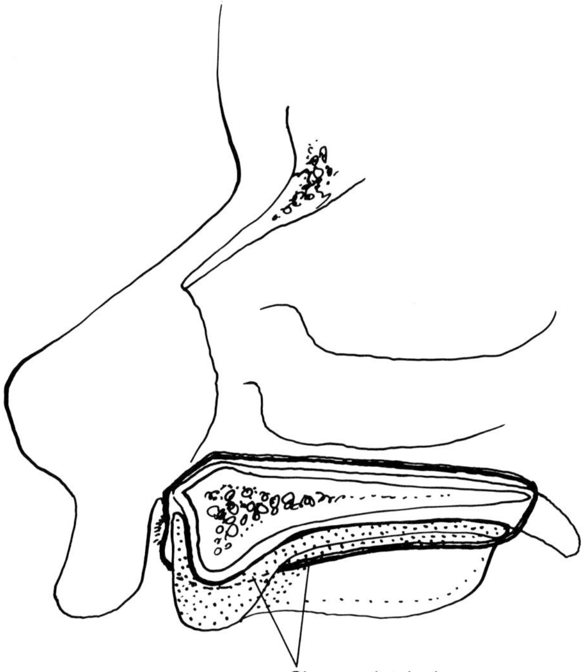

Figure 20-20. *A circumpalatal wire can be used to secure a maxillary denture to the maxilla.*

Caution must be used in placement of rigid fixation because of the comminuted tendency of these fractures and the resultant necrosis of bone with reckless dissection. Although circumvestibular incisions may provide good visualization, excessive subperiosteal dissection may be a problem. Because the structures to be supported are the zygomatic buttress and buttress of the piriform aperture, vertical incisions through the vestibule in these regions are the most advantageous.

Vertical vestibular incisions are made through mucosa, submucosa, and periosteum. Care must be taken to dissect subperiosteally from superior to and inferior to the fracture site, thus preventing entrance into the antrum. Bone plates are adapted, placed, and secured in position. For application of rigid fixation in higher level Le Fort fractures, additional incisions may be used. To accomplish this, an infraorbital lid incision may be made to gain access to the zygomaticomaxillary suture.

TRANSFIXATION WIRE. Kirshner wires and Steinman pins are not routinely used for fixation of midfacial fractures but do have special application. For grossly comminuted, unstable midfacial fractures that require fixation but are unamenable to open reduction, the rigid wire may be of assistance. This wire is used to "shish kebob" each of the individual bony units in order, while the surgeon manipulates the wire by hand.[28] These wires are also highly desirable for affixing splints transpalatally or transalveolarly. After the splint is positioned, the wire is driven through the outer flange of the splint through the alveolar bone and into the inner flange. Four quadrants provide a satisfactory stabilization.

The rigid wire may also be used to rigidly stabilize a maxilla if an intact zygoma exists.[29] Through a small mucoperiosteal incision made intraorally over the eminence, a wire is driven. It should engage two cortices. It is then contoured to rest against the arch bar and is secured by luting it with acrylic. This method of fixation may preclude the use of intermaxillary fixation (Fig. 20-21).

OPEN REDUCTION WITH IMMEDIATE BONE GRAFTING. Open reduction with immediate bone

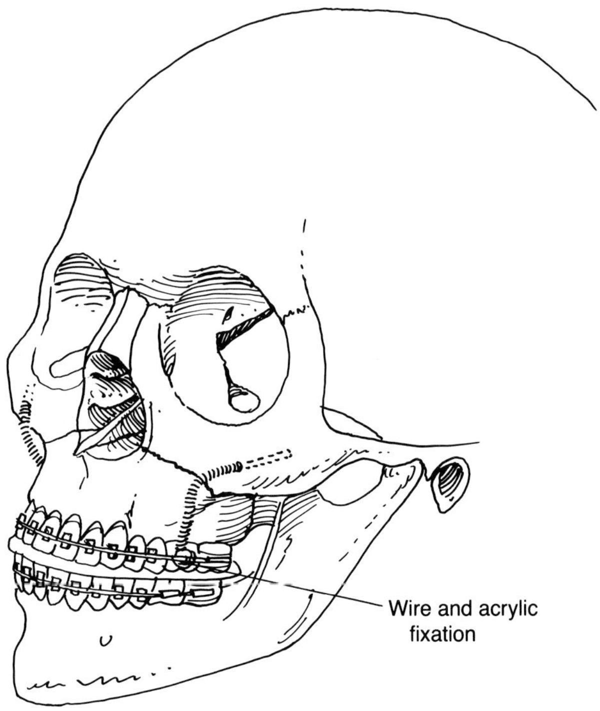

Figure 20-21. *A threaded Steinman pin driven through the zygomatic buttress and bent at right angles is secured to the arch bar with acrylic and wire ligatures. This method stabilizes the maxilla in an anteroposterior and superoinferior direction.*

grafting has been used in a manner similar to rigid fixation.[30] The principles behind this procedure are to provide support to the structural buttresses of the face. The surgical access gained is through the same incisions described for bone plating, i.e., by an infraorbital incision, coronal incision, and lateral brow incisions. Iliac crest corticocancellous grafts or split rib grafts are wired to the zygomaticomaxillary suture, infraorbital rim, zygomatic buttress, frontozygomatic suture, and, if a coronal incision is made, the zygomaticotemporal suture.

The advantages of this technique are that it provides additional support and replaces avulsed tissue. The disadvantages of the procedure are the morbidity of a second surgical site, increased surgical time, longer incisions, increased rates of infection, resorption, and necrosis of the bone grafts.

ISOLATED BONE SCREWS. Single bone screws are not often used but may aid unusual cases requiring skeletal fixation. They tend to be unsightly. Care must be used when placing the fixation so that dissimilar metals are not used, thereby creating a galvanic reaction. Screws may be placed in the frontal bone either at the zygomatic process or over the frontal sinus for suspension wires.[27] Screws also may be used to secure Gunning splints. When used, they must engage the outer flange of the splint or denture in four quadrants and be secured to good alveolar bone.

REMOVAL OF SUSPENSION DEVICES. Most fixation and suspension devices can be removed under local anesthesia supplemented with inhalation or intravenous sedation. Unless there is a high degree of suspicion that the wound is contaminated, antibiotic prophylaxis is not used routinely. An antiseptic mouth rinse such as chlorhexidine should precede the removal of the device. A mild analgesic is helpful in the postoperative phase.

External Fixation Devices

External fixation devices are indicated when a midfacial fracture coexists with bilateral subcondylar fractures of the mandible that are not amenable to open reduction, when there is gross comminution of both jaws that has resulted in loss of vertical dimension, or when anterior traction is required. Many types of head frames have been described with various techniques and modifications.[31–33]

The University of Tennessee head frame (Walter Lorenz Surgical Supply, Jacksonville, FL) is the most frequently used and is placed in the following fashion (Fig. 20-22). The occipitoparietal and frontoparietal sutures are palpated. The heights of bony contour are identified, taking care to avoid skull fractures. The region is prepared with an antiseptic solution and shaved free of hair. The aluminum head frame is then assembled with four cranial screw blocks centered over the heights of contour of the occipitoparietal and frontoparietal region. Cranial screws of an appropriate length are selected, and stab incisions are made in the scalp. A hemostat spreads the soft tissues, and the cranial screws are passively advanced until the stabilizing pin engages the outer cortex of the skull. Equal distance must be kept between the skull and frame at each screw. The screws are then secured with equal turns of opposite screws. The head frame

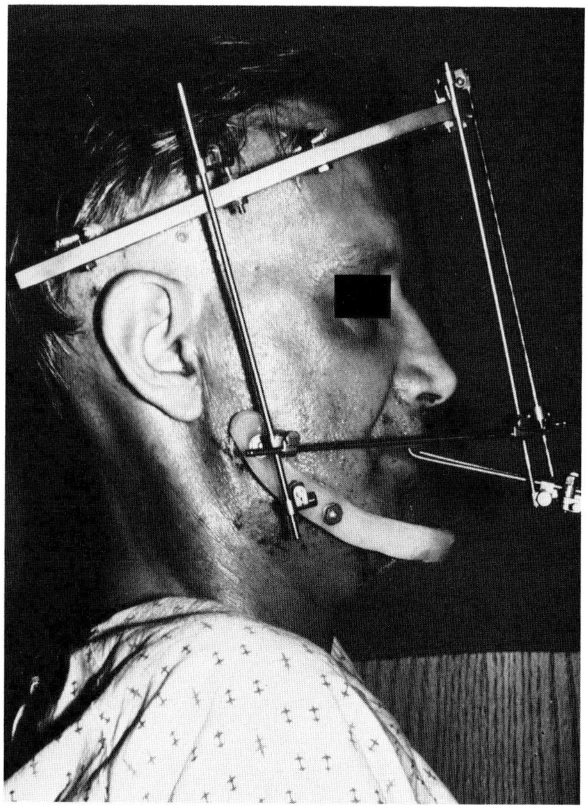

Figure 20-22. *An externally applied metal head frame is a valuable adjunct in holding the maxilla in a reduced anterior position while healing occurs. This is especially important with severely comminuted fractures in which direct wires or plates cannot be used.*

is then rocked to evaluate stability. One or two straight posts are secured to the anterior head frame, and traction rods are placed so that the maxilla may be secured.

Steinman pins or Kirschner's wires may be used to directly secure the maxilla. Traction rods may be luted to existing dentures or Gunning splints with acrylic. An acrylic occlusal wafer also may be fabricated to lute to the traction rod. The traction rods are then secured in three dimensions in space by double clamps.

Care must be taken not to advance the cranial screws so far that a skull fracture ensues. In addition, the cranial screws should be secured the day of the operation and then only once again 2 days later. Continued tightening during the month after fixation allows the cranial screw to cross both cranial tables and enter the skull. Care must be taken not to mix metals because galvanic responses have been reported.[34]

SPECIAL CONSIDERATIONS

Cerebrospinal Fluid Leak

The clinical appearance of a cerebrospinal fluid (CSF) leak after trauma to the maxilla is that of a thin blood-tinged liquid. When dry, two red lines, similar in appearance to railroad tracks, appear (Fig. 20-5). Generally, the CSF leak is through the cribriform plate of the ethmoid and stops spontaneously within 48 to 72 hours (Fig. 20-23). Varying opinions by the neurosurgical services exist regarding repair, antibiotics, steroids, and hyperosmotic agents. It is generally thought that early reduction of the displaced bony segments that caused the leak will not only reduce the fracture but obstruct the leak. If the leakage continues beyond 72 hours after reduction, an anterior craniotomy approach by a neurosurgeon may be required to gain access to the leak in the dura. This will be repaired with dura or fascia lata. The patient with facial fractures probably is being treated with a narrow-spectrum antibiotic directed at oral or nasal contaminants. Therefore no additional coverage for prevention of meningitis is necessary. Hyperosmotic agents or steroids to reduce cerebral edema or deter leakage are not indicated unless coincidental intracranial injury is noted. Under no circumstances should nasal packing be used to reduce the CSF flow. This may cause stagnation and retrograde flow of bacteria.

Traumatic Telecanthus

When a positive Furness test indicates severance of the medial canthal ligament with or without bony fragments attached and when intercanthal measurements are beyond the norm, a repair is indicated. Open re-

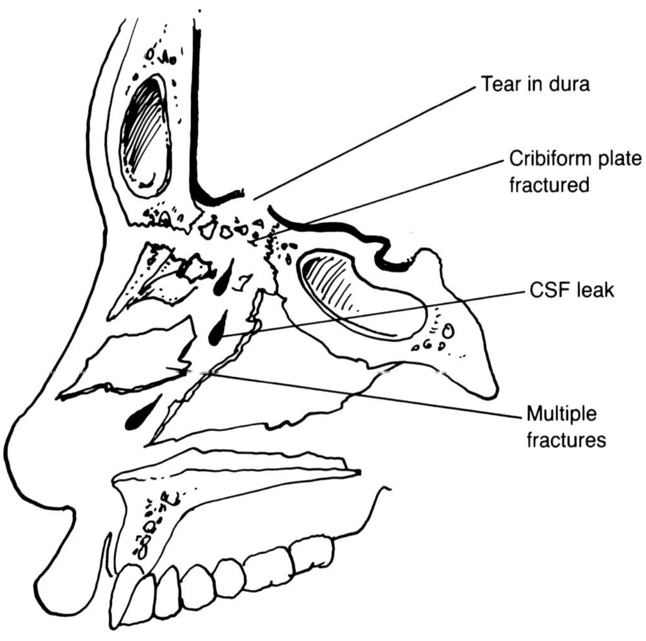

Figure 20-23. *Cerebrospiral fluid leaks are most commonly the result of a tear of the dura in the region of the cribriform plate, resulting in a rhinorrhea.*

duction is preferred. However, under certain circumstances, an older method may be used. This method is performed by fabricating two plates, ovoid in shape, from a lead sheet. A sternal puncture needle, is passed through the lead sheet, and the medial canthal ligament is grasped through the skin with an Adson forceps. The sternal puncture needle is passed through the skin, canthal ligament, associated fragment of the frontal process of the maxilla, nasal septum, opposite bony fragment, skin, pad, and plate. A 24-gauge stain-less steel wire is then placed through the sternal puncture needle, and the wire is pulled through. The needle is then repassed through in the same sequence so that both ends of the wire remain on one side. The same procedure is performed for the opposite canthus, and the wires are twisted simultaneously and secured. The position of the medial canthus must be visualized for proper inferior-superior position, as well as proper intercanthal dimension (Fig. 20-24). These may be removed in 4 weeks.

Avulsion Injuries

High-calibre, high-velocity gunshot wounds, blast injuries, and high-speed motor vehicle accidents with unrestrained victims cause the highest incidence of avulsion injury associated with maxillary fractures. The priority in these injuries is to preserve as much of the remaining tissue as possible. After administration of a narrow-spectrum antibiotic directed at oral and nasal contaminants, as well as tetanus prophylaxis, the wounds may be evaluated. Extensive irrigation may be used to remove debris, while hemostasis is achieved. Because of the collateral blood supply of the face, most tissues remain viable with even a small

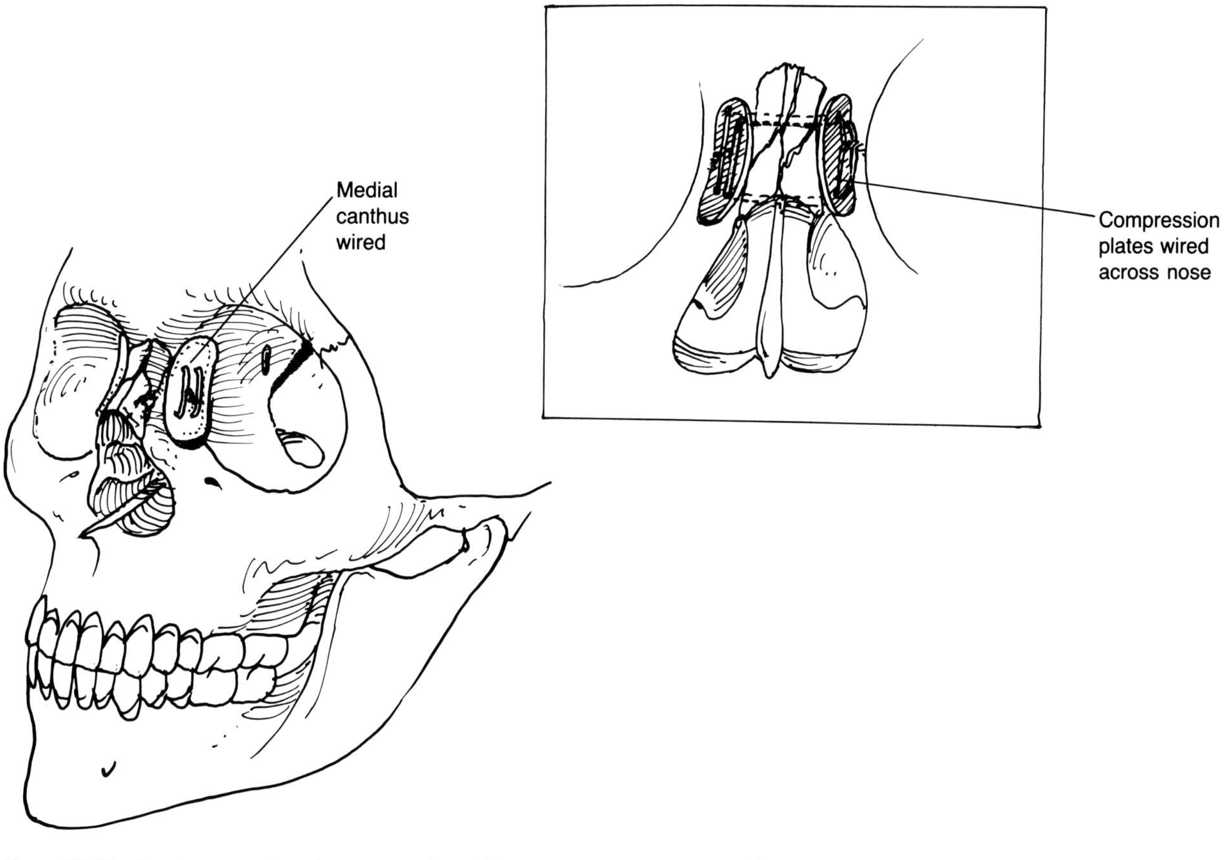

Figure 20-24. *Lead compression plates are used to aid in repositioning communited bony segments that remain attached to the medial canthal ligament. If the ligament is torn free from the bone, an open procedure is required to reattach it.*

isthmus of blood supply. Attention should next be directed at reassembling the bony segments. Voids in bone should be addressed with a secondary reconstruction. Multiple lacerations with comminuted fractures will have associated edema and significant venous congestion. This provides satisfactory blood supply to existing segments but not large bone grafts. Next, the soft tissue lacerations should be addressed. If advancement flaps can be performed, they should only be performed to cover exposed bone or to correct oronasal or oroantral fistulas. If too little soft tissue exists, flaps should not be advanced to jeopardize any further tissue; such repair should be addressed during a secondary reconstruction.

Geriatric Injuries

The geriatric patient suffering a LeFort injury poses a special concern. Additional medical illness and disabilities may make the use of general anesthesia a considerable risk. The surgeon should exercise judgment when cases of morbid medical conditions exist with minimally displaced fractures that are edentulous. A new prosthesis may be more efficacious than a reduction and fixation.

The anatomy of the geriatric maxilla is less vascular and has more pneumatized antra, less alveolar bone, and less dense trabeculation. Should a reduction and fixation be required, existing dentures may be modified by relining and affixing arch bars or intermaxillary fixation buttons. A Gunning splint also may be fabricated. Fixation for such a splint may be with circumzygomatic, anterior nasal spine, piriform aperture, or circumpalatal wires. Additional fixation methods include placement of Kirschner wires, Steinman pins, or long 2.5-mm screws through the stent into the thickest part of the alveolus, paranasal buttress, or zygomatic buttress.

Pediatric Maxillary Fractures

Pediatric maxillary fractures are infrequent. Because of the lack of pneumatization of sinuses, these fractures tend to be less comminuted than in the adult. No long-term studies with significantly large populations exist to determine what alterations in maxillary growth will occur. Consideration for fixation should be given to the contour and root length of the primary dentition.[35] The use of occlusal splints and skeletal fixation should be entertained.

COMPLICATIONS

Repair of trauma requires an altered anatomic condition, technical management by a surgeon, and healing by the host. Limitations in any of these areas may result in complication. Complications in maxillary fractures are infrequent and may be categorized as perioperative, perifixation, and postfixation.

Perioperative Complications

The most obvious postoperative complications are misplaced bone segments or fixation devices and are identified with clinical examination or postoperative radiographic examinations. A second surgical procedure will correct such complications.

Immediate postoperative blindness is a complication of the reduction of LeFort III fractures and occurs because of a retinal artery spasm, retrobulbar hemorrhage, or bone fragments impinging on the optic nerve.

Perioperative and postoperative airway embarrassment is unusual in cases of maxillary fracture alone. However, they may occur with extubation while the patient is obtunded, with a septal hematoma or nasal packing, and with excessively edematous soft tissues that do not allow breathing through the embrasures. Reintubation, opening nasopharyngeal airways, or merely discontinuing the intermaxillary fixation may be effective.

Postoperative hemorrhage occurs if arterioles and veins are not ligated in laceration repair, if inadequate bone reduction allows continued oozing, if an aneurysm is present, or if an artery is partially transected. Lacerations should be reexplored to control hemorrhage. Hematomas should be drained. Bone ooze requires re-reduction or bone wax. Major artery hemorrhage requires emergency tamponade, and if the source cannot be identified, an arteriogram is indicated.

Perifixation Complications

Infections may occur during the early postoperative period. They may occur from contaminated soft tissue lacerations or foreign bodies. Hematomas may cause secondary infection if not identified early. Acute sinusitis also may occur in the ethmoid, sphenoid, frontal, and maxillary sinus because fractures may obliterate or obstruct their ducts or ostea. In addition, odontogenic infections may occur from previously diseased dentition or from a fractured devitalized tooth. In each case the cause should be identified and eliminated. An incision and drainage should be performed. Narrow-spectrum antibiotics directed at the offending agent must be administered.

The most significant complication of a maxillary fracture is nonunion. In nonunion the bones move in all directions after a routine period of fixation. The causes are inadequate blood supply, inaccurate position, movement of segments, infection, and nutritional deficiencies.[36] When the cause is identified, correction may be addressed. After control of infections and correction of nutritional deficiencies, an osteotomy and bone graft may be performed. These procedures are discussed in greater detail elsewhere in the text.

Failed fixation and suspension devices must be identified clinically and confirmed radiographically. If these are critical to the treatment, they must be replaced.

Epiphora may be noted early in the postoperative phase. Higher level LeFort fractures may damage the nasolacrimal duct. If this injury is not identified at surgery and repaired, epiphora will result.

Symptoms of oronasal and oroantral communications should be identified during the fixation phase but are not addressed until after fixation. These occur with avulsion injuries in which inadequate tissue remained or with advancement flaps or segmentalized fractures in which the soft tissue repair has failed.

Postfixation Complications

Posttraumatic deformities of contour and mass should be addressed 3 to 6 months after the fracture repair. Infection around deeply implanted fixation devices may occur even years after placement. Local edema, erythema, warmth, and pain will be indicative of this problem. The removal of fixation devices is necessary, along with curettage of any associated infected granulation tissue. Posttraumatic sinusitis of the ethmoid, sphenoid, and frontal sinuses may be identified many months after trauma and are due to altered functions of the ostea and ducts in the nose. Scar tissue that replaces ciliated nasal epithelium may alter these functions. Mucoceles and polyps may be identified years after the traumatic episode.

REFERENCES

1. Haug RH, Prather J, Indresano AT. An epidemiologic survey of facial fractures and concomitant injury. J Oral Maxillofac Surg 1990; 48:926–932.
2. Turvey TA. Midfacial fractures: A retrospective analysis of 593 cases. J Oral Surg 1977; 35:887–891.
3. Matsanuga RS, Simpson W, Toffel DH: Simplified protocol for treatment of malar fractures. Arch Otolaryngol 1977; 103:535–538.
4. Kelly DE, Harrigan WF. A survey of facial fractures: Bellevue Hospital, 1948–1974. J Oral Surg 1975; 33: 146–149.
5. Adekeye EO. The pattern of fractures of the facial skeleton in Kaduna, Nigeria. Oral Surg Oral Med Oral Pathol 1980; 49:491–495.
6. Dingman RO, Natvig P. The Men of elder days. In: Dingman RO, Natvig P. Surgery of facial fractures. Philadelphia: WB Saunders, 1964; 29–35.
7. Drommer RB. The history of the LeFort I osteotomy. J Maxillofac Surg 1986; 14:119–122.
8. Moloney F. The origin of the LeFort I maxillary osteotomy: Cheever's operation. J Oral Surg 1981; 39: 731–734.
9. LeFort R. Etude experimentale sur les fractures de la machoire superiore. Review de Chirugie 1901; 23: 208–227.
10. LeFort R. Etude experimentale sur les fractures de la machoire superiore. Review de Chirugie 1901; 23: 360–379.
11. LeFort R. Etude experimentale sur les fractures de la machoire superiore. Review de Chirugie 1901; 23: 479–507.
12. Tilson HB, McFee AS, Soudah HP. The maxillofacial works of Rene LeFort. Houston, TX: The University of Texas Dental Branch, 1972.
13. Williams DL, Warwick R. Osteology. In: Williams DL, Warwick R, Gray's anatomy, ed. 36. Philadelphia: WB Saunders, 1980; 333–343.
14. Moss-Salentijn L. Anatomy and embryology. In: Blitzer A, Lawson W, Friedman W. Surgery of the paranasal sinuses. Philadelphia: WB Saunders, 1985; 13–15.
15. Turvey TA, Fonseca RJ. The anatomy of the internal maxillary artery in the pterygopalatine fossa: Its relationship to maxillary surgery. J Oral Surg 1980; 38: 92–95.
16. Kofke WA, Levy JH. Appendix. In: Kofke WA, Levy JH. Post-critical care procedures of the Massachusetts General Hospital. Boston: Little, Brown & Co, 1986; 527.
17. Freihofer HPM. Inner intercanthal and interorbital distances. J Maxillofac Surg 1980; 8:324–326.

18. Fenner CS. A case of fracture of the upper jaw. Dental Cosmos 1859; 1:383–384.
19. Chalian VA, Maxillofacial problems involving the use of splints and stents. In: Laney WR, Maxillofacial prosthetics: PSG Publishing Co, Littleton, MA, 1979; 216–219.
20. Adams WM. Internal wiring fixation of facial fractures. Surgery 1942; 12:523:540.
21. Thoma K. Methods of fixation of the jaws and their indications. Oral Surg 1948; 6:125–134.
22. Merville LC. Multiple dislocations of the facial skeleton. Maxillofac Surg 1974; 2:187–200.
23. Sherman MJ. Intraoral reduction of maxillary fractures by malar suspension. J Oral Surg 1955; 13:321.
24. Edwards JB. A modified technique for placement of circumzygomatic wires. Br J Oral Surg 1965; 2: 205–211.
25. Joy ED, McGaha LE, Bear SE. Facial elongation after treatment of horizontal fracture of the maxilla without vertical suspension. J Oral Surg 1969; 27:560–562.
26. Bowerman JE, Conroy B. Maxillofacial prosthetics. In: Rob C, Operative surgery head and neck, vol. I. Philadelphia: JB Lippincott, 1981.
27. Stoll P, Schilli W, Joos U. The stabilization of midface fractures in the vertical dimension. J Maxillofac Surg 1983; 11:248–251.
28. Brown JB, Fryer MP, McDowell F. Internal wire-pin fixation for fractures of upper jaw, orbit, zygoma and severe facial crushes. Plast Reconstr Surg 1952; 9: 276–283.
29. Bennett MA, Wolford LM. The maxillary step osteotomy and Steinman pin stabilization. J Oral Maxillofac Surg 1985; 43:307–311.
30. Manson PN, Crawley WA, Yaremchuk MJ, et al. Midface fractures: Advantages of immediate extended open reduction and bone grafting. Plast Reconstr Surg 1985; 76:1–12.
31. Crawford MJ. Appliances and attachments for treatment of jaw fractures. US Naval Med Bull 1943; 41: 1151–1157.
32. Irby WB, Gavin GP. A new head appliance for use in patients with maxillofacial injuries. J Oral Surg 1955; 13:297.
33. Georgiade N, Nash T. An external cranial function apparatus for severe maxillofacial injuries. Plast Reconstr Surg 1966; 38:142–146.
34. Bradley PF. Electrolytic action around bone pins in the "halo" head frame. Br J Oral Surg 1969; 7:69–70.
35. Rowe NL. Fractures of the jaws in children. J Oral Surg 1969; 27:497–507.
36. Rowe NL. Non-union of the mandible and maxilla. J Oral Surg 1969; 27:520–529.

21

Management of Zygomatic Complex Fractures

David H. Perrott
Leonard B. Kaban

The zygoma articulates with the frontal, sphenoid, temporal, and maxillary bones and contributes significantly to the strength and stability of the midface. The forward projection of the zygoma causes it to be injured frequently.[1] However, it is thick and strong (50 to 80 g of force is required to break it), and therefore the zygoma itself is rarely fractured.[4,5,7] The zygomatic arch may be fractured (a zygomaticotemporal fracture), or the zygoma may be separated from its four articulations, which is called a zygomaticomaxillary or zygomatic complex (ZMC) fracture. The commonly used terms *trimalar* or *tripod fracture* are therefore inaccurate. They reflect an inability to easily identify the orbital (zygomaticosphenoid) portion of the injury before the advent of computed tomography (CT).

The cause of zygomatic injuries varies with patient demographics and location of the reporting institution. Matsunaga at Los Angeles County/University of Southern California Medical Center found that a majority of the 1200 zygomatic fractures studied were the result of motor vehicle accidents (MVAs).[2] In contrast, Winstanley found that 85% of zygomatic fractures in Manchester, England, resulted from assault, a fall, or sporting injuries. Only 8% of fractures in this series involved MVAs.[3]

In this chapter, the anatomic features, diagnosis, treatment, and complications of zygomatic fractures are discussed.

SURGICAL ANATOMY

The zygoma has four projections, which create a quadrangular shape: the frontal, temporal, and lateral portions of the infraorbital rim and articulation with the maxilla, and the inferior projection or buttress. The zygoma articulates with four bones: the frontal, temporal, maxilla, and the greater wing of the sphenoid. A ZMC fracture includes disruption of the four articulating sutures: frontozygomatic, zygomaticotemporal, zygomaticomaxillary and the zygomaticosphenoid sutures (Fig. 21–1, A and B).

All zygomatic complex fractures involve the orbital floor, and therefore an understanding of orbital anatomic features is essential for those treating these injuries. The orbit is a quadrilateral pyramid that is based anteriorly. The lateral and medial walls converge posteriorly at the orbital apex. The roof is composed of the frontal bone and lesser wing of the sphenoid. The medial wall consists of the frontal process of the maxilla, the lacrimal bone, the orbital plate of the ethmoid, and a small portion of the sphenoid body (Fig. 21–1, C).

The orbital floor slopes inferiorly and is the shortest of the orbital walls, averaging 47 mm.[8] It is composed of the orbital plate of the maxilla, the orbital surface of the zygomatic bone, and the orbital process of the palatine bone. The lateral orbital wall is the

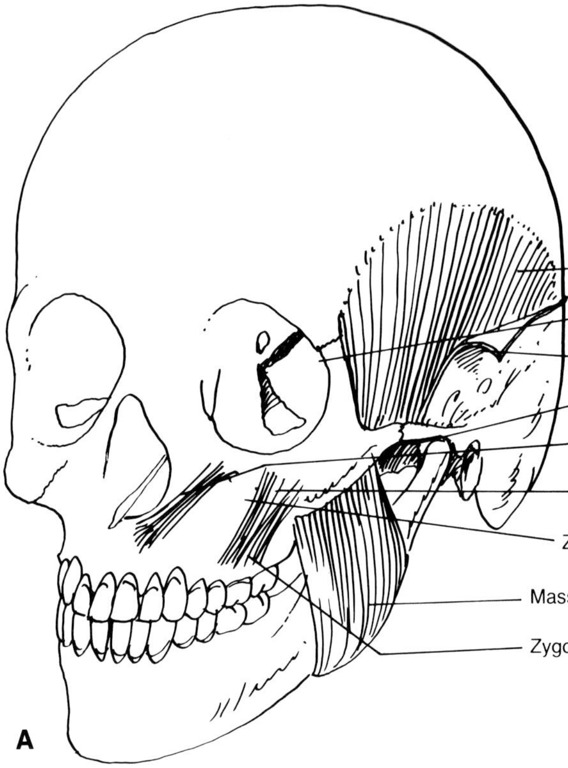

A

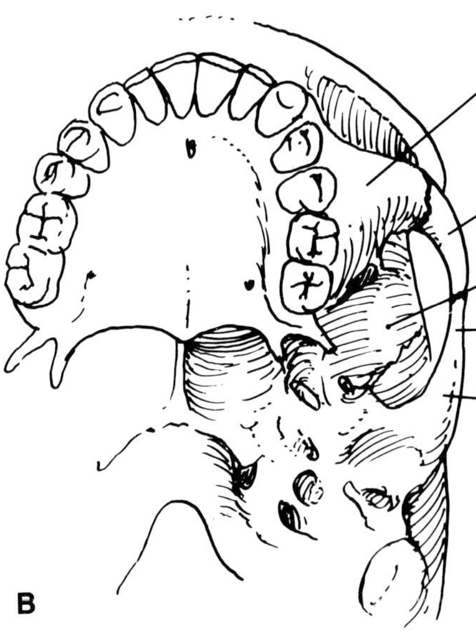

B

Figure 21–1. *(**A**) Relation of muscles and cranial bones to the zygomatic complex as seen in frontal or lateral view. (**B**) Relation of the skull to the zygomatic complex as seen from a submental view. (**C**) Relation of soft tissues, muscle, and nerves to the orbit as seen from a frontal view. (**D**) Frontal view of fascia and muscle attachment to the skull, zygomatic arch, and coronoid process.*

thickest and is formed by the zygomatic and sphenoid bones.

Isolated fractures of the zygomatic arch consist of three fracture lines: the zygomaticotemporal suture and sutures anterior and posterior to the articulation. This creates a V-shaped depression of the arch.

The sensory nerve associated with the zygoma is the second division of the trigeminal nerve. The zygomatic, facial, and temporal branches exit the foramina in the body of the zygoma and supply sensation to the cheek and anterior temporal region. The infraorbital nerve passes through the orbital floor and exits at the

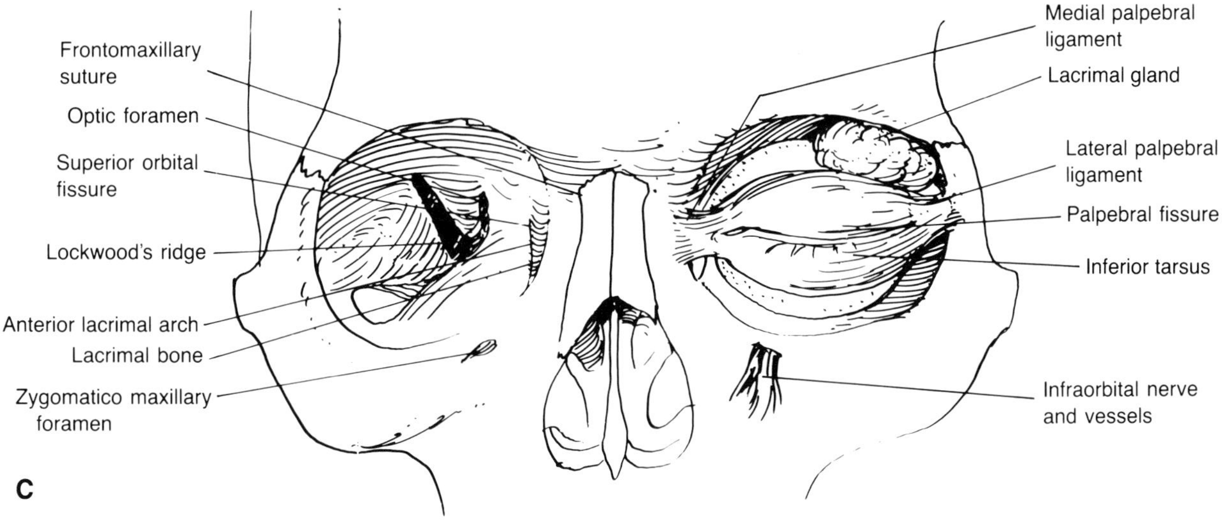

C

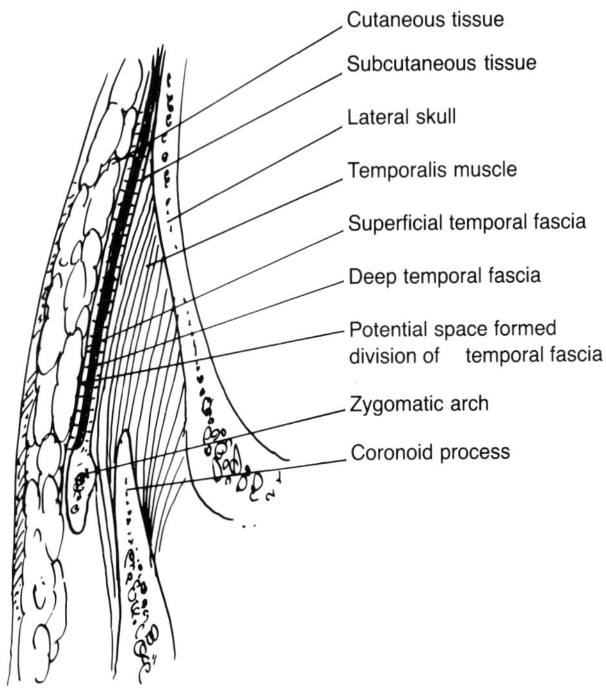

D

Figure 21–1. *(Continued)*

infraorbital foramen (Fig. 21–1, C). It provides sensation for the anterior cheek, lateral nose, upper lip, and maxillary anterior teeth. Muscles of facial expression originating from the zygoma include the zygomaticus major and labii superiorus muscles. They are innervated by cranial nerve VII. The masseter muscle attaches along the concave temporal surface of the zygoma and arch and is innervated by a branch of the mandibular nerve (Fig. 21–1, D).

The temporalis fascia attaches to the frontal process of the zygoma and zygomatic arch and is also innervated by a branch of the mandibular nerve. The fascia produces resistance to inferior displacement of a fractured fragment by the downward pull of the masseter muscle.

The position of the globe in relation to the horizontal axis is maintained by Lockwood's suspensory ligament. This attaches medially to the posterior aspect of the lacrimal bone and laterally to the orbital (Whitnall's) tubercle (which is 1 cm below the frontozygomatic suture on the inner aspect of the frontal process of the zygoma). The shape and location of the medial and lateral canthi of the eyelid is maintained by the canthal tendons. The lateral canthal tendon also attaches to Whitnall's tubercle. The medial canthal tendon has an attachment both to the anterior and posterior lacrimal crests. ZMC fractures are often accompanied by antimongoloid (downward) cant of the lateral canthal region caused by displacement of the tendon (Fig. 21–1, C).

GENERAL DIAGNOSTIC CONSIDERATIONS

Zygomatic fractures are not life-threatening and are usually treated after more serious injuries are stabilized and swelling has resolved (4 to 5 days after injuries).

Initial evaluation of the patient with a zygomatic fracture includes documentation of the bony injury and the status of surrounding soft tissue (eyelids, lacrimal apparatus, canthal tendons, and globe) and cranial nerves II to VI. Visual acuity and the status of the globe and retina should be established; an opthalmologist should be consulted.

History and Physical Examination

History

The nature, force, and direction of the injuring blow should be determined from the patient, witnesses, or both. A direct lateral blow often results in an isolated zygomatic arch or a medially and inferiorly displaced ZMC fracture. A frontal blow usually produces a posteriorly and inferiorly displaced zygomatic fracture.

The patient with a ZMC fracture complains of pain, periorbital edema, and ecchymosis. There may be paresthesia or anesthesia over the cheek, lateral nose, upper lip, and maxillary anterior teeth resulting from injury to the zygomaticotemporal or infraorbital nerves. This occurs in 18% to 56% of all patients with zygomatic trauma.[12-17] When the arch is medially displaced, the patient often complains of trismus. There is frequently epistaxis and diplopia may result from entrapment of extraocular muscles, displacement of the globe (enophthalmos), or both. This symptom usually becomes evident within 2 to 3 days after injury.[5]

Physical Examination

Ecchymosis and edema are the most common early clinical signs and are present in 64% of all zygomatic injuries (Fig. 21–2, A).[2] Depression of the malar eminence and infraorbital rim produce flattening of the cheek (Fig. 21–2, B). Downward displacement of the zygoma produces an antimongoloid slant to the lateral canthus, enophthalmos, and accentuation of the supratarsal fold of the upper eyelid. Lacerations in the facial region should lead the surgeon to suspect underlying fracture.

Palpation of the zygomaticofrontal suture, the entire 360° of the orbital rim, and the zygomatic arch should be carried out in an orderly fashion. Tenderness, a step-off, or separation at the sutures are indicative of a fracture. Intraorally, disruption at the zygomatic buttress area is palpable, and ecchymosis in the region of the canine fossa may be visible. The range of mandibular motion is evaluated to rule out impingement of the zygomatic arch on the coronoid process.

In isolated zygomatic arch fractures, a depression is observed and palpated anterior to the tragus (Fig. 21–3, A and B). Pain and decreased mandibular motion are commonly present in these injuries, whereas orbital signs are absent.

Figure 21–2. *24-year-old man who sustained a blow to the left cheek. (**A**) Frontal photograph illustrates typical findings of zygomatic complex fracture: periorbital ecchymosis, antimongoloid slant of the lateral canthus, and depression of the cheek. (**B**) Lateral view better illustrates marked cheek depression. (**C**) Waters'-view radiograph demonstrates fracture at the frontozygomatic suture, displacement of the zygoma, and a cloudy maxillary sinus. (**D**) Axial computed tomographic scan demonstrates depression of the zygoma and buckling of the posterior wall of the maxillary sinus. (**E**) Sagittal reconstruction of the orbit demonstrates no signs of orbital floor or wall disruption.*

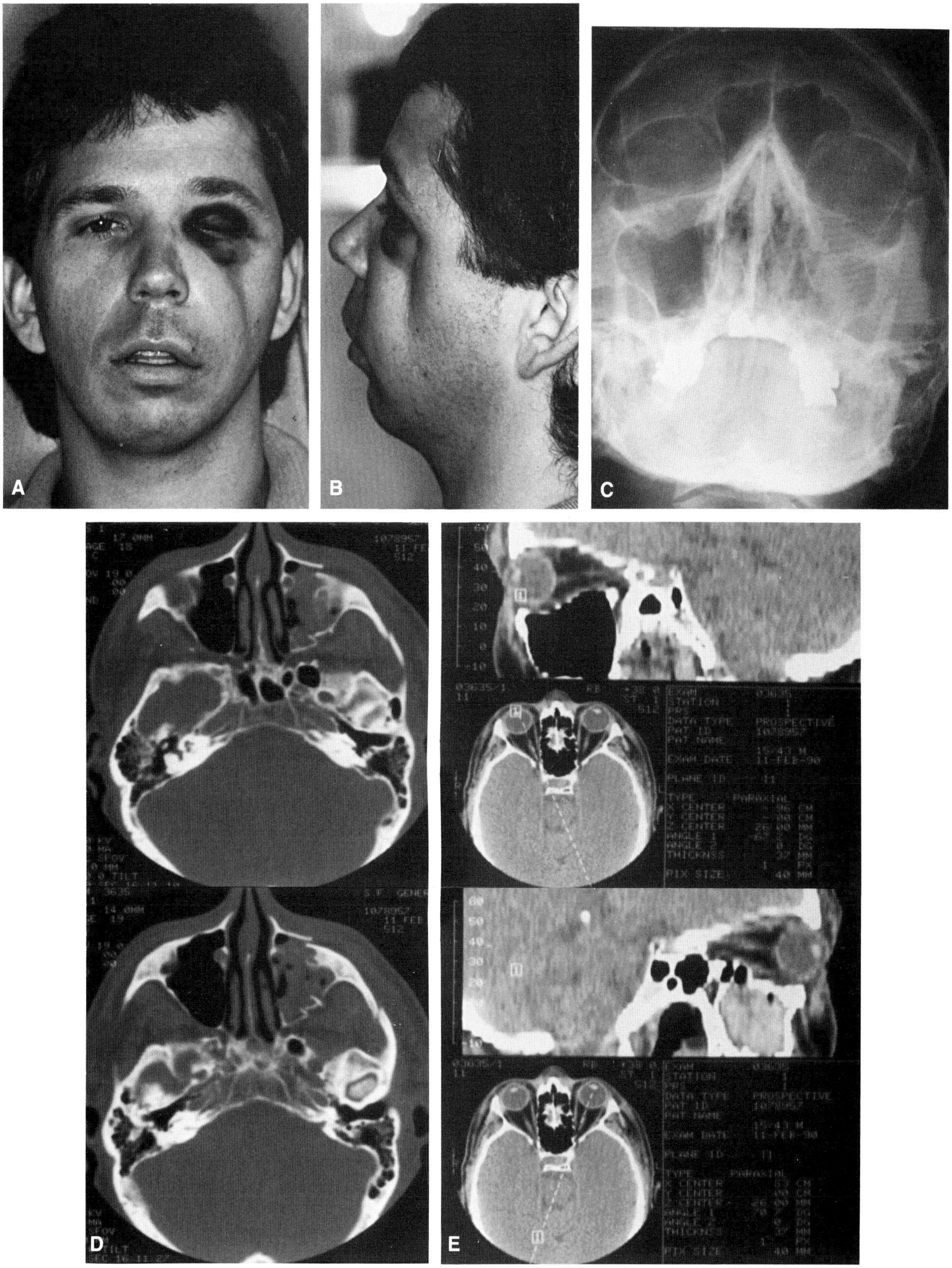
A
B
C
D
E
EXAM
STATION
DATA TYPE PROSPECTIVE
PAT ID
PAT NAME
EXAM DATE 11-FEB-90
PLANE ID 11
TYPE PARAXIAL
X CENTER
Y CENTER
Z CENTER
ANGLE 1
ANGLE 2
THICKNSS
PIX SIZE

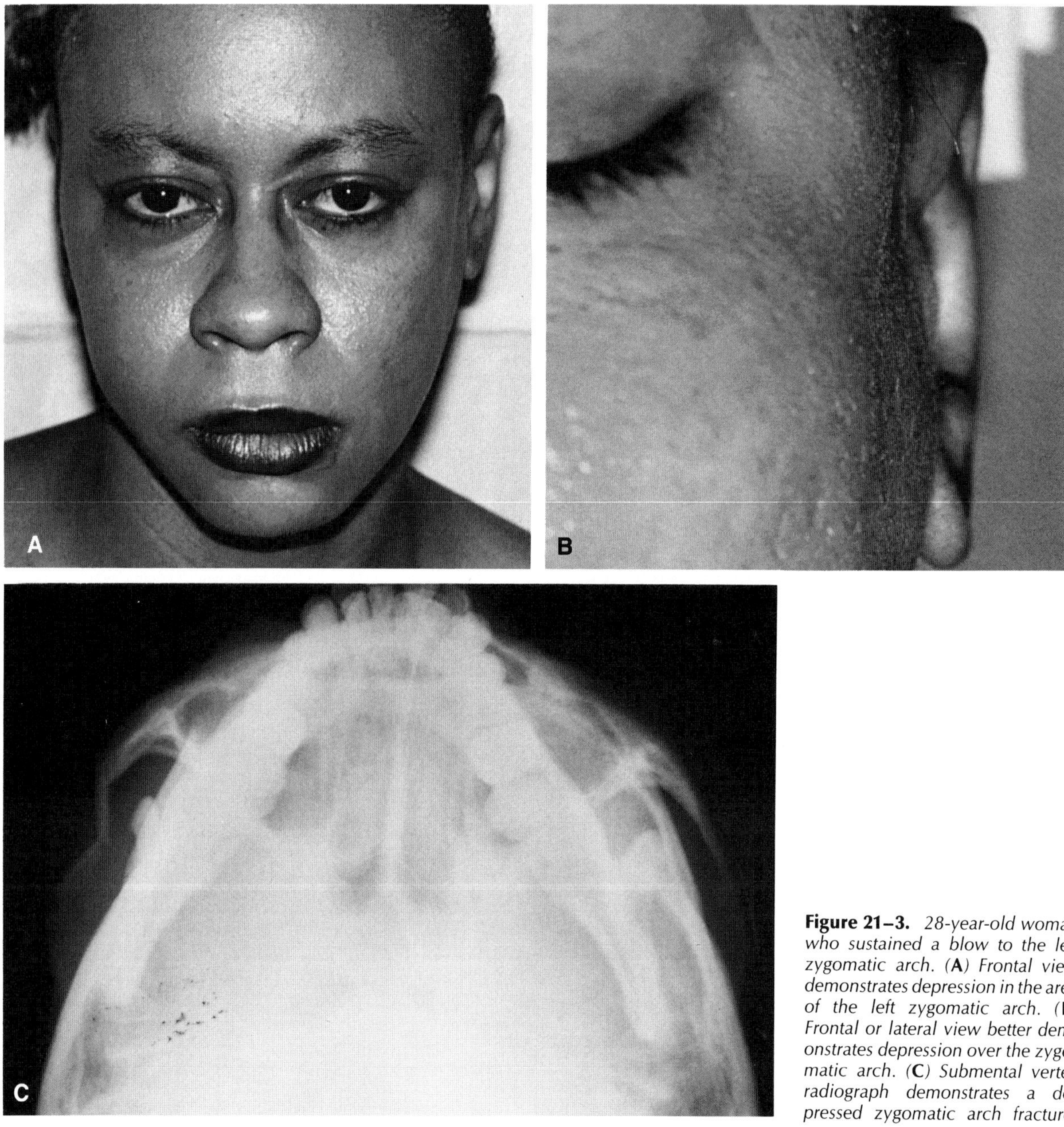

Figure 21–3. *28-year-old woman who sustained a blow to the left zygomatic arch. (**A**) Frontal view demonstrates depression in the area of the left zygomatic arch. (**B**) Frontal or lateral view better demonstrates depression over the zygomatic arch. (**C**) Submental vertex radiograph demonstrates a depressed zygomatic arch fracture.*

Evaluation of the eye includes documentation of visual acuity, pupillary response to light, funduscopic examination, ocular movement, and globe position. Limitation of motion of the extraocular muscles and enophthalmos may be noted if significant fractures of the orbital floor or medial or lateral walls are present. Lack of pupillary response and ptosis is present if cranial nerve III has been injured. Injuries to the optic nerve, retinal detachment, injury to the globe, hyphema, and lacrimal ducts should be ruled out.

Neurologic examination includes careful evaluation of all cranial nerves with special attention directed toward the second division of the trigeminal nerve and the nerves associated with the eye (cranial nerves III, IV, and VI).

Radiographs

The diagnosis of zygomatic fractures is usually established by the history and physical examination. Radiographs are helpful for confirmation and medicolegal documentation and, in some cases, to establish the extent of the bony injury.

Waters' View

The single best radiograph for evaluation of ZMC fractures is the Waters' view. It is a posteroanterior (PA) projection with the head positioned at a 27° angle to the vertical and the chin resting on the cassette. This projects the petrous pyramids off the maxillary sinuses, permitting visualization of the sinuses, lateral orbits, and infraorbital rims (Fig. 21–2, C). When this is combined with an erect Waters' view, a stereographic view of the fracture can be obtained. In patients who are unable to assume a face-down position, a reverse Waters' projection provides similar information.

Caldwell View

The Caldwell view is a posteroanterior (PA) projection with the face at a 15° angle to the cassette. This study is helpful in the evaluation of rotation (around a horizontal axis).

Submentovertex View

The submentovertex ("jug-handle") view is directed from the submandibular region to the vertex of the skull. It is helpful in the evaluation of the zygomatic arch and malar projection (Fig. 21–3, C).

Tomograms

Before the advent of computed tomography (CT), tomograms were commonly used for assessment of ZMC fractures and orbital displacement.[18-20] This study has been completely replaced by CT.

Computed Tomography

CT is frequently used for evaluation of patients with facial trauma.[20] Fractures undetected by standard radiographic examinations are often revealed by this technique and the anatomic features are clearly visualized because there is no superimposition of adjacent structures (Fig. 21–2, D and E). The advantages of CT are that it provides satisfactory resolution; that patient orientation and technique are standardized; that limited patient cooperation is required; and that images can be formatted in three dimensions and to preferentially show hard or soft tissue. By altering the density and thickness of the CT cuts, small bone fragments and soft tissue detail can be evaluated. Coronal views are particularly helpful in the evaluation of orbital floor fractures.[19] The disadvantages of CT are its expense; equipment is not available at all hospitals; it provides less resolution than standard radiographs; patients must remain motionless for 2 seconds during imaging; and artifacts from metal objects such as dental restorations obscures images.[20,21]

Classification of Fractures

In 1961 Knight and North classified zygomatic fractures by the direction of displacement on a Waters' view radiograph.[22] They classified 120 fractures into six groups, hypothesizing that stability after reduction might be related to the direction of displacement. The six groups are as follows (Fig. 21–4):

Group I: Nondisplaced fractures—Cases in which there is no clinical or radiographic evidence of displacement; no treatment is required.

Group II: Arch fractures—A pure fracture of the zygomatic arch. The classical three fracture lines produces a V-shaped deformity.

Group III: Unrotated body fractures—The cause is a direct blow to the zygomatic prominence. The zygoma is driven posteriorly and medially, producing a flattening of the cheek. A Waters' view indicates that the infraorbital rim is displaced inferiorly and medially at the buttress.

Group IV: Medially rotated body fractures—The cause is a blow from above the horizontal axis of the zygoma. The bone is driven medially, inferiorly, and posteriorly with rotation. The radiograph demonstrates displacement inferiorly at the infraorbital rim and either outward at the malar buttress or inward at the frontozygomatic suture.

Group V: Laterally rotated body fractures—The cause is a blow below the horizontal axis of the bone. The zygoma is displaced medially and posteriorly with lateral rotation. The radiograph indicates upward displacement at the infraorbital rim and lateral displacement at the frontozygomatic suture.

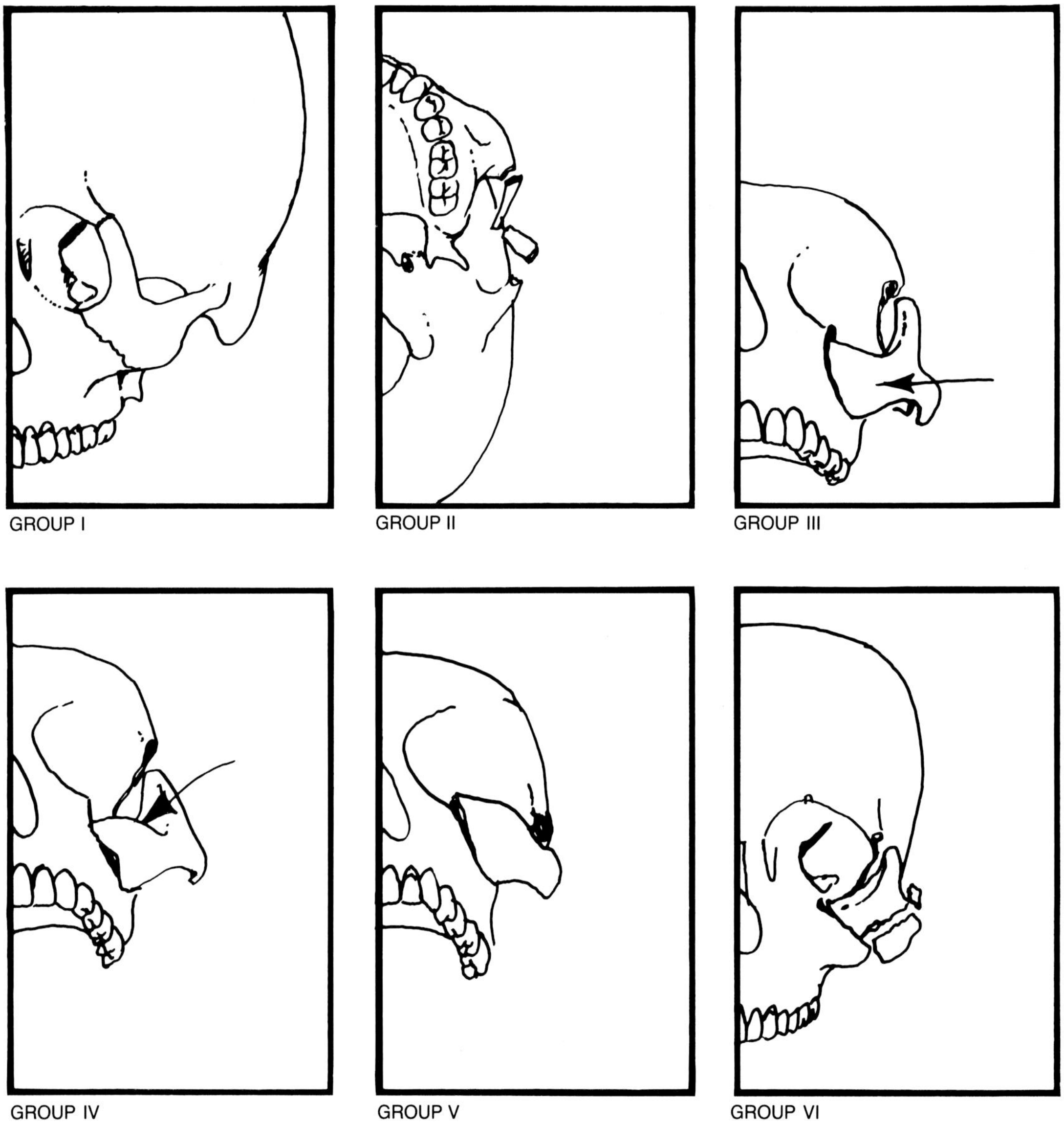

Figure 21–4. *The Knight and North classification for zygomatic fractures.* Group I: *Undisplaced fracture.* Group II: *Arch fracture only.* Group III: *Unrotated body fracture.* Group IV: *Medial rotated body fracture.* Group V: *Laterally rotated body fracture.* Group VI: *Complex fracture.*

Group VI: Complex fractures—These have additional fractures across the body of the zygoma.

In 1968 Rowe and Kiley modified the Knight and North classification. Additional consideration was given to integrity of the periosteal "envelope" of the bone and accuracy and adequacy of the bony apposition at the fracture interface.[6,23] In 1973 Yanagisawa evaluated 200 zygomatic fractures and modified the Rowe and Kiley classification.[24] Yanagisawa's classification addressed the additional component of rotation around longitudinal (sagittal or anteroposterior) and vertical planes. This modified classification had the following effects:

Groups I and II: Unchanged.
Group III: Medial or lateral rotation around a vertical axis.
Group IV: Medial or lateral rotation around a longitudinal axis.
Group V: Medial or lateral displacement without rotation.

Group VI: Isolated rim fracture.
Group VII: All complex fractures.

In 1978 Larsen and Thomson proposed a simplified classification method[25]:

Group I: Nondisplaced fractures requiring no treatment—During the initial evaluation, if there is any doubt about stability, reevaluation should occur 1 week after injury.
Group II: All fractures requiring treatment—The group is further divided into fractures that are stable and fractures that are unstable after reduction.

TREATMENT

Classification techniques, if they are accepted, are helpful to standardize terminology, to plan treatment, and to predict prognosis. However, the surgeon must individualize treatment based on a combination of sound clinical judgment, history, physical examination, and radiologic findings.

Management of ZMC and zygomatic arch fractures depends on the degree of displacement and the resultant aesthetic and functional deficits. Treatment may therefore range from simple observation of resolving swelling, extraocular muscle dysfunction, and paresthesia to open reduction and internal fixation of multiple fractures.

Zygomatic Arch Fractures

Minimally and nondisplaced zygomatic arch fractures may require no surgical correction. Because these injuries usually do not result in significant functional deficits, it may be appropriate to simply observe the patient.[30]

Duverney was the first surgeon to describe an operative technique for treatment of a fractured zygomatic arch.[26] He used intraoral finger pressure to elevate the depressed arch. Alternatively in this technique, the patient is instructed to bite on a block of wood, which results in temporalis muscle and tendon tension. This force, along with finger pressure in an outward direction, reduces the fracture.[26]

Fractures requiring an operation should be treated no later than 7 to 10 days following injury.[11] Beyond this time period, the fracture may be partially healed and difficult to reduce. In addition, irregularities at the edges of the bony fragments resorb and the fracture has a greater tendency to be unstable following reduction.

Goldthwaite (1924) was the first to describe an intraoral approach to the zygomatic arch through a stab wound in the buccal sulcus.[27] A sharp elevator is passed superiorly through the vestibule and behind the maxillary tuberosity and forward pressure is applied to reduce the arch.

Quinn modified this technique by making an incision in the mucosa at the level of the maxillary alveolus and extending it inferiorly along the anterior border of the ramus. The dissection continues along the lateral aspect of the coronoid process, ending at the level of the zygomatic arch at the site of the fracture. An elevator is placed between the coronoid processes and zygomatic arch, and the fracture is reduced.[28]

The standard technique for treatment of zygomatic arch fractures, first described by Gillies, Kilner, and Stone in 1927, can also be used to reduce ZMC fractures.[29] A temporal incision (2 cm in length) is made behind the hairline. The dissection continues through the subcutaneous and superficial temporal fascia down to the glistening white deep temporal fascia (Fig. 21–5, A). The temporal fascia is incised horizontally, and a sturdy elevator is inserted deep to the fascia, underneath the temporal surface of the zygoma. The elevator must pass between the deep temporal fascia and temporalis muscle or it will be lateral to the arch. The bone should be elevated in an outward and forward direction, with care taken not to put force on the temporal bone (Fig. 21–5, B). The arch should be palpated at all times as a guide to proper reduction. The wound is closed in layers.

Following reduction without internal fixation, the zygomatic arch may require temporary support to maintain its position. A Penrose drain or $\frac{1}{2}$-in strip gauze may be used to pack the temporal fossa deep to the arch. Alternatively, a urinary catheter may be placed medial to the arch and the balloon inflated to support the arch during the early phase of fracture healing. The pack or catheter is removed in 7 to 10 days.[11] External support techniques such as Kirschner's wire (K-wire) fixation or transcutaneous suspension from a halo or biphase appliance have also been described.[31] Although not a support technique, an aluminum foam–rubber-backed finger splint has been used to prevent the patient from placing undue force on the arch. The splint is formed into a U shape, taped to the face, and maintained for 3 to 5 days.[32]

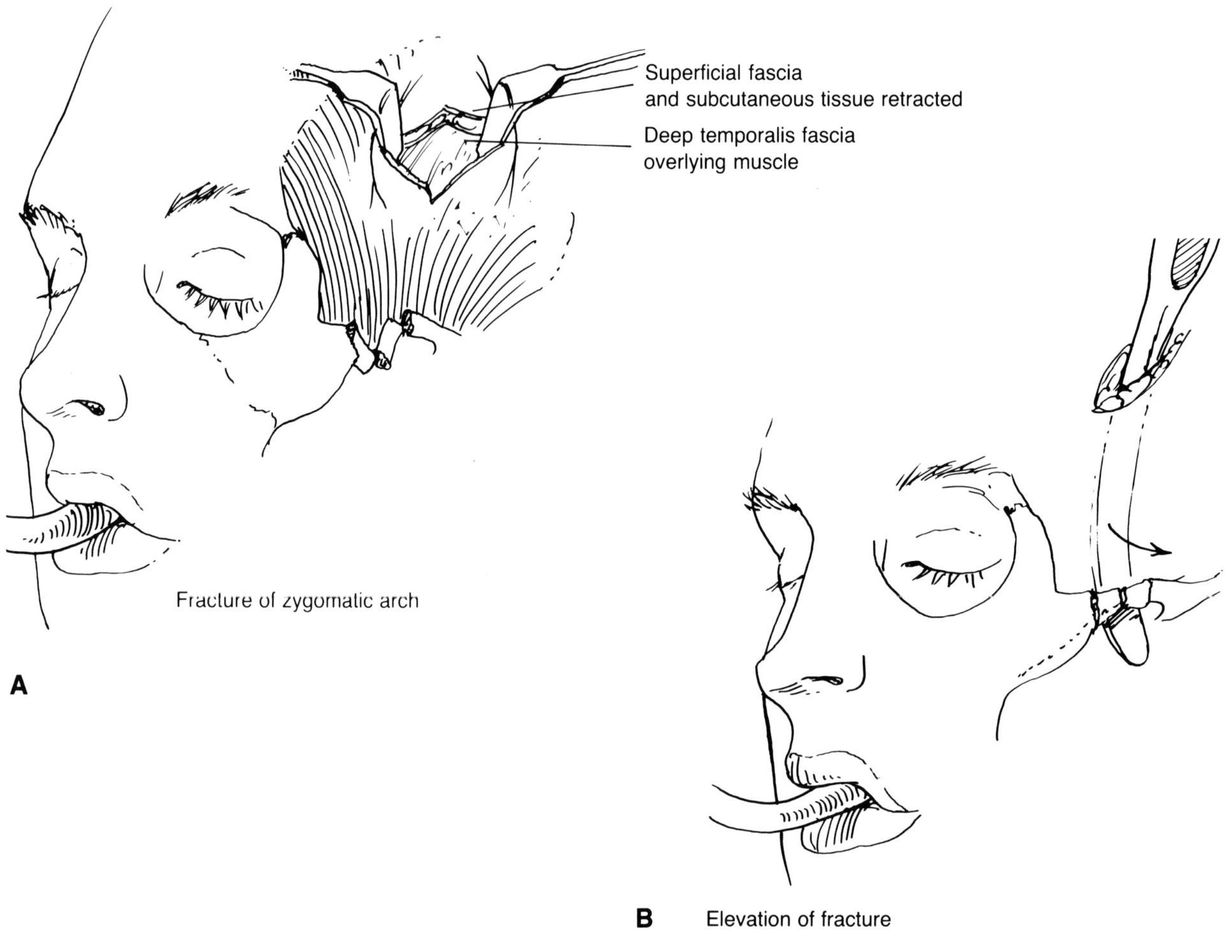

Figure 21–5. *Gillies' approach to reduce zygomatic arch fracture. (**A**) Temporal incision through subcutaneous and superficial fascia down to the deep temporal fascia. (**B**) Reduction of fracture with elevator.*

Open reduction with direct fixation is seldom necessary for treatment of zygomatic arch fractures. Direct fixation by intraosseous wires or miniplates is convenient when there is a laceration over the arch.

Zygomatic Complex

Nondisplaced ZMC fractures require no operative correction. The patient should be observed longitudinally for signs of displacement, extraocular muscle dysfunction, and enophthalmos after swelling resolves. Stable, minimally displaced ZMC fractures without significant clinical findings may require no treatment. The patient should be made to appreciate the risk of residual asymmetry of the cheek, orbit, and eyelid if the fracture is not reduced. Good documentation, including photographs, is recommended.[11]

It has been reported that 60% to 64% of zygomatic fractures will remain stable following reduction without fixation.[22,25] In contrast, Pozatek, Kaban, and Guralnick, using the Knight and North classification, found a larger percentage required stabilization to achieve optimal results.[6] Chuong and Kaban reported 85.5% of ZMC fractures treated by open reduction required fixation at the frontozygomatic suture, infraorbital rim, or both.[33]

Closed Reduction

Closed reduction of a ZMC fracture can be performed with an intraoral or extraoral approach. Intraorally, a

1-cm incision in the depth of the sulcus is made opposite the first and second molars. An elevator is directed posteriorly and superiorly under the zygoma, and force is applied in an upward and outward direction to reduce the fracture. Extraorally, the Gillies' approach may be used for closed reduction of the ZMC fracture in a manner similar to that described in treatment of zygomatic arch fractures. (Fig. 21–5).[29]

Poswillo described the use of an extraoral traction hook.[34] A stab incision is made about $\frac{3}{4}$ in below the lateral canthus of the eye. Through the incision, the point of the "malar" hook is introduced until it engages the displaced bone. The fracture is reduced by an upward and outward pull. Adequate reduction is determined by palpation. Rather than using a traction hook, others have advocated the use of a Carroll-Girard screw (Fig. 21–6). The instrument is introduced through a similar incision, screwed into the zygoma, and then used for reduction of the fracture.

Open Reduction

INCISIONS. Access and exposure for open reduction of a ZMC fracture are achieved through a lateral eyebrow or eyelid incision (frontozygomatic suture), a lower eyelid or infraorbital incision (infraorbital rim and orbital floor), and an intraoral vestibular incision (zygomatic buttress).

The frontozygomatic suture is palpated and then a 2.5-cm incision is made within the confines of the lateral eyebrow parallel to the superior lateral orbital rim (Fig. 21–7, A). Sharp dissection is continued to the fracture site. The eyebrow should not be shaved because the hair will not grow back. The lateral brow incision is the most common approach for access to the frontozygomatic suture.[36]

Chuong and Kaban have described the use of an upper eyelid incision (Fig. 21–7, B).[33] The incision is placed within the lateral aspect of the supratarsal fold. A 1.5-cm incision is usually adequate and rarely extends into the "crow's foot." Blunt dissection parallel to the orbicularis oculi muscle fibers separates them and exposes the frontozygomatic suture. The dissection is continued, superficial to the orbital septum and down to the periosteum over the lateral orbital rim. This incision provides more direct access to the frontozygomatic suture and results in a less noticeable scar.

To expose the infraorbital rim, a subciliary incision is made 1 to 2 mm below and parallel to the lower eyelash margin (Fig. 21–7, A). It should extend from just lateral to the punctum and then inferiorly in a natural skin fold. A skin flap is dissected to the level of the infraorbital rim. The fibers of the orbicularis oculi muscle are then separated to expose the rim. The periosteum is then incised and dissected off the rim to allow for exploration of the orbital floor (Fig. 21–8). This layered approach to the orbital rim is important. Failure to perform the dissection in this fashion may result in a higher incidence of ectropion. In addition, an incision below the tarsus is less likely to result in vertical shortening of the eyelid.[37]

Tessier described a conjunctival incision (Fig. 21–7, C).[38] The lower lid is retracted, and an incision is made below the lower border of the tarsus. Dissection is extended inferiorly, and a preseptal (superficial to the orbital septum) incision is used to expose the bone. Converse modified this approach by use of a retroseptal transconjunctival incision.[39] Converse's method allows dissection to the septum orbitale without herniation of the orbital fat. This technique often requires a lateral canthotomy for adequate exposure and reattachment of the ligament on closure.

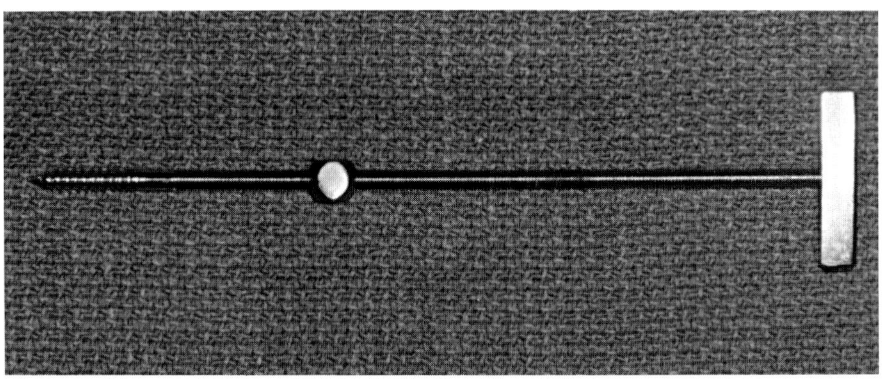

Figure 21–6. *Carroll-Girard screw.*

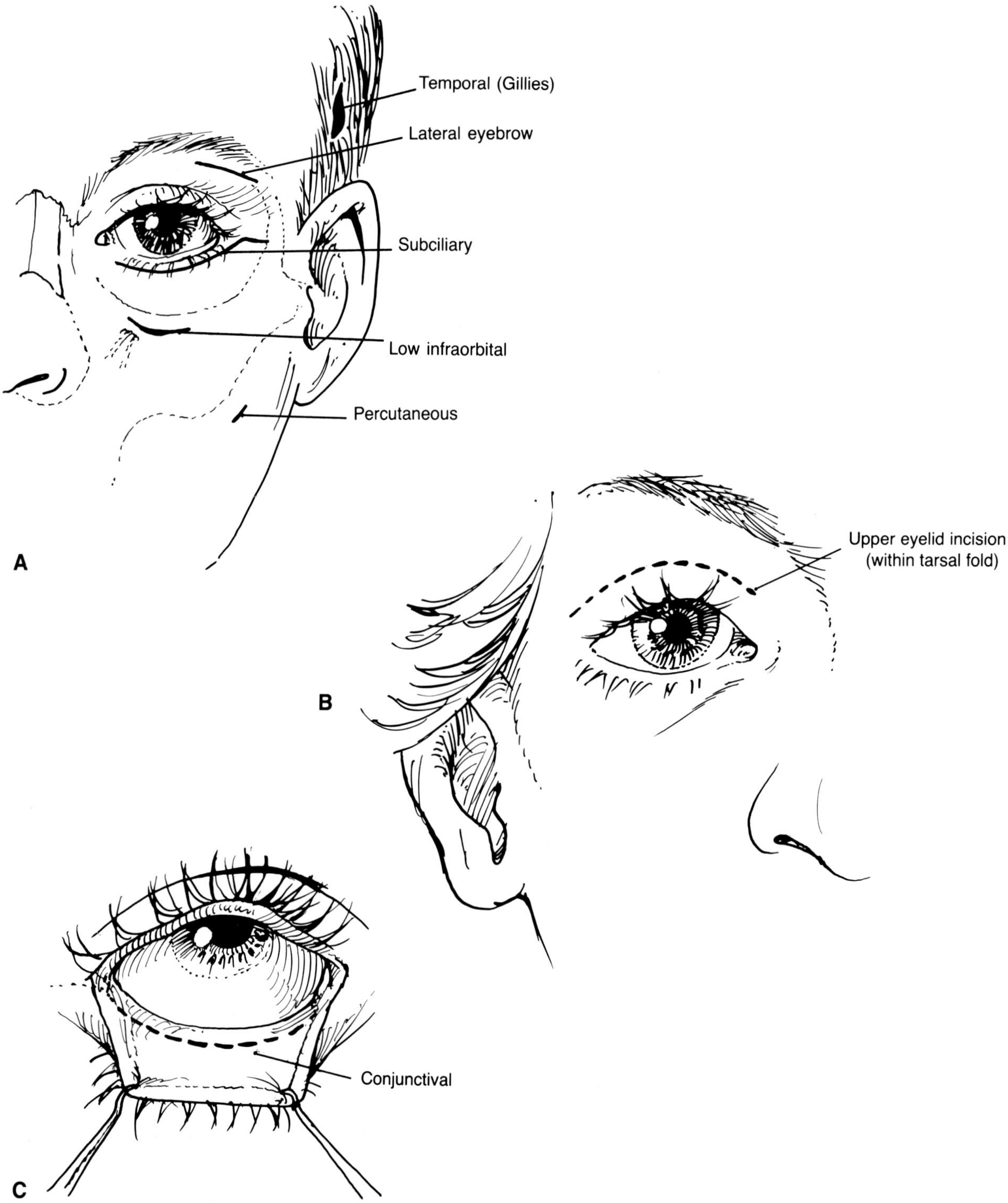

Figure 21–7. *Frontal view illustrating periorbital incision sites. (**A**) Illustrates five different periorbital incision sites for access to the orbital rim. (**B**) Upper eyelid incision within the lateral supratarsal fold. (**C**) Conjunctival incision within the lower border of the tarsus.*

The infraorbital incision is made approximately 5 mm below the lower lid margin through a natural skin fold (Fig. 21–7, A). The subcutaneous dissection is extended to the lower eyelid and then deepened through the orbicularis oculi muscle to the orbital rim. The periosteum is incised along the orbital rim and elevated from the orbital floor (Fig. 21–8). Layering the dissection helps to decrease scarring and fixation of the soft tissue to the bony orbital rim.

All three approaches to the infraorbital rim may result in potential complications, and the infraorbital incision may result in an unacceptable scar. The subciliary and conjunctival incisions may result in ectropion or entropion, respectively. Wray conducted a postoperative follow-up study of 45 subciliary and 45 conjunctival incisions.[37] Entropion was present in none of the subciliary incisions and in one of the conjunctival incisions. Ectropion was present in 19 of the subciliary incisions and none of the conjunctival incisions. Of the 19 patients with ectropion, 15 were transient. Ectropion that was present after 3 months demonstrated no further signs of improvement.

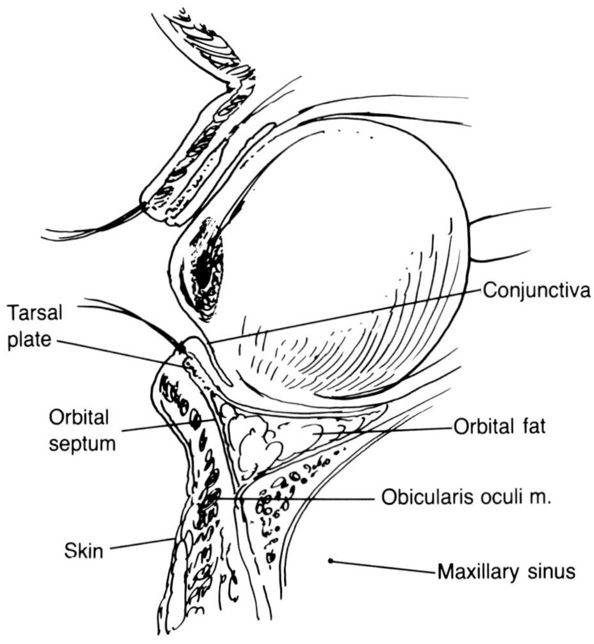

Figure 21–8. *Sagittal view of eye illustrating relation of conjunctiva, orbital septum and fat, and orbicularis muscle to the eye and infraorbital rim.*

In cases of severe zygomatic fractures or secondary correction of zygomatic deformities, access is limited with conventional incisions. To obtain adequate exposure, a coronal incision combined with a lower eyelid approach is recommended. The skin incision is made through a preauricular skin fold and extended into the temporal region to the top of the skull. The dissection is along the temporal fascia. As the superior orbital rim is identified, the dissection is continued into the orbit in a subperiosteal manner. For adequate exposure, the supraorbital nerve and vessel may need to be reflected, requiring bone removal from the foramen. The dissection is extended inferiorly to the zygomatic arch and medially to the lateral orbital rim. The facial nerve is protected within the flap. Although tunneling subperiosteally along the orbital floor is often possible, the anterior wall of the maxilla and orbital floor may need to be exposed through a lower eyelid incision.[10]

In summary, the frontozygomatic region should be exposed with a lateral eyebrow or upper eyelid incision. The incision of choice for the infraorbital rim and orbital floor is the subciliary incision. The dissection should be done in a layered fashion to avoid ectropion. An intraoral vestibule incision may be used for exposure of the buttress.

Fixation

DIRECT FIXATION. Wire osteosynthesis has been used extensively for stabilization of bone fractures and fragments. The frontozygomatic suture and infraorbital rim fracture may be secured with a 26-gauge wire. While drilling and passing the wire, care must be taken not to injure the globe. The infraorbital rim, if not comminuted, may be secured with 26-gauge wire. When the fracture is comminuted, the fragments can be maintained in position with 28-gauge wire.

The use of a K-wire for stabilization is advocated by Brown and Matsunaga.[40,41] The authors report a shorter opening time and fewer complications such as globe injuries and ectropion. Brown described a transnasal approach using a transnasal (.062) K-wire.[40] The wire was placed through the skin and body of the zygoma after reduction and extended into or through the opposite maxilla and zygoma for stabilization. The wire was cut, covered, then removed after 2 to 3 weeks. Matsunaga believed that the K-wire placed in the direction described by Brown allowed the muscles to rotate the zygoma in an eccentric fashion. He reduces the fracture through a Gillies' approach and stabilizes the fracture with a Steinmann pin.[41] The pin is driven in a transmalar direction, aiming obliquely through the sinus for a point on the hard palate approximately 2 cm posterior to the anterior nasal spine. This passage anchors the ZMC fragment eccentric to the usual axis of rotation, providing stability. The pin is cut flush to the skin and is removed after 6 weeks of healing.

Osteosynthesis of zygomatic fractures is now possible with the development of the miniplate.[46] The plates are small, low in profile, easily adaptable, and have sufficient strength to maintain stability. A variety of plate designs provides the surgeon with unlimited stabilization possibilities.

Miniplates can be placed at the frontozygomatic suture, buttress, and infraorbital rim. One miniplate may provide sufficient stabilization when the orbital floor is not severely fractured. The plate is placed extraorally at the frontozygomatic suture or intraorally at the buttress. Fracture stability is dependent on adequate reduction and secure placement of the plate. If the fracture remains unstable, more than one plate should be placed. One long or series of multiple plates are useful when the bone has been severely comminuted.

External pin fixation with a stabilizing bar has been used in the past. This technique is effective but often inconvenient for the patient and carries a small risk of infection around the pins.[31]

INDIRECT FIXATION. Indirect fixation techniques may also be used to stabilize the ZMC fracture. Jackson described the use of an antral balloon introduced into the maxillary sinus through a nasal antrostomy.[35] Jarabak used a urinary catheter through an oroantral approach.[43] With this approach, the orbital floor may be visualized and inadvertent displacement of bony fragments is less likely to occur. Gutman reported a successful outcome in 38 fractures using this technique.[44]

ZMC fractures that require treatment should undergo exploration of at least one fracture site, allowing the surgeon to judge the reduction. If doubts remain, further sites should be explored. Once reduced, wire osteosynthesis at the frontozygomatic suture and infraorbital rim or rigid fixation with a miniplate at the frontozygomatic, infraorbital rim, buttress, or a combination of these is recommended for stabilization.

Orbital Floor Considerations

A ZMC fracture includes injury to the orbital floor. Crumley reported a series of 324 orbital floor fractures in which 46% were associated with ZMC fractures.[9] Chuong and Kaban reported that orbital floor exploration was required in 58% of ZMC fractures requiring open reduction.[33] Clinical findings associated with orbital floor injuries include: enophthalmos, extraocular muscle dysfunction with an abnormal forced duction test, diplopia, and infraorbital paresthesia. When any of the signs are present, a CT scan should be obtained to document the status of the orbit.[6]

Fujiino et al. classified orbital floor injuries as linear and pure blow-out fractures.[45] A linear fracture occurs when the infraorbital rim is struck, displacing the orbital contents and floor posteriorly. The orbital septum is torn, herniating soft tissue into the maxillary sinus. When the force is removed, the orbital floor returns to its original position and the soft tissues are entrapped in the fracture site. Comminution of the orbital floor is produced by a force 10 times greater than that required for a linear fracture. Fragments are forced inferiorly into the sinus, producing bony discontinuity.

Treatment

The decision to explore the orbital floor is a difficult one to make, and the subject has produced considerable controversy in the literature.[9,31,33,47–49] It is important to remember that the degree of orbital floor disruption is often greater than that which appears on the radiographs. The indications for exploration of the orbital floor in the presence of a ZMC fracture include enophthalmos greater than 3 mm; limitation of extraocular muscle function; and a large orbital floor defect with herniation of soft tissue into the sinuses seen on CT scan or tomograms.

Access to the floor is accomplished by a subciliary, conjunctival, or infraorbital incision. Simple linear fractures may require only removal of entrapped tissue. Larger defects require reduction of the fragments and soft tissue from the sinus and reconstruction of the floor with a bone graft or implant. The orbital floor may be reconstructed with an autograft, allograft, or a prosthetic implant.[31] Autograft sources include the rib, the iliac crest, the calvaria, and ear or nasal cartilage. Allograft sources include lyophilized dura, the rib, the iliac crest, and cartilage. Alloplastic materials such as Teflon, Silastic, Marlex Mesh, and Gelfilm have been used successfully.[47]

The Role of Bone Grafting

Early bone grafting is limited to severe injuries in which there is loss of bone or extensive comminution. These ZMC fractures are often associated with other severe midface fractures that require treatment. Grafts may help to achieve anatomic reduction and stability, as well as to prevent soft tissue contraction.[50]

The asymmetry that results from inadequate reduction of a ZMC fracture may require bone graft contour augmentation (Fig. 21–9, A to C). Access is achieved through a coronal flap and craniofacial dissection.

Chuong and Kaban advocate the use of calvarial bone for ZMC reconstruction because it can be harvested through the primary incision and because early experimental and clinical studies indicate that there is less resorption than with iliac crest bone (Fig. 21–10, A and B).[33] Temporoparietal calvaria offers an excellent contour for reconstruction, and there is little postoperative morbidity. The bone graft is contoured to correct the asymmetry and is secured into position by either wire, suture, bone plates, or screws.

Postoperative Care

ZMC fractures violate the maxillary sinus. For this reason, antibiotics and decongestants are recommended. Penicillin is the antibiotic of choice (1 million U every 6 hours). A first generation cephalosporin (1 gm by IV tid) may be used in the presence of penicillin allergic patients. A decongestant such as pseudoephedrine (30 mg tid) is also used to clear the airway.

Incisions are observed carefully for signs of infection, and the eye is examined to document visual acuity and to rule out complications such as corneal abrasion. Postoperative radiographs (Waters', Submentovertex) are obtained to document reduction of the fracture.

COMPLICATIONS

Although complications of ZMC and zygomatic arch fractures are uncommon, the surgeon must recognize their signs and symptoms to provide appropriate care. The most serious complications involve the eye and surrounding structures.

Eye

Corneal Abrasion

Corneal abrasion or conjunctival irritation may occur as a result of the initial injury, operative trauma, or corneal or conjunctival desiccation. The patient usually complains of a "scratchy feeling" or "sand in the eye." If corneal abrasion is identified, topical antibiotics should be administered, an eye patch applied, and an ophthalmologist consulted.[31]

Retrobulbar Hemorrhage

This rare but severe complication may be the result of either the initial injury or the operative correction. Disruption of the retinal circulation may lead to irreversible ischemia and permanent blindness. In a review of 1405 ZMC fractures Ord reported a 0.3% incidence of postoperative retrobulbar hemorrhage with visual loss.[51] An emergent ophthalmologic consultation is necessary.

Superior Orbital Fissure Syndrome

This rare complication is the result of compression of the structures within the superior orbital fissure. Trauma and neoplasms are the two most common causes.[53]

Traumatic Hyphema

Trauma to the eye may result in bleeding into the anterior chamber—the area between the clear cornea and the colored iris. An ophthalmologist should be

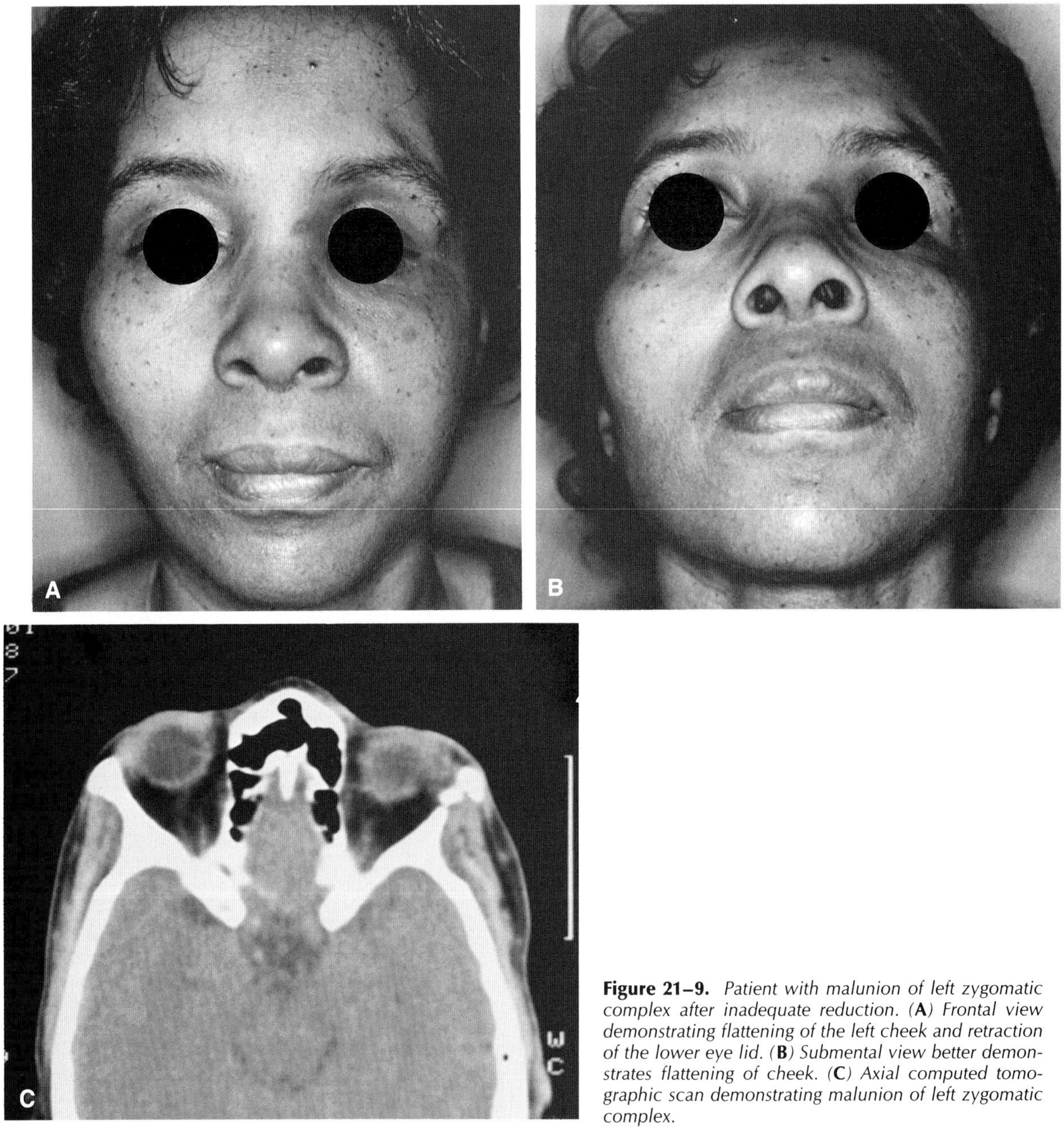

Figure 21–9. *Patient with malunion of left zygomatic complex after inadequate reduction. (**A**) Frontal view demonstrating flattening of the left cheek and retraction of the lower eye lid. (**B**) Submental view better demonstrates flattening of cheek. (**C**) Axial computed tomographic scan demonstrating malunion of left zygomatic complex.*

consulted. Initial treatment consists of a combination of bedrest, use of a cycloplegic agent, and eye-shield protection.

Other Eye Injuries

Other serious but uncommon eye injuries that may occur following a ZMC fracture include lens dislocation,[55] a ruptured globe,[55] retinal detachment,[55] and canalicular injuries.[56]

Neurosensory Deficiencies

The incidence of sensory alterations (loss of sensation or hyperesthesia) of the infraorbital nerve following zygomatic trauma ranges from 18% to 56%.[12-17] With-

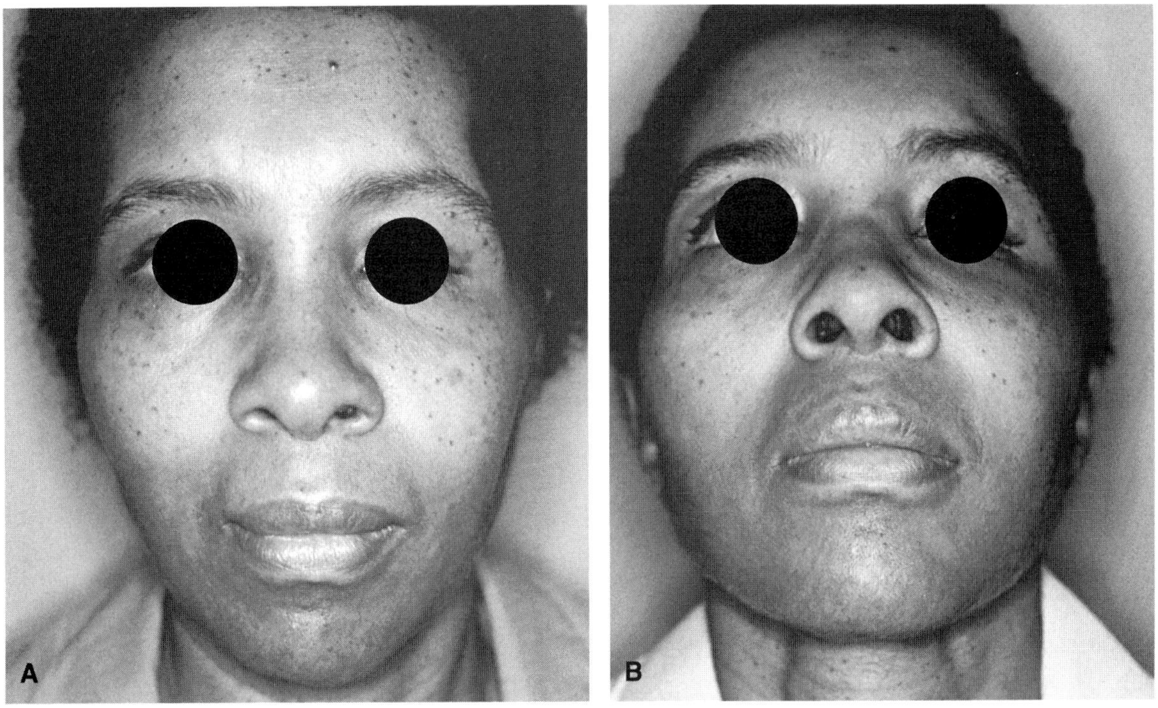

Figure 21–10. *Same patient as in Fig. 21-9, 24 months after calvarial bone graft to left zygomatic complex. (**A**) Frontal view demonstrating symmetry of orbits and periorbital soft tissues. (**B**) Submental view better demonstrates symmetrical appearance of cheeks.*

out special attention to the nerve, open reduction techniques provide no more restoration of function than closed techniques. Reports of sensory alterations in the nerve following open reduction range from 22% to 65% versus 20% to 40% for closed reduction.[13-15]

Proof is lacking, but it seems likely that entrapment of the nerve or perineural fibrosis is responsible for persistent deficits. Total anesthesia is usually tolerated better than hyperesthesia or dysesthesia, which may be very unpleasant.[32]

There is little evidence to suggest that late decompression has any therapeutic value. The occasional patient with severe dysesthesia, hyperesthesia, or debilitating anesthesia may benefit from surgical treatment. Exploration of the orbital floor through an extraoral approach should be done to remove any bone spicules or to decompress the nerve. Alternatively, an intraoral approach may be necessary to relieve scar tissue along the nerve, following its exit from the foramen. Results are disappointing, with recovery taking from 12 to 18 months. Should treatment be unsuccessful, destruction of the nerve by cryosurgery, alcohol, or peripheral neurectomy may be necessary.

Enophthalmos

Enophthalmos may be a noticeable and debilitating consequence of zygomatic fractures with a reported incidence of 5% to 26%. Treatment of this complication is difficult, and the results are poor. As high as 80% of treated patients have persistence of enophthalmos.[12,14,15,17] It appears that better results are achieved with early reduction of the orbital floor and soft tissue at the time of ZMC reduction.

Malunion and Asymmetry

Malunited fractures of the zygoma occur in varying degrees of severity. Although the majority of cases results in a cosmetic deficit, malposition of the bone can result in impairment of mandibular function. The reported incidence of asymmetry ranges from 3.6% to 27% of all ZMC fractures, but these numbers are based only on clinical judgment.[1,12,14,15,17]

The majority of malunited fractures of the zygoma result from failure to recognize the severity of the injury or an unstable reduction. Malunion that is recognized up to 6 weeks after injury may be corrected, using routine zygomatic reduction techniques.[56] Late corrective technique involves onlay grafts with autograft or homograft (iliac crest, rib, calvaria, cartilage, or dermal fat) or alloplastic materials and zygomatic ostectomy. Although alloplastic materials have been advocated, contours resulting from implants may be irregular, and there is a potential for migration and extrusion of the implant over time. For minor deformities, cartilage has proven effective. However, larger defects require the placement of bone or craniofacial repositioning. The use of calvarial bone and the surgical approach were discussed earlier in this chapter.

Success is dependent on an accurate assessment of the patient's contour requirement, an appropriate choice of procedure, and the material used. The use of three-dimensional reconstruction models can be useful to determine the necessary recontouring or repositioning of the zygoma.

Trismus

Limited range of mandibular motion may be a debilitating complication of zygomatic fractures. The most common cause is impingement of the zygomatic body on the coronoid process of the mandible. Trismus may also occur secondary to fibrous or fibroosseous ankylosis of the coronoid to the zygomatic arch.[11,52] Impingement of the zygoma or zygomatic arch on the coronoid process is identified by CT scan. Repositioning of the zygoma or zygomatic arch or coronoidectomy may be necessary to restore normal movement of the mandible.

SUMMARY

In this chapter, we discussed the surgical anatomic features, diagnosis, and treatment techniques for ZMC and zygoma arch fractures. A careful history, physical examination, and radiographic evaluation are critical to document the injury. Treatment should be planned using this information along with sound operative principles and techniques described in this chapter.

REFERENCES

1. Martin BC, Trabue JC, Leech TR. An analysis of the etiology, treatment and complications of fractures of the malar compound and zygomatic arch. Am J Surg 1956; 92:920.
2. Matsunaga RS, Simpson W. Simplified protocol for the treatment of malar fractures. Arch Otolaryngol 1977; 103:535.
3. Winstanley RD. The management of fractures of zygoma. Int J Oral Surg 1981; 10(s):235.
4. Edgerton MT Jr. Emergency care of maxillo-facial injury. In: Zuidema GD, ed. The management of trauma. Philadelphia: WB Saunders, 1979; 286.
5. Luce EA, Tubb TD, Moore AM. Review of 1000 major facial fractures and associated injuries. Plast Reconstr Surg 1979; 63(1):26.
6. Pozatek ZW, Kaban LB, Guralnick WC. Fractures of the zygomatic complex: An evaluation of surgical management with special emphasis on the eyebrow approach. J Oral Surg 1973; 31:141.
7. Banovetz JD, Duvall AJ. Zygomatic fractures: Symposium on maxillofacial trauma. Otolaryngol Clin North Am 1976; 9(2):499.
8. Rontal E, Rontal M, Guilford FT. Surgical anatomy of the orbit. Ann Otol Rhinol Laryngol 1979; 88:382.
9. Crumley RL, Leibsohn J, Krause CJ, Burton TC. Fractures of the orbital floor. Laryngoscope 1977; 87:934.
10. Shaw RC, Parsons RW. Exposure through a coronal incision for initial treatment of facial fractures. Plast Reconstr Surg 1975; 56:254.
11. Feinstein FR, Krizek TJ. Fractures of the zygoma and zygomatic arch. In: Foster CA, Sherman JE, eds. Surgery of facial bone fractures. New York: Churchhill Livingstone, 1987; 123.
12. Hotta HHA. Orbital fractures. Springfield, IL: Charles C Thomas, 1970.
13. Lund K. Fractures of the zygoma: A follow-up study of 62 patients. J Oral Surg 1971; 29:557.
14. Altonen M, Kohonen A, Dickhoff K. Treatment of zygomatic fractures: Internal wiring antral packing reposition without fixation. J Maxillofac Surg 1976; 4:107.
15. Hardt H, Steinhauser EW. Treatment results after zygomatic-orbital fractures. Schweiz Monatsschr Zahnheilkd 1976; 86:825.
16. Schiffer HP, Austerman KH, Busse H. Ophthalmological long-term effects of malar fractures. Klin Monatsbl Augenheilkd 1977; 171:567.
17. Larsen OD, Thomsen M. Zygomatic fractures: A follow up study of 17 patients. Scand J Plast Reconstr Surg 1978; 12:59.
18. Schultz RC. Fractures of the middle third of the face. In: Facial injuries. Chicago: Year Book Medical Publishers, 1988; 283.

19. Hammerschlag SB, Hughes S, O'Reiley GV, et al. Blowout fracture of the orbit: A comparison of CT and conventional radiography with anatomic correlation. Radiology 1982; 143:487.
20. Noyek AM, Kassel EE, Wortzman G, Jazrawy H, Greyson ND, Zizmor J. Contemporary radiologic evaluation in maxillofacial trauma. Otolaryngol Clin North Am 1983; 16(3):473.
21. Finkle DR, Ringler SL, Luttenten CR, Beernink JH, Peterson NT, Dean RE. Comparison of the diagnostic methods used in maxillofacial trauma. Plast Reconstr Surg 1985; 75(1):32.
22. Knight JS, North JF. The classification of malar fractures: An analysis of displacement as a guide to treatment. Br J Plast Surg 1961; 13:325.
23. Rowe NL, Killey HC. In: Fractures of the facial skeleton, ed 2. Edinburgh and London: E & S Livingstone, 1968.
24. Yanagisawa E. Symposium on maxillo-facial trauma. III. Pitfalls in the management of zygomatic fractures. Laryngoscope 1973; 83:527.
25. Larsen OD, Thomsen M. Zygomatic fractures. I. A simplified classification for practical use. Scand J Plast Reconstr Surg 1978; 12:55.
26. Smith HW, Yanagisawa E. Fracture-dislocations of zygoma and zygomatic arch. Arch Otolaryngol 1961; 73:68.
27. Goldthwaite RH. Plastic repair of depressed fracture of lower orbital rim. JAMA 1924; 82:628.
28. Quinn JH. Lateral coronoid approach for intra-oral reduction of fractures of the zygomatic arch. J Oral Surg 1977; 35:321.
29. Gillies HD, Kilner TP, Stone D. Fractures of the malarzygomatic compound, with a description of a new x-ray position. Br J Surg 1927; 14:651.
30. Dingman RO, Natvig P. In: Surgery of facial fractures. Philadelphia: WB Saunders 1964.
31. Rowe NL, Williams JL, ed. Fractures of the zygomatic complex and orbital. In: Maxillofacial injuries. Edinburgh: Churchhill-Livingstone, 1985; 435.
32. Thomson ERE. A simple zygomatic splint. Br Dent J 1983; 155:257.
33. Chuong R, Kaban LB. Fractures of the zygomatic complex. J Oral Maxillofac Surg 1986; 44:283.
34. Poswillo D. Reduction of the fractured malar by a traction hook. Br J Oral Surg 1976; 14:76.
35. Kackson WR, Abbey JA, Glanz S. Balloon technique for treatment of fractures of the zygomatic bone. J Oral Surg 1956; 14:14.
36. Converse JM, ed. The clinical management of facial injuries and fractures of the facial bones. In: Reconstructive plastic surgery, ed 2. Philadelphia: WB Saunders, 1977; 599.
37. Wray RC, Holtmann B, Ribaudo JM, Keiter J, Weeks PM. A comparison of conjunctival and subciliary incisions for orbital fractures. Br J Plast Surg 1977; 30:142.
38. Tessier P. The conjunctival approach to the orbital floor and maxilla in congenital malformations and trauma. J Maxillofac Surg 1973; 1:3.
39. Converse JM, Firmin F, Wood-Smith D, Friedland JAN. The conjunctival approach in orbital fractures. Plast Reconstr Surg 1973; 52:656.
40. Brown J, Barnard D. The trans-nasal Kirschner wire as a method of fixation of the unstable fracture of the zygomatic complex. Br J Oral Surg 1983; 21:208.
41. Matsunaga RS, Simpson W, Toffel PH. Simplified protocol for treatment of malar fractures. Arch Otolaryngol 1977; 103:555.
42. Kawamoto HK. Late posttraumatic enophthalmos: A correctible deformity? Plast Reconstr Surg 1982; 3:423.
43. Jarabak JP. Use of Foley catheter in supporting zygomatic fractures. J Oral Surg 1959; 17:39.
44. Gutman D, Laufer D, Neder A. The use of the Foley catheter in the treatment of zygomatic bone fracture. Br J Oral Surg 1965; 2:153.
45. Fujino T, Makino K. Entrapment mechanism and ocular injury in orbital blowout fracture. Plast Reconstr Surg 1980; 65:571.
46. Champy M, Lodde JP. Osteosynthesis of the external orbital cavity using screwed plates: Therapeutic indications and results. Revue Otoneuroopthalmologique 1976; 48:243.
47. Boudreau RG, Tidemann H. Reconstruction of the orbital floor using lyophilised dura: Report of a case. J Oral Surg 1976; 34:618.
48. Burres S, Cohn AM, Mathog RH. Repair of orbital blowout fractures with Marlex mesh and Gelfilm. Laryngoscope 1981; 91:1881.
49. Bartkowski SB, Krzystkowa KM. Blow-out fracture of the orbit: Diagnostic and therapeutic considerations and results in 90 patients treated. J Maxillofac Surg 1982; 10:155.
50. Gruss JS, MacKinnon SE, Kassel EE, et al. The role of primary bone grafting in complex craniomaxillofacial trauma. Plast Reconstr Surg 1985; 75:17.
51. Ord RA. Postoperative retrobulbar hemorrhage and blindness complicating trauma surgery. Br J Oral Surg 1981; 19:202.
52. Karlan M. Complications of malar fractures. In: Mathog R, ed. Maxillofacial trauma. Baltimore: Williams & Wilkins, 1984; 350.
53. Banks P. The superior orbital fissure syndrome. Oral Surg Oral Med Oral Pathol 1967; 24:455.
54. Kershner RM. Management of traumatic hyphema. Resident Staff Physician 1988; 34(1):107.
55. Waring GO. Eye emergency cookbook. Emerg Med 1979; 11:24.
56. Jackson ST. A new probe for silicone intubation of the lacrimal drainage system. Ophthalmic Surg 1980; 11:588.
57. Kellner MJ, Sher M, Stoopack JC. Extracapsular fibrous ankylosis of the mandible after open reduction of a zygomatic arch fracture: Report of case. J Oral Surg 1979; 37:665.

22

Management of Ocular and Orbital Trauma

Michael S. Hauser

The bony orbit contains many of the most functional and delicate structures within the facial skeleton. Unilateral loss of vision is disabling and total blindness is crippling. Orbital trauma must be approached with preservation of binocular vision as the primary goal whenever possible, and restoration and reconstruction of the bony facial skeleton as critically important but secondary goals.

A fracture of the bony orbit, antrum, or zygoma implies potential injury to the eye or periocular structures. Therefore, surgeons who restore the form and function of the facial skeleton must recognize the injury patterns of the eye and the ever present potential to damage a previously intact eye during treatment of a periocular fracture. Periorbital injuries are often best treated by a multidisciplinary approach. However, trauma to the eye proper or the extraocular muscle cone within the periorbital periosteum must be treated by an ophthalmologist. Although interdependent, diagnosis and treatment can be understood by separating the components as follows: bony orbit, periorbital soft tissues, periocular soft tissues, and the eye. This chapter will focus on understanding the individual components involved in orbital trauma.

ANATOMY OF THE ORBIT AND EYE

Diagnosis of orbital trauma and surgery of the region depend on a thorough understanding of the delicate anatomy involved. The orbital region can be broken down into four basic components: The bony orbit, the periocular soft tissues, the globe, and the protective soft tissue apparatus consisting of the lids and lacrimal apparatus. As is the case with facial anatomy in general, it is best learned by studying cadavers and skulls. The following descriptions can serve as a review to aid the reader in the understanding of the medical and surgical treatment of orbital trauma.

The Bony Orbit

The osteology of the orbit consists of a union of the following bones: zygoma, maxilla, lacrimal, ethmoid, frontal, palatine, and sphenoid (Fig. 22–1). The orbital rim is very solid and protects the eye from many injuries. The rim comprises the frontal bone superiorly and laterally, the zygomatic bone laterally and inferiorly, and the maxillary bone inferiorly and medially. Most lateral rim fractures occur at the frontozygomatic suture, and inferior fractures occur at the zygomaticomaxillary suture. The lacrimal sac is tucked into the medial rim between the maxillary and lacrimal bones. The resulting depression forms the anterior and posterior lacrimal crest. The infraorbital nerve and artery exit from the infraorbital foramen, which presents an area of weakness through which anterior rim fractures often occur.

The supraorbital rim is particularly solid and is infrequently fractured, although the frontal sinuses above it may be. The supraorbital nerve and artery

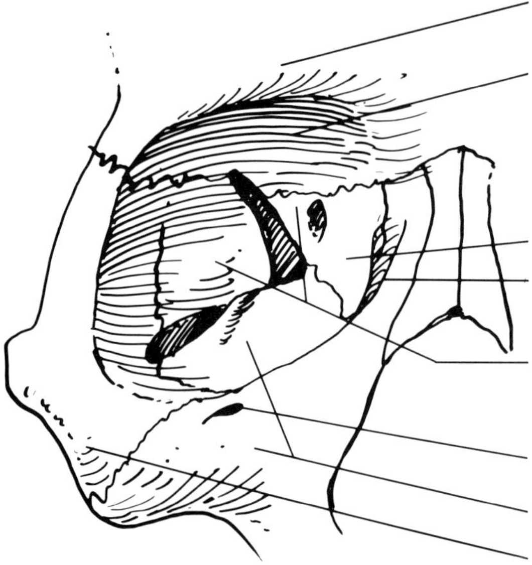

Figure 22–1. *Bony walls of the orbit. (Redrawn from Moore KL. Clinically Oriented Anatomy. Baltimore: Williams and Wilkins, 1985; 888)*

exit from a foramen at the supraorbital notch in the medial aspect of the superior orbital rim. Just posterior to the lateral orbital rim is the orbital tubercle (Whitnall's tubercle), which serves as the attachment for the lateral canthal tendon, and Lockwood's ligament, which suspends the eye.

The orbital walls form roughly a pyramid with the optic foramen at its apex. The medial walls are almost parallel, while the lateral walls diverge at about 45° from the midsagittal plane. The anteroposterior dimension of the orbit is about 4 cm. The medial wall is the thinnest wall (the "paper plate") of the ethmoid bone. Fortunately, it is bolstered by the many septae of the ethmoid sinus on its medial aspect, which provide some support and resistance to fractures. The lateral wall of the orbit lies between the superior and inferior orbital fissures at its posterior aspect. The greater wing of the sphenoid posteriorly and the zygoma anteriorly form the bulk of the wall. The lateral wall is relatively thick and is generally not susceptible to fracture.

The maxillary bone composes the majority of the floor of the orbit. It is most susceptible to fracture because it is relatively thin and forms the roof of the pneumatized maxillary sinus. The floor is further weakened by the infraorbital groove, which contains the infraorbital nerve.

The roof of the orbit is formed primarily by the frontal bone with a small contribution from the lesser wing of the sphenoid. The optic foramen which conducts the optic nerve transverses the roof at its most posterior aspect. The lacrimal gland sits in a fossa anterolaterally, and the trochlea fossa containing the "pulley" of the trochlea muscle is positioned anteromedially.

Orbital Apex

The confluence of the bony walls of the orbit forms the orbital apex. The anatomy of the apex is complex, in a large part due to the superior and inferior orbital fissures. The anterior border of the inferior orbital fissure is approximately 20 mm from the inferior orbital rim. Therefore, during orbital floor exploration, the dissection should not proceed more posteriorly than 20 mm. Structures traversing the inferior orbital fissure include the zygomatic nerve, the inferior orbital vein to the pterygoid plexus, and some parasympathetic nerves from the sphenopalatine ganglion. Posterior to the inferior orbital fissure is the foramen rotundum, which surrounds the maxillary division of the trigeminal nerve. This nerve joins with the infraorbital artery (terminal branch of the maxillary artery) and runs in the infraorbital sulcus immediately beneath the orbital floor terminating at the infraorbital foramen.

The superior orbital fissure runs obliquely between

the greater and lesser wings of the sphenoid. The nerves passing through the fissure are the lacrimal and frontal nerves (V), the trochlear nerve (IV), both divisions of the oculomotor nerve (III), the abducens nerve (VI), and the nasociliary nerve (V). The superior and inferior ophthalmic veins pass through the fissure as well. This group of neurovascular structures passes immediately from the cavernous sinus to the superior orbital fissure, which accounts for the ophthalmoplegia seen with trauma to either of these spaces.

The optic foramen is just medial to the superior orbital fissure and transmits the optic nerve and ophthalmic artery. Its axis is about 38° from the sagittal plane and is directed downward and outward. The optic foramen is about 45 mm posterior from the supraorbital notch. The muscular cone that surrounds the posterior globe forms a tendonous ring which inserts at the orbital apex. This ring surrounds the optic foramen and part of the inferior orbital fissure including the oculomotor and abducens nerves. The trochlear nerve runs outside the cone and is more vulnerable, thus increasing the risk of superior oblique muscle palsy.

The Periocular Soft Tissues

The structures within the bony orbit can be thought of as a globe surrounded by a muscular cone, in turn surrounded by protective fat and attached to the bony orbit by a complex system of suspensory ligaments and attachments. Lining the bony orbit is a layer of periosteum known as the periorbita, which becomes the orbital septum superiorly and inferiorly at the orbital rims as it extends into the eyelids. Interior to the periosteum is a layer of periorbital fat. The fat contains many fibrous septae, which can become trapped in blow-out fractures. The fat and periosteum outside of the globe and extraocular muscles are referred to as the extraconal space (Fig. 22–2). The intraconal space is formed by the combination of fascia that partially encapsulates the extraocular muscles and the muscular cone itself. Within the intraconal space are the optic nerve and intraconal fat.

The eye is supported within the orbit by a complex arrangement of fascia and ligaments. Lockwood's suspensory ligament supports the globe vertically and has medial and lateral attachments in a configuration somewhat like a hammock (Fig. 22–3). A fascial sheath, called Tenon's capsule, surrounds the globe posterior to the cornea and invests the extraocular muscles. Lateral and medial folds of Tenon's capsule form the lateral and medial check ligaments, which resist the posterior pull of the extraoccular muscles and help to anchor the globe (see Fig. 22–2). Some of this fascia fuses with the fascia surrounding the inferior rectus and the inferior oblique muscles to form the suspensory ligament. If the orbital floor is disrupted or absent, the suspensory ligament prevents the globe from dropping. If there is enophthalmos, it is due to loss of periorbital fat or posterior positioning of the globe.

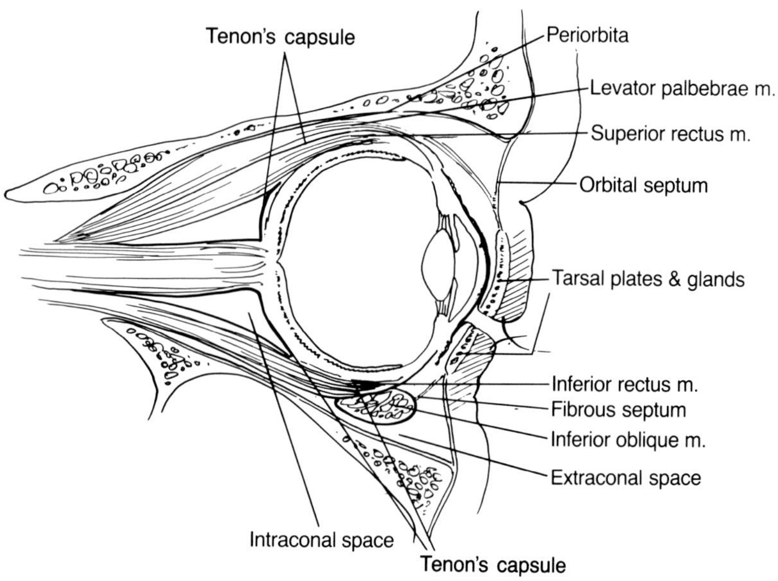

Figure 22–2. *Sagittal view of the orbital contents. (Redrawn with permission from Rowe N, Williams JI. Maxillofacial Injuries. London: Churchill Livingstone, 1985; 443)*

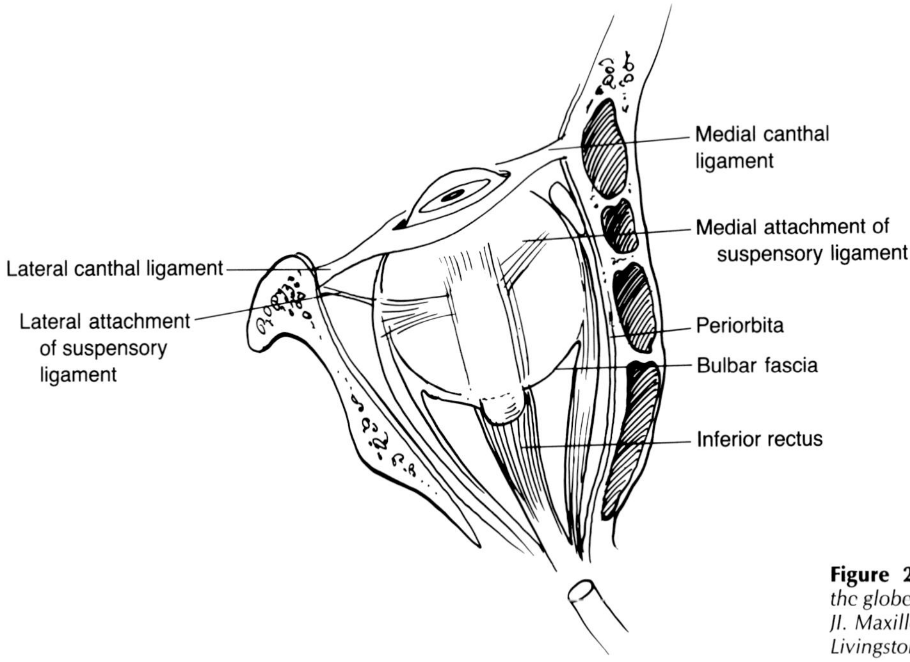

Figure 22–3. *Suspensory mechanism of thc globc. (Redrawn from Rowe N, Williams JI. Maxillofacial Injuries. London: Churchill Livingstone, 1985; 444)*

Extraocular Muscles

There are six extraocular muscles that form the muscular cone and move the globe. The eyes normally have the capability of moving along a vertical axis, horizontal axis, both axes simultaneously (oblique motion), or a rotational axis (torsion). The seventh extraocular muscle, the levator palpebrae superioris, runs immediately above the muscular cone and does not move the globe. The primary actions of the extraocular muscles are as follows:

Muscle	*Action*	*Innervation*
Lateral rectus	Abduction (away from the midline)	VI
Medial rectus	Abduction (toward the midline)	III
Superior rectus	Elevation, abduction, intorsion	III
Inferior rectus	Depression, abduction, extorsion	III
Superior oblique	Depression, abduction, intorsion	IV
Inferior oblique	Elevation, abduction, extorsion	III
Levator palpebrae superioris	Elevation of the upper lid	III

Figure 22–4 depicts the positions of gaze and the actions of the extraocular muscles. Pure elevation requires action of both the superior rectus and inferior oblique muscles simultaneously. Depression of the eyes involves contraction of the superior oblique and inferior rectus muscles. Horizontal and oblique gazes use primarily one extraocular muscle, although different muscles are used in opposite eyes to obtain conjugate gaze. Traumatically induced diplopia, or double vision, results when the eyes cannot move conjugately and light is focused on different points on the right and left retinae.

The Globe

A review of the basic gross anatomy of the eye itself allows the maxillofacial surgeon to assess the possible degree of injury to the eye and communicate appropriately with the ophthalmologist. The eye is the organ of visual perception and much of the functional anatomy and physiology of the midface is designed to protect and service the globe.

The eye itself is more or less round and projects about 3 mm anterior to the inferior and lateral orbital rims. A very thin conjunctival membrane (palpebral conjunctiva) coats the inner lid surfaces and the visible

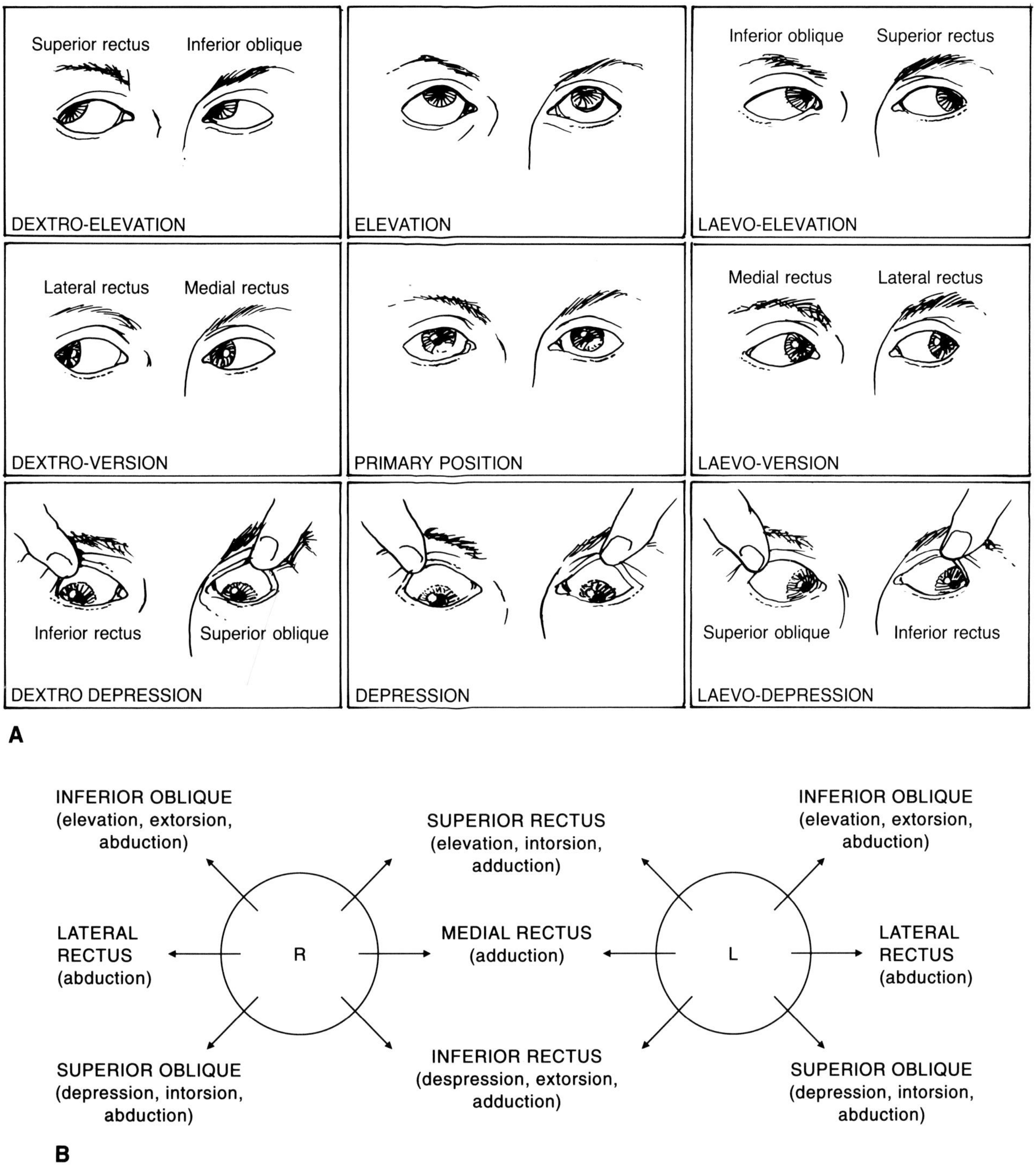

Figure 22–4. *(A, B) Movements of eye and actions by the extraocular muscles (Redrawn from Rowe N, Williams JI. Maxillofacial Injuries. London: Churchill Livingstone, 1985; 717)*

part of the eye up to the cornea (bulbar conjunctiva). The eyeball is about 2.5 cm in length and is surrounded by three layers: the fibrous, vascular, and retina layers from outside in (Fig. 22–5).

The sclera makes up the posterior five-sixths of the tough fibrous layer. The anterior portion of this layer is made up of the clear cornea. The cornea is largely responsible for light refraction and is continuous with the sclera. The cornea is very vulnerable to injury and drying out and should be protected during maxillofacial procedures.

The middle layer, which is vascular and pigmented, is composed of the choroid posteriorly and the ciliary body and iris anteriorly. The choroid contains an extensive venous plexus and capillary network. The anterior border of the choroid becomes the ciliary body, which secretes aqueous humor. The aqueous humor originates from the posterior chamber just posterior to the iris, flows to the anterior chamber between the cornea and iris, and drains at the iridocorneal angle into the canal of Schlemm. Obstruction of drainage is one cause of glaucoma. The pigmented iris is a diaphragm that projects from the ciliary body. The central aperture of the iris is the pupil. Inflammation of the iris and ciliary body from trauma commonly results in traumatic mydriasis (dilatation).

The lens is positioned posterior to the iris and is suspended by the ciliary zonule (suspensory ligament of the lens). The suspensory ligaments are attached peripherally to the ciliary processes. The lens is biconcave, avascular, and transparent. The capsule of the lens changes its degree of curvature to focus refracted light from the cornea to the retina. Since the lens is protected within the globe it is only infrequently traumatized. A lens can become detached from the zonular fibers and become displaced. Blunt trauma to the eye can result in lens opacification (traumatic cataract).

Posterior to the lens is the vitreous body comprising four-fifths of the eye. The vitreous is a clear gel and is not replaced as is aqueous humor. It supports the retina and lens and transmits light to the retina. Hemorrhage into the vitreous can occur from retinal or choroidal vessel rupture, which may block light perception.

The internal coat of the eye is the retina, which comprises an outer pigmented cell layer and an inner neural layer. Anteriorly the retina ends at the ciliary body; posteriorly it begins at the optic disk. The optic nerve enters the eye slightly towards its medial aspect and forms a distinct pale disk. The absence of photoreceptor cells in the disk creates a "blind spot." Vision is perceived in the retina and is most acute at the fovea centralis in the center of the yellow macula. The macula is lateral to the optic disk and in a more direct line with the visual anteroposterior axis of the eye.

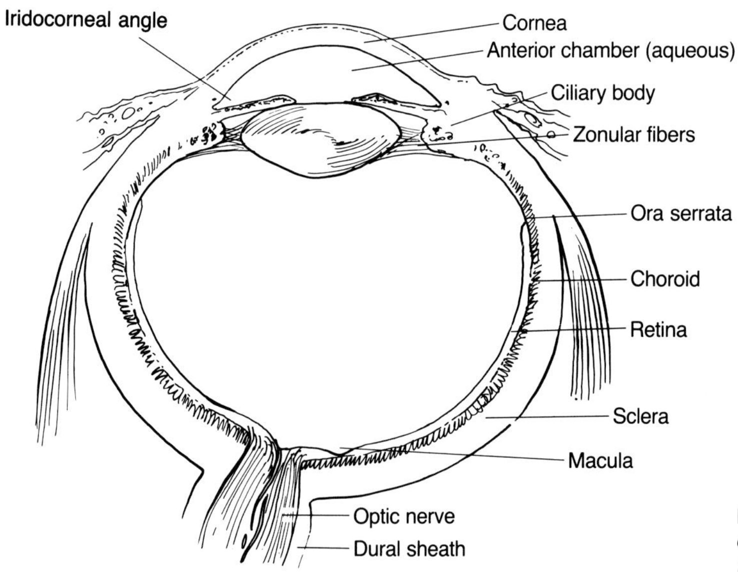

Figure 22–5. *Horizontal section of the eye. (Redrawn from Moore KL. Clinically Oriented Anatomy. Baltimore: Williams and Wilkins, 1985; 888)*

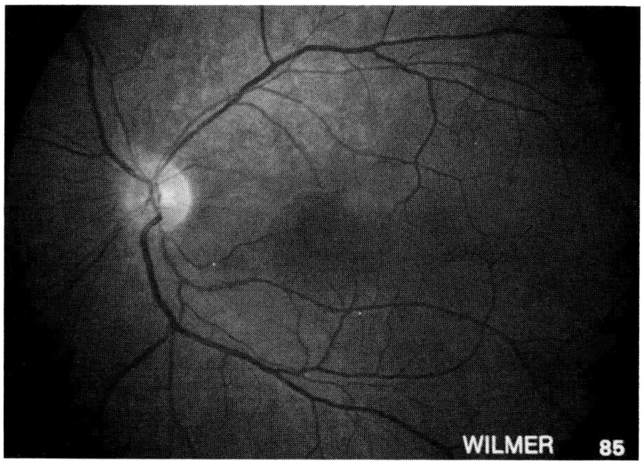

Figure 22–6. *Normal optic disk and retinal artery distribution; macula at center of field. (Courtesy of the Wilmer Eye Institute. Hirst LW, et al. Sights and sounds in ophthalmology, vol. 5. In: Ocular and Periocular Trauma. St. Louis: CV Mosby, 1984)*

The blood supply of the retina is through the central retinal artery which travels with the optic nerve. Retinal arteries and veins are directly visible on ophthalmoscopy, and the normal pattern emanating from the optic disk should be recognized (Fig. 22–6). A tear at the ora serrata (junction of the retina and ciliary body) is the most common type of traumatic tear and causes retinal detachment; it is referred to as diastesis. Since these tears occur at the very peripheral retina, they are difficult to detect.

ANATOMY OF THE LIDS AND ADNEXA

An understanding of eyelid anatomy is necessary in the clinical assessment of orbital injuries as well as in the approaches used for surgical repair. The lids and adnexa serve to protect the eye as well as lubricate and clean the corneal surface.

The eyelids are composed essentially of three layers (see Fig. 22–2): the outer layer is composed of skin; the middle layer contains the orbicularis oris muscle; and innermost is the tarsal plate, which is lined on its posterior aspect by very vascular palpebral conjunctiva. At the lid margin, posterior to the eyelashes, is the grey line, which is the mucocutaneous junction between skin and conjunctiva. The conjunctiva covers the entire posterior upper and lower lid surface and forms upper and lower fornicies where it turns to reflect onto the sclera (bulbar conjunctiva). Immediately anterior to the conjunctiva are the tarsal plates (tarsus), which give form and strength to the lids. They are composed of a fibrous connective tissue band about 2.5-cm wide and contain meibomian glands at the lid margin, which serve to lubricate the lashes to prevent sticking. Extending from near the proximal edge of each tarsal plate is an orbital septum, which is attached to periosteum of the orbital rim and, therefore, anchors the lids. Posterior to the orbital septum lies the periorbital fat and extraocular muscles. The superior tarsus has a thin smooth muscle called Müller's muscle, by which it attaches to the underside of the levator palpebrae superioris muscle. This muscle has clinical significance because of its sympathetic innervation. Interruption of this sympathetic nerve supply causes the ptosis seen in Horner's syndrome. This syndrome also causes miosis from unopposed parasympathetic action on the iris.

The upper eyelid is elevated by the levator palpebrae superioris, which runs in the superior aspect of the bony orbit and inserts near and anterior to the superior edge of the tarsal plate. This muscle is innervated by the oculomotor nerve (III). Therefore, a cranial nerve III palsy due to the herniation of the uncus from cerebral compression will result in upper lid ptosis as well as palsy of four of the extraocular muscles. The pupil progressively becomes fixed and dilated, since the pupillary constriction fibers of the oculomotor nerve become paralyzed.

The lower eyelid is similar in construction to the upper lid, except it does not have a depressor muscle analagous to the levator of the upper lid. Therefore, the lower lid remains more stationary than the upper lid as the lids open and close. The opening between the upper and lower lids is the palpebral fissure and should be nearly horizontal, except in the Mongolian race. The lids meet medially and laterally at a sharply defined angle called the canthus (Fig. 22–7). Occasionally an epicanthal fold is present medially (especially in Down's syndrome and the Mongolian race), whcih obscures the medial canthal angle and causes a rounding of the region. This must be differentiated from traumatic medial canthal tendon detachment, which results in blunting of the medial canthal angle.

The orbicularis oculi muscle is positioned between the skin of the eyelid and the tarsus and functions to circumferentially close the eyelids. It is innervated by cranial nerve VII and is used in active eye closure as

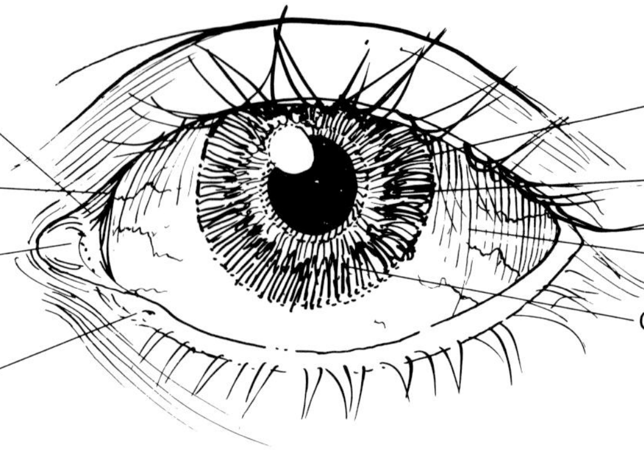

Figure 22–7. *Surface anatomy of the eye. (Redrawn from Moore KL. Clinically Oriented Anatomy. Baltimore: Williams and Wilkins, 1985; 892)*

well as reflex blinking. In nerve VII paralysis, the unopposed levator muscle of the upper lid prevents the eye from closing, which leads to corneal desiccation and excessive tearing. The orbicularis has thick fibers around the bony orbital rim for active eye closure and a very thin layer at the palpebral margin for gentle eye closure and blinking. A third portion of the orbicularis muscle surrounds the lacrimal sac behind the medial canthus. Contraction of the muscle compresses the lacrimal sac and activates the nasolacrimal drainage pump.

The eyelids and their associated muscles are attached to the bony orbit medially and laterally by the medial and lateral canthal tendons. These should be termed tendons as opposed to ligaments because they primarily insert muscles into bone. The lateral canthal tendon has superficial and deep heads, which insert at Whitnall's lateral orbital tubercle.

Medial Canthal Tendon

The intimate relation of the medial canthal tendon insertion and the nasolacrimal apparatus must be appreciated in order to accomplish a function repair of nasoethmoidal injuries. The medial canthus is a fibrous extension of the tarsal plates medially and anchors the eyelids after fusing with the orbicularis muscle and orbital septum (see Fig. 22–8). The medial canthal tendon has superficial and deep insertions. Superficially it inserts on the anterior lacrimal crest, which is part of the frontal process of the maxillary bone. The deep head inserts more posteriorly on the posterior lacrimal crest, which provides convexity to the eyelids. The medial canthus is surrounded on three sides by Horner's muscle (pretarsal portion of the deep orbicularis), which is part of the nasolacrimal drainage pump (Fig. 22–8).

Avulsion of a medial canthal tendon results in traumatic telecanthus. The medial canthi are normally 33 to 38 mm apart (roughly the width of one eye). This distance becomes increased in traumatic telecanthus. The medial canthal tendon may remain attached to the anterior and posterior lacrimal crests, but the comminuted bony fragments cause the tendon insertions to become displaced laterally. This condition should not be confused with congenital widening of the canthi seen in orbital hypertelorism such as that found in Apert's syndrome. In this condition, the bony orbits are positioned abnormally laterally from the midline, causing both medial and lateral canthi to be abnormally wide with respect to the opposite side.

The Nasolacrimal Apparatus

The nasolacrimal apparatus functions to drain the eye of tears. The tears originate from the lacrimal gland, which lies on the superolateral portion of the orbit in the lacrimal fossa of the temporal bone. The frontal bone is extremely thick in this region, so the lacrimal gland is rarely injured in orbital fractures. The gland secretes tears into the superior fornix of the conjunctiva, which are pooled in the inferior fornix and drain toward the lacrimal canaliculi in the eyelids. The canaliculi terminate as small punctae 8 to 10 mm from the lacrimal sac, which lies medial to the medial canthal tendon. The opening of the papillae are directed posteriorly toward the globe. The canaliculi run at right angles to their respective lid margins for about 2 mm before turning and traveling parallel to the lids as they head medially to the lacrimal sac (Fig.

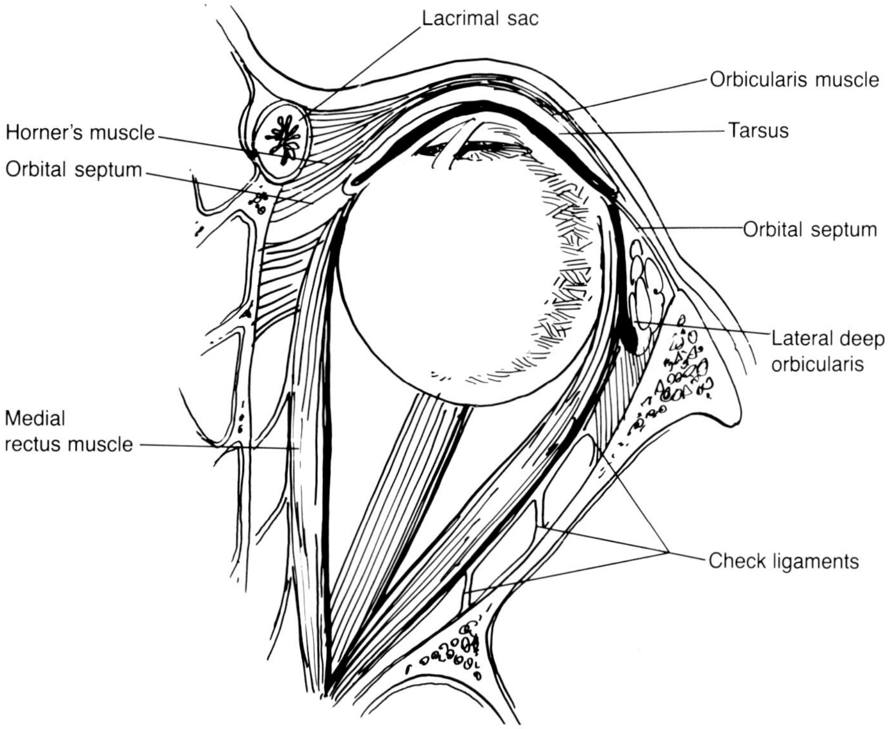

Figure 22–8. *Horizontal section of the orbit. The medial canthal tendon is just deep to this cut and it replaces Horner's muscle. (Smith BC. Ophthalmic Plastic and Reconstructive Surgery, vol. 1. St. Louis: CV Mosby, 1987; 33)*

22–9). The ducts are only 0.5 mm in width but can be dilated with small lacrimal duct probes if intubation is necessary in repair of injuries. Appreciation of the right-angle turns made by the lacrimal canaliculi will help the surgeon to canaliculate the ducts when repairing perforations of the nasolacrimal system.

The superior and inferior canaliculi form a common duct just before entering the lacrimal sac, which is just deep and superior to the medial canthal tendon. The lacrimal sac lies in the bony lacrimal fossa medially but has soft tissue attachments of the lacrimal fascia on its lateral aspect. The thicker anterior

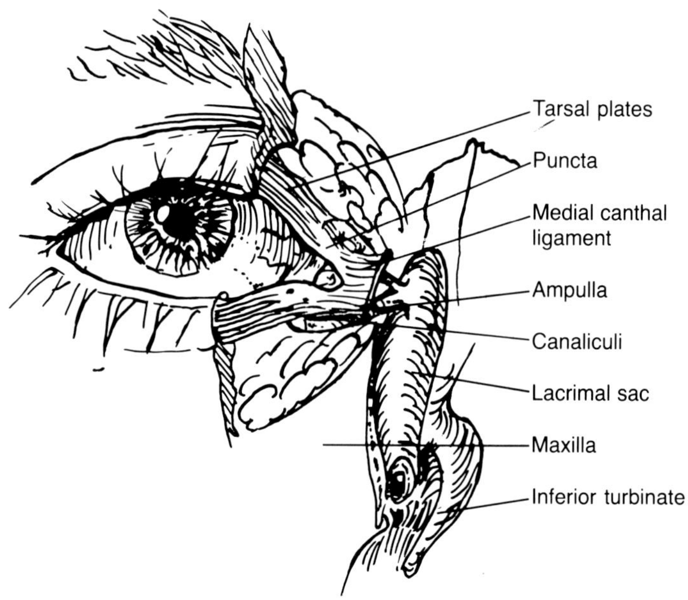

Figure 22–9. *The lacrimal drainage system. (Smith BC. Ophthalmic Plastic and Reconstructive Surgery, vol 1. St. Louis: CV Mosby, 1987; 23)*

limb of the medial canthal tendon inserts on the anterior lacrimal crest just anterior to the lacrimal sac. A smaller posterior limb of the tendon inserts deep to the lacrimal sac onto the posterior lacrimal crest and lacrimal fascia. The common canaliculus courses through the central portion of the medial canthal tendon. In reconstruction of the medial canthal region after trauma, emphasis is placed on reestablishing the anterior attachment of the medial canthal tendon and the nasolacrimal ducts, while the posterior tendon attachment is usually left unrepaired.

The lacrimal sac is continuous with the nasolacrimal duct, which lies entirely within bone and drains into the nose beneath the inferior turbinate. The common canaliculi join the lacrimal sac and nasolacrimal duct at a right angle, so that a probe or tube must make two right-angle turns along its pathway from the puncta in the lid to the nasal cavity. The lacrimal sac and nasolacrimal duct are approximately 30 to 32 mm long (Figs. 22–9 and 22–10).

Epiphora, or excessive tearing, can result from an increase in lacrimation (e.g., from corneal irritation) or interruption of the nasolacrimal drainage pump. Closure of the eyelids contracts the pretarsal portion of the orbicularis oculi (Horner's muscle), which creates negative pressure on the lacrimal sac, drawing tears away from the eye and into the canaliculi. Contraction of the muscles surrounding the ducts also serves to push fluid toward the sac and nasolacrimal duct. Failure of the nasolacrimal drainage pump can result from cranial nerve VII injury (paralysis of the orbicularis muscle), edema of the puncta or ducts, severance or avulsion of the medial canthal tendon with the common canaliculus, or disruption or blockage of the lacrimal sac or nasolacrimal duct. Postoperatively, epiphora may result from surgical edema from manipulation of the eyelids as well as distortion of the canalicular system. Assessment of patency of the lacrimal drainage system is advisable during repair of nasoethmoidal fractures or sharp trauma to the medial orbit. Late epiphora may develop if ectropion (eyelid eversion) causes contraction or malpositioning of the puncta.

DIAGNOSIS OF ORBITAL TRAUMA

Radiologic Examination

The radiologic diagnosis of orbital trauma is a sequential examination proceeding from screening films to computed tomography, if indicated. Generally, plain films of the orbit consisting of posteroanterior (Caldwell) views and a Water's projection are obtained initially. Occasionally 20° oblique views of the orbit are beneficial. The Caldwell view best demonstrates the orbital rims, frontal bone, and frontal and ethmoid sinuses (Fig. 22–11). The Water's view is excellent for

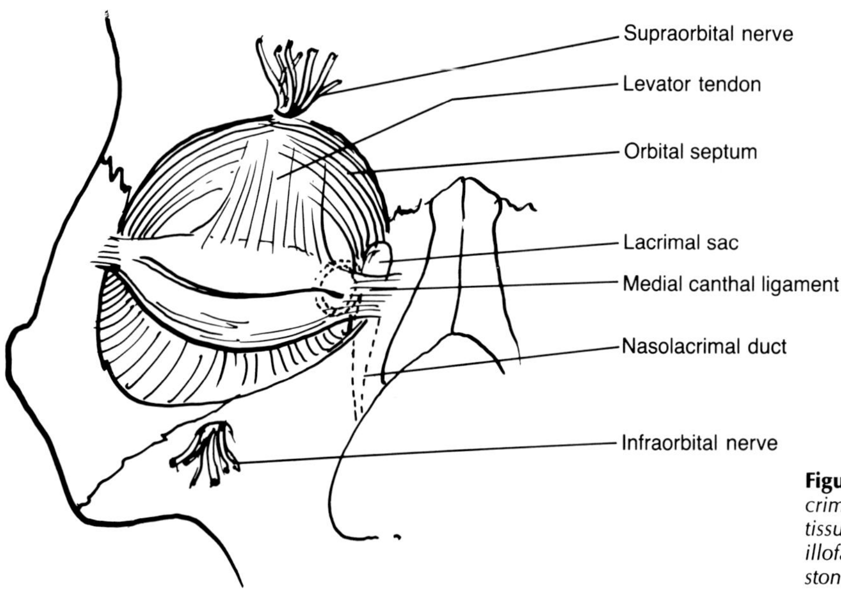

Figure 22–10. *Relationship of the nasolacrimal excretory system to the anterior soft tissues of the orbit. (Rowe N, Williams JI. Maxillofacial Injuries. London: Churchill Livingstone, 1985; 442)*

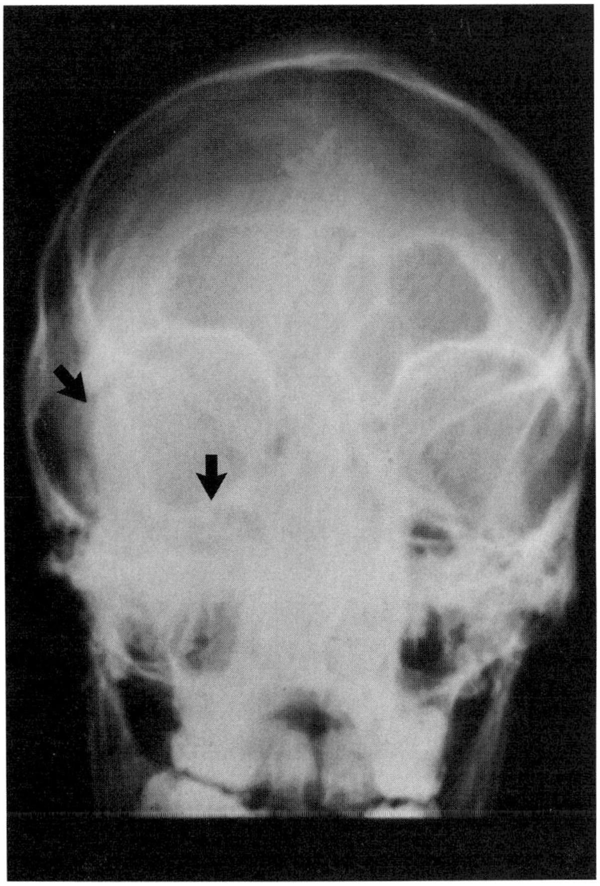

Figure 22–11. *Displaced fractures at the right frontozygomatic suture and infraorbital rim (Caldwell view).*

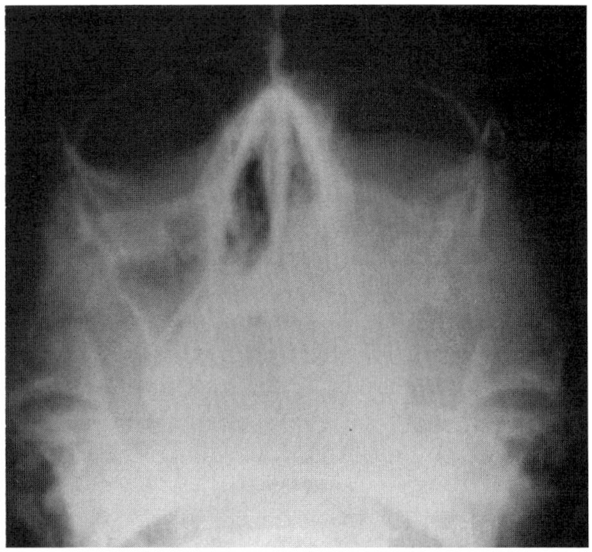

Figure 22–12. *Note the disruption of left infraorbital rim and clouding of maxillary sinus (Waters' view).*

imaging the inferior and lateral orbital rims, the maxillary sinus, the nasoethmoid region, and the zygomas (Fig. 22–12). Oblique orbital views best demonstrate the lateral rims and the sphenoid bone. From plain films it is possible to diagnose fractures of the medial, lateral, superior, and inferior orbital rims; gross depression of the orbital floor; opacification of the maxillary sinus, ethmoid and frontal sinuses; prolapse of orbital contents into the maxillary sinuses; or orbital emphysema.

Plain films in the orbital region are often difficult to interpret. The superimposition of skull structures can obscure fractures or be mistaken for fractures. Hemorrhage and edema can literally cloud the ability to distinguish structures accurately. Conventional tomography can improve the ability to distinguish and localize small fracture segments, especially of the orbital floor (Fig. 22–13). Several films can be obtained at 0.5-cm intervals in coronal and sagittal planes. Disadvantages of conventional tomography include its inability to differentiate soft tissue structures, such as prolapse of the inferior rectus muscle into the maxillary sinus, from a hematoma. Conventional tomograms often have significant blurring. The disadvantages of conventional tomography are essentially eliminated by the use of high-resolution computed tomography.

Computed tomography (CT) scans are generally obtained along an axial plane. Computed tomographic data can then be reformatted coronally or sagittally to provide additional information. Occasionally a direct coronal CT scan can be obtained, which offers much higher resolution and accuracy than a reformatted coronal CT. CT images reduce structure superimposition and allow more accurate identification of fractures, including small comminutions of the orbital rim, sinus walls, and medial and lateral orbital walls (Fig. 22–14). Often it is not possible to accurately visualize the orbital floor on CT, since the image generally runs parallel to the axial plane. However, bone fragments from the orbital floor can often be located on CT if the section is through the superior portion of the maxillary sinus.

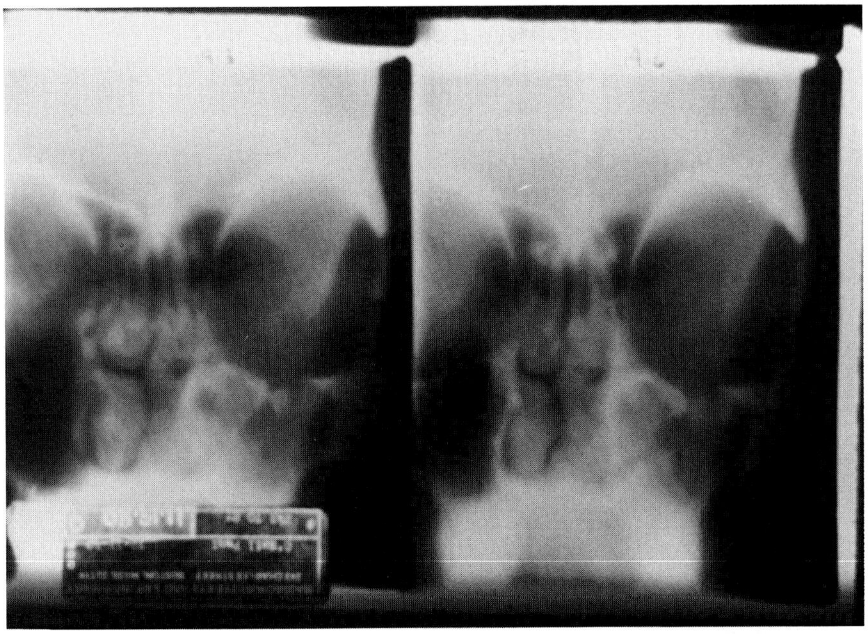

Figure 22–13. *Successive sections by conventional tomography show fragments of the left orbital rim and floor displaced inferiorly.*

CT offers a major advantage over conventional radiography in that it can be used to differentiate soft tissue structures. Accordingly, it is possible to visualize the globe ocular muscles, optic nerve, hematoma, abscess cavities, proptosis, and soft tissue edema or emphysema. The imaging density window can be altered to emphasize either bone or soft tissue densities. Duvall[1] states that conventional radiography and tomography tend to underestimate the degree of bony displacement and comminution found at the time of operation. The reconstructive surgeon can restore the traumatized structures based on an exact demonstration of the position of the various fragments as demonstrated by high resolution CT.[2] Bernardo et al.[3] compared conventional radiography, complex motion tomography, and computed tomography for evaluation of orbital trauma. Their findings support the superiority of CT over conventional modalities in the diagnosis of traumatized structures. Furthermore, patients they studied were exposed to from 17 to 20 roentgens at a given skin point per study for planar tomography versus only 4 roentgens during CT.[3]

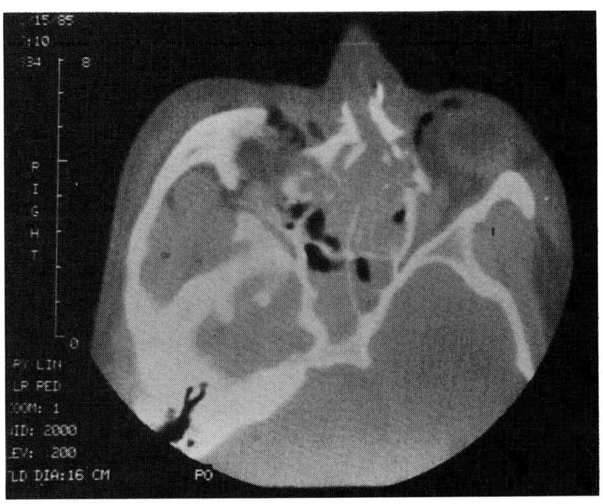

Figure 22–14. *Computed tomography section shows comminutions of the nasoethmoidal region with displacement of the medial wall into the retroorbital region.*

Orbital Blow-Out Fractures

The term blow-out fracture was proposed by Smith and Regan[4] after studying the mechanism of orbital wall fractures in cadavers. Blow-out fractures of the orbital walls are caused by sudden transmission of force applied to relatively noncompressible orbital soft tissues, which are surrounded by the very thin bones of the medial wall (lamina papyracea) and orbital floor.[4–6] Since water is noncompressible, increased hydrostatic pressure within the globe and periorbita tends to displace the delicate orbital floor inferiorly and medial wall medially (Fig. 22–15). Blow-out fractures result when a blunt object larger in diameter than the orbital rim strikes the rim and orbital contents simultaneously. Objects smaller than the orbital aperture are much more likely to penetrate or rupture the globe and orbital contents. A second theory involves a buckling effect on the orbital walls when force is applied to the orbital rim.[7] Less force is required to rupture the orbital wall buckling than from hydraulic pressure.[7]

The radiographic signs of orbital blow-out fractures as described by Zizmor et al.[8] are fragmentation of the orbital floor, displacement of the fragments, and prolapse of the orbital soft tissues into the maxillary sinus. Medial wall fractures are difficult to detect on plain films but are readily diagnosed by CT.

The clinical signs of blow-out fractures include periorbital ecchymosis and edema, diplopia in upward gaze and occasionally in the primary position, paresthesia or anesthesia of the infraorbital nerve, and enophthalmos. The orbital floor is very vulnerable along the infraorbital groove anterior to the inferior orbital fissure. This can result in inferior displacement and entrapment of the inferior rectus and the inferior oblique muscles or the surrounding fat tissue, with subsequent limitation of upward mobility of the globe. The clinical consequence of this limitation is diplopia on upward gaze. Diplopia can frequently result from orbital edema and hemorrhage without entrapment of the orbital muscles or fat. A forced duction test, which applies traction at the insertion of the inferior rectus, can be used to determine whether entrapment exists (Fig. 22–16).

Diplopia

The limited ocular mobility that follows a blow-out fracture as postulated by Putterman et al.[9] is due to edema, hemorrhage, or fat entrapment as opposed to muscle entrapment. They based their theory on research that showed positive forced direction tests with diplopia on upward gaze on traumatized patients who did not have blow-out fractures. Occular mobility returns as the edema and hemorrhage of the fat resolves or the fat stretches. Putterman, Smith, and Lisman have observed limitation of vertical eye motion when grasping posterior-inferior orbital fat during cosmetic blepharoplasty.[10] Koorneef[11] suggests that the fine tissue septae between fat and muscles becomes inhibited by the fracture. This concept is suggested by the often unusual ocular mobility patterns observed without gross entrapment of tissues.

Limitation of ocular motion can be detected by observing a patient's eyes as they follow an object through the positions of gaze. The degree of diplopia

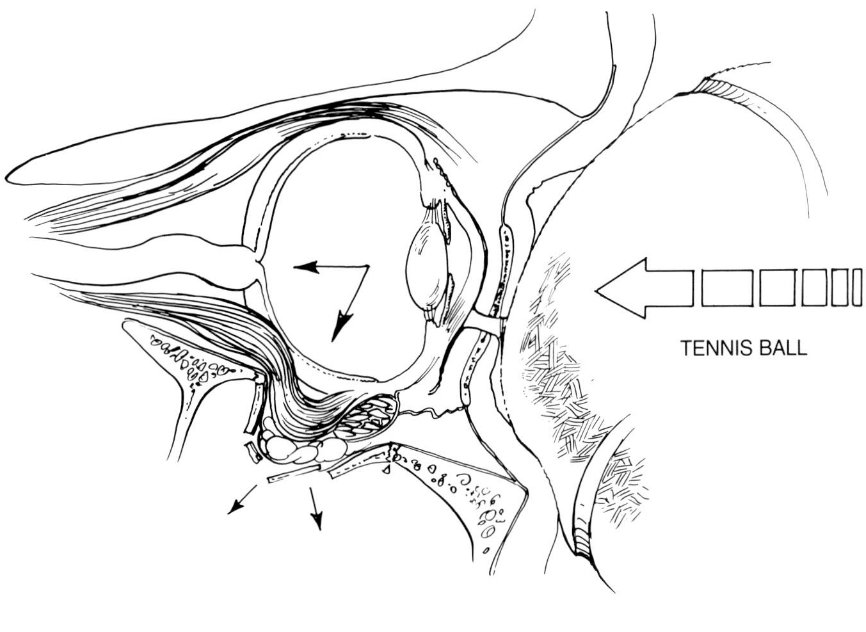

Figure 22–15. *Possible mechanism of blow-out fracture. (Smith BC. Ophthalmic Plastic and Reconstructive Surgery, vol. 1. St. Louis: CV Mosby, 1987; 476)*

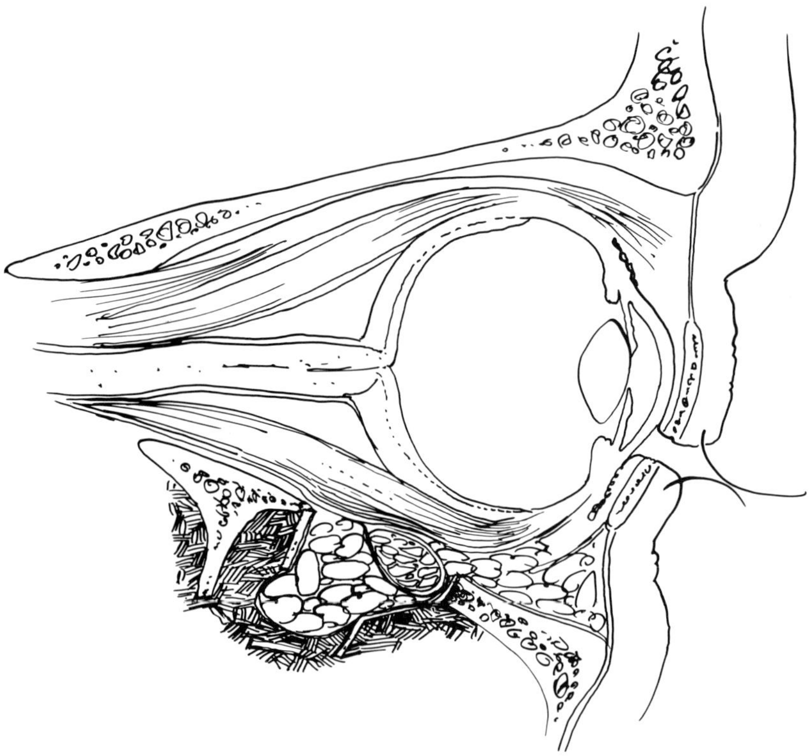

Figure 22–16. *Limitation of globe mobility due to hematoma or fat entrapment. (Smith BC. Ophthalmic Plastic and Reconstructive Surgery, vol. 1. St. Louis: CV Mosby, 1987; 479)*

can be documented and followed using the method of Smith[12] (Fig. 22–17). The examiner shines a small light at the patient who is initially looking in the primary gaze position. The light is moved to each of the gaze positions and the patient notes whether one light or two is seen. The regions of diplopia are marked on a square of paper resembling a television screen. The test is repeated several times per week for the first week and weekly thereafter. It is best repeated by the same examiner each time to maintain validity.[12] More sophisticated testing of gaze can be performed,[13,14] but discussion of the technique is beyond the scope of this text.

Enophthalmos

Enophthalmos is retrodisplacement of the globe. The globe is tethered by periocular muscles and connective tissues and surrounded by fat within the orbital bony pyramid. Enophthalmos can result from a change in the position of the globe due to loss of orbital fat or contraction of the supporting structures (Fig. 22–18). Outward displacement of orbital walls will increase orbital volume. Resulting enophthalmos can then occur because of the relative decrease in periocular soft tissues in an enlarged orbit. Experimentally, Parsons and Mathog[15] showed that 1 mm of displacement of the orbital floor resulted in a 0.4-ml increase in orbital volume, causing a 1.5-mm change in the global position.

The globe can become displaced if the fascial sling that attaches the orbit to the globe is disrupted. Mustarde[16] showed that displacement of Lockwood's suspensory ligament, which runs from Whitnall's tubercle on the lateral orbital rim to the bulbar sheath of the globe, will cause displacement of the globe. This is most often seen in displaced zygomaticomaxillary complex fractures. However, there can be orbital volume changes due to displacement of periorbital contents from the associated orbital floor fractures.

It is difficult to accurately assess what degree of enophthalmos is likely to result from any particular fracture. Hemorrhage, and especially edema, mask the degree of enophthalmos and may initially cause proptosis. Posttraumatic scarring and fat atrophy are

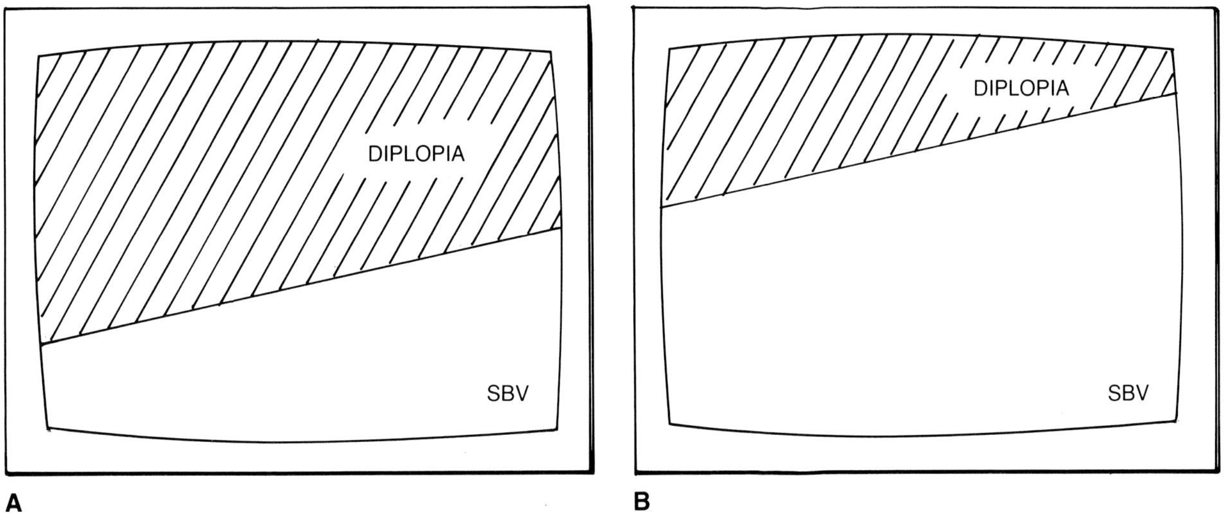

Figure 22–17. *Charting of diplopia and simultaneous binocular vision (SBV). (**A**) Partial resolution of diplopia (**B**) (Smith BC. Ophthalmic Plastic and Reconstructive Surgery. St. Louis: CV Mosby, 1987; 479)*

variable. Enophthalmos may present acutely if the orbit is enlarged and orbital contents are displaced. Conversely, enophthalmos can develop over several weeks or months if an initially enlarged orbital space is masked by edema or hematoma, giving a false impression of the degree of injury. Enophthalmos can also progress as trapped orbital fat atrophies or as orbital soft tissue scars down to the damaged orbital floor.

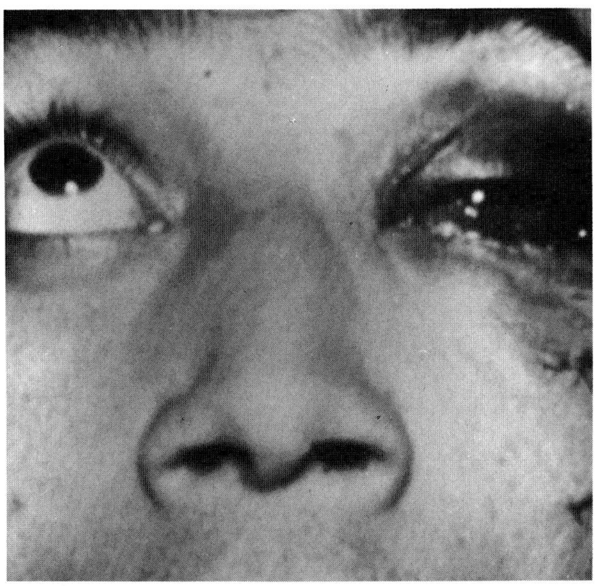

Figure 22–18. *This patient demonstrates enophthalmos and limitation of upward gaze on the left side. Note also periorbital ecchymosis and subconjunctival hemorrhage.*

Enophthalmos is not unique to orbital blow-out fractures. It frequently is associated with malar bone and orbital floor displacement depressed zygomatic complex fractures. This condition has been coined combined orbital trauma syndrome[17] by Stanley and Mathog. The resultant deformity is often striking with a flattened cheek bone, inferior and lateral globe displacement from lateral canthus displacement, orbital enlargement, and marked enophthalmos.

Clinically, enophthalmos of greater than 3 mm can usually be observed by the examiner (Fig. 22–18). The anterior projection of the involved globe can be compared to the contralateral globe projection as it relates to the adjacent supraorbital ridge or lateral rim. Soft tissue edema of the injured side often obscures the relative comparison between the globes. The palpebral fissure is narrowed from posterior global displacement. The interpupillary level is normally horizontal, but with enophthalmos there is usually inferior displacement of the globe resulting in a nonhorizontal interpupillary line. Relative drooping or ptosis of the upper lid may be noted from inferior or posterior globe displacement. An objective measurement of enophthalmos is made with a Hertel exophthalmometer. There are limitations with this instrument, and with complex orbital injuries a thorough ophthalmologic exam should be performed to rule out ocular injuries and to document visual loss or limitations. Appropriate films and CT scans should be obtained.

MANAGEMENT OF ORBITAL FLOOR FRACTURES, DIPLOPIA, AND ENOPHTHALMOS

Timing of Treatment

A question of when to intervene and surgically repair blow-out fractures with resultant enophthalmos or diplopia has caused some controversy. Putterman et al.,[18] Emery et al.,[19] and Koorneef[20] have proposed late surgical intervention. However, other investigators found that early intervention, usually within 2 weeks of injury, provides the most satisfactory results.[21–27] Due to the difficulties encountered in successfully treating late diplopia and less satisfactory results in treating long-standing enophthalmos, Putterman et al.[27] unequivocally recommend that significant diplopia or enophthalmos be explored surgically if not resolved in 1 to 2 weeks. A short delay of 1 to 2 weeks allows resolution of most edema and hematoma. Forced duction testing is easier to perform after resolution of edema. Enophthalmos that was initially masked by edema generally becomes more apparent. Diplopia persisting after a week or two is unlikely to be attributed to edema.

When surgical intervention is indicated to repair displaced facial bones, especially the zygoma, it is advantageous to treat enophthalmos, diplopia, or orbital floor fractures simultaneously and often much earlier than at 1 to 2 weeks. This is not to imply that all zygomatic bone reductions necessitate exploration of the orbital floor, even though the orbital floor is routinely fractured as part of the zygomatic complex. With an intact periorbita, and no clinical or radiographic evidence of loss of orbital contents, orbital exploration should rarely be necessary after zygomatic repair. A forced duction test performed after fixation of the orbital rim can be done to verify freedom of the inferior rectus muscle. Orbital exploration poses risks of blindness, periocular nerve or muscle damage, infection, bleeding, scarring, and corneal injury, and, therefore, should be undertaken only when known clinical problems exist and not as a routine measure following zygoma elevation.

Surgical Treatment of Orbital Fractures

Orbital fractures necessitating surgical treatment are, in general, those exhibiting persistent diplopia after 2 weeks, clinically detectable enophthalmos after edema has subsided, clinical depression or elevation or displacement of the orbital rims, traumatically induced cosmetic deformities, orbital fractures that are components of displaced nasoethmoidal or zygomatic fractures, and radiographically (or CT) evident orbital floor fractures with displacement or prolapse or orbital contents. Concomitant injury to the globe or visual apparatus should be assessed and treated by the ophthalmologist.

Injuries to the lateral orbital rim can be approached several different ways depending on the extent of the injury, associated injuries, and cosmetic considerations. When the eyebrow is of average size and quality, an incision in the lateral eyebrow parallel to the superolateral orbital rim and angled obliquely so as not to cut across eyebrow hair shafts is acceptable (Fig. 22–19). The soft tissues in this region are quite pliable, allowing excellent access to the frontozygomatic suture even though the incision is not placed directly over the bone suture. The eyebrow should not be shaved, since regrowth of the hairs can be unpredictable and infection is very unlikely despite the presence of hair. This incision is minimally detectable when healed. A lateral supratarsal incision can be

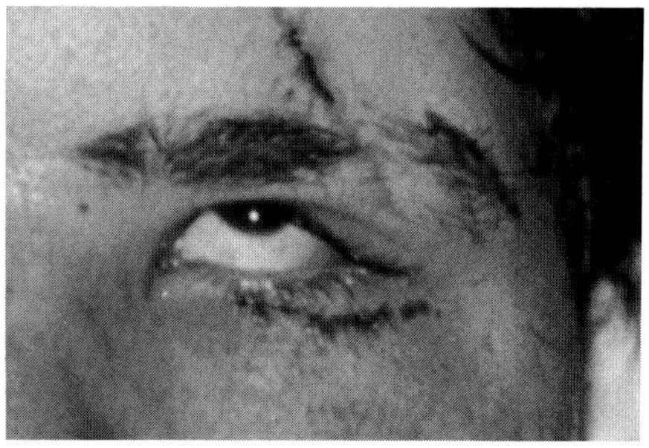

Figure 22–19. *Left lateral brow incision and subciliary incision were made. Note lack of entrapment of the left eye after surgical repair of the fractured orbit. The forehead laceration was sustained at the time of the fractures.*

placed in the superior palpebral fold and provide access to the lateral orbital rim. This incision may be the approach of choice in patients with very fine or fair eyebrow hair. For extensive upper midface injuries, a coronal flap provides outstanding access to the lateral rim.

Access to the fracture site is gained by reflecting the skin to expose the thin layer of connective tissue and periosteum below. A knife or a cautery unit can incise through these tissues to the bone. It is rare to encounter significant blood vessels, and major sensory or motor nerves do not cross the surgical site. A small periosteal elevator is used to strip the periosteum. It is easier to work from superior to inferior because the frontal bone is normally stable. Once the fracture is located, the periosteal incision can be extended inferiorly to expose the frontal process of the zygomatic bone. The fracture is reduced and, if unstable, is fixated with a 24- to 26-g wire. This region is not under function so that rigid bone plating and compression are not necessary. Bone plates in this region can sometimes be palpable and may be removed at a later date. A bone plate[28] is desirable when there are multiple comminutions; the plate can span the tiny fragments to stabilize the larger pieces. In noncomminuted fractures, wire should be used in a direct or figure-of-8 fashion and both ends directed into the posterior aspect of the rim with the pigtail tied posteriorly. This technique results in very minimal palpable foreign body at the lateral rim.

The inferior orbital rim, as well as the orbital floor, can be approached numerous ways. The most satisfactory method is probably the subciliary incision placed 2 to 3 mm below the lower lid lashes, parallel to them or in a crease if one exists (Fig. 22–20). The incision heals with minimal scarring and ectropion. The most direct approach is to place the incision over the inferior orbital rim. However, the incision is not hidden by the lashes as well as with the subciliary and occasionally is unsatisfactory if the scar binds down to the orbital rim and periosteum immediately below it. A conjunctival incision[29] placed in the fornix with a lateral canthotomy provides a completely hidden incision (Fig. 22–21). However, ectropion may be more common with an incision so close to the lid margin and access to the rim appears more difficult.

The subciliary incision is marked with a fine marker about 3 mm below the cilia extending across the entire lower lid. A very small amount of anesthetic with

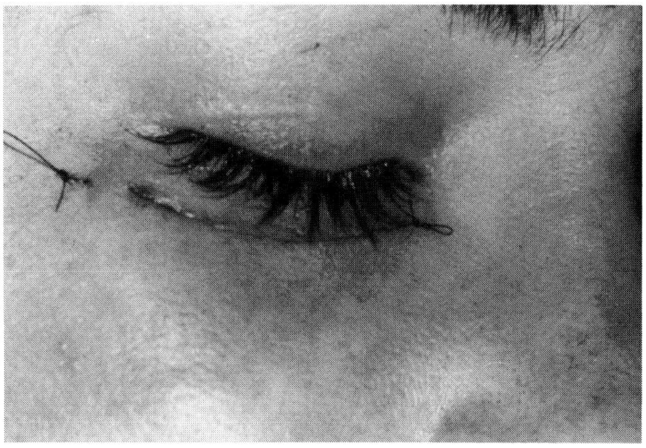

Figure 22–20. *Subciliary incision was made in a fine skin crease about 3 mm from the lower lashes.*

vasoconstrictor is injected subcutaneously so as not to balloon or distort this delicate tissue. The incision is made with a blade down to, but not through, the orbicularis oculi muscle (Fig. 22–22). A small double-skin hook placed at the superior and inferior skin margins provides excellent retraction. The next step is to dissect the subcutaneous layer from the underlying muscle down to the level of the intraorbital rim. This is done by blunt dissection with fine, slightly blunted, tipped scissors such as Stevens scissors. This step is facilitated when the surgeon operates from the head of the table and the scissors are held with the tips down so the curve of the scissors conforms to the curvature of the muscle layer and the underlying tarsal plate. When the level of the orbital rim is reached, the muscle fibers are spread parallel to the rim until the periosteum is visualized. The periosteum is incised with a blade at or below the edge of the orbital rim where it joins with the floor.

When exploration of the orbital floor is to be performed, the orbital floor periosteum (periorbita) is dissected superiorly with a small periosteal elevator. Sweeping from medial to lateral while proceeding posteriorly is effective. When the orbital floor is very comminuted, it is easier to elevate the periosteum from a solid medial or lateral segment of the orbit and proceed to the midorbit where the fractures usually are found. As the dissection proceeds posteriorly, a malleable retractor can be inserted to gently elevate the periosteum with the overlying globe and soft tissues from the floor. Excessive or continuous pressure

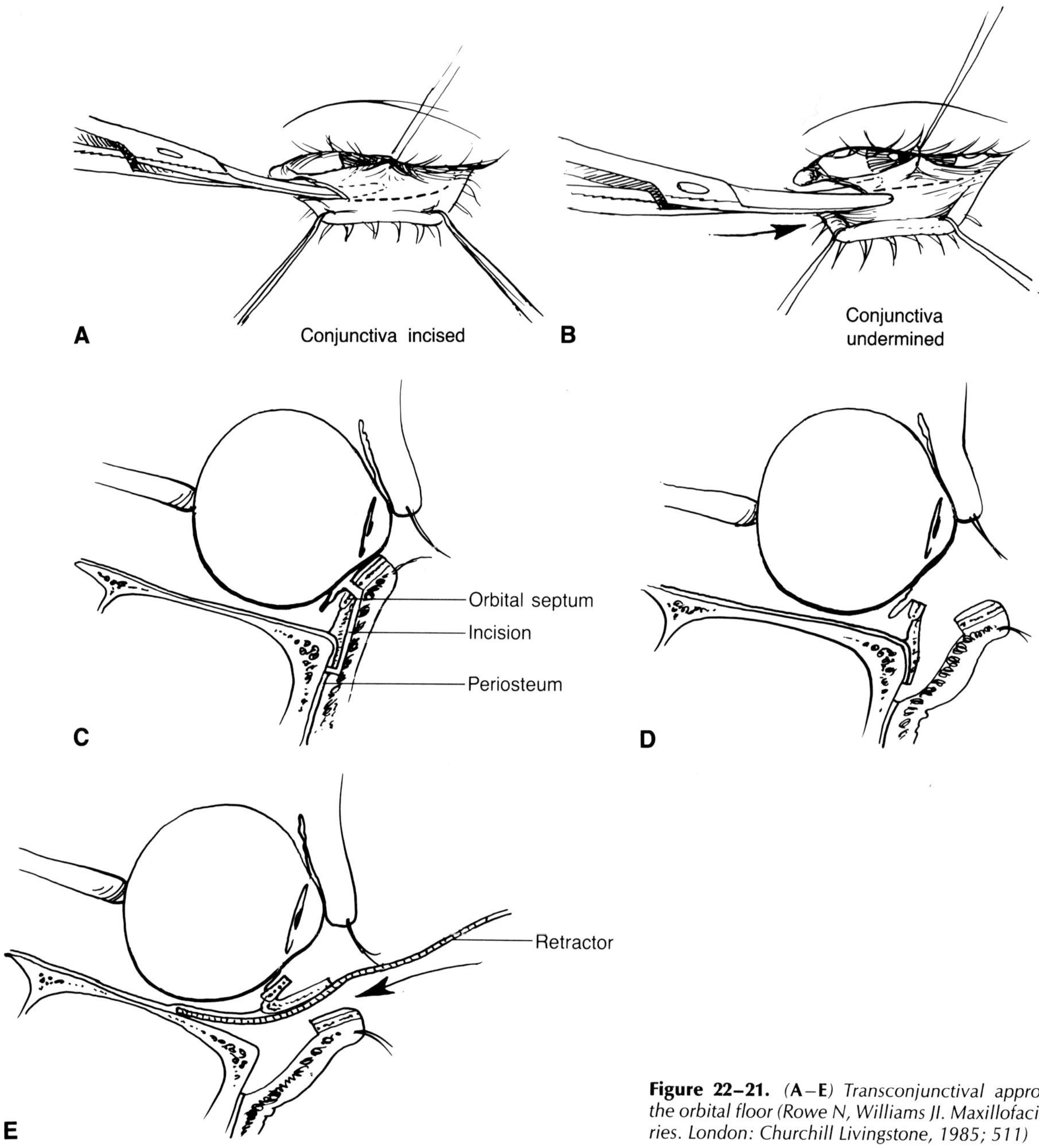

Figure 22–21. *(***A–E***) Transconjunctival approach to the orbital floor (Rowe N, Williams JI. Maxillofacial Injuries. London: Churchill Livingstone, 1985; 511)*

should not be exerted on the globe. Posteriorly the periosteum should not be dissected farther than 20 mm from the orbital rim to avoid the inferior orbital fissure and the structures contained within.

At this point, an examination of the bones of the orbital floor is accomplished. Fragments are usually displaced inferiorly into the maxillary sinus in those orbits exhibiting diplopia, enophthalmos, or radiographic evidence of displacement. Occasionally, fragments are displaced medially. A fine, single-skin hook is very effective in elevating orbital floor fragments out of the sinuses. When the periorbita has been interrupted, periorbital fat, connective tissue septae, and possibly muscle may be displaced into the antrum. These tissues are freed from the defect with blunt dissection and elevated back into the orbit. The bony

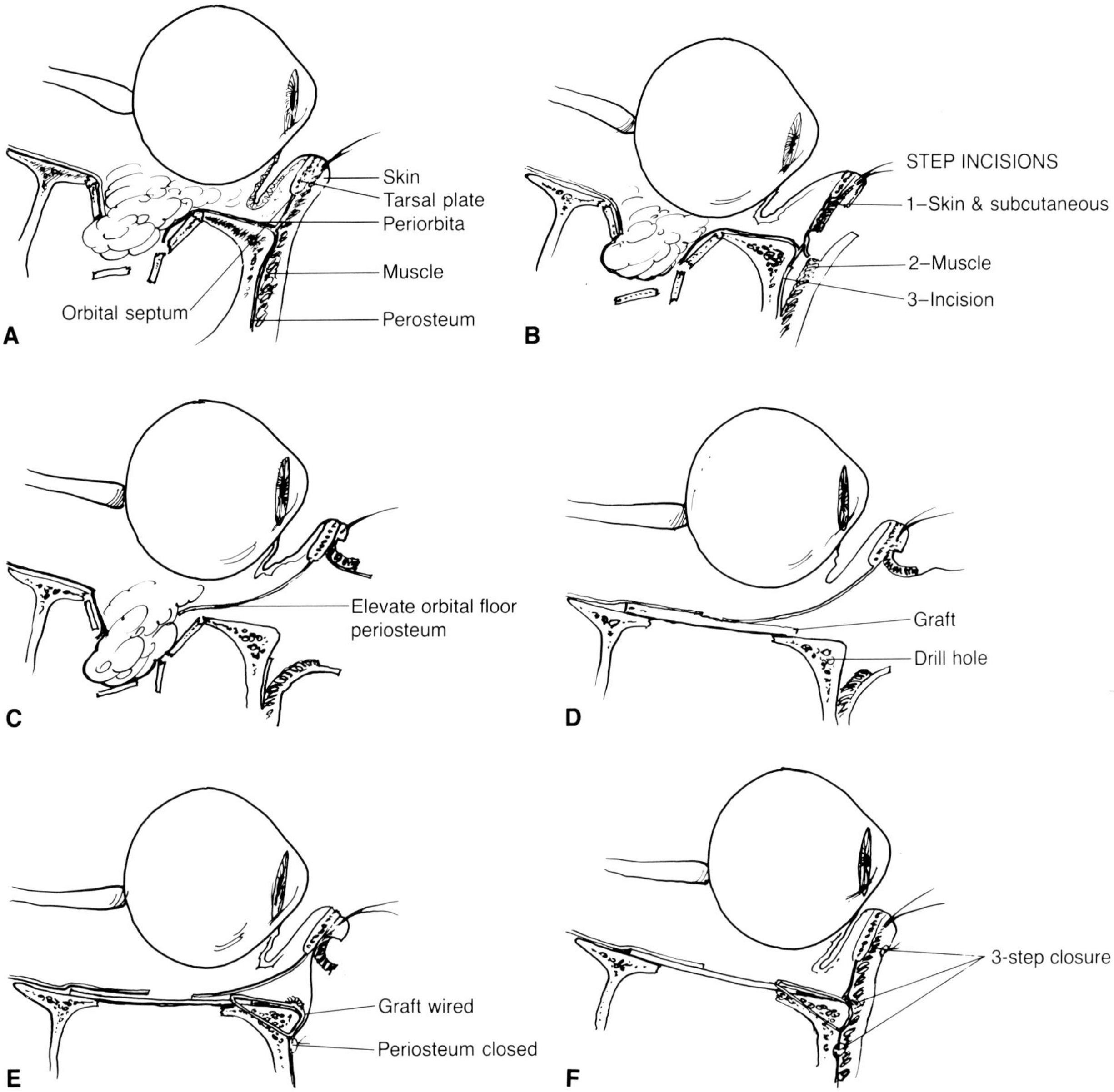

Figure 22–22. *(**A–D**) Subciliary approach and dissection for repair of orbital floor fracture (Rowe N, Williams JI. Maxillofacial Injuries. London: Churchill Livingstone, 1985; 513)*

fragments of the orbital floor may be attached and will then elevate with the soft tissue. If exploration is performed early (1 to 2 weeks) these tissues are much less likely to be atrophied or scarred into the antrum. A forced duction test is performed with a toothed tissue pickup to verify that entrapped soft tissues have been adequately released and that the globe can elevate.

When the dissection is complete, the inferior orbital rim should be reduced and fixated. In the case of a noncomminuted fracture that is relatively stable after reduction, a direct or figure-of-8 wire (26 to 28 g) is adequate (Fig. 22–23). Comminuted or unstable fractures are more satisfactorily stabilized with a small bone plate[28] (Fig. 22–24). On occasion, the bone plate will become palpable or annoying to the patient necessitating removal.

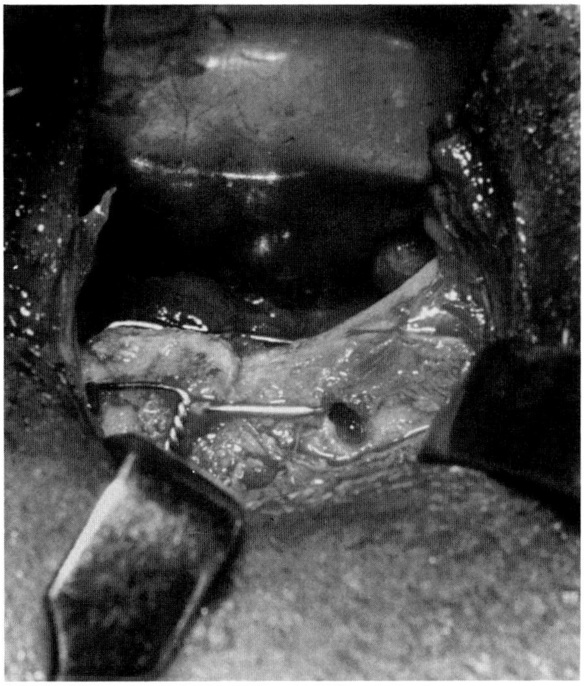

Figure 22–23. *Direct wire osteosynthesis of noncomminuted infraorbital rim fracture.*

The surgeon must determine whether or not additional reconstruction is necessary to restore the orbital floor. Comminuted fragments that have been returned to and maintain their pre-traumatic position need no further intervention if the periorbita is intact. Should a defect remain in the orbital floor, or should the fragile bones tend to prolapse back into the sinus, mechanical support of the orbital floor is indicated. Alloplastic material such as Teflon, Silastic, or Marlex mesh are commonly employed (Fig. 22–25). Bone grafts and autografts can be used, as will be discussed. The implant is cut to size to span the defect from its medial and lateral aspects. The implant should be no longer than necessary in its anteroposterior dimensions so as not to encroach on the inferior orbital tissue or optic nerve or the orbital rim. The implant is usually wider anteriorly than posteriorly and parallels the dimensions of the bony orbit. Implants should be fixed so they do not extrude. A 28-g wire or resorbable suture can be used to secure the anterior aspect of the implant to the posterior aspect of the inferior orbital rim (Fig. 22–26). The Marlex mesh is particularly easy to secure, and the mesh allows some ingrowth of adjacent tissue to immobilize the implant. Alternatively, a small lip can be made in an alloplastic

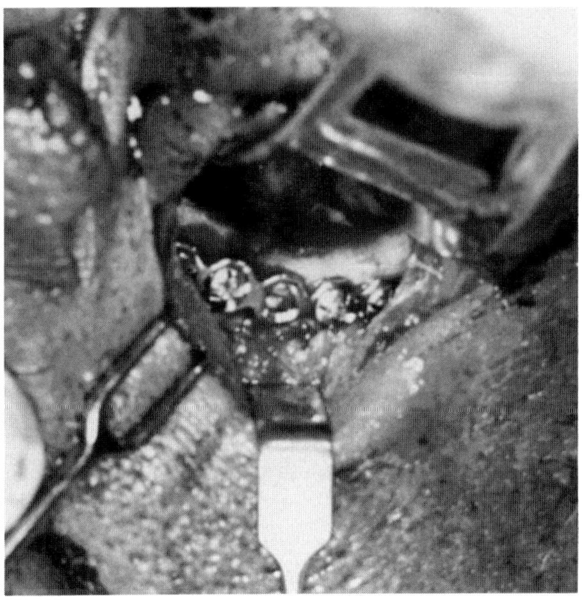

Figure 22–24. *Bone plate reconstruction of infraorbital rim.*

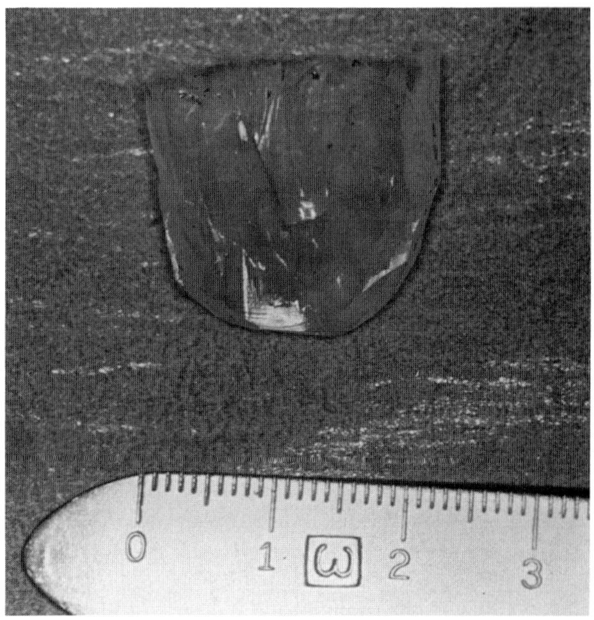

Figure 22–25. *Silastic alloplastic graft has been contoured to reconstruct the orbital floor.*

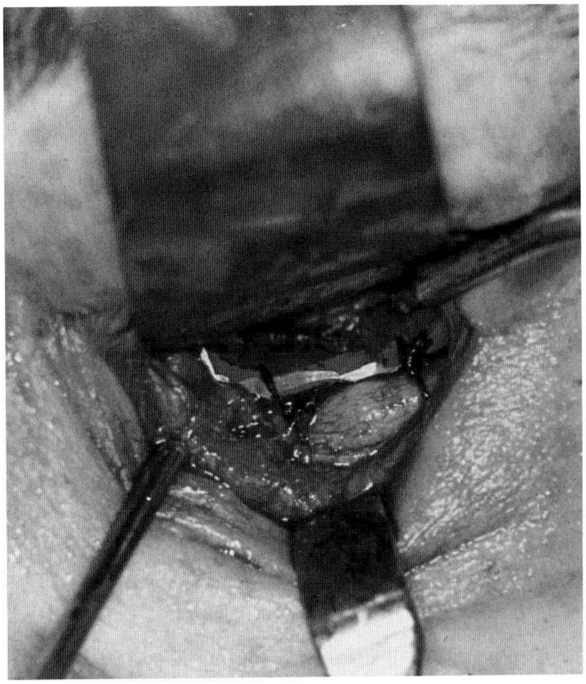

Figure 22–26. *Silastic graft is secured to inferior orbital rim by resorbable sutures.*

implant by placing two cuts into the anterior aspect of the implant and bending the lip inferiorly to engage in the fracture site.[30] This mechanically prevents extrusion and has the advantage of keeping the implant further away from the orbital rim and lid margin.

After reconstruction of the orbital floor by any means it is important to assess the condition of the infraorbital nerve. The nerve is often visible within the defect of the floor and should not be compressed by large bone fragments or graft materials. Fractures extending through the inferior orbital rim generally extend through the infraorbital foramen and frequently cause paresthesia of the infraorbital nerve. Compression or distortion of the nerve by reduction at the rim will reduce the chances of adequate sensation returning to the region.

Before closure, reassessment of enophthalmos and globe entrapment is done. Increased graft support or thickness may be necessary if additional globe elevation is desired. Forced duction is done in the inferior and possibly lateral and medial conjunctive fornices to prove that the globe is free of interferences.

Repair of the incision is accomplished in layers. Resorbable material such as 3-0 chronic catgut can be used to close the periosteum. This step is advocated to ensure proper positioning of the lower eyelid and to allow graft material to be covered. The thin muscular layer can be closed with a few resorbable sutures or left open, since the orientation of the muscular incision allows the tissues to close passively. There are multiple satisfactory ways of closing the skin incision. A "baseball" suture of 6-0 nylon is technically the easiest method but is somewhat difficult to remove. Interrupted nonabsorbable sutures present the same postoperative difficulty. A running horizontal dermal suture affords excellent closure and is very easy to remove. It can be difficult to place due to the skin in the region. The use of 6-0 plain gut placed in a "baseball" fashion provides a rapid and excellent cosmetic result and it does not require removal since it dissolves in 3 to 5 days.

Postoperatively the vision in both eyes should be checked and compared to the preoperative baseline. This can be difficult because of edema. If there is any question of decreased visual acuity, an ophthalmologist should be consulted. Examination of the retina has been recommended to assess the adequacy of retinal perfusion, especially if an antral pack is used which may compress the afferent blood supply to the retina.[31] Topical ophthalmic antibiotic drops can be employed in cases of severe edema to prevent infection, which can occasionally result from stasis. The lacrimal apparatus will function normally once the edema subsides. The pumping action of the lids and the lacrimal pump flush pathogens from the inferior fornix. If the lids function properly, antibiotics offer no benefit. Periorbital infection after the surgical repair of fractures is rare. Empirically, antibiotics are recommended if graft material is used in the orbital floor, since it is in contact with the antrum. Penicillin has historically been very effective, although a drug with a broader spectrum such as amoxicillin-clavulanic acid (Augmentin) to cover potential sinus pathogens, including anaerobes, H-influenza, and staphylococcus, can be considered.

Graft Materials for Orbital Floor Reconstruction

At least four methods of rebuilding the orbital floor are commonly employed. These include repositioning of the displaced bones (see previous discussion), use of alloplastic graft material such as Marlex mesh, Silastic, and Teflon (see previous discussion); autogenous bone grafts; and homografts such as lyophilized dura.

Materials used for grafting must be biocompatible, adaptable, contourable, and capable of maintaining strength and position. Autogenous bone is the ideal material for implantation except that a donor operation is required. The bone can be harvested from the inner table of the iliac crest or the outer cortex of cranial bone. Autogenous bone is not rejected by host tissues and unites with adjacent bare bone; it is the preferred method when bone is necessarily going to be harvested to treat concomitant problems. Rowe[32] suggests that autogenous bone is preferable when restoring defects greater than 1.5 cm in diameter, since there is often an insufficient bone margin on which an alloplast can rest. Autogenous bone is used when the orbital rim is grafted simultaneously with the orbital floor.

Homografts of banked bone can be used in lieu of autogenous bone to provide a framework for host bone replacement.[33] Banked cadaveric bone is widely successful in orthopedic and maxillofacial applications and has the advantage of avoiding a donor site harvest operation. A recent disadvantage has been patient reluctance to accept donor materials from anonymous donors due to the fear of acquiring human immunodeficiency virus infection. Lyophilized dura has been used as a homograft for orbital floor reconstruction.[34–36] Waite and Clanton[36] state that lyophilized dura is close to the ideal implant because of its strength, adaptability, ease of suturing across the defect, biocompatibility with and replacement by host connective tissue, lack of migration, absence of infection, prepackaged shapes appropriate for orbital reconstruction, nonimpingement on orbital structures, and greater allowable margin for error in placement over other graft materials.[36] It may not be suitable for large defects because dura, although tough, is not rigid. Since it is thin it is not suitable to connect enophthalmos. Creutzfeld-Jakob disease transmission through infected dura mater is of concern, although there is not conclusive evidence for this.[37]

Antral Packing

The orbital floor can be reconstructed and supported from below by the use of an antral pack placed through a Caldwell-Luc approach. When the bone of the orbital floor is present yet sagging into the maxillary sinus, elevation and support from below is satisfactory. Rowe[38] states that an antral pack can support the orbital floor if the orbital rim is intact or has been repaired, the bone comprising the antral roof is present, and the antral floor is stable. When the bone has been lost, a graft is used to bridge the defect and reconstruct the orbital floor (Fig. 22–27). If diplopia is present, the orbital floor should be explored directly in order to elevate fat, connective tissue, and possibly muscle out of the defect and back into the orbit. Trapdooring may prevent full return of orbital contents only if the antral approach is used. The antral pack is recommended primarily to elevate and stabilize a depressed, highly commuted antral floor in the absence of diplopia or enophthalmos. The antral pack will allow the repositioned comminutions to remain attached to periosteum as they heal and to prevent enlargement of the globe and the possibility of late enophthalmos.

The surgical approach to the antrum is the Caldwell-Luc approach. A bone window is made large enough to admit a finger and also to allow enough light for visual inspection. Prolapsed orbital tissues are palpated and gently pushed superiorly. A forced duction is done to ascertain that entrapment has not occurred as a result of the floor elevation. The antrum is packed with half-inch iodoform gauze soaked in deodorizing compounds such as benzoin, balsam of Peru, or Whitehead's varnish. After 3 weeks a nasal antrostomy is created to allow egress of the packing. The packing must not be overcompressed posteriorly or superiorly, since the optic foramen is immediately above this region. The pupillary levels should be compared as well as the lateral projection of the corneas to prevent overstuffing of the pack. Visual acuity and checking of retinal blood flow by fundoscopic examination is advisable to ensure that overcompression of the orbit has not occurred. Antibiotics can be used empirically while the packing is in place to prevent sinusitis. Removal of antrostomy packing is extremely unpleasant and usually painful for patients. Intravenous sedation or ultralight general anesthesia may be advisable for many patients. Occasionally bleeding occurs after pack removal, possibly due to adherence of the pack to granulation tissue at the sinus periphery. A temporary nasal pack will tamponade persistent bleeding and allow a clot to form. Another approach[38] to pack removal is to elevate the lateral flap slightly under local anesthesia and pull out the care-

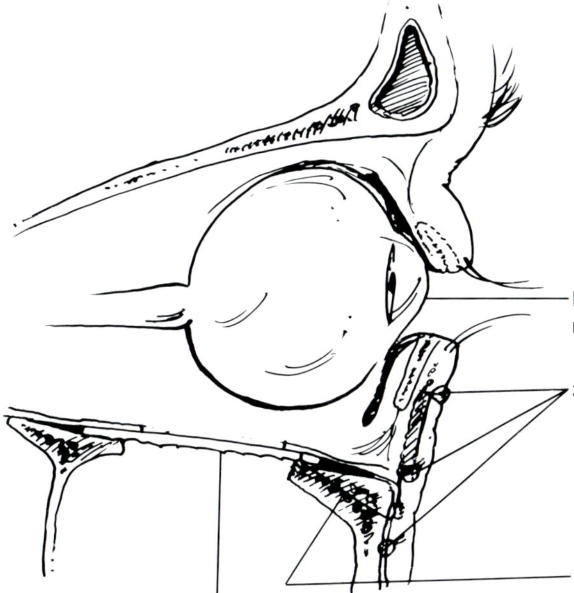

Figure 22–27. *Diagram shows a bone graft used to reconstruct a large defect in the orbital floor. (Rowe N, Williams JI. Maxillofacial Injuries. London: Churchill Livingstone, 1985; 517)*

fully layered pack. The flap is then resutured. No nasal antrostomy is used in this technique.

Some surgeons advocate the use of an antral balloon or a Foley catheter to support the antral roof.[39] The antrum is exposed and inspected by the lateral approach while the catheter is placed through and let out of a nasal antrostomy. An antral balloon does not allow selective control of pressure within the antrum and has more limited application than the pack. A possible advantage of an inflatable balloon over a pack is that more fluid can be added postsurgically if this is deemed clinically desirable. Care must be taken to avoid compression of the globe, retinal blood supply, and optic nerve.

Early Complications of Orbital Repair

Complications following orbital repair encompass the spectrum of problems following treatment of any facial fracture such as infection or malunion, but occasionally they are manifest as untoward sequelae of the visual apparatus. It is therefore of utmost importance to establish a clearly documented presurgical baseline as to the trauma victim's vision, ocular mobility, degree of enophthalmos, diplopia, pupillary reflex, and the appearance of the retina. In this section, discussion will be of complications unique to the orbit. General complications associated with trauma and fractures are discussed elsewhere in this text.

In the treatment of periorbital fractures, preservation of vision takes precedence over restoration of the bony anatomy, gaze, or enophthalmos. Certain complications can lead to vision loss and must be recognized early:

Optic nerve compression Central retinal artery occlusion
Retrobulbar hemorrhage
Superior orbital fissure syndrome
Cavernous sinus syndrome
Orbital apex syndrome

Although definitive treatment of ocular or retrobulbar complications is accomplished by the ophthalmologist, the maxillofacial surgeon must recognize the signs and symptoms of impending or present complications in order to institute emergency therapy and consultation. Fortunately, the complications listed are extremely rare and, when present, are usually the result of the traumatic injury as opposed to surgical intervention.

Optic Nerve Compression

The optic disk is the distal extension of the optic nerve, and any interruption in nerve transmission along this pathway prevents visual impulse transmission to the brain. The optic foramen transmits the optic nerve through the lesser sphenoid wing. The nerve is then contained within the globe within the muscular cone where it is usually protected from bony displacement. However, extensive fractures on rare occasion could extend back to involve the optic foramen. Fortunately, fracture lines usually stop anteriorly at the inferior orbital fracture so that elevation of the orbital floor, or zygoma, does not alter the borders of the optic foramen.

Contusion or compression of the optic nerve will cause decreased visual acuity. Progressive worsening is consistent with compression of the nerve secondary to edema or hematoma. Although the fundus of the eye may be normal, pallor of the optic disk develops.[40] Trauma may result in shearing forces along the optic nerve, which disrupt the vascular supply in the optic canal causing ischemic necrosis.[41] When the optic nerve is compressed the visual changes are delayed and progressive, whereas when the nerve is contused the visual loss is apparent and maximized immediately.[42] A compressed nerve can be decompressed, but intervention cannot improve a contused nerve.[42] CT scanning of the orbit and optic canal can be helpful in diagnosis in conjunction with serial clinical examinations. Clearly, ophthalmologic consultation is indicated for evaluation and treatment of suspected optic nerve compression or contusion.

Central Retinal Artery Occlusion

The central retinal artery is a branch of the ophthalmic artery that runs within the dural sheath of the optic nerve. Just posterior to the globe, it pierces the optic nerve and enters the eye with the nerve at the optic disk. This artery essentially supplies the retina. Occlusion of this artery may occur from optic nerve compression, shearing, or hematoma. Thrombosis or embolism can occlude the artery as can external pressure on the lids or periocular compression within the bony orbit. Clinically there is total loss of vision, which may be intermittent initially in compression injuries. Fundascopically, optic disk pallor, narrowed arterioles, and a cherry red spot at the macula are observed. The prognosis is very poor and blindness of the involved eye is expected.

Retrobulbar Hemorrhage

Retrobulbar hemorrhage can result from orbitofacial trauma and, infrequently, secondary to surgical repair of such injuries. An extensive study by Ord[43] showed that 0.3% of the patients studied developed retrobulbar hemorrhage after treatment of orbital fractures (zygomatic complex). Those who had evacuation of the retrobulbar hemorrhage had improvement of their vision while those left unevacuated lost vision in the involved eye.

Retrobulbar hemorrhage should be suspected in patients complaining of ocular pain made worse with eye movement, decreasing vision, and diplopia. Clinical examination is usually positive for marked proptosis and subconjunctual hemorrhage. The globe loses its retrobulbar cushion and becomes hard. The intraocular pressure measured by tonometry increases (15 mm is normal). Compression of the vascular structures causes retinal artery constriction and optic disk pallor. Compression causes dilation of the pupil and loss of its ability to constrict appropriately to light. The consensual light reflex is preserved as long as the optic pathway from the injured eye remains functional. Dilation of the pupil must be distinguished from other causes such as brain stem compression of the ocular motor nerve, instillation of dilating eyedrops for ocular examination, and traumatic mydriasis.

Posterior to the globe a muscular cone is formulated by the six extraocular muscles. Within the cone are the ophthalmic artery and its branches. This muscular cone is a closed compartment except for a small opening at its posterolateral border. Rupture of a blood vessel within the compartment causes pressure to rise within the cone and results in compression of the posterior globe containing the optic nerve and disk, retina, and choroid.

Treatment of retrobulbar hemorrhage involves medical and surgical therapies. Rowe[44] recommends early initiation of the following medical therapy:

1. Intravenous mannitol (200 ml, 20% solution) to promote reduction of vitreous and aqueous humor by encouraging systemic dehydration
2. Intravenous acetazolamide (Diamox) 500 mg to reduce humor production
3. Papaverine 40 mg IV to reduce vascular spasm of the vessels supplying the eye
4. Intravenous steroids such as hydrocortisone 100 mg or megadose steroids such as dexamethasone phosphate (Decadron) 3 to 4 mg/kg, followed by 1 to 3 mg/kg every 6 hours as advocated by Anderson et al.[45]

Failure to respond to medical therapy after 15 to 20 minutes is an indication for surgical intervention,[44] although some surgeons wait 12 hours to assess the response to megadose steroids.[45] Although a comprehensive review of the surgical approaches to the treatment of retrobulbar hemorrhage is beyond the scope of this chapter, a brief synopsis will follow.

The basic concept of surgical decompression is release of pressure from hematoma of the retroorbital region. Should the hematoma lie beneath the periorbita, reopening the infraorbital incision will allow access for decompression and hemostasis. Intraconal hematoma is drained by opening the muscular cone laterally between the inferior rectus and lateral rectus muscles. Surgery of the intraconal space should be performed by an eye surgeon. The antral roof can be removed, if necessary, to gain access to the posterior inferior muscular cone or orbital floor. Division of the orbital septum may be necessary to release hemorrhage from the extraconal space if an incision to expose the orbital floor has not been made previously. Intraarterial papaverine (40 mg) has been injected into the supraorbital artery after surgical exposure to successfully reduce spasm of the central retinal artery.[46]

Superior Orbital Fissure Syndrome

Infrequently the neurovascular structures that pass through the superior orbital fissure of the posterior orbit become compressed or contused from fracture or hematoma in the fissure (greater sphenoid wing). The clinical presentation of the superior orbital fissure syndrome is a result of the physiologic consequences of injury to the anatomical structures that pass through the fissure (Fig. 22–28). Ophthalmoplegia is due to palsy of cranial nerves III, IV, V, and VI. Ptosis of the lid results from cranial nerve III injury. The pupil dilates because the parasympathetic nerve supply carried on the oculomotor nerve is blocked, resulting in unbalanced sympathetic activity. The ophthalmic division of cranial nerve V (V_1) with its frontal and nasociliary branches becomes dysfunctional, giving rise to forehead anesthesia and loss of the corneal reflex. Pupillary constriction to light is absent because the oculomotor nerve is affected on the ipsilateral side. On the opposite side the reflex constriction is present, since the contralateral oculomotor nerve is intact as is light perception in the involved eye. Obstruction of the ophthalmic veins and lymphatics can cause proptosis and edema. Radiographically, displacement of the greater wing of the spheroid or narrowing of the superior orbital fissure can be seen. CT scanning better demonstrates the bony relationships in the posterior orbit as well as hematoma.[47]

Treatment of superior orbital fissure syndrome is generally by observation and may take up to one year to resolve.[48] Rowe[49] recommends that, if surgical intervention is necessary to treat zygomaticoorbital fractures, 10 to 14 days should elapse to allow clot organization. Elevation of the orbital floor is unwise because it may further compress the involved neurovascular structures or compromise the optic nerve nearby.[49]

Cavernous Sinus Syndrome

The clinical presentation of cavernous sinus syndrome is essentially the same as the superior orbital fissure syndrome (ophthalmoplegia, lid ptosis, dilated pupil, cutaneous anesthesia of V_1) with the additional finding of maxillary nerve (V_2) sensory loss. The V_2 crosses the cavernous sinus but does not enter the superior orbital fissure.

Traumatically induced aneurysms occasionally oc-

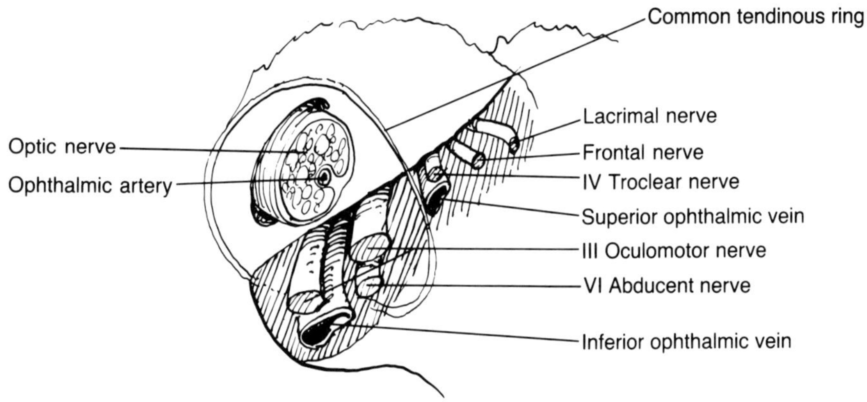

Figure 22–28. *Contents of the superior orbital fissure. (Rowe N, Williams JI. Maxillofacial Injuries. London: Churchill Livingstone, 1985; 450)*

cur in the internal carotid artery within the cavernous sinus and may result in a carotid-cavernous sinus fistula.[50] The clinical presentation may be that of cavernous sinus syndrome with a bruit over the orbit. Also present may be ocular injection, lid swelling, diplopia, pulsatile exophthalmos, arteriolization of conjunctival veins, conjunctival sclerosis, and elevated intraocular pressure.[51] Such injuries are uncommon but have been reported following midface trauma.[52] High-resolution CT scanning and angiography are used in diagnosis and in treatment[53] (embolization). The therapeutic objective in treating a carotid cavernous fistula is prevention of blindness secondary to retinal or optic nerve ischemia and glaucoma.

Orbital Apex Syndrome

At the apex of the bony orbit exists the superior orbital fissure and the optic canal containing the optic nerve and ophthalmic artery. A fracture in this region or a significant hematoma will present with signs and symptoms similar to retrobulbar hematoma and superior orbital fissure syndrome. This extremely severe condition is very uncommon and little has been reported on it.

Late Complications of Orbital Fractures

In addition to complications seen with midface fractures such as poor reduction, wound infection, infected grafts, enophthalmos, diplopia, and retrobulbar complications, the orbital region presents many additional complications unique to the orbit. Included among them are late development of enophthalmos or diplopia, ectropion, entropion, displacement of the lateral or medial canthal tendons, lid ptosis, and injury to the lacrimal apparatus.

Late Enophthalmos and Diplopia

The primary goal in the treatment of orbital fractures is the restoration or preservation of normal anatomy and physiology of the orbital region. Early treatment best preserves this goal, but treatment failures do occur owing to infection, lack of patient compliance, extensive scarring, technical problems, and massive tissue loss, among others. The residual problem confronting the surgeon is usually enophthalmos or diplopia.

Late enophthalmos is approached somewhat differently than immediate posttraumatic enophthalmos in that the surgeon is usually confronted with a stable but enlarged orbit containing scarred and atrophied periorbital soft tissues. Enophthalmos becomes cosmetically obvious at 3 mm,[54] and if more severe it can interfere with vision from obstruction by the orbital rim. Late diplopia may be due to reentrapment of periocular soft tissues, muscle atrophy, scar formation, or intrinsic muscle or nerve dysfunction. Muscles or nerves may be irreversibly injured.

Treatment of late enophthalmos and diplopia is more difficult than early repair. Many methods of restoring globe position have been performed, including the use of alloplastic implants,[55,56] autogenous grafts of bone,[57–60] homografts of dura,[61] osteotomy of the zygoma,[62] and combination of the above procedures.[63]

Mathog et al.[64] published a study of 38 cases with long-term follow-up after correction of late enophthalmos (Fig. 22–29). Almost two-thirds of their patients had orbital reconstruction 6 months to 2 years after injury. In their method a combination of three incisions (infraciliary, medial canthus, and lateral brow) is used to expose the inferior, medial, and superolateral orbital walls.[64] The medial pocket[65] is limited posteriorly by the posterior ethmoid artery, superiorly by the trochlea, and inferiorly by the lacrimal groove. The dissection may cause bleeding from the anterior ethmoid artery, which is controlled by pressure. The incision is placed halfway between the caruncle of the eye and the nasal dorsum. Bleeding from the angular vessels is controlled by cautery. The lacrimal collecting system and the medial canthal tendon are avoided inferiorly. This approach allows 280° of access but avoids the optic nerve, ophthalmic artery, superior orbital fissure, and tendineus ring. Bone grafts from the iliac crest, ribs, or cranium are contoured and placed appropriately around the orbit subperiosteally to overcorrect the defect by 1 to 2 mm.[63] The grafts are placed strategically to move the globe in the intended direction. Inferiorly placed grafts elevate the globe, posterior superior grafts move the globe anteriorly, and medially positioned grafts push the globe laterally. Stable postoperative globe position within 1 to 2 mm of the opposite eye is possible. Those patients exhibiting diplopia had complete resolution or improvement of the diplopia.[64]

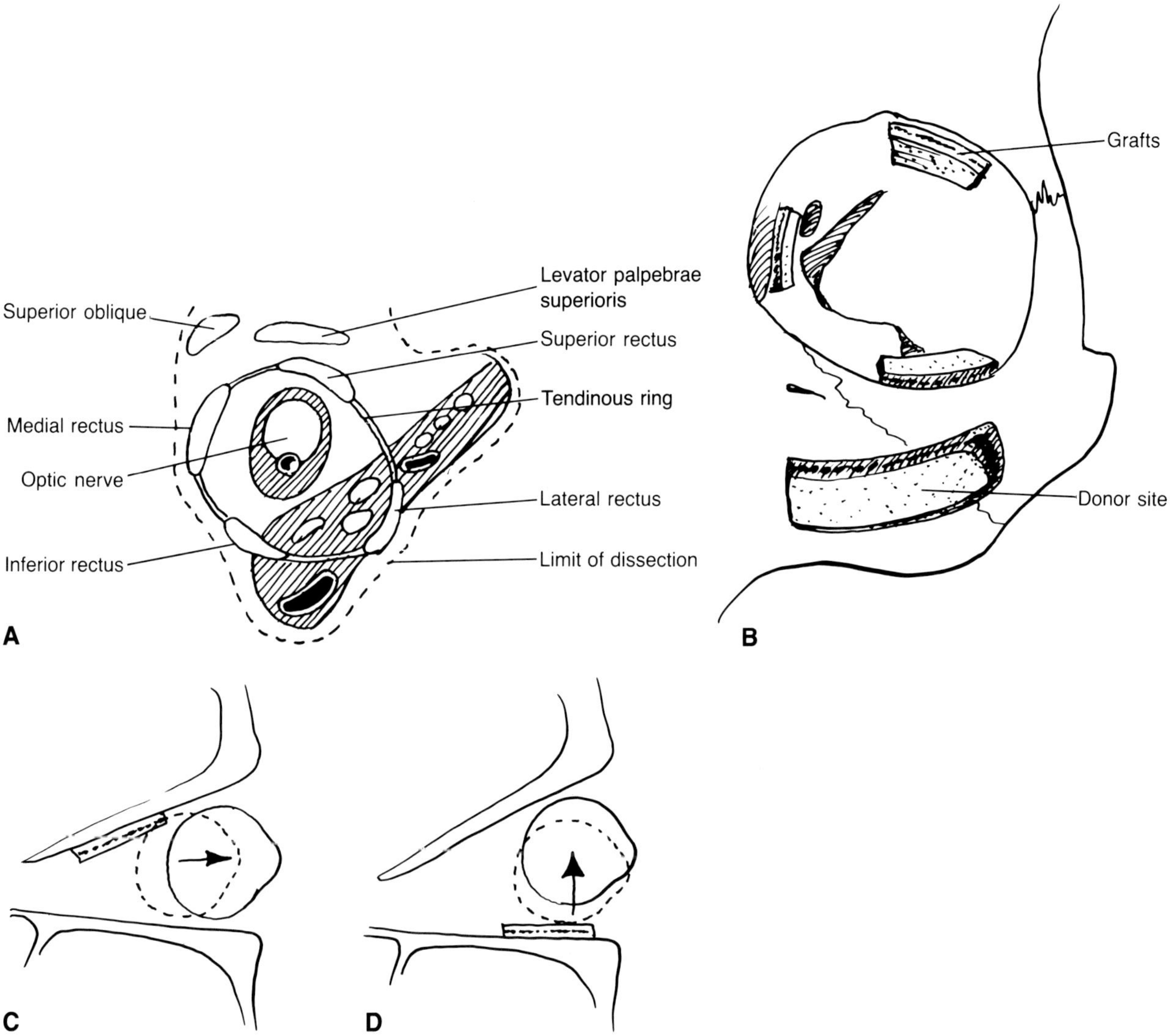

Figure 22–29. *Correction of late enophthalmos and diplopia by iliac bone grafts. (**A**) The limit of the dissection. Dissection allows 270° of access to the orbit. (**B**) Position of various bone grafts. (**C**) Superiorly positioned graft causes anterior movement of the globe. (**D**) Elevation of the globe by grafting the orbital floor. (Mathog RH, et al. Surgical correction of enophthalmos and diplopia. Arch Otolarynyol Head Neck Surg 1989; 115:172)*

Ectropion

Ectropion is a drooping or eversion of the lower eyelid as a result of lower lid laxity, canthal tendon laxity, or cicatrix formation from scarring. Ectropion can also be congenital or develop with aging. In the context of this chapter, this complication can arise from primary trauma to the lower lid apparatus or as a result of unfavorable healing from infraorbital incisions. A well placed infraciliary incision, which is appropriately stepped through the various layers, seems least likely to result in unfavorable scar contracture (Fig. 22–30). Medial or lateral canthal tendon laxity or displacement may worsen the degree of ectropion. Sophisticated techniques for correction of ectropion have been developed by oculoplastic surgeons and are be-

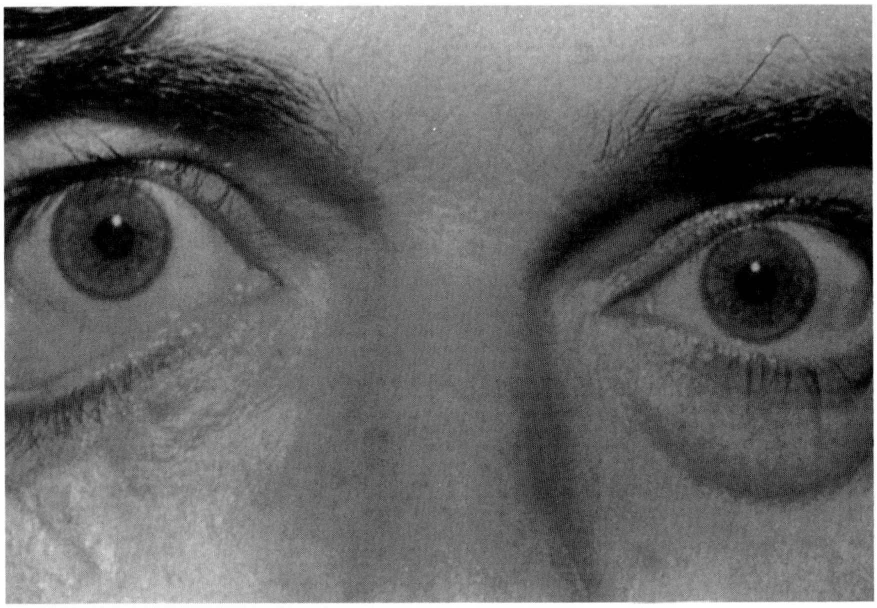

Figure 22–30. *Ectropion of the right lower lid secondary to scarring. (Spalton HJ. Atlas of Clinical Ophthalmology. London: Gower, p. 2.5)*

yond the scope of this chapter. Bosniak[66] has outlined the techniques graphically and the reader is referred to his work.

Entropion

Entropion is an inversion of the lid margin resulting in cilia or eyelashes brushing the globe or conjunctiva. In trauma or surgery, it may occur if the tarsal plate, orbital septum, and lid retractor relation is disturbed. In addition to the cosmetic deformity, there can be ulceration of the cornea, conjunctivitis, and keratitis. Careful surgical dissection, as described previously, will minimize disturbance of the tarsal plate and orbital septum. Entropion can be predictably corrected by imbrication of the lower lid retractors.[67,68]

Medial Canthal Tendon and Lacrimal Apparatus Injuries

The medial canthal tendon is often displaced or separated in fractures involving the medial orbital wall. Nasoethmoidal injuries may cause lateral displacement of the medial canthal tendon on one or both sides and result in traumatic telecanthus. When the tendon remains attached to its bony insertion, proper reduction and fixation of the fractures will restore the tendon. If the tendon has separated from its insertion, it must be mechanically joined to its counterpart on the opposite side. This can be accomplished using nonabsorbable sutures such as 3-0 polyester on a very small needle so as not to pull through the free end of the tendon. The suture can be placed in a figure-of-8 fashion with both ends brought to the stable side and secured over a button, or directly to the lacrimal bone on the opposite side if access is available. The intercanthal distance should be 33 to 38 mm, and overcorrection is desired since postoperative widening is common. Transnasal wiring is necessary when bilateral nasoethmoidal fractures result in telecanthus.

In certain fractures, lacerations, and avulsion injuries such as dog bites, the medial canthal tendon is severed. Direct reapproximation of the severed ends can be accomplished with 4-0 nonabsorbable suture. The lateral end can also be attached to periosteum or affixed directly to bone with a wire loop if the avulsion is at the bone-tendon interface.

The medial canthal tendon has two insertions into bone, one anterior and the other posterior. Between the heads courses the main lacrimal canaliculus, which is formed as the superior and inferior canaliculi join. The canaliculus is damaged in medial canthal injuries, and lacrimal drainage must be reestablished or epiphora results. Laceration in the medial canthal region is likely to lacerate the lacrimal drainage canaliculus whereas blunt trauma is much less likely to tear the canaliculus. A torn tear duct must be reconstructed over an appropriate stent,[69] and some authors recommend reanastomosis under the microscope with microsuture material (9-0 monofilament).

When the medial canthal tendon has been bluntly injured or displaced, it should be assumed that the lacrimal drainage system has been damaged. The superior and inferior puncta should be examined and if the drainage system is clinically not functioning, the superior and inferior canaliculi should be probed with lacrimal probes and very fine 1-mm silastic tubing can be threaded through each canaliculus and brought out into the nose and the free ends tied (Fig. 22–31). A small loop of tubing will be visible passing between the superior and inferior puncta. While the tubing remains in place, epiphora will be evident since the tube occludes the ducts. Upon removal of the tubing, the lacrimal apparatus should remain cannulized and functional. Mustarde[70] recommends removing the tubing after 2 weeks and then probing the canaliculus twice a week for 3 weeks to reduce stricture formation. A silicone tube with swaged lacrimal probe devised by Jackson[71] can be threaded through the inferior and superior puncta and tied to allow the free end to fall into the nose. Jackson recommends removing the tubing at 3 months.[71]

Lateral Canthal Injury

Displacement of the lateral canthus of the eye occurs with displacement of the frontal process of the zygomatic bone because the bone contains Whitnall's tubercle to which the canthus is attached. It is unusual for the tendon to separate from its bony origin and, therefore, the lateral canthal tendon is appropriately restored to its proper position upon accurate reduction and fixation of the zygomatic complex. The medial and lateral canthi are essentially on the same plane and should be compared with the opposite eye. In cases of severely comminuted orbital trauma, it may not be possible to reduce all of the bony segments exactly. Visual judgment is needed to establish the appropriate canthal position. As a rule of thumb, the distance between the medial and lateral canthi of the eye is the same as the distance between the two medial canthi. It is recommended that the whole face be exposed during midface or orbital surgery to allow visual comparisons with the opposite side.

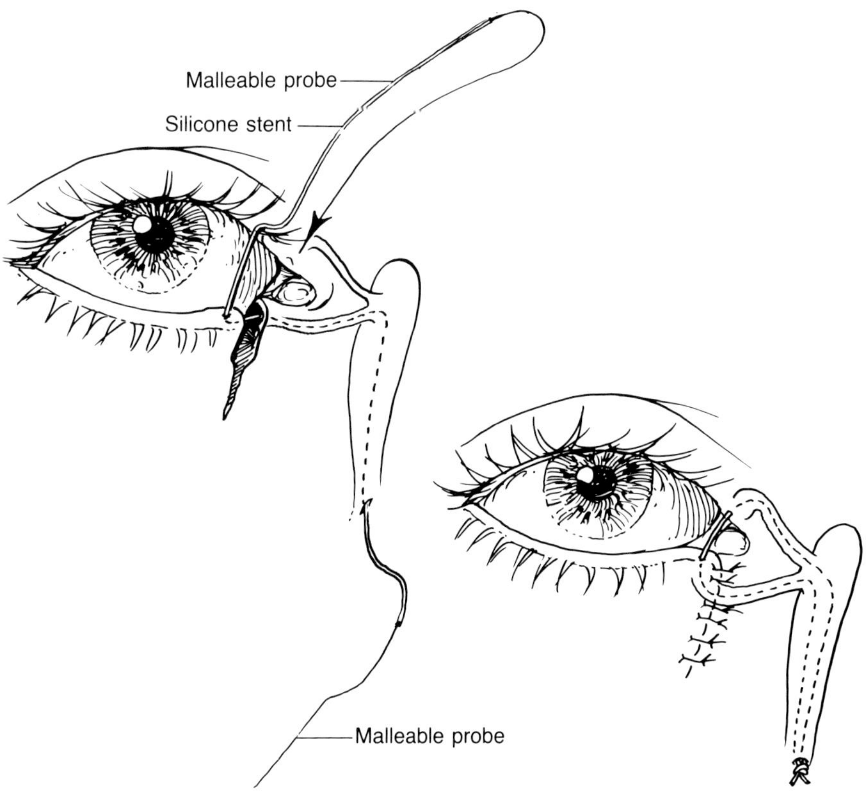

Figure 22–31. *Reconstruction of the nasolacrimal drainage ducts using silastic tubing onto a malleable duct probe. (Rowe N, Williams JI. Maxillofacial Injuries. London: Churchill Livingstone, 1985; 533)*

The lateral canthus forms a sharp, clearly defined point as the superior and inferior lids meet. If the tendon insertion is displaced medially or severed, the canthus will become blunt or rounded. In the unusual case of an avulsed lateral canthal tendon, the ends should be reapproximated using a 4-0 mattress suture of nonabsorbable material.[72] If the tendon is severed at the bone, it can be joined to the periorbita above Whitnall's tubercle. A lacerated canthus can be restored by using the method of Garber et al.[72] by placing a 6-0 silk double-armed suture through the grey line of the upper lid 2 mm above the torn canthus and brought out through the skin along the lateral orbital rim. The other arm is passed through the grey line of the lower lid 2 mm from the laceration and also brought out through the skin of the lateral rim. The orbicularis and subcutaneous layer is closed with fine absorbable suture, and the skin is closed with 6-0 silk. The suture passing through the gray line is now tied over a small cotton bolster and can be removed in 10 to 14 days. This suture acts to pull the canthus laterally and recreates the acute angle of the canthus.

Eyelid Repair

Repair of lacerated eyelids is an application of anatomical repositioning of delicate functional structures. This section focuses on repair of the lacerations that the maxillofacial surgeon may be faced with, especially in conjunction with multiple maxillofacial injuries and fractures. Repair of lid deformities and late reconstruction of the eyelids is best accomplished by specialists and is beyond the scope of this chapter.

The basic principles of wound repair must be meticulously adhered to when repairing eyelids because this soft tissue is uniquely under function, and even minor unsatisfactory scarring results in both functional and cosmetic compromise. The eye itself can become compromised if lid function is incomplete. Particular principles, such as closure without tension, elimination of dead space, proper orientation of flaps parallel to orbicularis fibers when possible, subcutaneous undermining, and exact approximation of layers are crucial.

Lacerations, especially in full-thickness injuries involving the margin of either lid, are best repaired in three layers. General anesthesia is preferred to minimize tissue distortion from local anesthesia. Reflex blinking by an awake patient during application of instruments and sutures will make repair difficult and possibly unsatisfactory. Loupe magnification or use of the operating microscope allows much more accurate suture placement. A protective corneal shield will help prevent corneal abrasion from instruments, needles, or suture material during repair.

Repair of the lid can be accomplished using the method of Mindlin et al.[73] (Fig. 22–32). Preparation of the wound edge is accomplished by squaring the full thickness with a very small blade. The lash line, meibomian glands, and grey line are used as anatomical landmarks for alignment. The meibomian glands are an extension of the tarsal plate. The grey line represents the fascial layer between the inner and outer lid surfaces (mucocutaneous junction) and is situated between the lash line and the meibomian gland orifices. A 6-0 silk suture is placed at the level of the meibomian glands. When the free margin of the lid is even and the lash line is anatomically continuous on either side of the wound, the meibomian line suture is tied. The second suture is placed just anterior to the mucocutaneous junction of the posterior free wound margin. The third suture is placed in the lash line with care taken to avoid suturing the lashes. The ends of the two more posterior sutures are tied to the knot of the anterior lash line suture to direct the free knot ends away from the cornea. The tarsal plate is then approximated using 5-0 or 6-0 absorbable suture placed from the anterior aspect about one-half the depth of the tarsus to avoid the cornea. Skin sutures are then placed. It is not necessary to suture the conjunctiva. The lid margin should be slightly everted at repair so notching does not occur as a result of wound contracture. Skin sutures are removed after 3 or 4 days and the lid margin sutures at 7 to 9 days.

The upper and lower lid margins are repaired using similar techniques.

OCULAR INJURIES

Each year there are 2.4 million eye injuries,[74] and between 20,000 and 68,000 of these injuries threaten vision.[75,76] Trauma to the eye can occur in conjunction with other maxillofacial trauma, as isolated injuries, or as a result of periorbital surgery such as orbital floor exploration. Therefore, it is imperative for the maxillofacial surgeon to evaluate the eyes in the presence of midface trauma. Sharp trauma, such as explo-

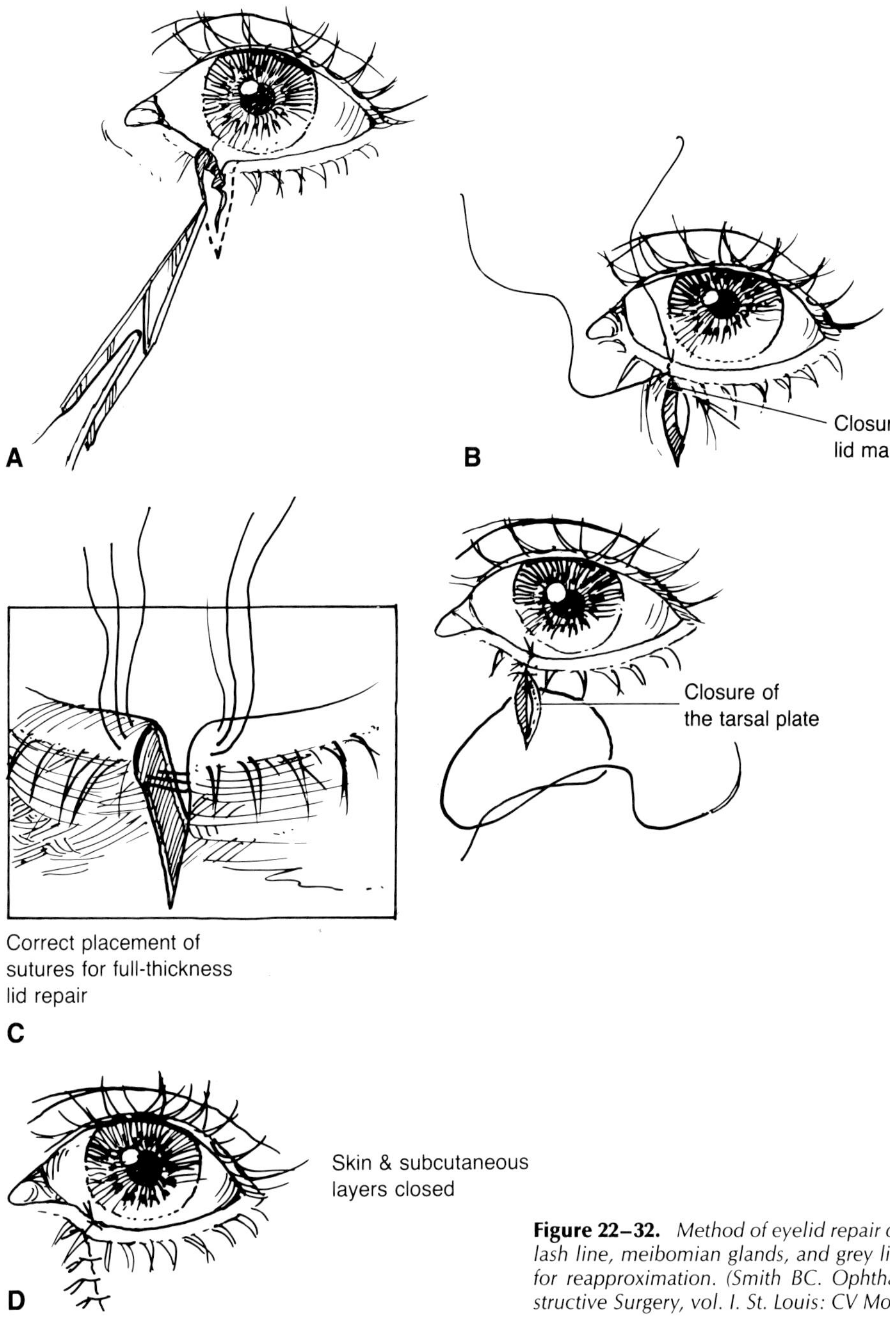

Figure 22–32. *Method of eyelid repair described by Mindlin. The lash line, meibomian glands, and grey line are used as landmarks for reapproximation. (Smith BC. Ophthalmic Plastic and Reconstructive Surgery, vol. I. St. Louis: CV Mosby, 1987; 432, 433)*

sions or windshield injuries, increase the probabilities for eye injury and ocular foreign bodies and must not be overlooked.

The primary eye function is vision, so visual acuity should be tested in both eyes after basic measures for all trauma patients have been accomplished. A history of the accident can alert the examiner to the possibility of blunt injury, globe laceration, or presence of a foreign body. In cases of chemical injury, the eye is flushed with copious irrigation before vision is tested.

A standard eye chart can be used to check acuity: a less satisfactory alternative which may be necessary in the multiple trauma patient is use of the pocket eye chart. Corrective lenses should be used or, if they are absent, the patient's uncorrected vision must be compared to the tested vision. If vision is decreased from the patient's normal baseline, the cause must be sought. The scope of the problem may range from edema of the lids, conjunctiva, or cornea, which requires minimal treatment; to mechanical interruptions in vision such as hemorrhage of the anterior chamber, dislocation of the lens, or globe laceration; to failure to perceive visual stimuli from retinal injuries or optic nerve trauma.

After vision testing, the eye is inspected and examined from anterior to posterior. The eyelids are examined for lacerations, function, and contour, especially with respect to the canthi. A lid laceration may imply a globe laceration below it. The conjunctiva, cornea, and sclera are evaluated next. Bright red subconjunctival hemorrhage is very common in midface trauma, is usually innocuous, and resolves in a few days without treatment. The bright red appearance is due to the ability of the subconjunctival blood to absorb oxygen through the very thin, air-permeable conjunctiva. Beneath the bulbar conjunctiva lies the tough white sclera which encloses the globe. Subconjunctival hemorrhage, however, can be associated with rupture of the globe and a tear of the sclera. Dark pigments seen on the sclera may be the choroid or ciliary body exuding through a scleral dehiscence. Edema of the conjunctiva, known as chemosis, is very common after trauma. It often signifies more serious underlying injuries, such as orbital fracture or scleral perforation.

Rupture of the Globe

Rupture of the globe is a true ocular emergency and must be diagnosed early to prevent irreversible damage. Rupture allows extravasation of the intraocular contents (Fig. 22–33). Hyphema, or blood in the anterior chamber, implies serious intraocular injury and is often present in globe rupture. Eccentricities in the shape of the pupil are seen with uveal prolapse. The lens of the eye is normally black to visual inspection or red on ophthalmoscopy. A hazy or white pupil should alert suspicion of trauma to the lens, which causes hydration of the lens with an opaque quality to

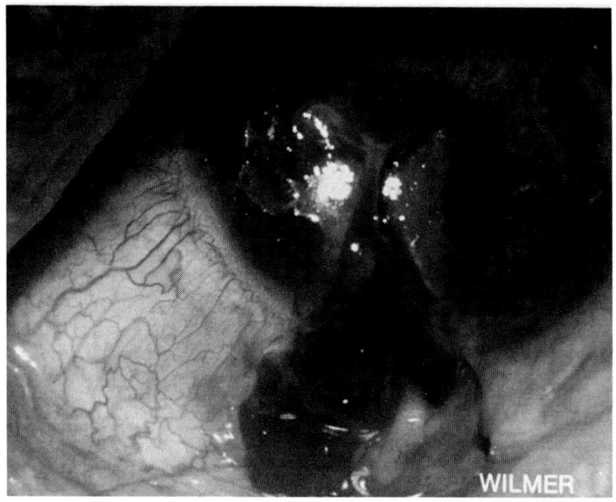

Figure 22–33. *Laceration of the cornea and sclera with exposure of the iris from glass injury. (Courtesy of the Wilmer Eye Institute. Hirst LW, et al. Sights and sounds in ophthalmology, vol. 5. In: Ocular and Periocular Trauma. St. Louis: CV Mosby, 1984)*

it. Traumatic cataract formation may be seen within a few hours after injury or may take months to develop.

When a ruptured globe is diagnosed, or even strongly suspected, the basic therapeutic principle is to stop all manipulation of the globe, including field of gaze testing or repair of lacerations. The eye must be protected without pressure, since a pressure patch can extrude eye contents. Simply taping the eye or applying a plastic eye shield, such as the type often used to protect the eye under drapes for general anesthesia, is adequate. Topical antibiotic drops should be applied and, in general, ophthalmic gentamycin is adequate.[77] Empiric administration of systemic antibiotics is given to prevent endophthalmitis. Parenteral gentamycin and cephalosporin in combination offer broad coverage and good intraocular penetration.[78]

The eye is repaired by an ophthalmologist as soon as possible with microsurgical techniques. A CT scan to assess for foreign bodies can be obtained. The prognosis depends on the quality of repair, the timing, and the degree of corneal scarring. Scarring of the cornea within the visual axis has a poorer prognosis for adequate vision. A ruptured globe rarely causes a granulomatous inflammation called sympathetic ophthalmia in the opposite eye, which can cause serious loss of vision in the nontraumatized eye. To prevent this, enucleation of a nonsalvagable eye is often performed early.

Hyphema

Hyphema, or blood in the anterior chamber, can result from blunt or penetrating trauma to the eye (Fig. 22–34). Twenty-five percent of hyphemas are associated with lens, iris, choroidal, or retinal injuries. Even hyphema without associated ocular damage is dangerous because rebleeding into the anterior chamber can cause acute elevation of interocular pressure, an ocular emergency. Rebleeding occurs between 3% and 33% of the time.[79] The bleeding is felt to be from a vessel in the ciliary body or iris. Blood degradation products can opacify the cornea and significantly reduce vision on a long-term basis.

Treatment of hyphema usually involves strict bed rest with the head of the bed elevated to prevent rebleeding and to allow the blood in the anterior chamber to settle dependently. However, a prospective study[79] of 137 patients comparing strict bed rest, sedation, and bilateral patching to a regimen of ambulation, no sedation, and patching of the traumatized eye found no significant differences in outcome. Hospital admission is still warranted for daily ocular examination and tonometry to measure intraocular pressure. A cycloplegic to dilate the pupil is usually administered to increase comfort. Cyclopentolate or atropine drops are effective cycloplegics. The injured eye should be patched. Antifibrinolytic agents, such as aminocaproic acid, appear to reduce the incidence of rebleeding.[80,81] The dose range is 50 mg/kg every 4 hours to a maximum of 30 g per day.

Should intraocular pressure rise above 25 mm Hg, medical therapy is administered to lower the pressure. Timolol, a beta blocker, 1 drop every 12 hours is the first-line drug to lower intraocular pressure. Other regimens include acetazolamide and hyperosmotic agents, such as mannitol. Persistent elevation of intraocular pressure or blood staining of the cornea are indications for ophthalmologic surgery;[82] however, the risk of rebleeding as a result of surgery must be weighed against potential benefits.

Chemical and Thermal Burns

Chemical burns to the face often involve the eyes and constitute a true emergency. Vision is not checked initially, since immediate initiation of irrigation is critical. Topical anesthetic is applied to relieve pain and make irrigation more tolerable. Any available IV solution is administered through tubing and dripped into the eye with the lids held apart for effective flushing. A cycloplegic, such as cyclopentolate 1% is given along with topical antibiotics. The eye is patched and the patient is referred to an ophthalmologist. Chemical burns not treated immediately result in an opaque or porcelainized ocular surface that does not permit vision (Fig. 22–35)

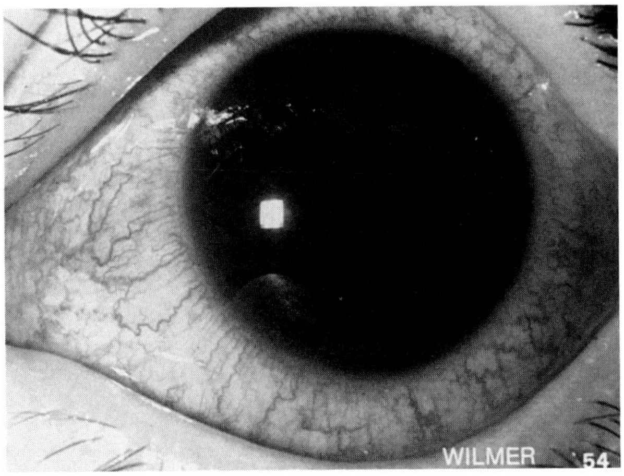

Figure 22–34. *Hyphema. Blood fills anterior chamber and obscures the iris and pupil. (Courtesy of the Wilmer Eye Institute. Hirst LW, et al. Sights and sounds in ophthalmology, vol. 5. In: Ocular and Periocular Trauma. St. Louis: CV Mosby, 1984)*

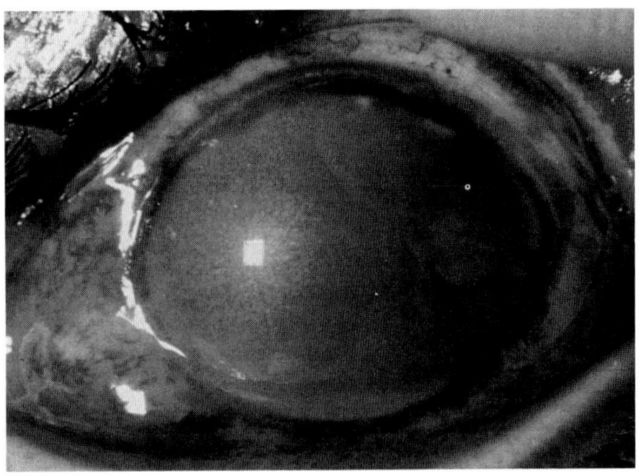

Figure 22–35. *Alkalai burn with severe corneal and conjunctival loss. (Courtesy of the Wilmer Eye Institute. Hirst LW, et al. Sights and sounds in ophthalmology, vol. 5. In: Ocular and Periocular Trauma. St. Louis: CV Mosby, 1984)*

Thermal burns to the ocular surface are less common than chemical burns because reflex closure of the lids protects the eye. Epithelial abrasion is common from burns and is treated like any other corneal abrasion. Thermal burns can prevent lid closure and result in desiccation of the eye. The eye should be kept moist with artificial tear solutions and patched until further ophthalmologic consultation is available. Burns can scar the lid mechanism and cause cicatricial ectropion, entropion, and trichiasis (ingrowth of eyelashes).

Corneal Abrasions

Abrasions of the cornea are usually a result of a foreign body trapped under the upper lid, but not infrequently occur iatrogenically during maxillofacial procedures. During oral procedures especially, the eyes are usually covered by drapes. Manipulation of the head along with partial opening of the eyelid increases the potential of the drapes rubbing the corneal surface. In general, all patients undergoing oral and maxillofacial procedures should have the eyes lubricated with appropriate ophthalmic ointment and the lids taped securely shut without pressure. Clear plastic eye shields with peripheral adhesive are excellent when the midface must be visualized, such as during a maxillary osteotomy. Towels or drapes can be safely secured over the eye shields for most oral procedures.

Corneal abrasion presents with several of the following symptoms: eye pain, tearing, photophobia, blurred vision, and lid spasm. Most patients complain of a sensation of a foreign body in the eyes even without any. The pain is typically increased upon blinking.

Examination of the eye requires patient cooperation and instillation of a topical anesthetic, such as tetracaine 1% solution, affords pain relief and permits a more thorough examination. The upper lid is pulled down and out and is everted over a cotton-tipped applicator while the patient maintains a downward gaze. Large abrasions can often be seen with penlight illumination, but a slitlamp permits a much more detailed examination under focused light and magnification. Fluorescein dye is applied to the surface of the eye to outline the abrasion. Fluorescein stains only the abraided stroma of the eye and is repelled by intact epithelial membranes. Sterile strips of paper impregnated with fluorescein are briefly applied to the inferior fornix of the eye at the conjunctival fold of the lower lid. The moist surfaces dissolve the fluorescein on the strip, causing orange staining of the eye and lid. Under ultraviolet light the fluorescein appears green. The tearing of the eye washes away the dye from the corneal surface except for abraded areas, which attack the hydrophilic dye and appear as green defects or scratches. Nonembedded foreign bodies, if present, can be removed with a moist cotton swab from the undersurface of the lid or the ocular surface. Embedded bodies are generally removed by an ophthalmologist.

The corneal epithelium has excellent regenerative capacity and treatment is based around prevention of complications. The mainstay of treatment is gentle pressure patching to prevent lid motion and further irritation of the corneal surface. Most ophthalmologists recommend use of broad-spectrum topical antibiotic ointment prior to patching, such as gentamycin, erythromycin, tobramycin, neosporin, or polysporin. Some patients have reflex irritation of the iris and ciliary body (iridocylitis) and are more comfortable after instillation of a cycloplegic such as cyclopentolate 1%. Topical anesthetics should not be given to the patient to administer at home, since they retard wound healing and cause corneal inflammation (keratitis).[83] Medications containing steroids must be avoided to prevent viral infection of an injured cornea and because herpetic keratitis often presents with the symptoms of a corneal abrasion.[84] The corneal epithelium usually heals in 24 to 48 hours, after which time the patch can be removed and the eye reexamined.

Corneal abrasions require prompt treatment, not only to relieve pain but to prevent bacterial corneal ulceration. A corneal ulcer can be detected by the grey, yellow, or white appearance of infection and by positive fluorescein staining, since the epithelium is absent. White blood cells may fill the anterior chamber of the eye (hypopyon). Because of the direct risk to vision, these patients are hospitalized and treated with frequent topical application of broad-spectrum antibiotics until the ulcer epithelializes.

Injuries of the Iris, Lens, and Posterior Segment

Trauma to the eye or orbit can be accompanied by persistent dilitation (traumatic mydriasis) or constriction (miosis) of the pupil. The condition resolves spontaneously after several days. The mydriatic pupil reacts minimally to light. Traumatic mydriasis must be distinguished from other causes of pupillary dilitation such as oculomotor nerve injury, brain stem compression, and topical mydriatic medications such as atropine and cyclopentolate. Traumatic iritis is also sometimes seen after eye trauma. Inflammation of the iris and ciliary body may cause intense pain in the eye without the presence of a foreign body or corneal abrasion. This condition is usually treated with a cycloplegic for patient comfort and occasionally topical steroids.

Lens Dislocation

Blunt trauma to the eye can result in a host of other ocular injuries, which will be briefly mentioned. The lens can be subluxated from its zonular fibers or completely dislocated into the vitreous chamber or anterior chamber (Fig. 22–36). Anterior dislocation can cause acute pupillary block glaucoma and is an emergency. This type of dislocation should be suspected if trembling of the iris is observed while the patient moves the eyes back and forth. Posterior dislocation of the lens into the vitreous chamber is managed after inflammation subsides.

Vitreous Hemorrhage

Bleeding into the vitreous, the jelly-like substance between the lens and retina, can be caused by blunt globe trauma. Retinal tears and damage to ciliary body or choroid vessels are the usual sources of blood. The blood accumulates over time. It may be impossible to view the retina, so it is recommended that all patients with blunt trauma to the globe have the fundus examined with pupil dilated.[85] Ultrasound and CT scanning can be used to diagnose detachments and foreign bodies. Most vitreous hemorrhages resorb over time.

Retinal Detachment

Traumatic retinal detachments can result from a break in the retina at the time of injury, which then slowly separates over time. A previously diseased retina is prone to separation. The common symptoms of retinal detachment are a defect in a peripheral visual field, flashes of light, or showers of black specks. The retinal tears are often too peripheral to be detachable by ophthalmoscopy (Fig. 22–37). Again, ultrasonography or CT scanning can help make the diagnosis. Treatment is usually by photocoagulation or a cryosurgery.

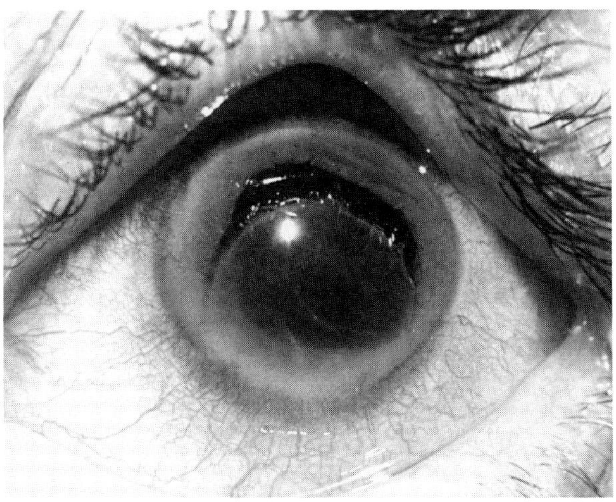

Figure 22–36. *Dislocation of the lens into the anterior chamber. (Courtesy of the Wilmer Eye Institute. Hirst LW, et al. Sights and sounds in ophthalmology, vol. 5. In: Ocular and Periocular Trauma. St. Louis: CV Mosby, 1984)*

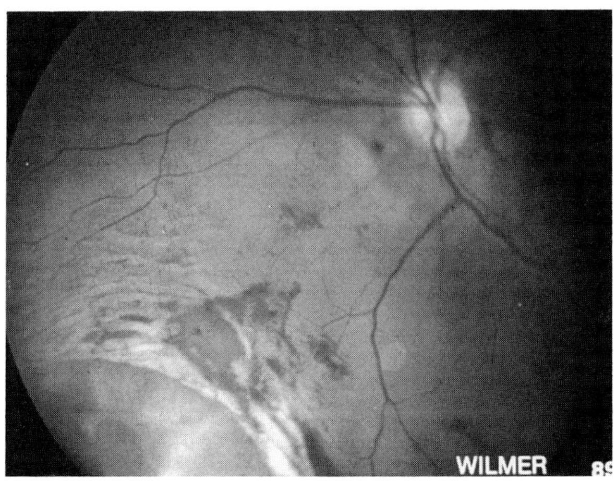

Figure 22–37. *Retinal detachment inferonasally from a BB-gun injury. (Courtesy of the Wilmer Eye Institute. Hirst LW, et al. Sights and sounds in ophthalmology, vol. 5. In: Ocular and Periocular Trauma. St. Louis: CV Mosby, 1984)*

The potential for serious consequences of untreated ocular injuries must not be overlooked in the face of other maxillofacial injuries. Early consultation with an ophthalmologist cannot be overemphasized.

REFERENCES

1. Duvall AJ, Banovetz JD. Maxillary fractures. Otolaryngol Clin 1976; 1:489.
2. Kassel EE, et al. Radiology and orbital pathology. In: Smith BC. Ophthalmic Plastic and Reconstructive Surgery, vol 1. St Louis: CV Mosby, 1987:173.
3. Bernardo N, Leban SW, Williams F. A comparison of radiographic treatment methods for evaluation of the orbit. J Oral Maxillofac Surg 1988; 46:844.
4. Smith B, Regan WE. Blow-out fractures of the orbit: Mechanism and correction of internal orbital fracture. Am J Ophthalmol 1957; 44:73.
5. Nesi FA, Spoor TC. Orbital fractures. In: Smith BC. Ophthalmic Plastic and Reconstructive Surgery, vol 1. St Louis: CV Mosby 1987:476.
6. Converse JM, Smith B. Blow-out fracture of the floor of the orbit. Trans Am Acad Ophthalmol Otolaryngol 1960; 64:676.
7. Fujino T, Makino K. Entrapment mechanism and ocular injury in orbital blow-out fractures. Plast Reconstr Surg 1980; 65:571.
8. Zizmor J, et al. Roentgen diagnosis of blow-out fractures of the orbit. Am J Roentgenol 1962; 87:1009.
9. Putterman AM, Stevens T, Urist MJ. Non-surgical management of blow-out fractures of the orbital floor. Am J Ophthalmol 1974; 77:232.
10. Putterman AM, Smith BC, Lisman RD. Blow-out fractures. In: Smith BC. Ophthalmic Plastic and Reconstructive Surgery, vol 1. St Louis: CV Mosby, 1987; 477.
11. Koorneef L. Current concepts on the management of orbital blow-out fractures. Ann Plast Surg 1982; 9:185.
12. Putterman AM, Smith BC, Lisman RD. Blow-out fractures. In: Smith BC. Ophthalmic Plastic and Reconstructive Surgery, vol 1. St Louis: CV Mosby, 1987; 478.
13. Lancaster WB. Detecting, measuring, plotting, and interpreting ocular deviations. Arch Ophthalmol 1939; 22:867.
14. Putterman AM, Stevens T, Urist MJ. Non-surgical treatment of blow-out fractures of the orbital floor. Am J Ophthalmol 1974; 77:232.
15. Parsons G, Mathog RH. Orbital wall and volume relationships. Arch Otolaryngol Head Neck Surg 1988; 114:743.
16. Mustarde JC. The role of Lockwood's suspensory ligament in preventing downward displacement of the eye. Br J Plast Surg 1968; 21:73.
17. Stanley RB, Mathog RH. Elevation and correction of combined orbital trauma syndrome. Laryngoscope 1983; 93:856.
18. Putterman AM, Stevens T, Urist MJ. Non-surgical treatment of blow-out fractures of the orbital floor. Am J Ophthalmol 1974; 77:232.
19. Emery JM, Van Noorden GK, Schernitzauer DA. Orbital floor fractures: long-term follow-up of cases with and without surgical repair. Trans Am Acad Ophthalmol Otolaryngol 1971; 75:802.
20. Koorneef L: Current concepts of the management of orbital blow-out fractures. Am Plast Surg 1982; 9:185.
21. Converse JM, Smith B, Obear M, et al. Orbital blow-out fractures: A ten year survey. Plast Reconstr Surg 1967; 39:20.
22. Hawes MJ, Dortzbach RK. Surgery on orbital floor fractures: Influence on time of repair and fracture size. Ophthalmology 1983; 90:1066.
23. Sacks CA, Friedland JA. Orbital floor fractures: Should they be explored early? Plast Reconstr Surg 1979; 64:190.
24. Hakelius L, Pontein B. Results of immediate and delayed surgical treatment of facial fractures with diplopia. J Maxillofac Surg 1973; 1:150.
25. Nesi F, LoVecchi J, Mathog RH. Orbital blow-out fractures. In: Mathog RH, ed. Maxillofacial Trauma. Baltimore: Williams & Wilkins, 1984:319–327.
26. Dulley B, Fells P. Long term follow-up of orbital blow-out fractures with and without surgery. Mod Prob Ophthalmol 1975; 14:467.
27. Putterman AM, Smith BC, Lisman RD. Blow-out fractures. In: Smith BC, ed. Ophthalmic Plastic and Reconstructive Surgery, vol 1. Philadelphia: CV Mosby, 1987:477.
28. Schilli W. Treatment of Zygoma fractures. Oral Maxillofac Clin North Am 1990; 2:161–164.
29. McCord CD, Moses JL. Exposure of the inferior orbit with fornix incision and lateral canthotomy. Ophthalmic Surg 1979; 10(6):53.
30. Smith B, Putterman AM. Fixation or orbital floor implants: Description of a simple technique. Arch Ophthalmol 1970; 83:598.
31. Hotte HH. Orbital fractures. In: Rowe NL, Williams JLI. Maxillofacial Injuries, vol 1. London: Churchill Livingstone, 1985:520.
32. Rowe NL. Fractures of the zygomatic complex and orbit. In: Rowe NL, Williams JLI. Maxillofacial Injuries, vol 1. London: Churchill Livingstone, 1985:515.
33. Luhr HG. Die Primare Rekinstruction von Orbitabodendefekten nach Trauma and Tumoroperation. Zahn Mund Kieferheilkinde 1971; 57:1.
34. Boudreau RG, Tideman H. Reconstruction of the orbital floor using lyophilized dura. J Oral Surg 1976; 34:618.
35. Ianetti G, D'Areo F. The use of lyophilized dura in reconstruction of the orbital floor. J Maxillofac Surg 1977; 5:58.
36. Waite P, Clanton J. Orbital floor reconstruction with lyophilized dura. J Oral Maxillofac Surg 1988; 46:727.
37. Prichard J, Thadoni V, Kalb R, et al. Rapidly progressive dementia in a patient who received a cadaveric dura-matter graft. JAMA 1987; 257:1036.

38. Rowe NL. Fractures of the zygomatic complex and orbit. In: Rowe NL, Williams JLI. Maxillofacial Injuries. Vol 1. London: Churchill Livingstone, 1985:507.
39. Jackson WR, Abbey JA, Glantz S. Balloon technique for treatment of fractures of the zygomatic bone. J Oral Surg 1956; 14:14.
40. Davis WH, Nevius RC, Elliott JH. Optic atrophy after ocular contusion. Am J. Ophthalmol 1972; 73:278.
41. Savino PJ, Harbour R. Neuro-ophthalmic manifestations of trauma. In: Smith BC. Ophthalmic Plastic and Reconstructive Surgery, vol 1. St Louis: CV Mosby, 1987:311.
42. Savino PJ, Harbour R. Neuro-ophthalmic manifestations of trauma. In: Smith BC. Ophthalmic Plastic and Reconstructive Surgery, vol 1. St Louis: CV Mosby, 1987:312.
43. Ord RA. Post-operative retrobulbar hemorrhage and blindness complicating trauma surgery. Br J Oral Surg 1981; 19:202.
44. Rowe NL. Fractures of the zygomatic complex and orbit. In: Rowe NL, Williams JLI. Maxillofacial Injuries, vol 1. Edinburgh: Churchill Livingstone, 1985: 526–528.
45. Anderson RL, Panje WR, Cross CE. Optic nerve blindness following blunt forehead trauma. Ophthalmol 1982; 89:445.
46. Varley E, Holt-Wilson A, Watson P. Acute retinal artery occlusion following reduction of a fractured zygoma and its successful treatment. Brit J Oral Surg 1968; 6:31.
47. Manfredi SJ, Raji MR, Sprinkle PM, et al. Computerized tomographic scan findings in facial fractures associated with blindness. Plast Reconstr Surg 1981; 68:479.
48. Bowerman JE. The superior orbital fissure syndrome complicating fractures of the facial skeleton. Br J Oral Surg 1969; 7:1.
49. Rowe NL. Fractures of the zygomatic complex and orbit. In: Rowe NL, Williams JLI. Maxillofacial Injuries, vol 1. Edinburgh: Churchill Livingstone, 1985:530.
50. Waga S. Marikava A. Fujimoto K. Carotid cavernous fistula associated with traumatic aneurysm of the internal carotid artery. Surg Neurol 1972; 9:367.
51. Savino PJ, Harbour R. Neuro-ophthalmic manifestations of trauma. In: Smith BC. Ophthalmic Plastic and Reconstruction Surgery, vol. 1. St Louis: CV Mosby, 1987:322.
52. Rogers R, Epker BN. Carotid cavernous sinus fistula accompanying mid-facial fractures. J Oral Surg 1972; 30:429.
53. Debrum G, et al. Treatment of 54 traumatic carotid-cavernous fistulae. J Neurosurg 1981; 55:678.
54. Fells P. Acute enophthalmos. Eye 1982; 102–88.
55. Borghouts JM, Otto AJ. Silicone sheet and bead implants to correct deformity of inadequately treated orbital fractures. Br J Plast Surg 1978; 31:254.
56. Burres S, Cohn AM, Mathog RH. Repair of orbital blowout fractures with Marlex mesh and Gelfilm. Laryngoscope 1981; 91:1881.
57. Mathog RH, Hillstrom MD, Nesi FA. Surgical correction of enophthalmos and diplopia: A report of 38 cases. Arch Otolaryngol Head Neck Surg 1989; 115:169.
58. Rowe NL. Fractures of the zygomatic complex and orbit. In: Rowe NL, Williams JLI. Maxillofacial Injuries, vol 1. Edinburgh: Churchill Livingstone, 1985:518.
59. Roncevic R, Malinger B. Experience with various procedures in the treatment of orbital floor fractures. J Maxillofac Surg 1981; 9:81.
60. Mathog RH, Nesi F, Smith B. Post-traumatic enophthalmos and diplopia. In: Mathog RH, ed. Maxillofacial Trauma. Baltimore: Williams & Wilkins, 1983.
61. Iannetti G, D'Areo F. The use of lyophilized dura in reconstruction of the orbital floor. Maxillofac Surg 1977; 5:58.
62. Kawamoto HK. Last post-traumatic enophthalmos. A correctable deformity. Plast Reconstr Surg 1982; 69:423.
63. Manson PN, Raus EJ, Iliff NT. Deep orbital reconstruction of correction of post-traumatic enophthalmos. Clin Plast Surg 1987; 14:113.
64. Mathog RH, Nesi F, Smith B. Post-traumatic enophthalmos and diplopia. In: Mathog RH, ed. Maxillofacial Trauma. Baltimore: Williams & Wilkins, 1984:329.
65. Mathog RH. Traumatic enophthalmos. In: Smith BC. Ophthalmic Plastic and Reconstructive Surgery, vol I. St Louis: CV Mosby, 1987:498.
66. Bosniak S. Ectropion. In: Smith BC. Ophthalmic Plastic and Reconstructive Surgery, vol 1. St Louis: CV Mosby, 1987:562.
67. Schaefer AJ. Variation in the pathophysiology of involutional entropion and its treatment. Ophthalmic Surg 1983; 14(8):653.
68. Jones LT, Reeh, MJ, Wobig JL. Senile entropion: A new concept for correction. Am J Ophthalmol 1972; 74:327.
69. Beyer CK. Canalicular injuries. Clin Plast Surg 1978; 5:547.
70. Mustarde JC. Repair and reconstruction. In: The Orbital Region, ed 2. London: Churchill Livingstone, 1980.
71. Jackson ST. A new probe for silicone intubation of the lacrimal drainage system. Ophthalmic Surg 1980; 11:588.
72. Garber PF, MacDonald D, Beyer-Machule CK. Management of trauma to the eyelids. In: Smith BC. Ophthalmic Plastic and Reconstructive Surgery, vol 1. St Louis: CV Mosby, 1987:450.
73. Mindlin AM, Nesi FA, Silver B, Lisman RD. Basic concepts in eyelid repair. In: Smith BC. Ophthalmic Plastic and Reconstructive Surgery, vol 1. St Louis: CV Mosby, 1987:431.
74. National Society to Prevent Blindness: Fact Sheet. New York: National Society to Prevent Blindness, 1980.
75. Feist RM, Farber MD. Ocular trauma epidemiology. Arch Opthalmol 1989; 107:503.
76. Glynn RJ, Seddon JM, Berlin BM. The incidence of eye injuries in New England adults. Arch Opthalmol 1988; 106:785.
77. Deutsch TA, Feller DB. Paton and Goldberg's Man-

agement of Ocular Injuries, ed 2. Philadelphia: WB Saunders, 1985:180.

78. Deutsch TA, Feller DB. Paton and Goldberg's Management of Ocular Injuries, ed 2. Philadelphia: WB Saunders, 1985:189.
79. Read T, Goldberg MF. Comparison of medical treatment of traumatic hyphema. Trans Am Acad Ophthalmol Otolaryngol 1974; 78:799.
80. McGetrick JJ, Jampol LM, Goldberg MF, et al. Aminocaproic acid decreases secondary hemorrhage after traumatic hyphema. Arch Ophthalmol 1983; 101:1031.
81. Watkins G, et al. Aminocaproic acid in traumatic hyphema. J National Med Assoc 1984; 66(6):484.
82. Chu W. Ocular trauma. In: Smith BC. Ophthalmic Plastic and Reconstructive Surgery, vol 1. St Louis: CV Mosby, 1987:274.
83. Epstein DL, Paton D. Keratitis from misuse of corneal anesthetics. N Engl J Med 1968; 279:396.
84. Deutsch TA, Feller DB. Patton and Goldberg's Management of Ocular Injuries, ed 2. Philadelphia: WB Saunders, 1985:127.
85. Deutsch TA, Feller DB. Patton and Goldberg's Management of Ocular Injuries, ed 2. Philadelphia: WB Saunders, 1985:204.

23

Nasal and Nasoorbital Ethmoid Fractures

Michael F. Zide

NASAL FRACTURES

Nasal bone fractures are the most common facial bone injury, composed of approximately 40% of all facial fractures.[1,2] Diagnosis can often be made by clinical evaluation alone if edema is not present. Proper treatment results from an understanding of the component parts involved in each individual fracture. In some patients, closed reduction performed in the emergency room will suffice. In others, however, swelling must be allowed to subside before treatment is undertaken. In addition, some patients may require open reduction, septal correction, or nasal packing.

Inadequate diagnosis or improper treatment of nasal fractures can lead to a wide spectrum of nasal and oropharyngeal complaints caused by altered physiologic conditions. These range from cosmetic problems and airway obstruction to chronic crusting, snoring, sinusitis, synechiae, and an increased incidence of throat infections. In children, nasal fractures may result in delayed growth and development of the midface.

ANATOMY

External

Skin

The skin overlying the nose varies in thickness and laxity in the upper, as opposed to the lower, nose. The upper nose is composed of thin, loose skin that extends toward the orbits. During injury, easy dissection of blood occurs beneath this skin and is responsible for the black eyes associated with a broken nose. Likewise, this skin can swell to several times its normal size shortly after injury, making diagnosis and accurate reduction more difficult.

The skin over the lower nose is usually thicker and more fixed. The lower alar cartilages are intimately attached to this skin, hence these cartilages are often injured or deformed when laceration occurs. This adherent skin also makes inflammatory conditions or injection of local anesthetic extremely painful because of the tenseness and consequent pressure on the underlying nerves. Likewise, the more sebaceous the nature of the skin (as is found in the lower nose), the more difficult it is to leave an inconspicuous scar on it.

Bone

The piriform rim is made up of the maxillary and nasal bones. At the root of the nose, the nasal bones articulate with the frontal bone, the perpendicular plate of the ethmoid bone, and the frontal processes of the maxilla (Fig. 23–1).

In children and in those who receive severe frontal injuries, the nasal bones may disarticulate at this frontonasal suture line. For the majority, however, fracture of the nasal bones usually occurs where the radix starts to widen out and the bone is thinner. This point is several millimeters below the frontonasal suture (Fig. 23–2). In fact, at the frontonasal suture, the nasal bones are relatively thick and strong and to

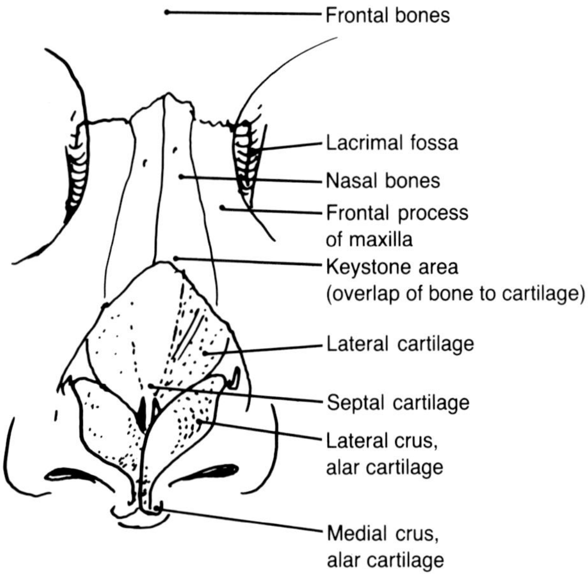

Figure 23-1. *Frontal view of the nose.*

some degree are supported underneath by the frontal bone. In addition, an isolated nasal bone fracture involving only the paired nasal bones is rare. Usually, the lateral supporting struts (i.e., the frontal processes of the maxilla) fracture as well. In a severe nasoorbital ethmoid (NOE) fracture, these bones and the perpendicular plate of the ethmoid bone, the cartilaginous septum, are fractured.

Nature has provided a series of stress points or pillars of defense. In the nose, the first stress point is the isthmus of the nasal bones. It is fortunate that fractures tend to occur here rather than at the nasofrontal suture under which is the cribriform plate, the base of the skull, and the dura. The secondary stress points are at the nasofrontal suture and the lacrimal bones. Hence, NOE fractures usually break through the floor of the frontal sinus and are "shock absorbed" at the lacrimal bones. Once again, the brain and the globe are offered some form of protection.

Cartilage

There are two main sets of cartilage on the outer nose. The paired upper lateral cartilages are attached to the underside of the distal nasal bones. These form the structural support of the middle third of the nose and are intimately adherent to the septum in the midline. These cartilages are often fused with the septum in their upper third and are firmly held in place by an overlying fascial sheet. In the open rhinoplasty approach, these cartilages may be separated in the midline to provide access for upper septal reconstruction. In most nasal fractures, these cartilages remain bonded to the nasal bones, but severe trauma can displace or telescope their position in relation to the nasal bone (the keystone area) and septal cartilage. When a nasal bone fracture is reduced properly, the cartilages

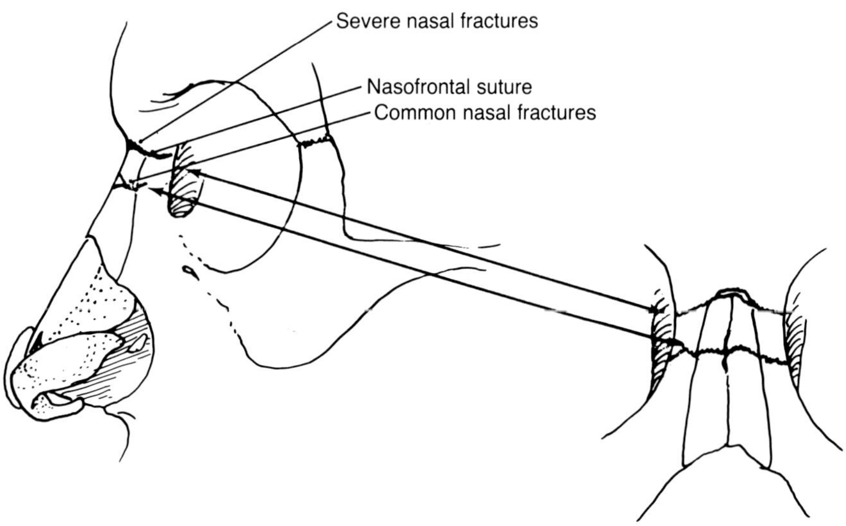

Figure 23-2. *Common nasal fractures often occur several millimeters below the nasion in the thinner area of the nasal bones. Severe nasal fractures may disarticulate the nasal bones from the frontal bone, and there may be other osseous or cartilaginous injuries as well.*

should return to proper position, but severe disarticulation can lead to an inverted Y-shaped deformity.

The paired lower lateral cartilages (also called *alar*, which means "winged" in Latin) have medial and lateral crura ("legs"). These cartilages, along with the septum, form the support of the lower third of the nose. The most protuberant anterior portion of these alar cartilages occurs where the cartilages rotate medially and lends form to the tip of the nose to an area called the *dome*. These cartilages frame the external nares (Fig. 23–1).

Internal

Septum

The septum is the central support of the nose. The anterior portion is cartilaginous and semirigid. The posterior portion is rigid and bony.

The cartilage of the septum joins the flexible membranous septum at its anterior caudal border. Behind this, the septal cartilage usually sits in the groove of the nasal crest of the maxilla, a common area of disruption. The cartilaginous septum articulates with the bony septum. The bony septum includes the perpendicular plate of the ethmoid posteriorly and the vomer bone inferiorly. Inferiorly, the bony septum joins the nasal crest of the maxilla and palatine bones (which may be considered part of the bony septum) (Fig. 23–3).

CLASSIFICATION

Several classifications of nasal injuries have been proposed as an aid in understanding the details of the fractured nose and the rationale for therapy.[3,4]

Adult

Unilateral

The adult unilateral fracture occurs from a lateral blow of moderate force. The nasal bone and frontal process of the maxilla are fractured (Fig. 23–4). The middle of the nose is solid and the septum is undamaged. A variant of this fracture is the medial maxillary fracture, which involves the medial portion of the orbital rim.

Bilateral: Simple

The bilateral fracture occurs from significant force and involves both nasal bones and both frontal processes

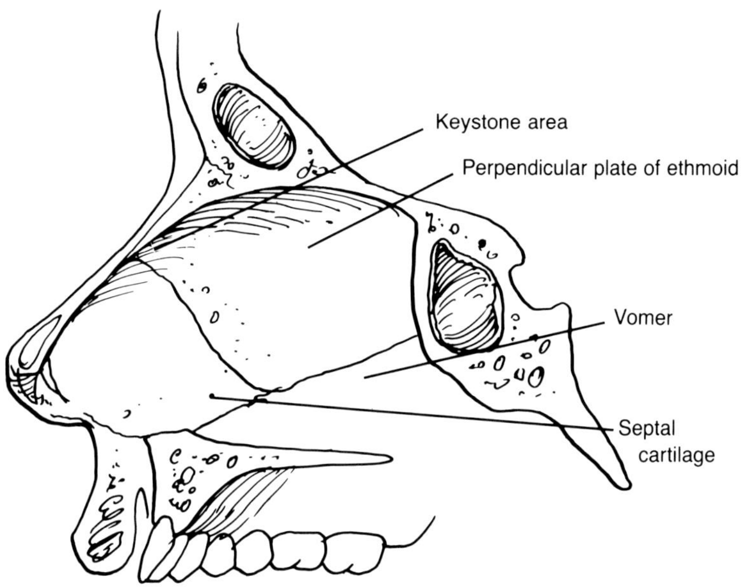

Figure 23-3. *The nasal septum is composed of the ethmoid, vomer, vomer bones, and septal cartilage.*

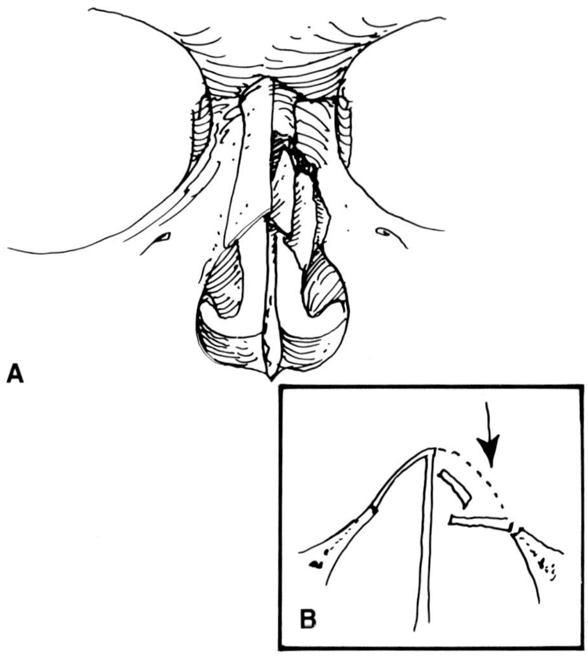

Figure 23-4. *(**A** and **B**) Unilateral nasal fracture involving the nasal bone and a portion of the frontal process of the maxilla.*

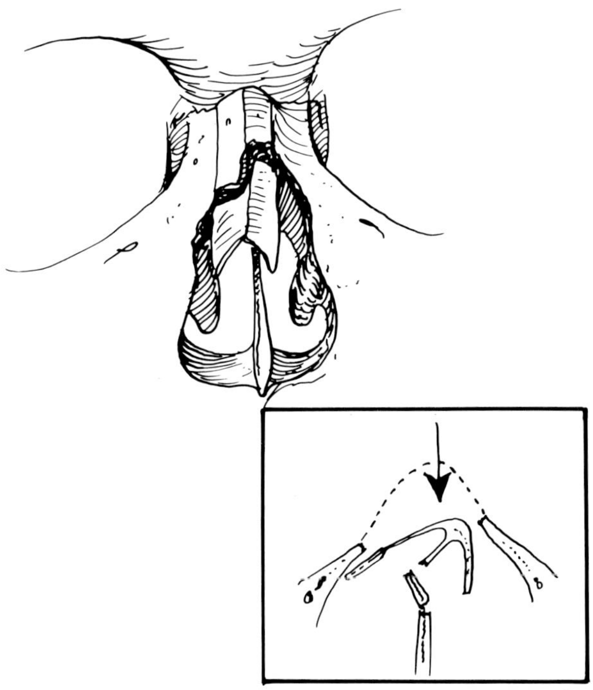

Figure 23-6. *Bilateral fracture with depression or telescoping of segments. This fracture will have to be elevated and perhaps supported in a proper position.*

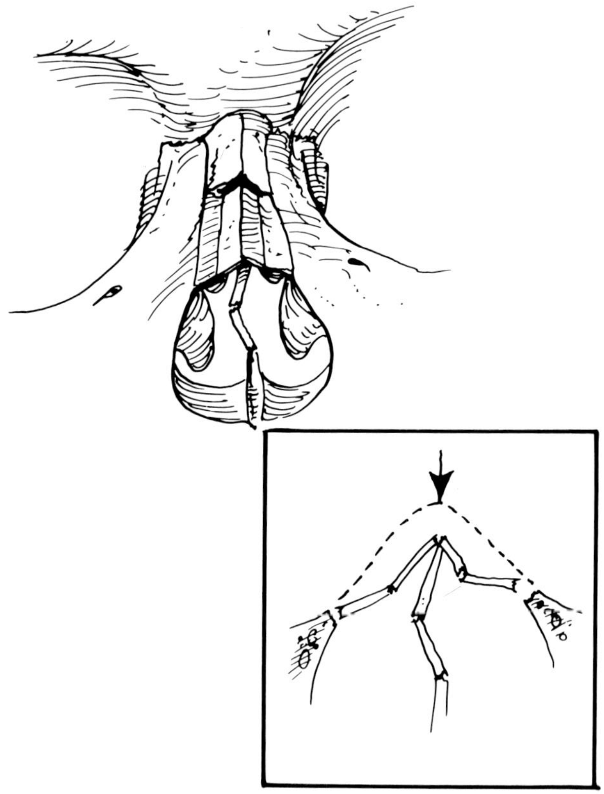

Figure 23-5. *Bilateral nasal fracture; simple. There is minimal to no telescoping. Often digital manipulation in the emergency room may push this nose over to its original position.*

of the maxilla (Fig. 23–5). The septum, which is similar to a tent pole, is shifted laterally with the bones. The bony shift is usually not great (less than one half of its width from the midline), and therefore the septum is usually only buckled.

This fracture involves minimal to no telescoping of bones, merely a lateral shifting of the nose.

Bilateral: complex

BILATERAL WITH TELESCOPING OR DEPRESSION OF BONY SEGMENTS (Fig. 23–6). If the force of injury has exceeded the bending capacity of the cartilageinous septum, then the septum may be dislocated or fractured and the nasal bones or frontal processes are telescoped.

BILATERAL WITH SEPTAL DISLOCATION OR FRACTURE (Fig. 23–7). When the nose is shifted more

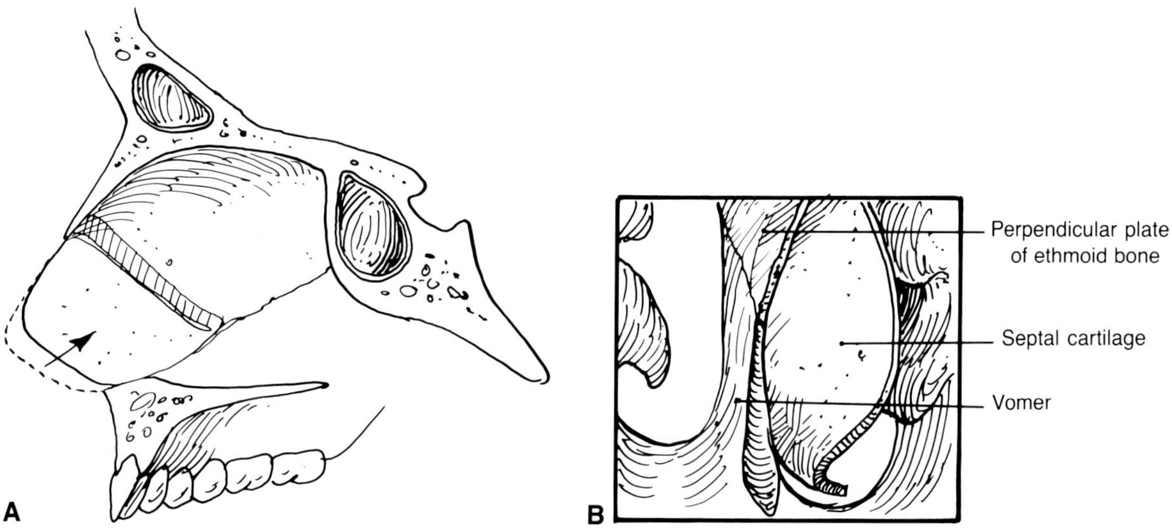

Figure 23-7. *(**A**) The bilateral fracture may cause buckling or disarticulation of the nasal septum. (**B**) The septal cartilage is displaced from its articulation with the vomer to a posterior position.*

than one half of its width from the midline, the septal injury may be more than a bend or buckle.[4] Dislocations or fractures may occur at the nasal crest of the maxilla, showing an obvious spur into the floor of the nose. Dislocation may also occur at the junction of the vomer and the perpendicular plate of the ethmoid.[5] Failure to recognize and to deal with the associated septal injury is the most common reason for unacceptable or poor therapeutic results.

These fractures can be vertical, as well as horizontal, and can leave cartilaginous ridges, which are associated with the deviated nose. Fractured segments can overlap and cause septal thickening and distortion. The nose may then be shortened and the columella retracted as a result of this telescopic overlap. Special treatment of this problem may be indicated.

Approximately 90% of fractures involve lateral forces. Frontal forces and depressed fractures, although less common, may involve major septal injury.

BILATERAL WITH MEDIAL MAXILLARY FRACTURE (Fig. 23–8). The medial maxillary fracture may oc-

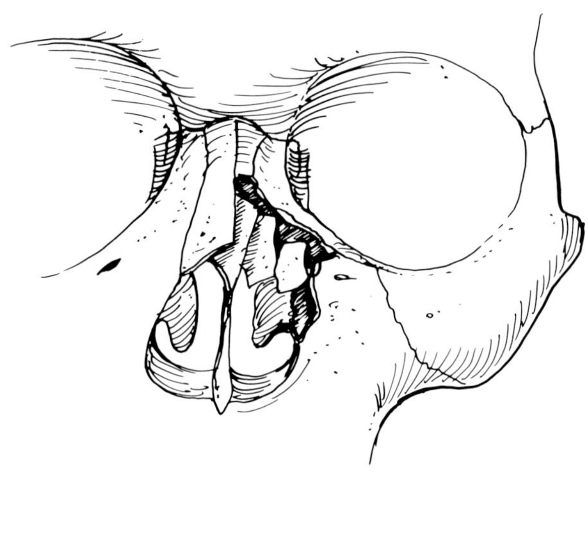

Figure 23–8. *Medial maxillary fracture involves more than the frontal process of the maxilla and the nasal bones. The orbital rim is frequently fractured.*

cur with a unilateral fracture, a bilateral fracture, or associated bony facial injuries. Clinical examination may reveal lacrimal sac injury, as well as some of the signs associated with orbital fractures. Symptoms include infraorbital and labial paresthesia, hypesthesia to the anterior teeth, and a cloudy sinus on Waters' view radiograph.

The patient may complain of nasal obstruction, which is located high in the nose even after resolution of swelling.

Septum Alone

A direct blow to the lower two thirds of the nose can produce an isolated septal injury and leave the nasal bones intact (Fig. 23–9). In children, the elastic nature of the nasal bones may allow direct impact to the upper third of the nose, causing deformation of the bones without fracture. The nasal bones may spring back unfractured, leaving an isolated septal injury or hematoma. This injury must be noted because "as the septum goes, so goes the nose."

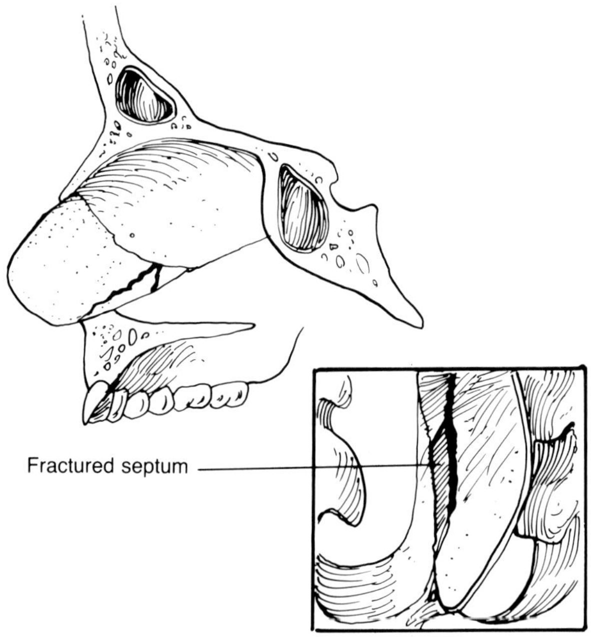

Figure 23-9. *Isolated septal fracture.*

Childhood
(Fig. 23–10)

The same type of fractures that occur in adults can occur in children. In addition, the open-book type of fracture may occur because the nasal bones are not fused in the midline until after adolescence. Upper lateral cartilages may be detached from the nasal bones.

The midfacial bones of children are small compared with the larger skull size and are much more giving, or elastic, than adults. Therefore children with major midfacial injuries also have a disproportionately high percentage of intracranial injury. This lower incidence of midfacial fracture probably also is due to decreased levels of sinus pneumatization.

Childhood nasal fractures are often greenstick in nature, with linear fractures common in the young

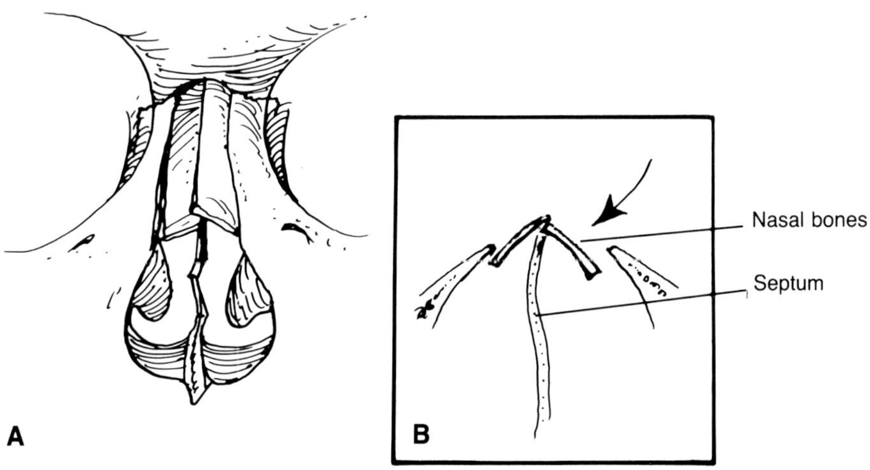

Figure 23-10. *(**A**) A childhood fracture is often the classic open-book fracture. (**B**) The nasal bones may disarticulate from the septum, as well as from the frontal processes of the maxilla.*

adult. Those contrast with the comminution that may occur in the more brittle bones of the elderly.

CLINICAL HISTORY AND EVALUATION

The clinical history surrounding a patient's nasal injury is important. Some worthwhile questions to ask are the following:

1. Has there been a change in the appearance of your nose since the injury?
2. How long has it been since the injury?
3. Have you ever had your nose broken before?
4. Have you ever had nasal surgery before?
5. Could you breathe through both sides of your nose before the injury?
6. What were you hit with?
7. Do you have any nasal allergies, sinusitis, and so forth?
8. Were you knocked out?
9. Do you have any good photos of yourself taken before the injury?
10. Do you use intranasal drugs? Cocaine? Afrin?

The physical examination should be the same systematic one used for all injured patients, ultimately honing into the area of concern. When swelling is present, the decision to admit the patient into the hospital may be based on priorities unrelated to the nasal fracture, such as loss of consciousness or associated injuries.

Examination of the nose should evaluate the following:

Skin: open wounds, subcutaneous emphysema, and intercanthal distance.
External bones and cartilage: Examine for depression or deviation of dorsum, tip, or columella, crepitus, tenderness, and swelling.
Intranasal (after suction): Examine for mucosal tears, cerebrospinal fluid (CSF) leak, septal hematoma, airway obstruction, septal spurs or distortion, epistaxis, and turbinate size.
Associated injuries: Examine for fractures of the orbital or frontal region, lacrimal injuries, basilar skull fracture, and sinus drainage.

The nasal history and a complete examination may be unobtainable in some patients, particularly children. Children may require sedation or general anesthesia for examination purposes.

RADIOGRAPHS

It has been estimated that 10% to 47% of clinically obvious nasal fractures are difficult to confirm radiographically.[7] Suture lines and vascular patterns complicate diagnoses and produce many false-positive and false-negative results unless correlated with clinical information.[8,9] Although it is true that most if not all therapeutic decisions regarding nasal fractures have not been influenced by the radiographic presentation,[10,11] radiographs should not be deemed useless. Some believe that, even if the nose looks straight but the radiographs show displacement the nose should be manipulated to prevent poor results from late diagnoses.[9]

The radiographs of choice are the lateral nasal (a dental occlusal film can be used for this purpose), frontal, and Waters' views. The lateral radiograph should be assessed for separation or depression. The frontal view may show alignment problems of the bony septum and the shape of the piriform rim. The Waters' view reveals symmetry or asymmetry with other facial bones, the frontal process of the maxilla displacement, cartilaginous septal displacement, and concurrent orbital fractures.

TREATMENT

Emergency Room Treatment

Although opinions differ, most surgeons believe that only certain types of nasal fractures are amenable to emergency room therapy. These are the unilateral and bilateral fractures, which present with minimal or no telescoping and minimal septal injury. Late fractures, fractures in children, and fractures which, by their nature, may involve possible open reduction merit operating room conditions with ideal instrumentation and lighting. Even in somewhat swollen patients, early manipulation may be beneficial, but deferral is an acceptable choice.

Timing of Treatment

Nasal reduction done in the emergency room (ER) is best performed before the onset of severe swelling or distortion, which could limit accurate anatomic assessment of the reduction. In most cases this is around 4 to 6 hours from the onset of injury. If swelling is a problem, then a delay of 4 to 6 days in the adult and 3 to 5 days in children is worthwhile, assuming that septal hematoma, CSF leak, or other mitigating factors are not present.

Because of related injuries, it often may be necessary to wait more than 2 weeks before treatment is begun in some adults. In these cases, however, the surgeon must be prepared to perform a refracture or osteotomy (open manipulative therapy) to remobilize the nose. In children, fibrosis sets in after 3 to 5 days, depending on the age of the child. However, these fractures can still be reduced.[6]

Treatment of Fractures

Treatment of nasal fractures must be based on accurate and specific diagnosis of the components of the injury. Every surgeon agrees on the value of adequate lighting, anesthesia, suction, and mucosal vasoconstriction. Each surgeon should choose those instruments that best fit his purpose. One surgeon may choose to elevate all nasal fractures with the back of a knife handle, whereas another might use a Walsham, Boise, or dental elevator sheathed in rubber tubing. However, the Asch forceps is the most common choice for septal elevation or manipulation.

Lacerations of the nose should be definitively treated after the bony injury is reduced. This may involve tacking the edges until open exploration and definitive plastic closure is possible under operating room conditions. Primary closure of nasal wounds can probably be performed safely on most wounds within 36 hours.

Treatment of Fractures by Type

Unilateral

Cocaine (4% to 10% and a maximum of 250 mg) is placed on cottonoids or packing; one piece is placed high in the radix and one behind the middle turbinate on the affected side. These are left in place for 10 minutes and removed. Next, the fractured segment may be elevated. Bimanual palpation and clinical examination will assess the proper position. In the case of instability, a rolled piece of Telfa covered with antibiotic ointment or a piece of Adaptic may be placed high in the nose. A suture is placed through the pack to avoid loss of the pack, which is left in for 2 to 5 days. The suture can be taped to the nose or placed through the nostril rim. Expanded Merocel packing (Fig. 23–11) may also be helpful because support packs tend to become soft and dislodge easily.

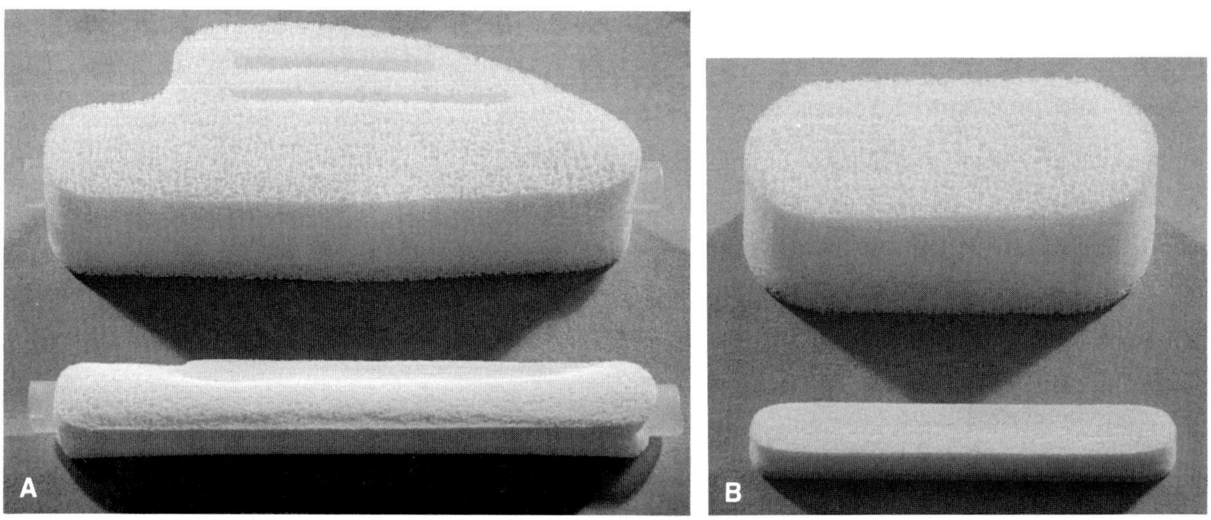

Figure 23-11. *(**A** and **B**) Expanding Merocel-type of packs. Airway tubes are noted in the Doyle-type of packing.*

Bilateral: Simple

The occasional bilateral fracture without telescoping can sometimes be manipulated back into the midline position without local anesthesia, using thumb pressure or an internal instrument with local blockade. Emergency room care alone is often possible. It is probably worthwhile to place an external splint to prevent reinjury and to maintain midline stability. Internal packing is rarely needed.[12]

In younger patients in whom the fracture line is of the greenstick variety and in fractures that are treated up to 2 weeks after injury, the facture line may have to be reosteotomized to shift the bones back into the midline. These latter types are not amenable to the emergency room, despite their simple appearance.

Bilateral with Telescoping

When the side of the bony infracture involves overriding bones, the telescoped bone will have to be repositioned (elevated) before reduction. In most of these cases the septum can be manipulated back to the midline in a closed fashion.

The standard closed reduction, long advocated as safe and effective,[13] is described in this section. Closed reduction does not produce routinely good results, unless the septum is minimally injured.[14,15] Whereas many surgeons might argue that closed reduction methods have withstood the test of time, recent publications lend credence to the proposition that closed reduction of some septal injuries produces too high a percentage of disfigurement.[18,19]

A prospective publication reports on acceptable late results for patients treated with closed manipulation of nasal fractures. Patients viewed their results as satisfactory 83% of the time when, according to the surgeon, acceptable results occurred much less frequently (51%).[20]

Local anesthesia for closed reduction involves the use of 4% to 10% cocaine placed on each side (maximum dose of 250 mg). The first anesthetic pack is placed high in the nose to anesthetize the anterior ethmoidal branches of the opthalmic nerve; the second is placed behind the middle turbinate to anesthetize the internal nasal branches of the maxillary nerve that exits the sphenopalatine foramen. A third swab may be used to paint the walls of the nose before the injection. A 5- to 10-minute period is required before manipulation. Local anesthesia containing xylocaine with epinephrine (1:100,000) is infiltrated subcutaneously over the dorsum, bilaterally in regions of the infraorbital foramina, along the columella to the nasal spine, and (if necessary) at the supratrochlear foramina. It is helpful to mix hyaluronidase (Wydase) with the local anesthesia to aid in diffusion and edema reduction.

Manipulation involves placement of a Boise elevator into the nostril on the depressed side after measurement of the appropriate depth of placement outside, along the lateral surface. The elevator should only be placed into the nose at that depth from the alar rim to the ipsilateral canthus. The nose is then elevated and bimanually shifted to the midline. An alternative method may involve grabbing the septum high in the nose with an Asch forceps and manipulating the nose and septum back into the midline.

Minimal septal displacement or buckling may be noted at this time; however, the airways are patent. A clinical decision to stabilize the septum in its reduced position is valid. Often a small piece of cartilage will need to be removed to allow for passive repositioning.

To maintain the septum in position, the following methods are suggested. The first technique involves the placement of silicone (Doyle type) splints, which are sutured in place. The second involves the use of a quilting stitch on a straightened 4-0 chromic needle, the end of which has been knotted to eliminate the need to tie a suture deeply in the nose. An external splint is then placed with one of several methods, using some combination of the following layers:

Layer one: Micropore paper tape placed in an overlapping fashion and held on by tincture of benzoin or Mastisol.
Layer two: Adhesive tape, moleskin, or Telfa as a buffer (Some newer splints have Velcro.)
Layer three: Plaster, Aquaplast, or an aluminum splint (Fig. 23–12, A and B)

Bilateral with Septal Dislocation or Fracture

Depressed nasal fractures and nasal fractures that are the result of severe force cause septal dislocations and fractures not amenable to closed reduction.

In these fractures, local anesthesia is infiltrated under the mucoperichondrium on the left-hand side of the septum for a right-handed surgeon. A hemistransfixion incision is then made in the right nostril

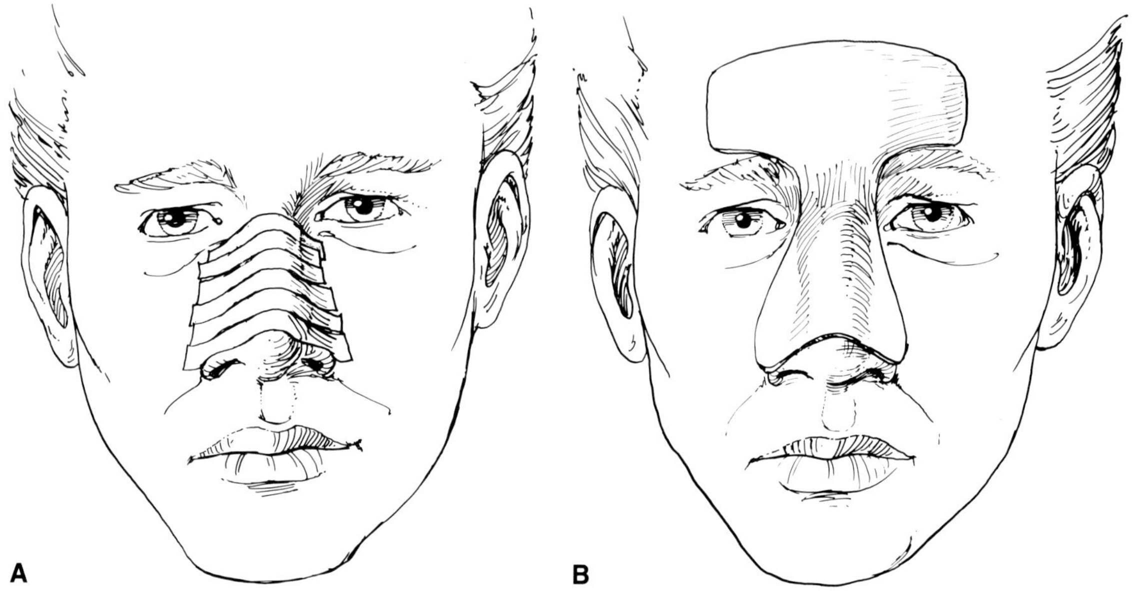

Figure 23-12. *(**A** and **B**) The outer cast of the nose is used to protect the nose and to keep mobile bones in the midline of the face. Tape is applied first, followed by an outer layer of plaster or similar material.*

and tunneling is begun on the left septum under the mucoperichondrium. A left inferior mucoperiosteal tunnel is then begun on the floor of the nose on the left, and these two tunnels are connected.

Under direct vision, overlapped segments then may be trimmed (Fig. 23–13) or the inferior caudal edge of the septum can be trimmed to allow passive settling into the nasal crest of the maxilla. Occasionally it is helpful to drill a hole (or insert a Kirschner's wire [K-wire] or small Keith needle) into the anterior nasal spine to hold the septum in place (Fig. 23–14). A figure-of-8 suture holds the anterior septum in place. Rarely is it necessary to perform any major resection of the superior bone of the perpendicular plate of the ethmoid. This could cause nasal bone collapse. Cartilage and bone removal usually incorporates the reverse C- or L-shaped articulation of the septal cartilage with the vomer. The anterior supporting strut is left inviolate. In patients who have had any significant time interval between the injury and surgical repair, scoring of the septum may be needed to eliminate bone memory. Note that a scored septum deviates back toward the intact side.

Silastic sheeting coated with an antibiotic ointment commonly is used to sandwich the septum. These are sutured through the septum with 3-0 catgut and left for 7 to 14 days. Although antibiotics may not be needed for routine fracture reduction, it is recommended to administer antibiotics to the patient until all foreign material is removed from the nose.

When open reduction of the bony injuries is con-

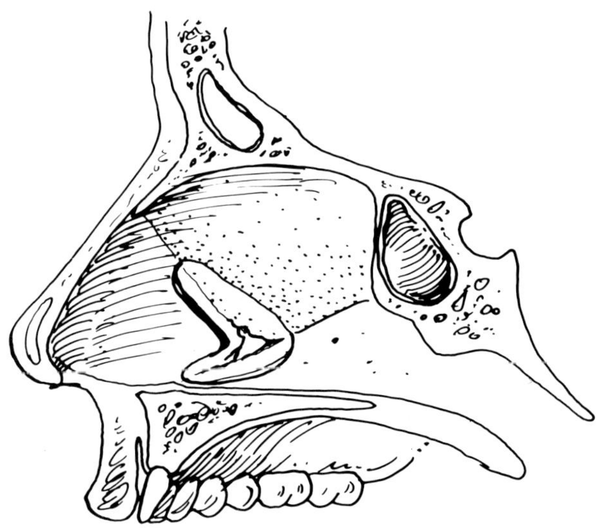

Figure 23-13. *An area of overlapping cartilage may have to be trimmed to allow passive settling of the septum. The inverted* L *or* C *reveals the most common area for this trimming.*

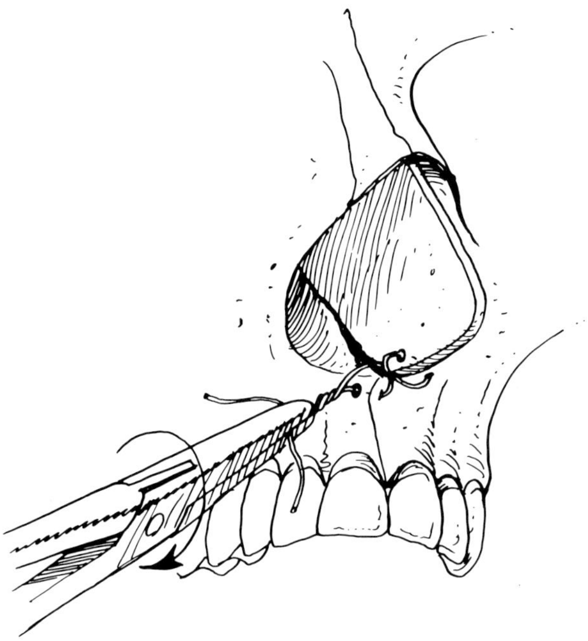

Figure 23-14. *A figure-of-8 wire is placed onto the anterior nasal spine to hold a malpositioned septum in the proper midline position.*

templated, it is done before the septal reduction. Two methods are acceptable: a blind and a direct method.

The first technique involves a small internal piriform rim incision and blind insertion of the guarded osteotomes to completely refracture any lateral fracture sites, just as if a rhinoplasty were being done.

The direct open method[36] uses the intercartilaginous incision in the internal nares. Scissors dissection is then accomplished just above the upper lateral cartilages, nasal bones, and frontal processes of the maxilla. An Aufrecht speculum may allow for palpation or direct vision of the fracture lines. An instrument is then placed into the incision to assess mobility of the bones. Refracture with an osteotome may be necessary and a Walsham forceps may be placed under the skin flap to mobilize the bones into position.

Medial Maxillary Fracture

This is perhaps the only injury that may be missed without a Waters' view radiograph. Treatment involves elevation of the frontal process of the maxilla on the affected side. If patients with medial maxillary fracture are treated relatively early, experience has shown that open reduction is rarely needed (Fig. 23–15). High and low internal packing may be used if there is instability.

Septum Alone

Treatment of partly or fully unstable septal injuries is discussed in the section on bilateral fractures with septal injury or dislocation. Some additional comments are warranted.

Once a septum has been placed into proper position, it must fibrose in that position so that new cartilaginous memory is obtained. This takes 5 to 7 days. Numerous devices for benign packing modalities such as nasal tampons have been used effectively. Iodoform gauze must be considered an outmoded technique.

Childhood

Nasal fractures often occur in children. Although adequate reduction of isolated nasal bone fractures causes no disturbance of nasal growth, late deformity or bulging of bone may occur at the fracture site. One paper reports that 71% of pediatric fractured noses treated by closed manipulation left no residual deformity, symptoms, or breathing difficulties.[16] Brain and Rock[16a] have shown that nasal injuries in childhood with or without the loss of septal cartilage may nevertheless lead to a loss of nasal projection during adult life. Osteotomies or fractures of the nasal bones themselves did not have any effect on subsequent nasal growth.

Generally, adult principles of nasal fracture treatment also apply to children. Septal hematomas must be evacuated and occasionally packed for 1 or 2 days and the child should be administered antibiotics. Septal dislocations are treated in an open reconstructive technique, if possible, with an aim toward conservatism and minimal disturbance of the vomerine maxillary suture.

SUMMARY

The term *broken nose* can actually mean any one of a wide range of nasal injuries. Primary care should be instituted in the emergency room according to some investigators, whereas others believe that an observation period of several weeks and full rhinoplastic techniques, or "planned delayed treatment," is the better choice.[17]

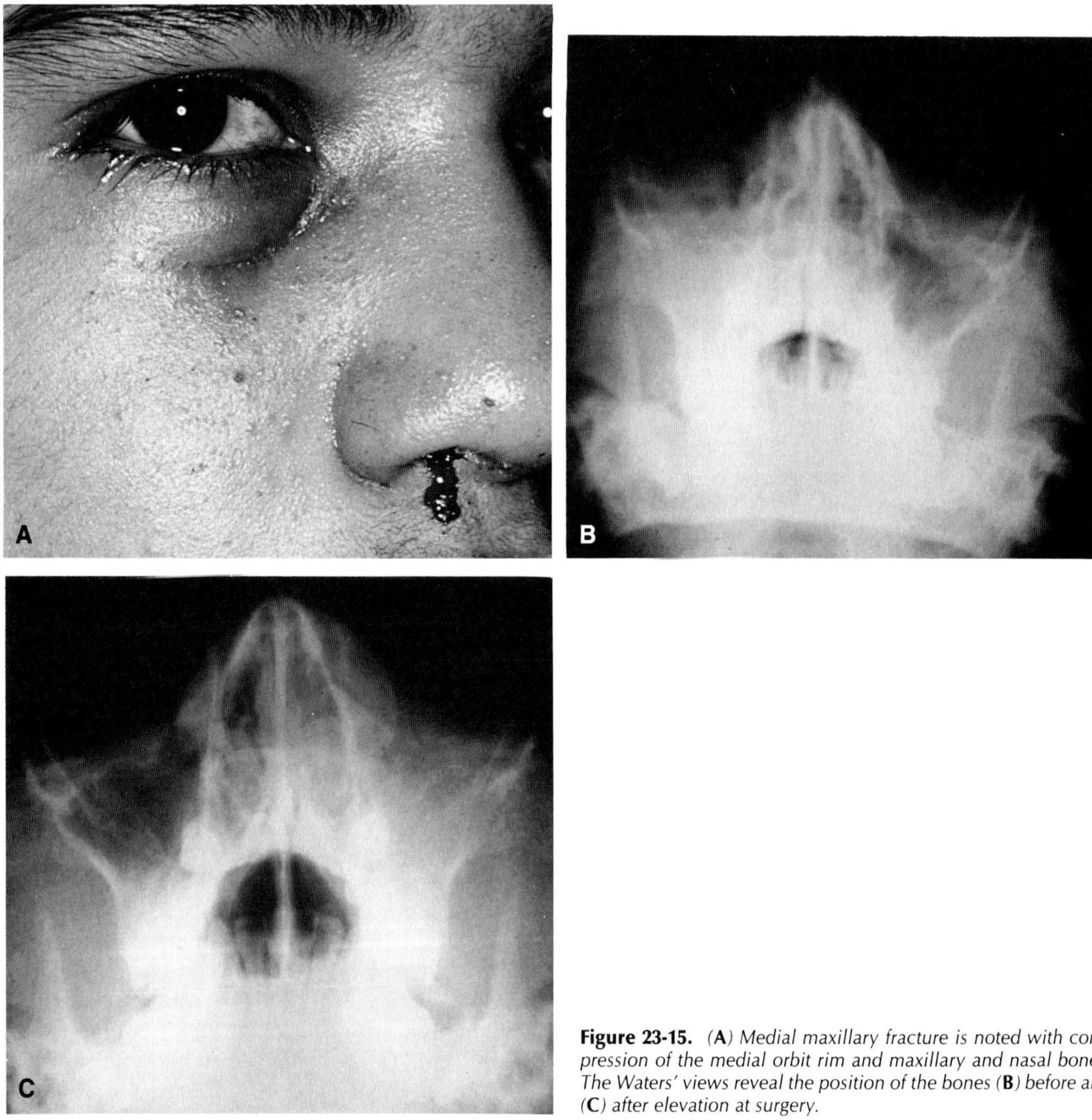

Figure 23-15. *(**A**) Medial maxillary fracture is noted with compression of the medial orbit rim and maxillary and nasal bones. The Waters' views reveal the position of the bones (**B**) before and (**C**) after elevation at surgery.*

NASOORBITAL ETHMOID FRACTURES

Severe forces to the nasofrontal or midfacial area produce fractures that are seen by many specialists.[25] Immediate or early interdisciplinary intervention has been shown to be the standard for acceptable results.

In the past the complexity of these nasoorbital injuries often led to mediocre results, even in the hands of experienced surgeons. Current radiographic techniques, aggressive early treatment with primary bone grafting, and the use of advanced craniofacial access methods with miniplate fixation have improved results dramatically.

Anatomy

Bony Anatomy

The medial walls of the orbit begin behind the frontal processes of the maxilla. The thin lacrimal bone and the frail lamina papyracea in the anterior portion provide meager resistance to crushing trauma in this area.

Higher up, the frontoethmoid suture represents the level of the cribriform plate and the crista galli. Once fractured, intimate attachment of the dura in this area can lead to CSF leak and loss of the sense of smell, two classic problems associated with NOE fractures. Total anosmia does not occur because of the presence of glands in the tongue and pharynx. Two foramina are present along this suture line: the anterior ethmoidal foramen, through which courses the nasociliary nerve and anterior ethmoidal artery, and the posterior ethmoidal foramen, which transmits a vessel and nerve of the same name.

Further posterior along the medial orbital wall, the optic nerve exits through the body of the sphenoid bone, 3.5 to 5 mm behind the posterior ethmoidal foramen in a line parallel with the two foramina.

Interorbital Space (Fig. 23–16)

The nasofrontal suture is the continuation of the frontoethmoid suture and corresponds to the plane of the base of the skull or frontal sinus. The interorbital space is bounded laterally by the medial wall of the orbits. In the middle is the perpendicular plate of the ethmoid and nasal septum. The anterior wall is composed of the paired nasal bones, the frontal processes of the maxilla, and the nasal processes of the frontal bone.

The ethmoid air cells within the interorbital space occupy the upper half of the lateral wall of the nasal fossa. The dimensions of the anterior end of the ethmoid labyrinth are approximately 2.5 cm vertically and 1 cm transversely. The pyramidal shaped sinus measures 3.5 to 5 cm from front to back.

The ethmoid air cells drain into the middle meatus. The frontal sinus, which is embryologically a direct extension of the ethmoid air cells, also drains there through its nasofrontal duct. The nasofrontal duct is located in the posterior medial floor of the frontal sinus at the junction of the ethmoid and nasal portions of the floor. The length of the duct may vary from a couple of millimeters to a centimeter, and it courses through the anterior ethmoids into the middle meatus or just anterior to the middle turbinate. Occlusion or untreated injury of the drainage apparatus is the forerunner to obstructive mucoceles or pyoceles, even years after the injury.

Frontal Bone and Sinus

The frontal bone is composed of the larger, vertical upper forehead portion and a horizontal lower portion that makes up the bilateral supraorbital ridges and the roofs of the anterior orbital and nasal cavities. The nasal process of the frontal bone lies beneath the paired nasal bones and frontal processes of the maxilla. This structural support causes most isolated nasal fractures to occur several millimeters below the nasofrontal suture line, at the thinner nasal bone isthmus. The horizontal portions of the frontal bone are separated by the ethmoid air cells, medially.

In children the frontal sinus begins to appear on radiographics around the age of 6 years, but it is not clinically significant with regard to facial trauma until the age of 10 to 12 years when pneumatization commences.[21] About 10% of the population have only a unilateral frontal sinus, and in 4%, no frontal sinus is visible on radiographs.

Medial Canthal Tendon

There are three portions to the orbicularis oculi muscle: the orbital, the preseptal, and the pretarsal. The pretarsal portions of the upper and lower lids unite at the canthus to form the medial canthal tendon.

The medial canthal tendon may be subdivided into a superficial portion and a deeper portion with the lacrimal sac in between. The superficial portion has two "legs"[22] and inserts into the frontal process of the maxilla. The deeper section (also known as Horner's muscle, or the pars lacrimalis) attaches to the posterior lacrimal crest (Fig. 23–17).

Injuries to the nasoorbital ethmoid area may cause avulsion of the tendons from the bone or, more commonly, fractures of bone that contain the attachments of the tendons.

CLINICAL EXAMINATION

The patient with a nasoorbital ethmoid injury has all the classic signs of nasal fracture and may also possess the following signs:

1. Flattened bridge of the nose
2. Edematous eyelids, periorbital ecchymosis, and subconjunctival hemorrhage
3. CSF leak
4. Hyposmia

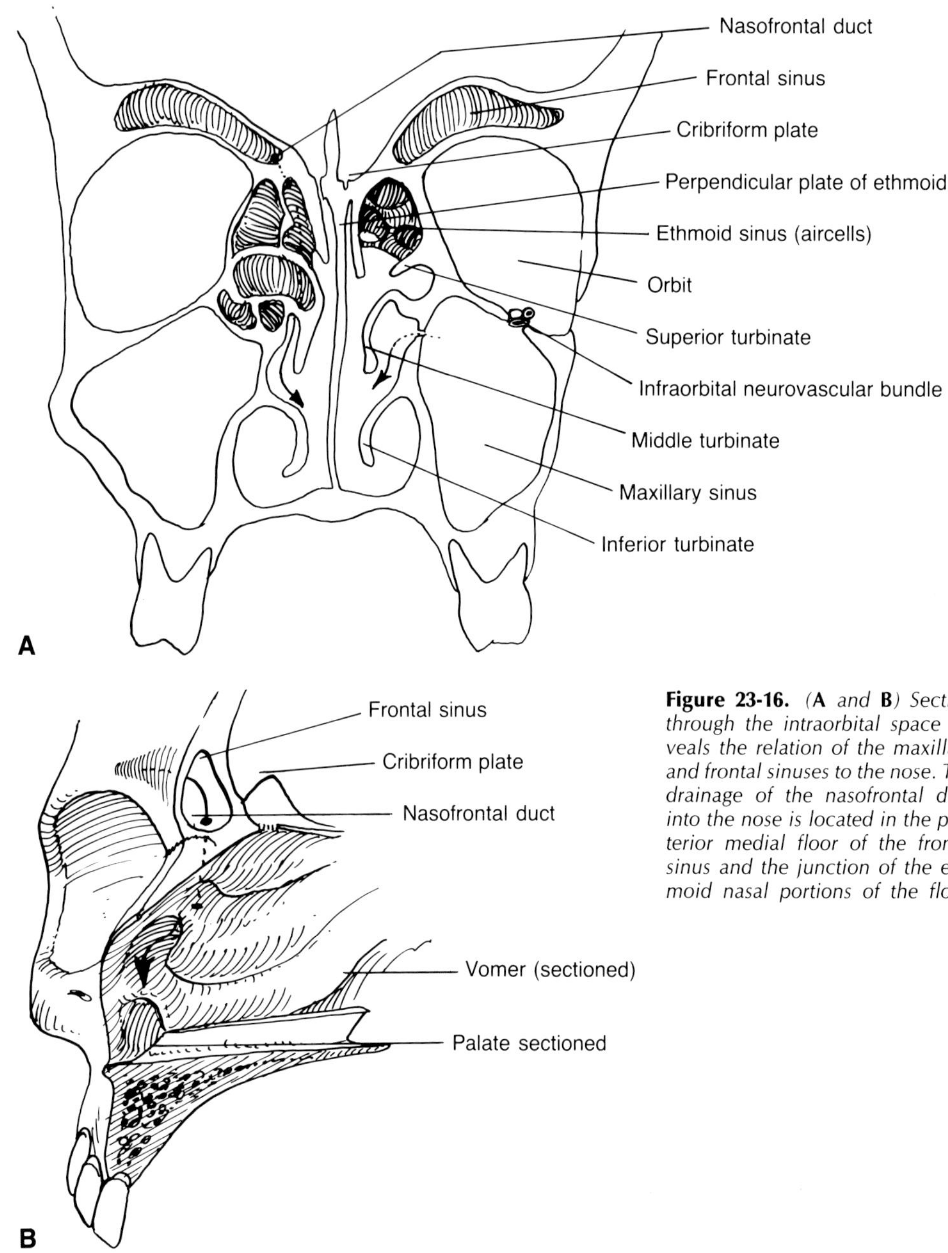

Figure 23-16. *(**A** and **B**) Section through the intraorbital space reveals the relation of the maxillary and frontal sinuses to the nose. The drainage of the nasofrontal duct into the nose is located in the posterior medial floor of the frontal sinus and the junction of the ethmoid nasal portions of the floor.*

5. Widened intercanthal measurement (called *traumatic telecanthism*)
6. Rounded lacrimal lake (i.e., increased canthal angles)
7. Associated facial or skull fractures

Two tests aid in the clinical diagnosis of instability of the canthal tendons. The first is the "bowstring" test, in which the lid is pulled laterally while the tendon area is palpated (Fig. 23–18).[23] The second is the bimanual examination. In this test the surgeon places a Kelly clamp high in the nose, tipping it directly beneath the medial canthal tendon. Gentle lifting with contralateral finger palpates the canthal tendons and allows for an assessment of the instability of the tendon attachment and, hence, the necessity for open reduction (Fig. 23–18).[24]

Open injuries to this area necessitate evaluation of the lacrimal apparatus. Ophthalmologic evaluation is a critical part of the basic examination, as is neurologic evaluation.

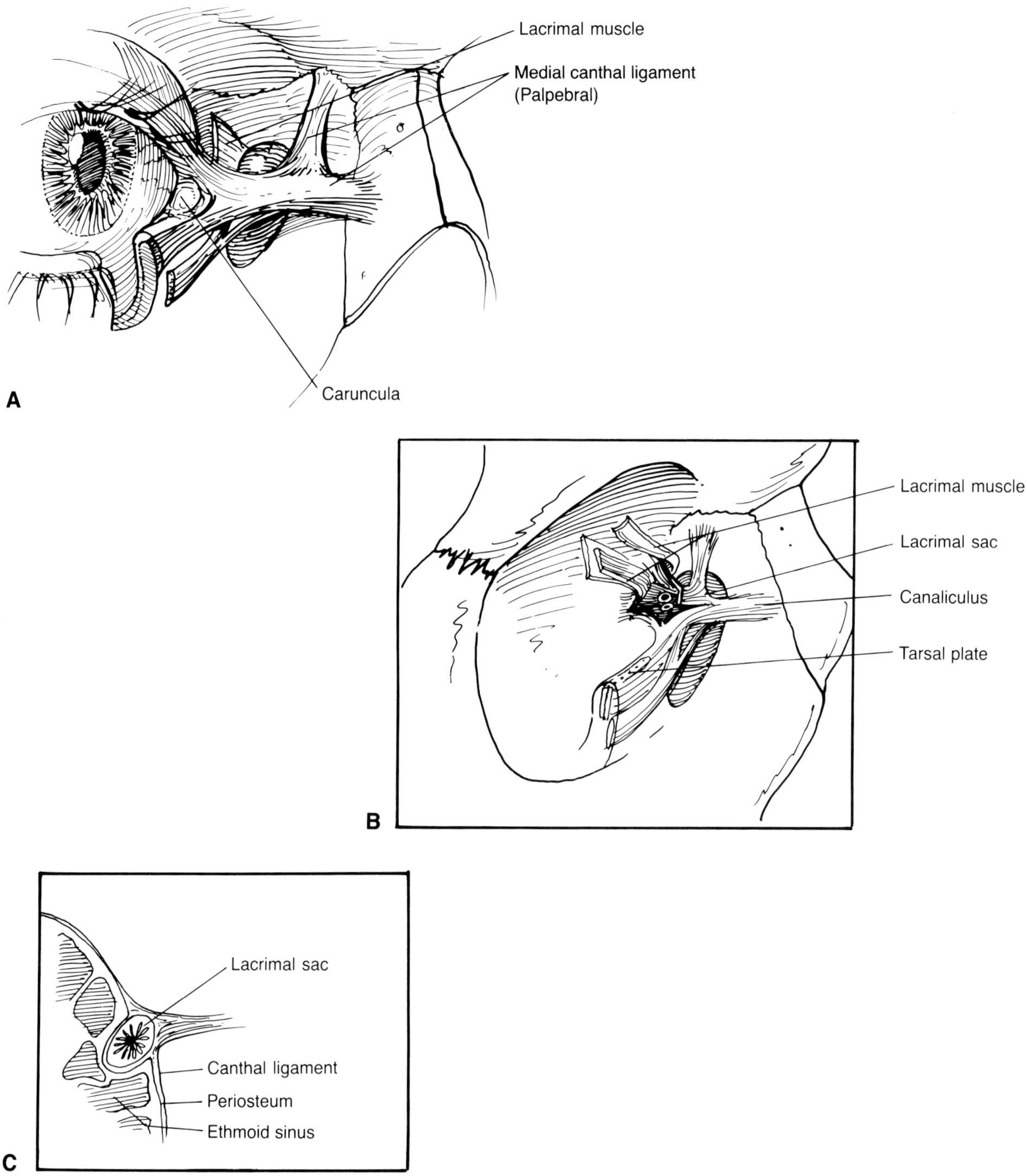

Figure 23-17. *(**A–C**) Medial canthal anatomy. Understanding the relation of the legs of the mediocanthal tendon is critical to repair of the nasal orbital ethmoid fracture. (Courtesy of Dr. Barry Zide, NYU Medical Center)*

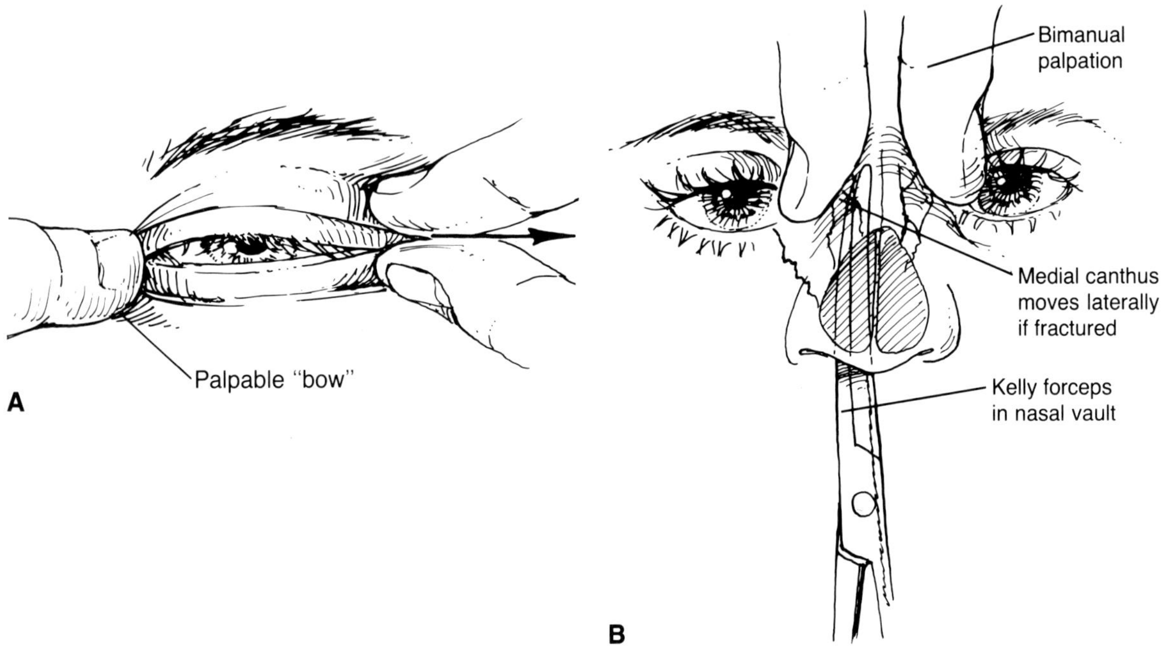

Figure 23-18. *The two evaluations of the medial canthal tendon involve the (**A**) bowstring test, which is done clinically before surgery, and the (**B**) instability test, which is done during surgery.*

CLASSIFICATION

As previously stated, there are several classifications of nasal fractures. Two of these are more specific toward the NOE fracture.[26,27] NOE fractures are usually telescoped or laterally spread. When telescoping occurs, the nose appears short and the tip may be elevated. The nasofrontal angle is deepened, and telecanthus might be present. The medial palpebral fissure maintains its almond shape. A step or separation at the nasofrontal suture appears obvious in the lateral radiographs of the head. The nasal bones and frontal processes of the maxilla sustained the force of the injury and were driven posteriorly.

Direct anterior force produces lateral spreading, and the nose appears flattened and wide. In severe telecanthism, measurements of more than 36 mm in white adults (with accountability toward known racial and age parameters [normal = 30 ± 2 in white adults]) may be present. The medial palpebral fissure is rounded, and there may be epicanthal folds, which often are not noted until swelling resolves. Radiographically, the bones are fragmented and splayed. Air may be present in the orbits and the maxillary sinuses may be clouded. The nasal bones, frontal processes of the maxilla, and lacrimal bones and lamina papyracea may be fractured. Orbital, lacrimal, and other types of craniofacial injury are commonly present.

RADIOGRAPHIC EXAMINATION

Waters' view may indeed be pathognomonic of NOE fracture, but other confirming evidence of injury must also be sought. Soft tissue swelling is significant, the sinuses may be clouded, and orbital blow-out and other facial or cranial fractures may be present. The fracture of the nose is at the nasofrontal suture line (Fig. 23–19).

In the past many surgeons operated on NOE fractures having seen only the facial series of radiographs, believing that all the bones that could be operated on were visualized. The true complexity of the injury suggests, however, that tomograms or (preferably) a CT scan should be performed to identify all fracture lines, as well as the degree of orbital and cranial injury (Fig. 23–20). If the patient has a suspected cervical spine injury, tomograms of the orbits may substitute for the CT scans because coronal CT scans must be obtained with the head tilted back. The

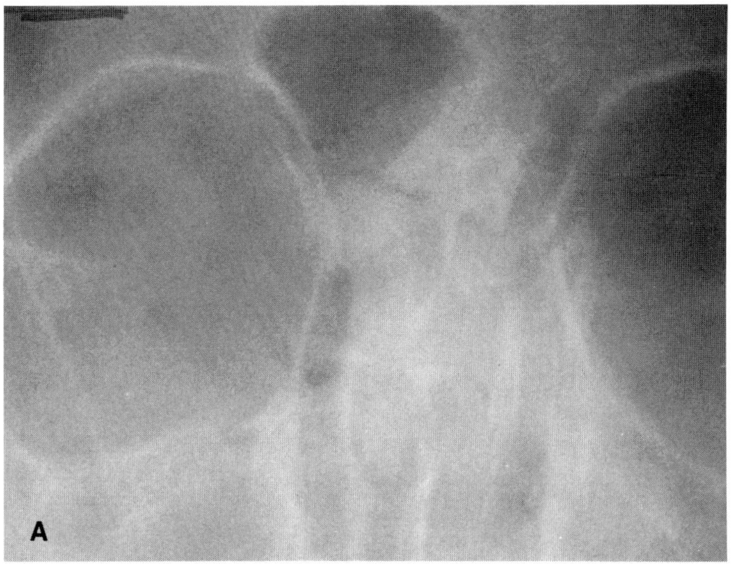

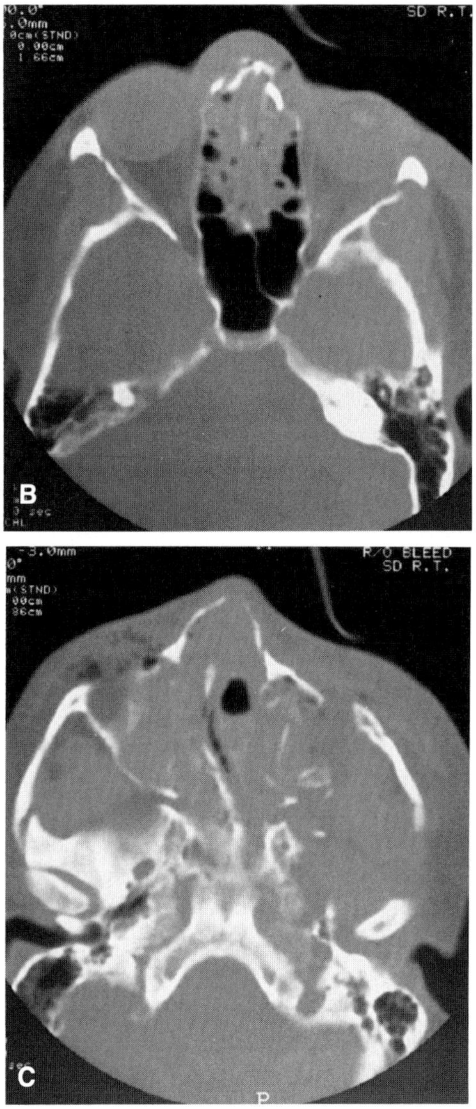

Figure 23-19. (**A–C**) *Comparison of Waters' view and computed tomographic (CT) scans reveal that additional information can be obtained at different levels from the CT scan. The CT scan is much more diagnostic of comminution patterns and internal injuries.*

frontonasal duct patency cannot be well evaluated, however, by CT scan.[28]

TREATMENT

Timing of Repair

Definitive surgery should be undertaken immediately, if possible. Repair in children should be early because fibrosis causes the bones to stick, making mobilization more difficult. However, delays are often required because of concomitant injuries (e.g., many patients have an open injury from the initial accident). If delay is significant, it is often helpful to reformat the CT scan images into a three-dimensional picture before the surgery.

Some surgeons allow for a short observation period to permit swelling to resolve significantly; to allow for appropriate consultations; and to obtain more definitive radiographic imaging. Early repair should be performed, especially if the patient must advance to the operating room for other associated injuries. Studies on maxillofacial trauma have suggested that patients

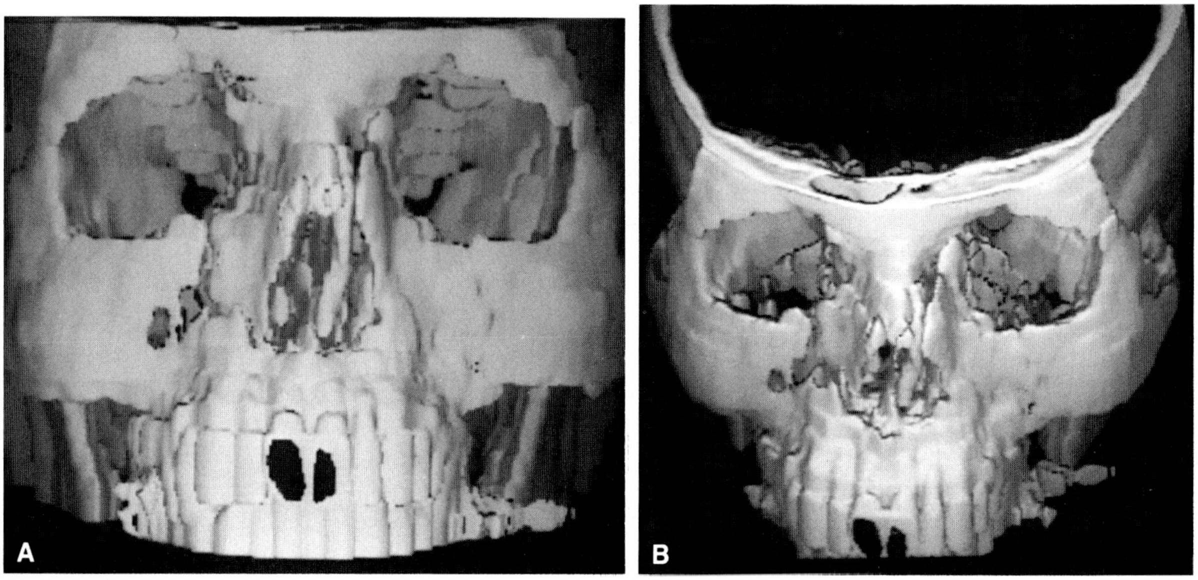

Figure 23-20. *(**A** and **B**) Computerized reconstructions of a nasal orbital ethmoid injury. Three-dimensional imaging may show the scope of the fracture more clearly. Increased details can be perceived using very small pixel sizes.*

with neurologic trauma can usually undergo acute surgery without fear of neurologic exacerbation. Likewise, the fear that it is unwise to treat extremity fractures at the same time as maxillofacial injuries because of bacterial seeding has never been substantiated.

It is not always possible to delay definitive surgery until all consultants have seen the patient and reviewed the studies relevant to their areas of expertise. The maxillofacial surgeon, who is often a coconsultant, also may assess the injuries (by rapid judicious clinical and radiographic methods) in sufficient detail to formulate a proper sequence of surgery. After all consultations are completed, integration of an acceptable interdisciplinary plan can evolve, the timing of which is dictated by patient priorities.

Open Versus Closed Reduction

Occasionally, closed reduction is applicable in the patient with a telescoped type of fracture. Care must be taken to assess disruption of the nasal septum and stability of the fractured segments and the medial canthal tendons. In patients who receive closed reduction of the nasal bones, open septal reconstruction with removal of any bony septum should be limited so that support of the nasal dorsum is not compromised.

Open reduction is a much more predictable mode of therapy for the majority of NOE fractures and should be the treatment of choice for patients with open injuries or canthal displacement or instability and for patients with laterally spread fractures.

Sequence of Surgery

The sequence of most maxillofacial surgery should be "from the bottom up and from the sides in." In patients with NOE fractures and accompanying LeFort fractures, arch bars should be applied first, and the upper jaw should be disimpacted and placed in a reduced state before approaching the NOE fracture. Next, the surgeon's attention is turned to the larger bones (e.g., zygoma and frontal bones), which can be anatomically reduced and stabilized. Obviously, the key to correct tendon placement resides in the proper placement of the frontal process of the maxilla (Fig. 23–21).

If the entire midface is crushed, exposure through a bicoronal flap is recommended to view the width of the midface. In this situation, reduction and stabilization starts from the zygomas. The zygomaticofrontal sutures and, perhaps, the zygomatic arches are plated. Intraoral zygomatic buttress exposure and plating may help if comminution is not present. Bone grafts

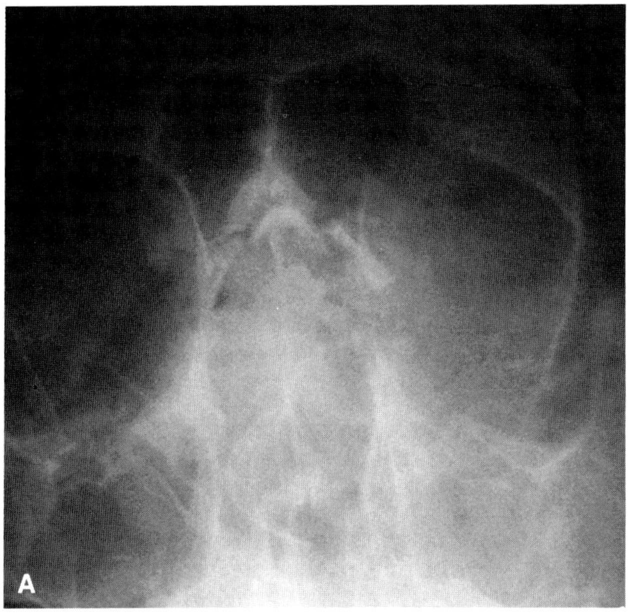

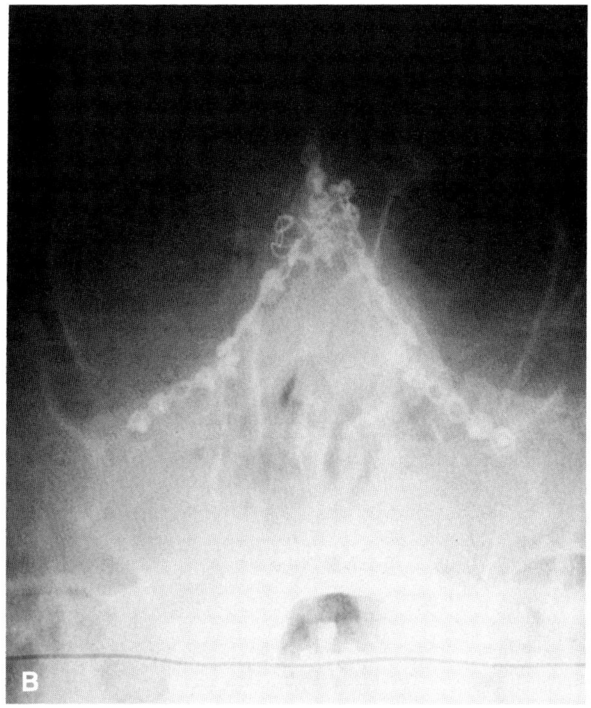

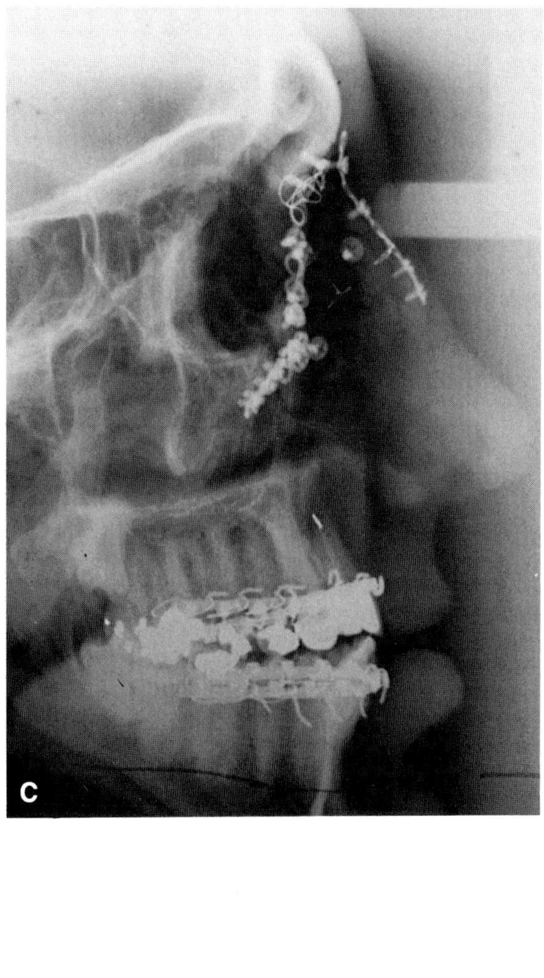

Figure 23-21. *(**A**) A Waters' view revealing a massive nasoorbital ethmoid injury with widening of the frontal processes of the maxilla. (**B**) The key to construction of this fracture is maintaining proper continuity of the frontal process of the maxilla with the nose. (**C**) The finishing touches of this type of fracture correction involve a central plate from the frontal bone on top of and through the nasal bones, holding them in proper position.*

may be necessary to stabilize the midface. Next, the nasofrontal suture and, subsequently the infraorbital rims, if involved, are exposed. Medial orbital reconstruction with grafts may be necessary. The last part of the procedure involves the reduction and stabilization of the larger and then the smaller pieces of the nasoethmoid complex. Primary bone grafting works well here.

If only the NOE complex is fractured, reduction starts at the more bulky nasofrontal suture. Infraorbital rim exposure is usually needed to aid in anatomic reduction as the surgery proceeds inwards. The final surgical maneuver involves reduction and stabilization of the medial canthal tendons with or without bone attached to them. This surgery may require revision (and often does) (Fig. 23–22).

Access to the Nasoorbital Ethmoid Area

Often the initial injury has provided access to the area by an open laceration. Frequently the surgeon may need to extend the wound. Lengthening is gained by using relaxed skin tension lines (Fig. 23–23).[29]

When the skin in the area is not violated, local incisions are best avoided in favor of the bicoronal ap-

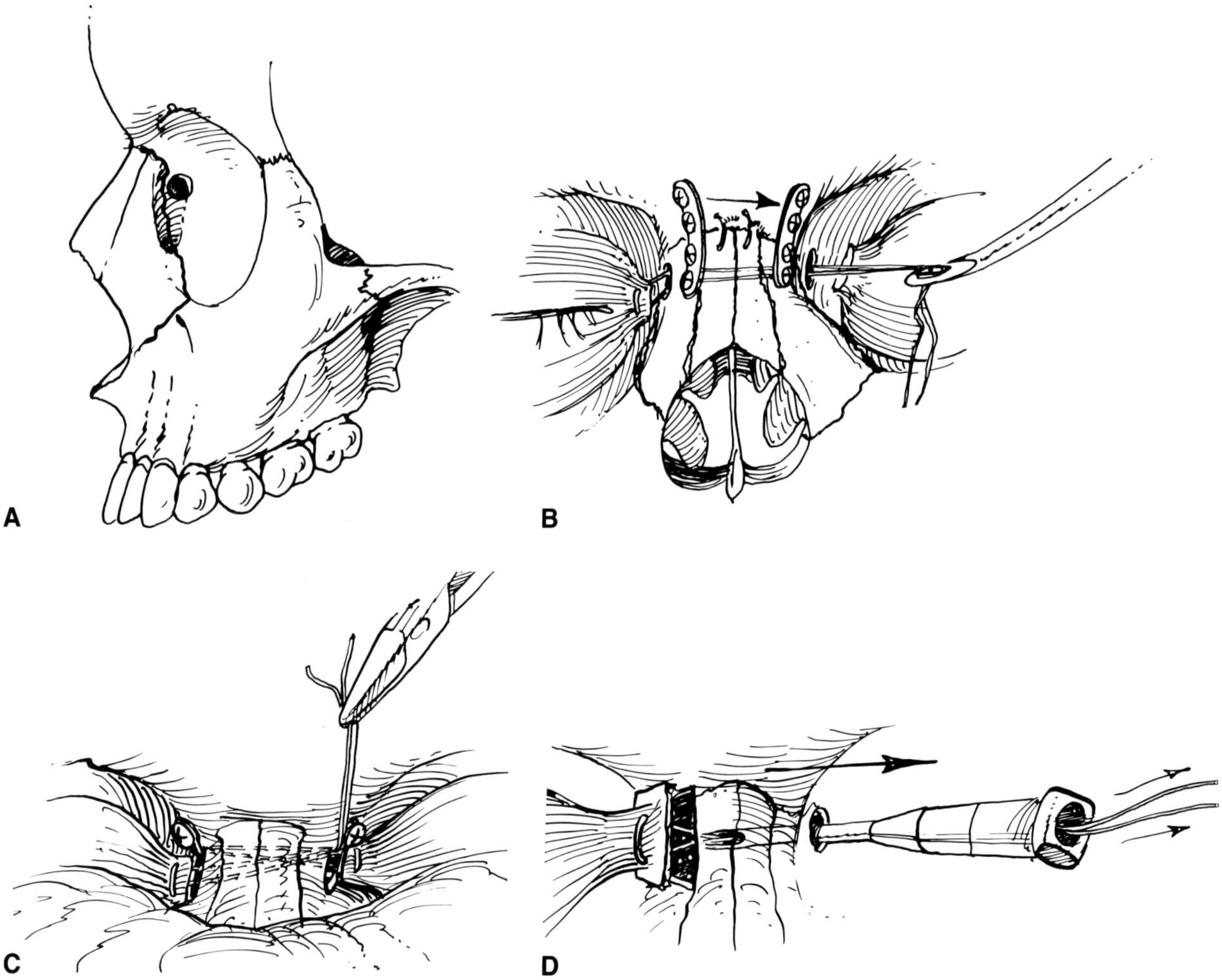

Figure 23-22. *(**A**) The correct positioning hole for the medial canthal tendon if it is avulsed. Note that it is posterior and medial and corresponds primarily to the posterior leg of the medial canthal tendon. (**B**) This tendon is being pulled in. Overcorrection is usually almost impossible. The further posterior this hole is made, the more medial the tendon should be pulled as the medial orbit slopes laterally. After the tendon is pulled into its hole, the wire is then ligated onto a screw or plate on the opposite side. (**C**) Ligating a wire onto a screw. (**D**) A repair of a primary injury. Note that the tendon should not be avulsed from a piece of bone if at all possible. Best results are obtained if the tendon remains attached so that the bone can be pulled into its normal anatomic position.*

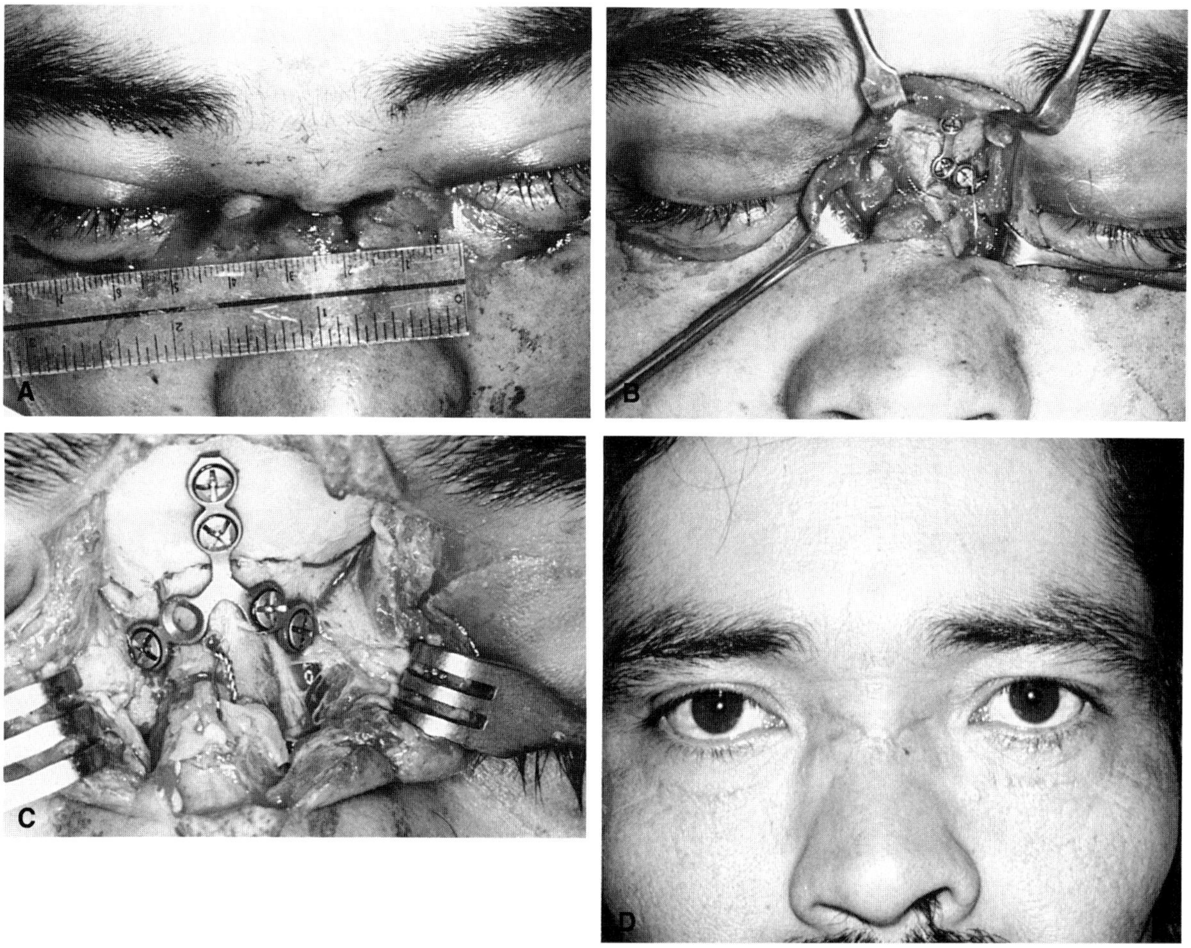

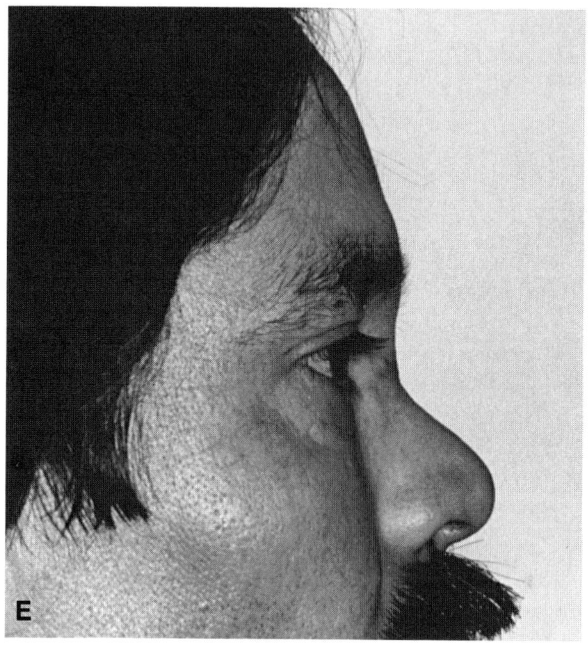

Figure 23-23. *(**A**) An open nasoorbital ethmoid injury with telecanthism measuring 50 mm. (**B**) The open treatment of this fracture with use of an* L *plate. (**C**) Another equivalent fracture with the use of a* Y *plate. Under the inferior screw on the patient's left, the medial canthal tendon is attached to a bony segment on the frontal process of the maxilla. (**D**) Good healing in the frontal view. (**E**) Good nasal projection in the lateral view at 3 months. Secondary dorsal augmentation would be a good option.*

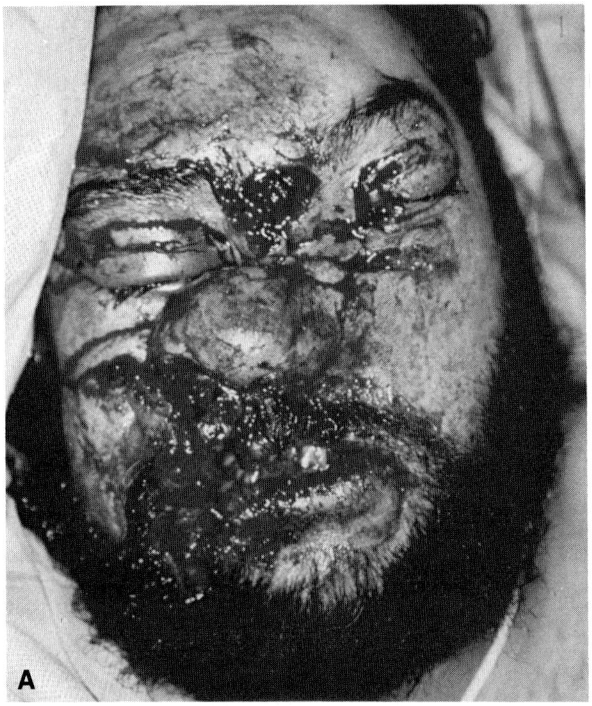

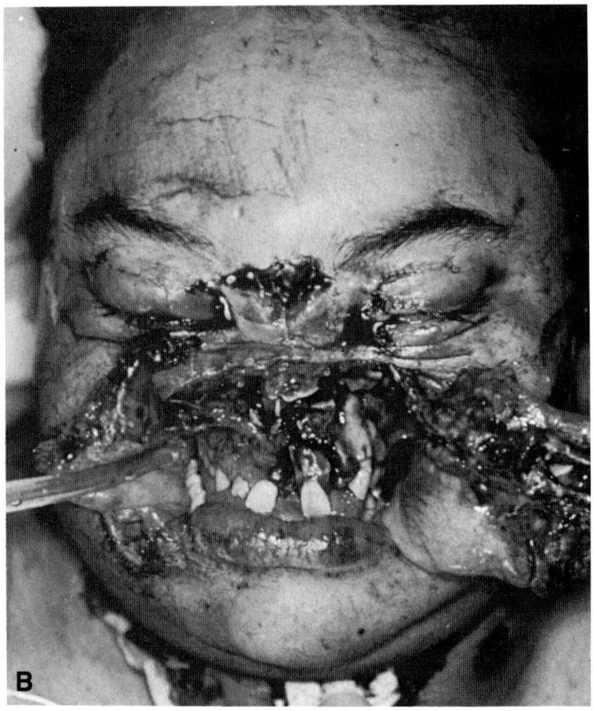

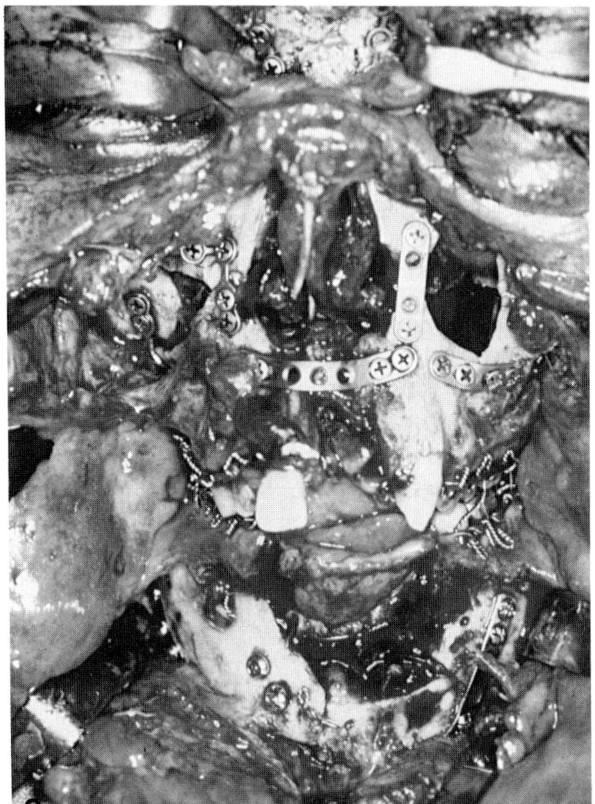

Figure 23-24. *(**A**) The severity of a midfacial fracture is revealed here. Note that there are two soft tissue injuries, one in the nasal dorsal area and the other through the upper lip. (**B**) The comminution of the midface. (**C**) The open plating and wiring and screwing, as indicated, with primary bone grafts were necessary in this case and were harvested to fill out the defects. (**D**) The nasoorbital ethmoid area reconstructed with plates. (**E**) The postoperative appearance approximately 4 months later with a prosthetic eye in place on the patient's right. (Courtesy of Dr. Richard Finn, Dallas VA Hospital, Department of Oral and Maxillofacial Surgery)*

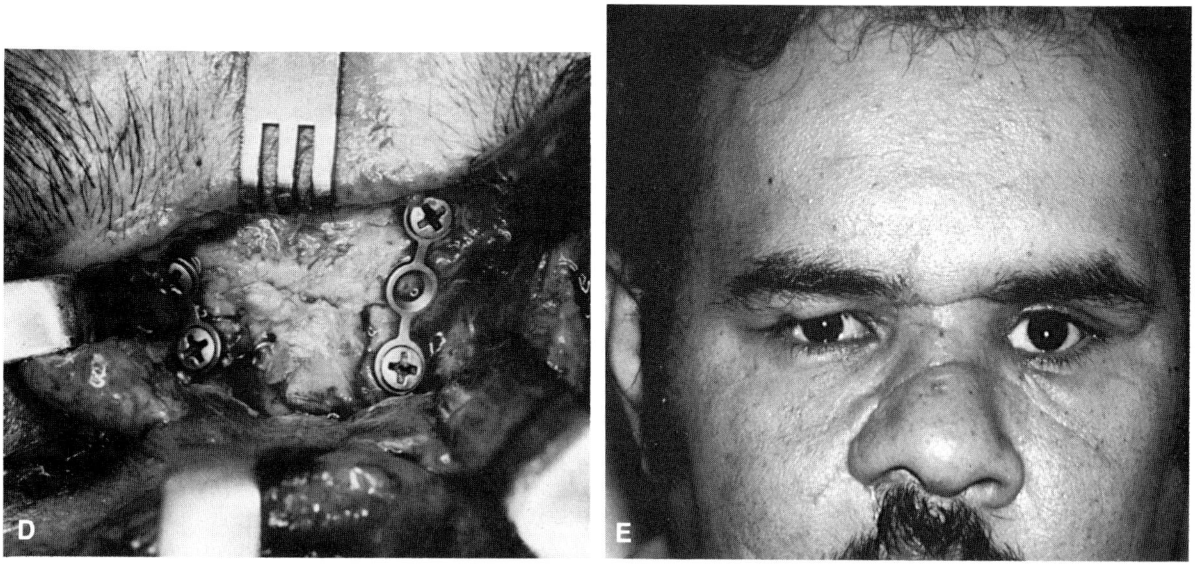

Figure 23-24. *(continued)*

proach, although various local incisions have been used with some aesthetic success.

Presently, one of three types of exposures are used: a coronal flap, a midline vertical incision no higher than the glabella, or extension of existing lacerations. The "open-sky" technique is not used because it leaves obvious webbed scars. The choice of one technique over another is made based on such variables as preexisting scars; amount of swelling; size, texture, and color of the eyebrows; age and character of the patient; hairline; and severity of the injury.

The coronal flap is ideal for exposing zygomatic and midfacial fractures. Incisions should be made in the directions of the hair follicles. Added access is made by incising the periosteum over the glabella, vertically from under the flap. An older male might be better served by direct exposure through relaxed skin tension lines or within camouflaging structures. However, even balding men have excellent scars after a bicoronal flap, as long as two layer closures with eversion are performed.

Primary Bone Grafting

In most cases in which large segments of bone are reducible and can be stabilized, primary bone grafts are not needed. Exceptions must be known so that the patient gives consent before surgery and the surgeon is prepared for the event.

Primary bone grafts may be used for rigid support or to fill in continuity defects in the following circumstances:

1. Comminution of bones does not allow for the use of usual modalities to hold the nose or midface in proper position (Fig. 23–24).
2. Comminution of the medial orbital wall or rim interferes with stable reduction.
3. Enophthalmos may be a consequence from herniation of orbital tissues.
4. A bony continuity defect, which would interfere with the aesthetic or functional result, is present.
5. A stable structure to transfix a medial canthal tendon from the opposite side is needed.

The surgeon should always use autogenous material as his first choice. Calvarial bone may be readily available through a preexisting coronal flap. Contour and pliability make split rib grafts a good choice for medial orbital walls. Iliac crest bone or calvarium works well for dorsal nasal grafting, and it may be screwed or plated into position. Alloplastic materials such as silastic or polyethylene have been used successfully, as long as they are contoured and secured properly. They are generally a successful substitute for small quantities of lost bone inside the orbit, but are not as useful as a primary onlay in facial trauma reconstruction.

Reestablishment of the Medial Canthal Tendons

After the reduction and stabilization of the bony injuries, the medial canthal tendons must be assessed. Often, the anterior legs of the tendon have been simultaneously replaced when the frontal processes of the maxilla (or a portion thereof) were stabilized. Even small pieces of bone can be held in place fairly readily with the correct bending of a malleable miniplate. The mimiplate fixation in the frontonasal area has virtually replaced a wide spectrum of methods and devices for canthal attachment, such as bone pitons, external head frames, and plaster caps. Miniscrews have afforded a means of rigidly fixating a central graft to "tent out" the entire midfacial area.

If the tendon has been avulsed or if the bone attachment is too small for fixation, a canthopexy is indicated. When canthopexy is considered, some anatomic points must be understood. If the posterior portion, and the anterior portion, of the ligament is avulsed, reattachment of the anterior attachment alone to the frontal process of the maxilla will not produce an acceptable result because the tendon will splay anteriorly onto the nose and the definition of the medial eye area will be lost. Therefore, when the entire tendon is avulsed, it should be attached more posteriorly and superiorly behind the lacrimal crest. Also, the medial orbital wall slants posterolaterally deeper into the orbit. The tendon must be grasped closer to the lacrimal lake or punctum to compensate for this slant. In essence, the same length of anterior tendon that would be fine if replaced at the anterior position (frontal process of the maxilla) is too long if placed more posteriorly.

Unilateral canthopexy is performed in the following manner. Adequate exposure of the lacrimal apparatus and medial orbital wall is obtained, and the tendon is secured with a monofilament suture, preferably of 28- to 30-gauge stainless steel wire or braided wire (because it can be tied). Monofilament can be wrapped around a screw.

Usually, there is a defect at the medial orbital wall, just above and posterior to the posterior lacrimal crest. If this hole is not present, a 5-mm hole is made. From the contralateral side, a passage is made toward this hole. Methods include drilling and passage of an autopsy, Keith needle, or awl with which to retrieve the wire attached to the ligament on the ligament side. A simple (and always available) method involves the use of an 18-gauge needle with an internal doubled over 30-gauge wire to retrieve to tendon wires (Fig. 23–22). The canthus is then pulled into the ligament hole and the wire is attached to an anchor on the contralateral side. The anchor can be a plate, screw, bone graft, or stable superior orbital rim. One interesting reported method uses an intranasal button as the tendon anchor.[31] Before the final tightening of the ligament sutures, all primary repairs to the lacrimal apparatus should be accomplished.

A controversy exists over the best method of bilateral canthal tendon repair. The preferred technique is to wire and stabilize each lateral canthal tendon to a separate stable anchoring point. If additional support is desired, the ligaments may be wired to each other with a separate wire close to the punctum. The final result should always be measured with calipers on the operating table. The use of lead plates on plastic buttons is superfluous because these do not add tendon support. A standard nasal splint is suggested, but tape alone may be adequate.

Even when early open repair is performed well, a large percentage of patients may benefit from additional surgery. Examples of postrepair surgery include correction of the nasolacrimal obstruction, onlay grafting, or revisional canthopexy. When these are needed, the entire periorbita must be mobilized to allow for adequate repositioning of the tendon and mobile lid structures.

High-speed vehicular injury may cause associated frontal bone and sinus injuries, even with the use of padded dashboards and shoulder harnesses.

Secondary Deformities

Secondary problems associated with NOE fractures may include telecanthus, lacrimal apparatus disruption, or neurologic problems. Characteristics of telecanthism are a flat nasal dorsum, rounded medial canthal area, and increased intercanthal distance (ICD). The normal ICD is 32 mm (the ICD is larger in nonwhite adults and often less in many white adults). Other cosmetic or functional problems indicating correction are epiphora, palpebral deformity, and soft tissue webbing (Fig. 23–25).

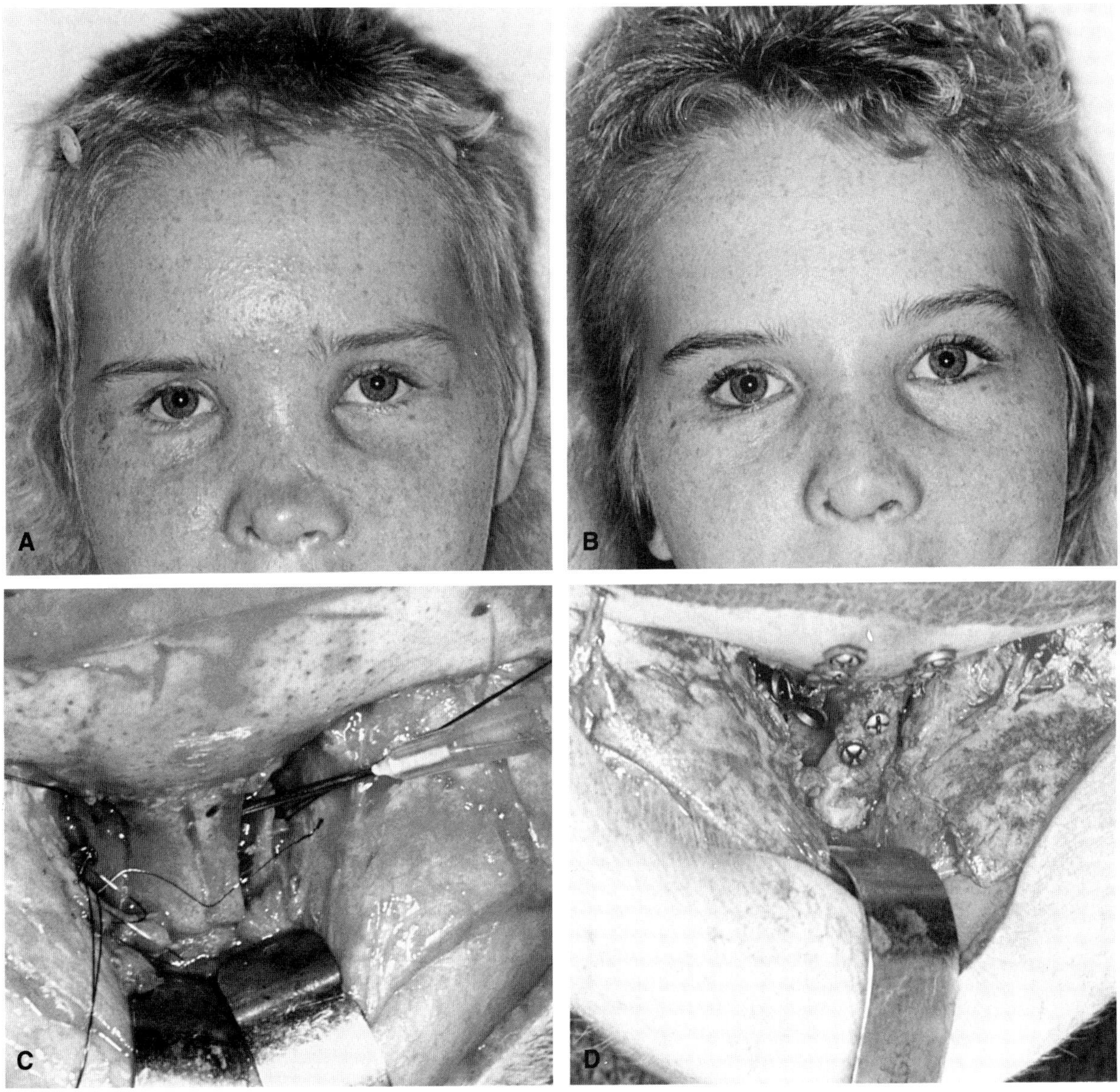

Figure 23-25. *(**A**) Classic traumatic telecanthism of a midfacial fracture after approximately 7 to 8 weeks. The nasal dorsum is indistinct and rarely used buttons are noted within the patient's hairline. (**B**) The 3-month result after appropriately osteotomizing the medial canthal area, performing medial canthopexies, and nasal onlay grafting. (**C**) Surgery, performed through a coronal flap. The frontal processes of the maxilla are osteotomized and turned inward. Subsequently, an 18-gauge needle is used to pass Burnel-type tendon wires to hold the medial canthal tendons in place. (**D**) Two screws through an onlay bone graft to the dorsum. Two screws are necessary to hold this onlay rigidly and to prevent untoward resorption.*

A distinction must be made about whether only the tendons are detached or whether the bones and associated tendons are splayed. In the first case, camouflaging might be possible with isolated soft tissue surgery or by drilling a hole into the posterior lacrimal crest and stabilizing the tendon on a more posteromediosuperior position. In the second instance, the patient requires osseous nasal narrowing and canthal repositioning, a much more complex surgical procedure. Onlay nasal dorsal grafting may also improve the cosmetic result.

Reconstructive canthopexy is done through the bicoronal incision. Intercanthal wires are passed transnasally. The tendons, with or without the associated bone, are reduced. The periorbital (and lateral canthal tendon) of the globe may need to be detached with the tendon to allow for medial movement. Final stabilization is done by contralateral bone or screws.

Although nasolacrimal and neurologic sequelae are possible complications of NOE fractures, a discussion of these is beyond the scope of this chapter.

SUMMARY

Aggressive management of NOE fractures with direct or bicoronal exposure and with the aid of CT is now an accepted norm.

REFERENCES

1. Lundin K, et al. One thousand maxillofacial and related fractures at the ENT Clinic at Gothenberg: A two year prospective study, Acta Otolaryngol 1972; 75:359–361.
2. Illum P, Kristensen S, Jorgensen K, Pedersen CB. Role of fixation in the treatment of nasal fractures. Clin Otolaryngol 1983; 8:191.
3. Stranc MF, Robertson GA. A classification of injuries of the nasal skeleton. Ann Plast Surg 1979; 2(6)468–474.
4. Murray JAM, Maran AGD. A pathological classification of nasal fractures. Injury 1986; 17:338–344.
5. Close LG, Meyerhoff W. Nasal fractures in surgery of facial bone fractures. In: Foster CA, Sherman JE, eds. New York: Churchhill Livingstone, 1987; 29.
6. Goode RL, Spooner TL. Management of nasal fractures in children. 1972; 11:9:526–529.
7. Murray JAM, Maran AGD. The treatment of nasal injuries by manipulation. J Laryngol Otol 1980; 94: 405–1410.
8. Altreuter RW. Facial form and function: Films versus physical examination. Ann Emerg Med 1986; 15: 240–244.
9. Colton JJ, Beekhuis GJ. Management of nasal fractures. Otolaryngol Clin North Am 1986; 19:73–85.
10. Delacey GJ, et al. The radiology of nasal injuries: Problems of interpretation and clinical relevance. Br J Radiol 1977; 50:412.
11. Clayton MI, Lesser THJ. The role of radiography in the management of nasal fractures. J Laryngol Otol 1986; 100:797–801.
12. Stucker FJ, Ansel DG. A case against nasal packing. Laryngoscope 1978; 88:1314.
13. Cottle MH. Nasal surgery in children. Eye Ear Nose Throat 1951; 30:32.
14. Kern EB. Acute nasal trauma in rhinoplasty problems and controversies. In: Rees TD, Baker DC, Tabbal, N, eds. St. Louis: CV Mosby Co, 1988; 392–396.
15. Drumhell DH. Acute nasal trauma. Int Rhinol 1970; 8:161.
16. Chmielik M, Gutkowska A, Kossouska E, Praglowska B. Nasal fractures in children. Int J Pediatr Otolaryngol 1986; 11:1–4.
16a. Brain DJ, Rock WP. The influence of nasal trauma during childhood on growth of the nasal skeleton. J Laryngol Otol 1983; 97:917–923.
17. Colton JJ, Beekhuis GJ. Management of nasal fractures. Otolaryngol Clin North Am 1986; 19:1:73–85.
18. Farrior R. Management of late sequelae of nasal fractures in maxillofacial trauma. In: Mathog RH, ed. Maxillofacial trauma. Baltimore: Williams and Wilkins, 1984; 266–279.
19. Clark WD, Stiernberg CM. Early aggressive treatment of nasal fractures. Ear Nose Throat 1986; 65:65–67.
20. Dickson MG, Sharpe DT. A prospective study of nasal fractures. J Laryngol Otol 1986; 100:543–551.
21. Gross C. Pathophysiology and evaluation of frontoethmoid fractures. In: Mathog RH, ed. Maxillofacial trauma. Baltimore: Williams and Wilkins, 1984; 280–287.
22. Zide BM, McCarthy JG. The medial canthus revisited: An anatomical basis for canthopexy. Am J Plast Surg 1983; 11:1–9.
23. Furnas DW, Bircoll MJ. Eyelash traction test to determine if the medial canthol tendon is detached. Plast Reconstr Surg 1973; 52:315.
24. Paskert JP, Manson PN. The bimanual examination for assessing instability in naso-orbital ethmoid injuries. Plast Reconstr Surg 1989; 83:1:165–167.
25. Swearinger JJ. Tolerances of the human face to crash impact. Oklahoma City: Federal Aviation Agency, 1965.
26. Gruss JS. Nasal-ethmoid-orbital fractures: Classification and role of primary bone grafting. Plast Reconstr Surg 1985; 75:303.
27. Duvall AJ, Foster CA, Lyons DP, Letson RD. Medial canthoplasty: Early and delayed repair. Laryngoscope 1981; 91:173.
28. Heller EM, Jacobs JB, Holliday RA. Evaluation of the frontonasal duct in frontal sinus fractures. Head Neck Surg 1989; 11:46.

29. Borges A. In: Holt, Regan, eds. Facial scars.
30. Callahan A, Callahan MA. Fixation of the medial canthal structures: Evolution of the best method. Ann Plast Surg 1983; 11:3:242–245.
31. Duvall HA, Foster CF, Lyons DP, Letson RD. Medial canthoplasty: Early and delayed repair. Laryngoscope 1981; 91:173.
32. Sataloff RT, et al. Surgical management of the frontal sinus. Neurosurgery 1984; 15:593.
33. Luce EA. Frontal sinus fracture: Guidelines to management. Plast Reconstr Surg 1987; 80:500.
34. Merville LC, Real JP. Fronto-orbito nasal dislocations: Initial total reconstruction. Scand J Plast Reconstr Surg 1981; 15:287.
35. Gruss JS, Phillips JH. Complex facial trauma: The evolving role of rigid fixation and immediate bone graft reconstruction. Plast Surg Clin North Am 1989; 93.

24

Management of Fractures of the Frontal Bone and Sinus

Richard H. Haug

Fractures of the frontal bone, although infrequent, may have devastating complications because of their proximity to the brain, eyes, and nose. Fractures of the frontal region range in incidence from 5% to 15% of all facial fractures.[1-5] The majority are caused by motor vehicle accidents and predominantly affect males.[1,6,7] There is essentially equal distribution between fractures of the supraorbital rim and frontal sinus.[3] As frontal bone fractures most frequently occur in the multiply injured trauma patient, a thorough physical examination of the patient is required before definitive treatment.

ANATOMY AND PHYSIOLOGY

Embryology

The frontal bone is an intramembranous bone that develops from two paired structures, which begin to ossify at the eighth or ninth week in utero. The frontal processes of the squamous regions are the sites of initial ossification, which progress to the orbital, squamous, and ultimately, the frontal and temporal faces by the 12th week. The metopic suture in the midline closes during the second year of life.[8] The forehead is displaced anteriorly by sutural growth, inner table resorption, and outer table deposition.[9] The frontal sinus develops from the ethmoid air cells as a mucosal pocket in or near the frontal recess.[10] Initial pneumatization begins at the fourth month in utero. Secondary pneumatization begins at 6 months to 2 years of life and develops laterally and vertically. The sinus is radiographically identifiable at 6 years of age.[11] The majority of pneumatization is completed by 14 to 16 years of age, and it continues until age 40.

Osteology

The frontal bone is shaped as a concave disk with a horizontal table forming the orbital rim. From the nasion, the bone extends approximately 12.5 cm superiorly, 8.0 cm laterally, and 5.5 cm posteriorly. Two frontal tuberosites are noted lateral to the midline and superior to the supraorbital rim. The thickest area of the bone is the supraorbital rim from the frontozygomatic process to the nasal bones. The ethmoid plate is bound on three surfaces along the floor of the frontal bone in the midline. As the floor of the frontal bone extends laterally, it becomes concave and forms the orbital roof. The supraorbital and frontal foramen are located at the most superior portion of the orbital rim.[12]

Paired triangular sinuses are found within the frontal bone. These are asymmetric and separated by a frontal septum. The average height of the sinuses is 32 mm, with a width of 26 mm.[11,12] The surface area is

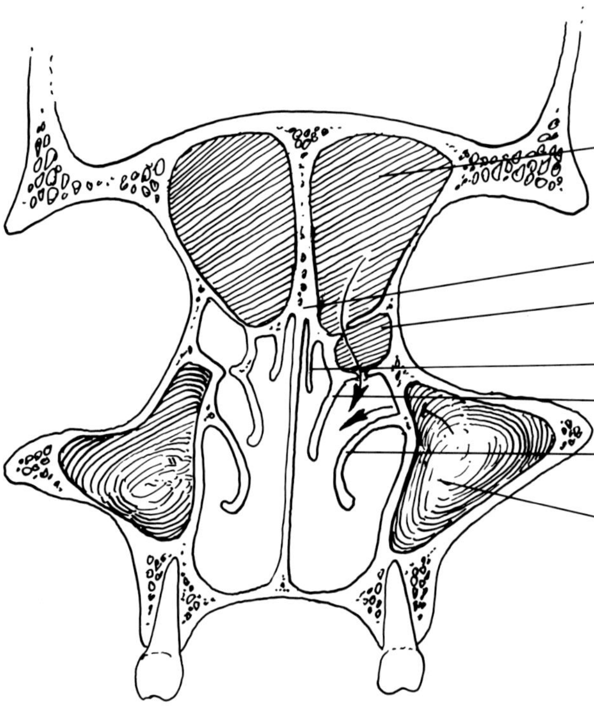

Figure 24–1. *Frontal bone and frontal sinus showing the relation of the nasofrontal duct and nose.*

approximately 720 mm.[13] The frontal bone is thinnest in the region of the glabella at the anterior wall and floor of the sinus. The duct of the frontal sinus empties into the ethmoid air cells or the middle meatus of the nose (Fig. 24–1).

Vessels and Nerves

The arterial blood supply to the frontal sinus is from the supraorbital and anterior ethmoid arteries. The frontal bone is supplied by the supraorbital, anterior superficial temporal, anterior cerebral, and middle meningeal arteries.[8,12]

Venous drainage is transosseous through the anastomosis of vessels of the subcutaneous, orbital, and intracranial structures. The supratrochlear, supraorbital, superficial temporal, frontal diploic, superior ophthalmic, and superior sagittal sinus are the major vessels of drainage.[8,12]

The supraorbital nerve supplies the frontal sinus, whereas innervation to the frontal bone is by small nerves that follow arterioles.[8,12]

Physiology of the Sinus

The entire surface area of the frontal sinus is covered with respiratory epithelium ranging in thickness from 0.07 mm to 2.0 mm.[10,14] The mucosa consists of pseudostratified ciliated epithelium, mucus-producing goblet cells, a thin basement membrane, and a thin lamina propria that contains seromucous glands.[14] Animal, as well as human, research shows that in a healthy state there is a blanket of mucin overlying the epithelium. The cilia flow at 250 cycles per minute.[10] The mucin blanket flows in a spiral fashion from a medial to lateral direction and is slowest at the roof and fastest at the nasofrontal duct.[15] The mucin empties at the nasofrontal duct at a rate of 5.0 g/cm^2.[10] It is the physiologic characteristics of the sinus and the status of the nasofrontal duct that

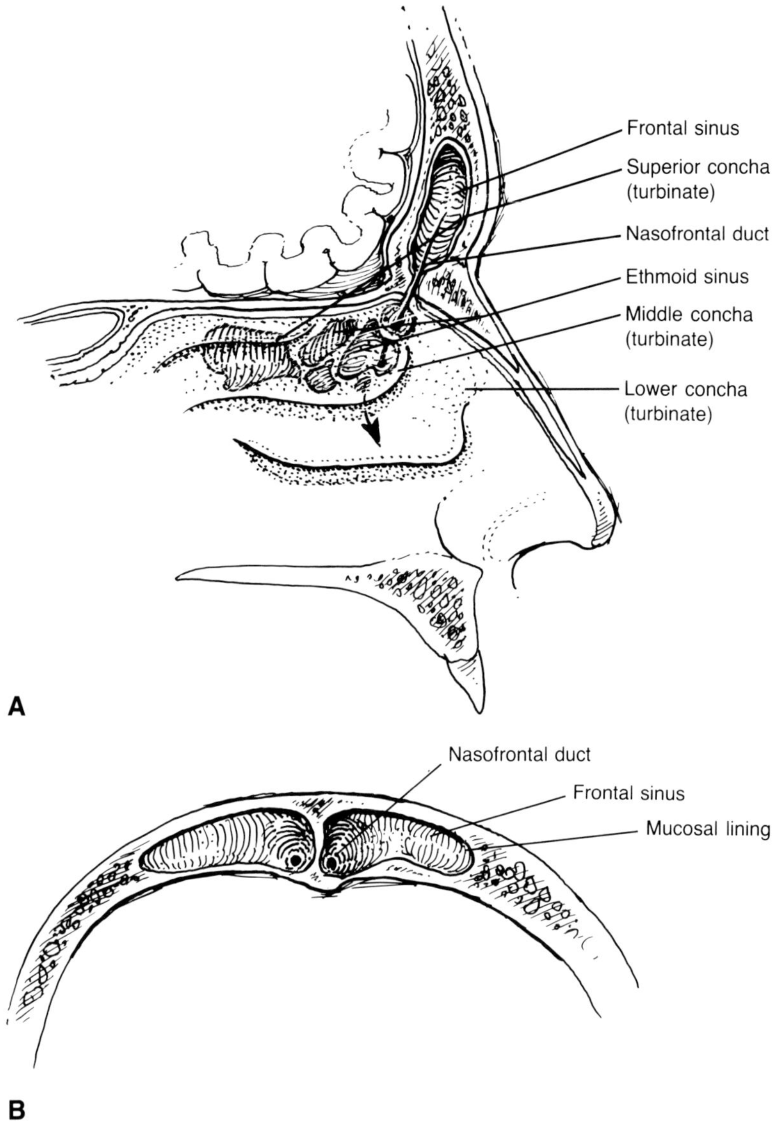

Figure 24–2. *(**A**) Lateral view of the normal nasofrontal duct. (**B**) Superior view of the normal nasofrontal duct.*

dictates the treatment of the frontal sinus in trauma (Fig. 24–2, A and B).

Adjacent Structures

The osseous structures that abut the frontal bone are the lacrimal and ethmoid inferiorly, the sphenoid inferiorly and posteriorly, the parietal posteriorly and superiorly, the zygoma laterally, the nasal bones anteriorly, and the maxilla anteriorly and inferiorly. The internal concave surface of the frontal bone forms the anterior cranial fossae that houses the brain. The floor the frontal bone outlines the roof of the orbit. The convex outer table is bound by the scalp and the frontalis, orbicularis, and procerus muscles. The ethmoid air cells and nasal apparatus are situated inferiorly. It is the damage to these adjacent structures that causes many of the complications associated with frontal bone fractures.

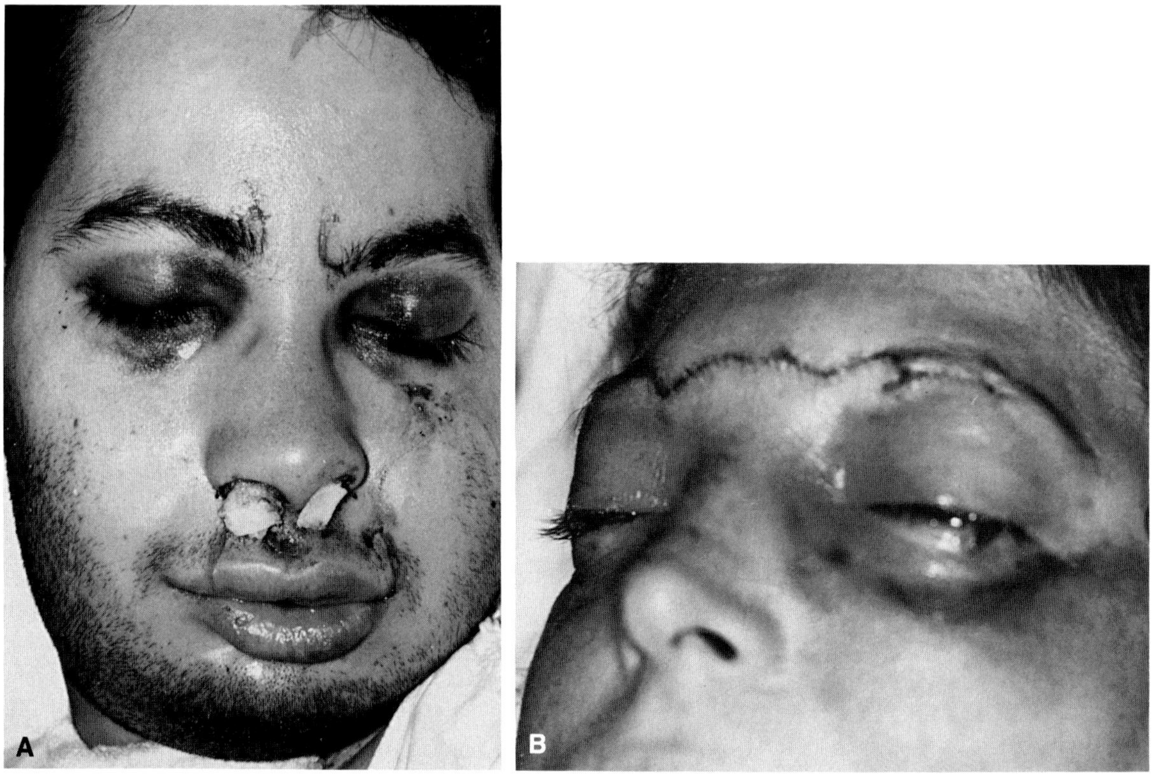

Figure 24–3. *(**A** and **B**) Typical appearance of patients with frontal sinus fractures. Note periorbital ecchymosis and lacerations.*

DIAGNOSIS

Clinical Findings

The most common finding associated with frontal bone fractures is periorbital ecchymosis (Fig. 24–3).[16-20] When the bone bleeds and periosteum is interrupted, blood leaks into the adjacent facial planes resulting in periorbital ecchymosis. Through this same mechanism, subconjunctival hemorrhage may be present. If the nose or zygoma are unaffected, subconjunctival hemorrhage is diagnostic for a frontal bone fracture.

Soft tissue lacerations in the region of the glabella and supraorbital rims are the second most common feature found (Fig. 24–3).[16-20] Depression of the bone with flatness and cosmetic deformity are noted if the patient is examined early. After the first hour and up to 5 days later, edema may be significant enough to hide the contour depression. Tenderness may be elicited over the fractured region and crepitation of underlying bony fragments will be found by palpation.[16-20] If the wound is compounded, bony fragments of the outer table and the presence of foreign bodies may be noted. If the impact was severe or penetrating, a cerebrospinal rhinorrhea may result. Interruption of the dura or cribriform plate causes a cerebrospinal fluid (CSF) leak.[16-20] A definitive diagnosis can be made by harvesting this fluid and comparing it with the patient's serum for glucose and chloride. If 0.1 cc can be harvested, a chloride concentration less than serum (95 mEq/L) and a glucose concentration higher than serum (120 mg/100 mL) confirms the presence of CSF.

If fragments of bone are depressed into the orbit, exophthalmos, proptosis, or ptosis may be noted. A depressed injury also causes restricted ocular movement if the superior rectus muscle, superior oblique muscle, or trochlear are damaged.[19-20] Interruption of the roof of the orbit may alter conduction along the supraorbital nerve. The skin over the forehead along the distribution of the supraorbital nerve may be anesthetic or paresthetic.

Imaging

After the patient is stabilized and a clinical examination is performed, radiographs may be obtained to confirm the clinical impression of fractures of the frontal bone or sinus.[21] A Waters' view is valuable in evaluating both middle third and upper third facial fractures. In this view, the orbits are well visualized and the frontal sinus is highlighted. Separation of the supraorbital rims and comminution of the frontal sinus may be noted (Fig. 24–4). The Caldwell, or reverse Townes, view is an ideal radiograph for localizing the frontal sinus but is not routine on most facial bone series and requires a specific request. The lateral radiograph of the face or skull includes the region of the glabella (Fig. 24–5). Depressed fractures of the anterior table in this region will be well visualized, but injury to the posterior table and nasofrontal duct are difficult to assess.

Laminar tomograms in the sagittal plane can help to identify the condition of both anterior and posterior tables (Fig. 24–6). In addition, the floor of the sinus and roof of the orbit may be examined. This modality is poor for examining the nasofrontal duct.

Although conventional plane radiographs may confirm a suspicion of frontal bone injury, computed tomography (CT) is unsurpassed in the evaluation of the frontal bone and frontal sinus injuries (Fig. 24–7).[22–24] The practitioner would be remiss in not using CT because treatment plans for specific injuries vary greatly and the need for neurosurgical consultation might be overlooked. Serial axial sections help to adequately identify anterior table fractures and displacement. They also reveal posterior wall injury, degree of dis-

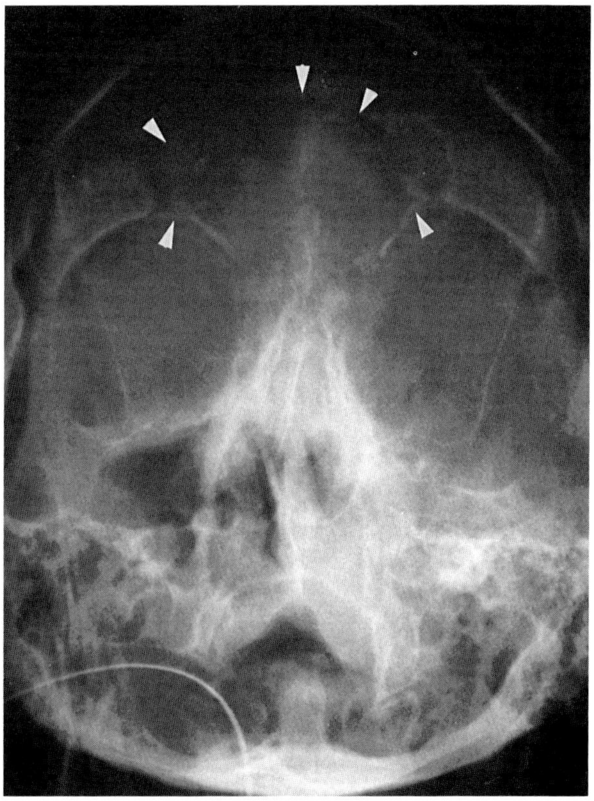

Figure 24–4. *Radiograph illustrating multiple fractures of the frontal sinus and medial supraorbital rim* (arrows).

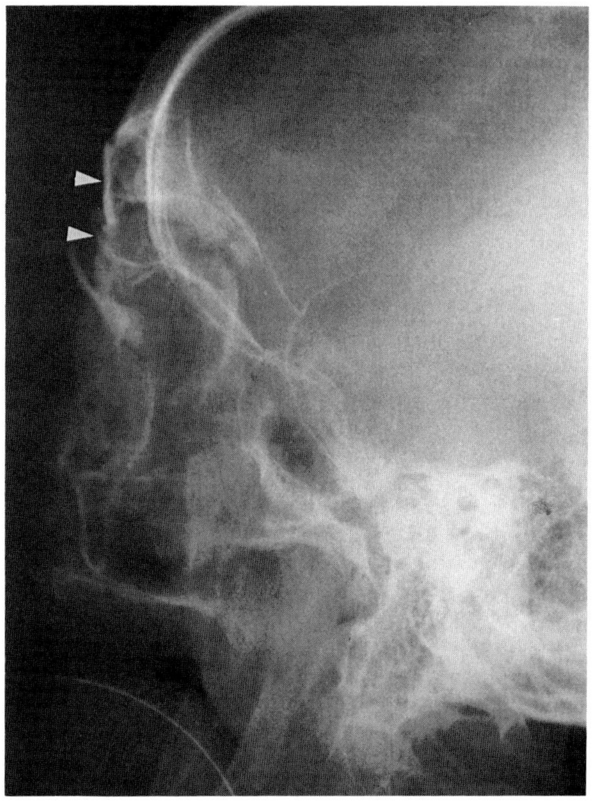

Figure 24–5. *Lateral radiograph illustrating displaced anterior wall of the frontal sinus* (arrows).

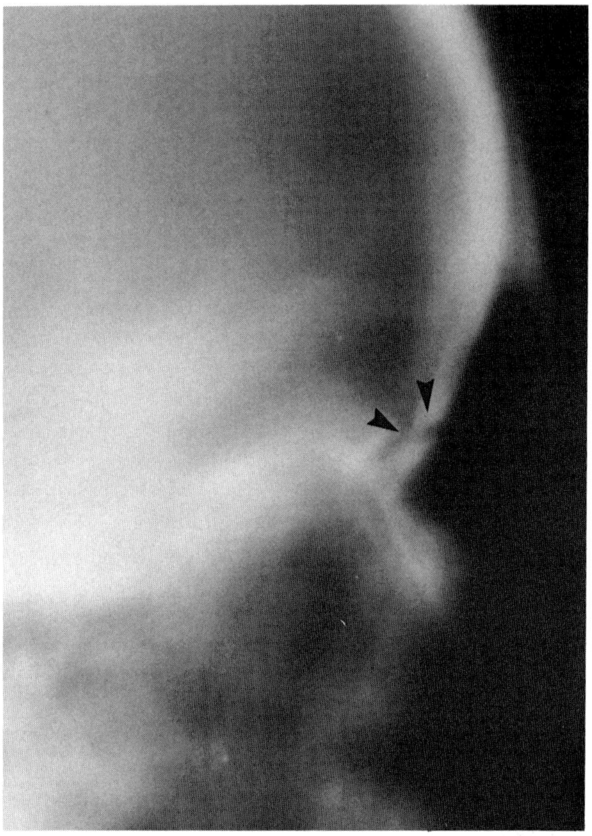

Figure 24–6. *Tomograph illustrating displaced posterior wall frontal sinus fracture (arrows).*

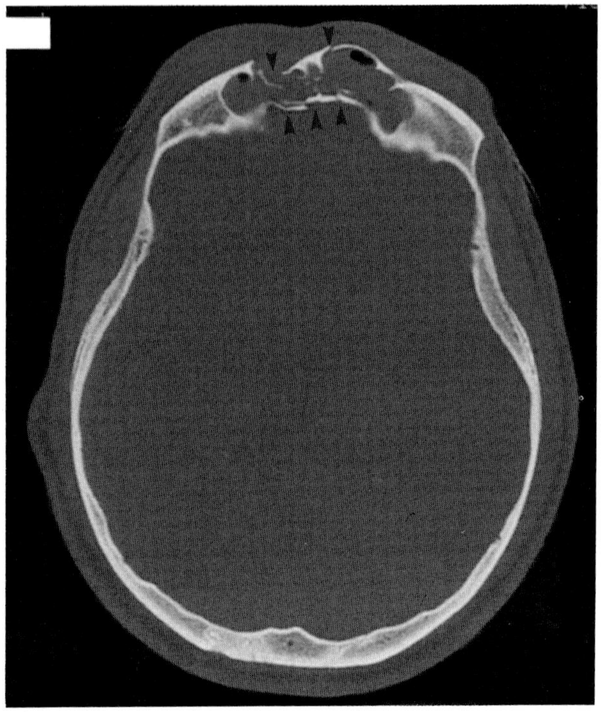

Figure 24–7. *Axial computed tomography (CT) identifying displaced anterior and posterior wall fractures (arrows).*

placement, and resultant intracranial damage. Coronal sections help to identify the displacement of the frontal bone into the orbit.[23] These sections also can disclose damage to the cribriform plate and adjacent ethmoid air cells. Only limited information can be obtained about the status of the nasofrontal duct. Noninvasive techniques fall short in evaluating this structure. If the floor of the sinus is interrupted, open exploration and examination are warranted.

Nasofrontal Duct Patency

Nasofrontal duct obstruction should be considered with medial supraorbital rim fractures, frontal bone fractures with nasoethmoidal components, and whenever there is a CSF leak.[25] It is these situations that mandate open evaluation.

The method of surgical access depends on the presence and type of concomitant injuries and their management. A bicoronal flap is indicated when a neurosurgical repair is required or when access to the zygomas and nasal bones are necessary (Fig. 24–8). An open-sky approach is useful in the repair of associated nasoethmoid injury.[26] The gull-wing incision permits access to the supraorbital rims, and to the frontal sinus. The butterfly incision has the advantage of providing access to the supraorbital rims, nasoethmoidal complex, and frontal sinus. The Sewall incision may be used for elevation of simple depressions. Existing lacerations may be modified to resemble any of these incisions for access. After gaining access through the anterior table of the sinus, the cavity is irrigated, suctioned, and visualized. The paired nasofrontal ducts on either side of the septum, along the posterior wall and lateral to the septum, are visualized (Fig. 24–2).[27–29]

Next, an 18-gauge $1\frac{1}{2}$-inch Teflon angiocatheter may be inserted into the duct to evaluate patency

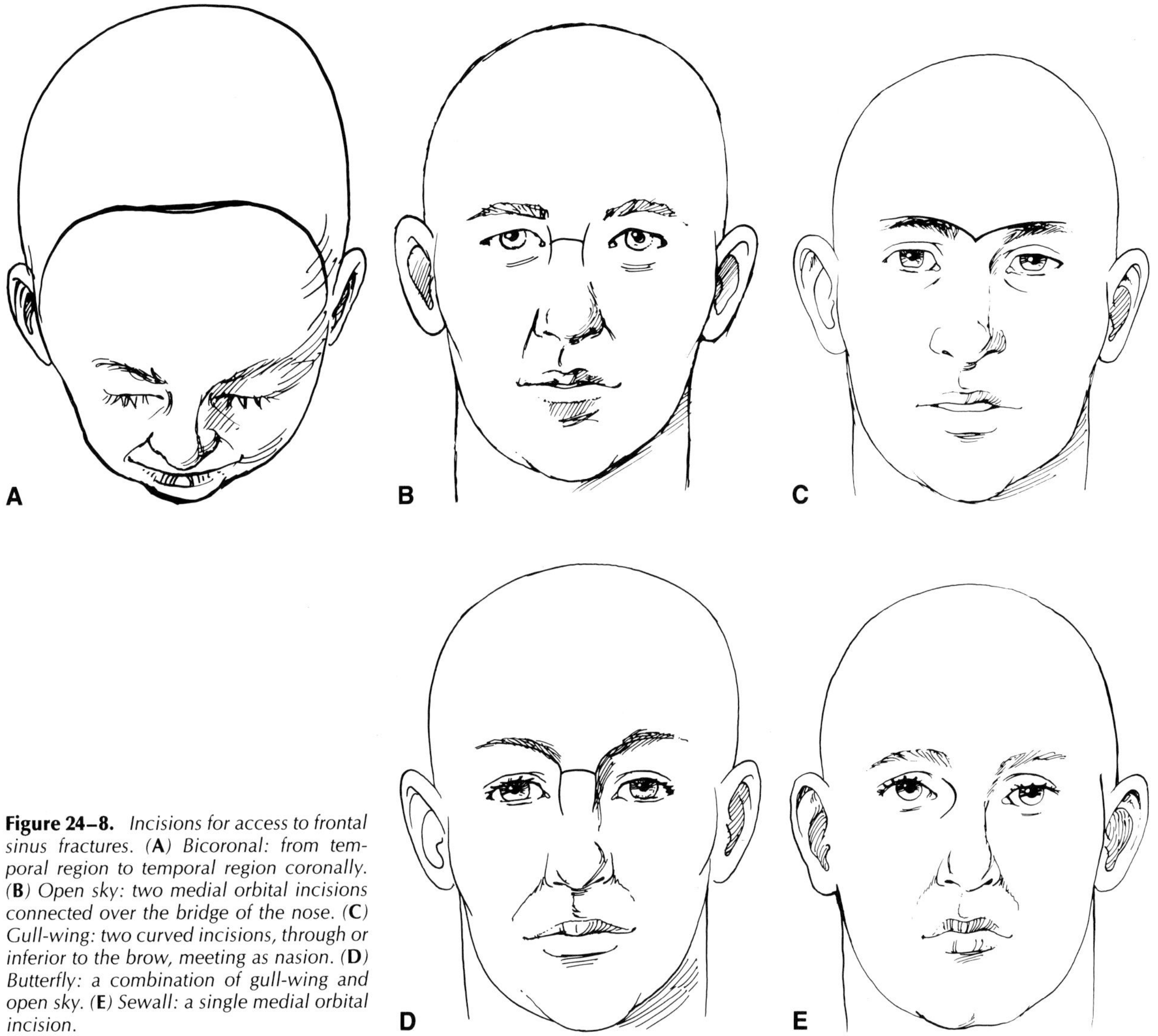

Figure 24–8. *Incisions for access to frontal sinus fractures. (**A**) Bicoronal: from temporal region to temporal region coronally. (**B**) Open sky: two medial orbital incisions connected over the bridge of the nose. (**C**) Gull-wing: two curved incisions, through or inferior to the brow, meeting as nasion. (**D**) Butterfly: a combination of gull-wing and open sky. (**E**) Sewall: a single medial orbital incision.*

(Fig. 24–9). Methylene blue may be introduced into the catheter and identification of the thin blue liquid under the medial turbinate is diagnostic of a patent duct.[27,29] This requires direct visualization through the nasal aperture with a nasal speculum. The drawback of methylene blue is that it soils the remainder of the anatomic field when mixed with blood. This makes further visualization of the anatomic structures difficult.

Lipiodol may be injected into the catheter and radiographic evidence of dye in the nose will verify patency of the duct.[29] Any interruption or deviation of the duct may be identified. The drawback of this method is that C-arm fluoroscopy is required in the operating room. If additional radiographs are required, spillage of the radiopaque dye will obstruct visualization.

Flourescein dye is another alternative that does

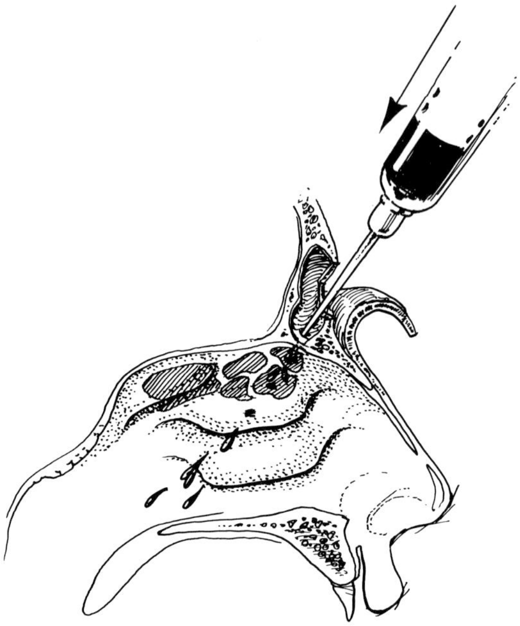

Figure 24–9. *Technique of identifying a patent nasofrontal duct. A Teflon catheter is placed into the remnants of the duct and dye is introduced. Free flow of droplets under the medial concha indicates patency.*

not have the drawbacks of the two previous methods. With the operating room lights dimmed, the dye is introduced. An ultraviolet light source will cause fluorescence and the patency can be verified. The fluorescein liquid is clear, water-soluble, and radiolucent.

TREATMENT

Displaced Frontal Bone Fractures

Simple frontal bone fractures that involve anterior and posterior tables require neurosurgical consultation. If the fracture is depressed or neurologic injury is suspected, this situation should be managed by the neurosurgeon.[30]

A significant degree of force is necessary to fracture the cranial vault, and neurologic injury may be caused by the concussion of the impact and not merely the displacement of the fractured segment. Linear nondisplaced fractures may be treated by observation alone. Even depressed fractures may remain unelevated and be treated with observation, if neurologic injury is not suspected. Complications of simple frontal bone fractures are most frequently caused by intracranial hemorrhage and contamination through overlying lacerations.[30]

Epidural hematoma is the most dramatic complication of nondepressed linear skull fractures. Depressed skull fractures may tear the dura, directly injure the brain with fragments, and cause focal cortical damage. Hemorrhage through venous sinuses and diploe and contamination from overlying lacerations are the principal concerns. Treatment consists of observation, CT imaging, repair of lacerations, control of intracranial hemorrhage when present, and antibiotic therapy.[30]

Supraorbital Rim Fracture

The supraorbital rim is the strongest portion of the frontal bone. Great impact is required to cause fracture and displacement. These fractures are most often compounded by overlying skin laceration or communication with the frontal sinus. If compounded, patients with these fractures should be placed on a narrow-spectrum antibiotic regimen directed at cutaneous and sinus contaminants. If these fractures are complicated by a sinus fracture, their treatment will be dictated by the management of the sinus.[1,3]

Simple nondisplaced fractures without sinus communication may be treated with observation alone. All displaced fractures should be treated by open reduction. Access may be obtained through any of the incisions illustrated in Figure 24-8 or by extension of existing lacerations to resemble these incisions. The simple supraorbital rim fracture may be elevated with a periosteal elevator, in a manner similar to a wedge or shoehorn. Frequently, the bones will snap into place. If the bone segments do not remain in place, the overlying periosteum may be sutured together to stabilize them. If displacement persists, direct stabilization of the segments with thin-gauge stainless steel wire or with low-profile bone plates is adequate. The soft tissues may then be closed.[1,3] Postoperative radiographs should be obtained to confirm reduction.

Anterior Table Fracture

The thinnest area of the frontal bone is in the region of the glabella, and thus the anterior wall of the frontal sinus is highly susceptible to fracture. Simple greenstick or nondisplaced anterior wall fractures require no operative treatment.[31] Antibiotic therapy in conjunction with systemic decongestants aid in the prevention of sinusitis. Soft tissue injuries may be addressed. A sinus series of radiographs may be taken at 1 week and 6 months after trauma to identify post-traumatic mucocele.

Displaced anterior table fractures require open reduction. Perioperative parenteral antibiotics and systemic decongestants should be administered.[31–34] Lacerations may be used for surgical access or extended to resemble the incisions in Fig. 24–8 (Figs. 24–10 and 24–11). An attempt should be made not to strip the periosteum from the outer table.[35] Free segments should be salvaged and identified. Even if contaminated, segments of bone may be cleansed and used for reconstruction as free grafts.[36] The sinus should be irrigated, suctioned dry, and inspected. Special attention should be given to the sinus floor and patency of the nasofrontal duct. The posterior wall should be inspected for previously undetected fracture. If the posterior wall and floor are free of injury, the pieces of the anterior wall may be replaced. Fixation by suturing of the periosteum may be adequate. If not, thin-gauge stainless steel wire or low-profile bone plates will be adequate.[35–37] Frequently, voids in the anterior wall are encountered after reconstruction. This may be addressed by an onlay bone graft, silastic patch, or room temperature curing methyl methacrylate

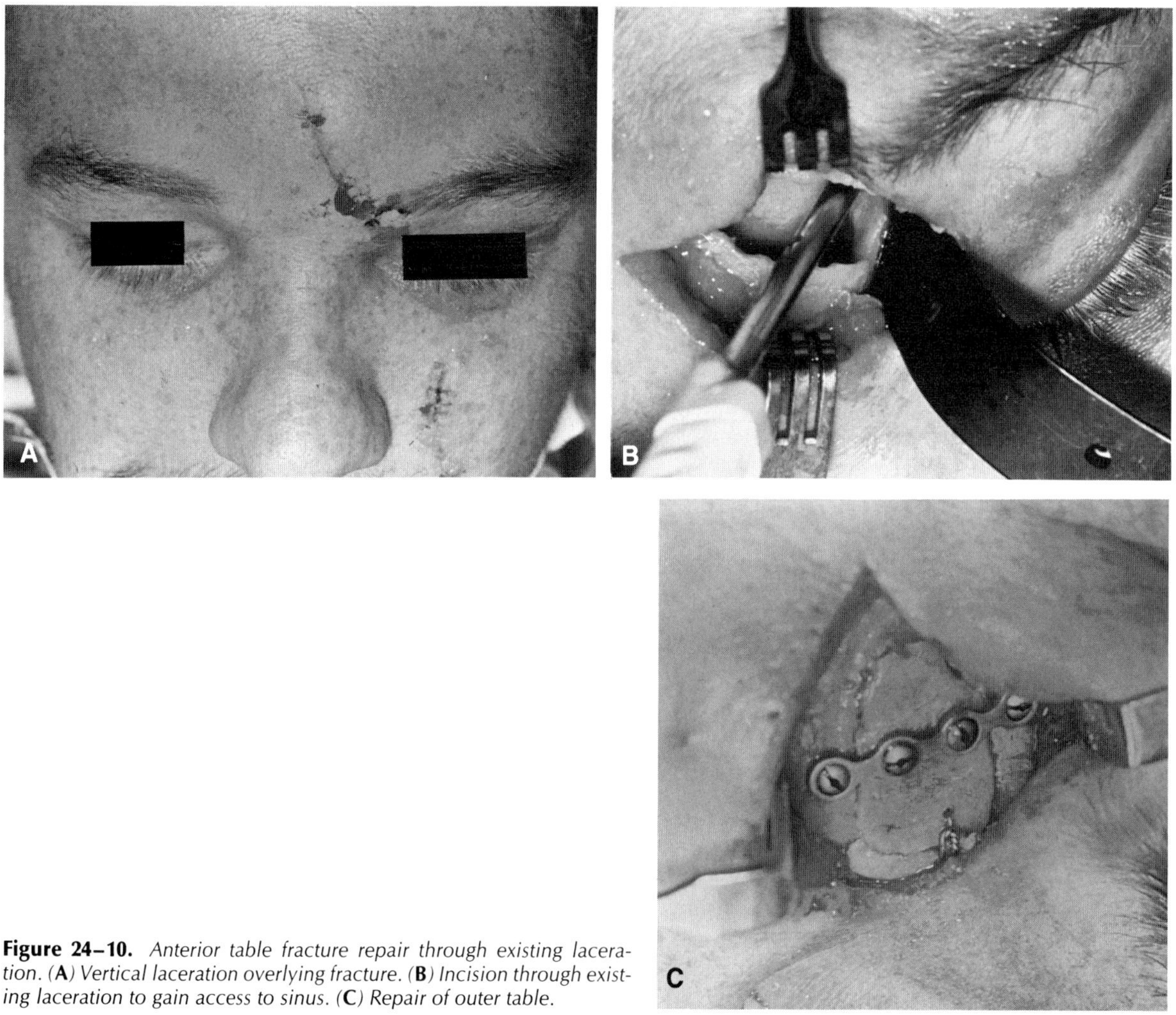

Figure 24–10. *Anterior table fracture repair through existing laceration. (**A**) Vertical laceration overlying fracture. (**B**) Incision through existing laceration to gain access to sinus. (**C**) Repair of outer table.*

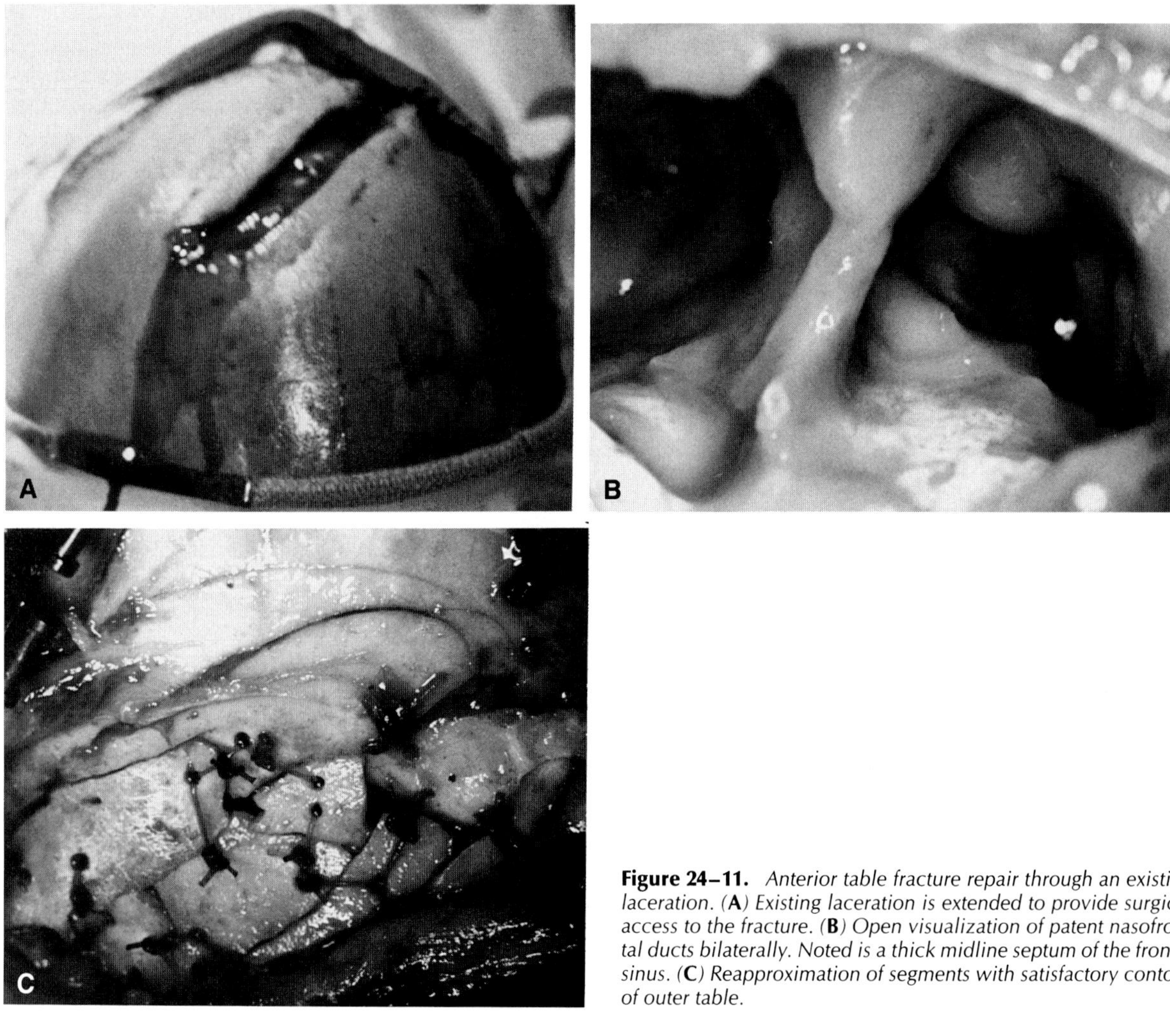

Figure 24–11. *Anterior table fracture repair through an existing laceration. (**A**) Existing laceration is extended to provide surgical access to the fracture. (**B**) Open visualization of patent nasofrontal ducts bilaterally. Noted is a thick midline septum of the frontal sinus. (**C**) Reapproximation of segments with satisfactory contour of outer table.*

(cranioplast). The soft tissue injuries may then be repaired.

Sinus Floor Injury

Fractures of the nasoethmoid complex, supraorbital rim, and frontal sinus floor can all interrupt the patency of the nasofrontal duct. Although displacement of the frontal bone into the orbit or anterior cranial fossae may produce devastating neurologic injury, it is damage to the nasofrontal duct that causes the most frequent and the broadest range of complications. It is the condition of the nasofrontal duct that essentially dictates treatment beyond osseous repair.[25,38,39]

Systemic decongestants and intravenous antibiotics are indicated in frontal sinus floor injury. The Sewall, open-sky, butterfly, and gull-wing incisions, or existing lacerations may provide an approach for exploration and inspection of the sinus floor. After reflection of the soft tissue flap and removal of bone, the floor should be inspected and the nasofrontal duct examined for patency. If the floor is grossly comminuted without hope of reconstruction, the duct should be obstructed and the sinus obliterated.

Great variability exists in the path of the nasofrontal duct. It may empty as an orifice into a labyrinth of ethmoid air cells or by a tortuous duct into the middle meatus. Cannulization is difficult but possible. Historically, cannulization of the existing duct or creation

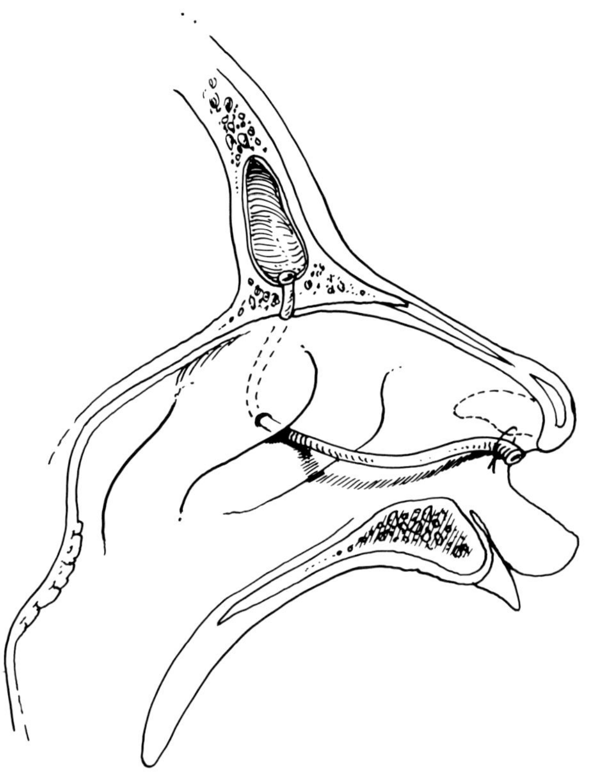

Figure 24–12. *Creation of new nasofrontal duct with a No. 16 silastic tube.*

of a new duct has been performed with silastic, tantalum, plastic, and gold tubes that can remain in place for 7 to 10 days.[40]

The simplest method of treatment is creation of a new duct. After reflection of the osteoplastic flap, the obstructed nasofrontal duct is identified. A trephine is then placed into the obstructed duct until it enters the ethmoid air cells or middle meatus. A No. 16 to No. 24 silastic or polyethylene tube is placed from the base of the frontal sinus into the nose. A pull-out suture is placed through the tube and attached to the alar rim for removal 7 to 10 days later (Fig. 24–12).[40]

Serial radiographs are taken 1 week after surgery and then every 6 months to identify postoperative complications.

Posterior Table Fracture

It is the posterior table sinus fracture that has the most devastating consequences because of its proximity to the anterior cranial fossae. Treatment is directed at management of the initial damage and prevention of infection.[41] There are three subclassifications of posterior sinus wall fractures: nondisplaced, displaced, and displaced with gross neurologic injury (Table 24–1). Each of the subclassifications will invariably have an associated anterior wall penetration. Each is treated differently, and each requires neurosurgical consultation or joint neurosurgical-oral and maxillofacial surgical management.

Because of the high probability of neurosurgical intervention, access to the posterior wall fracture should be obtained through bicoronal incisions (Fig. 24–8).[33,34] Intravenous antibiotics should be administered before surgery and for 1 week after surgery.

A bicoronal flap should be considered even when treating the simple nondisplaced posterior sinus fracture. The anterior table should be removed for visual access and the pieces identified by number and shape on a map. These segments may be stored in normal saline-soaked gauze. The sinus is then irrigated and suctioned dry, and the posterior wall may be inspected for the extent of injury. Displacement of the fracture, CSF leak, entrapment of sinus membranes, and dural tears should be identified. If no significant injury exists and the nasofrontal duct is patent, the anterior table may be replaced and fixed and the soft tissue injuries repaired. A sinus series of radiographs should be taken 1 week after surgery and every 6

Table 24–1. *Classification of Frontal Bone Fractures*

- Linear frontal bone fractures
  - Nondisplaced
  - Displaced
- Supraorbital rim fractures
  - Nondisplaced
  - Displaced
  - Displaced involving frontal sinus or nasoethmoid complex
- Frontal sinus fractures
  - Anterior wall
    - Nondisplaced
    - Displaced
  - Posterior wall
    - Nondisplaced
    - Displaced
    - Displaced with gross neurologic injury
  - Floor of sinus fracture
    - Patent nasofrontal duct
    - Compromised nasofrontal duct

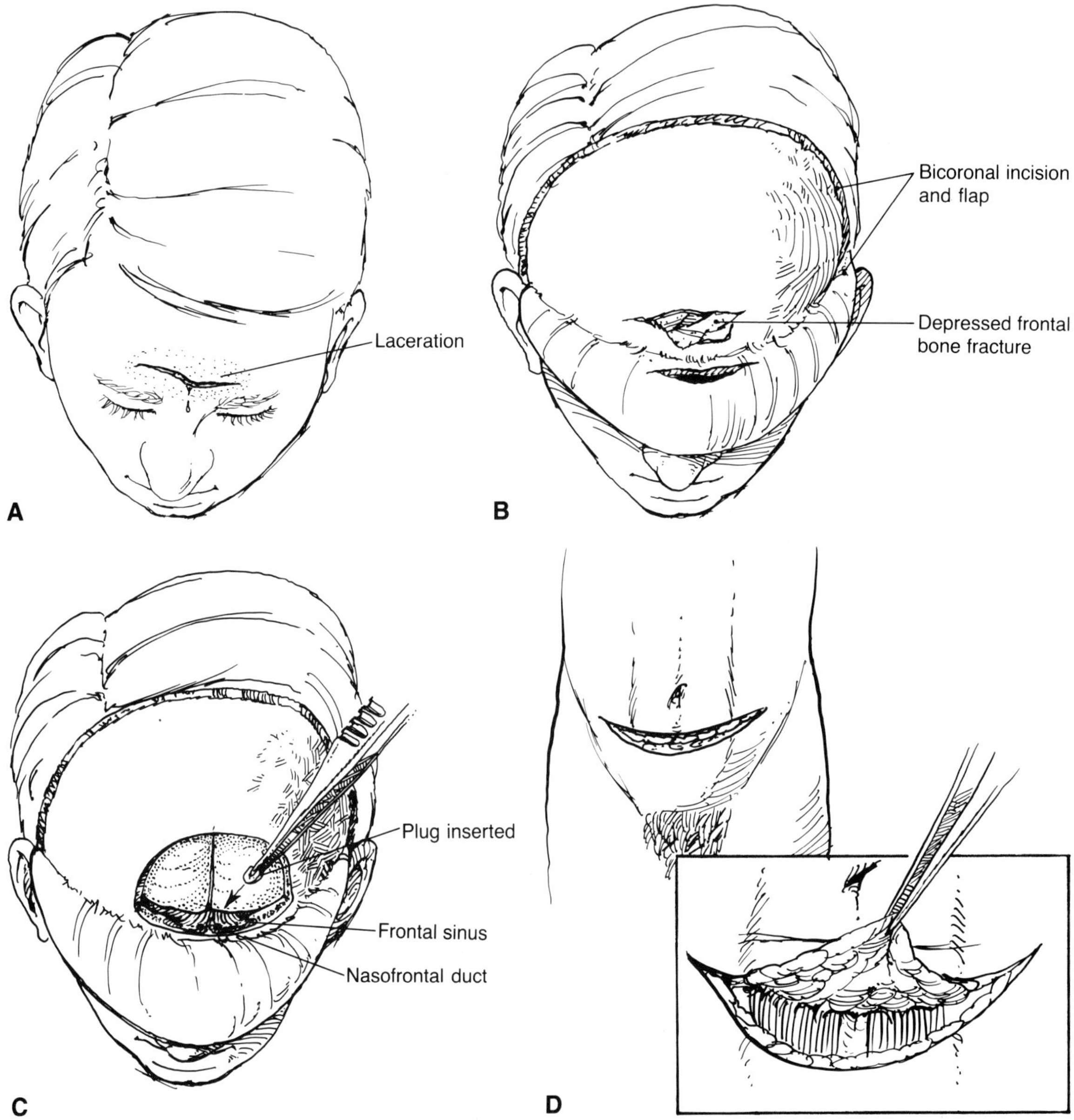

Figure 24–13. *Sinus obliteration. (**A**) Patient before surgical procedures. (**B**) Bicoronal flap reflection exposing fracture. (**C**) Obliteration of nasofrontal duct. (**D**) Harvest of free fat from abdominal wall. (**E**) Obliteration of sinus with fat. (**F**) Repair of anterior wall.*

months for 5 years to identify postoperative sinusitis, mucocele, and pyocele.

The displaced posterior table fracture requires neurosurgical management or joint oral and maxillofacial and neurosurgical treatment. Because of the potential need for a craniotomy, a bicoronal flap should be reflected (Fig. 24–13 B). The anterior wall should be removed, identified by number and shape, recorded on a map, and stored in normal saline-soaked gauze. The posterior wall then is examined, and the dura inspected for lacerations. Most lacerations are linear and may be sutured to obtain a watertight seal. The fracture may be reduced or the displaced segment removed.

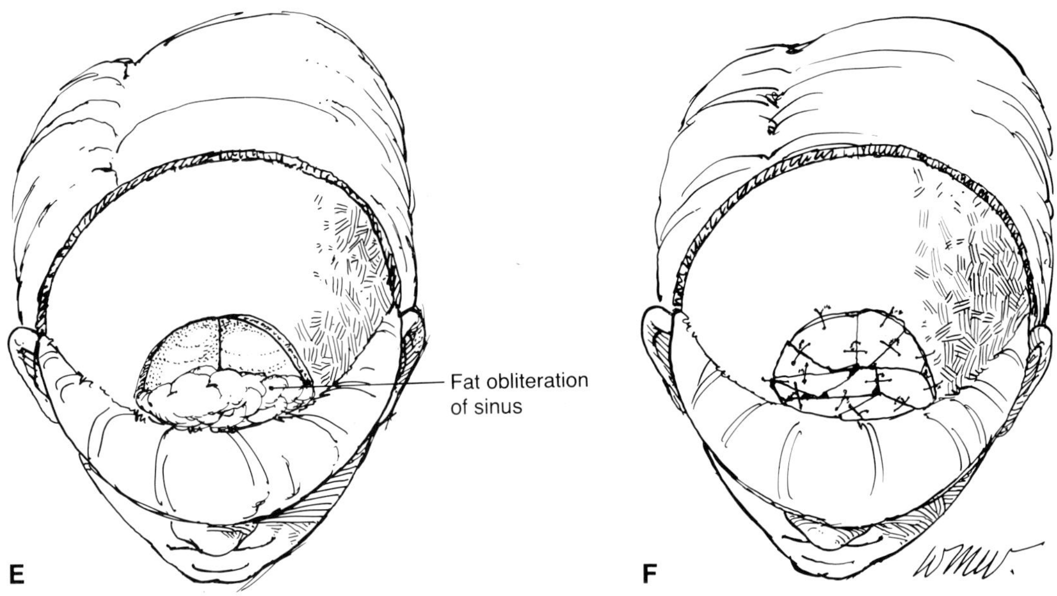

Figure 24–13. *(continued)*

Therapy is next directed at prevention of infection by obliteration of the sinus. Historically, a multiplicity of materials have been used, including glass wool, Teflon, bone, cartilage, muscle, gelfoam, Surgicel, acrylic, and fat.[41–48]

Fat may be harvested by liposuction or as a free graft.[48] A free graft is best obtained at the abdominal wall (Fig. 24–13 D). The skin is prepared with an antiseptic cleansing agent, an incision is made through the skin of the anterior abdominal wall inferior to the umbilicus and an adequate volume of fat is harvested.

Strict attention must be given to meticulous removal of all of the mucosal elements from the walls, cul de sacs, septae, and fragments.[38,43–45] Failure to remove such elements may result in mucoceles or pyoceles. The mucosa is then reflected down into the nasofrontal duct and the orifice is obstructed by local bone or muscle (Fig. 24–13 C). The harvested fat is then placed into the sinus and packed until full (Fig. 24–13 E). The outer table is then reassembled and restored as in the simple anterior wall fracture (Fig. 24–13 F). Serial radiographs are taken to identify sinusitis and mucocele or pyocele, which may develop many years later.

The most serious of the frontal sinus injuries is a penetrating injury through the posterior wall. This type of injury should be managed by a neurosurgeon with oral and maxillofacial surgical assistance. The treatment of choice is cranialization. The classic cranialization procedure requires removal of posterior and anterior tables to provide sinus decompression for subsequent expansion of the swollen brain and elimination of potential sources of infection.

The sinus is exposed in the usual fashion, the posterior wall inspected, and loose fragments excised (Fig. 24–14 A). All sinus membrane is removed. The entire posterior table and all irregularities of the sinus are smoothed with an acrylic bur (Fig. 24–14 B). The mucosa of the nasofrontal duct is inverted into the duct, and temporalis muscle is used to occlude it. Necrotic brain is excised, and the dura is repaired with fascia lata, dermis, or by direct suture (Fig. 24–14 C). The anterior table is then reconstructed (Fig. 24–14 D). Decompression of the sinus allows for swelling of the brain. Hard tissue protection of the brain is provided by the anterior table. There is no compromise in contour.[6]

COMPLICATIONS

Complications of frontal bone injury vary in severity and may occur many years after the incident. The major types of complication are those that occur directly at the time of injury, those of an infectious nature, and chronic problems.

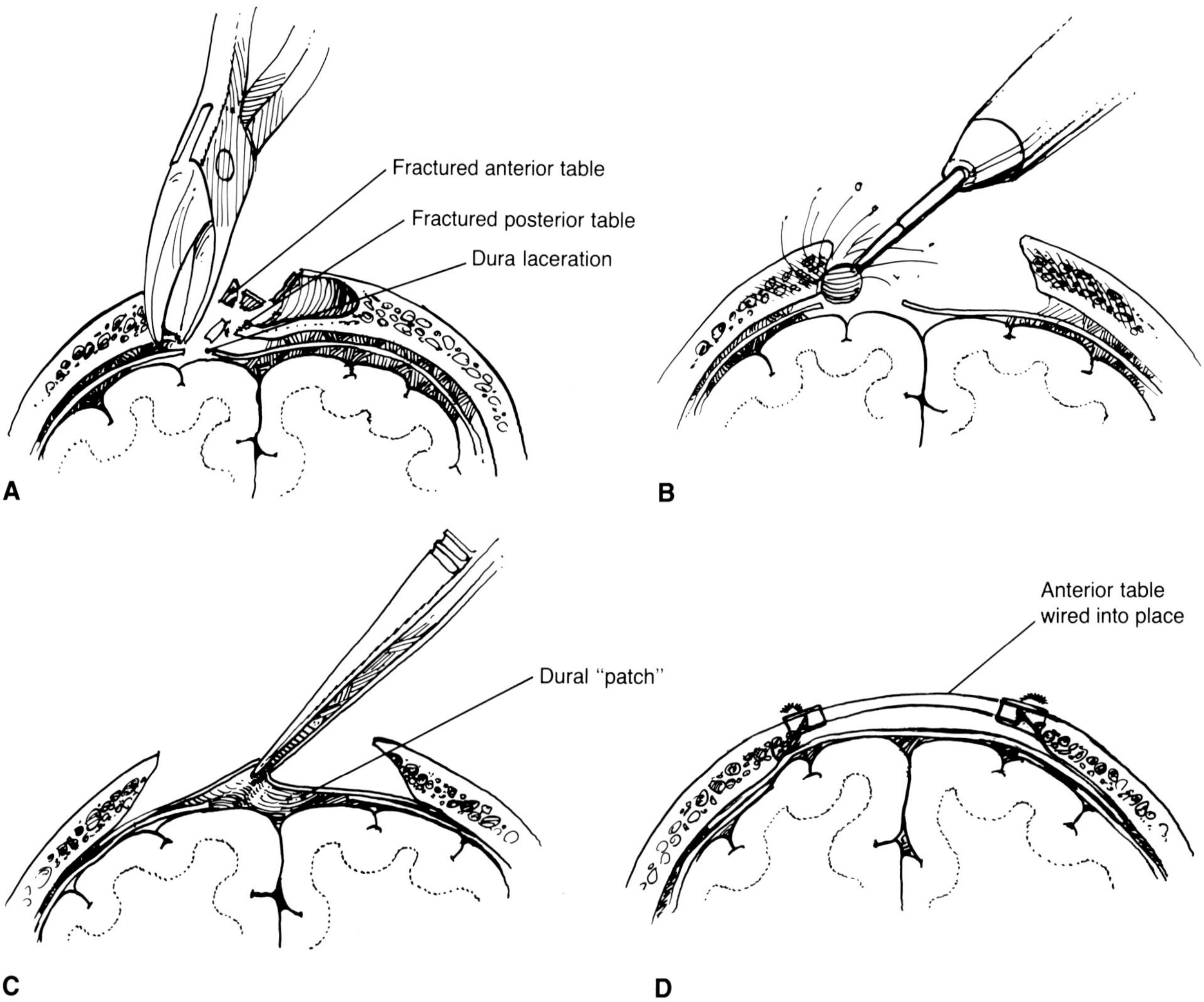

Figure 24–14. *Cranialization procedure. (***A***) Removal of posterior table. (***B***) Recontouring of irregularities. (***C***) Repair of dura. (***D***) Reconstruction of outer table.*

The most devastating complications are neurologic problems resulting from displacement or penetration of the frontal bone.[49] These injuries range from death to concussion. Displacement of the floor of the frontal bone can cause orbital damage. The most frequent ocular complication is diplopia. Damage to the superior rectus and superior oblique muscles or trochlea results in a limited range of motion. Severance of the supraorbital nerve by the injury or during reflection of the osteoplastic flap leaves a permanent anesthesia over the distribution of the forehead.[50] Trauma of the floor of the frontal sinus or displacement of the medial supraorbital rim may cause a CSF leak. Generally, reduction of the fractures corrects this problem. If persistent, neurosurgical repair is indicated.

Infectious complications most frequently arise from occlusion of the nasofrontal duct or contamination by penetrating foreign bodies. The most frequently encountered infection is meningitis,[47] and it usually occurs secondary to penetration and contamination. With occlusion of the nasofrontal duct and accumulation of blood in the sinus,[51–53] an environment is created that is conducive to anaerobic bacterial growth. Frontal sinus abscesses spread by direct extension through small fractures of the frontal bone or through transosseous anastomotic vessels. The result is brain

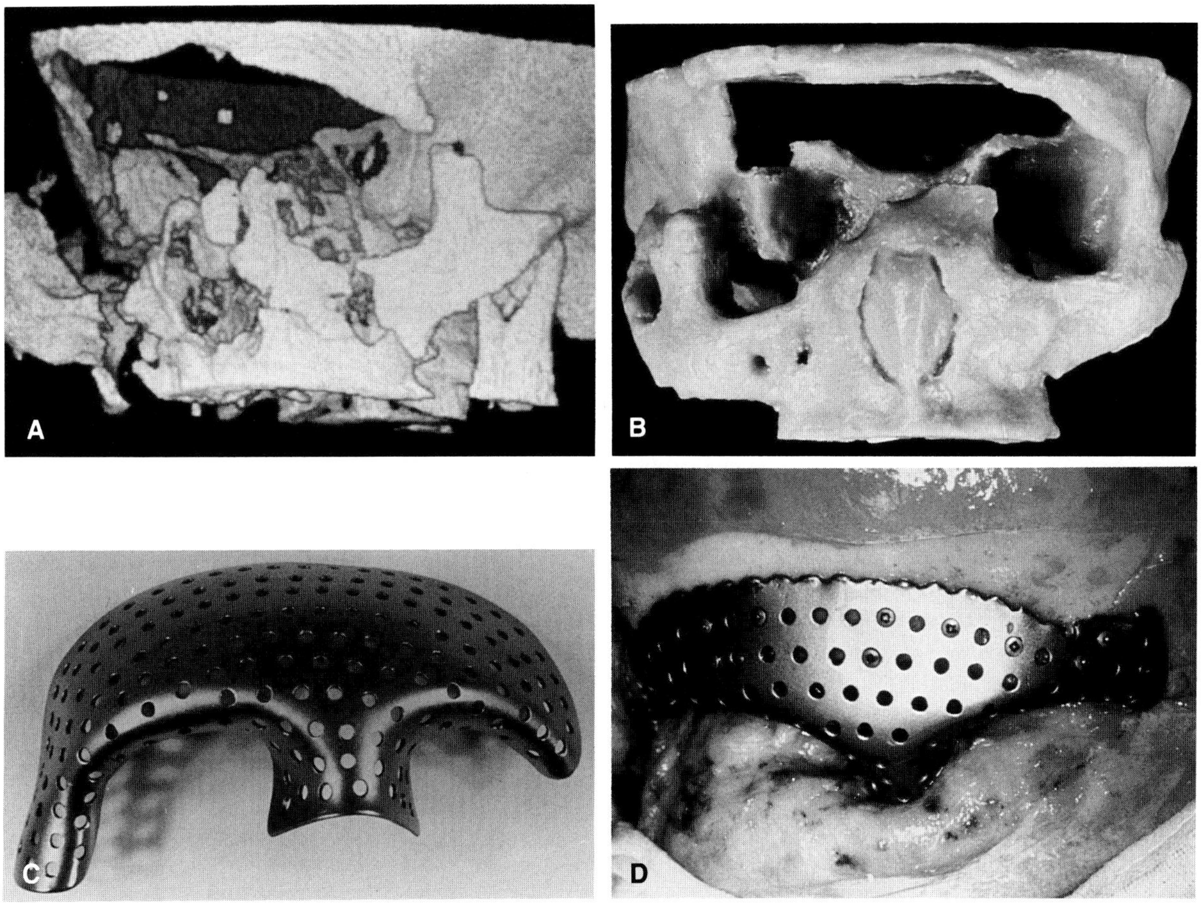

Figure 24–15. *CAD-CAM one-stage reconstruction. (**A**) Three-dimensional computed tomograph. (**B**) Model fabricated from image. (**C**) Prosthesis fabricated from model. (**D**) Prosthesis inserted.*

abscess, meningitis, cavernous sinus thrombosis, and (if long-term) osteomyelitis.

Mucoceles are the most common chronic problems.[39,54–56] Respiratory mucosa trapped between fracture segments or left behind during obliteration procedures may continue to grow. This continued growth may form mucoceles or pyoceles. The size of the growth will determine how much damage occurs to adjacent bone and neurologic tissue. For this reason, long-term serial sinus radiographs are taken after surgery. Mucoceles and pyoceles may develop up to 15 years later.

Chronic pain and headache may be persistent without identifiable cause.[53] Cosmetic deformity consisting of contour deficits and irregularities stem from multiple causes. Bone lost at the time of injury may not be noticed for months. Osteomyelitis with subsequent debridement leaves voids in bone. Even if properly treated at the time of injury, remodeling may leave irregularities.

CORRECTION OF POSTTRAUMATIC DEFORMITY

At 6 months to 1 year after the initial surgical correction, secondary deformities of the frontal bone may be addressed. Contour defects result from failure to fully elevate depressed fractures, from voids in bone lost at the time of the trauma, and from infection. A multiplicity of materials have been used to correct contour defects. These include bone from adjacent calvarium, ilium, or rib, cartilage, titanium, stainless steel, silastic, methyl methacrylate, hydroxyapatite granules, silver, Vitallium, Teflon, Dacron, nylon, polyethylene, and aluminum.[57,58]

The procedures for correcting such defects involve one-stage indirect prosthetic techniques, two-stage techniques, single-stage direct techniques, or computer-generated single-stage techniques.[59–61]

The one-stage indirect technique requires that an impression be taken of the defect through the skin. The impression negative is then filled with plaster to form a positive image on which an onlay prosthesis may be fabricated. Acrylic, polyethylene, tantalum, titanium, and cobalt chromium prostheses may be fabricated with this technique. A full-thickness flap is then reflected and the prosthesis secured.

The two-stage technique requires that a full-thickness flap be reflected initially. An impression is then taken directly of the defect. The wound is closed and laboratory procedures and materials are used as in the direct technique. Another full-thickness flap is reflected and the prosthesis is inserted. Although this procedure requires a second operation, the fit of the prosthesis is more intimate.

The single-stage direct technique requires that a full-thickness flap be reflected beyond the margins of the defect. Onlay cartilage or bone grafts then may be secured if an autograft is desired. Otherwise, an acrylic resin may be used. The bone is moistened and acrylic is mixed and placed on a glass or Teflon slab and rolled to a uniform thickness. It is placed directly over the bone and covered with a sheet of separating foil. The full-thickness flap is replaced to ensure proper contour and again reflected. Copious amounts of irrigation are then used to keep the material from causing thermal damage to the skull. The flap is then replaced and sutured.

Improvements in computer design and technology have now enabled the fabrication of prostheses for one-stage reconstructions. A two-dimensional CT scan is taken of the patient before surgery.[61] A computer-aided design—computer-aided manufacturer (CAD–CAM) then is used to create a model of the frontal bone and defect. A prosthesis may be created from silastic, acrylic, vitalium, or hydroxyapatite-coated metals (Fig. 24–15). At surgery, the prosthesis is inserted as described for the other single-stage techniques.

REFERENCES

1. Schultz RC. Supraorbital glabellar fractures. Plast Reconstr Surg 1970; 45:227–233.
2. Onishi K, Nakajima T, Yoshimura Y. Treatment and therapeutic devices in the management of frontal sinus fractures. J Craniomaxillofac Surg 1989; 17:58–63.
3. Schultz RC. Frontal sinus and supraorbital fractures from vehicle accidents. Clin Plast Surg 1975; 2:93–106.
4. McHugh HE. Treatment of fractures of the frontal and ethmoid sinuses. Laryngoscope 1958; 68:1616–1640.
5. May M, Ogura JH, Schramm V. Nasofrontal duct in frontal sinus fractures. Arch Otolaryngol 1970; 92:534–538.
6. Donald PJ. Frontal sinus ablation by cranialization. Arch Otolaryngol 1982; 108:142–146.
7. Whited RE. Anterior table frontal sinus fractures. Laryngoscope 1979; 89:1951–1955.
8. Salentijn LM. Anatomy and embryology. In: Blitzer A, Lawson W, Friedman W, eds. Surgery of the paranasal sinuses. Philadelphia: WB Saunders, 1985; 5, 15–19.
9. Enlow D. The facial growth process. In: Enlow D, ed. Handbook of facial growth, ed 2. Philadelphia: WB Saunders, 1982; 152.
10. Goodale RL. The rationale for frontal sinus surgery. Laryngoscope 1965; 75:981–987.
11. Brown WAB, Molleson TI. Enlargement of the frontal sinus. Ann Human Biol 1984; 11:221–226.
12. Williams P, Warwick R. The paranasal sinuses. In: Williams P, Warwick R, eds. Gray's anatomy, ed 36. Philadelphia: WB Saunders, 1980; 332–334, 1148–1149.
13. Urken ML, Som PM, Lawson W, et al. The abnormally large frontal sinus. I. A practical method for its determination based upon an analysis of 100 normal patients. Laryngoscope 1987; 97:602–605.
14. Tos M, Mogensen C, Novotny Z. Quantitative histologic features of the normal frontal sinus. Arch Otolaryngol 1980; 106:143–148.
15. Dolezal RF, Baker SR. Mucociliary flow in the canine frontal sinus. Ann Otolaryngol Rhinol Laryngol 1983; 92:78–80.
16. Holt GR. Ethmoid and frontal sinus fractures. Ear Nose Throat J 1983; 62:33–42.
17. Sataloff RT, Sariego J, Meyers DL, et al. Surgical management of the frontal sinus. Neurosurgery 1984; 15:593–596.
18. Lanigan DT, Stoelinga DJ. Fractures of supraorbital rim. J Oral Surg 1980; 38:764–770.
19. Miller, SH, Lung RJ, Davis TS, et al. Management of fractures of the supraorbital rim. J Trauma 1978; 18:507–512.
20. Rowe NL, Kiley HC. The surgical anatomy, diagnosis, and treatment of fractures of the nasal region, frontal sinus and paranasal air sinus. In: Rowe NL, Kiley HC, eds. Fractures of the facial skeleton, ed 2. Baltimore: Williams & Wilkins Co., 1970.
21. Newman MH, Travis LW. Frontal sinus fractures. Laryngoscope 1973; 83:1281–1292.
22. Schatz CJ, Becker TS. Normal CT anatomy of the paranasal sinuses. Radiol Clin North Am 1984; 22:107–118.
23. Noyek AM, Kassel EE. Computed tomography in frontal sinus fractures. Arch Otolaryngol 1982; 108:378–379.

24. Kassel EE, Noyek AM, Cooper PW. CT in facial trauma. J Otolaryngol 1983; 12:2–15.
25. Stanley RB, Becker TS. Injuries of the nasofrontal orifices in frontal sinus fractures. Laryngoscope 1987; 97:728–231.
26. Converse JM, Hogan UM. Opensky approach for reduction of naso-orbital fractures. Plast Reconstr Surg 1970; 46:396–398.
27. Hybels RL. Posterior table fractures of the frontal sinus. II. Clinical aspects. Laryngoscope 1977; 87:1740–1745.
28. Work WP. Trauma to frontal sinuses. Arch Otolaryngol 1954; 59:54–64.
29. Pollak K, Payne EE. Fractures of the frontal sinus. Otolaryngol Clin North Am 1976; 9:517–522.
30. Becker DP, Miller JD, Young HF, et al. Diagnosis and treatment of head injury in adults. In: Youmans JR, ed. Neurological surgery. Philadelphia: WB Saunders Co. 1982; 1904–1907.
31. Levine SB, Rowe LP, Keane WM, et al. Evaluation and treatment of frontal sinus fractures. Otolaryngol Head Neck Surg 1986; 95:19–22.
32. Nichols RD, Ford CN, Szymanoski. Systematic evaluation and management of fractures of the frontal sinus. Trans Am Acad Ophth Otol 1973; 77:ORL 429–ORL433.
33. Denneny JC, Davidson WD. Combined otolaryngological and neurosurgical approach in treating sinus fractures. Laryngoscope 1987; 97:633–637.
34. Peri G, Chabannes J, Menes R, et al. Fractures of the frontal sinus. J Oral Maxillofac Surg 1981; 9:73–80.
35. McGrath MH, Smith CJ. A simple method to maintain reduction of unstable fractures of the frontal sinus. Plast Reconstr Surg 1988; 68:948–949.
36. Nadell J, Kline DG. Primary reconstruction of depressed frontal skull fractures including those involving the sinus orbit and cribiform plate. J Neurosurg 1974; 41:200–207.
37. Nichols RD. Treatment of frontal sinus fractures. In: Mathog RH. Maxillofacial trauma. Baltimore: Williams & Wilkins, 1984; 288–296.
38. Hybels RL, Newman MH. Posterior table fracture of the frontal sinus. I. An experimental study. Laryngoscope 1976; 86:171–179.
39. Schenk NL, Rauchback E, Ogura JH. Frontal sinus disease. II. Development of the frontal sinus model: Occlusion of the nasofrontal duct. Laryngoscope 1974; 84:1233–1247.
40. Porto DD, Duvall AJ. Long term results with nasofrontal duct reconstruction. Laryngoscope 1986; 96: 858–862.
41. Larabee WF, Travis LW, Tobb HG. Frontal sinus fracture: Their suppurative complications and surgical management. Laryngoscope 1980; 90:1810–1813.
42. Failla A. Operative management of injuries involving the frontal sinus. Laryngoscope 1968; 78:1833–1852.
43. Dickinson JT, Capic JA, Kameron DB. Principles of frontal reconstruction. Laryngoscope 1969; 79:1019–1075.
44. Valenzela C. Treatment of traumatic disease of the frontal sinus by adipose implant obliteration. Laryngoscope 1967; 77:1695–1705.
45. Goodale RL, Montgomery WW. Technical advances in osteoplastic frontal sinusectomy. Arch Otolaryngol 1964; 79:522–529.
46. Goodale RL, Montgomery WW. Experiences with osteoplastic anterior wall approach to the frontal sinus. Arch Otolaryngol 1958; 60:271–283.
47. Sessions RB, Alford BR, Stratton C, et al. Current concepts of frontal sinus surgery: An appraisal of the osteoplastic flap-fat obliteration operation. Laryngoscope 1972; 82:918–930.
48. Denneny JC. Frontal sinus obliteration using liposuction. Otolaryngol Head Neck Surg 1986; 95:15–18.
49. Treachnor FR. Intracranial complications of fractures of skull involving frontal sinus. JAMA 1927; 88:987–989.
50. Lindorf HH. A contribution on revisional and drainage of the frontal sinus by osteoplastic operation. J Maxillofac Surg 1986; 14:34–39.
51. Schenck NL, Tomlinson MJ. Frontal sinus trauma: Experimental reconstruction with proplast. Laryngoscope 1977; 87:398–407.
52. Ogura JH, Watson RK, Jurema AA. Frontal surgery: Use of mucoperiosteal flap for reconstruction of a nasofrontal duct. Laryngoscope 1960; 70:1229–1243.
53. Duvall AJ, Porto DP, Lyons D, et al. Frontal sinus fractures. Arch Otolaryngol Head Neck Surg 1987; 113:933–935.
54. Larson CH, Adkins WY, Oscuthorpe JD. Posttraumatic frontal and frontoethmoid mucoceles causing reversible visual loss. Otolaryngol Head Neck Surg 1983; 91:691–694.
55. Abramson AL, Eason RL. Experimental frontal sinus obliteration: Long term results following removal of mucous membrane lining. Laryngoscope 1977; 87: 1066–1073.
56. Goodale RL. Obliteration of the frontal sinus. Ann Otolaryngol Rhin Laryngol 1965; 74:831–840.
57. McNulty JS. Frontal sinus reconstruction with bone or cartilage grafts. Ear Nose Throat 1986; 65:512–516.
58. Zide MF, Kent JN, Machado L. Hydroxylapatite cranioplasty directly over dura. J Oral Maxillofac Surg 1987; 45:481–486.
59. Remsen K, Lawson W, Biller H. Acrylic frontal cranioplasty. Head Neck Surg 1986; 9:32–41.
60. Conroy B. Maxillofacial prosthetics and technology. In: Rowe NL, Williams JL. Maxillofacial injuries. New York: Churchill Livingstone, 1985; 869–998.
61. Kaplan EN. 3-D CT images for facial implant design and manufacture. Clin Plast Surg 1987; 14:663–675.

25

Gunshot Wounds

David W. Shelton

Trauma is the leading cause of mortality in the United States for persons between the ages of 1 and 38 years. Second only to motor vehicle accidents as a source of morbidity and mortality from trauma, more than 33,000 Americans lose their lives each year as a result of injury inflicted by firearms.[1,2] Statistically, firearm deaths closely approach the totals reported for cancer of the breast and diabetes mellitus.[3] Moreover, firearms presently rank as the nation's eighth leading cause of death.[4–6] Nearly one million firearm deaths occurred during the half century of 1933 to 1982, excluding those occurring from military conflicts and legal action.[7,8]

SOURCES OF INJURY BY FIREARMS

In 1982, the most recent year for which complete and reliable data are available, there were 33,000 firearm deaths in the United States and they may be categorized in the following manner.[9]

16,575	suicides
13,841	homicides
1756	unintentional/accidental
540	intent undetermined
276	legal action

There are approximately 15 firearm-related deaths per 100,000 U.S. population per year compared with about 20 deaths per 100,000 U.S. population per year for motor vehicle accidents.[10–12]

Mortality alone fails to convey the overall impact of injuries inflicted by firearms. Although there is no data reference demonstrating the types and number of nonfatal injuries resulting from firearms, nonfatal firearm injuries greatly outnumber firearm deaths, perhaps by as much as 3 to 1.[13] The National Center for Health Statistics lists 155,000 nonfatal gunshot injuries for 1972.[14] For the same year there were 29,000 firearm deaths; a ratio of more than five nonfatal firearm injuries for each firearm fatality.[15]

BALLISTIC CONSIDERATIONS

With reference to firearms the science of ballistics is generally divided into three separate but related components. Internal ballistics is concerned with events that take place from the time the firing pin strikes the cartridge primer until the bullet makes its exit from the muzzle of the weapon. Included in this area are such considerations as rate of burn of the propellant substance, accumulation of gas pressures within the ignition chamber, and rate of twist of the bore rifling.

External ballistics addresses those factors that influence the behavior of the bullet in its flight from the weapon to the target. In essence, it is largely the design of the bullet, its shape, or the manner in which its mass is distributed and other related factors that determine just how much of its acquired kinetic energy (KE) is eventually delivered to the target.

Terminal ballistics encompasses the examination of bullet behavior on impact and the evaluation of energy transfer to the target media. Although such factors as specific gravity of various substances, retardation, velocity change in passage through media, wound volume, and other factors are measurable and calculable, other phenomena related to wound severity are less predictable, especially in living human tissues.

In the evaluation and management of gunshot injuries, the most critical aspects of ballistics are the external and terminal components. It is in these areas that the interested clinician will acquire an enhanced appreciation of the forces at work and the mechanisms operative in the production of the wound with which he or she is confronted.

The energy of a missile or bullet expressed in units of measurements represents an attempt to quantify its lethal potential. In effect, the most efficient bullet is one that dissipates the greatest amount of its energy within the target object. Several theories have been advanced in attempting to explain and predict tissue damage resulting from gunshot injuries. Unquestionably, the theory that is most widely applied to the study of ballistics and that appears to be most consistent with the performance of missiles in both air and target media is the kinetic energy theory.

Kinetic Energy

A functional understanding of the explosive effect of a high-velocity missile at impact lies largely in an appreciation of the terms: force, work, and energy, especially kinetic energy.[16]

A force (F) acting on a given mass (m) for a specified period of time (t) produces in the mass a velocity (v):

$$F = m \times v/t$$

Work is done in overcoming a resistance (or force of static inertia) to impart velocity to the mass. A near equivalent quantity of work is therefore required to bring the mass to rest. In translocating the mass through a distance (d) the amount of work (W) done is:

$$W = F \times d$$

Because the distance is the product of the rate of travel and the time over which the travel occurred (1/2v being the average velocity):

$$d = 1/2v \times t$$

The product F × d thus becomes:

$$(m \times v/t)\,(1/2v \times t)$$

Or:

$$W = \frac{m \times v^2}{2}$$

Because the work accomplished by the force in imparting acceleration to the mass represents a capacity to perform an equal amount of work upon coming to rest, it is indeed energy in motion. This form of energy is recognized as kinetic energy (KE).

Considering the flight of a bullet, for example, it must be remembered that the force vector exerted by gravity (g) produces a downward deviation in the translocational vector of the bullet and thus a derogating effect on kinetic energy. Therefore:

$$KE = \frac{m \times v^2}{2g}$$

Significance of Velocity as a Determinant of Kinetic Energy

From the expression for kinetic energy, it is readily apparent that the single most important determinant of kinetic energy is velocity. All else being equal, kinetic energy is doubled when mass is doubled but quadrupled when velocity is doubled. The significance of velocity as a determinant of kinetic energy is illustrated in Table 25–1 and Figure 25–1, A through E.

Table 25–1. *Comparison of .22 Caliber Rifles*

Caliber	*Bullet Wt (grains)*	*Muzzle Velocity (ft/second)*	*Energy (ft lbs)*
.22 (Long rifle)	40	1150	117
.222 (Hornet)	45	2100	892
.223 (M-16 A1)	55	3240	1282
Ratio of increase (between long rifle and M-16)		2.82	10.96

(Modified from Matumas E. In: American Ammunition and Ballistics. *Tulsa, OK: Winchester Press, 1979; 13–14, 52–53)*

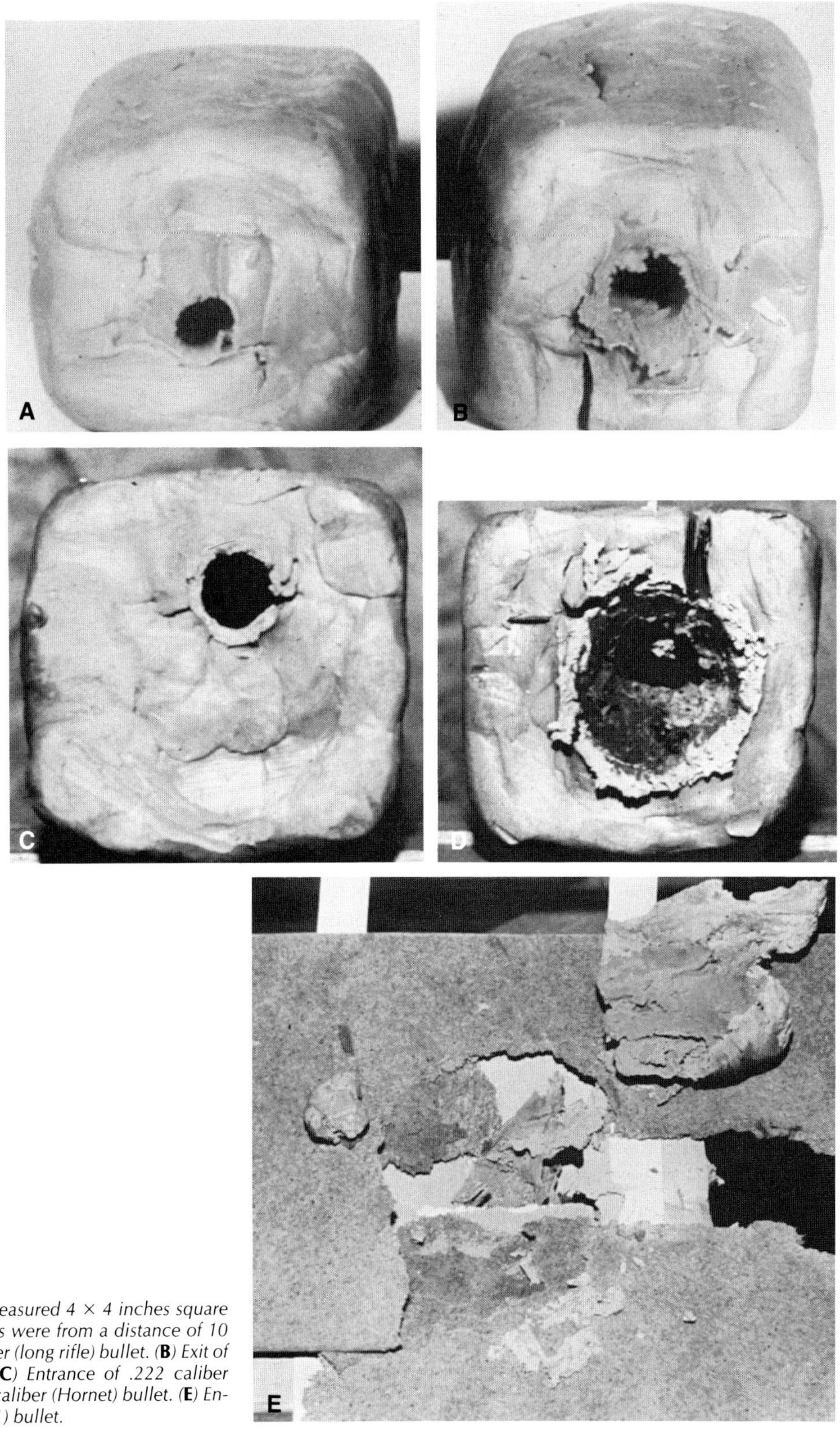

Figure 25–1. *All clay blocks measured 4 × 4 inches square and 8 in in length. All bullet hits were from a distance of 10 meters. (**A**) Entrance of .22 caliber (long rifle) bullet. (**B**) Exit of .22 caliber (long rifle) bullet. (**C**) Entrance of .222 caliber (Hornet) bullet. (**D**) Exit of .222 caliber (Hornet) bullet. (**E**) Entrance and exit of .223 (M-16 A1) bullet.*

Energy Dissipation

Although it is clear that velocity is the most important consideration in the generation of kinetic energy and, hence, striking energy, there are some other significant considerations that greatly influence the nature of the wound which is produced.

In the final analysis, lethality in gunshot wounds is determined by the amount of striking energy that is dissipated within the target substance. Kinetic energy dissipation within target media can be calculated from the velocity loss as the missile passes through the target media, i.e., v_1 (entrance velocity) minus v_2 (exit velocity). Tissue disruption and destruction correlates with energy dissipation. Energy dissipation is a function of retardation.

Retardation

The term *retardation* refers to those factors that cause expenditure of the kinetic energy of the bullet by resisting its forward progress. As discussed previously, many factors in living tissues involved in retardation are neither measurable nor calculable and have never been elucidated.[17] Much of our knowledge of bullet retardation is derived from experimental studies that have been done in ballistic gelatin, water, various plastic media, and of course, animal tissue.[18-20]

This particular aspect of ballistics, specifically terminal or wound ballistics, concerns itself with the movement and behavior of the bullet within the target medium and is at once fascinating, complex, and beyond the scope of the present review. In essence and in any medium, including air, retardation varies according to the density of the retarding medium, the diameter of the missile, and the square of its velocity. It varies inversely with the mass of the missile because the greater mass has the greater momentum. Retardation may be expressed as:

$$R = P\frac{Dv^2}{m}$$

when R equals retardation; P, density of retarding medium (specific gravity); D, diameter of missile; v^2, velocity of missile; and m, mass.

Table 25–2 demonstrates the correlation between tissue specific gravity and wound severity (Table 25–2). The influence of increasing the diameter of the missile on wound severity is illustrated in Table 25–3 and Figure 25–2, A through D.

Table 25–2. *Correlation Between Tissue Specific Gravity and Wound Severity Produced by High-Velocity Bullets*

Tissue	Specific Gravity	Severity of Wound
Fat	0.80	Moderate
Skin	1.09	Marked
Lung	0.40	Minimum
Bone	1.11	Extreme

(From DeMuth WE. J Trauma 1966; 6 : 222)

CHARACTERISTICS OF MAXILLOFACIAL GUNSHOT WOUNDS

Low-Velocity Missile Wounds

Missiles traveling at velocities below 2000 ft per second are classified as low velocity and exhibit a behavior in the tissues that is different from higher velocity missiles. Examples are those fired from handguns, low-velocity rifles, shotguns, and most missile fragments (Table 25–4).

Characteristically, the low-velocity missile wound has an entrance but no exit. The entrance wound may appear small and clean cut or ragged and ugly as a result of yawing or tumbling of the bullet, which is retained either intact or separated from its jacket (when such ammunition is used) or simply fragmented within the tissues (Fig. 25–3). When hard tissues are struck; fracture, comminution, and even displacement of segments of bone may be produced, but external avulsion does not ordinarily occur with this type of missile wound. Regional blood vessels and nerves, as well as other structures such as salivary glands and ducts, may be damaged (Fig. 25–4, A to D).

High-Velocity Missile Wounds

Missiles traveling in excess of 2000 ft per second are classified as high velocity (although some references employ the value of 2500 ft per second).[21] Examples

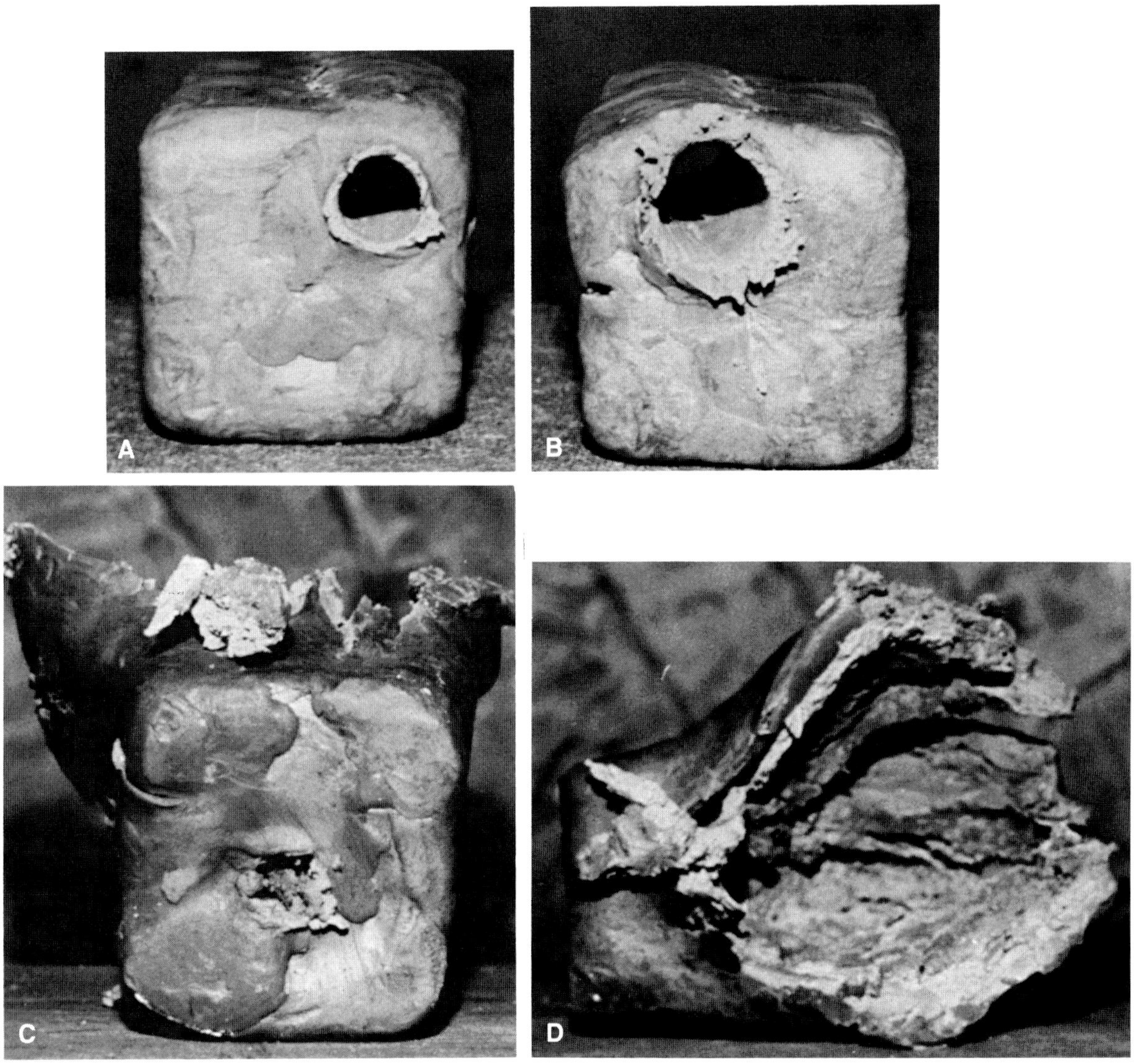

Figure 25–2. *All clay blocks measured 4 × 4 inches square and 8 in in length. All bullet hits were from a distance of 10 meters.* (**A**) *Entrance of .38 caliber standard bullet.* (**B**) *Exit of .38 caliber standard bullet.* (**C**) *Entrance of .38 caliber hollow point–soft nose bullet.* (**D**) *Exit and wound volume of .38 caliber hollow point–soft nose bullet.*

Table 25–3. Correlation Between Bullet Diameter and Wound Volume*

Bullet Type	Diameter Entry Wound	Diameter Exit Wound	Wound Volume
Military (full jacket)	0.75 cm	2.0 cm	23.5 cm
Hunting (expanding)	0.75 cm	12.5 cm	917.0 cm
Ratio of increase		6.25	39.02

* *150 gr.; .30 cal.; 2900 ft/sec, fired through dog thorax.*
(DeMuth WE. J Trauma 1966; 6:222)

Table 25–4. Handgun Striking Energy

Caliber	Bullet Wt (grains)	Muzzle Velocity (ft/second)	Striking Energy (ft pounds)
.22 Short	29	1045	70
.25 Auto	50	810	73
.32 Long revolver	98	705	115
.38 SW	145	685	150
.38 Special + P	158	915	294
.45 Auto	230	810	335
.357 Magnum	125	1450	583
.44 Magnum	240	1350	970

(Modified from Matumas E. In: American Ammunition and Ballistics. Tulsa, OK: Winchester Press, 1979; 13, 91–92)

are those fired from rifles, machine guns, and other missile fragments that are generated by explosions and are moving at a very high velocity. Although most such missile fragments are endowed with high–initial-velocities, the poor ballistic properties of these fragments cause this extreme initial velocity to rapidly diminish so that actual striking energies are greatly reduced.

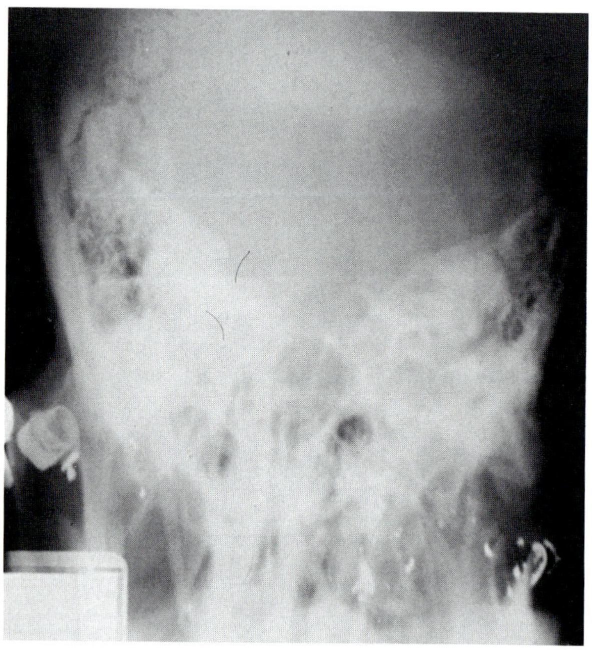

Figure 25–3. *Low-velocity gunshot wound in which the bullet, entering on the left, is fragmented throughout the tissues and the bullet jacket is in the condylar region on the right.*

Characteristically, the high-velocity missile produces a small, clean cut entrance wound, passes through the victim, and if the missile does not strike calcified tissues, creates a somewhat larger exit wound. Destruction may be surprisingly minimal or, depending on the design and velocity of the bullet and the bulk or thickness and density (specific gravity) of the tissues struck or perforated, it may be severe.

The track of this missile, which decelerates rapidly and thus transfers its energy to the tissues, will be rapidly surrounded by a water vapor filled cavity larger than the size of the missile as the substance into which it has impacted is flung away from the missile path. The cavity then collapses and undergoes several repetitions of alternate expansion and collapse, which diminish in magnitude until the target mass finally comes to rest. The entire process occurs within the span of a few microseconds. It is during this cavitation phenomenon that foreign debris and contamination is drawn into the wound in addition to that which is driven in directly by penetration of the missile. Surrounding tissues are devitalized, blood vessels and nerves are torn or destroyed, and bone is fractured, often even when it is not struck directly.

If the missile impacts bone and teeth it is often disintegrated and the exit wound is massive and explosive. Bone and soft tissue avulsion is common, and extensive regional damage is produced frequently by radiation of impact energy throughout the sutured facial skeleton and by generation of secondary missile

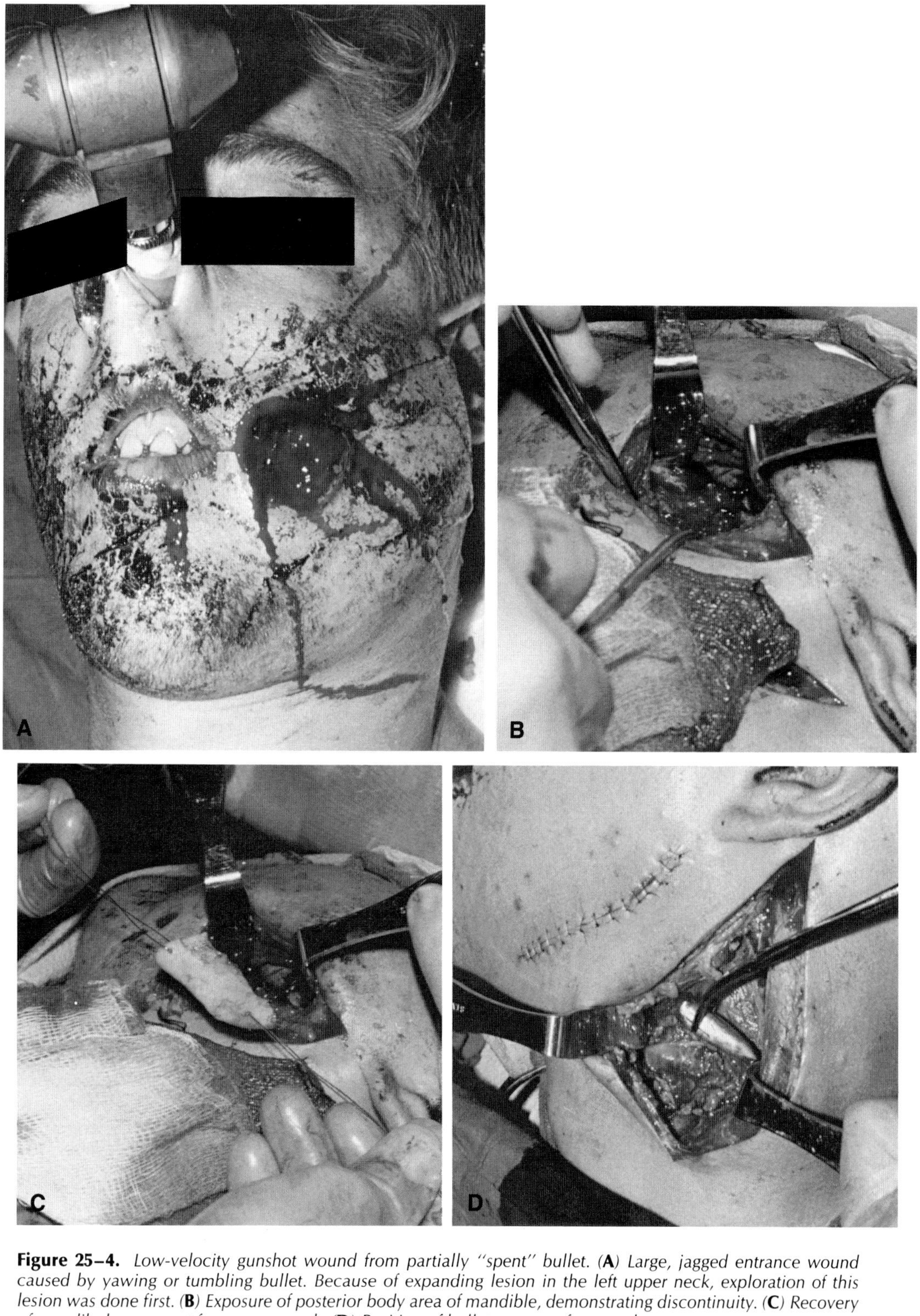

Figure 25–4. *Low-velocity gunshot wound from partially "spent" bullet. (**A**) Large, jagged entrance wound caused by yawing or tumbling bullet. Because of expanding lesion in the left upper neck, exploration of this lesion was done first. (**B**) Exposure of posterior body area of mandible, demonstrating discontinuity. (**C**) Recovery of mandibular segment from upper neck. (**D**) Position of bullet recovery from neck.*

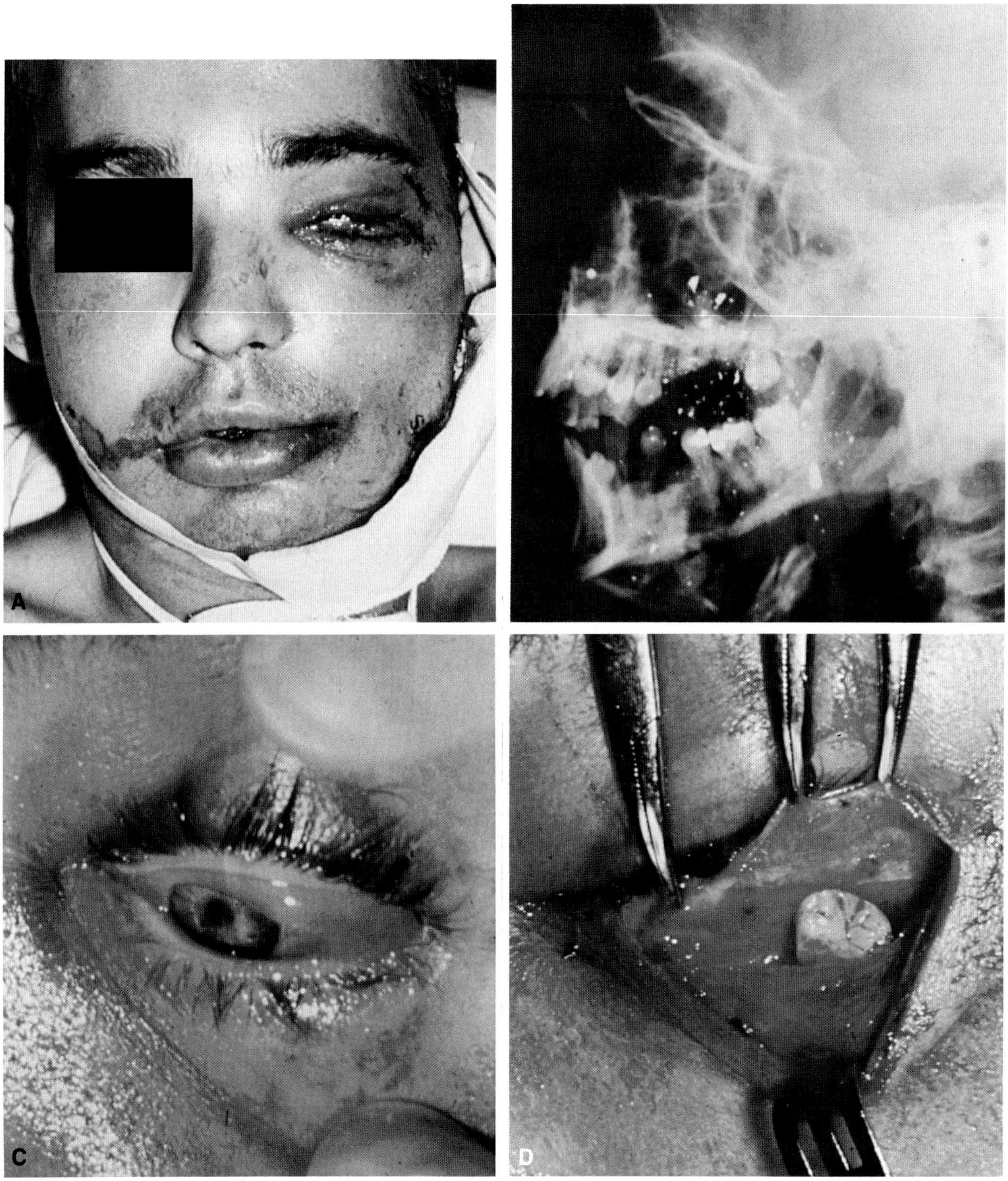

Figure 25–5. *High-velocity gunshot wound. (**A**) Entrance wound was on the patient's right cheek. The bullet struck the maxilla on the right, traveled across the oral cavity, and impacted the mandible on the left. Notice the periorbital ecchymosis and edema about the left orbit. (**B**) Lateral skull radiograph demonstrating avulsion of the mandible on exit side. (**C**) Chemosis of the left eye. (**D**) Recovery of the crown of a mandibular tooth during exploration of the left orbital rim and floor.*

fragments, especially tooth crowns, amalgam and gold dental restorations, and fixed or removable partial denture prostheses.

On radiographic examination, minute traces of the primary missile frequently are seen scattered throughout the wound but the intact missile is not seen. The result of hard and soft tissue avulsions is also apparent (Fig. 25–5A–D).

Shotguns

The shotgun was originally designed to be used on small and fast moving game, e.g., flying birds. Accordingly, its basic design incorporates a long barrel, the inside surface of which is smooth. The shell contains one to hundreds of lead pellets, which are propelled at velocities of 1000 to 1500 ft per second.[22] The shotgun shell also contains a plastic cap that holds the shot in place. In contact or close range wounds inflicted by a shotgun, these materials are frequently propelled into the tissues.

Several factors are operative in determining the severity of shotgun wounds, the most important of which is the range, or distance, over which the wound was incurred. Table 25–5 classifies and summarizes shotgun wounds.

Rubber and Plastic Bullets

Rubber and plastic bullets were introduced for use in subduing unruly crowds and controlling riots with the hope of inflicting less destructive wounds. However, these missiles are capable of producing serious injury, including depressed skull fractures and death.[23] However, it is true that the lower mass of these missiles results in lesser momentum and thus lower penetrating capacity on impact.

Devastator Bullets

Devastator bullets or exploding bullets have been in existence since the Civil War. Originally, the tip of the bullet was hollowed out and the explosive (fulminate of mercury) was placed into the leading point of the bullet and sealed over. On impact, the explosive detonated, resulting in enhanced dissipation of the bullet energy within the target. Presently, lead oxide is used as the explosive. There is a high-failure rate of devastator bullets fired into tissue, presenting a risk of explosion later and therefore a danger to healthcare providers.[24]

BB and Pellet Guns

These pneumatic devices occasionally pose problems for the surgeon. Muzzle velocities exceeding 100 ft per second have been demonstrated.[25] Random and careless use of airguns not infrequently leads to loss of vision and, occasionally, loss of life.

Missile Embolization

Movement or migration of bullets and missile fragments may occur in any vessel or between potential tissue spaces. A number of case reports of this phenomenon are documented in the literature. The incidence of vascular embolism reported at autopsy is 1.1%.[26]

Table 25–5. *Classification of Shotgun Wounds*

Range	Injury	Mortality (%)
Type I: Long (> 12 m)	Penetrates only subcutaneous tissue and deep fascia	0–5
Type II: Close (> 5 m, < 12 m)	Penetrates beyond deep fascia	15–20
Type III: Point blank (< 5 m)	Extensive tissue damage	85–90

(Ordog GJ. In: Ordog GJ, ed. Management of gunshot wounds. *New York: Elsevier, 1988; 47)*

Lead Intoxication

Lead intoxication is a well documented, albeit rare, complication of lead bullet wounds in which the bullet or its fragments remain lodged in tissue—typically in bones, synovial joints, or a pseudocyst.[27] Signs and symptoms of lead intoxication may occur acutely or several years after the gunshot wound.[28]

Manifestations may encompass elevated concentrations of lead in plasma and urine, proteinuria, anemia, colic, and encephalopathy. The range of severity may include death.[29] In cases of of plumbism, the bullet or lead fragments should be removed. If located within a joint space, initial treatment should be removal because of increased risk of lead poisoning and the likelihood of progressive destruction of the joint.[30] Extensive exploration for the bullet or fragment at the time of initial surgery or after recovery from the injury is usually contraindicated because of the rarity of this complication. It is sufficient to apprise the patient of this remote possibility.[27]

EARLY DEFINITIVE MANAGEMENT

After the airway has been secured, bleeding has been controlled, and appropriate intravascular volume restitution has been initiated, laboratory studies should be obtained. A neurologic and ophthalmologic examination are carried out. A careful neck examination for any suggestion of hematoma or other injury should be done. It is important to gather all possible information about the type and caliber of the weapon, type of ammunition, and range and time of wounding.

Early Medical Management Considerations

Laboratory studies should include a complete blood count, electrolyte count, blood gas analysis, and urinalysis. Blood should be cross-matched for any patient in which the wound is severe and additional significant blood loss is anticipated, for patients in whom vasular injury is suspected, and especially for patients who exhibit signs and symptoms consistent with an acute blood loss approaching 30% of the circulating blood volume. Tetanus prophylaxis is given and intravenous antibiotic administration is started. At the present time, the antibiotics of choice are ticarcillin and clavulanic acid (Timentin). Antibiotic therapy is maintained for a minimum of 10 days. Any change in the antibiotic regimen should be based on the clinical course and culture and sensitivity information.

Clinical Examination

Although a clinical examination is performed on initial contact with the patient, a thorough, detailed reexamination of the wound under anesthesia is recommended for all gunshot wounds of the face before beginning any surgical manipulations. This is especially true in massive, avulsive types of wounds (Fig. 25–6). Concomitant with the examination of the wound, copious amounts of irrigation should be employed. Such irrigations wash away blood clots and debris, enabling the surgeon to more accurately identify, super-

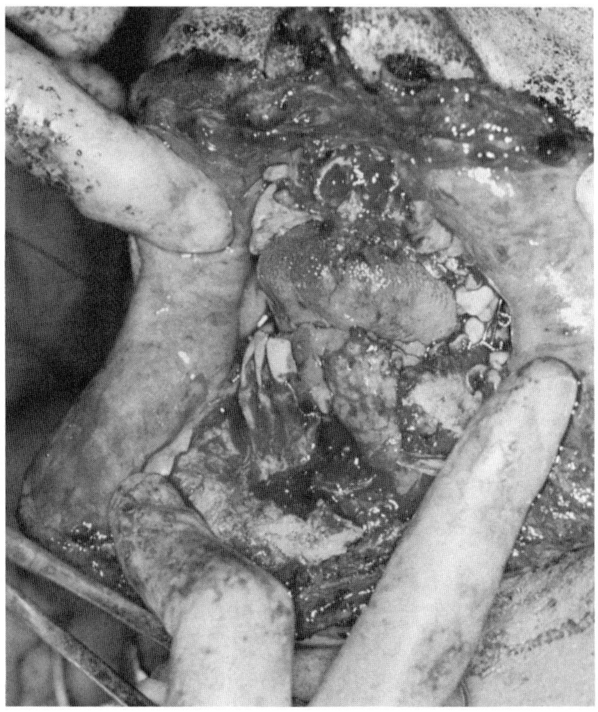

Figure 25–6. *Massive, avulsive gunshot wound caused by a high-velocity missile. This is the type of wound in which a detailed examination under anesthesia before definitive surgical repair, as described in the text, is indicated.*

ficially debride, and visualize the condition of the bone, soft tissues, and other structures, e.g., salivary glands, salivary gland ducts, and nerves. Overall assessment of the wound is thus enormously enhanced.

Good research data and abundant clinical evidence indicates that irrigation with pulsating jet-lavage techniques and incorporation of antibiotics in the irrigant is beneficial in both debridement and in reducing the bacterial inoculum.[31] Irrigation with pulsating jet-lavage devices with saline to which 50,000 U of bacitracin has been added is recommended.

The actual examination then proceeds in the following manner:

1. *Eye:* Careful attention is devoted to the eye, if there is a question of ocular injury, an opthalmologist is consulted. If the globe is penetrated and, especially, if uveal tissue is involved, the affected eye will generally require enucleation.[32,33]
2. *Bone:* It should be determined how much of the mandible and maxilla is involved in the injury.
3. *Teeth:* It should be determined whether sufficient teeth remain to establish dental occlusion and to allow for alignment and stabilization of the jaws.
4. *Soft tissue:* The following determinations must be made: the amount of buccal and labial mucosa that has been lost; the presence or absence of adequate mucosal tissue to obtain intraoral bone coverage and a watertight closure without tension; whether any of the tongue is missing; the amount of the lips that has been lost; the status of the salivary glands and ducts; the amount of nasal structures that remain.
5. *Sinuses:* The extent of damage to the paranasal sinuses must be evaluated.
6. *Facial nerves:* The amount of facial soft tissues remaining for primary closure should be determined. From the initial presenting examination, some assessment of the status of the facial nerve also can be made.

An examination of this type will serve to fix in the surgeon's mind what the problems are and will assist in the formulation of a predefined treatment plan.

Imaging

Plane film radiographs should be obtained initially. Computed tomography (CT) is often useful, indeed mandatory in given situations, as are other studies (Fig. 25–7A–D). However, such time consuming and costly studies are not necessary in each and every case (Fig. 25–8). If there is a question of vascular injury (e.g., a bullet in the area of a major vessel) or evidence of a hematoma or expanding lesion, contrast vascular studies are indicated, if time permits (Fig. 25–9A–D).

The early definitive management of maxillofacial gunshot wounds consists of debridement, stabilization, and immobilization of fractured bones, watertight closure of intraoral mucosa, primary closure of soft tissues where possible, and the prevention of infection. An orderly and systematic approach to these injuries proceeds in the following manner.

Bone and Teeth

Conservation of as much bone as possible is indicated in wounds and injuries of the maxillofacial region. As a general rule, only that bone which washes freely away with copious irrigation should be removed. No bone that has appreciable soft tissue attachment should be picked from the wound (Fig. 25–10A,B). However, the surgeon occasionally will encounter grossly soiled and contaminated bone in the wound. In these situations, it is necessary to exercise judgment while always keeping in mind the basic concept of conservation of as much bone as possible. Involved teeth that are fractured, exposing the pulp, and that are of no particular strategic value in immobilizing the fractured bone should be treated appropriately or removed. However, under no circumstances should such teeth be removed if they are firmly attached to fractured and mobile bony segments; the removal of these involved teeth could be at the expense of the loss of significant bone segments. Such teeth should be left in place and treated appropriately or attended to after the situation becomes more clarified. It is reasonable to extirpate the pulps of such teeth if appropriate instruments are available.

Stabilization of fractured bone is by direct interosseous wiring or rigid fixation whenever practical. Multiple and comminuted fractures of the mandible and midfacial bones, those appropriately described as a "bag of bones," are most often best managed in a closed fashion by digitally molding into the most accurate alignment and stabilizing in an appropriate manner. Intraoral splint stabilization may be highly effective in selected cases. Given adequate laboratory

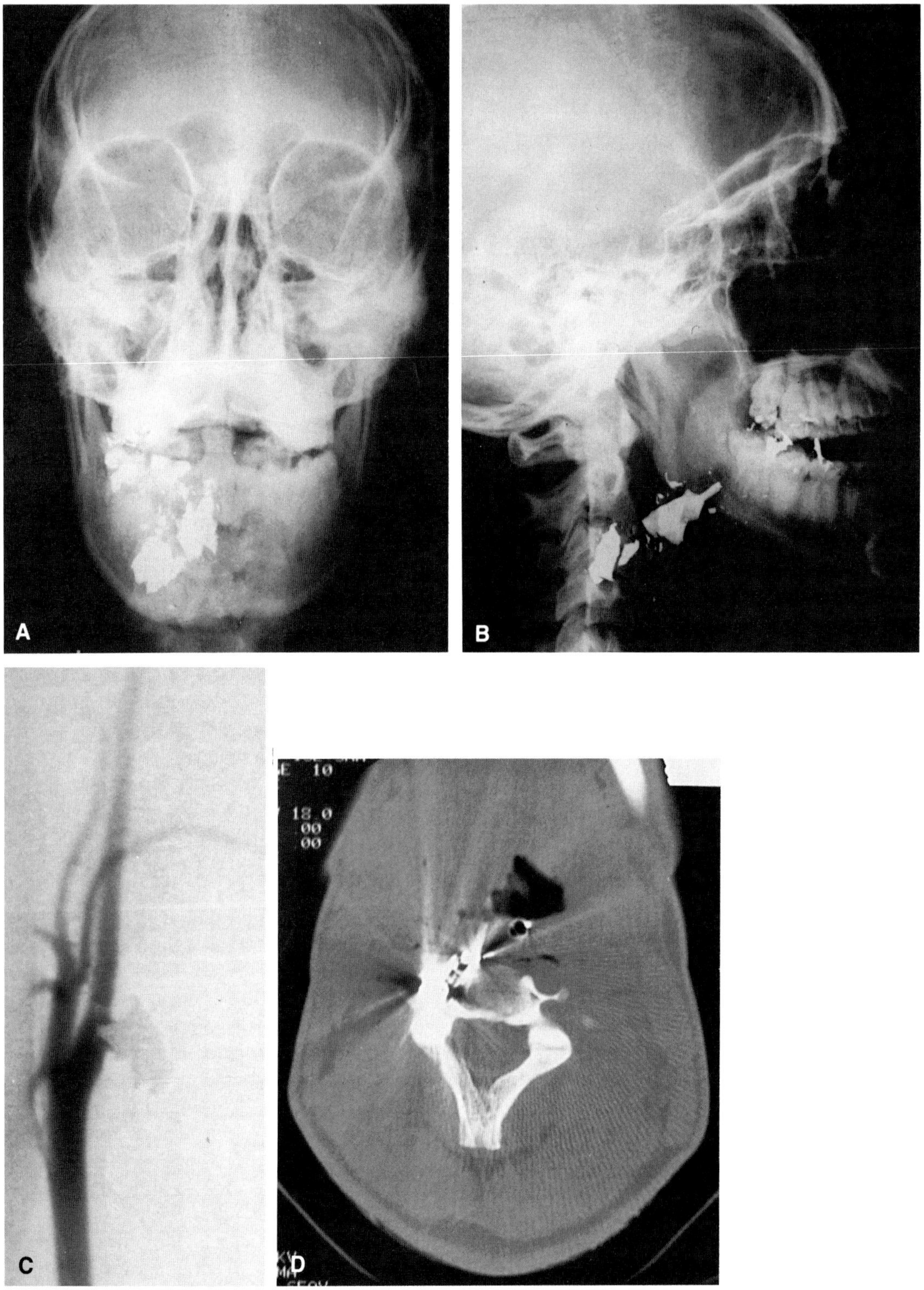

Figure 25–7. *Low-velocity gunshot wound in which additional special studies were clearly indicated. (***A** *and* **B***) PA and lateral plane radiographs indicating bullet fragment located precariously near major vessels in neck. (***C***) Subtraction arteriograms indicating no obvious vascular injury and good flow in the right external and internal carotid arteries. (***D***) CT scans indicating the bullet fragment lodged in the body of the fourth cervical vertebra. There was no neurologic deficit.*

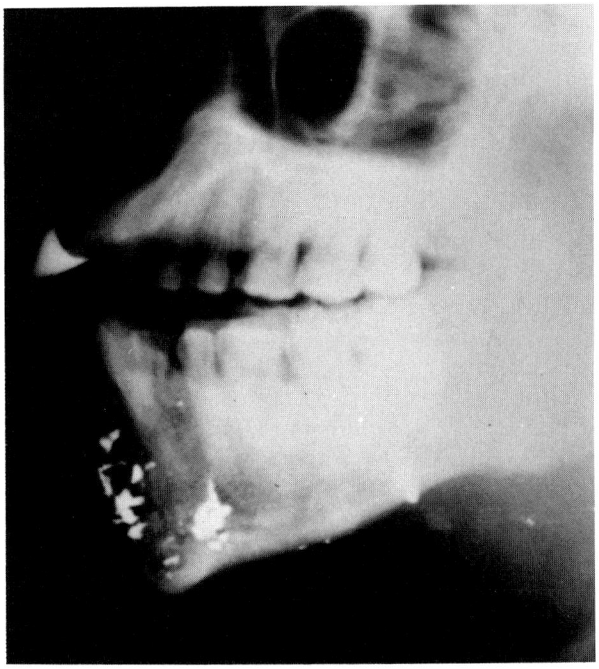

Figure 25–8. *Low-velocity gunshot wound resulting in minimally displaced fracture of the mandible. No further imaging required.*

facilities and ancillary personnel, construction of such splints may be done intraoperatively and certainly preoperatively when time permits. They are often useful in bimaxillary and multiple facial fracture cases, especially for alignment and stabilization of fractured alveolar segments and in cases involving sagittal fractures of the maxilla. When the construction of intraoral splints is not possible because of logistic reasons or anatomic considerations, the external biphase splint is useful. This is especially true in cases involving bony avulsion in the mandible.

There are other options in the early definitive management of bony avulsive injuries resulting from gunshot wounds. These include various preformed metallic meshes, segments of various types of tray devices, preformed plates and bars, and autogenous and homogeneous bone grafting. All of these modalities have the advantage of avoiding a bulky external device and are infinitely more comfortable for the patient. In the case of immediate bone grafting, particularly autogenous bone grafting, it may be the only treatment the patient requires—at least for reestablishment of mandibular continuity.

As attractive as these techniques may be, they also have some limitations.

1. There must be quantitatively and qualitatively adequate soft tissue to permit watertight intraoral and extraoral primary closure. All closures must be tension free. Moreover, during healing, there will be wound contracture. Closure under tension and wound contracture often leads to dehiscence of implanted materials and significant postoperative wound complications with increased morbidity.
2. The wound must be treated as early after injury as possible (especially if primary bone grafting is undertaken).
3. The techniques are inadvisable in grossly and highly contaminated wounds.
4. The patient must be in otherwise good general health.
5. There must be no problem with maintaining a good tissue Po_2 (hematocrit 30% or greater).
6. There must be no contraindication to maintaining the patient under general anesthesia for the additional time required to accomplish the procedure at the time of initial debridement and definitive management of the wound.

Kirshner's and Steinman pins may also be driven through bone fragments to assist in maintaining alignment. With this technique, however, it is possible to "fix" the fragments in malposition, and unless two or more pins are used, little resistance is offered against forces tending to torque the reduction, particularly in the mandible. In the midfacial skeleton, fracture fragments should be reduced and stabilized with miniplates or interfragmentary wiring. However, packings may be placed under the nasal bones and in the maxillary sinuses to support grossly comminuted fractures. Various pneumatic devices are available for use in the maxillary sinus and function well.

Both implosion (upward fracture) and so-called blow-out (explosion or downward fracture) of the orbital floor may occur. The former are not uncommon in medium- and high-velocity missile wounds passing through the maxillary sinuses, presumably as a result of missile kinetic energy; the latter occurs more commonly with lower velocity blunt trauma. In the course of initial wound treatment, if it becomes necessary to surgically open the maxillary sinus or the orbital rim (and they are not already exposed), this also provides ample opportunity to investigate the orbital flow. Herniated periorbital contents should be reduced into the confines of the bony orbit and supported with

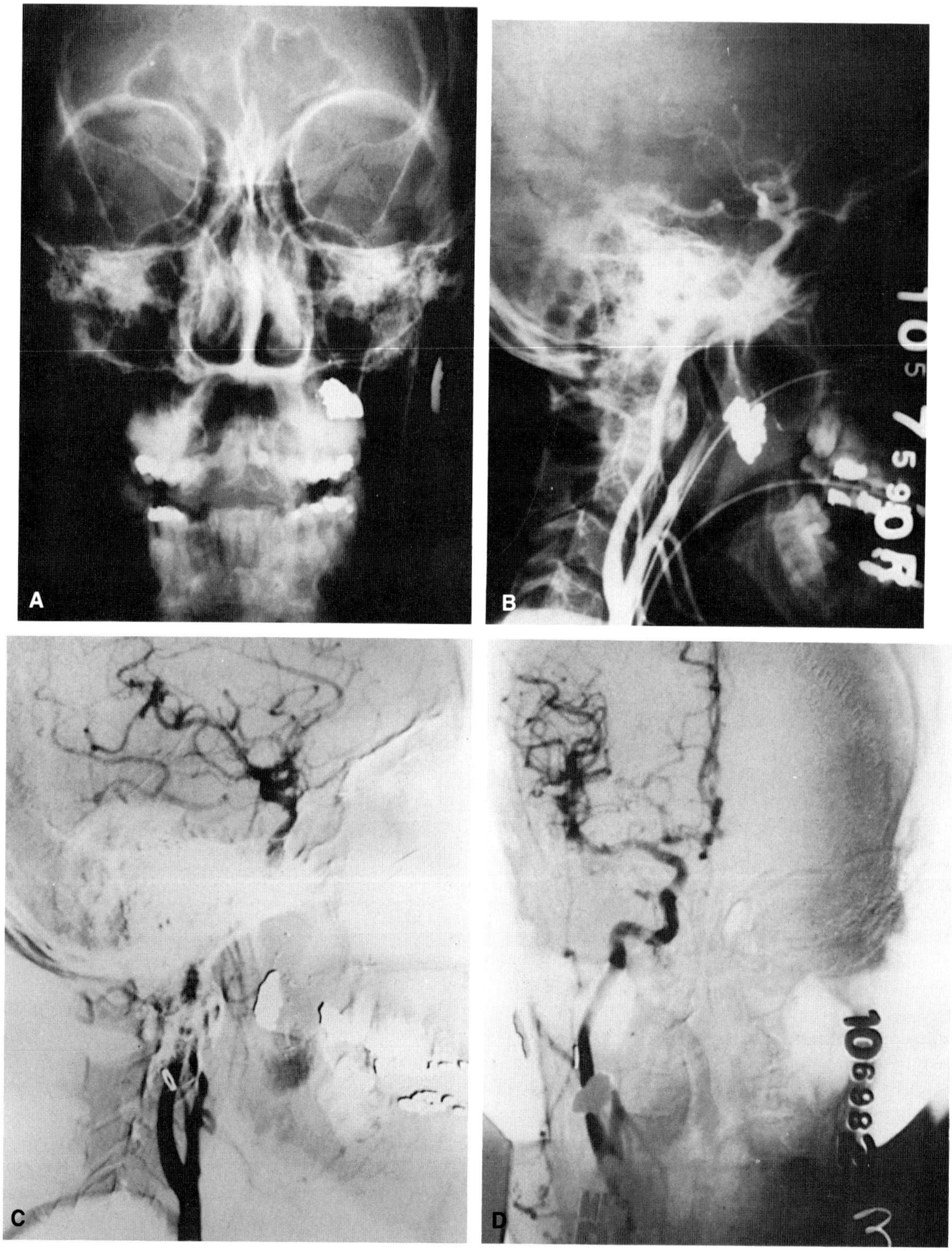

Figure 25–9. *Low-velocity gunshot wound with acute hemorrhage from palatal entrance site 8 days after injury. Lesion was a rupture of a traumatic aneurysm of the right external carotid artery treated by a detachable balloon catheter technique. (***A***) PA radiograph demonstrating position of bullet. (***B***) Lateral skull radiograph with contrast in right common carotid artery indicating possible arterial injury. (***C*** and ***D***) Subtraction arteriograms clearly showing injury to the right external carotid artery.*

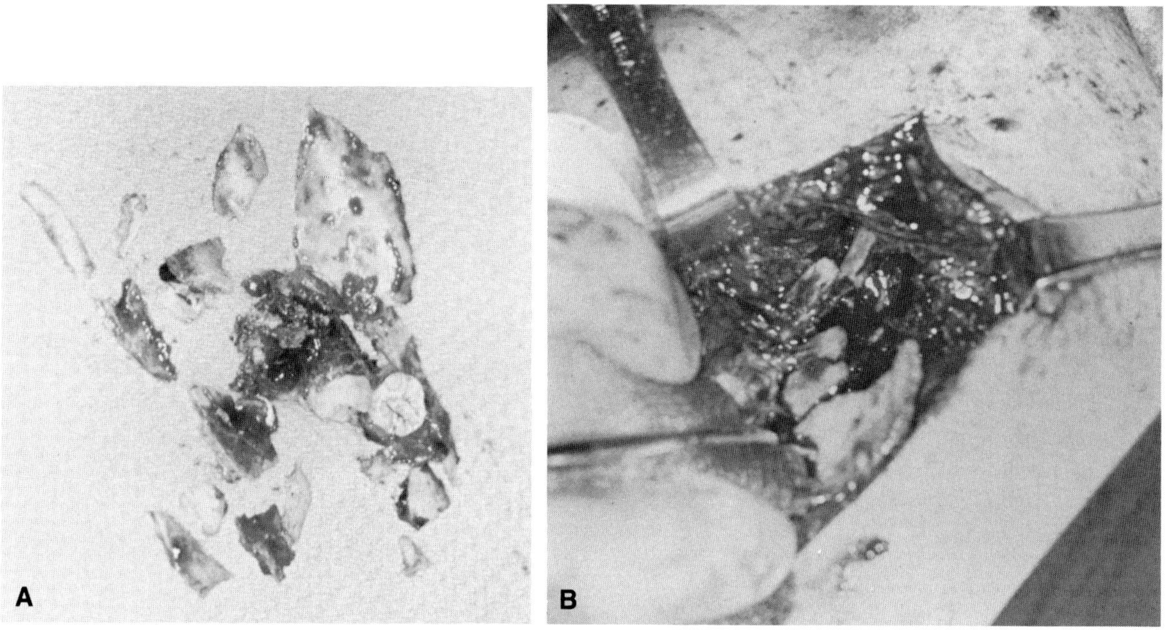

Figure 25–10. *Through-and-through high-velocity gunshot wound. (**A**) Bone and teeth fragments that were freely washed from the wound. (**B**) Remaining bone, although significantly fractured and comminuted, has appreciable soft tissue attachment and is left in place.*

an appropriate implant if necessary. The implant should be of sufficient size to rest on intact bone throughout as much of its periphery as possible. In those cases which are treated with closed techniques (e.g., in grossly fragmented and comminuted bony structures), the orbital floor may be supported transantrally by packing or placement of a pneumatic device. However, these techniques do not yield results as positive as a direct orbital floor implant.

Wounds in which avulsion of bone has occurred present challenging problems in early definitive management. In the mandible, if the avulsed segment is not extensive and if the adjacent stumps are not splintered, it is possible to split the distal or proximal stump of bone sagittally, thus mobilizing a sufficient length of corticocancellous material to span the gap and reestablish continuity. Such a maneuver must be done with the mandibular condyles in centric relation within the glenoid fossa in the base of the temporal bone and the teeth immobilized in centric occlusion. If the avulsed segment is larger or the potential donor sites are splintered, other means of spanning the defect or stabilization must be employed.

Avulsion of osseous substances in the maxilla and midfacial region is usually best managed by closing over or packing the defect and deferring treatment to later reconstruction. Although immediate bone graft reconstruction is most certainly possible and feasible in selected avulsive missile wounds of the face, it is subject to all of those conditions previously discussed.

As a general principle, in the repair of missile-induced fracture fragments of the facial skeleton, the mandible is initially reconstituted. It then serves as the base for fixating, in proper position, the intervening bony structures to the most superior stable point or points. Intermaxillary fixation with the mandibular condyles in centric relation within the glenoid fossa and with the teeth fixed in centric occlusion, as mentioned previously, are the keys to successful reduction. Intermaxillary fixation is then achieved by any of several appropriate methods.

Missile wounds involving the paranasal sinuses are best managed initially by irrigation, washing them free of debris, loose and devitalized bone, and blood clots, and by closure with appropriate drainage where necessary, e.g., the frontal sinus. Management of a frontal sinus injury must be individualized and the patency of its drainage is of special concern.

Soft Tissue: Ducts and Nerves

Primarily because of the abundant blood supply in the maxillofacial region, primary closure of soft tissues is the treatment of choice. Soft tissue approximation begins intraorally, where watertight closure is achieved using a horizontal mattress suturing technique. It is frequently necessary to undermine and mobilize intraoral mucosa to effect such closures without tension. Closure under tension results in separation of wound edges and dehiscences. Irrigation before closure should be copious, and every effort should be made to obtain the best possible hemostasis. All bone must be covered.

Severed ducts (e.g., parotid and submandibular) should be cannulated and the cannula sewn in place (Fig. 25–11A–C). The object is to route the saliva into the mouth, thus reducing the incidence of cutaneous salivary fistulae. It is possible to repair by suture the parotid duct if there has been negligible avulsion of the structure. This is best done under magnification and is more time consuming. The results of the two methods appear to be equally effective. If the investing tissues of the parotid gland have been opened and the gland itself has been damaged, it should be appropriately washed and minimally debrided (if indicated) and covered over by suturing the remaining investing and regional tissues. Salivary pseudocysts and cutane-

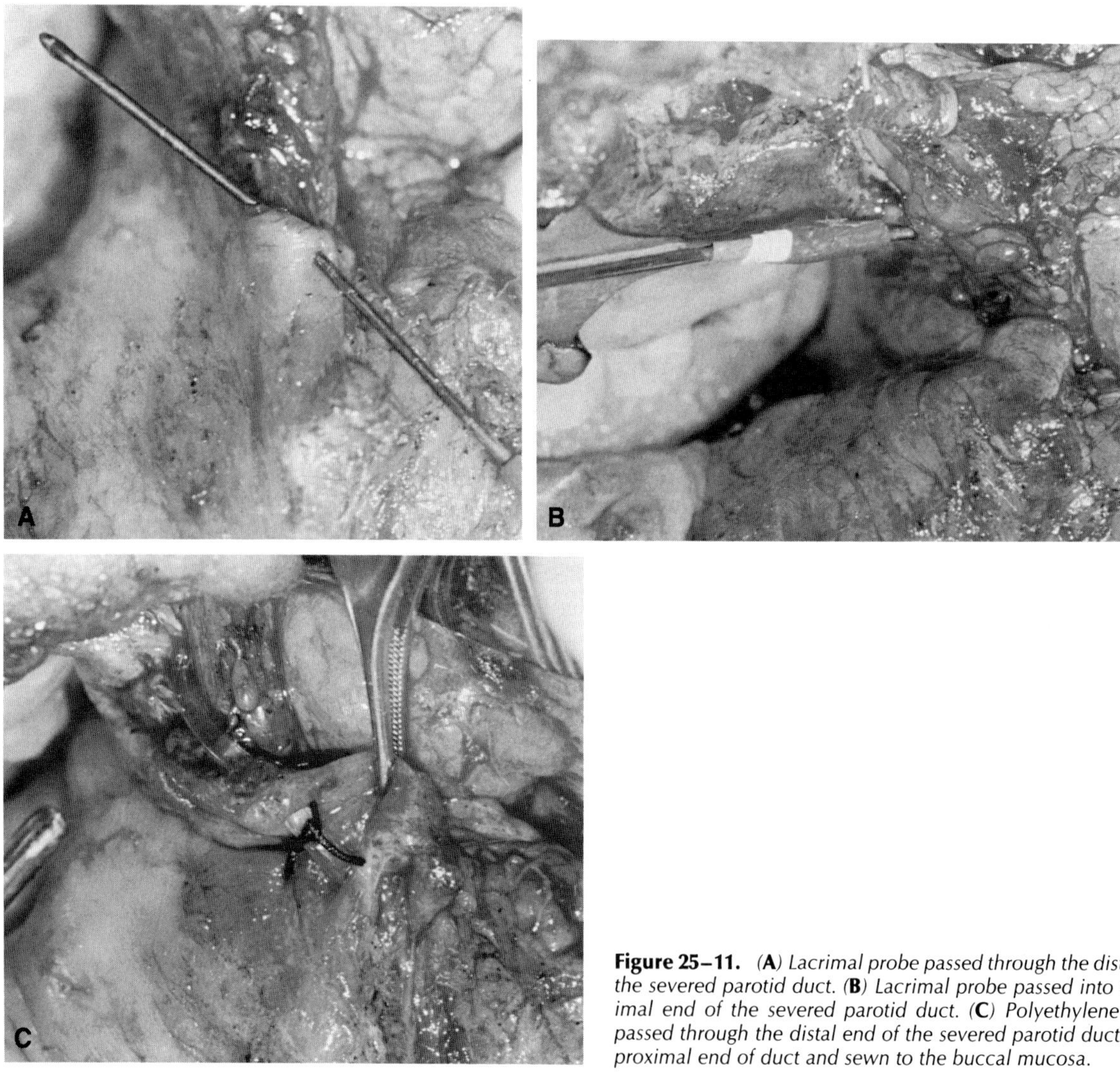

Figure 25–11. *(**A**) Lacrimal probe passed through the distal end of the severed parotid duct. (**B**) Lacrimal probe passed into the proximal end of the severed parotid duct. (**C**) Polyethylene catheter passed through the distal end of the severed parotid duct and into proximal end of duct and sewn to the buccal mucosa.*

ous salivary fistulae are complications that may be seen after surgery following injury to the parotid gland. Should these complications occur, they most often respond to simple drainage and conservative patient follow-up without the use of antisialogogue or radiation therapy.

When the submandibular duct has sustained significant damage, it may be brought up to the floor of mouth mucosa and sewn in place or the egress of saliva may simply be allowed to seek a path into the mouth. If there has been significant damage to the submandibular gland, especially in open wounds, the preferred course of action is removal of the gland. Establishing drainage intraorally from this dependent structure is fraught with problems and its removal is of no clinically significant consequence.

If any part of the facial nerve is severed or avulsed proximal to a line joining the lateral canthus of the eye and the antegonial notch of the mandible, primary repair or grafting is inadvisable. Instead, the nerve stumps are tagged with a small metallic vascular clip to facilitate their location radiographically and surgically at the time of later repair. A demarcation of injury does not occur for several days.[34] For the nerve to regain its regenerative capacity, for the epineurium to become firm enough to hold sutures, and for the definition of extent of cicatrix to be excised, a waiting period of 2 to 6 weeks is recommended.[34] Nerve injuries distal to the vertical line do not require repair because spontaneous regeneration is likely. The final phase in primary closure is reapproximation of the deep layers, eliminating any dead space, and finally, closure of the skin. Wounds in which the soft tissues are grossly disrupted with ragged margins are sometimes confusing to repair. As mentioned, conservation is the watchword and only deeply discolored tissue pedicles that do not regain normal color following blanching under finger pressure should be considered for excision. Skin margins are trimmed only to establish nonbeveled approximation. Known points of reference are tacked initially (e.g., the vermilion of the lip, the hairline of the eyebrow, and the ala or columella of the nose).

Limited soft tissue avulsions are managed by undermining skin margins to achieve closure with no or very little tension. When larger quantities of tissue loss preclude tension-free closure by simple undermining, it is best to resist the temptation to mobilize adjacent tissues for transpositional or rotational flaps to close the defect. It is generally better to delay such maneuvers until the regional tissues and the wound margins are well demarcated. A free full- or split-thickness skin graft may be used at the time of initial surgery to provide cover. These grafts not only act as a biologic dressing but frequently survive in a very favorable fashion quantitatively. Yet another option is simply to dress the defect with fine mesh gauze and permit secondary epithelization to occur. This produces the least desirable result, and it is better to interrupt the secondary epithelization process after 3 to 5 days with a split-thickness or full-thickness skin graft applied over the then available bed of granulation tissue. Split-thickness skin grafts may also be meshed to achieve expansion and to facilitate adaptation to the contours of the defect.

When soft tissue avulsions involve an orifice (e.g., the lips or the nares), the mucosa is sutured to the skin and the defect is deferred to later reconstruction (Fig. 25–12A,B). However, in some cases it may be possible to replace the ala of the nose with a portion of the helix of the ear.

Eyelid injuries represent special and unique problems with considerable postoperative implications. Those involving the lid margins, cannaliculi of the nasolacrimal apparatus (which, if involved, must be cannulated), levator muscle, and tarsus require highly accurate closure and detailed repair, preferably under magnification. Avulsion injuries of the eyelids may require canthopexy or halving procedures. Hyphema and penetrating and other injuries to the ocular globe must be meticulously searched for in examination. Such injuries mandate ophthalmologic consultation, particularly in cases involving avulsive injuries of the eyelids and trauma to the ocular globe.

Prevention of Infection

Primary indications for placement of drains in maxillofacial wounds are the need to prevent hematoma formation and the presence of significantly contaminated wounds. Those wounds in which multiple missile fragments have been retained and those that have undergone a delay in treatment are especially vulnerable. It often is a matter of judgment on the part of the surgeon; however, if one is to err it is better to do so on the side of drain placement.

Pressure dressings following completion of surgical

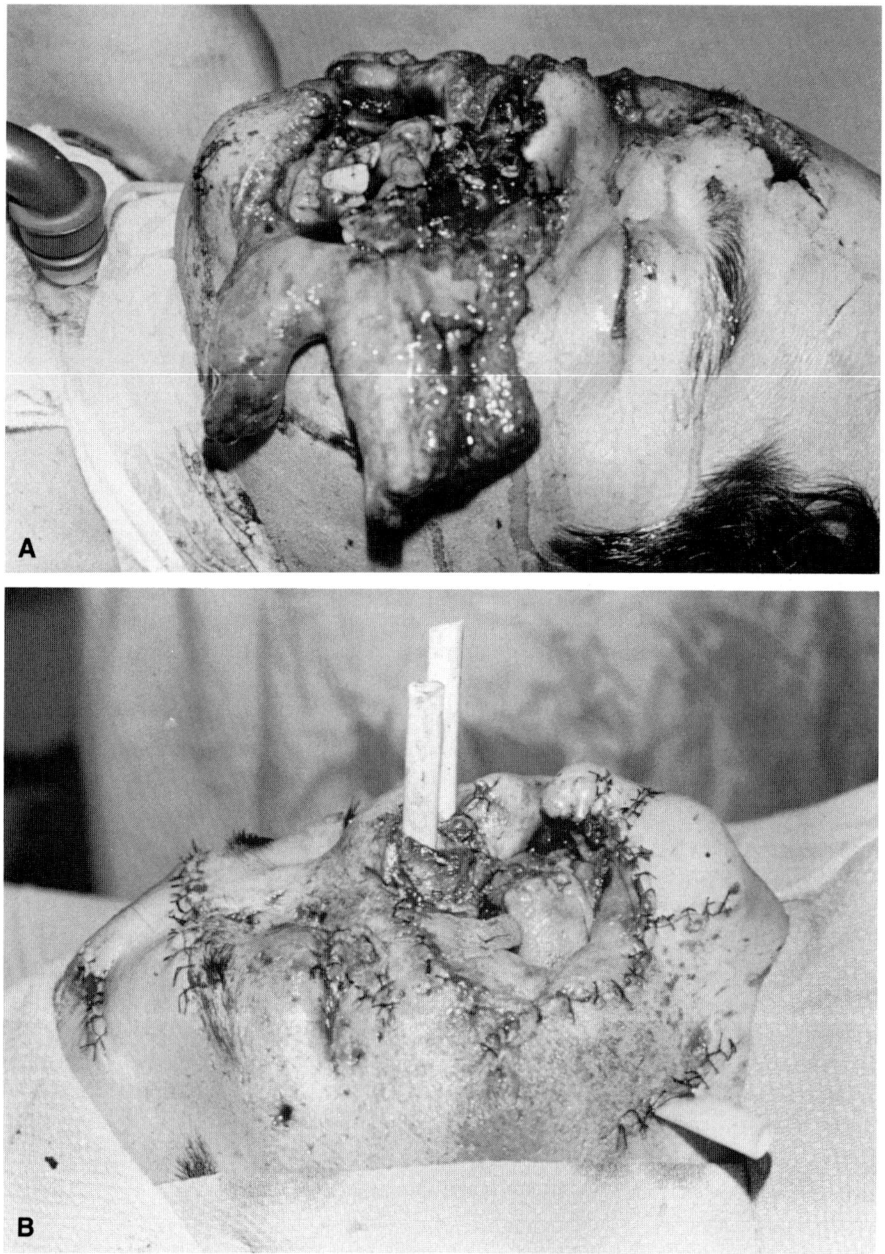

Figure 25–12. *(**A**) Soft tissue avulsion involving a portion of the cheek and the oral commissure. (**B**) Mucosa sutured to the skin margin. Defect deferred to later reconstruction.*

procedures are helpful to assist in achieving hemostasis, preventing hematoma formation, and supporting the repairs. Their use in controlling edema must be evaluated in light of their potential to produce airway difficulties by forcing the swelling inwards. All maxillofacial gunshot wounds are contaminated injuries, especially high-velocity gunshot wounds. The sources of contamination are multiple and varied. Both the entrance and the exit wounds are sources of microbes and foreign bodies, as are the mouth, pharynx, nose, and paranasal sinuses. All patients with these injuries should be given antibiotics. It is important to remember that the microbiologic condition of the wound varies according to a number of factors. Among these factors are:

1. Geographic location
2. Type of debris soiling the wound
3. Time interval between wounding and treatment
4. Type of weapon that produced the wound

Initial therapy, therefore, must often be empirical. Antibiotic use unquestionably plays a major role in the prevention of infection of these injuries; but of no less importance is early and appropriate surgical debridement, copious irrigation, fixation and immobilization of injured tissues, detailed wound closure, drainage where indicated, and maintenance of clean dressings, nutrition, and circulating fluid volume, with due consideration given to oxygen carrying capacity.

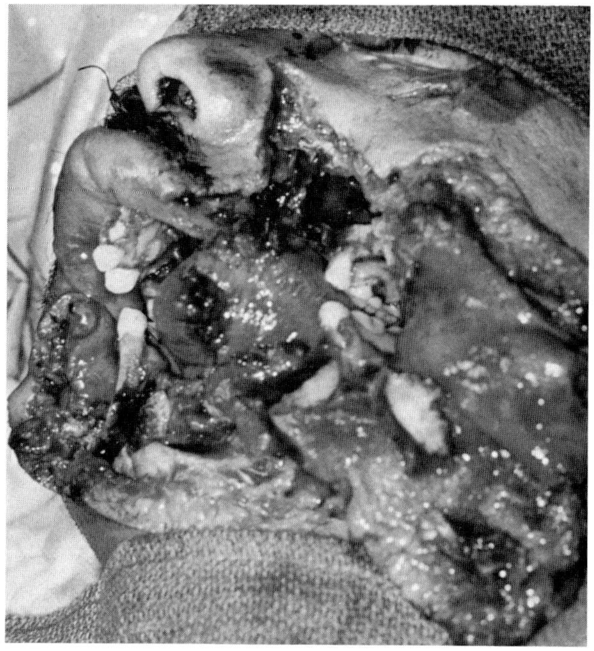

Figure 25–13.

ILLUSTRATIVE CASE REPORT

A 23-year-old male was shot at close range with a low-velocity hollow point .45 caliber bullet. The bullet struck the right anterior mandible, resulting in avulsion of a significant portion of the anterior mandible and a lesser portion of the anterior maxilla, as well as extensive laceration and some avulsion of the soft tissues in the region of the chin (Fig. 25–13). Posteroanterior and lateral radiographs reveal residual bullet fragments confined to the anterior mandibular region, as well as bony avulsion (Figs. 25–14 and 25–15). After intubation in the emergency room, tracheostomy was performed in the operating room. Intersegmental wiring then was done in the mandible and maxilla. The remaining teeth were placed into intermaxillary fixation, thus aligning the mandibular segments, and immobilized in place using an external biphase appliance (Fig. 25–16). Intraoral closure was achieved in a water-tight fashion, followed by deep closure and primary skin closure. There was inadequate soft tissue in the chin region for primary closure (Fig. 25–17). A split-thickness skin graft was used to cover the deficient area over the chin (Fig. 25–18). Posteroanterior and submento vertex plane film radiographs demonstrate the position and alignment of the mandible and maxilla achieved at surgery (Figs. 25–19 and 25–20).

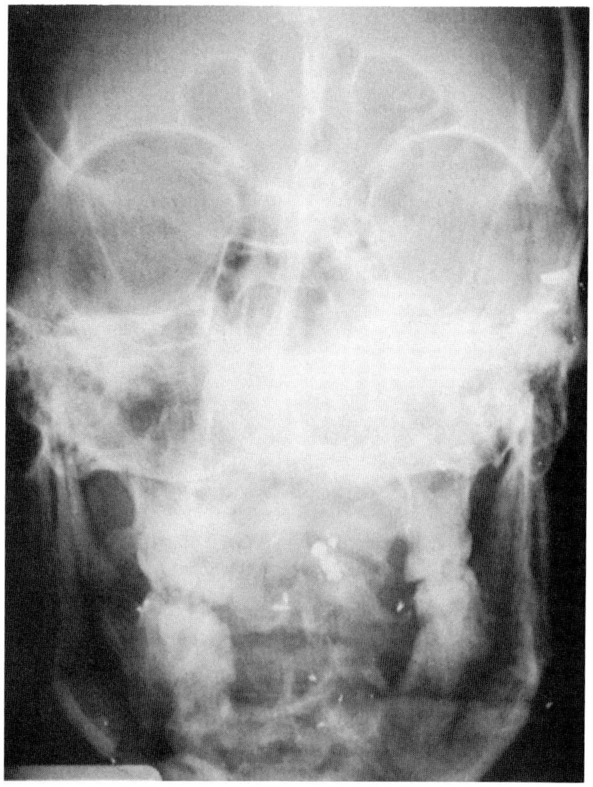

Figure 25–14.

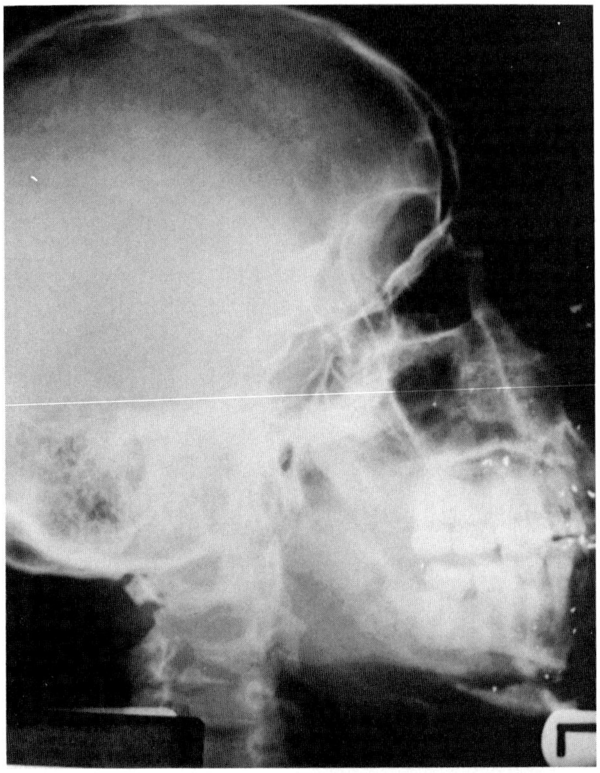

Figure 25–15.

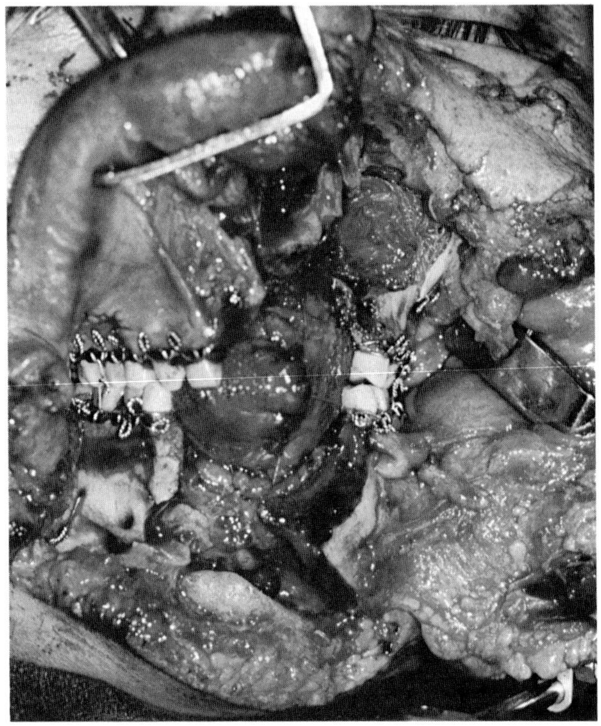

Figure 25–16.

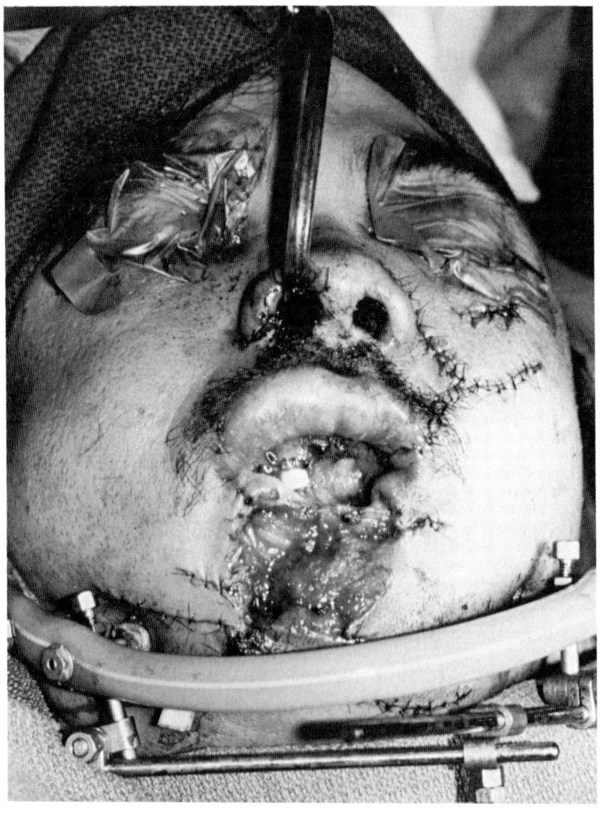

Figure 25–17.

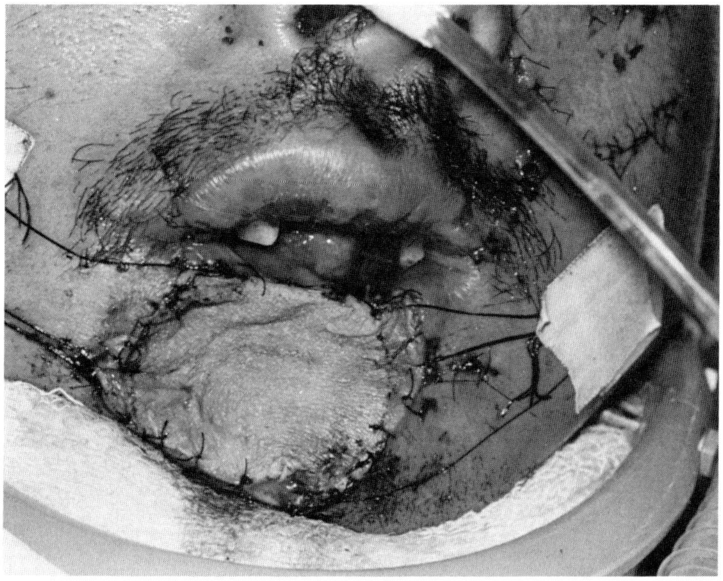

Figure 25–18.

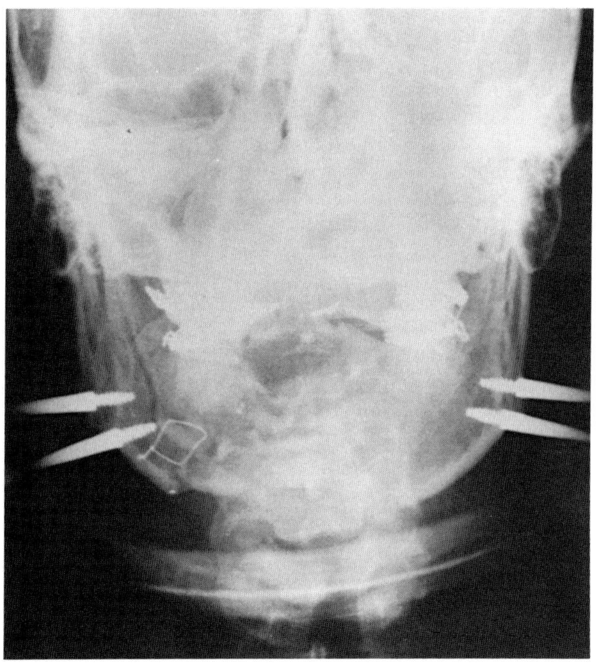

Figure 25–19.

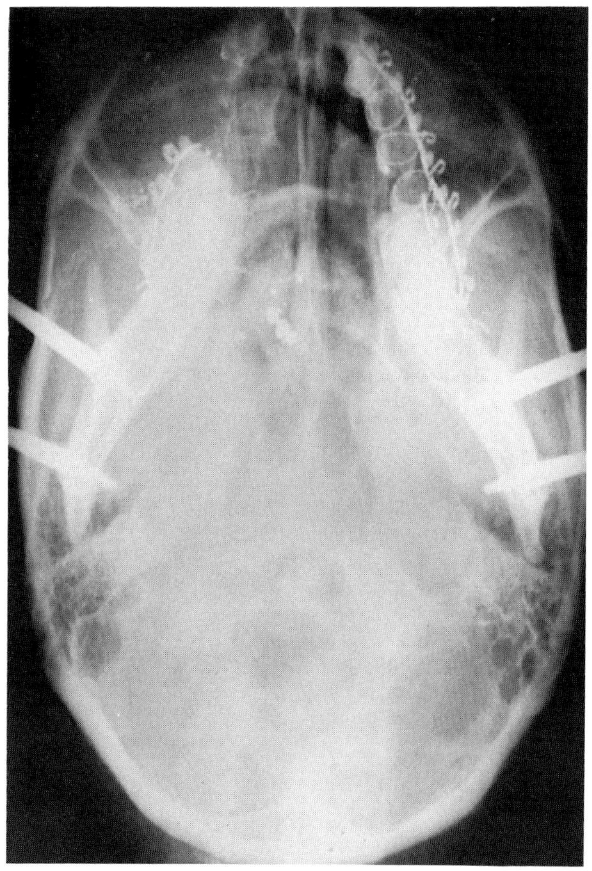

Figure 25–20.

Acknowledgement

Figures 25–1 A–E and 25–2 A–D used by permission from Swan KG, Haycock CE, Levine MG. Gunshot Wounds. College of Medicine and Dentistry of New Jersey, New Jersey Medical School, Newark, New Jersey.

REFERENCES

1. Trunkey DD. Trauma. Sci Am 1983; 249: 28.
2. National Research Council. Injury in America: A continuing public health problem. Washington, DC: National Academy Press, 1985.
3. National Center for Health Statistics. DHHS publication 85–1120. Monthly Vital Statistics Report 33 (suppl 9): 00, 1984.
4. Alexander GR, Massey RM, Gibbs T. Firearm related fatalities: An epidemiologic assessment of violent death. Am J Public Health 1985; 75: 165.
5. Fatteh A, Troxler D. The gun and its victims: A study of 1024 firearm fatalities in North Carolina during 1970. NC Med J 1971; 32: 489.
6. Wintemute GJ, Teret P, Kraus JF. The epidemiology of firearm deaths among residents of California. West J Med 1987; 146: 374.
7. Mahler AJ, Fielding JE. Firearms and gun control: A public health concern. N Engl J Med 1977; 297: 556.
8. Garen J. Firearms as a cause of death in the United States. J Trauma 1987; 27: 532.
9. National Center for Health Statistics. Rockville, MD: The Center, 1982.
10. Baker SP, O'Neil B, Karpf RS. In: The injury fact book. Lexington, MA: Lexington Books, 1984.
11. Shields P, Greenya J. In: Guns don't die, people do. New York: Arbor House, 1981; 172.
12. U.S. Department of Commerce. Statistical abstracts of the United States: ed. 104. U.S. National Center for Health Statistics—Vital statistics of the United States. Rockville, MD: 1984; 83.
13. Iskrant AP, Joliet PV. In: Accidents and homicide. Cambridge, MA: Harvard University Press, 1968.
14. National Center for Health Statistics. Persons injured and disability days by delayed type and class of accident: United States, 1971–1972. Rockville, MD: The Center, 1976.
15. National Center for Health Statistics. Vital and Health Statistics of the United States, vol. 2, part A. Rockville, MD: The Center, 1976.
16. Shelton DW, Albright CR. Study in wound ballastics. J Oral Surg 1967; 25: 341.
17. DeMuth WE. Bullet velocity and design as determinants of wounding capability. J Trauma 1966; 6: 222.
18. Jauhari M, Bandyopadhyay A. Wound ballistics: An analysis of a bullet in gel. J Forensic Sci 1976; 21: 616.
19. Callender GR, French RW. Wound ballistics. Milit Surgeon 1935; 77: 177.
20. Herget CM. In: Bowers WF, ed. Wound ballistics: Surgery of trauma. Philadelphia: JB Lippincott Co, 1953; 494.
21. Emergency War Surgery. Washington DC: USGPO, 1975: 10.
22. Swan KG, Swan RC. In: Gunshot wounds: Pathophysiology and management. Chicago: Yearbook Medical Publishers Inc, 1989; 16.
23. Swan KG, Swan RC. In: Gunshot wounds: Pathophysiology and management. Chicago: Yearbook Medical Publishers Inc, 1989; 17.
24. Eckert WG. Exploding bullets. Am J Forensic Med Pathol 1981; 2: 103.
25. Reddick EJ, Carter PL, Bickerstaff L. Airgun injuries in children. Ann Emerg Med 1985; 14: 1108.
26. Chapman AJ. Wandering missiles: Autopsy study. J Trauma 1984; 24: 634.
27. Swan KG, Swan, RC. Wound ballistics. In: Gunshot wounds: Pathophysiology and management. Chicago: Yearbook Medical Publishers Inc, 1989; 18.
28. Selbst SM, Henretig F, Fee MA, et al. Lead poisoning in a child with a gunshot wound. Pediatrics 1986; 3: 413.
29. Linden MA, Manton, WI, Stewart RM, et al. Lead poisoning from retained lead bullets: Pathogenesis, diagnosis, and management. Am Surg 1982; 3: 305.
30. Grogan DP, Buckholz RW. Acute lead intoxication from a bullet in an intervertebral disc space: A case report. J Bone J Surg 1981; 63A: 1180.
31. Bhaskar SN. Pulsating water jet devices in debridement of combat wounds. Milit Med 1971; 136: 264.
32. Barnes K, ed. Medical and surgical history of the war of the rebellion, 1861–1865. Washington: Government Printing Office, 1875; 342.
33. Makley TA, Azar A. Sympathetic ophthalmia: A long term follow-up. Arch Ophthalmol 1978; 96: 257.
34. White JC. Timing of nerve suture after a gunshot wound. Surgery 1960; 48: 946.

26

Sequencing of Care for Multiple Maxillofacial Injuries

Louis G. Mercuri
Mark J. Steinberg

The management of the patient with multiple maxillofacial injuries is complicated by the complex relation of the maxillofacial structures (Fig. 26–1). Proper sequencing of treatment is critical. Multiple maxillofacial injuries must be appropriately timed and sequenced in a logical manner to ensure an optimal surgical outcome. The goals of this chapter are to discuss the proper sequencing of treatment in these difficult and challenging cases and to present some basic surgical principles for the maxillofacial surgeon to follow in the definitive management of such cases.

TIMING OF THE PROCEDURE

The management of a traumatized patient can be divided into five general phases of care (Table 26–1). The concepts of resuscitation and stabilization are discussed elsewhere. In sequencing treatment for multiple maxillofacial injuries, it is critical to be able to differentiate injuries needing immediate operation from those that can be delayed.

Immediate operation may be indicated as a means of initially stabilizing a patient rather than of providing definitive treatment; therefore, those procedures that require more extensive evaluation are delayed to a later date when the patient is systemically stable. Occasionally, the immediate operation can be the definitive procedure. The following are indications for immediate operation in patients with maxillofacial injuries:

Inability to maintain an adequate airway
Severe hemorrhage
Large open wounds
Coincidental surgical procedure being performed

Airway compromise, common in severe maxillofacial injuries, may require immediate operation to temporarily reduce the fractured facial bones encroaching on the airway. Frequently the establishment of a surgical airway is necessary to facilitate later surgical procedures. Severe bleeding from fractured bony segments may also necessitate immediate surgery to ligate associated major vessels or to reduce the segments and thus control the hemorrhage. Large open wounds should not be left open or delayed until definitive management. These wounds should be judiciously debrided and closed in a layered fashion early. Wounds that are to be used later for access to repair fractures may be closed in a temporary manner.

Occasionally, the multiply injured patient is taken to surgery immediately by another service to manage a concomitant injury. It is advantageous to debride and stabilize maxillofacial injuries and even take dental impressions while the patient is anesthetized for

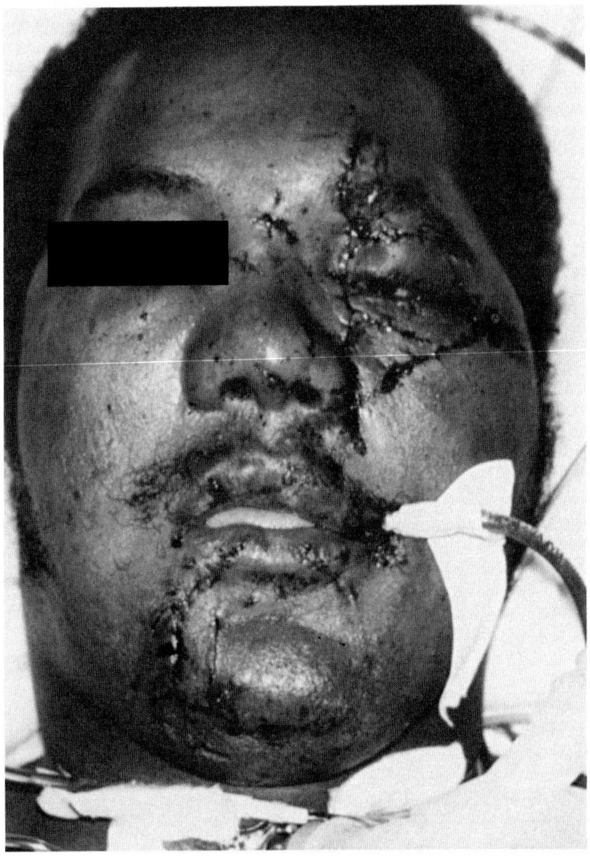

Figure 26–1. *Typical appearance of severe facial trauma. Patient is in need of evaluation and sequencing of treatment. (Courtesy of Dr. A. Thomas Indresano, Cleveland Metropolitan General Hospital, Cleveland, Ohio)*

the other procedure. However, if appropriate imaging studies, consultations, or splints have not yet been secured, it is not advisable to perform definitive procedures simultaneously with another procedure. Although it may be tempting to operate simultaneously in order to minimize anesthesia time, procedures performed in haste without proper evaluation and planning frequently require revision or reoperation at a later date.

Table 26–1. Phases of trauma care

1. Resuscitation
2. Immediate operation
3. Stabilization
4. Delayed operation
5. Recovery

Definitive treatment of maxillofacial injuries can be delayed in the face of severe compromising concomitant systemic trauma. Facial fractures that do not involve cranial structures can be satisfactorily treated up to 2 weeks after injury.[1] Patients having cranial injury or neurologic symptoms should be operated on as soon as their condition is stable. Delaying the definitive procedure allows for accurate evaluation of the injuries, promotes proper planning of the surgical procedure, and allows for correction of blood volume, electrolyte, and nutritional deficits. Resolution of facial edema during this time can aid in the evaluation of the injury and simplify the surgical procedure. Appropriate radiographs, other imaging studies, and consultations with other services can be obtained during this time, and splints and other appliances can be constructed.

PATIENT EVALUATION

Physical Examination

The force of the blow that is necessary to create severe facial injuries must be considered significant enough to have potentially caused concomitant injury to the central nervous system (brain, brain stem, spinal cord), and severe injuries to one or more other body parts (chest, abdomen, pelvis, extremities). The surgeon presented with such complex maxillofacial injuries must be alert to the potential of not only the obvious but also of occult injuries to other systems of the body.

A detailed systematic examination should be carried out on the patient with multiple maxillofacial injuries so as not to miss any of the injuries clinically. The clinical examination in such a patient will often provide more information to the surgeon than the radiographs, which were hastily made on admission to the emergency department and usually are of very poor diagnostic quality; therefore, the importance of a very systematic maxillofacial examination as soon as the patient is stable. This examination should be documented with not only a verbal written description but also with drawings of both the soft and hard tissue injuries (Fig 26–2). This is extremely helpful in the preparation of the treatment plan and in dictation

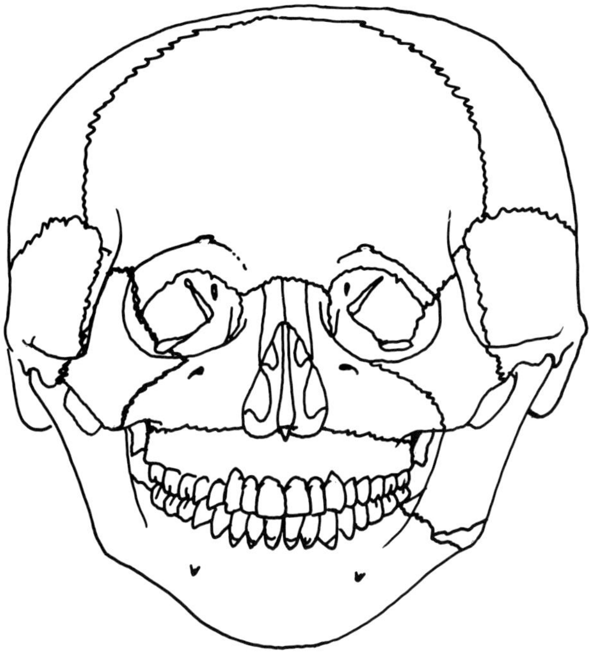

Figure 26–2. *Illustration of facial skeleton shows schematic representation of multiple fractures that were identified from composite radiographic studies.*

for hospital and office records and preparation for deposition, because many of these cases will involve personal injury litigation at some time in the future. Photographs are an excellent means of documenting the preoperative soft tissue injuries.

Work-up

Once the patient has been stabilized systemically and a detailed maxillofacial physical examination is completed and documented, the treatment plan can be prepared using the basic principles for the treatment of maxillofacial injuries presented in prior chapters. Synthesis of these aforementioned principles into one plan is all that is needed in these cases.

Data from the detailed physical examination must be confirmed and correlated with diagnostic radiographic images. As mentioned previously, often initial films are hastily made and consequently of poor quality and must be remade as dictated by the careful and thorough physical examination. The patient shown to be stable enough systemically to proceed with surgery or who requires immediate treatment of the maxillofacial injuries may be taken to the operating room immediately, often leaving no time to remake the radiographs, which only emphasizes further the importance of a thorough physical examination.

Radiographs

Plain films should be ordered as dictated by the physical examination. Because of the complexity of the bony anatomy of the maxillofacial skeleton more sophisticated imaging studies yield better information related to the bony architecture and its disruption by injury than do the plain films. The patient with multiple maxillofacial injuries will often have concomitant head injury, for which computed tomography (CT) will have been done to examine intracranial structures (Fig. 26–3). Many times these examinations are done as a series over days to look for resolution or worsening of an intracranial process. It is very reasonable to request that the radiologist carry one or more of these subsequent studies into and through the maxillofacial region in order to capture in the bone window the normal and disrupted bony architecture. The views most commonly obtained are axial, but coronal and sagittal reconstructions may also be obtained during the same examination (Fig. 26–4).

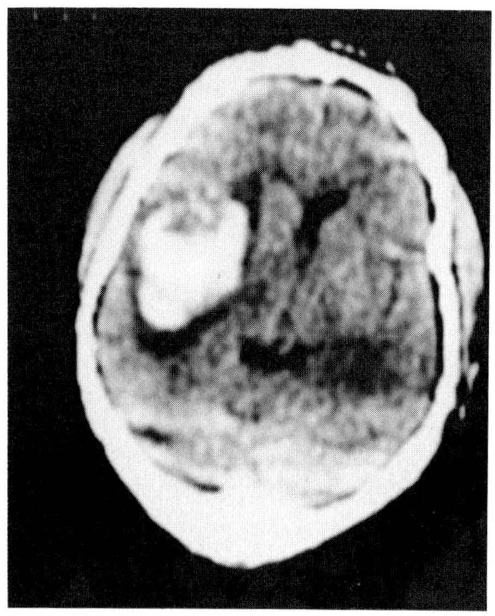

Figure 26–3. *CT examination of brain shows right subdural hematoma. (Courtesy of Dr. A. Thomas Indresano, Cleveland Metropolitan General Hospital, Cleveland, Ohio)*

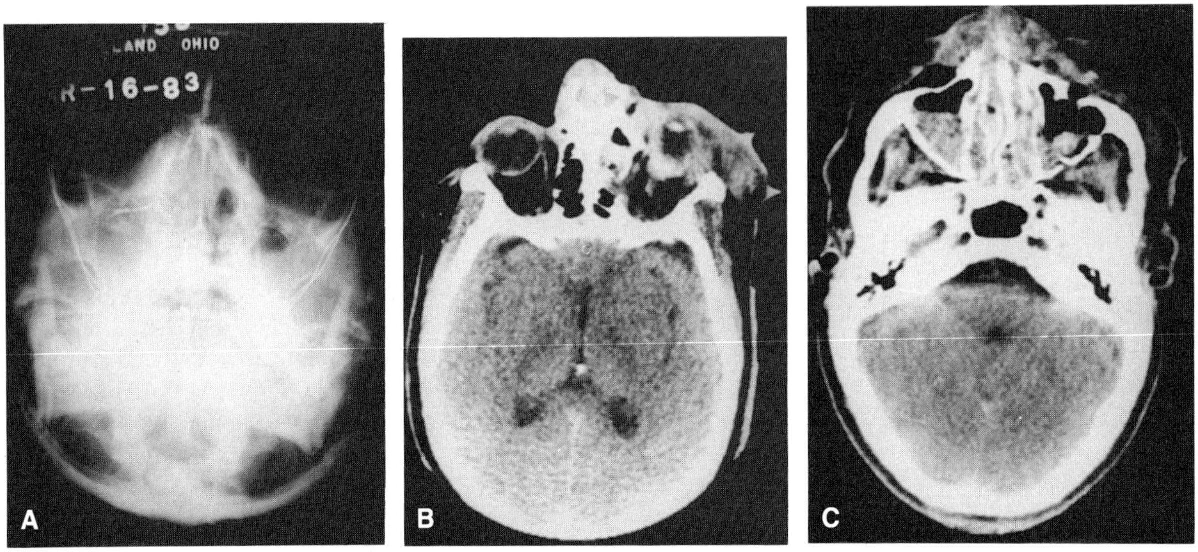

Figure 26–4. *(***A***). Typical Water's view of facial fractures has limited diagnostic value and must be supplemented. (***B***,* **C***) CT cuts with bony window clearly show multiple facial bone fractures. (Courtesy of Dr. A. Thomas Indresano, Cleveland Metropolitan General Hospital, Cleveland, Ohio)*

Three-dimensional CT imaging[2,3] (Fig. 26–5) and computer generated models of the facial skeleton can be useful in complex cases. These modalities add another dimension in the visualization of the bony injuries, which can aid the surgeon to evaluate and reconstruct complicated fractures. Despite the technical and diagnostic limitations of CT imaging in the patient with multiple maxillofacial injuries, it may provide added information as a treatment plan is developed, especially when a systemic problem leads to a delay in treatment.[3]

Tomography is also an adjunct to treatment planning. Once again, such studies are time consuming and are not indicated in the immediate surgery case,

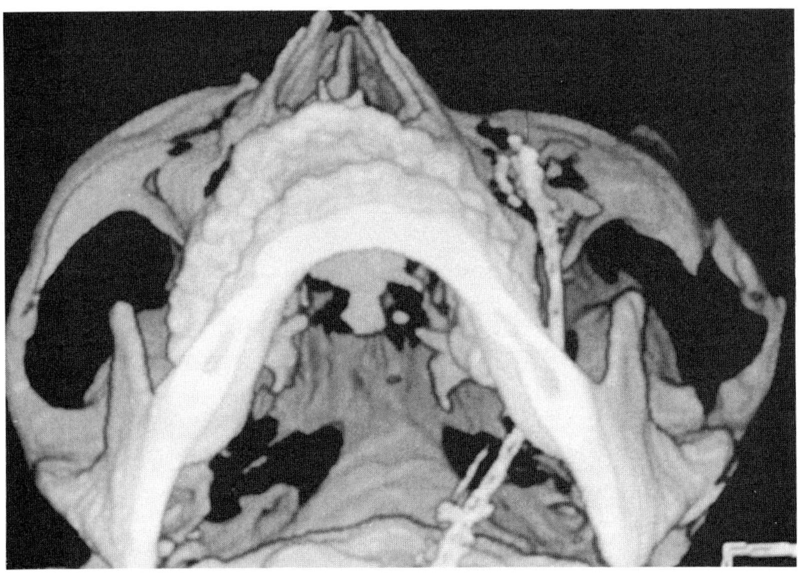

Figure 26–5. *Three-dimensional CT reconstruction is rotated by computer to show the zygomatic arch from below. (Courtesy of Dr. Richard Haug, Cleveland Metropolitan General Hospital, Cleveland, Ohio)*

but they can be used much in the same manner as CT scans are used in cases in which treatment must be delayed. The controversy of CT versus tomograms is usually resolved by the availability of each, the physical condition of the patient, and the preference of the surgeon.[4] Magnetic resonance imaging (MRI) has gained popularity as an imaging study in most areas of medicine, but its utility in maxillofacial traumatology has yet to be elucidated, because the portrayal of bone on the MRI image is not as distinctive as in the other imaging techniques. Also, MRI may be contraindicated in such cases, especially where there is the possibility of the presence of free metallic foreign bodies in the soft tissue of the face or periorbitally (e.g., due to gunshot wound, high-speed motor vehicle accident).

Imaging studies are not a substitute for a thorough, well-documented physical examination in the treatment of the patient with multiple maxillofacial injuries.

Dental Impressions

The multiply injured patient presents the surgeon with a complex reconstruction problem from the start. The basic principles used in the treatment of maxillofacial injuries dictate that the repair begin with an intact mandible as a base upon which to build the maxilla and other facial bones. The second and most important principle is that the key to the repair or reconstruction of the maxillofacial skeleton is the occlusion of the teeth. Therefore, it is often valuable that some documentation of the occlusion of the patient is obtained in the form of study models. Such models are useful in determining the exact position of displaced segments of both the maxilla and mandible attached to teeth, and they draw on the surgeon's knowledge of wear facets of the teeth and occlusion. They are useful in the construction of acrylic stents and splints and in future as records of the preoperative condition of the patient or as reference for any further secondary reconstructive procedures.

Photographs

The use of preoperative photographs (Fig. 26–6) as a form of documentation and data for treatment planning has been mentioned. Preinjury photographs of the patient obtained from the family can be helpful in determining the patient's preinjury appearance and the presence of any preexisting maxillofacial problems such as congenital telecanthism, hypertelorism, apertognathia, prognathism, retrognathism, and nasal deviation. Knowledge of any such preexisting conditions will make repair and reconstruction much easier.

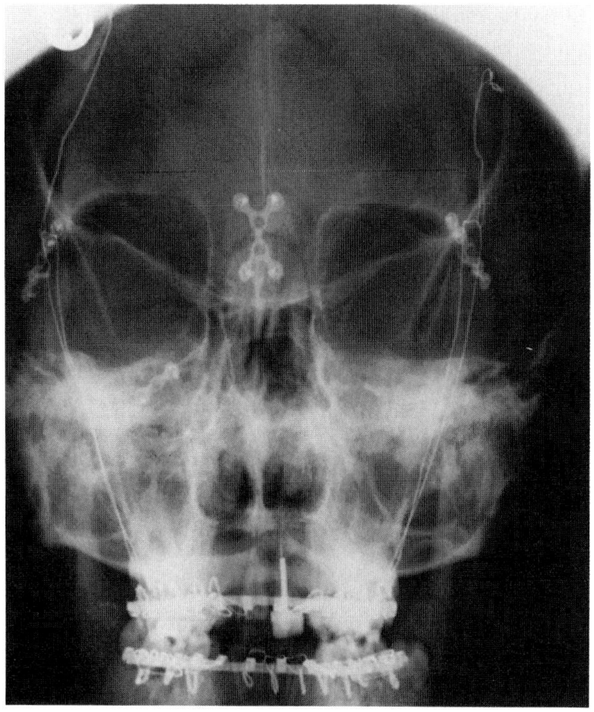

Figure 26–6. *Radiograph is of a patient with multiple facial fractures including LeFort I, bilateral zygoma, nasoethmoidal, and nasal bone fractures. This patient was treated in the sequential fashion outlined in this chapter, working from bottom to top.*

Consultations

The patient with multiple maxillofacial injuries will have sustained a devastating injury through a traumatic incident involving a high velocity impact to the facial region of the head. The incidence of neurologic, ophthalmologic, chest, abdomen, and extremity involvement in such injuries is high. Therefore, after initial clearance by the various consultative services, the maxillofacial surgeon must be particularly sensitive to any systemic physical findings that might be indicative of occult damage to any of these systems. The maxillofacial surgeon must use consultations in all areas to manage the multiply injured patient both preoperatively and postoperatively.

TREATMENT PLANNING

Formulation of the Data Base

Once the physical examination and work-up are completed and any necessary consultations obtained, all this information can be put together to formulate a treatment plan. Having a clear picture of the patient's hard and soft tissue injuries aids the surgeon in planning the surgical approaches and sequencing the procedure. All of the above goes into the formulation of the data base, which is the key step in the preparation of the treatment plan in these complex cases. The information that should be obtained is summarized in Table 26–2.

The most important piece of information is the location and extent of all injuries. From the detailed examination and imaging studies, a schematic illustration can be mapped on a diagram of the skull (see Fig. 26–2). This diagram not only serves to document the nature and extent of the injuries but also aids the surgeon in the determination of surgical approaches to and repair of the fractures or defects.

Another factor that must be considered is the identification of any deficits in the hard and soft tissues involved in the injury, and their location. Management of these defects will have significant bearing on the surgical plan. Minor soft tissue deficits may be addressed by simple advancement of adjacent tissues. A severe soft tissue loss, however, may necessitate consideration of a regional or distant flap to cover the defect. This might influence the incision placement and design and, therefore, must be taken into account before beginning the procedure. Soft tissue deficits also include nerve transection or avulsion. A decision to reanastomose or graft nerve tissue, either as an immediate or delayed procedure, must be incorporated into the overall surgical strategy.

Table 26–2. Data base for multiple maxillofacial injuries

- **I.** Fractures
  - A. Location
  - B. Extent
  - C. Other structures involved
- **II.** Tissue deficits
  - A. Soft tissue loss
    1. Skin
    2. Mucosa
    3. Nerve
  - B. Bone loss
    1. Extent
    2. Tissue cover
  - C. Tooth loss
    1. Vertical height problem
    2. Splint or prosthetic problem

Loss of bone resulting in bony defects may be managed in either an immediate or delayed fashion. Small bony defects with adequate soft tissue coverage may be grafted immediately. An example of this would be a cranial bone graft that reconstructs the floor of the orbit or orbital rim of a fractured zygoma. Harvesting the cranial bone can be done by a bicoronal flap, which would also facilitate the reduction of the zygoma fracture. Large bony defects or defects with poor soft tissue cover are best treated in a delayed fashion. Discontinuity defects are managed by maxillomandibular fixation or internal or external fixation devices. The definitive bone grafting procedure can be accomplished as a secondary procedure.

The loss of teeth is usually addressed at a later stage in the management of the trauma patient. Such deficits can be reconstructed secondarily, but because tooth loss may affect the primary repair surgery it should be considered before the procedure. The ability to relate the maxilla to the mandible may be lost in situations of gross multiple tooth loss. Additionally, loss of posterior teeth may mean loss of vertical dimension. This is of great importance in cases involving mandibular condyle fracture. Establishment of a proper vertical dimension with splint construction is essential in such cases. The use of study models is a valuable adjunct to such cases.

Careful assessment of all the defects requiring repair will generate a list of possible needs for the planned surgery (Table 26–3). Such needs might include autologous grafts (i.e., bone or nerve) or alloplastic devices. The surgeon must know what material is available before performing surgery. Alloplastic devices such as reconstruction plates and prosthetic condyles may have to be special ordered. Autologous grafts frequently require harvesting from a distant site. Informed consent must be obtained for the harvesting of all contemplated grafts. Consideration of these points and the formation of a data base will assist the surgeon in planning a complicated procedure.

Table 26–3. *Possible needs at the time of surgery*

- **I.** Bone grafts
  - A. Local
    - 1. Calvarial
    - 2. Mandible
      - a. Inferior border
      - b. Symphysis
    - 3. Maxilla, lateral wall
- **II.** Soft tissue
  - A. Grafts
    - 1. Skin graft
    - 2. Mucosal graft
    - 3. Fat graft
    - 4. Nerve graft
  - B. Flaps
    - 1. Local
    - 2. Distant
- **III.** Alloplastic devices
  - A. Bone plates
  - B. Bone trays
  - C. Implants
  - D. External fixators, halo devices
  - E. Dental splints

It will also help eliminate surprises and the need for later revision procedures.

Once a data base has been formulated and a treatment plan developed from it, the surgical execution of that plan can then be undertaken. The specific surgical procedures are well described in other sections of this text.

General Treatment Principles

The sequencing of the multiple components of the surgical procedure is guided by two main principles: bottom to top and inside to outside.

Bottom to Top

The maxillofacial surgeon should approach the repair and reconstruction of the maxillofacial skeleton as an architect would the construction of a building. There must be a solid foundation on which to build the upper floors. In the case of the maxillofacial region, the solid foundation is the intact mandible and the upper floors are all of the maxillofacial structures that lie cephalad of the mandible. The patient with multiple maxillofacial injuries must have the unstable or compromised mandible completely stabilized in both its horizontal and vertical planes prior to reduction and fixation of the mid- and upper facial structures.

Observing the principles of mandibular fracture repair the maxillofacial surgeon must stabilize this component of the injury first. Proper vertical height must be reestablished. In situations where vertical height is lost secondary to bilateral mandibular fractures, open reductions or splint fabrication may be necessary to restore appropriate facial height. One of the relative indications for open reduction of a mandibular condyle fracture is bilateral condyle fractures in association with midfacial fractures.[5]

Once the mandible is stabilized, the unstable, displaced, or segmented maxilla is brought into its appropriate relation to the mandible by using the occlusion of the teeth for that specific patient. At this point, the advantage of the dental impressions and study models can be appreciated. The surgeon can determine from the wear facets on the teeth preoperatively the specific occlusion in each case, resulting in a less tedious intraoperative course. In addition, by knowing ahead of time that there may be an instability in that specific patient's occlusion, the surgeon can construct a splint as an interocclusal wafer to add stability to the fixation. Once the maxilla has been fixated to the stabilized mandible, attention can be directed to any zygomatic, naso-orbital-ethmoidal or frontal compromise present.

Zygomaticomaxillary fractures can be easily related and fixated to the stabilized maxilla. Frontal and supraorbital rim fractures can then be reduced based on the position of the frontozygomatic and frontomaxillary sutures that have been established from the stabilized zygoma and maxilla. Naso-orbital-ethmoidal complexes can now be related to the reduced maxilla and frontal bones. Nasal fractures are treated at the completion of these other fractures (see Fig. 26–6).

Like an architect, the maxillofacial surgeon has followed a logical and planned course in the repair and reconstruction of the maxillofacial skeleton, from the stable base of the mandible to the top of the head.

Inside to Outside

In multiple maxillofacial injuries, closure of the soft tissues should proceed from the bone or oral cavity outward toward the skin. Lacerations of the pharynx, tongue, and palate should be closed prior to placing the patient in maxillomandibular fixation. Lacerations of the lips and buccal mucosa are best repaired after the patient is placed in maxillomandibular fixation. The stretching of the tissues during placement of the arch bars and dental wires is usually sufficient to reopen wounds that were previously closed. The oral mucosa of a through-and-through wound must be debrided and repaired. There is no indication for leaving the oral mucosa open and closing just the dermis and skin of the face in such a wound.

The surgeon should carry out a thorough examination of the soft tissue injuries associated with the multiple maxillofacial injuries. This is best carried out after the patient has been anesthetized. This examination can be facilitated by the use of copious irrigation with a sterile isotonic solution, which acts as a mechanical debridement not only for potential foreign bodies but also blood clots and organisms. Once the soft tissue wounds have been irrigated and explored, care must be taken not to condemn injured tissue to instrument debridement at this point. Such debridement should be done after it has been determined that the associated laceration cannot be used for entry to repair the bony discontinuity, or after the laceration has been used to gain access for bony repair or reconstruction. All lacerations should be thoroughly irrigated, debrided, and closed only after all bony surgery has been completed.

Frequently the traumatic laceration may be used or extended to approach the fracture. In cases in which the traumatic lacerations do not provide convenient access for bony repair or reconstruction, the surgeon must determine access to the facial skeleton by using the appropriate incisions for the specific bony injuries. Incision design and location is guided by the overall treatment plan in an effort to do as much as possible through a minimal amount of esthetically placed incisions. For example, the bicoronal incision approach is a convenient and efficient means of access in multiple maxillofacial injuries that involve the naso-orbital-ethmoidal complex alone or with the zygomaticomaxillary complex; the frontal or supraorbital bones; or the use of cranial bone as a bone graft.

Multiple maxillofacial trauma cases at first glance appear complex and difficult to treat. However, they are actually a conglomeration of many smaller procedures that are commonplace in oral and maxillofacial surgical practice. It is crucial that the surgeon be able to coordinate and properly sequence these procedures to achieve the optimal result in these cases. The development of a step-by-step treatment plan prior to surgery and adherence to the general principles of maxillofacial trauma will facilitate the treatment of these cases.

REFERENCES

1. Irby WB. Facial Trauma and Concomitant Problems, ed 2. St Louis: CV Mosby, 1979.
2. DeMarino DP, Steiner E, Poster RB, et al. Three dimensional computed tomography in maxillofacial trauma. Arch Otolaryngol Head Neck Surg 1986; 112:146.
3. Gillespie JE, Quale AA, Barker G. Three-dimensional CT reformations in the assessment of congenital and traumatic cranio-facial deformities. Br J Oral Maxillofac Surg 1987; 25:171.
4. Bernardo N, Leban SG, Williams FA. A comparison of radiographic treatment methods for evaluation of the orbit. J Oral Maxillofac Surg 1988; 46:844.
5. Zide MF, Kent JN. Indications for open reduction of mandibular fractures. J Oral Maxillofac Surg 1983; 41:89.

27

Diagnosis and Management of Pediatric Craniomaxillofacial Fractures

Jeffrey C. Posnick

Facial fractures are generally managed according to the dictum "form follows function." The goal therefore is to reestablish the bony anatomic condition and apply fixation measures adequate enough to allow for bony healing and rapid return of normal function.

When the patient is considered too ill to undergo ideal facial fracture management, endotracheal intubation or tracheostomy may be needed to bypass the airway and a nasogastric tube inserted or gastrostomy performed to replace oral feedings. Fortunately these measures are rarely required.

When options for fracture fixation are available, the method used is determined by the patient's total treatment plan. It must be individualized to accommodate the overall healing of each facial fracture and the timely restoration of normal upper airway breathing, swallowing, and chewing, especially in the medically compromised patient.

CONSULTATION

Appropriate, early, preoperative consultation is essential for good patient management. Patients with multiple-system trauma and facial injuries must first be assessed by a pediatric trauma surgeon. This surgeon will suggest additional consultations and clear the patient for repair of facial fractures as indicated.

Whenever cranial base fractures, cranial vault fractures, or intracranial (brain) trauma has occurred, neurosurgical consultation is mandatory. If orbital fractures or eye trauma has occurred or if any operative manipulation of the orbit is planned, an ophthalmologic consultation is essential. If the facial nerve, nasolacrimal apparatus, or Stensen duct of the parotid gland has been lacerated, consultation with a microsurgeon should be arranged. If the dentition has been injured or the occlusion changed from the preinjury state, a surgeon with dental expertise should be involved.

Once a decision has been made to perform an examination under anesthesia or undertake more definitive surgical intervention, discussion should follow with the consulting anesthesiologist and operating room nursing staff. They can then ensure that the necessary instrumentation is available at the time of operation.

EARLY MANAGEMENT OF PEDIATRIC PATIENTS WITH MULTIPLE-SYSTEM TRAUMA

The general principles for resuscitating multiple-trauma patients are well described in the *Advanced Trauma Life Support Course of the American College of Surgeons*.[54] Early treatment is divided into four phases: primary survey, initial resuscitation, secondary survey, and definitive treatment. Although the systematic approach is useful in caring for pediatric patients, there are differences between pediatric and adult patients that must be kept in mind.

Facts to Remember When Managing Pediatric Trauma

1. Children have a much larger body surface area to mass ratio and are therefore more prone to develop hypothermia.
2. Children swallow air when they are injured or frightened, especially when they have an intraabdominal injury, and will therefore have gastric dilation.
3. Abdominal girth and the volume of the peritoneal cavity in children and infants are relatively small. Significant intraabdominal bleeding usually leads to a change in girth.
4. Infants are nose breathers, and their air passages are relatively narrow.
5. The chest wall in children is very pliable, and major thoracic injuries may exist with few external signs of trauma.
6. Children may maintain normal or borderline blood pressure levels despite significant hypovolemia because of their ability to constrict their vascular bed.

Practical Considerations

Airway Management

The establishment and maintenance of an adequate airway are fundamental to the management of acutely traumatized patients. The preferred method is endotracheal intubation with cervical spine control. The size of tube needed is roughly determined by the size of the child's external nares or fifth finger. Appropriately sized laryngoscope blades for intubation are also critical.

Venous Access

In urgent circumstances, a saphenous vein in the groin may be used for access. When rapid vascular access is required in children with circulatory collapse or cardiac arrest, intraosseous infusion may be used as an initial alternative to standard intravenous cannulation during the early phase of resuscitation. The intraosseous needle is inserted into the marrow cavity of the proximal tibia in children under 5 years of age and into the distal tibia in children over 5 years of age.

EPIDEMIOLOGY OF PEDIATRIC FACIAL FRACTURES

Of 336 pediatric patients who sustained facial fractures, 113 sustained concurrent injuries to other body regions, the distribution of which is shown in Table 27–1. In this study 55 patients had associated head trauma and of these, 22 (40%) sustained skull fractures.[1] Another 17 had associated ocular injuries, including six with blind eyes, six with eyes with reduced visual acuity, and two with eyes with residual diplopia. Only one patient had associated cervical spine injury. The high incidence of head and ocular trauma and low incidence of cervical spine and abdominal trauma are interesting because they contrast with observations in adults with facial trauma. Nearly one third of the fractures were the result of motor vehicle accidents (MVAs) (Table 27–2).

The facial fractures were broken down by region as follows: orbit, zygoma, nose, midface, and mandibular and dentoalveolar (Table 27–3). The most frequently injured region was the nose (38%) and the mandible (32%). Single fractures were seen in 23 subjects, 42 had multiple fractures at a single site, and 60 had multiple fractures at multiple sites (e.g., mandible, maxilla, and zygoma). A breakdown by region of the mandibular fractures sustained is shown in Table 27–4, demonstrating that the most frequently injured is the condylar region (40%). Associated soft-tissue injuries, mostly consisting of facial abrasions and lacerations, occurred in 25% of the patients.

Table 27–1. Injuries Associated with Pediatric Facial Fractures

Associated Injuries	Number
Head	55 (49%)
Ocular	17 (15%)
Cervical spine	1 (1%)
Thorax	5 (4%)
Abdomen	4 (4%)
Extremity	22 (19%)
Other	9 (8%)

n = 113

(Smith KA, Posnick JC, et al. Facial fractures in the pediatric population: Ten years experience. In: Proceedings of the 43rd Annual Meeting of the Canadian Society of Plastic Surgeons, June 1989; 1)

Table 27–2. Etiology of Pediatric Facial Fractures

Etiology	Number
Vehicle/passenger	60 (18%)
Vehicle/pedestrian	33 (10%)
Bicycle	22 (7%)
Fall	53 (16%)
Sport	65 (19%)
Altercation	28 (8%)
All-terrain vehicles	6 (2%)
Other	69 (20%)

n = 336
(Smith KA, Posnick JC, et al. Facial fractures in the pediatric population: Ten years experience. In: Proceedings of the 43rd Annual Meeting of the Canadian Society of Plastic Surgeons, June 1989; 1)

Numerous review articles, book chapters, and incidence studies on the subject of pediatric facial fractures are available.[2–12,14–19]

SURGICAL ANATOMY

Maxillofacial trauma is much less common in younger children than in adolescents or adults. The comparative immunity of children to facial fractures is a result of environmental, physical, and craniofacial anatomic factors.[19]

Before the age of 5 years most children live a relatively protected existence in which close parental supervision provides a safeguard to their spontaneous, curious spirit and general lack of caution.[17] Although falls are frequent, they usually occur from minimal heights and the momentum gained by the child's small body is of a low velocity. As a result, the low-impact force can usually be absorbed by the generally well-padded skin, elastic skeleton, and cartilaginous growth centers between the bones.

Table 27–3. Regions Fractured in Pediatric Facial Injuries

Region	Number
Orbit	57 (12%)
Zygoma	32 (7%)
Nose	175 (38%)
Midface	27 (6%)
Mandibular	148 (32%)
Dentoalveolar	25 (5%)

n = 464
(Smith KA, Posnick JC, et al. Facial fractures in the pediatric population: Ten years experience. In: Proceedings of the 43rd Annual Meeting of the Canadian Society of Plastic Surgeons, June 1989; 1)

Table 27–4. Pediatric Mandible Fractures

Region	Number
Condyle	58 (39%)
Ramus	15 (10%)
Coronoid	1 (1%)
Angle	16 (11%)
Body	17 (11%)
Parasymphysis/symphysis	41 (28%)

n = 148
(Smith KA, Posnick JC, et al. Facial fractures in the pediatric population: Ten years experience. In: Proceedings of the 43rd Annual Meeting of the Canadian Society of Plastic Surgeons, June 1989; 1)

After 5 years of age, children become active at school, begin to play contact sports and ride a bicycle, and travel more often in automobiles. Height, weight, and muscular development increase and are often combined with a more competitive and physical manner that leads to more frequent falls from greater heights, with a resultant increase in direct facial trauma.

For the first several years of life, the cranium is relatively large with a prominent forehead. The orbits are also well developed, closely following brain and cranial growth. This period is marked by a lack of maxillary and ethmoid sinus development, as well as by limited dental development. As a result, there is minimal downward projection of the face in infancy and early childhood. These factors result in a high skull-to-face ratio, leaving the frontal bones, brain, upper orbits, and eyes more exposed to trauma, whereas the facial bones are relatively protected (Fig. 27–1).

From the time of birth until skeletal maturity, the size of the cranium increases fourfold and that of the facial bones increases tenfold. Approximately 85% to 90% of cranial vault and orbital growth is complete by the age of 5 years. In contrast, the jaws are small at

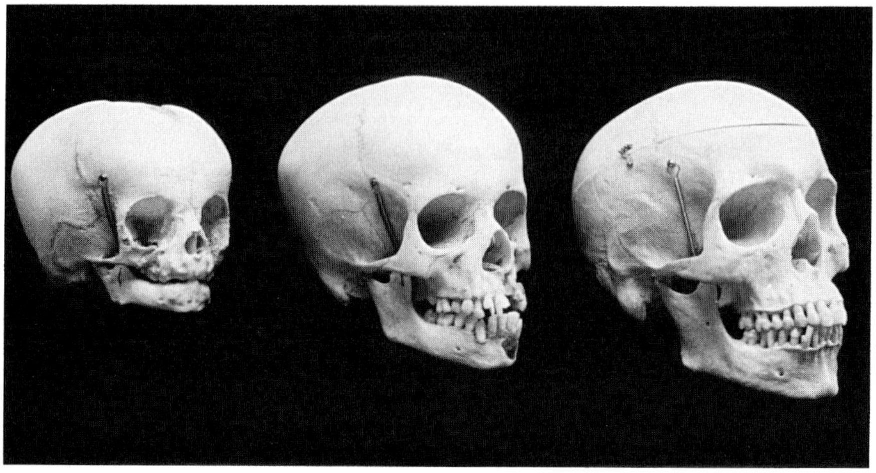

Figure 27–1. *Dry skulls of various ages demonstrated in oblique view. Ages of skulls are approximately 6 months, 11 years, and 20 years. (Posnick JC. Role of plate and screw fixation in the treatment of paediatric facial fractures. In: Yaremchuk MJ. Rigid Fixation of the Craniomaxillofacial Skeleton. England: Butterworth, 1992)*

birth, throughout infancy, and during much of childhood. The maxilla is not separated from the cranial base by well-pneumatized air sinuses as it is in later life. The condylar process of the mandible is well vascularized; its neck is thick and short, making the mandible a strong region in comparison with its thin shape and limited strength later in childhood and adolescence. The mandible and maxilla grow rapidly in childhood with a high ratio of cancellous to cortical bone. This results in greater elasticity in the jaws and in more greenstick and nondisplaced fractures than are seen in adulthood. In children, the periosteum is extremely osteogenic, leading to early bony union and active remodeling of the healed bone.

During the first few years of life, the developing permanent teeth are incompletely formed and the ratio of tooth to bone is relatively low. Later, in the mixed deciduous and permanent dentition phase, this ratio changes. The resulting high tooth-to-bone ratio weakens the mandible and encourages fracture through the developing tooth crypts. In adults, a linear pattern is usually seen in mandibular fractures, whereas in children the fracture line is often irregular, as the bone shears between the crypts of the developing teeth.

Later in childhood and adolescence, the development of the maxillary and other paranasal sinuses produces areas of weakness and is a major factor in the shift of facial bone fractures towards the zygomatic bones and LeFort (midface) fractures.

AIRWAY MANAGEMENT

The first step in managing a traumatized patient is to ensure a patent airway. An adequate spontaneous or assisted airway must be established and maintained throughout fracture healing.

When an artificial airway is required, endotracheal intubation is almost always possible and in pediatric patients is preferred to a tracheostomy. A tracheostomy with its associated complications is performed only as a last resort.[20,21] Possible indications for tracheostomy include long-term management of central nervous system (CNS) impairment, management of a direct tracheal injury, a need to maintain adequate pulmonary toilet, and situations in which the larynx cannot be intubated using endotracheal procedures.

PRINCIPLES OF TREATMENT BY REGION

Cranial Vault and Supraorbital Ridge Fractures

These injuries are more common in the infant or young child (less than 5 years of age) when craniofacial injury does occur.

Thorough evaluation using computed tomography (CT) scanning, neurosurgical assessment, and ophthalmologic consultation must be performed. Unless direct lacerations provide adequate exposure for fracture treatment, a coronal incision is usually made. A thorough subperiosteal dissection of the fracture region with complete exposure out to the region of normal anatomic structures is generally required. Fixation is achieved using either direct interosseous wires or miniplates or microplates as indicated. When bony defects are present, primary bone grafting using autogenous cranial bone is preferred to secondary bone grafting. A combined procedure is carried out with the neurosurgeon if intracranial exposure is required as part of the trauma management or if exposure is needed for fracture reduction.

Nasofrontoethmoid Fractures

These injuries can occur at any age and generally result from direct trauma at the level of the frontonasal suture.

Preoperative assessment, incisions, and dissection for nasofrontoethmoid fractures are similar to those required for cranial vault and orbital ridge fractures. Plate-and-screw internal fixation and primary cranial bone grafting are employed to achieve and maintain anatomic reduction and adequate fixation to permit bone healing in the preinjury location. If the medial canthal ligament is displaced, it is usually attached to a bone fragment. If at all possible, the medial canthal ligament–bone fragment unit is repositioned and immobilized without using a direct medial canthopexy procedure. Formal medial canthopexies often contribute to an unnatural appearance. During the periorbital dissection and fracture reduction process, it is essential to avoid iatrogenic injury to the nasolacrimal apparatus.

When the frontal sinus is injured, anterior table fractures should be anatomically repositioned and stabilized if a cosmetic deformity would otherwise result. If the fracture components are severely comminuted, it is often preferable to harvest cranial bone graft and replace the injured region. Depending on the extent of sinus fracture, the mucous membranes may require debridement with maintenance of a patent nasofrontal duct. If the posterior table of the frontal sinus is also fractured, neurosurgical consultation is needed to determine whether it is necessary to remove the posterior table and obliterate the nasofrontal duct (cranialization of the sinus). The possible growth disturbance to the supraorbital ridge must be considered if the frontal sinus is injured or debrided at an early age.

LeFort I, II, and III Fractures

LeFort fractures generally occur in older children and adolescents and should be treated with open reduction and internal fixation as required to achieve anatomic restoration (Fig. 27–2). Closed reduction is often preferred in the younger child to avoid injury to the unerupted permanent dentition.

The use of a maxillary circumvestibular mucosal incision gives excellent exposure to fractures through the zygomatic buttress, anterior maxillary wall, and piriform nasal aperture regions. Fracture is often through the infraorbital neurovascular foramen with resulting paresthesia to the upper lip, lateral nasal, and cheek skin. When access to the combined areas of the zygomatic arch, frontozygomatic suture, and supraorbital ridge regions is required, a coronal incision is generally preferred. Occasionally a subciliary, upper eyelid and intraoral incision are combined to avoid the coronal approach.

The goal of midface and zygomatic fracture fixation in children is to restore normal anatomic position of the skeleton and immobilize the segments for fracture healing.[22] This is frequently accomplished with bone grafts, the use of direct wires, and miniplate or microplate and screw fixation, as in adults.

Zygomatic Complex Fractures

A zygomatic complex (ZMC) fracture denotes a fracture through the frontozygomatic suture, zygomatic buttress, infraorbital rim, and zygomatic arch. With displacement of the ZMC fracture, the orbital floor and lateral orbital wall are also fractured.

The most common physical findings in a ZMC fracture are periorbital ecchymosis, numbness over the zygomatic arch, and subconjunctival hemorrhage. Treatment is similar to that in adults. If a comminuted zygomatic arch fracture is associated with a ZMC fracture, a coronal incision is frequently combined with intraoral incisions to give full exposure for reduction and fixation.

When minimally displaced or incomplete ZMC

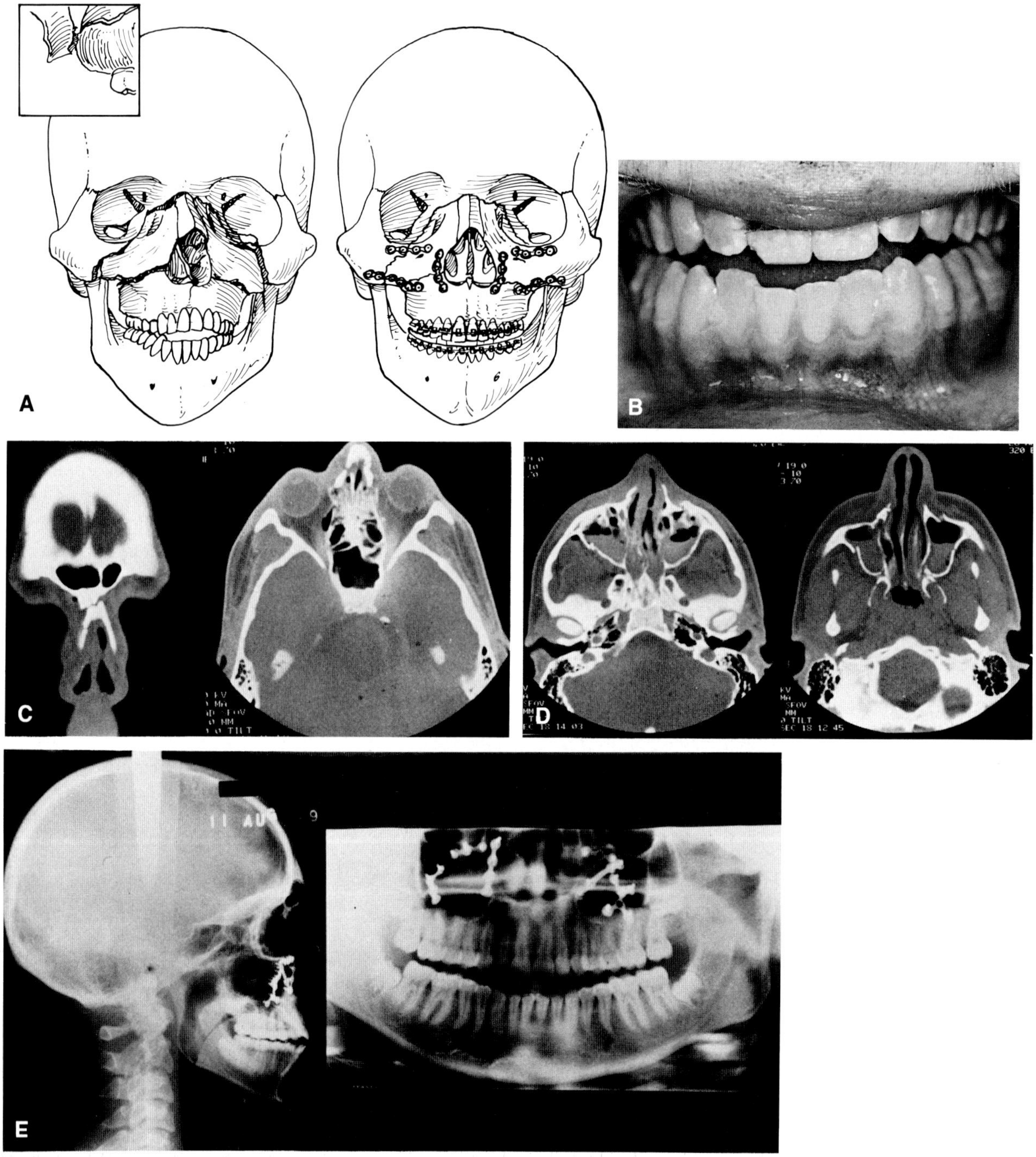

Figure 27–2. *A 14-year-old boy who sustained combined LeFort I and II fractures with bilateral orbital floor blow-out fractures when he was kicked in the face. (**A**) Illustration of location of fractures, reduction, and methods of fixation. (**B**) Occlusal view demonstrating open bite caused by the fracture. (**C**) Computed tomographic (CT) scan demonstrating nasofrontal bone separation and comminuted medial orbital walls. (**D**) CT scan demonstrating fractures through anterior and posterior maxillary walls. (**E**) Postoperative plain radiographs demonstrating location of miniplate and screw fixation. (**F**) Full face view 2 years after surgery. (**G**) Occlusal view 2 years after surgery. (**B–G** from Posnick JC. Role of plate and screw fixation in the treatment of paediatric facial fractures. In: Yaremchuk MJ. Rigid Fixation of the Craniomaxillofacial Skeleton. England: Butterworth, 1992)*

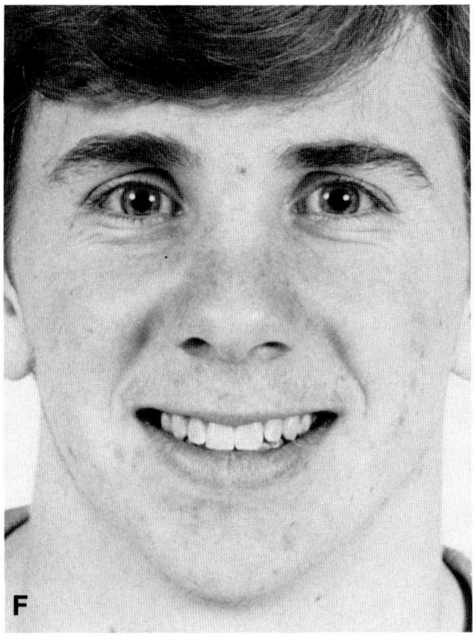
F

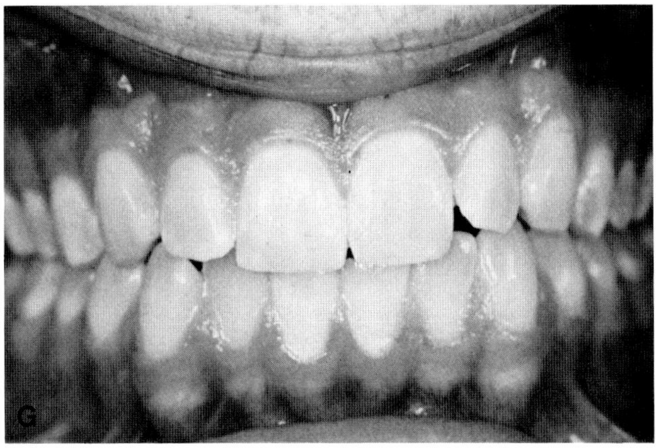
G

Figure 27–2. *(continued)*

fractures occur, local incisions (i.e., lateral brow, subciliary, and intraoral) can be used to gain needed exposure and avoid a coronal incision.

Blow-Out Fractures

Blow-out fractures may occur as isolated events involving one or more orbital walls. They may also be associated with more complex fractures (i.e., nasofrontoethmoid, cranial vault-supraorbital ridge, ZMC, LeFort II, or LeFort III). A thorough ophthalmologic assessment is mandatory and an adequate CT scan with coronal cuts is essential for complete orbital evaluation.

It is important to visualize all four orbital walls on the preoperative CT scan to be certain that all blow-out (Fig. 27–3) or blow-in fractures are recognized and treated with appropriate soft tissue repositioning and bony reconstruction to regain the preinjury intraorbital volume. When frontoorbital fractures occur, a blow-in fracture of the orbital roof commonly results and may be overlooked, thus requiring secondary reconstruction. Manson has outlined the mechanism of injury, surgical anatomic status, and general indications for surgical intervention in blow-out fractures.[23] Because the complications of entrapment, enophthalmus, and diplopia are difficult to treat later, early evaluation, recognition of patients at high risk, and surgical intervention are mandatory.

If left untreated, blow-out fractures heal rapidly in children and result in scar cicatrization of the herniated orbital contents. When indicated, early exploration, followed by intraorbital soft tissue repositioning and reconstruction of orbital walls to appropriate dimensions and volume, is preferred.

Nasal Fractures

The growth of the nasal septum is often considered a major factor in midface development.[24,25] In theory, severe trauma to this region in childhood could retard normal growth, resulting in a saddle nose and total midface deficiency. However, the nasal area is the most frequently fractured part of the face in children, and yet, extensive midface growth retardation is rarely documented. Moreover, Tulasne and Tessier have described cases of orbital hypertelorism in which patients underwent nasal septal resection at a young age. Follow-up study to adulthood showed no resulting midface collapse.[26]

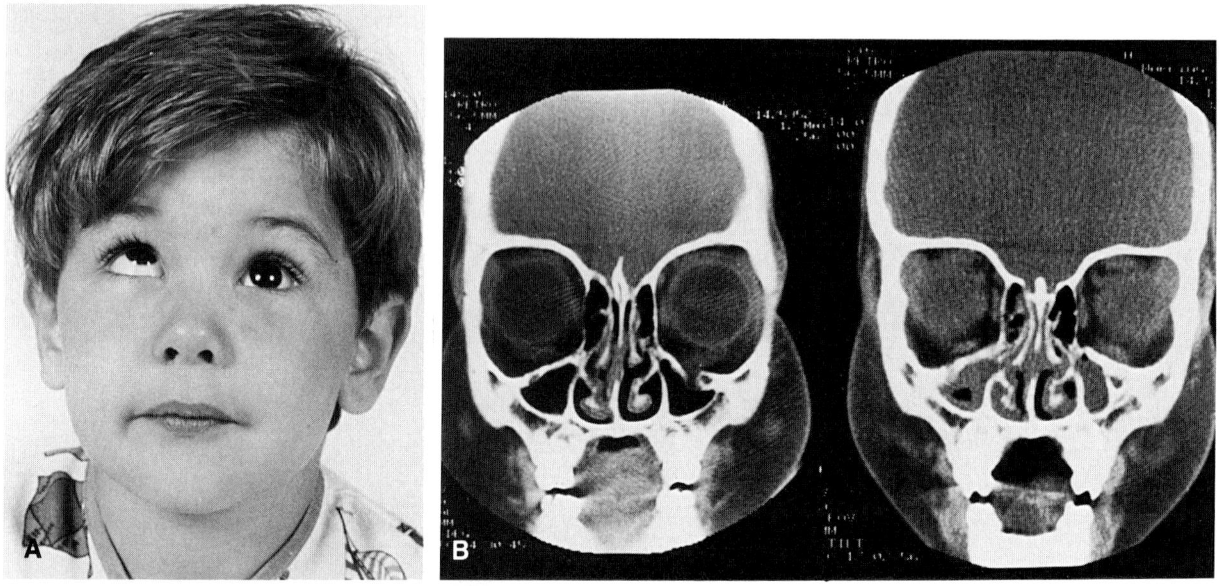

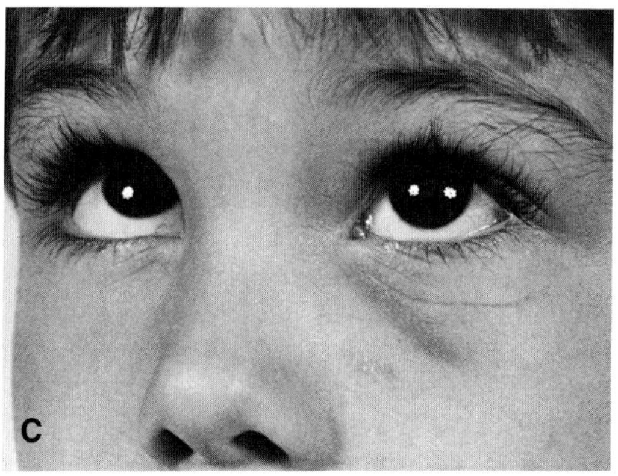

Figure 27–3. *A 4-year-old boy sustained an isolated orbital floor blow-out fracture with entrapment of the inferior rectus muscle through the orbital floor defect. He underwent explorative surgery with repositioning of the orbital contents back into the orbit. Reconstruction of the orbit floor defect was with split cranial grafts taken from the temporoparietal region. (**A**) Frontal view with eyes in upward gaze demonstrating left inferior rectus entrapment. (**B**) Two-dimensional coronal computed tomographic scan through midorbits demonstrating left orbital floor defect before and after reconstruction. (**C**) Close-up view early after reconstruction demonstrating improved upward gaze ability. (Posnick JC. Role of plate and screw fixation in the treatment of paediatric facial fractures. In: Yaremchuk MJ. Rigid Fixation of the Craniomaxillofacial Skeleton. England: Butterworth, 1992)*

Nasal fractures are often treated but then ignored as unimportant, and as a result, late deformity with functional symptoms is frequently seen. Late problems from malunion include a deviated pyramid, nasal dorsal "hump," and septal deformity with resulting partial nasal obstruction. The most serious pitfall in treating nasal fractures is the failure to recognize those extending outside the nose.[13] Adjacent fractures may include the maxilla, orbit, frontal sinus, or frontal bone regions.

The residual malalignment of nasal bones despite surgical manipulation may be masked by edema. Laterally deviated greenstick fractures are the most common in the pediatric population. If closed reduction is carried out, completion of the fracture by manipulation to avoid the problem of incomplete reduction is suggested.

A septal hematoma after nasal trauma is more likely to occur in children than in adults. This complication must be watched for and drainage instituted once it is identified if septal necrosis and perforation is to be prevented or limited.

PRINCIPLES OF MANDIBLE FRACTURE REPAIR

Mandibular fractures in children present a changing anatomy that in some ways resembles that in the adult.[27-31] Fracture patterns are affected by the fact that the child's mandible is filled with teeth in various stages of development. Injury to the developing tooth buds may result not only from the trauma of the fracture but also from overzealous and misdirected open reduction techniques.

In theory, either the primary or the mixed dentition can present obstacles to the application of surgical arch bars and intermaxillary fixation (IMF). However, once one becomes familiar with the variations in dentition, arch bars can be placed and IMF carried out with relative certainty, even in 2-year-old children. Circumandibular, circumzygomatic, infraorbital, and piriform aperture wires can be used as needed for extra support (Fig. 27–4).

When internal fixation techniques are required, either direct interosseous wire fixation or mini or micro plate-and-screw fixation must be applied carefully so that drill holes are located at or close to the mandibular inferior border to avoid the developing teeth.

In general, loose teeth and alveolar fractures should be supported with surgical immobilization until bone union has occurred (4 to 6 weeks).[32–34] It is rarely adequate to treat dentoalveolar fractures with a soft diet alone. If the involved primary teeth are almost ready to come out naturally and are not attached to alveolar bone, extraction is a better procedure than reduction.

The general principles of treating mandibular fractures are the same in children and adults: fixation of the bony fragments in their preinjury pattern with the teeth in their preinjury occlusion and the establishment of stabilization until bone union has occurred. Children have some flexibility in regard to occlusion; when the primary teeth exfoliate and the permanent teeth erupt, minor discrepancies in occlusion may be self-correcting or at least amenable to orthodontic alignment.

As a result of the greatly increased osteogenic potential of the mandible, union will occur rapidly and the fragments become sticky within the first week. For these reasons early definitive treatment is indicated. Specific treatment recommendations depend on the type of fracture (i.e., greenstick or complete), its location (e.g., condyle, body), age of the patient, presence of other facial fractures, and presence of other associated systemic injuries and illnesses. Efforts must be made not only to normalize occlusion but also to prevent impairment of the developing dentition and preserve temporomandibular joint (TMJ) mobility; otherwise, mandibular range of motion could be restricted and growth distortions could occur.

Condylar Process

The treatment of fractures of the mandibular condylar process remains controversial.[35–53] Most authors advocate a conservative approach, whereas a few prefer a more frequent use of open reduction techniques.[52,53]

The condylar head is an important growth center of the mandible, the final facial bone to complete its normal growth and development. Its growth is generally complete in girls by the age of 14 to 16 years and in boys by the age of 16 to 18 years. Injury to the condylar head before these ages may lead to growth retardation with resulting facial asymmetry and malocclusion.

It is likely that the condylar growth center does not maintain a constant low level of activity but rather experiences high-growth rates at specific times.[18] From birth to 12 years of age, the face undergoes continual growth but its velocity varies with age. Growth is very rapid up to 6 months of age, relatively slow from 6 months to 4 years, rapid again between 4 and 7 years, and then slower between 9 and 15 years of age. The last facial growth phase, between 15 and 19 years of age, primarily affects the mandible. Condylar injury (fracture or compression) before the age of 3 years will likely result in significant mandibular growth distortion but after 12 years of age will have little effect on growth.[18] Between these ages, a wide spectrum of effects may be seen.

Secondary growth distortion may occur in adjacent regions following mandible distortion. This is most commonly seen in the maxilla, with canting of the occlusal plane and shifting of the maxillary dental midline off the facial midline. Growth distortions may be seen in the nasal septum, nasal bones, zygoma, and even the orbit. When a condylar fracture occurs in early childhood and goes unrecognized, the whole side of the face may appear hypoplastic and be confused with hemifacial microsomia.

When considering condylar fractures and their treatment, it is important to recognize that not all these fractures are the same. They may be either intracapsular or extracapsular, displaced or nondisplaced, open or closed, low–condylar neck or high–condylar

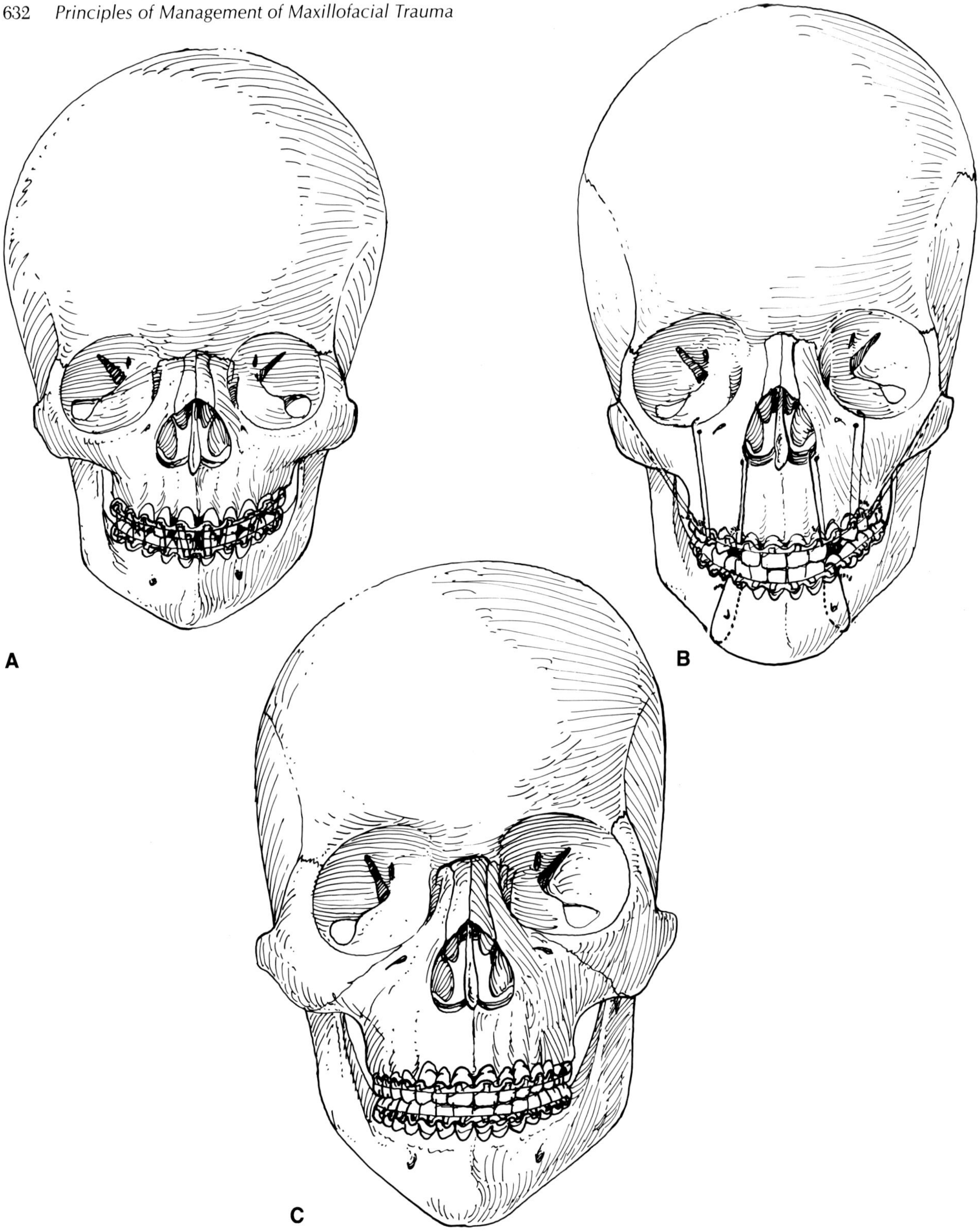

Figure 27–4. *Illustration of three skulls of various ages ([**A**] 2 years, [**B**] 6 years, and [**C**] 12 years of age). Different methods of direct wire fixation are demonstrated. These include arch bars and intermaxillary fixation, circumandibular, circumzygomatic, infraorbital, and piriform sinus skeleton fixation.*

neck, medial or lateral pole fractures. When a complete fracture of the condylar process occurs, the fracture segment is generally dislocated anteriorly and medially. Dislocation of the segment results directly from spasm of the lateral pterygoid muscle, which originates on the lateral pterygoid plate and inserts on the condylar head.

Dislocation of the condylar fragment is accompanied by a loss of posterior facial height on the affected side, with resulting premature contact of the posterior teeth on the fracture side. With wide vertical opening or protrusive excursion, the mandible shifts to the side of the fracture.

On radiographic examination the fragment may be visualized in its displaced location. The surgeon, who wants to restore anatomic status and function, is therefore tempted to suggest open reduction and internal fixation on a regular basis. However, the treatment options for condylar process fractures should vary depending on the location of the fracture. For example, intracapsular fractures of the condylar head and high–condylar neck fractures are both poor candidates for open reduction and internal fixation (ORIF). Low–condylar neck fractures (extending into the ramus) may be suitable for ORIF, but unfortunately they make up only a small proportion of condylar fractures. Overzealous attempts at surgical exploration with combined preauricular-coronal, submandibular, and intraoral incisions for condylar exposure, fracture reduction, and fixation often result in incomplete fracture reduction, devascularization of the condylar head, and injury to branches of the facial nerve. Furthermore, it has not been clearly demonstrated that a lower incidence of growth disturbance, TMJ ankylosis, or malocclusion can be achieved through open reduction techniques than through the use of more conservative treatment measures. It may be that the growth-center injury from the blunt trauma and ischemia resulted in irreversible growth arrest.

Indications for Open Reduction of Condyle Fractures

The indications for open reduction of fractures of the condyle in children are: lateral displacement of the proximal fracture segment, with cosmetic deformity or a decrease in range function; presence of a foreign body in the joint capsule; fracture with dislocation into the middle cranial fossa or temporal fossa with clinical disability; inability to open or close the mouth because of mechanical blockage of the fractured segments; and a low–condylar neck fracture with displacement or dislocation (Fig. 27–5). In addition, if internal fixation is to be performed, then the assumptions are that the fracture is extracapsular and its location low in the condylar neck; the condylar head is not split; functional disability would be likely without ORIF; and use of the ORIF technique will limit functional disability.

Bilateral condylar fractures with or without midface fractures are not in themselves indications for ORIF unless the above indications are met. If the conservative approach is selected for condylar fracture treatment, IMF may be useful for patient comfort, encouraging soft tissue healing, relieving muscle spasm, and limiting the conversion of greenstick or minimally displaced fractures into a complete or fully displaced fracture. Approximately 2 weeks of IMF is enough to accomplish these goals and yet allow early range of motion to limit the likelihood of developing TMJ ankylosis.

When a condyle fracture is present and IMF needs to be limited, the fixation technique for additional fractures must be carefully selected. For example, if parasymphyseal and condylar fractures have occurred, a more stable form of internal fixation (miniplates and screws) may be selected for the parasymphyseal fracture so that IMF can be released early, as would be preferred for the condylar fracture.

It is important to look for a condylar fracture in the growing patient who has sustained facial trauma.[48] Not only can TMJ ankylosis occur as an early complication (Fig. 27–6), but long-term follow-up will be required by the surgeon and orthodontist to monitor growth and development. Later, some patients will require a combined orthodontic and surgical approach (i.e., LeFort I osteotomy, bilateral sagittal split osteotomies of the mandible, and genioplasty) to restore facial contour and occlusion.

Body Fractures of the Mandible

Because body fractures of the mandible usually have favorable muscle force, closed reduction with IMF will suffice. In very young patients or in situations of simple greenstick or nondisplaced fractures, a soft

(text continues on page 637)

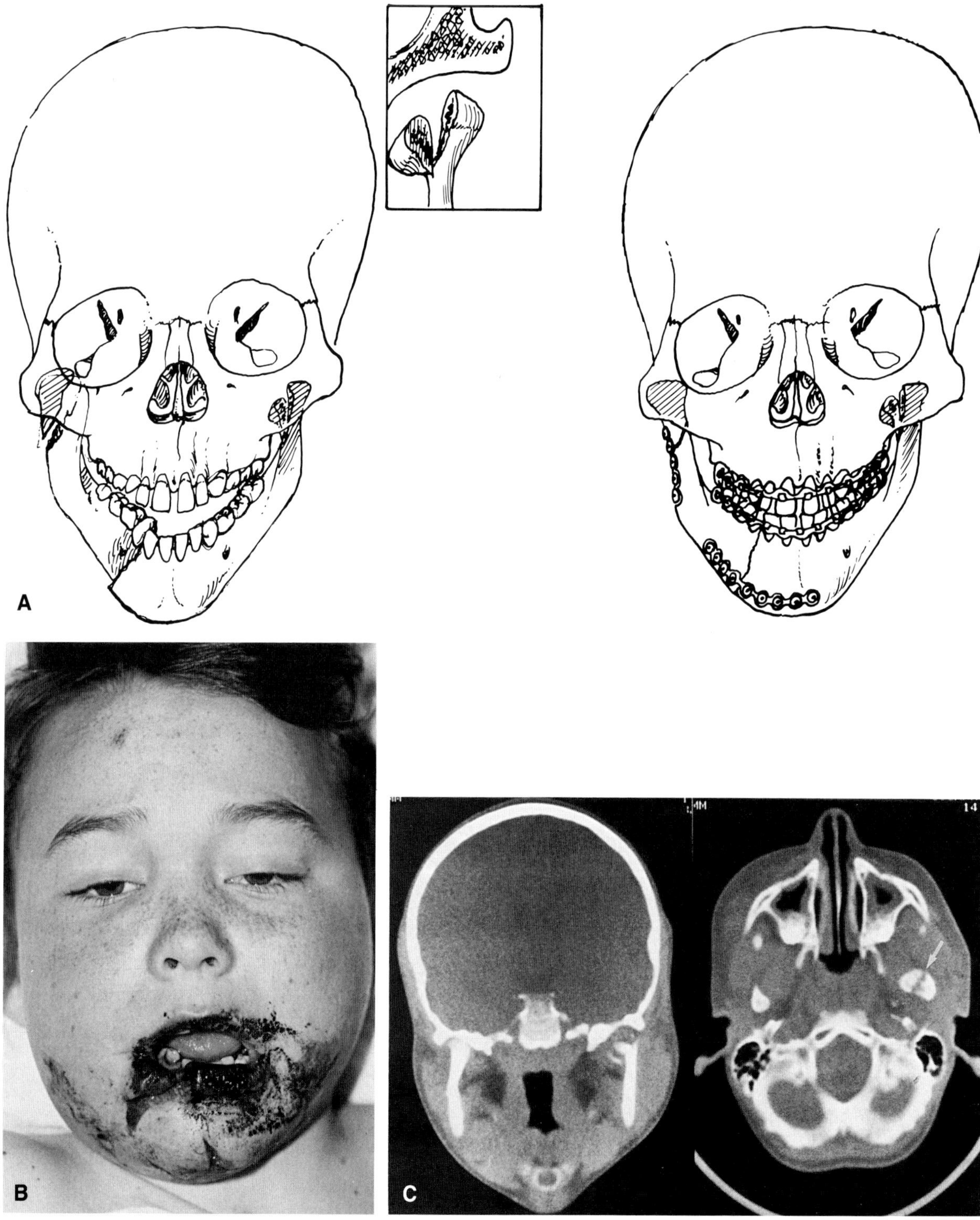

Figure 27–5. *An 11-year-old boy who sustained multiple facial trauma including a left intracapsular condyle fracture, a right low condylar neck fracture, a right parasymphyseal fracture of the mandible, dentoalveolar injuries, and multiple facial lacerations. (**A**) Location of fractures, reduction, and method of fixation. (**B**) Frontal view of face before fracture reduction. (**C**) Computed tomographic (CT) scan demonstrating left intracapsular condyle fracture (**arrow**) and right condylar neck fracture. (**D**) CT scan demonstrating displaced right parasymphyseal fracture. (**E**) Intraoral view of displaced right parasymphyseal fracture of mandible. (**F**) Intraoral view of reduced right parasymphyseal fracture of mandible. (**G**) Postoperative panorex demonstrating good reduction of fractures. (**H**) Six months later with 40 mm of vertical opening. (**I**) Occlusal view 6 months after injury.*

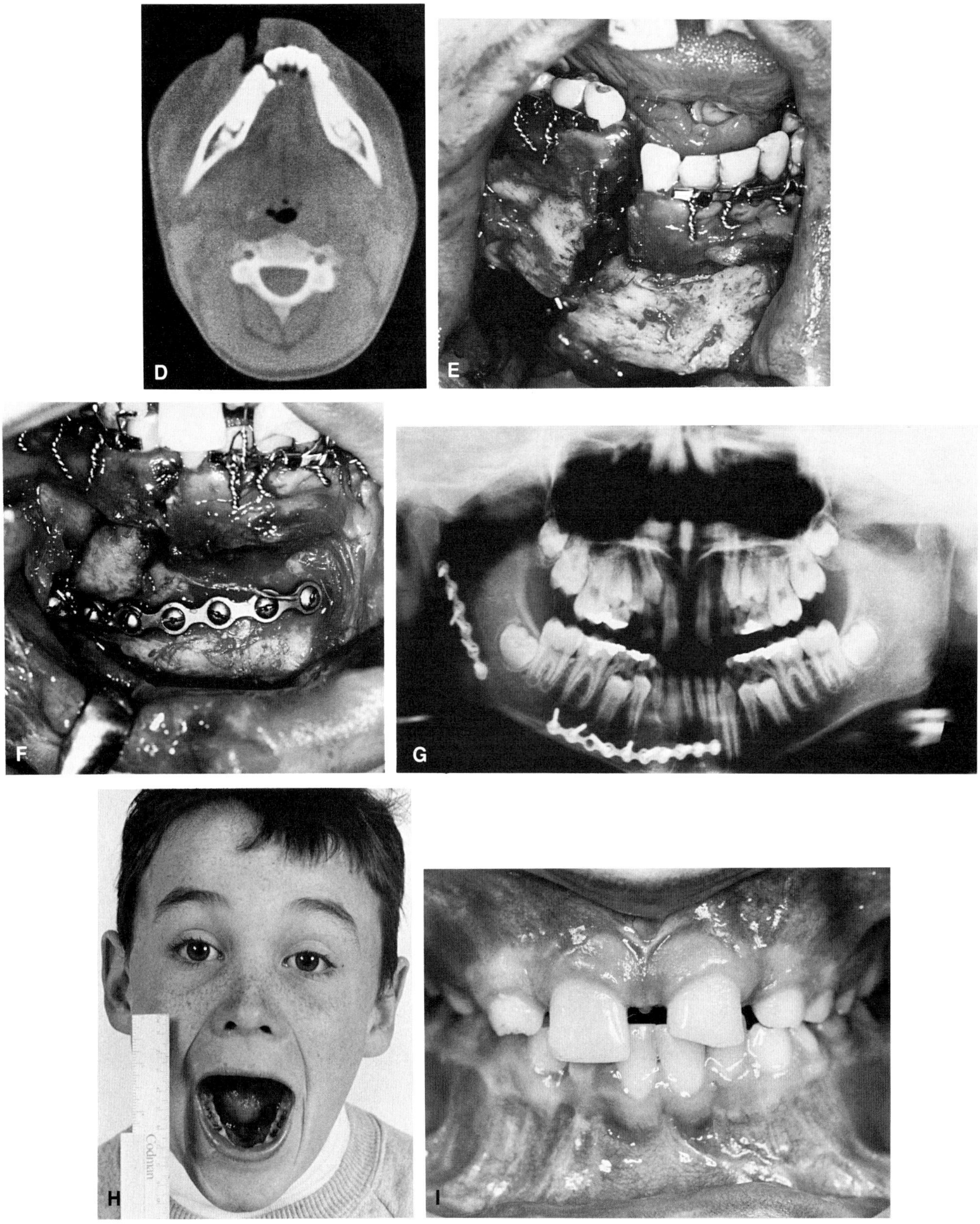

Figure 27–5. *(continued)*

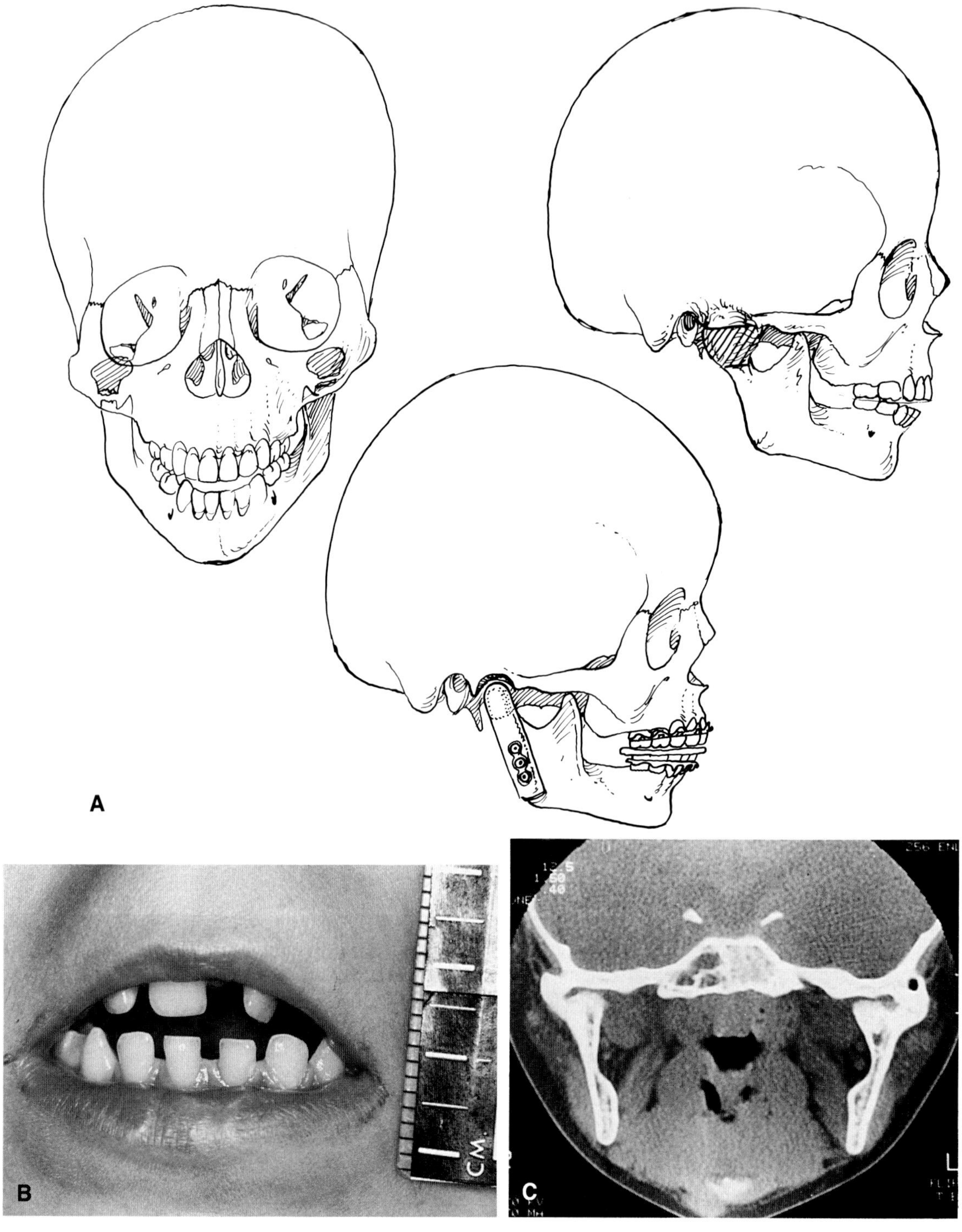

Figure 27–6. *A 5-year-old girl with bilateral intracapsular condyle fractures of the mandible resulting in bilateral TMJ ankylosis. (**A**) Illustration of bilateral TMJ fusion to zygomatic arches. Reconstruction with costochondral grafts stabilized with miniplates and screws. (**B**) Maximum vertical opening of 2 mm. (**C**) Coronal computed tomographic scan demonstrating bilateral bony fusion of condyles to zygomatic arches and glenoid fossa. (**D**) Costochondral rib graft being inset through coronal incision to reconstruct ascending ramus-condylar head. (**E**) Intraoperative view through Risdon incision demonstrating costochondral graft fixed to mandible with miniplate and screws. (**F**) Frontal view demonstrating adequate vertical opening. (**G**) Panorex 1 year after reconstruction demonstrating costochondral rib grafts with miniplate fixation. (**B–G** from Posnick JC. Role of plate and screw fixation in the treatment of paediatric facial fractures. In: Yaremchuk MJ. Rigid Fixation of the Craniomaxillofacial Skeleton. England: Butterworth, 1992)*

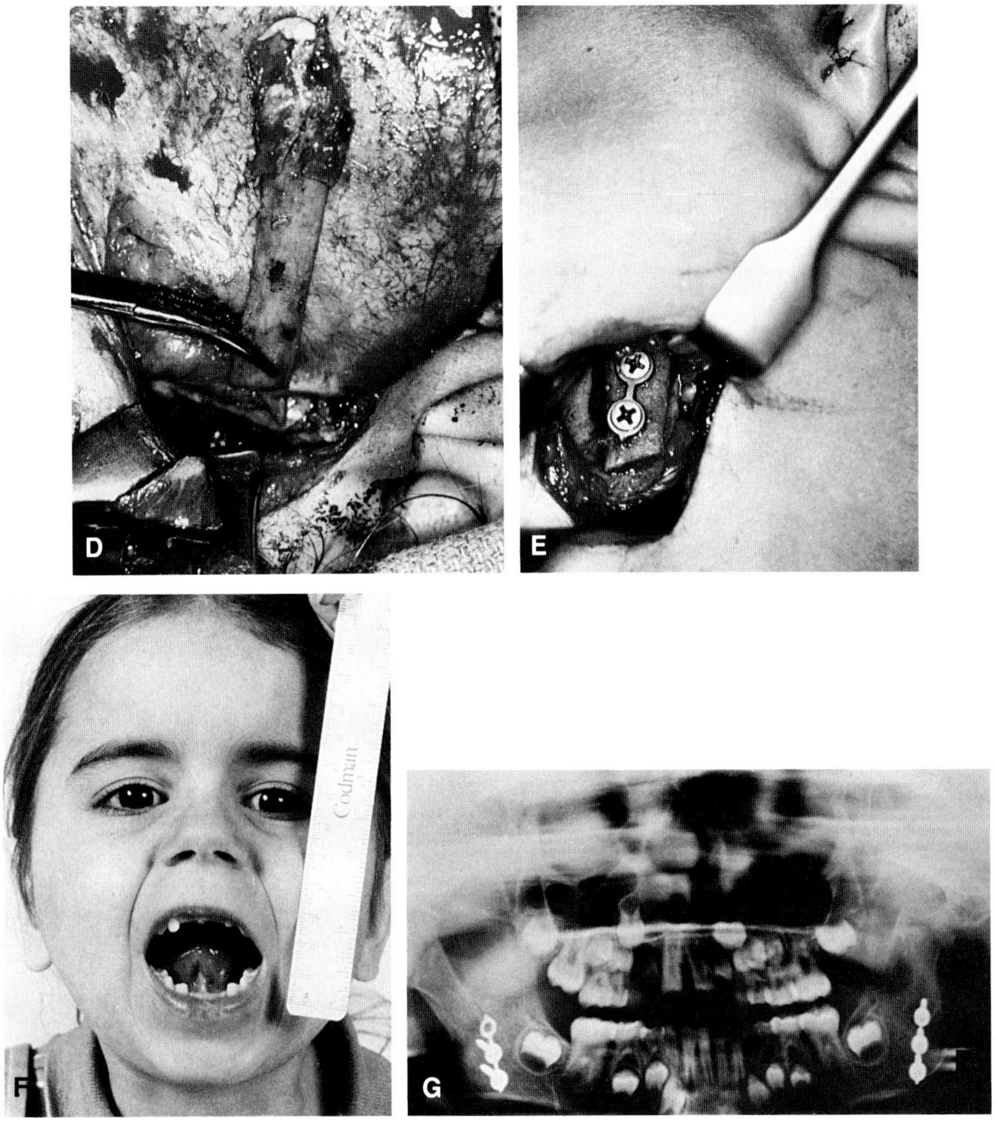

Figure 27–6. *(continued)*

diet alone may provide adequate treatment, but close follow-up is required.

Parasymphyseal and Symphyseal Fractures

Even with closed reduction and IMF techniques, the muscle forces on parasymphyseal fractures tend to displace the fracture during the healing process. Often a small gap occurs between the two teeth adjacent to the fracture site, most commonly the lateral incisor and canine tooth. In the primary or early mixed dentition a minor gap may be self-correcting. If the parasymphyseal fracture is seen in association with other facial fractures, such as a condylar fracture, a more stable form of fixation (e.g., miniplate-and-screw fixation) is preferred to allow for early mobility of the condylar fracture and limit problems of TMJ ankylosis.

Dentoalveolar Fractures

Anterior teeth may bear the brunt of accidental injury, along with their supporting alveolar bony structures.[32–34] Individual teeth may be loosened, partially or totally avulsed, or impacted. A single panoramic view may be useful, but for greater detail, additional intraoral occlusal or periapical films may be required. It is advisable to repair tooth and alveolar damage before definitive care of facial or lip lacerations because intraoral manipulations frequently disturb delicate suturing.

Minor luxations without complete laceration of the periodontal ligaments may not require splinting if the teeth can be easily returned to a stable position. Teeth that have been significantly loosened should be returned to their normal position in the alveolar arch and stabilized as soon as possible because return to a stable anatomic position after hematoma formation can be difficult. Controlled digital force is required to accomplish reduction.

Reimplantation of avulsed teeth should be regarded as a temporary measure, but it may prove useful. The teeth usually become reattached, although late root resorption or ankylosis may occur.

Methods of stabilizing dentoalveolar fractures involve acrylic splints, wires, and arch bars. The acid-etch technique is now becoming popular. Regardless of the stabilization technique selected, the splint must meet specific criteria; these include being easily fabricated, maintaining only passive force on the teeth, not injuring cemented surfaces of the tooth roots, not irritating the soft tissues, allowing normal occlusion to be maintained, permitting good oral hygiene, allowing access for subsequent endodontic treatment, and being easily removable.

ILLUSTRATIVE CASE REPORTS

Case 1

(See Figure 27–5)

An 11-year-old boy sustained multiple facial trauma—including a left intracapsular condyle fracture, a right condylar neck fracture, a right parasymphyseal fracture of the mandible, and multiple facial lacerations—when the all-terrain vehicle in which he was riding overturned.

Erich arch bars were applied under general anesthesia to stabilize his dentoalveolar fractures. His jaws were then wired together in their preinjury occlusion. He underwent ORIF of the right parasymphyseal fracture of the mandible with application of a titanium miniplate at the inferior border of the mandible through an intraoral incision. The low–condylar neck fracture was also treated with ORIF by means of a miniplate placed through a submandibular incision. The jaws were wired together, and the wires kept in place for 1 week after surgery, when progressive physiotherapy was instituted. This patient has maintained a good range of motion without evidence of ankylosis or major occlusal discrepancies.

Case 2

(See Fig. 27–2)

A 14-year-old boy sustained combined LeFort I and LeFort II fractures with bilateral orbital floor blow-out fractures resulting in an anterior open-bite deformity when he was accidentally kicked in the face during a high-school soccer game.

He underwent surgery during which Erich arch bars were placed on the upper and lower jaw. Maxillary circumvestibular, intraoral, and bilateral lower eyelid incisions were made to expose the fractures. Tessier disimpaction forceps were placed, and the midface fractures were reduced. IMF was then applied to achieve the preinjury occlusion. Through the intraoral and lower lid incisions, bone miniplates were placed vertically at each zygomatic buttress and piriform aperture and horizontally at each intraorbital rim. After orbital exploration and repositioning of orbital contents, split cranial bone grafts were harvested and placed to reestablish the orbital floors. When IMF was released intraoperatively, the occlusion was found to be stable.

Case 3

(See Fig. 27–3)

A 4-year-old boy sustained blunt trauma to his left eyeball when he fell and struck the edge of a table. He sustained an isolated orbital floor blow-out with entrapment of the inferior rectus muscle through the orbital floor defect. He was not seen until 6 weeks after the original injury. At this time, exploration was carried out through a lower eyelid incision, and the orbital contents were repositioned. The orbital floor defect was reconstructed with autogenous split cranial bone harvested through a small left temporal incision. A forced duction test carried out during the operation confirmed improved and adequate range of motion. His preoperative diplopia resolved.

Case 4

(See Fig. 27–6)

A 5-year-old girl sustained bilateral intracapsular condyle fractures of the mandible when she fell down a flight of stairs, a year before she was seen clinically. She was unable to open her mouth more than 2 mm. A CT scan confirmed the presence of bilateral ankylosis of the condyles to the zygomatic arches and glenoid fossa.

She underwent surgery, and two costochondral rib grafts were harvested from the right chest. Coronal and bilateral Risdon neck incisions were made. The ankylosis was identified through the coronal incision. Both an oscillating and a reciprocating saw were used to excise the bony ankylosed condylar heads, and the glenoid fossa was carefully cleaned out. Range of motion of the mandible improved immediately to 35 mm.

The harvested costochondral rib grafts were inset and secured to the residual ascending rami of the mandible with bone miniplates. During the operation, the occlusion was checked but the jaws were not found to be unsatisfactory. The patient remained on a blender diet for 6 weeks but range of motion was encouraged. One year later, she maintained a good vertical opening.

SUMMARY

Differences in the pattern of craniomaxillofacial fractures between children and adults must be recognized to provide appropriate treatment. Whenever possible, the pediatric trauma patient should be evaluated, treated, and monitored at a pediatric hospital by a surgeon familiar with the management of pediatric patients.

Facial fractures in children may go unrecognized as a result of incomplete communication with the patient, inadequate radiographic examination in the fussy child, or late presentation of the patient by the family. Late sequelae are common, even when appropriate and prompt treatment is instituted. These are a consequence of growth retardation and distortion secondary to the trauma event and treatment rendered.

Long-term follow-up by appropriate practitioners is essential to the monitoring of facial growth and development. Intervention at appropriate intervals may minimize growth distortions and maximize the functional, psychologic, and aesthetic results for both patient and family.

Acknowledgment

This chapter was prepared with the assistance of Medical Publications, The Hospital for Sick Children.

REFERENCES

1. Smith KA, Posnick JC, et al. Facial fractures in the pediatric population: Ten years experience. In: Proceedings of the 43rd Annual Meeting of the Canadian Society of Plastic Surgeons, June 1989; 1.
2. Adekey EO. Pediatric fractures of the facial skeleton: A survey of 85 cases from Kaduna, Nigeria. J Oral Surg 1975; 38:355–358.
3. Bales CR, Randal P, Lehr HB. Fractures of the facial bones in children. J Trauma 1972; 12:56–66.
4. Bernstein L. Maxillofacial injuries in children. Otolaryngol Clin North Am 1974; 2:397.
5. Carroll MJ, Hill CM, Mason DA. Facial fractures in children. Br Dent J 1987; 163:23–26.
6. Freif MG, Baden E. Management of fractures in children. J Oral Surg 1954; 12:129.
7. Fortunato MA, Fielding AF, Guernsey LH. Facial bone fractures in children. Oral Surg 1982; 53:225–230.
8. Graham GG, Peltier JR. The management of mandibular fractures in children. J Oral Surg 1960; 18: 416–423.
9. Hall RK. Injuries of the face and jaws in children. Int J Oral Surg 1972; 1:65–75.
10. Hall RK. Facial trauma in children. Austr Dent J 1974; 19:336–345.
11. Kaban LB, Mulliken JB, Murray JE. Facial fractures in children: An analysis of 122 fractures in 109 patients. Plast Reconstr Surg 1977; 59:15–20.
12. Maniglia AJ, Kline SN. Maxillofacial trauma in the pediatric age group. Otolaryngol Clin North Am 1983; 16:717–730.
13. Manson PN. Skull and midface injuries. In: Mustarde JC, Jackson IT, eds. Plastic surgery in infancy and childhood; ed 3. New York: Churchill Livingston, 1988; 317–345.
14. McCoy FJ, Chandler RA, Crow ML. Facial fractures in children. Plast Reconstr Surg 1966; 37:209–215.
15. McGraw BL, Cole RR. Pediatric maxillofacial trauma. Otolaryngol Head Neck Surg 1990; 116:41–45.
16. Ramba J. Fractures of facial bones in children. Int J Oral Surg 1985; 14:472–478.
17. Rowe NL. Fractures of the facial skeleton in children. J Oral Surg 1968; 26:505–515.
18. Schultz RC. Facial trauma in children. In: Marshall DK, ed. Facial injuries, ed 3. Chicago: Year Book Medical Publishers, 1988; 471–491.
19. Nahum AM. The biomechanics of maxillofacial trauma. Clin Plast Surg 1975; 2:59–64.

20. Bridges CP, Ryan RF, Longenecker CG, Vincent RW. Tracheostomy in children: A twenty-year study at Charity Hospital in New Orleans. Plast Reconstr Surg 1966; 37:117–120.
21. Crysdale W, Kohli-Dang N, Mullins GC, et al. Airway management in craniofacial surgery: Experience in 542 patients. J Otolaryngol 1987; 16:207–215.
22. Ousterhout DK, Vargervik K. Maxillary hypoplasia secondary to midfacial trauma in childhood. Plast Reconstr Surg 1987; 80:491–498.
23. Manson PN, Clifford CM, Su CT, Iliff NT, Morgan R. Mechanisms of global support and posttraumatic enophthalmos. I. The anatomy of the ligament sling and its relation to intramuscular cone orbital fat. Plast Reconstr Surg 1986; 77:193–202.
24. Bergland O, Borchgrevink H. The role of the nasal septum in midfacial growth in man elucidated by the maxillary development in certain types of facial clefts: A preliminary report. Scand J Plast Reconstr Surg 1974; 8:42–48.
25. Moss ML, Bromberg BE, Song IC, Eisenman G. The passive role of nasal septal cartilage in mid-facial growth. Plast Reconstr Surg 1968; 41:536–542.
26. Tulasne J-F. Maxillary growth following total septal resection in teleorbitism. In: Caronni EP, ed. Craniofacial surgery. Boston: Little, Brown & Co, 1985; 176–189.
27. Khosla VM, Boren W. Mandibular fracture in children and their management. J Oral Surg 1971; 29:116.
28. Lehman JA Jr, Saddawi ND. Fractures of the mandible in children. J Trauma 1976; 16:773–777.
29. MacLennan WD. Injuries involving the teeth and jaws in young children. Arch Dis Child 1957; 32:492–494.
30. Morgan WC. Pediatric mandibular fractures. Oral Surg 1975; 40:320–326.
31. Moos K, El-Attar A. Mandible and dental injuries. In: Mustarde JC, Jackson IT, eds. Plastic surgery in infancy and childhood, ed 3. New York: Churchill Livingstone, 1988; 345–364.
32. Andreasen JO, Ravn JJ. The effect of traumatic injuries to primary teeth on their permanent successors. II. A clinical and radiographic follow-up study of 213 teeth. Scand J Dent Res 1971; 79:284.
33. Gelbier S. Injured anterior teeth in children: A preliminary discussion. Br Dent J 1967; 123:331–335.
34. Lu M. Reimplantation of avulsed anterior teeth in patients with jaw fractures. Plast Reconstr Surg 1973; 51: 377–383.
35. Anderson MF, Alling CC. Subcondylar fracture in young dogs. Oral Surg Oral Med Oral Pathol 1965; 19: 263–268.
36. Boyne PJ. Osseous repair and mandibular growth after subcondylar fractures. J Oral Surg 1967; 25:300–309.
37. Campbell RL, Moore RF. Fractured condyle in a 3-month-old infant. Oral Surg 1975; 40:45.
38. Chalmers J, Lyons C: Fractures involving the mandibular condyle: A post-treatment survey of 120 cases. J Oral Surg 1947; 5:45.
39. Coccaro PJ: Restitution of mandibular form after condylar injury in infancy (a 7-year study of a child). Am J Orthodont 1969; 55:32–49.
40. Gilhauus-Moe O. Fractures of the mandibular condyle in the growth period. Stockholm: Scandinavian University Books, 1969.
41. Kaplan SL, Mark HI. Bilateral fractures of the mandibular condyles and fracture of the symphysis menti in an 18-month-old child: Two year preliminary report with a plea for conservative treatment. Oral Surg 1962; 15:136–147.
42. Leake D, Doykos J III, Habal MB, Murray JE. Long-term follow-up of fractures of the mandibular condyle in children. Plast Reconstr Surg 1971; 47:127–131.
43. MacLennan WD, Simpson W. Treatment of fractured mandibular condylar processes in children. Br J Plast Surg 1965; 18:423–427.
44. Proffitt WR, Vig KW, Turvey TA. Early fractures of the mandibular condyles: Frequently an unsuspected cause of growth disturbances. Am J Orthod 1980; 78: 1–24.
45. Rakower W, Protzell A, Rosencrans M. Treatment of displaced condylar fractures in children: Report of cases. J Oral Surg 1961; 19:517–521.
46. Rowe NL. Mandibular joint lesions in infants and adults. Int Dent J 1960; 10:484.
47. Schettler D, Rehrmann A. Long-term results of functional treatment of condylar fractures with the long bridle according to A. Rehrmann. J Maxillofac Surg 1975; 3:14–22.
48. Thomson HG, Farmer AW, Lindsay WK. Condylar neck fractures of the mandible in children. Plast Reconstr Surg 1964; 34:452–463.
49. Walker RV. Traumatic mandibular condylar fracture dislocations: Effect of growth in the Macaca Rhesus monkey. Am J Surg 1960; 100:850–863.
50. Walker DG. Mandibular condyle: Fifty cases demonstrating arrest in development. Dent Practitioner (Bristol) 1957; 7:160–168.
51. Winstanley RP. Collapse of the condylar head of the mandible in children and subsequent ankylosis. Br J Oral Surg 1978; 16:3–11.
52. Zide MF, Kent JN. Indication for open reduction of mandibular condyle fractures. J Oral Maxillofac Surg 1983; 41:89.
53. Zide MF. Open reduction of mandibular condyle fractures: Indications and technique. Clin Plast Surg 1989; 16:69–76.
54. American College of Surgeons. Advanced Trauma Life Support Course. Chicago: American College of Surgeons, 1989.

Index

Page numbers followed by *f* indicate figures; those followed by *t* indicate tabular material.

B

C

D

J

K

L

N

P

Q

R

S

T

U

V

ISBN 0-397-51232-5

90000

9 780397 512324